MW00981786

Instructional Course Lectures Shoulder and Elbow

Instructional Course Lectures Shoulder and Elbow

Edited by
Jon J.P. Warner, MD
Chief, The Harvard Shoulder Service
Professor of Orthopaedic Surgery
Department of Orthopaedics
Harvard Medical School
Boston, Massachusetts

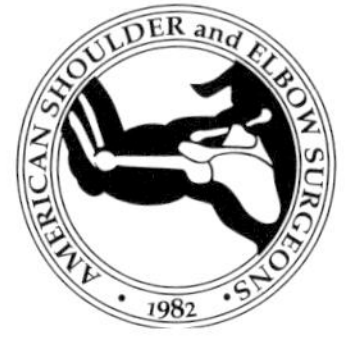

Developed with support from
American Shoulder and Elbow Surgeons

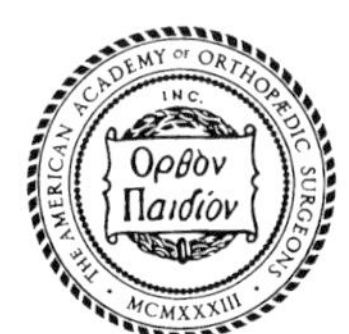

Published by the
American Academy
of Orthopaedic Surgeons
6300 North River Road
Rosemont, IL 60018

American Academy of Orthopaedic Surgeons

The material presented in the *Instructional Course Lectures Shoulder and Elbow* has been made available by the American Academy of Orthopaedic Surgeons for educational purposes only. This material is not intended to present the only, or necessarily best, methods or procedures for the medical situations discussed, but rather is intended to represent an approach, view, statement, or opinion of the author(s) or producer(s), which may be helpful to others who face similar situations.

Some drugs or medical devices demonstrated in Academy courses or described in Academy print or electronic publications have not been cleared by the Food and Drug Administration (FDA) or have been cleared for specific uses only. The FDA has stated that it is the responsibility of the physician to determine the FDA clearance status of each drug or device he or she wishes to use in clinical practice.

The FDA has expressed concern about potential serious patient care issues involved with the use of polymethlymethacrylate (PMMA) bone cement in the spine. A physician might insert the PMMA bone cement into vertebrae by various procedures, including vertebroplasty and kyphoplasty. Orthopaedic surgeons should be alert to possible complications.

PMMA bone cement is considered a device for FDA purposes. In October 1999, the FDA reclassified PMMA bone cement as a Class II device for its intended use "in arthroplastic procedures of the hip, knee and other joints for the fixation of polymer or metallic prosthetic implants to living bone." Some bone cements have recently received marketing clearance for the fixation of pathological fractures of the vertebral body using vertebroplasty or kyphoplasty procedures. Orthopaedic surgeons should contact their manufacturer for the FDA-clearance status. The use of a device for other than its FDA-cleared indication is an off-label use. Physicians may use a device off-label if they believe, in their best medical judgment, that its use is appropriate for a particular patient (eg, tumors).

The use of PMMA bone cement in the spine is described in Academy educational courses, videotapes and publications for educational purposes only. As is the Academy's policy regarding all of its educational offerings, the fact that the use of PMMA bone cement in the spine is discussed does not constitute an Academy endorsement of this use.

Furthermore, any statements about commercial products are solely the opinion(s) of the author(s) and do not represent an Academy endorsement or evaluation of these products. These statements may not be used in advertising or for any commercial purpose.

Some of the authors or the departments with which they are affiliated have received something of value from a commercial or other party related directly or indirectly to the subject of their chapter.

First Edition

ISBN 0-89203-389-4
Library of Congress Cataloging-in-Publication Data

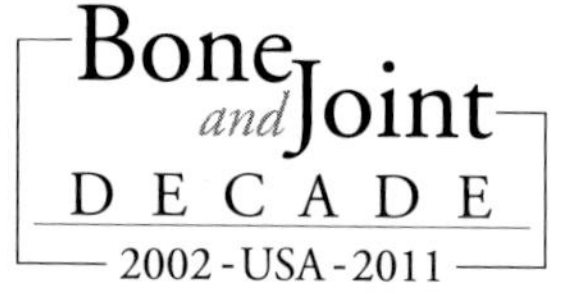

Editorial Board

Contributors

Christopher H. Allan, MD
Assistant Professor
Department of Orthopaedics
University of Washington School of Medicine
Seattle, Washington

David W. Altchek, MD
Associate Attending Surgeon
The Hospital for Special Surgery
New York-Presbyterian Hospital
New York, New York

James R. Andrews, MD
Chairman of the Board
Alabama Sports Medicine and Orthopaedics Center
American Sports Medicine Institute
Birmingham, Alabama

April Armstrong, BSc, PT, MD, FRCSC
Fellow, Shoulder and Elbow Service
Department of Orthopaedic Surgery
Barnes-Jewish Hospital
St. Louis, Missouri

Craig M. Ball, FRACS
Shoulder and Elbow Specialist
Waitemata Health
North Shore Hospital
Auckland, New Zealand

Keith M. Baumgarten, MD
Resident
Orthopaedic Surgery
Washington University
St. Louis, Missouri

James B. Bennett, MD
Clinical Professor
Orthopedic Surgery
University of Texas Health Science Center, Houston
Houston, Texas

Louis U. Bigliani, MD
Chief, The Shoulder Service
Department of Orthopaedic Surgery
College of Physicians and Surgeons
Columbia University
New York, New York

Julie Y. Bishop, MD
Shoulder Fellow
Department of Orthopaedics
Mt. Sinai School of Medicine
New York, New York

Theodore A. Blaine, MD
Fellow, The Shoulder Service
Department of Orthopaedic Surgery
College of Physicians and Surgeons
Columbia University
New York, New York

Dory Boyer, MD

John J. Brems
Department of Orthopaeic Surgery
Cleveland Clinic
Cleveland, Ohio

Stephen S. Burkhart, MD
Clinical Associate Professor
Department of Orthopaedic Surgery
University of Texas Health Science Center
San Antonio, Texas

Wayne Z. Burkhead, Jr, MD
W.B. Carrell Memorial Clinic
University of Texas Southwestern Medical School
Dallas, Texas

Raymond M. Carroll, MD
Clinical Instructor
Department of Orthopaedic Surgery
Georgetown University
Washington, DC

Michael G. Ciccotti, MD
Associate Professor
Director of Sports Medicine
Department of Orthopaedic Surgery
Rothman Institute at Thomas Jefferson University
Philadelphia, Pennsylvania

Robert H. Cofield, MD
Professor of Orthopaedics
Mayo Medical School
Chair, Department of Orthopaedics
Mayo Clinic
Rochester, Minnesota

Mark S. Cohen, MD
Associate Professor
Director, Hand and Elbow Program
Director, Orthopaedic Education
Department of Orthopaedic Surgery
Rush-Presbyterian-St. Luke's Medical Center
Chicago, Illinois

Brian J. Cole, MD
Associate Professor
Director, Cartilage Restoration Center at Rush
Departments of Orthopaedic Surgery and Anatomy and Cell Biology
Rush University Medical Center
Chicago, Illinois

Edward V. Craig, MD
Professor of Clinical Orthopaedics
Hospital for Special Surgery
Cornell Medical College
New York, New York

R. Alexander Creighton, MD
Assistant Professor
Department of Orthopaedics
University of North Carolina at Chapel Hill
Chapel Hill, North Carolina

Konstantinos Ditsios, MD
Orthopaedic Surgeon
Health Services Department
Organising Committee for the Olympic Games, Athens 2004
Athens, Greece

Jeffrey R. Dugas, MD
Clinical Instructor in Orthopaedic Surgery
Alabama Sports Medicine and Orthopaedic Center
American Sports Medicine Institute
Birmingham, Alabama

Anil K. Dutta, MD
Houston Hand and Upper Extremity Center
University of Texas Medical School
Houston, Texas

Larry D. Field, MD
Co-Director, Upper Extremity Service
Mississippi Sports Medicine and Orthopaedic Center
Jackson, Mississippi

Evan L. Flatow, MD
Lasker Professor and Interim Chair
Department of Orthopaedics
Mount Sinai School of Medicine
New York, New York

Michael Q. Freehill, MD
Fellow, The Shoulder Service
Department of Orthopaedic Surgery
College of Physicians and Surgeons
Columbia University
New York, New York

Leesa M. Galatz, MD
Department of Orthopaedic Surgery
Washington University School of Medicine
St. Louis, Missouri

Thomas J. Gill, MD
Instructor in Orthopedic Surgery
Department of Orthopedic Surgery
Massachusetts General Hospital
Boston, Massachusetts

Douglas T. Harryman II, MD
Codman Associate Professor
Department of Orthopaedics
University of Washington
Seattle, Washington (deceased)

Richard J. Hawkins, MD, FRCSC
Clinical Professor, Department of Orthopaedics
University of Colorado
Team Physician, Denver Broncos
Orthopaedic Consultant, Steadman Hawkins Clinic
Vail, Colorado

Patrick R.L. Hayes, MD
Chief, Shoulder Service
Department of Orthopedic Surgery
National Navy Medical Center
Bethesda, Maryland

Laurence D. Higgins, MD
Associate Professor
Chief, Sports Medicine
Co-Director, The Harvard Shoulder Service
Department of Orthopaedics
Brigham and Women's Hospital
Harvard Medical School
Boston, Massachusetts

Robert N. Hotchkiss, MD
Chief, Hand Service
Hospital for Special Surgery
New York, New York

Mark R. Hutchinson, MD
Associate Professor
Orthopaedics and Sports Medicine
Head Team Physician
University of Illinois at Chicago
Chicago, Illinois

Joseph P. Iannotti, MD, PhD
Professor and Chairman
Department of Orthopaedic Surgery
Cleveland Clinic Foundation
Cleveland Clinic Lerner School of Medicine
Cleveland, Ohio

Mary Lloyd Ireland, MD
President and Orthopaedic Surgeon
Kentucky Sports Medicine
Lexington, Kentucky

Rolando Izquierdo, MD
Fellow, The Shoulder Service
Department of Orthopaedic Surgery
Columbia-Presbyterian Medical Center
New York, New York

Laith M. Jazrawi, MD
Sports Medicine Fellow
Department of Orthopaedics
American Sports Medicine Institute
Birmingham, Alabama

Jesse B. Jupiter, MD
Director, Orthopaedic Hand Service
Professor, Orthopaedic Surgery
Massachusetts General Hospital
Harvard Medical School
Boston, Massachusetts

Graham J.W. King, MD
Associate Professor
Department of Surgery
University of Western Ontario
London, Ontario, Canada

Steven Klepps, MD
Shoulder Fellow
Mt. Sinai Department of Orthopedics
New York, New York

Young W. Kwon, MD, PhD
Assistant Professor
Department of Orthopaedic Surgery
New York University-Hospital for Joint Diseases
New York, New York

Cyrus J. Lashgari, MD
Orthopaedics and Sports Medicine
Anne Arundel Medical Center
Anapolis, Maryland

Gregory N. Lervick, MD
Fellow
Center for Shoulder, Elbow, and Sports Medicine
Department of Orthopaedic Surgery
Columbia-Presbyterian Medical Center
New York, New York

William N. Levine, MD
Assistant Professor of Orthopaedic Surgery
Columbia Center for Shoulder, Elbow and Sports Medicine Columbia-Presbyterian Medical Center
New York, New York

Ian King Yeung Lo, MD, FRCSC
Assistant Professor, Surgery
University of Calgary
Calgary, Alberta, Canada

Thomas R. Lyons, MD
Fellow
Mississippi Sports Medicine and Orthopaedic Center
Jackson, Mississippi

Guido Marra, MD
Assistant Professor
Department of Orthopaedic Surgeons
Loyola University Medical Center
Maywood, Illinois

Gary Matthys, MD
Fellow
Harvard University
Boston, Massachusetts

George M. McCluskey III, MD
Director, Southeastern Shoulder Institute
McCluskey Orthopaedic Surgery, PC
Columbus, Georgia

Michael D. McKee, MD, FRCSC
Associate Professor, Division of Orthopaedic Surgery
Department of Surgery
St. Michael's Hospital and the University of Toronto
Toronto, Ontario, Canada

Michael J. Medvecky, MD
Chief Resident
Department of Orthopaedic Surgery
New York University Hospital for Joint Diseases
New York, New York

Michael H. Metcalf, MD
Fellow
Mississippi Sports Medicine and Orthopaedic Center
Jackson, Mississippi

Peter J. Millett, MD
Associate Surgeon
Shoulder and Sports Medicine
Steadman Hawkins Clinic
Vail, Colorado

Anthony Miniaci, MD, FRCSC
Professor of Surgery
Department of Orthopaedic Surgery
Toronto Western Hospital
Toronto, Ontario, Canada

Bernard F. Morrey, MD
Emeritus Chairman
Professor of Orthopaedics
Mayo Clinic
Rochester, Minnesota

Michael J. Moskal, MD
Fellow
Upper Extremity Sports Medicine
Mississippi Sports Medicine and Orthopaedic Center
Jackson, Mississippi

Gregory P. Nicholson, MD
Assistant Professor of Orthopaedic Surgery
Rush University Medical Center
Midwest Orthopaedics at Rush
Chicago, Illinois

Frank B. Norberg, MD
Fellow in Sports Medicine
Mississippi Sports Medicine and Orthopaedic Center
Jackson, Mississippi

Tom R. Norris, MD
Department of Orthopaedics
California-Pacific Medical Center
San Francisco, California

Shawn W. O'Driscoll, PhD, MD, FRCS
Professor of Orthopaedic Surgery
Department of Orthopaedic Surgery
Mayo Clinic and Foundation
Rochester, Minnesota

Nader E. Paksima, DO
Clinical Instructor, Hand Service
Department of Orthopaedic Surgery
New York University Hospital for Joint Diseases
New York, New York

Michael L. Pearl, MD
Clinical Instructor of Orthopaedics
University of Southern California
Shoulder and Elbow Surgeon
Kaiser Permanente Medical Center
Los Angeles, California

Wesley P. Phipatanakul, MD
Department of Orthopedics
California-Pacific Medical Center
San Francisco, California

Derek Plausinis, MD
Fellow in Shoulder and Elbow Surgery
Department of Orthopaedic Surgery
New York University-Hospital for Joint Diseases
New York, New York

Matthew L. Ramsey, MD
Associate Professor of Orthopaedic Surgery
Chief, Shoulder and Elbow Service
Penn Orthopaedic Institute
University of Pennsylvania School of Medicine
Philadelphia, Pennsylvania

David Ring, MD
Department of Orthopaedic Surgery
Massachusetts General Hospital
Boston, Massachusetts

Charles A. Rockwood, Jr, MD
Professor and Chairman Emeritus
Department of Orthopaedics
University of Texas Medical School and Health Science Center
San Antonio, Texas

Anthony A. Romeo, MD
Associate Professor
Department of Orthopaedics
Rush-Presbyterian-St. Luke's Medical Center
Chicago, Illinois

Marc R. Safran, MD
Associate Professor
Chief, Section of Sports Medicine
Department of Orthopaedic Surgery
University of California at San Francisco
San Francisco, California

Felix H. Savoie III, MD
Co-Director, Upper Extremity Service
Mississippi Sports Medicine and Orthopaedic Center
Jackson, Mississippi

Marius M. Scarlat, MD
Acting Instructor
Department of Orthopaedics
University of Washington
Seattle, Washington

Joel Shapiro, MD
Shoulder and Elbow Fellow
Department of Orthopaedic Surgery
Hospital for Joint Diseases
New York, New York

Walter G. Stanwood, MD
Clinical Fellow, Shoulder, Elbow and Sports Medicine
Department of Orthopaedic Surgery
Columbia-Presbyterian Medical Center
New York, New York

Erica Rowe Urquhart, MD, PhD
Orthopedic Surgery Resident
Department of Orthopedics
Hospital for Special Surgery
New York, New York

Jon J.P. Warner, MD
Chief, The Harvard Shoulder Service
Professor of Orthopaedic Surgery
Department of Orthopaedics
Harvard Medical School
Boston, Massachusetts

Russell F. Warren, MD
Surgeon-in-Chief
Hospital for Special Surgery
Professor of Surgery, Orthopaedics
Cornell Medical College
New York, New York

Gerald R. Williams, Jr, MD
Chief, Shoulder and Elbow Service
Associate Professor,Orthopaedic Surgery
University of Pennsylvania
Philadelphia, Pennsylvania

Riley J. Williams III, MD
Assistant Professor, Sports Medicine and Shoulder Service
Hospital for Special Surgery
Weill Cornell Medical College
New York, New York

Michael A. Wirth, MD
Associate Professor of Orthopaedics
Orthopaedics Shoulder Department
University of Texas Health Science Center at San Antonio
San Antonio, Texas

Melissa A. Yadao, MD
Sports Medicine Fellow
Mississippi Sports Medicine and Orthopaedic Center
Jackson, Mississippi

Ken Yamaguchi, MD
Professor of Orthopaedic Surgery
Chief, Shoulder and Elbow Service
Department of Orthopaedic Surgery
Washington University School of Medicine
Barnes-Jewish Hospital
St. Louis, Missouri

Joseph D. Zuckerman, MD
Professor and Chairman
Department of Orthopaedic Surgery
New York University Hospital for Joint Diseases
New York, New York

Preface

The Instructional Course Lectures (ICL) series of the American Academy of Orthopaedic Surgeons (AAOS) remains one of the most respected resources in orthopaedics for providing timely, relevant information about the treatment of musculoskeletal problems. Thus, I am honored to have been asked to organize a volume dedicated to the shoulder and elbow. Our knowledge of diagnosing and treating shoulder and elbow problems has grown exponentially over the past several decades. This growth is timely because problems in this region are second only to problems of the spine and knee. This single volume represents current thinking about these problems since the beginning of the new millennium.

ICL Shoulder and Elbow includes 43 articles organized into eight sections, five of which focus on shoulder problems and three on elbow. The shoulder sections address instability and superior labrum injuries, rotator cuff disease, degenerative disease, fractures, and miscellaneous conditions. For the elbow, sections address ligament and sports injuries, degenerative conditions, and fractures.

I invited seven internationally respected clinicians to review and comment on these articles. These surgeons not only have extensive clinical experience in the area assigned, but they are also scientists who have consistently demonstrated that they evaluate our current understanding of shoulder and elbow problems in the context of questions that remain to be answered. Thus, their perspectives both clarify current knowledge and highlight a number of important questions.

Dr. Brian Cole is an international expert in the management of shoulder ligament injuries whose clinical experience in treating traumatic labral lesions of the shoulder is unparalleled. He provides a succinct summary and critical analysis of a series of articles on throwing injuries, labrum tears, and injuries to the skeletally immature shoulder.

Dr. Laurence Higgins has extensive experience in the management of rotator cuff disease. His insightful review considers the spectrum of rotator cuff disease described in these articles, including open and arthroscopic rotator cuff repair and the role of tendon transfers.

In my section on degenerative conditions of the shoulder, I review articles that broadly consider these problems and their treatment, not only with conventional arthroplasty but also with the more controversial joint-preserving approaches in younger patients with arthritis. My experience over the past 15 years has given me an appreciation for the challenges of relieving pain and restoring function in patients with arthritis.

Dr. Evan Flatow supplies an excellent review of the management of shoulder fractures. His depth of experience and insight in this clinical area are matched only by his sharp analytical wit, which is evident in his review. He skillfully points out the common pitfalls associated with fracture management and the very exciting recent developments of minimally invasive osteosynthesis.

Dr. Peter Millett has extensive experience treating complicated shoulder problems, and he shares these insights in his review. This section should be especially interesting to surgeons who wish to better understand problems of the shoulder because the conditions described in this section are among the least frequently encountered in clinical practice, specifically refractory shoulder stiffness, nerve injuries of the shoulder, sternoclavicular joint injuries, and complications of shoulder surgery.

Dr. Marc Safran has a special interest in elbow ligamentous problems that he has cultivated through clinical experience and biomechanical research. He provides an excellent summary of the articles on elbow arthroscopy, ligamentous injuries of the elbow, and other problems that affect the throwing athlete.

Dr. Ken Yamaguchi is an internationally recognized authority in the management of degenerative problems of the elbow. He considers a superb group of articles that together must be one of the best dissertations on degenerative elbow problems in the orthopaedic literature. Joint salvage through arthroplasty is considered along with relevant anatomic concerns and arthroscopy.

Finally, Dr. Matthew Ramsey is a renowned educator and author who lectures both nationally and internationally on the topic of elbow trauma. The articles in his section consider the range of traumatic problems that affect the elbow, including instability and fracture. He carefully assists the reader in navigating this difficult subject by highlighting the important points of each article.

I feel privileged to have been asked to organize ICL Shoulder and Elbow and to coordinate the reviews of these very gifted clinicians, educators, and scientists. This volume represents an important reference for the most current approaches to problems of the shoulder and elbow. Even with my day-to-day experience in managing complex problems of the shoulder and elbow, I have learned a great deal by reading these excellent papers. I believe that residents, general orthopaedic surgeons, and shoulder and elbow specialists will want to add this volume to their personal library as well.

I would also like to thank the AAOS Publications Department for organizing this volume, and especially Lynne Shindoll, Managing Editor, for finalizing the editing of these reviews.

Jon J.P. Warner, MD
Editor

Contents

Section 1 Shoulder Instability and Labrum Injuries

Section 2 Rotator Cuff Injuries

Section 3 Degenerative Diseases About the Shoulder

Section 4 Shoulder Fractures

Section 5 Miscellaneous Conditions About the Shoulder

Section 6 Elbow Arthroscoy and Sports Medicine

Section 7 Degenerative Diseases About the Elbow

Section 8 Trauma About the Elbow

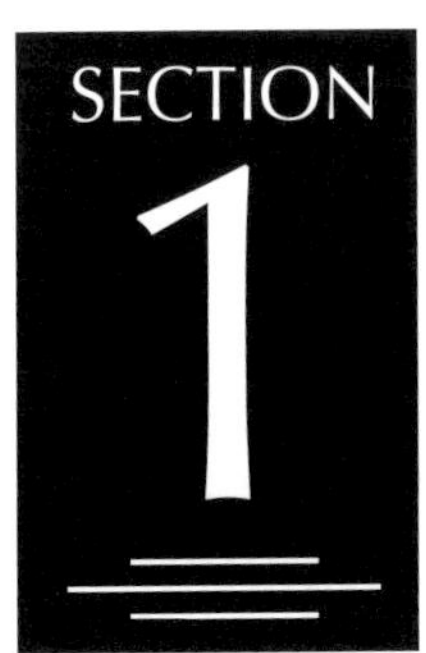

Shoulder Instability and Labrum Injuries

Shoulder Instability and Labrum Injuries

This section on the management of shoulder instability provides an overview with specific consideration for the spectrum of disease as it affects the immature athlete through the high-level competitive thrower. Specifically, this series of articles provides highly informative reviews on the following topics: (1) throwing injuries in the skeletally immature athlete; (2) the arthroscopic treatment of instability, with discussions relevant to the outcomes of arthroscopic versus open management; (3) the management of superior labral anterior and posterior lesions, and internal impingement in the overhead throwing athlete, and (4) the management of multidirectional instability, with specific focus on arthroscopic stabilization in patients with bidirectional or greater patterns of glenohumeral instability. These articles collectively provide a foundation for the arthroscopist interested in managing the entire spectrum of shoulder instability, in addition to the specific concerns related to the skeletally immature upper extremity.

Hutchinson and Ireland provide an excellent review on overuse and throwing injuries in the skeletally immature athlete. Their article is timely, given the increased demands placed on our skeletally immature athletes arising from family and contemporary competitive pressures. Unique to the skeletally immature athlete is Little Leaguer shoulder and elbow, osteochondritis dissecans of the elbow, epicondylitis, and distal radial epiphysitis. Most commonly as sports medicine specialists, we are often less adept at managing overuse and physeal injuries in the immature athlete given the relatively low incidence of these problems compared to the adult population. This article provides a comprehensive overview of these problems originating in the shoulder, elbow, forearm, wrist, and hand as they relate specifically to throwing injuries in the skeletally immature athlete. It is likely that this article will become a reference for years to come, given the thoroughness of the overview.

My colleagues and I wrote an article reviewing the arthroscopic treatment of anterior glenohumeral instability. This comprehensive review of the pathoanatomy specific to shoulder instability links the unique aspects of the anatomy to the specific concerns of arthroscopic management. Contemporary biomechanics are reviewed, as are the bases for currently used evaluation methods, including specific findings at the time of the examination under anesthesia and diagnostic arthroscopy. The basic principles of arthroscopic repair and the specific steps required to perform these techniques also are described and amply illustrated as a "how to" in successfully performing arthroscopic stabilization in patients with anterior glenohumeral instability.

As a complement to the previous article, the status of arthroscopic versus open treatment of anterior instability is summarized by Armstrong and associates. These authors supply a thorough literature review, illustrating how contemporary treatment of shoulder instability, including imbrication and labral stabilization, can yield results that rival or exceed those of open stabilization techniques. This ongoing controversy is discussed openly in an objective fashion, allowing readers to draw their own conclusions based on contemporary literature.

Jazrawi and associates provide a thorough review of the management of superior labral anterior and posterior lesions, as well as internal impingement in the overhead throwing athlete. This article describes the often very confusing intricacies of superior labral anterior and posterior pathology (SLAP lesions). This condition represents an extremely complex pathophysiology in a challenging and physically demanding patient group. A review of the pathophysiology of internal impingement is provided, as is a clear treatment algorithm that considers both surgical and nonsurgical treatment options as mainstays of definitive management in this patient group.

In the next article on the management of multidirectional instability, Lo and associates emphasize the surgical decision making required to evaluate patients who present with a confusing picture of pain, with or without episodes of frank instability. They also discuss open, arthroscopic, and thermal management of this diverse patient group with a graphic overview of the specific steps required to perform these techniques.

Finally, Metcalf and associates complement Lo and associates' review by describing arthroscopic stabilization of patients with multidirectional instability. This article provides an overview of the management of labral lesions, explains the role of the rotator interval and the effects of excessive capsular redundancy, and describes specific management techniques for the pathoanatomy associated with this condition.

With the volume of evidence supporting the use of arthroscopy in the management of intra-articular glenohumeral pathology, a thorough understanding of the athlete, from youth through adulthood, is critical to strengthen the armamentarium of the arthroscopic shoulder surgeon. The techniques described in these articles, which emphasize proper kinematics about the shoulder, convey the basic principles required to better understand glenohumeral instability and the skeletally immature athlete. The contemporary results reported and discussed in each article clearly support the more widespread application of arthroscopic techniques when proper indications are followed.

Brian J. Cole, MD, MBA
Associate Professor
Department of Orthopaedic Surgery
and Anatomy and Cell Biology
Rush University Medical Center
Chicago, Illinois

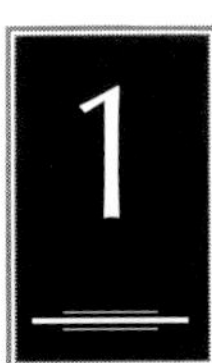

Overuse and Throwing Injuries in the Skeletally Immature Athlete

Mark R. Hutchinson, MD
Mary Lloyd Ireland, MD

Abstract

Over 25 million children participate in school-sponsored sports, and an additional 20 million participate in extracurricular organized sports. Over the past decade, increased intensity of training, more pressure for success, new opportunities for structured play, and more organized advanced leagues and traveling teams have led to a corresponding increase in overuse injuries in the skeletally immature athlete. Perhaps the classic sports model for overuse injuries of the upper extremity is baseball. Throwing sports contribute to an increased incidence of elbow and shoulder injuries that might be related to intensity of training, throwing mechanics, and poor conditioning, including core strength. Specific areas of concern regarding overuse injuries in young athletes include such diagnoses as little leaguer's shoulder, little leaguer's elbow, osteochondritis dissecans of the elbow, tennis elbow, and distal radial epiphysitis. Ultimately, overuse injuries, and particularly physeal injuries, should be suspected in any young athlete who has pain in the upper extremity. Comparative bilateral radiographs are the rule in workup.

Compared with adult athletes, the skeletally immature athlete has unique issues regarding treatment and injury patterns. Poor technique or mechanics that increase loads across the physis make the skeletally immature developing athlete prone to injury. Coordination and physical skills are dynamically changing. When performed properly and with gradual progression of intensity, strength training for children and adolescents is a safe undertaking.[1] Nonetheless, acute changes in intensity or weight place the growing physis at increased risk of injury. Although the weak link in the young athlete is generally considered to be the physis, muscle-tendon, ligament, and other bone injuries can occur secondary to acute trauma or overuse. Injury to the physis can cause long-term disability, deformity, or shortening. Each potential physeal injury should be evaluated with comparison views of the opposite extremity. The contribution each physis has to total growth and the timing of appearance and closure of the growth plates should also be determined (Figs. 1 and 2). **(DVD-4.1)**

Acute Injury/Overuse Injury

Acute injuries occur secondary to a single traumatic event or a catastrophic failure of structure. Fractures of the upper extremity are a common injury; the most common site is the distal radius physis, followed by the distal humerus and the fingers[2-4] (Table 1).

An apparently acute injury can occur in the presence of chronic problems or pathologic processes that reduce the young athlete's threshold for injury. If the energy involved in the injury mechanism is not consistent with the severity of the injury in the young athlete, heightened suspicion for an underlying process is warranted. Fortunately, fractures through unicameral bone cysts usually lead to healing of both fracture and cyst and allow for full return to sport (Fig. 3).

Overuse injuries in children imply some activity or demand that resulted in repetitive load and stress to the immature skeleton.[5,6] This scenario may be secondary to stresses that were too great, too frequent, or advanced too quickly. The physis is susceptible to overuse leading to pain, widening, weakened bone strength, and growth abnormalities. Muscle-tendon units may have elevated risk of overuse injuries in the actively growing child because as the bone lengthens, the muscle-tendons have to stretch to keep up. This relative tightness and related poor flexibility place young athletes at increased risk of muscle-tendon strains, avulsion injuries, and muscle tears. Fortunately, chronic tendon breakdown

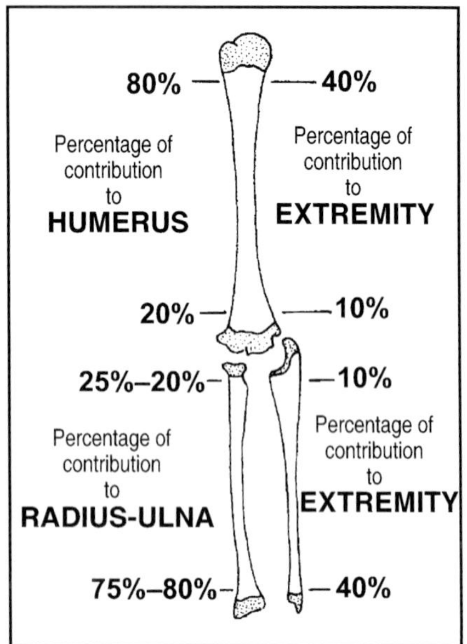

Fig. 1 Percentage of contribution to specific bone is shown on the left, and percentage of contribution to the entire upper extremity is shown on the right.

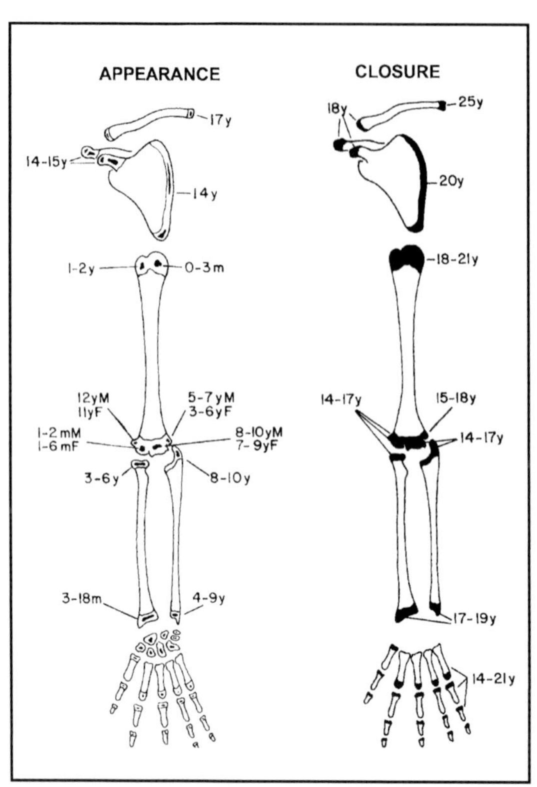

Fig. 2 The times of appearance *(left)* and closure *(right)* of the secondary ossification centers of the upper extremity. y = years, m = months, M = males, F = females.

Table 1
Epiphyseal Fracture Rates: Upper Extremity

	Ogden		Peterson		Neer	
	n	%	n	%	n	%
Distal Radius	197	43.1	98	48.5	1,096	61.5
Distal Humerus	108	23.6	20	9.9	332	18.6
Distal Ulna	13	2.8	12	5.9	136	7.6
Proximal Radius	12	2.6	1	0.5	124	7.0
Proximal Humerus	41	9.0	22	10.9	72	4.0
Phalanges	55	12.0	39	19.3		
Metacarpals	9	2.0	10	5.0		
Proximal Ulna	9	2.0			21	1.2
Proximal Clavicle	8	1.7				
Distal Clavicle	5	1.1				
Total	457	100	232	100	1,781	100

(Reproduced with permission from Andrews JR, Zarins B, Wilk KE (eds): *Injuries in Baseball.* Philadelphia, PA, Lippincott-Raven, 1998, p 261.)

(tendinosis) occurs less frequently in children than adults because of less repetitive motions. A club-level 50-year-old tennis player would have had many thousands more backhands than a 16- to 18-year-old elite player, which explains the reduced incidence of tennis elbow in the younger age group.

Changes in equipment and rules that target safety have the potential to somewhat reduce the risk of acute traumatic injuries of children in sport. However, the best opportunity to reduce the total number of injuries in youth sports is training in correct technique for the particular sport. In Little League baseball, acute traumatic fractures are commonly related to contact with the ball, a base, or another player rather than throwing. Helmet use and breakaway bases have been proven to reduce injury. Overuse arm pain is very common in young baseball pitchers.[7] Interventions targeted to reduce overuse injuries in young throwers have included limiting the total number of innings allowed per week and total pitch counts. Unfortunately, quality long-term follow-up studies regarding the efficacy of such interventions are unavailable. Further prospective research is needed to evaluate the effect of the safety interventions suggested not only for baseball but for all childhood sports.

The Shoulder

The differential diagnosis of shoulder complaints in the skeletally immature

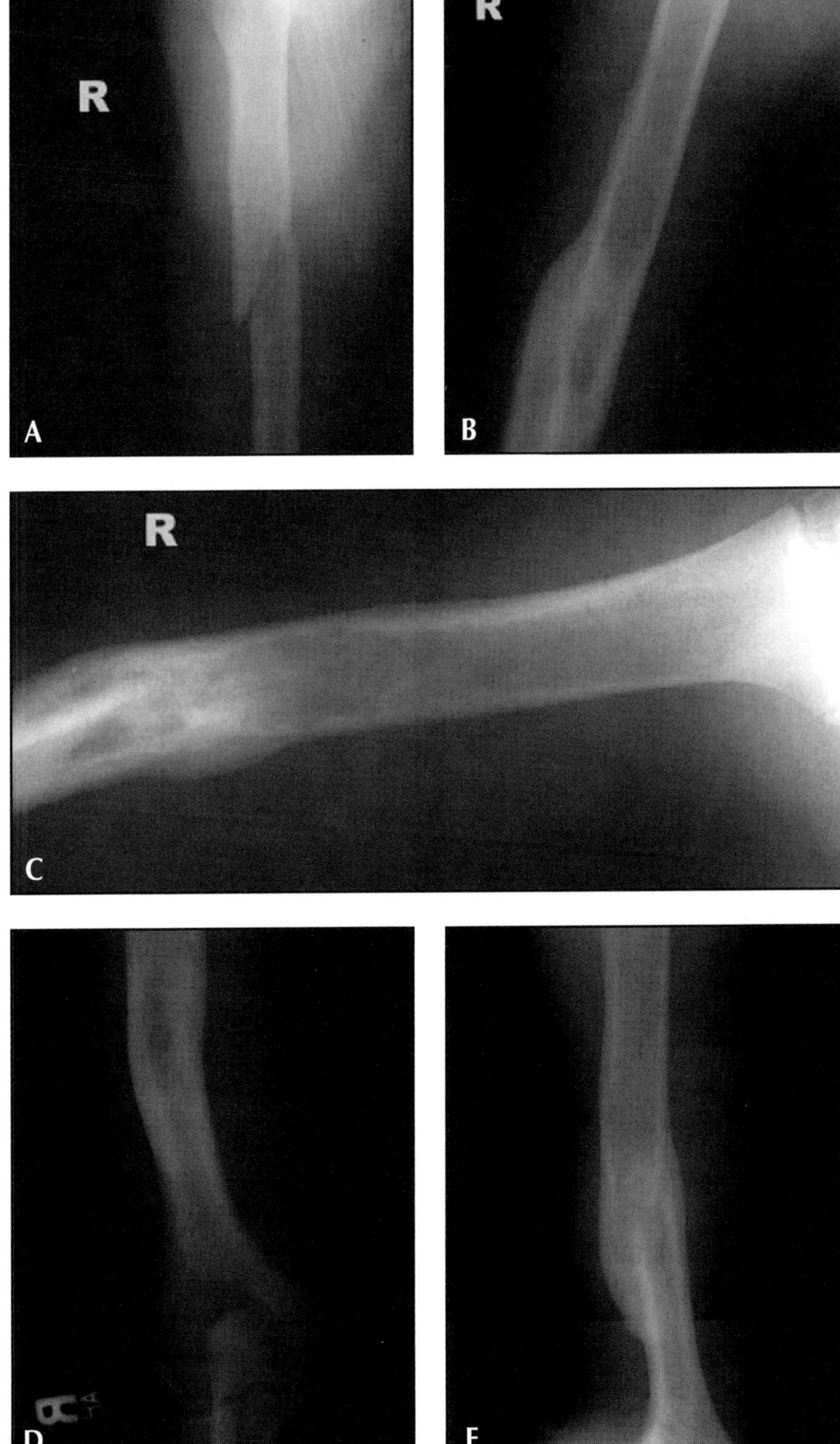

Fig. 3 A, Diaphyseal humerus fracture in an 11-year-old pitcher who felt acute pain in his arm. At 2 months, the unicameral bone cyst can be more clearly seen in the AP (**B**) and lateral (**C**) views. **D** and **E,** Follow-up radiographs show complete healing of the fracture and healing of the cyst.

shoulder includes little leaguer's shoulder (a physeal injury of the proximal humeral physis), osteochondrosis of the proximal humerus, instability, and impingement.[8-11] In general, impingement of the rotator cuff is a disease pattern that occurs secondary to chronic overuse. It is much more common in older athletes because of the higher number of repetitions and stresses to which these athletes' shoulders have been exposed. Young athletes may sustain rotator cuff injuries and strain secondary to repetitive loading or an acute traumatic event; however, signs and symptoms of classic impingement should raise concern about underlying instability. Traumatic injuries such as fractures and dislocations can also occur.[12,13]

Overthrowing the shoulder with associated poor mechanics places increased forces across the anterior capsule and shoulder joint. Children should be taught to throw with proper mechanics, including good foot push-off, solid and strong core stability, and trunk rotation. Proper throwing technique will allow the athlete to achieve the same speed as his or her cohorts without placing pathologic energy demands on the shoulder. Recurrent anterior loads in the cocking phase of throwing have been associated with labral detachments and capsular stretching in older athletes. A young athlete's shoulder is exposed to similar forces and is prone to similar failure if repetitions are too frequent or loads too high. More commonly, however, the weak link in the young thrower's shoulder is the physis and not the capsuloligamentous structures.[14]

Little leaguer's shoulder is a term coined by Dotter[15] in 1995 regarding the relatively common complaint of proximal shoulder pain in Little League pitchers. It is commonly correlated with a stress fracture of the proximal humeral physis. The more innings pitched and greater total number of pitches thrown per week results in an increased risk of arm pain.[16]

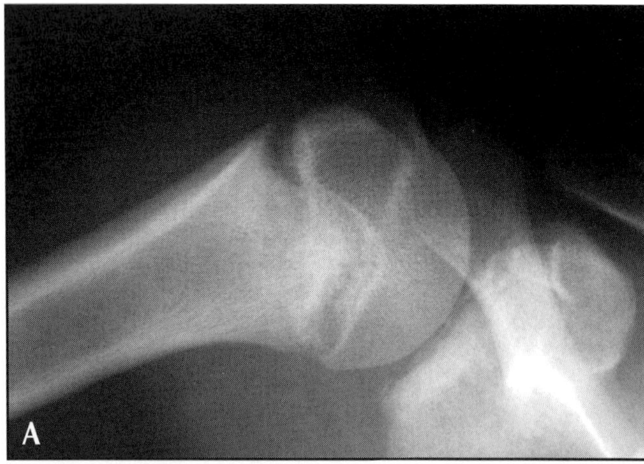

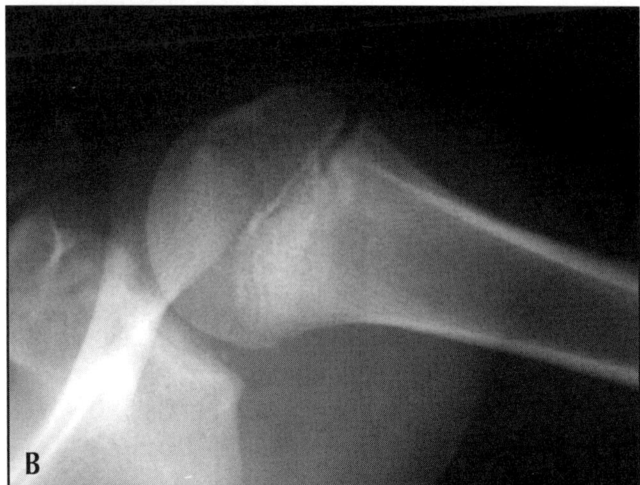

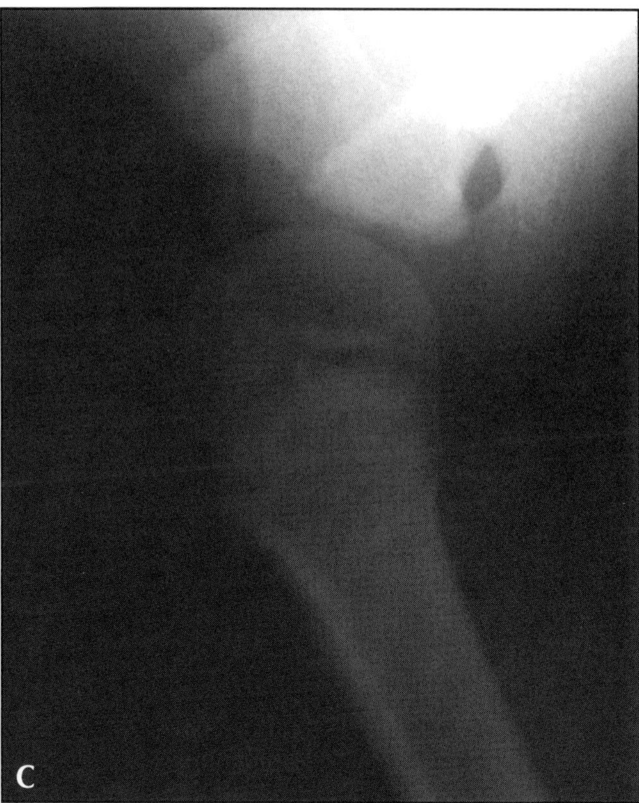

Fig. 4 A, Radiograph of a 14-year-old baseball pitcher who developed pain a month prior to radiographs that show stress fracture of the proximal humeral epiphysis. **B,** The opposite side demonstrates the normal undulating proximal humeral epiphyseal plate. **C**, Axillary lateral view of the right shoulder shows the lysis at the metaphysis across the epiphyseal plate suggestive of stress injury.

Overuse and poor technique have also been implicated as contributing causes. The athlete complains of pain over the proximal humerus that is worse with extremes of motion. Direct palpation over the physis is usually very painful. Percussion at the elbow may also exacerbate pain. Onset is usually gradual, although the athlete will occasionally be able to describe a single pitch that brought on the initial complaints of pain. Evaluation should always include comparative imaging studies of the opposite side because subtle physeal widening may easily be missed (Fig. 4).

Treatment is based on the patient's age, symptoms, and amount of displacement or angulation. With over 4 years remaining for expected skeletal growth, angulations of 45° with well over 50% displacement can be expected to remodel. With increasing skeletal maturity or greater deformity, closed reduction and percutaneous pinning may be indicated. Fortunately, most proximal physeal injuries in throwers are subtle with minimal displacement. A sling is used for comfort until symptoms resolve. Early range of motion is allowed but return to sports activity should be delayed for at least 3 to 4 months to prevent recurrence. When the athlete does return to sports activity, progression of intensity and number of pitches should be gradual. A knowledgeable coach should evaluate the athlete's mechanics and throwing style. The parents should be counseled to count the number of pitches and not just the number of innings to reduce the risk of overuse and recurrence.

Proximal humeral osteochondrosis was described by Adams in 1966.[17] It is a rare problem that is in the family of osteochondroses including osteochondritis dissecans of the elbow, Legg-Calvé-Perthes disease of the hip, Sever's disease of the calcaneus, and Osgood-Schlatter's disease of the knee. It is likely a vascular phenomenon, exacerbated by overuse in an athlete, that has some genetic predisposition. Imaging studies will reveal fragmentation of the proximal humeral epiphysis. Treatment for nondisplaced fragments is rest and a reduction of stresses about the shoulder. Throwers should refrain from throwing until symptoms resolve.

Acromioclavicular and sternoclavicular injuries are relatively rare in children, accounting for only 15% of all clavicle injuries and with the medial clavicle injuries accounting for less than 1%. Injuries are usually physeal and not ligamentous. Isolated ligamentous injury is virtually unheard of before age 13 years.[18,19] Treatment is generally conservative to allow the physis to remodel. A sling is usually adequate, although some authors prefer a figure-of-8 swathe. If severe displacement is present, acromioclavicular joint injuries or posterior sternoclavicular dislocations with associated impingement on vital structures should be reduced or (in the case of a posterior sternoclavicular joint fracture/dislocation) converted to an anterior dislocation.

The Elbow

Overuse and throwing injuries about the skeletally immature elbow can be categorized as acute versus chronic or by mechanism of injury. Classification by mechanism of injury is particularly helpful in creating a thorough differential diagnosis to make the most accurate diagnosis (Table 2). Determining the onset and type of injury (acute, chronic, or acute-on-chronic) cannot only guide the expected prognosis but also assist in avoiding missing an underlying factor or cause.[20,21] Further subclassification involving anatomic compartment (medial, lateral, and posterior) will help ensure that associated injury patterns are not missed. A specific diagnosis is important to guide treatment and to better advise the athlete regarding return to play. The term little leaguer's elbow, coined by Brogdon and Crow in 1960,[22] is nonspecific and can account for a myriad of conditions related to the pathologic forces of the immature elbow when throwing. This term should be avoided as a specific diagnosis.

During throwing, compression forces occur laterally, and tensile forces occur medially (Fig. 5, *A*). Tensile forces can cause injuries over the medial, lateral, or posterior aspects of the immature elbow. Medial tension can lead to muscle strains of the flexor muscles, collateral ligament injuries, and avulsions of the medial epicondyle. Lateral tension can lead to muscle strains and tendinosis of the extensor muscles. Posterior tension can lead to avulsion or apophysitis of the olecranon apophysis. Compression forces in throwing or weight bearing, including radial head hypertrophy, radial head fractures, osteochondritis dissecans, and capitellar fractures, have been implicated in causing changes in the lateral compartment of the elbow (Fig. 5, *B*). Posterior compression or impingement can lead to olecranon spurring or loose bodies.

For the skeletally immature throwing athlete, the common injury pattern is a blend of mechanisms called valgus-extension overload. During the cocking and acceleration phases of throwing, the medial structures of the elbow are placed in tension and the lateral structures are placed in compression, potentially leading to injury. In the follow-through phase of throwing, the elbow is locked in extension, leading to stresses on the olecranon, triceps, and olecranon fossa. Laxity in the medial structures, in turn, leads to impaction of the medial border of the olecranon in the olecranon fossa. In addition to these findings, chronic clinical findings can include an increased valgus carrying angle, flexion contractures, pain with throwing, medial epicondyle hypertrophy or fragmentation, and trochlear or olecranon fragmentation.[9,23-26]

Osteochondritis Dissecans

Osteochondritis dissecans, usually seen in patients age 10 to 14 years, is vascular compromise of the capitellum that has been related to repetitive compressive forces. Panner's disease is a similar appearing osteochondrosis that presents in patients age 4 to 8 years.[27] Segmentation of cartilage and subchondral bone is seen on radiographs. Osteochondritis dissecans is more common in males but that

Table 2
Differential Diagnosis of Elbow Injuries of the Immature Skeleton

- Medial
  - Acute
    - Avulsion fracture medial humeral epicondyle
    - Flexor/pronator strain
    - Fracture trochlea/distal humerus
    - Ulnar collateral ligament sprain
    - Ulnar nerve subluxation (Neuritis)
  - Chronic
    - Fracture medial epicondyle
    - Ulnar neuropathy
    - Ulnar nerve subluxation
    - Medial humeral epicondylitis
    - Traction spurs coronoid process
    - Valgus extension overload
    - Ulnar collateral instability
- Lateral
  - Acute
    - Osteochondritis dissecans capitellum
    - Osteochondral fracture capitellum
    - Avulsion fracture lateral humeral epicondyle (Apophysis)
    - Fracture capitellum/distal humerus
    - Anterior subluxation radial head
    - Fracture proximal radius
    - Fracture radial head—dislocation radial head
  - Chronic
    - Lateral humeral epicondylitis
    - Radial head hypertrophy/ overdevelopment
    - Loose bodies
    - Osteochondritis dissecans capitellum
    - Osteochondritis radial head
- Posterior
  - Acute
    - Olecranon fracture
    - Olecranon apophysitis
    - Olecranon spur with fracture
    - Triceps strain
    - Olecranon bursitis
    - Dislocation
  - Chronic
    - Olecranon traction apophysitis
    - Olecranon spurs
    - Loose bodies
    - Synovitis
    - Posteromedial spurs
    - Valgus extension overload
- Anterior
  - Acute
    - Biceps strain
    - Distal physeal humerus fracture
  - Chronic
    - Loose bodies
    - Adhesions
    - Synovitis
    - Capsular sprain

(Reproduced with permission from Andrews JR, Zarins B, Wilk KE (eds): *Injuries in Baseball.* Philadelphia, PA, Lippincott-Raven, 1998, p 291.)

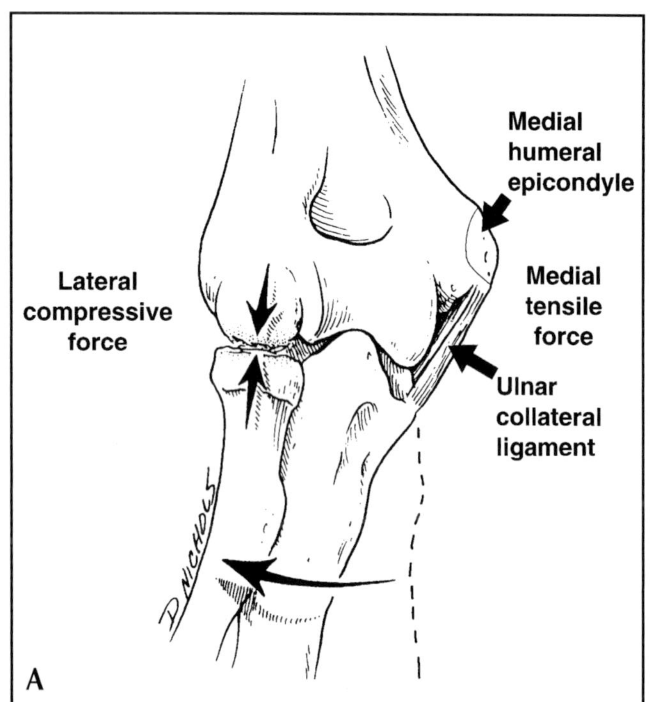

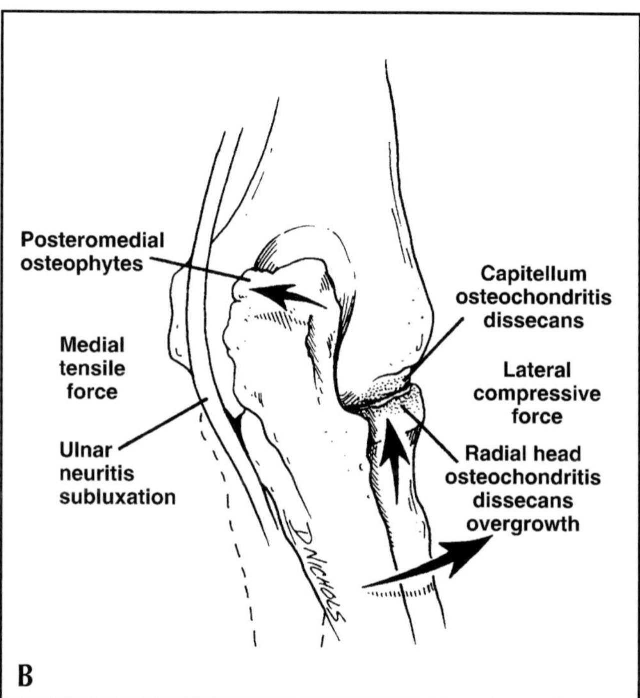

Fig. 5 Forces at the elbow are compression on the lateral side and tension of the medially side. The ulnar collateral ligament attaches lateral to the medial humeral epiphysis. When skeletally immature, medial forces cause medial humeral epicondyle stress fracture rather than ulnar collateral ligament sprain as seen in adults **(A)**. In chronic conditions, as these forces continue, the medial tensile forces result in ulnar neuritis or subluxation, posterior medial osteophytes. Laterally, the compressive forces result in osteochondritis dissecans of the capitellum, radial head overgrowth and joint incongruity **(B)**. (Reproduced with permission from Andrews JR, Zarins B, Wilk KE (eds): *Injuries in Baseball.* Philadelphia, PA, Lippincott-Raven, 1998.)

may be because of demand and total number of boys throwing compared with girls rather than an absolute genetic predisposition. Age is also a factor, and the earlier maturity of females may be relatively protective. Athletes will complain of pain on the lateral aspect of the elbow in 90% of cases. Other symptoms include loss of motion (55% of patients), symptoms of locking (less than 20%), and an acute onset (14%).[28]

Treatment of osteochondritis dissecans and Panner's disease is guided by the age of the patient, radiographic appearance of an unstable fragment, and the presence of loose bodies. Panner's disease is generally self-limited, does not create loose bodies, and rarely causes long-term problems. Treatment for Panner's disease, therefore, is symptomatic. Young athletes with Panner's disease should be restricted from axial stresses and valgus loading of the elbow (no gymnastics and no throwing).

Varying stages of osteochondritis dissecans exist, ranging from cystic changes to unstable but retained fragments to fragmentation and loose bodies. In general, the earlier the presentation the better the prognosis. As patients with osteochondritis dissecans approach maturity, healing potential diminishes and surgery becomes more likely. The presence of loose bodies and elbow locking is a strong indication for arthroscopy and removal of loose bodies. Once floating free, the fragments can rarely be returned to their bed and should be removed. Athletes with fragmentation and loose bodies may present with elbow pain and locking (Fig. 6, *A*). The capitellum should be carefully evaluated as a potential source of other loose fragments or for the presence of exposed subchondral bone that might be treated with marrow stimulation techniques (Fig. 6, *B* and *C*). Locking, as a symptom, is not always present even when loose bodies are present. The most common presenting complaint is pain with a loss of motion, especially extension. **(DVD-4.2)**

Specific guidelines in treatment of osteochondritis dissecans lesions can be controversial. Fundamentally, the best option is always to save the athlete's native cartilage.[9,21] Cystic changes and stable fragments should be allowed to heal without surgical intervention by reducing axial or valgus stresses until the fragment has healed. Temporary immobilization can reduce symptoms, but long-term immobilization can lead to stiffness. When evidence of healing is delayed or the patient is resistant to conservative treatment, anterograde drilling that does not violate the chondral surface has been suggested to improve circulation to the region.

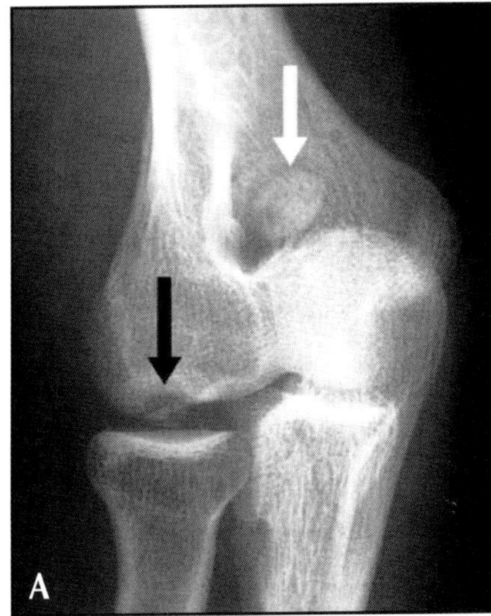

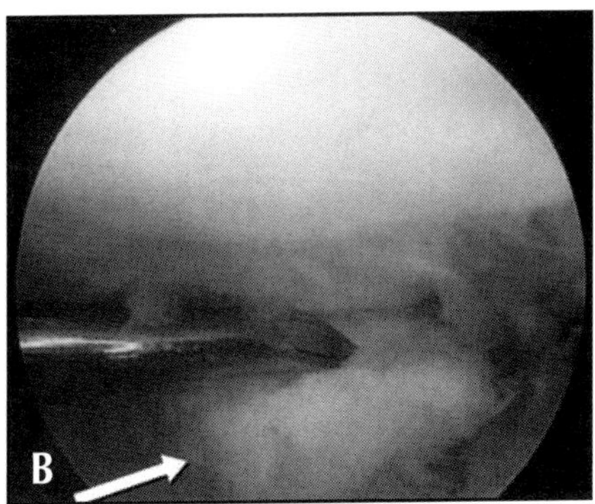

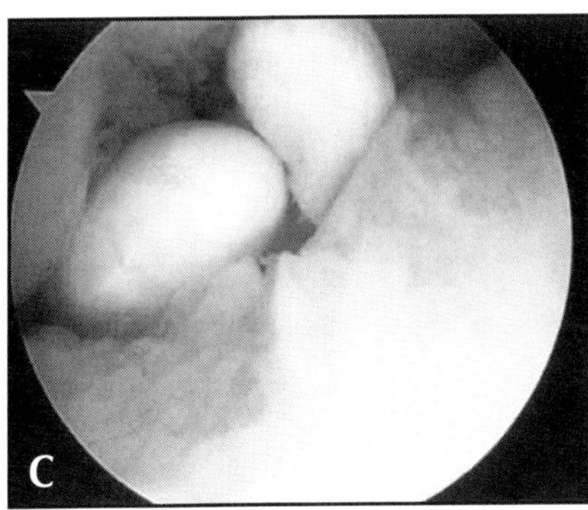

Fig. 6 A, Loose bodies are evident in the olecranon fossa (*white arrow*), and an osteochondritis dissecans lesion is seen at the capitellum (*black arrow*). **B,** Arthroscopic view shows a loose fragment of the capitellum (*arrow*) that required débridement and two loose bodies in the posterior compartment. **C,** Débridement only and no marrow stimulation technique on the capitellum was necessary in this pitcher.

Unstable fragments that remain in their chondral bed can be seen on radiographs and confirmed on MRI as having a fluid line beneath the chondral fragment (Fig. 7). Confirmation of an unstable fragment by MRI should include visualization of an actual chondral defect. Unstable fragments require surgical intervention in an attempt to save the in situ fragment. If the fragment can be elevated, the base is débrided or drilled to encourage a bleeding base for healing. Fixation of the fragment in the past has included anterograde Kirschner wires, small AO screws with subsequent screw removal, and bone pegs. Complications ranging from loss of fixation to fragmentation of the fragment and iatrogenic tibial chondral damage have been described. More recently, headless, variably threaded, metal screws (Accutrac, Acumed, Hillsboro, OR) or Herbert-Whipple screws) can apply some compression at the site and have been used with some success. The fragment must be large enough to tolerate the screw and have a bony component large enough to allow the screw to be recessed but still hold onto the fragment. Current trends of fixation have also included bioabsorbable pins or tacks that reduce or eliminate the need for a second surgery to remove

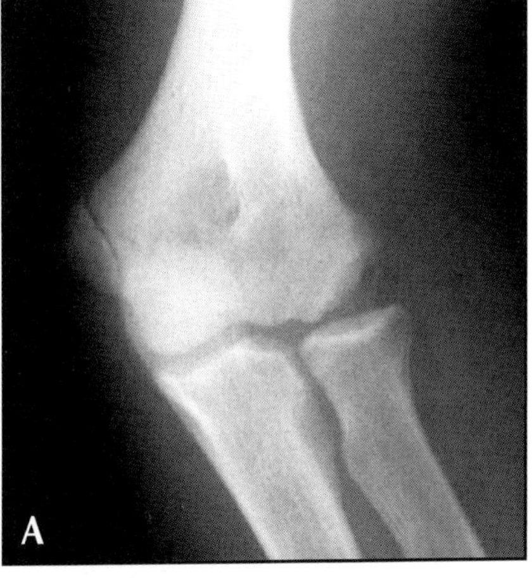

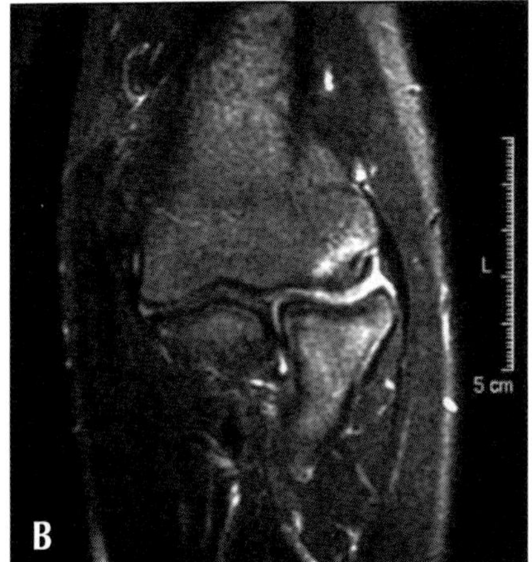

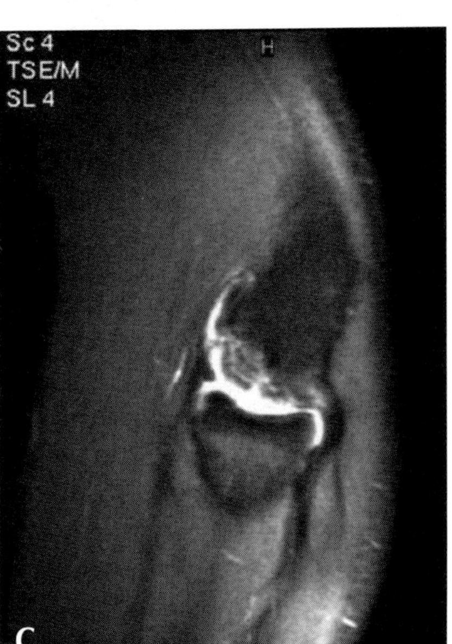

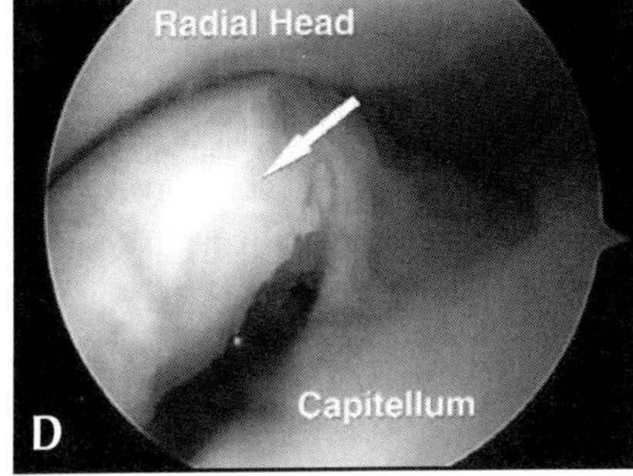

Fig. 7 A, AP radiograph in this left-hand–dominant baseball pitcher reveals osteochondritis dissecans lesion of the capitellum with open medial humeral epiphysis. MRI scan of coronal **(B)** and sagittal **(C)** views confirm the depth of the lesion and fragmentation of the articular cartilage. **D,** Arthroscopically, the capitellar piece was almost all cartilaginous (*arrow*).

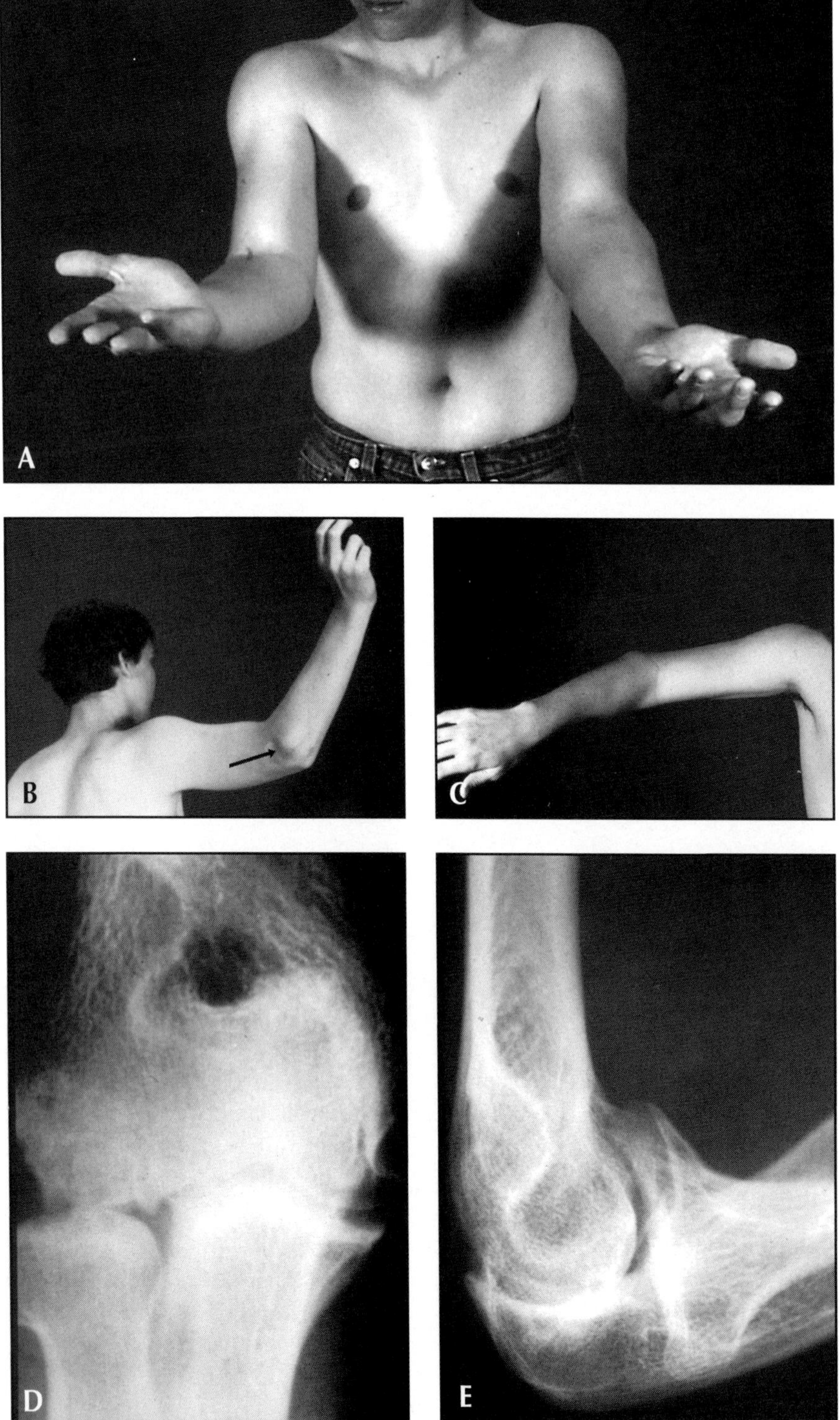

Fig. 8 A former high-school pitcher with painful limited motion of his right elbow, 40° of flexion contracture **(A)** and loss of pronation **(B)**. The radial head is quite prominent (*arrow*) **(C)**. AP lateral radiographs show an irregular capitellum with overgrowth of the radial head **(D)** and spurring of the coronoid anteriorly and joint incongruity **(E)**.

hardware. When the fragment is loose and unsalvageable, the loose piece should be removed. The defect that remains in the capitellum may remodel but many surgeons will drill or marrow-stimulate this region in the hope of covering it with fibrocartilage. Chondral transplants have also been attempted.

The long-term prognosis for displaced osteochondritis dissecans fragments, especially in the older athlete with less than 2 years until skeletal maturity, is guarded. The loose fragments or irregularly shaped capitellum can lead to early arthrosis, stiffness, and dysfunction (Fig. 8). It is in the best interest of the young athlete to be steadfast in restrictions for nondisplaced fragments and aggressive in the treatment of retained stable or unstable fragments to reduce the risk of long-term morbidity.

Medial Epicondylitis and Epicondyle Avulsions

Tension over the medial structures of the elbow can lead to muscle strains, tears of the medial collateral ligament, and avulsion of the medial epicondyle. As stated earlier, the weak link in the skeletally immature athlete is the physis; therefore, medial collateral ligament tears are rare in comparison to adult throwers, and medial epicondyle avulsions are more common in young athletes. Increased risk of medial epicondyle injuries have been correlated with overuse and the total number of pitches an athlete throws per week. An association with a sidearm or curveball throwing technique has also been argued but with less scientific support. Acute trauma can occur; nonetheless, most young athletes can provide a history of medial elbow pain that preceded the ultimate failure. Chronic stresses can lead to chronic changes and hypertrophy (Fig. 9).

Diagnosis is confirmed by localized tenderness, and comparative views of the opposite elbow should always be obtained. Treatment for nondisplaced fractures is symptomatic and may include a short period of immobilization (1 to 3 weeks) followed by early range of motion.[20] Protection against valgus forces and avoidance of resisted flexor strengthening is recommended until symptoms have subsided. As with little leaguer's shoulder, return to throwing should be avoided for 3 months to avoid recurrence; return to sports activity should be slow and progressive. Cross-training focused on core strengthening and stabilization is encouraged throughout the course of treatment. Technique evaluation by a quality pitching coach may also be of benefit to avoid recurrence.

The treatment of displaced fractures is somewhat more controversial.[9] Clearly any fragment that is incarcerated into the joint should be extricated and fixed. Most authors would agree that fragments displaced greater than 1 cm should also be fixed.[29-31] The treatment of minimally displaced fractures is less clear. They may heal with solid bone union but commonly heal with a fibrous union. When fibrous union occurs, high-level throwers, gymnasts, and power lifters may experience chronic pain, weakness, and dysfunction. Therefore, in these select athletes, internal fixation may be the best choice. Perhaps the greatest challenge is identifying the high-level thrower. The determination of surgical intervention in these cases must be made on an individual basis. When a posterior elbow dislocation occurs, some damage to the medial collateral ligament or avulsion of the medial epicondyle invariably occurs. Careful examination should include assessment of neurovascular function and imaging studies before and after reduction and imaging studies to evaluate displaced or intra-articular fragments (Fig. 10).

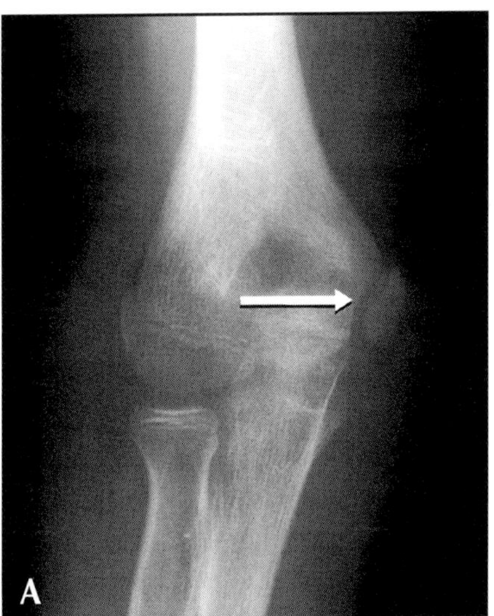

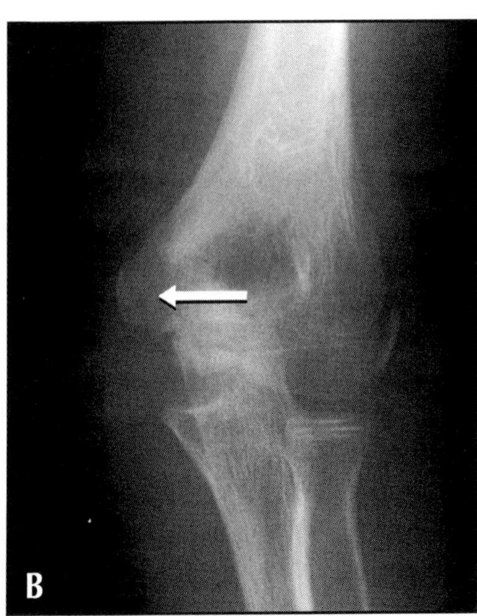

Fig. 9 A, Widening of the medial humeral epicondyle plate and overgrowth are evident in this right elbow (*arrow*). **B,** The nondominant side medial humeral epicondyle is smaller without the radiolucency at the epiphysis (*arrow*).

Tennis Elbow

Tension injuries over the lateral aspect of the elbow occur with the lead hand in hitting sports such as baseball and golf but are most commonly associated with the backhand motion in tennis. While ligamentous injuries are possible, the most common site of pathology is just distal to the lateral epicondyle in the extensor carpi radialis brevis muscle. Pain is exacerbated by extreme wrist flexion with the arm extended and resisted wrist extension. Tennis elbow is more common in adults than children.[32] Over 50% of club-level adult players have had some complaints of lateral elbow pain, whereas fewer than 10% of all boys and girls playing national-level tennis have lateral elbow complaints. Again, tendinosis of the extensor carpi radialis brevis is a problem of chronic overuse, and the young athlete has not yet had enough exposure and repetitions. The incidence of tennis elbow has also been related to grip size (larger being protective), string tension (tighter being worse), racquet size (larger head with bigger sweet spot being protective), and backhand technique (two-fisted being protective).[33]

Treatment is generally symptomatic with rest, ice, deep friction massage, and extensor stretches. Equipment and technique modification may also be helpful in reducing the rate of recurrence. Cross-pressure straps or taping can also be helpful. Nonsteroidal anti-inflammatory drugs should be used cautiously in children. Steroid injections in the skeletally immature athlete should be avoided, and surgical release is rarely if ever necessary or suggested.

Olecranon Apophysitis and Avulsions

Repetitive forceful extension leads to traction along the triceps tendon through the apophysis of the olecranon.[20,21] When the elbow is locked in full extension (follow-through and deceleration phases of throwing), further extension stresses can lead to shear forces across the apophysis. Both tension and shear forces can lead to physeal irritation, widening, or complete failure (avulsion). Like avulsions of the medial epicondyle of the elbow in throwers, complete avulsions in young athletes are associated with overuse and are commonly preceded by a prodrome of achy pain.

Treatment for nondisplaced fractures or olecranon apophysitis is rest, a temporary splint or sling for comfort, and reduction in extension stresses until

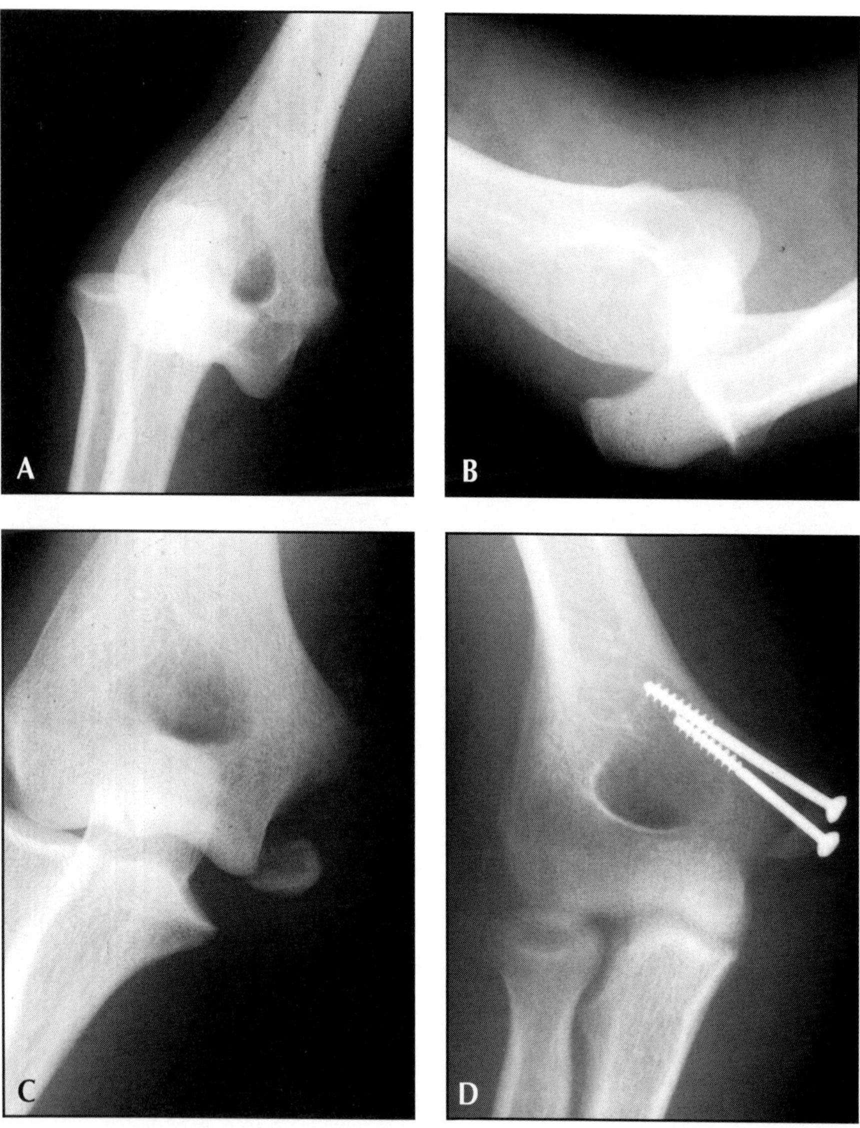

Fig. 10 Posterolateral elbow dislocation occurred in players sliding headfirst into base in AP **(A)** and lateral **(B)** views. **C,** The medial humeral epicondyle displaced fracture is not seen until reduction views. **D,** Open reduction and internal fixation and repair of the capsular injury was performed.

healed. Even after symptoms have resolved, athletes should not return to forceful throwing or upper extremity weight-bearing activities for 2 to 3 months to reduce the risk of recurrence. Displaced fractures imply an extensor mechanism in discontinuity and should be fixed with screws, pins, or tension band technique. Athletes who continue to throw despite an olecranon physeal injury can develop nonunion or resistance to an attempted course of conservative treatment[34,35] (Fig. 11). Surgical fixation can speed healing and time to return to sport.

Olecranon Bursitis and Posterior Olecranon Impingement

If comparative radiographs fail to reveal changes at the olecranon apophysis and the patient has no tenderness over the apophysis, olecranon bursitis or posterior olecranon impingement may be present in young athletes with posterior elbow pain. Olecranon bursitis is usually an obvious diagnosis, with swelling in the soft tissues superficial to the olecranon. The condition is commonly associated with acute or chronic repetitive trauma to the dorsal aspect of the elbow. Radiographs are usually negative but may reveal soft-tissue swelling or calcific densities in the bursa. Treatment is conservative with ice, anti-inflammatory medications, compression wrapping, and elbow pads for return to play. Aspiration and steroid injection have been recommended prior to the need for bursectomy in resistant cases. Any injections or surgeries attempted in this area should be done with caution because of the elevated risk of infection. Perioperative antibiotics are recommended for all surgical bursectomies.

If careful inspection of the radiographs reveals intra-articular loose bodies in the posterior compartment of the elbow or spurs on the medial border of the olecranon, the working diagnosis is likely posterior olecranon impingement. Athletes will generally present with a loss of full extension and pain with forced extension. A locking sensation is good evidence of an intra-articular loose body. Initial treatment begins with optimization of full extension. The presence of intra-articular loose bodies is a good indication for an elbow arthroscopy and removal of the loose bodies. The medial olecranon spur can be débrided at the same time. The prognosis after a simple arthroscopic débridement is guarded. The presence of posterior olecranon spurring and loose bodies is generally a secondary sign of valgus-extension overload. The integrity of the medial collateral ligament should be assessed with physical examination, stress radiographs, and possibly CT or MRI with contrast. Although young throwing athletes may experience improvement with arthroscopic débridement, they are unlikely to return to competitive throwing unless all components of pathology are addressed.

The Forearm, Wrist, and Hand

Although the classic upper extremity regions of concern for the skeletally immature athlete involve the shoulder and elbow, injuries related to overuse and throwing can also affect the forearm, wrist, and hand. Overuse problems of the forearm are rare in children and uncommon in throwing athletes. Activities such as gymnastics that demand weight bearing on the upper extremities are more prone to forearm complaints. Chronic exertional compartment syndrome of the forearm has been reported in skeletally mature collegiate gymnasts but not in children. Stress fractures and stress injuries to the radius and ulna have presented as forearm splints in skeletally mature and immature athletes. Radiographs are commonly negative, but bone scans may reveal diffuse or focal bone changes consistent with periostitis or stress fracture, respectively. Treatment is always conservative, beginning with reduced stresses and loading. Some athletes have returned to competition early with forearm splinting. Nonsteroidal anti-inflammatory agents are discouraged because they may impede the progress of bone healing. As is the case for all stress fractures, the presence of eating disorders is a possibility, and the athlete should be screened with an evaluation of nutrition and energy balance.

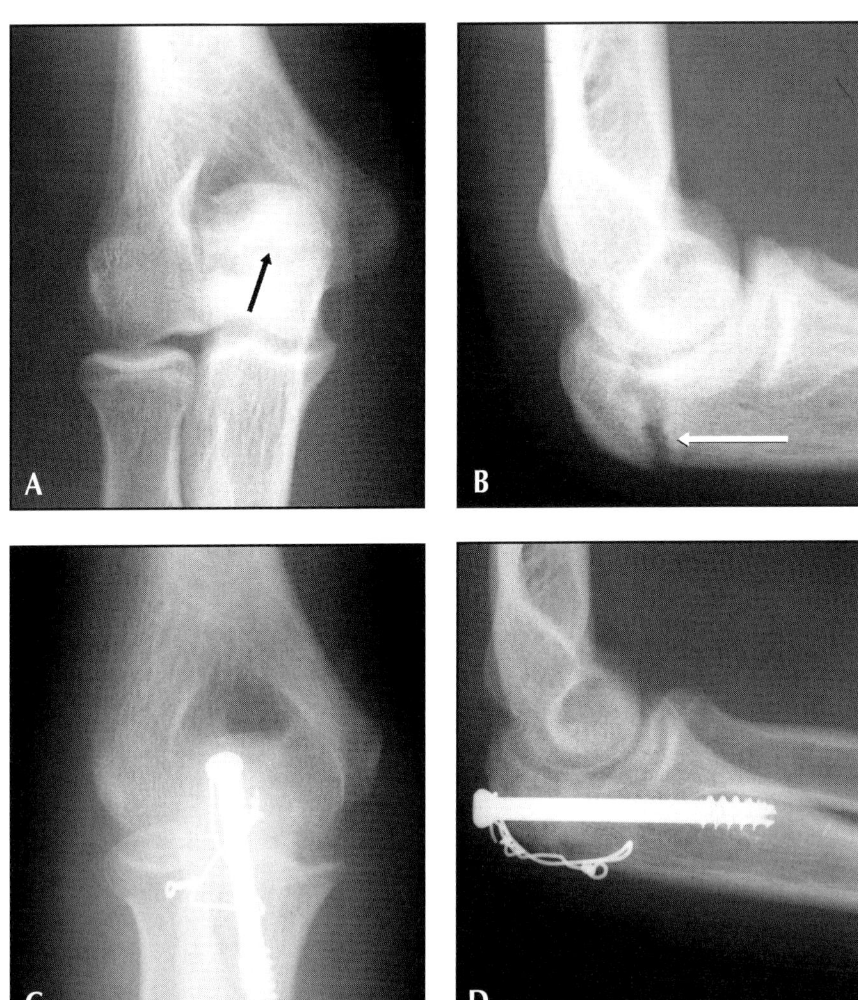

Fig. 11 Continued olecranon pain in this pitcher was caused by olecranon nonunion of the apophysis (*arrows*) as seen in AP (**A**) and lateral (**B**) views. The same views (**C** and **D**) show the result of open reduction and internal fixation with tension band wiring and screw placement.

The most common overuse injury at the level of the distal radius and wrist in young athletes is distal radius epiphysitis.[36-38] Pain on the dorsal aspect of the wrist with extension and weight bearing is the major complaint. Comparative radiographs will reveal an asymmetric widening of the distal radial physis. Continued stresses could lead to permanent deformity, radial shortening, and an ulnar positive wrist. These are nondisplaced fractures, and surgery is never necessary. Treatment is based on reduction of stresses. When the athlete is asymptomatic, a gradual progressive return to sport may begin; taping or bracing of the wrist will protect against the extremes of dorsiflexion.

Less common injuries about the wrist in young athletes include carpal tunnel syndrome, Kienböck's disease (lunatomalacia), and tears of the triangular fibrocartilaginous complex.[39] Only two cases of a purely ligamentous wrist injury in skeletally immature athletes have been reported. Physeal injuries or carpal stress fractures are more common. The most common carpal bone injured in all athletes is the scaphoid, and this injury should be suspected in athletes with wrist pain, reduced flexibility, and pain in the anatomic snuff box. Even when radiographs are negative, temporary immobilization is recommended until bone scans or repeat radiographs at 2 weeks are negative. Injuries to the metacarpal and phalanges in young athletes are frequently physeal. Comparison should be made to adjacent physis and to the opposite hand.

Summary

Overuse and throwing injuries that occur in the skeletally immature athlete can lead to long-term disability and deformity. Therefore, it is imperative to encourage prevention when possible and early recognition of all injuries to prevent progression to a more serious stage. Early recognition can be aided by a high index of suspicion and a dedication to perform complete evaluations, which should always include radiographs of the contralateral side for the skeletally immature patient.

Young athletes usually want to continue sports participation and may play through pain to please their parents, coaches, or peers. Education of athletes, coaches, and parents that pain in young athletes is a key symptom that should not be ignored is important. These athletes can be protected from progression or more serious injury by early clinical evaluation, appropriate radiographs, accurate diagnosis, and tailored care and rehabilitation programs. Fortunately, for a majority of overuse and throwing injuries in the skeletal immature athlete, conservative treatment, thorough rehabilitation, and gradual progressive retraining and reconditioning will allow a full and safe return to sport.

References

1. Guy JA, Micheli LJ: Strength training for children and adolescents. *J Am Acad Orthop Surg* 2001;9:29-36.
2. Ogden JA (ed): *Skeletal Injury in the Child*, ed 2. Philadelphia, PA, WB Saunders, 1990.
3. Peterson CA, Peterson HA: Analysis of the incidence of injuries to the epiphyseal growth plate. *J Trauma* 1972;12:275-281.
4. Neer CS II, Horwitz BS: Fractures of the proximal humeral epiphysial plate. *Clin Orthop* 1965;41:24-31.
5. Micheli LJ: Pediatric and adolescent musculoskeletal sports injuries, in Teitz CC (ed): *Scientific Foundations of Sports Medicine*. Toronto, Canada, BC Decker, 1989, pp 329-343.
6. Outerbridge AR, Micheli LJ: Overuse injuries in the young athlete. *Clin Sports Med* 1995;14:503-516.
7. Lyman S, Fleisig GS, Waterbor JW, et al: Longitudinal study of elbow and shoulder pain in youth baseball pitchers. *Med Sci Sports Exerc* 2001;33:1803-1810.
8. Ireland ML, Satterwhite YE: Shoulder injuries, in Andrews JR, Zarins B, Wilk KE (eds): *Injuries in Baseball*. Philadelphia, PA, Lippincott-Raven, 1998, pp 271-281.
9. Ireland ML, Hutchinson MR: Upper extremity injuries in young athletes. *Clin Sports Med* 1995;14:533-569.
10. Patel PR, Warner JP: Shoulder injuries in the skeletally immature athlete, in Micheli LJ (ed): *Adolescent Sports Medicine*. Philadelphia, PA, Lippincott-Raven, 1996, pp 99-101.
11. Patterson PD, Waters PM: Shoulder injuries in the childhood athlete. *Clin Sports Med* 2000;19:681-692.
12. Hovelius L, Augustini BG, Fredin H, Johansson O, Norlin R, Thorling J: Primary anterior dislocation of the shoulder in young patients: A ten-year prospective study. *J Bone Joint Surg Am* 1996;78:1677-1682.
13. Paletta GA Jr: Treatment of glenohumeral instability in the pediatric athlete. *Op Tech Sports Med* 1998;6:213-216.
14. Wilkins KE, Curtis RJ: Shoulder injuries, in Stanitski CL, DeLee JC, Drez D Jr (eds): *Pediatric and Adolescent Sports Medicine*. Philadelphia, PA, WB Saunders, 1994, pp 262-278.
15. Dotter WE: Little leaguer's shoulder: A fracture of the proximal epiphysial cartilage of the humerus due to baseball pitching. *Guthrie Clin Bull* 1953;23:68-72.
16. Carson WG Jr, Gasser SI: Little Leaguer's shoulder: A report of 23 cases. *Am J Sports Med* 1998;26:575-580.
17. Adams JE: Little league shoulder: Osteochondrosis of the proximal humeral epiphysis in boy baseball pitchers. *Calif Med* 1966;105: 105:22-25.
18. Eidman DK, Siff SJ, Tullos HS: Acromioclavicular lesions in children. *Am J Sports Med* 1981;9:150-154.
19. Winter J, Sterner S, Maurer D, Varecka T, Zarzycki M: Retrosternal epiphyseal disruption of the medial clavicle: Case report and review in children. *J Emerg Med* 1989;7:9-13.
20. Bradley JP: Upper extremity: Elbow injuries in children and adolescents, in Stanitski CL, DeLee JC, Drez D Jr (eds): *Pediatric and Adolescent Sports Medicine*. Philadelphia, PA, WB Saunders, 1994, pp 242-261.
21. Gerbino PG, Waters PM: Elbow injuries in the young athlete. *Op Tech Sports Med* 1998;6: 259-267.
22. Brogdon BG, Crow NE: Little leaguer's elbow. *AJR Am J Roentgenol* 1960;83:671-675.
23. Ireland ML, Hutchinson MR: Elbow injuries, in Andrews JR, Zarins B, Wilk KE (eds): *Injuries in Baseball*. Philadelphia, PA, Lippincott-Raven, 1988, pp 283-306.
24. Whiteside JA, Andrews JR, Fleisig GS: Elbow injuries in young baseball players. *Phys Sportsmed* 1999;27:87-92.
25. Pappas AM: Elbow problems associated with baseball during childhood and adolescence. *Clin Orthop* 1982;164:30-41.
26. Chen FS, Rokito AS, Jobe FW: Medial elbow problems in the overhead-throwing athlete. *J Am Acad Orthop Surg* 2001;9:99-113.
27. Panner HJ: A peculiar affection of the capitulum humeri, resembling Calve-Perthes disease of the hip. *Acta Radiol* 1929;10:234-242.
28. Schenck RC Jr, Goodnight JM: Osteochondritis dissecans. *J Bone Joint Surg Am* 1996;78:439-456.
29. Ireland ML, Andrews JR: Shoulder and elbow injuries in the young athlete. *Clin Sports Med* 1988;7:473-494.
30. Micheli LJ: Elbow pain in a little league pitcher, in Smith NJ (ed): *Common Problems in Pediatric Sports Medicine*. Chicago, IL, Year-Book Publishers, 1989, pp 233-241.
31. Woods GW, Tullos HS: Elbow instability and medial epicondyle fractures. *Am J Sports Med* 1977;5:23-30.
32. Hutchinson MR, Laprade RF, Burnett QM II, Moss R, Terpstra J: Injury surveillance at the USTA Boys' Tennis Championships: A 6-yr study. *Med Sci Sports Exerc* 1995;27:826-830.
33. Marx RG, Sperling JW, Cordasco FA: Overuse injuries of the upper extremity in tennis players. *Clin Sports Med* 2001;20:439-451.
34. Torg JS, Moyer RA: Non-union of a stress fracture through the olecranon epiphyseal plate observed in an adolescent baseball pitcher: A case report. *J Bone Joint Surg Am* 1977;59: 264-265.
35. Pavlov H, Torg JS, Jacobs B, Vigorita V: Nonunion of the olecranon epiphysis: Two cases in adolescent baseball pitchers. *AJR Am J Roentgenol* 1981;136:819-820.
36. Gerbino PG II: Wrist disorders in the young athlete. *Op Tech Sports Med* 1998;6:197-205.
37. Zetaruk MN: The young gymnast. *Clin Sports Med* 2000;19:757-780.
38. Morgan WJ, Slowman LS: Acute hand and wrist injuries in athletes: Evaluation and management. *J Am Acad Orthop Surg* 2001;9:389-400.
39. Lovallo JL, Simmons BP: Hand and wrist injuries in Stanitski CL, DeLee JC, Drez D Jr (eds): *Pediatric and Adolescent Sports Medicine*. Philadelphia, PA, WB Saunders, 1994, pp 262–278.

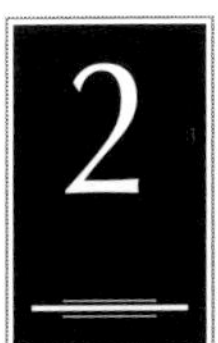

Arthroscopic Treatment of Anterior Glenohumeral Instability: Indications and Techniques

Brian J. Cole, MD, MBA
Peter J. Millett, MD, MSc
Anthony A. Romeo, MD
Stephen S. Burkhart, MD
James R. Andrews, MD
Jeffrey R. Dugas, MD
Jon J.P. Warner, MD

Abstract

The arthroscopic treatment of anterior glenohumeral instability is becoming increasingly accepted as a viable treatment option because reported success rates parallel those of open stabilization techniques. This improved success rate is largely the result of advances in surgical techniques and technology. An improved understanding of the pathoanatomy associated with shoulder instability and continuing education initiatives have also been instrumental in expanding the indications for arthroscopic stabilization of the unstable shoulder. Important considerations during arthroscopy include identifying all pathology, mobilizing soft tissue, enhancing the local biology to promote soft-tissue healing to bone or to itself, securing anatomic fixation, and respecting the healing period during postoperative rehabilitation efforts. Principal contraindications include significant bone deficits and the inability to repair capsular avulsions or rupture. Adherence to these basic principles should lead to excellent results with arthroscopic stabilization of the unstable shoulder.

Arthroscopy is becoming increasingly accepted as a viable treatment option for anterior glenohumeral instability. Despite early reports of variable recurrence rates, arthroscopic techniques have now evolved significantly largely as a result of improved understanding of the associated pathoanatomy, improved patient selection, simplified techniques, and advanced technology. The major advantages of arthroscopic repair over traditional open repair include the ability to identify and treat concomitant pathology, lower morbidity and decreased pain, shorter surgical time, and improved cosmesis. Some surgeons believe that patients who undergo arthroscopic repair of anterior glenohumeral instability have an easier functional recovery with greater returns in motion compared with patients undergoing traditional open repair. Finally, some of the inherent risks of open repair procedures, such as postoperative subscapularis rupture, are virtually eliminated.

One or more of the authors or the departments with which they are affiliated have received something of value from a commercial or other party related directly or indirectly to the subject of this chapter.

Anatomy of Shoulder Stability

Although the diverse stabilizing structures of the glenohumeral joint have been previously described in detail elsewhere,[1] a brief review here will provide a foundation for the discussion to follow. Because the large spherical head of the humerus articulates with the relatively small and shallow glenoid, the glenohumeral joint requires several mechanisms that maintain stability and allow for a large range of motion. Static and dynamic stability are provided by the combined effects of the capsuloligamentous structures, the rotator cuff, the scapular stabilizers, and the biceps muscle. In the midrange of motion, the principal stabilizers are the rotator cuff and biceps tendons, which dynamically stabilize the humeral head through concavity-compression within the glenoid socket. The ligamentous structures function at the extremes of rotation, preventing excessive rotation and translation.

The labrum increases the depth and surface area of the bony glenoid. Its principal function is to increase the depth of the glenoid socket and to act as a "chock block" to prevent the head from rolling over the anterior edge of the glenoid. It consists of a fibrocartilaginous ring that attaches to the glenoid articular cartilage.[2] Above the glenoid equator, the labrum is relatively mobile; below the glenoid equator, the labrum is more tightly attached to the glenoid articular cartilage. The labrum also provides an attachment site for the glenohumeral ligaments and the tendon of the long head of the biceps. Virtually all labral lesions, especially those below the glenoid equator, are thought to be associated with glenohumeral instability.

The role of the capsule and ligaments in shoulder stability is complex and depends on the position of the joint and the direction of the applied force. The inferior glenohumeral ligament complex is the primary static check against anterior, posterior, and inferior translation between 45° and 90° of glenohumeral elevation. The superior and middle glenohumeral ligaments limit anteroposterior and inferior translation in the middle and lower ranges of elevation as the arm approaches the adducted position.

The rotator interval region between the supraspinatus and subscapularis tendons provides stability against inferior and posterior translations, particularly when the arm is adducted and externally rotated. Evidence suggests that this may be a normal variant present at birth and is only a relative contributor to instability in the symptomatic patient with excessive inferior or posterior translation that is not eliminated despite correction of other existing pathology.[3]

The rotator cuff and long head of the biceps brachii enhance stability by increasing compression across the glenohumeral joint, thereby increasing the loads required to translate the humeral head. This is particularly apparent in the midranges of motion where the capsuloligamentous structures are more lax. The scapulothoracic stabilizers help to position the glenoid beneath the humeral head. Dysfunction in any of these stabilizers can lead to symptoms of instability. Proprioceptive mechanisms help to coordinate and time this system and are restored after instability surgery.

The articular surfaces also play a key role in stability. Articular version, negative intra-articular pressure, and adhesion-cohesion all enhance shoulder stability. In general, each of these factors plays a relatively small role in the pathogenesis of shoulder instability, although bone loss, particularly on the glenoid, can be significant enough to warrant surgical correction and remains the principal contraindication to arthroscopic shoulder stabilization.

Pathoanatomy

Labrum

Disruption between the anterior labrum and the glenoid below the equator is termed a Bankart lesion. Because the inferior glenohumeral ligament complex is the major static stabilizer when the shoulder is positioned in abduction and external rotation, a capsulolabral separation in this area effectively destabilizes the glenohumeral joint. Furthermore, the normal stabilizing effect of the rotator cuff compressing the humeral head into the glenoid socket is diminished when the labrum is separated from the glenoid rim. The Bankart lesion, which is considered the essential pathoanatomic lesion, is present in about 90% of all traumatic anterior shoulder dislocations. Because of its essential stabilizing functions, the labrum must be anatomically restored in patients with instability.

In some patients, the labrum heals in a medialized position (anterior labrum periosteal sleeve avulsion lesion).[4] When this occurs, the labroligamentous complex must be mobilized surgically and released from the glenoid and underlying subscapularis so that it can be reattached at its correct anatomic insertion. When the labrum is repaired to the glenoid, the suture anchors should be placed 1 to 2 mm onto the "face" of the glenoid to restore the concavity and to ensure that the labrum can perform its essential biomechanical functions.[5,6] Currently, the use of multiple anchors (ie, three to four) with multiple sutures providing multiple fixation points is preferred. It is also important that the anchors are placed at least down to the 5 o'clock position. This sometimes necessitates a "5 o'clock portal" to give a proper angle of approach for insertion of the anchors.[7] At the conclusion of the repair, the glenoid concavity should be visibly extended and a buttress or "bumper" effect should be achieved, as is present in the uninjured shoulder.

Above the glenoid equator, labral

anatomy may be quite variable, and a loose attachment below the biceps tendon may be a normal variant (ie, a sublabral foramen). Injuries to the superior labrum with associated destabilization of the biceps insertion may occur with shoulder instability. Both experimental and clinical studies have provided a rationale for arthroscopic repair of these superior labral injuries when treating instability.[8,9] The variations in superior labral anatomy may pose challenges in determining whether a patient's anatomy is a variant of normal or an abnormal labral detachment. In general, a loosely attached superior labrum with a smooth cartilage transition is a variant of normal and not a labral separation. True labral injury is associated with failure of the origin fibers of the superior labrum, cartilage injury at the margin of the labral attachment, synovitis, and/or extension of the tear into the biceps tendon itself. In the setting of shoulder instability, such tears of the superior labrum should always be repaired.

Ligaments

In addition to the Bankart lesion, recurrent dislocations can also cause stretching of the glenohumeral capsule and ligaments. This plastic deformation occurs from repetitive loading. Although identification of this stretch injury or laxity of the ligaments may be difficult, failure to address this component of the instability when performing an arthroscopic repair may contribute to failure of the procedure. Indeed, in some series, higher failure rates have been attributed to this error. If the middle or inferior glenohumeral ligament complex is stretched, then the joint volume will be increased, and the joint will be susceptible to instability on that basis even with an intact labrum.[6,10]

Actual macroscopic midsubstance failure of the capsule or failure at the humeral insertion (humeral avulsion of glenohumeral ligament) is uncommon but appears to constitute a relative contraindication to arthroscopic repair because of the technical difficulty associated with repairing such an injury. Although it is technically possible to repair this condition arthroscopically, direct repair with capsule repair and reinsertion appears to be more reliable through an open approach.

Insufficiency of the rotator interval may be responsible for failures in some series. This interval is usually involved if there is a large inferior component to the instability, particularly when the arm is in adduction and external rotation.[11] Rowe and Sakellarides[12] originally pointed out that the capsule may be absent or deficient in this area, and these authors and others recommended closure at the time of open instability repair.[3,11] The defect may represent either an injury or, more likely, a relative dysplasia of the ligaments of this region. When the defect is recognized arthroscopically, repair by overlapping the capsular region between the anterior edge of the supraspinatus and proximal edge of the subscapularis is the preferred method.

Rotator Cuff

When the rotator cuff is injured, its concavity-compression effect is diminished. Rotator cuff injury in younger patients usually occurs in the setting of repetitive overload. In such patients, the tear results from eccentric overload of the tendon and represents a secondary injury to the tendon from the recurrent instability. Full-thickness tears of the rotator cuff after a traumatic dislocation are uncommon in patients younger than 40 years but should be suspected in those who continue to have weakness and pain 3 weeks after a traumatic anterior dislocation. In this setting, careful physical examination and early soft-tissue imaging studies will discern the presence and configuration of the rotator cuff tear. Generally, tears of the superior cuff can be repaired arthroscopically at the same time as the instability. Significant tears of the subscapularis can also be repaired arthroscopically, although this does require considerable technical skill, and a traditional open repair is certainly an acceptable option.

Bone

Bone deficiency is a significant cause for the failure of arthroscopic Bankart repairs. Burkhart and De Beer[13] reported on a group of 194 patients who had undergone arthroscopic Bankart repair of the shoulder. One hundred one of these patients were contact athletes. These authors found that when the patients had no significant bone defects (173 patients), the recurrence rate was 4%. However, when patients had significant bone defects (21 patients), the recurrence rate was 67%. Contact athletes with significant bone defects had an 87% recurrence rate, whereas contact athletes without bone defects had a 6.5% recurrence rate.

Three types of bone lesions are found in patients with anterior instability: (1) glenoid erosion (also known as inverted pear glenoid morphology) (Figure 1); (2) the engaging Hill-Sachs lesion (Figure 2); and (3) the nonengaging Hill-Sachs lesion[13] (Figure 3).

Glenoid Erosion The normal glenoid is broader inferiorly than superiorly (pear-shaped). Because the glenoid resists both axial and off-axis loads, significant bone loss results in a shorter arc through which the gle-

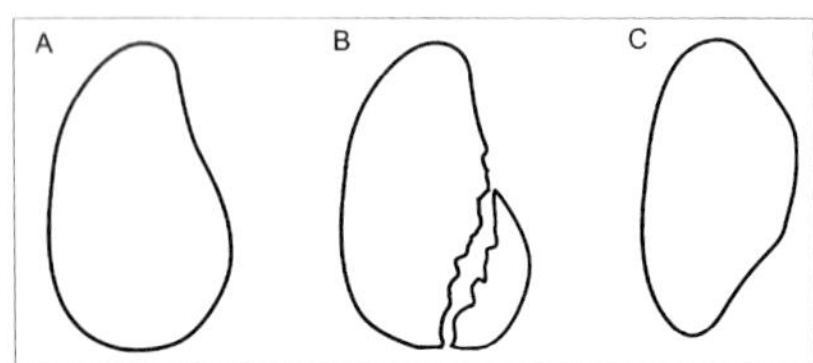

Figure 1 The normal glenoid and the inverted-pear glenoid morphology. **A,** The normal shape of the glenoid is that of a pear, larger inferiorly than superiorly. **B,** An acute bony Bankart fracture can create an "inverted pear" configuration. **C,** Erosion of the anterior glenoid can also create this configuration.

noid can resist these loads. Furthermore, the glenoid resists shear by rim loading. If part of the rim is lost (as the result of a labral tear, fracture, or erosion, for example), then it cannot effectively resist shear. When a large bony Bankart lesion is present or when glenoid erosion occurs from multiple dislocations, the glenoid loses its normal anatomic configuration and assumes the shape of an inverted pear (Figure 1). Anatomic studies have shown that the inverted pear morphology always involves more than a 25% loss in diameter.[13,14]

Burkhart and associates[14] have also shown that the glenoid bare spot is the center of a circle defined by the margins of the anterior, posterior, and inferior glenoids, and therefore it is useful as a reference to gauge how much bone has been lost, particularly in a patient with erosive bone loss from chronic recurrent anterior dislocations. The bare spot is visible in virtually all patients and is best viewed through an anterosuperior viewing portal. Significant bone loss, with greater than a 25% loss of the inferior diameter of the glenoid, is a contraindication for arthroscopic repair because of an unacceptably high recurrence rate among such patients, particularly active individuals and contact athletes. In such cases, an open approach with bone grafting of the anteroinferior glenoid is preferred. Alternatively, coracoid transfer procedures offer acceptable treatment options.

Hill-Sachs Lesion When the glenohumeral joint dislocates, the Hill-Sachs defect can occur at a variety of angles as determined by the position of the humerus at the time of dislocation. Some Hill-Sachs lesions will "engage" the anterior glenoid rim when the glenohumeral joint is in a position of abduction and external rotation. Burkhart and De Beer[13] have described these as engaging Hill-Sachs lesions, in which the long axis of the humeral bone defects aligns parallel to the anterior glenoid rim when the shoulder is in a position of abduction and external rotation. Such fracture configurations have been found to be particularly prone to recurrent dislocation and subluxation after arthroscopic repair (Figure 2).

With the nonengaging Hill-Sachs lesion, the long axis of the Hill-Sachs defect diagonally crosses glenoid rim with the arm in abduction and external rotation so that it never "engages" the glenoid rim (Figure 3). In these types of defects, there is a continuous smooth articular contact throughout the range of motion. Such shoulders with nonengaging Hill-Sachs lesions are not at significant risk for recurrence when repaired arthroscopically, and therefore patients with these types of humeral lesions are good candidates for arthroscopic repair.

Evolution of Arthroscopic Repairs

The failure rate after open repair is generally less than 10%; this is benchmark against which arthroscopic repairs must be compared.[15-18] Historically, the literature has classified failures of instability repair as those that develop recurrent instability (ie, the shoulders of patients become too loose). However, there is scant mention in the literature of failures of instability repair that are too tight, resulting in stiffness, loss of motion, and late degenerative changes. It is important to remember that stiffness does not equal stability, and that there is significant danger in soft-tissue overconstraint. In addition, the early literature describing the results of open stabilization consists of largely retrospective series with relatively poor results in terms of returning athletes back to their original level of play. In addition, early reports fail to describe patients who have persistent apprehension or recurrent subluxation despite open stabilization procedure.

Variations in surgical indications, surgical techniques, and definitions of success and failure make comparisons across series difficult. Recent prospective studies of arthroscopic stabilization techniques have reported failure rates as low as those reported in the best open repair series, with a high rate of return to sporting activities[10,19-29] (Table 1).

Johnson[30] first introduced arthroscopic repair with metal staples in 1982; subsequent reports, however, demonstrated unacceptable recurrence rates as high as 33%. This technique has largely been abandoned because of the relatively high complication rates (between 5% and 10%) related principally to the hardware. Transglenoid sutures were introduced by Morgan and Bodenstab[31] and popularized by Caspari and Savoie.[7] Success rates of 90% have been reported,[32,33] but other authors do not report comparable success rates.[34-36] The major advantage of this technique was the multiple points of fixation for the labrum. It also allowed the surgeon to address capsular laxity by shifting the capsule

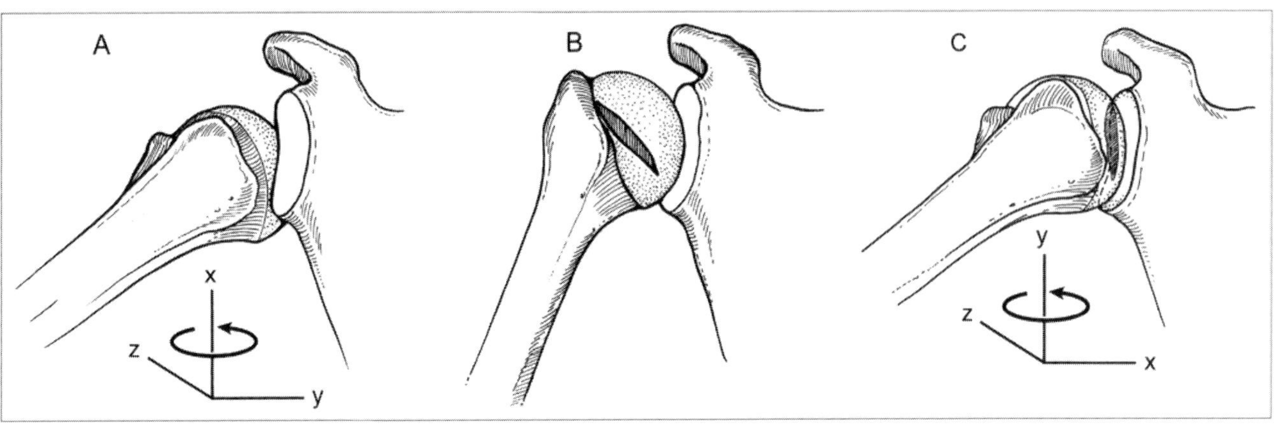

Figure 2 The engaging Hill-Sachs lesion. **A,** This impaction fracture is created when a glenohumeral dislocation occurs with the humerus in abduction and external rotation. **B,** Schematic showing the orientation of the osseous defect, which is more horizontal. **C,** Schematic showing the "engagement" of the defect on the anterior glenoid in a functional position of abduction and external rotation.

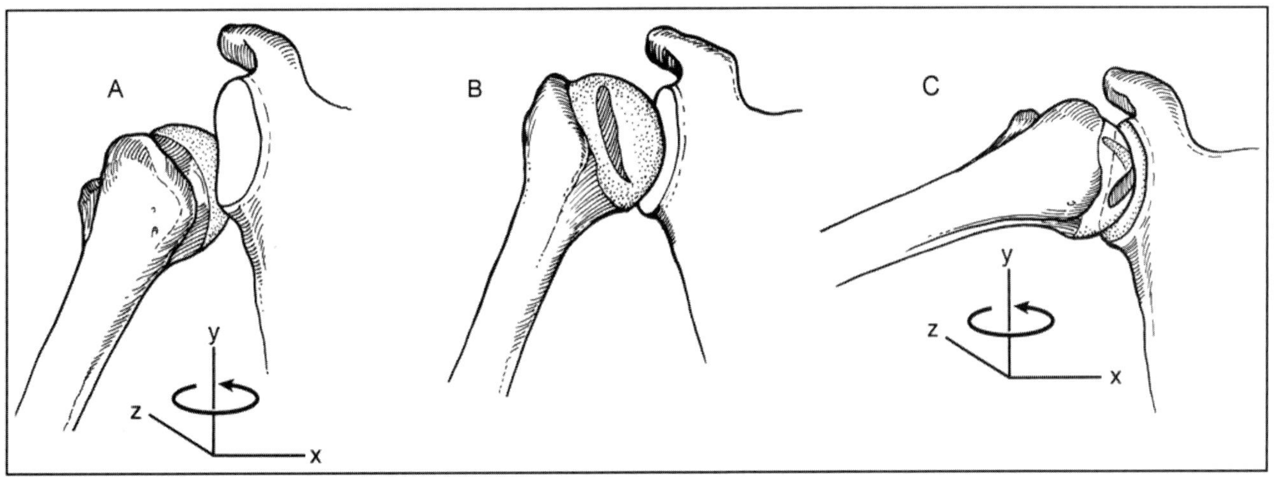

Figure 3 The nonengaging Hill-Sachs lesion. **A,** This impaction fracture is created when a glenohumeral dislocation occurs with the humerus in adduction. **B,** Schematic showing the orientation of the osseous defect on the humerus, which is more vertical. **C,** Schematic showing that the defect does not engage the anterior glenoid in a functional position of abduction and external rotation.

superiorly and medially on the glenoid rim. The major disadvantages were the technical difficulty and the transscapular drilling that placed the suprascapular nerve in jeopardy.

To obviate some of these concerns, Speer and associates[37] introduced a bioabsorbable (polyglycolic acid) single-point transfixing implant for intra-articular labral repair (Suretac, Acufex Microsurgical, Norwood, MA). Initial enthusiasm was tempered when recurrence rates up to 21% were reported. Recent experience has suggested that recurrence rates can be decreased to less than 10% if the procedure is limited to those with isolated Bankart lesions and no capsular injury.[38-41] Disadvantages of this technique include the inability to address concomitant capsular laxity and the potential for a synovial reaction to the polyglyconate of the implant, which may occur in up to 6% of patients.[42,43]

Modern Suture Anchor Repairs

Repair techniques that use suture anchors have become the most commonly used arthroscopic repair method. This is also the authors' preferred method of repair. The method was first described by Wolf,[10] who reported using a metal anchor and tying knots with absorbable sutures. In 1994, Snyder[44] mod-

Table 1
Arthroscopic Reconstruction Using Suture Anchors

Author(s)	No. of Patients	Mean Follow-up (months)	Recurrence (%)	Comments
Wolf[10]	50	"short"	0	
Belzer and Snyder[19]	37	22	11	13% reported "apprehension"
Hoffman and Reif[20]	30	24	11	
Guanche et al[21]	25	27	33	Comparative series
Bacilla et al[22]	40	30	7	High-demand patients
Sisto and Cook[23]	27	47	13	Refined indications
Field et al[24]	50	33	8	Comparative series
Gartsman et al[25]	53	33	8	"Rx all pathology"
Cole and Romeo[26]	32	26	0	3 to 4 anchors per shoulder
Mishra and Fanton[27]	42	28	7	Radiofrequency augmentation
Kim et al[28]	58	39	10	Comparative series
Abrams et al[29]	61	35	6.6	

Table 2
Comparison of Same Surgeon Arthroscopic Versus Open Stabilization (Varied Techniques)

Authors	No. of Patients (Arthroscopy/Open Stabilization)	Mean Follow-up (Months)	Recurrence (%) (Arthroscopy/Open Stabilization)
Geiger et al[45]	16/8	23/24	43/8
Guanche et al[21]	25/12	27/25	33/8
Steinbeck and Jerosch[46]	30/32	36/40	17/6
Field et al[24]	50/50	33/30	8/0
Cole and Warner[47]	37/22	52/55	24/18
Karlsson et al[48]	66/53	32	15/10
Sperber et al[49]	30/26	13/10	23/12
Kim et al[28]	30/58	39	10/10

ified the technique with the use of permanent sutures. Although in the past 10 years several series have reported failure rates ranging between 0 and 33%[10,19-29] (Table 1), recent comparative studies of arthroscopic suture anchor technique and open stabilization report recurrence rates of less than 10%[21,24,28,45-49] (Table 2). Compared with transglenoid repair techniques, suture anchor repair techniques allow for knots to be tied in the joint arthroscopically, thus avoiding the risk of and need for a posterior incision. Newer implant designs allow for suture repair using anchors without knots, thus eliminating knot tying altogether.

Patient Selection

When considering arthroscopic shoulder stabilization, patient selection is critical, and the patient's history, motivation, and goals must be considered. The relative contraindications to arthroscopic stabilization, including significant bone loss, humeral avulsions of the glenohumeral ligaments, capsular insufficiency (revisions), and the inability to achieve stability by an all-arthroscopic technique, must also be considered.

Evaluation

History and Physical Examination

A thoughtful and detailed history and physical examination are the most important tools in the evaluation of anterior glenohumeral instability. Historical information includes details surrounding the onset, duration, and frequency of symptoms. Discerning the traumatic nature of instability and ruling out any volitional component is critical to the ultimate success in treating traumatic anterior glenohumeral instability. The arm position at the time of the initial injury and the methods required to reduce the dislocation give clues to the extent of the intra-articular pathology. The response to previous treatment, including rehabilitation and activity modification, should be determined. The patient should also be asked comprehensive questions regarding the nature and location of the pain and disability. Catching or audible "clicks" or "pops" may suggest a displaced labral tear. For example, patients who sustain sudden severe trauma with the arm positioned in abduction and external rotation are likely to have a Bankart lesion, whereas patients with recurrent subluxations from repetitive overhead activities such as pitching are likely to have a significant component of capsular laxity contributing to their instability.

Patient age and activity level are

critical to predicting the natural history and risk of recurrence. Patients younger than 20 years and those who participate in contact sports are at the highest risk for recurrence (approaching 90% to 95%). There is particular interest in using immediate arthroscopic stabilization to treat young athletes with an initial anterior glenohumeral dislocation.[38,39] Advantages include optimal pathology with good quality tissue and minimal collateral tissue damage in patients with a high likelihood of recurrence without surgery despite immobilization. Patients with recurrent anterior glenohumeral instability despite attempts at physical therapy or a willingness to modify their activities are also deemed candidates for surgical intervention. Although the literature reports high failure rates among athletes who participate in collision sports and undergo arthroscopic stabilization for anterior glenohumeral instability, specific attention to the entire spectrum of pathoanatomy identified at surgery is likely to lead to a satisfactory result.

Careful motor and sensory evaluation of the axillary nerve should be performed to exclude an injury. In older patients, weakness may indicate a rotator cuff tear. The presence of muscle atrophy and ligamentous laxity should be noted. Although it may be difficult to clinically assess laxity of the joint because of muscle guarding, side-to-side comparisons should be made for both the degree and direction of glenohumeral translation. In the appropriate setting, provocative testing, particularly testing for apprehension with a relocation maneuver, can be virtually diagnostic for anterior glenohumeral instability.[50] Inferior laxity should be assessed with a sulcus sign. Although the degree of a normal sulcus sign is quite variable, a painful sulcus sign suggests inferior instability. Furthermore, a large sulcus sign that persists when the adducted arm is externally rotated suggests insufficiency of the rotator interval capsular region.

Radiographic Evaluation

Radiographic evaluation may include plain radiographs, MRI, and CT. An appreciation for concomitant glenoid fractures, large Hill-Sachs lesions, and other bony abnormalities will be helpful in determining whether arthroscopic or open stabilization is the appropriate surgical approach. Determining coexisting pathology (ie, rotator cuff tears), the degree of capsular laxity, and the extent of labral pathology is also helpful in selecting the appropriate surgical procedure. Recent studies demonstrate that magnetic resonance arthrography is more than 90% sensitive and specific in detecting inferior labral ligamentous lesions.[51,52] CT can effectively demonstrate the size of associated glenoid fractures or erosions and impression fractures of the humeral head. It is also useful to determine the orientation of the glenoid to exclude hypoplasia and version abnormalities. CT arthrography can also be used to demonstrate soft-tissue pathology such as capsular or labral detachment and excessive capsular redundancy.[53,54]

Arthroscopic Repair

General Principles

Surgical tenets include the reattachment of the anteroinferior labrum along with the reestablishment of proper tension in the inferior glenohumeral ligament complex. Capsular laxity is addressed by superior and medial shift of the capsule. If the capsulolabral suture repair does not seem to decrease all of the capsular laxity, capsular plication or thermal capsulorrhaphy can be used as adjuncts. If there appears to be insufficiency of the rotator interval region with persistent inferior laxity, then this region should be plicated as well. Finally, an associated tear of the superior labrum should also be repaired. In the rare instances in which a midcapsular rupture or an avulsion of the humeral insertion of the glenohumeral ligament is encountered, conversion to an open reconstruction may be required. **(DVD 49.1)**

Instrumentation

Various commercial instruments are available, and choices are typically based on surgeon experience and familiarity. Appropriately sized disposable cannulas are necessary to accommodate the instrumentation required for glenoid preparation, suture passage through soft tissue, and arthroscopic knot tying. Typically, 5- and 8-mm cannulas are used. Most commercially available cortical anchors have pullout strengths that exceed the ultimate failure strength of the suture, knot, and soft-tissue interface. Thus, the limiting factors are the suture-tissue interface and the security of the arthroscopic knots. Once the anchor has been placed in the tissue, several different types of devices can be used to retrieve the suture and place it through the capsule and ligaments. Some of these devices pierce the ligaments and labrum and then retrieve the suture, and others use a suture loop that is placed through the tissue. This suture loop then serves as a shuttle for the actual suture from the anchor. Surgeon preference again determines which device is used, although it is the authors' opinion that shuttling devices seem to be more flexible and gentler on delicate tissues.

After the sutures are passed through the tissues, arthroscopic knots are tied. This requires an arthroscopic knot pusher. Although some knot pushers allow the individual suture limbs to be pushed away from each other, thus tensioning the knot, others are simply straight pushers that allow a sliding knot or a half-hitch knot to be slid down a post. If a transfixing device is used, then all of the required instrumentation is part of the insertion of this device.

Anesthesia and Positioning

Interscalene regional anesthesia, general anesthesia, or a combination of both may be used. Regional nerve blocks decrease narcotic requirements and aid in early postoperative pain relief. Either the beach chair or lateral decubitus position may be used. The beach chair position is efficient and conversion to an open approach is easier with the patient in this position compared with the lateral decubitus position. Access to the capsule may be limited compared with the lateral decubitus position, which uses traction on the arm to improve access to the axillary pouch and posterior recess.

Examination Under Anesthesia

Examination under anesthesia should be performed with side-to-side comparisons, and range of motion and the degree and direction of humeral head translation should be documented. Typically, anterior translation over the glenoid rim with (2+ instability) or without (3+ instability) spontaneous reduction is considered abnormal. The sulcus between the inferolateral border of the acromion and the greater tuberosity is measured in centimeters using an inferior displacement force with the arm in different positions of rotation to evaluate capsular laxity and the rotator interval.[55]

In general, the examination under anesthesia confirms the diagnosis established through careful history taking and physical examination. Stability testing with the arm in different positions of abduction will help identify regions of labral or capsular pathology. For example, increased inferior translation when the arm is adducted and externally rotated indicates laxity of the inferior capsule and the rotator interval. Even if translation does not appear to be significantly increased, a Bankart lesion may still be discovered. Thus, correlation with history and preoperative examination is important.

Diagnostic Arthroscopy

The shoulder is prepared for surgery and draped in a sterile manner, and the bony landmarks are carefully marked. A standard posterior portal is established. A systematic evaluation of the glenohumeral joint will demonstrate concomitant pathology including anterior labral detachments, capsular injuries, articular cartilage damage (glenoid and/or Hill-Sachs lesion), superior labrum from anterior to posterior lesions, and rotator cuff tears.

The quality and integrity of the anterior capsuloligamentous structures is determined by observing these structures in different positions of arm rotation while probing and grasping. In general, when the shoulder is placed in a position of abduction and external rotation, the inferior glenohumeral ligament should tighten while the humeral head remains in the glenoid. If an anterior force is applied to the humerus, the humeral head will move anteriorly on the glenoid (arthroscopic drawer). Although the humeral head may move to the anterior edge of the glenoid when the arm is in adduction, there should be no appreciable anterior translation when the shoulder is in abduction and external rotation.

The drive-through sign is the ability to pass the arthroscope easily from posterior to anterior and then into the axillary pouch. This is indicative of capsular laxity and further delineates the extent of this laxity. A complete diagnostic arthroscopy is performed with the arthroscope placed in both the anterior and posterior portals. Special attention is paid to the rotator interval, superior labrum, rotator cuff, articular cartilage, and reciprocal tightening of the glenohumeral ligaments, especially with the arm abducted and externally rotated. The labrum is evaluated circumferentially for signs of frank detachment or medial healing along the scapular neck. Detachment of the labrum with healing medially on the scapula (anterior labrum periosteal sleeve avulsion lesion) may be difficult to recognize, but it usually appears as a bare glenoid rim with the capsular attachment based medially. It results from repetitive dislocations that strip the capsulolabral attachments from their anatomic origin and push them medially along the scapular neck. This is a condition that must be recognized as the entire capsulolabral sleeve must be mobilized surgically and repaired to the anatomic insertion at the margin of the glenoid rim.

Portals

Two anterior portals (superior and inferior) are established using an outside-in technique with a spinal needle (Figure 4). These portals function as utility portals for instrument passage, glenoid preparation, suture management, and knot tying. It is important to separate these anterior cannulas widely so that access in the joint is not a problem. Therefore, a 5- or 6-mm cannula is initially placed in a vertical orientation so that it enters the joint just underneath the biceps ten-

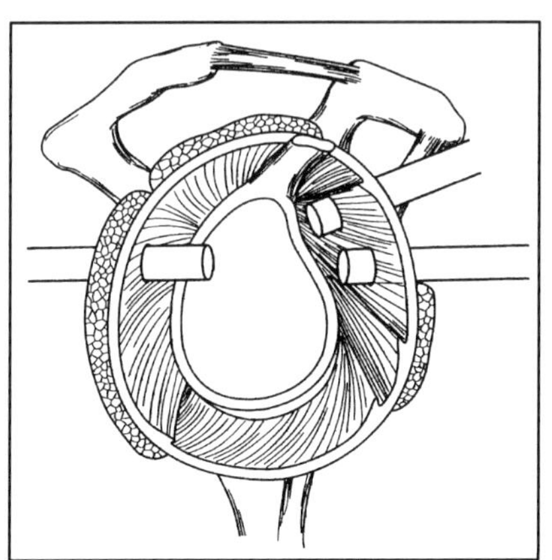

Figure 4 Schematic of the portals used for arthroscopic instability repairs. Note the relationship of the two anterior portals to the biceps and subscapularis tendons. (Reproduced with permission from Cohen B, Cole B, Romeo A: Thermal capsulorrhaphy of the shoulder. *Oper Tech Orthop* 2001;11:38-45).

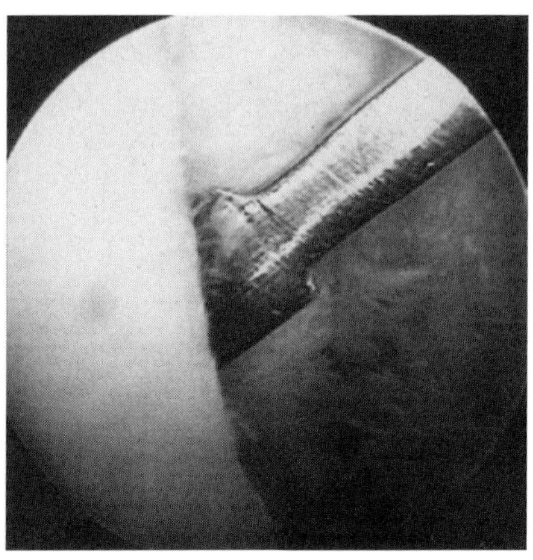

Figure 5 Intra-articular view showing a knife rasp used to mobilize the capsulolabral sleeve. It is important to elevate the tissues until the underlying subscapularis muscle is seen. (Reproduced with permission from Cole BJ, Romeo AA: Arthroscopic shoulder stabilization with suture anchors: Technique, technology, and pitfalls. *Clin Orthop* 2001;390:17-30.)

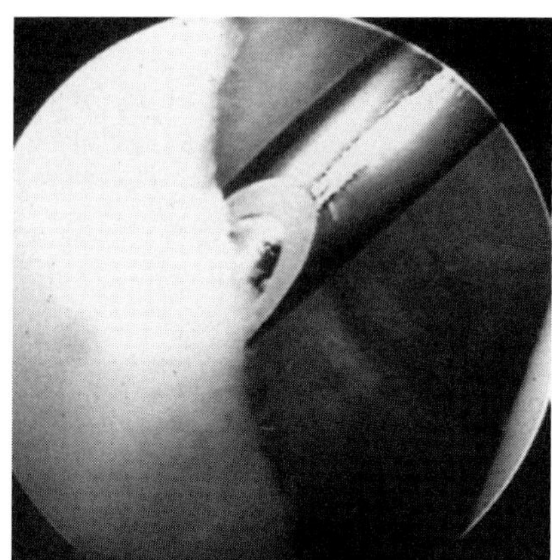

Figure 6 An arthroscopic shaver or burr should be used to decorticate the anterior and inferior glenoid surface to achieve an optimal surface for healing. (Reproduced with permission from Cole BJ, Romeo AA: Arthroscopic shoulder stabilization with suture anchors: Technique, technology, and pitfalls. *Clin Orthop* 2001;390:17-30.)

don. This anterosuperior cannula is usually at a 90° angle to the arthroscope. The second cannula is 8 mm in diameter and is placed in the orientation as low as possible in the rotator interval, typically entering just superior to the subscapularis tendon. The proper angle for each portal should be assessed using an outside-in technique with a spinal needle to confirm orientation. The lower, larger cannula is usually placed 1 cm inferior and lateral to the palpable coracoid process so that it enters the joint just over the subscapularis tendon, aiming slightly lateral to medial. This allows the first anchor to be placed at the 5 o'clock position on the clock face of the glenoid (for a right shoulder) with the proper medial orientation. Alternatively, a trans-subscapularis approach can be used to improve inferior access.

Glenoid Preparation and Anchor Placement

The 30° arthroscope can be placed in the posterior viewing portal as well as in the anterosuperior portal while working instruments are placed in the anteroinferior portal. In some instances, it is helpful to use a 70° arthroscope to see over the glenoid rim while mobilizing the capsulolabral sleeve. The capsulolabral complex is mobilized off the glenoid neck inferiorly to the 6 o'clock position using electrocautery or a radiofrequency device. A periosteal elevator or knife rasp may also be useful (Figure 5). It is especially important to mobilize the capsulolabral sleeve so that it is freely mobile and can be shifted superiorly and laterally to the glenoid rim. This often requires it to be released from the glenoid neck until the muscle fibers of the underlying subscapularis are seen. Either a motorized hooded burr or shaver may be used to decorticate the anterior and inferior glenoid neck (Figure 6). The abrasion of the juxta-articular scapula should continue approximately 1 to 1.5 cm medial to the articular cartilage and extend all the way to the inferior glenoid (6 o'clock).

Anchors are placed on the articular rim through the anteroinferior cannula at an angle of approximately 45° to the frontal plane to avoid articular penetration and to minimize the risk of inadvertent medial placement along the scapular neck. Anchor placement is from inferior to superior, with the first anchor placed at approximately the 5 o'clock position. Suture passage and knot tying are done after each anchor is placed and before subsequent anchor insertion. Anchor placement may be facilitated by a toothed or serrated cannulated drill guide that maintains the juxta-articular anchor position and by predrilling if necessary. Anchors are generally either metal or bioabsorbable polymers. More recently, anchor technology that allows for suture repair without knots has been developed. This design permits the suture to be captured in the end of the anchor once the suture has been passed

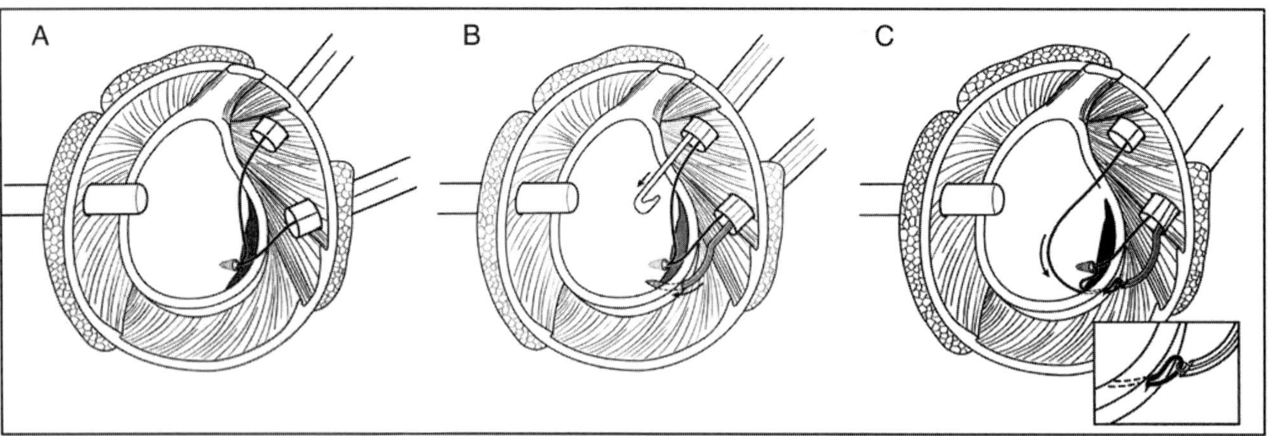

Figure 7 Schematic showing the placement of the first anchor and passage of the sutures. **A,** Using the anteroinferior portal, the first anchor is placed low (5 o'clock) on the glenoid and at the articular margin. A crochet hook is used to separate the two sutures between the two cannulae. **B,** A penetrating shuttling device is placed through the anteroinferior cannula and is passed through the capsulolabral tissues. The arrows indicate the direction of insertion. The capsulolabral tissue is penetrated laterally and inferiorly to the anchor so that the capsule will be shifted medially and superiorly. **C,** The suture in the anterosuperior cannula is retrieved with the shuttling device and is passed through the capsulolabral complex (inset). For knot tying, this limb will then become the post suture so that the knot will rest on the capsulolabral side of the repair. The arrow indicates the direction in which the suture is pulled. (Reproduced with permission from Romeo A, Cohen B, Carreira D: Traumatic anterior shoulder instability. *Oper Tech Orthop* 2000;8:188-196.)

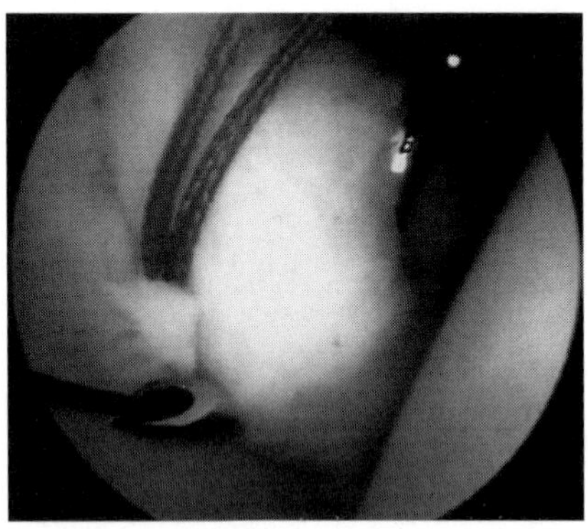

Figure 8 A suture hook (Linvatec) is passed through the capsulolabral tissues. A shuttle relay (Linvatec) device is then passed into the joint so that the suture from the anchor can be shuttled through the tissue. (Reproduced with permission from Cole BJ, Romeo AA: Arthroscopic shoulder stabilization with suture anchors: Technique, technology, and pitfalls. *Clin Orthop* 2001;390:17-30.)

through the tissue. It is then placed into a predrilled hole and impacted until the capsulolabral tissue is pulled securely against the glenoid rim, thus avoiding all of the steps of knot tying.

Following anchor placement, assessment of anchor security, suture slippage, and knot security is performed. Most surgeons use No. 1 or No. 2 braided, nonabsorbable material or prolonged absorbable, braided suture because of its strength and handling properties, which allows for secure knots that do not slip.

Anterior Glenohumeral Reconstruction

The first anchor is critical in establishing proper capsular tension (Figure 7). After mobilization of the capsulolabral periosteal sleeve as described above, the first anchor is placed at the articular margin at least as low as the 5 o'clock position. One limb of the suture from this anchor is retrieved through the superior cannula as this will be transported through the capsule with a device placed through the inferior cannula. A crochet hook or other retrieving device can be used for this step. If possible, it is important to transport the suture that comes out of the anchor on the inferior or medial surface. This will prevent the suture from twisting on itself and will thereby permit easier knot tying with a sliding knot. A hooked device or punch device (eg, the Arthex Suture Lasso, Arthex, Naples, FL or the Spectrum Soft-Tissue Repair System, Linvatec, Largo, FL) is placed through the capsule medial and inferior to the lowest anchor so that the entire inferior glenohumeral ligament is shifted superiorly and laterally (Figure 8). The hook can be pulled when it is in the tissue to confirm the quality of the bite and the tension in the inferior glenohumeral ligament. Tension can also be assessed with a soft-tissue grasper placed through the superior portal while pulling on the hook in the inferior glenohumeral ligament. The labrum should be included in this suture loop so that it will be repaired when the capsule is shifted and repaired. The suture retrieval device is usually placed through the inferior glenohumeral ligament about 1 cm inferior and slightly medial to the lowest anchor.

If a suture shuttle device or punch device (Caspari punch) is used, then a shuttle relay (Linvatec) is placed through the device and retrieved out of the superior cannula. Alternatively, a monofilament suture (2-0) can be placed, either as a loop or as a single strand to shuttle the suture. If it is retrieved as a loop, it is used to shuttle the suture limb from the anchor back through the capsulolabral tissue. If it is a single limb, it is simply tied to the suture limb from the anchor, which is then shuttled through the tissue. The shuttle relay device is used in the same manner. When transferring suture, it is important to watch carefully to prevent inadvertently unloading the suture from the anchor. Placing a hemostat on the suture limb remaining within the anteroinferior cannula and visualizing the limb during transfer is the most effective way to prevent this from occurring. Alternatively, the eyelet on the anchor can be observed as the suture is pulled; if the sutures are moving at the eyelet, the wrong end of the suture is being pulled.

The suture limb that exits the anterosuperior cannula is the suture that will ultimately pass through the soft tissue. This is called the post suture because the sliding arthroscopic knot will move down this limb. It is important to choose this limb as the post because the knot will then sit on top of the tissue and not underneath it. It is preferable to have the knot on the capsulolabral side.

The sequence of steps involved with knot tying begins by placing the knot pusher on each individual limb and passing it down into the joint to make sure there is no tangling or twisting of the suture limbs. Most surgeons prefer to tie a sliding knot first. This allows the knot to be securely placed, tensioning the tissue. This may be a sliding knot that does not lock (ie, Duncan loop) or a self-locking knot (eg, Bunt line half-hitch, Roeder, or Weston). The knot is "set" by placing a hemostat between the two limbs just distal to the knot and eliminating the slack within the suture loops against the post.

Placing a knot pusher on the post limb and pushing the knot down the post while simultaneously pulling the knot into the joint minimizes suture trauma and reduces the risk for suture failure. Subsequently, several alternating half-hitch, nonsliding knots are advanced down the post guided by the knot pusher. While the first sliding knot is placed by pulling on the post and pushing on the knot, the subsequent half-hitch knots are pulled into the joint by placing the knot pusher just past the half hitch so it pulls on the suture bringing the knot down into the joint. The knot is then tightened by using a past pointing technique with the knot pusher. Alternating the posts and the direction of each half hitch maximizes knot security. The ends are cut, leaving a 3-mm tail. These steps are repeated for each subsequent anchor (Figure 9).

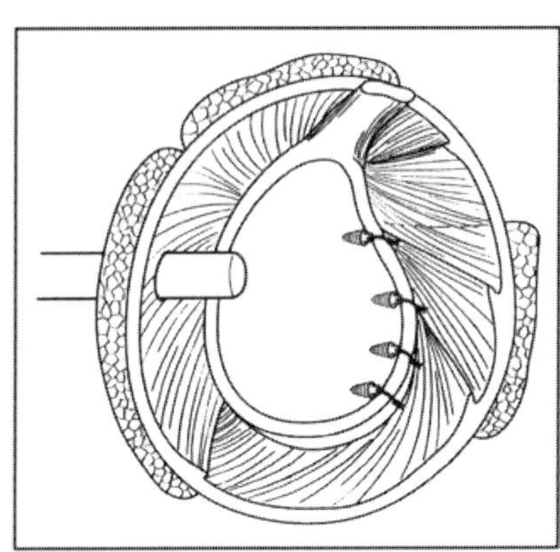

Figure 9 Schematic showing the completed anterior capsulolabral repair with three to four anchors placed sequentially from inferior to superior. (Reproduced with permission from Romeo A, Cohen B, Carreira D: Traumatic anterior shoulder instability. *Oper Tech Orthop* 2000;8: 188-196.)

Rotator Interval

If the shoulder demonstrates persistent inferior or inferoposterior translation after repair of the labrum and inferior and middle glenohumeral ligaments, rotator interval closure should be considered. The arm should be placed in slight external rotation to avoid restriction of this motion postoperatively. A curved suture hook or spinal needle is placed through the anterosuperior cannula or percutaneously through the portal without the cannula and advanced through the healthy tissue capsular immediately adjacent to the supraspinatus tendon. The suture hook is advanced inferiorly through the capsular tissue adjacent to the subscapularis tendon and a No. 1 monofilament is advanced through these two tissue regions.

If it is difficult to grasp sufficient tissue with a single pass of the suture hook, an alternative method involves the percutaneous placement of a suture grasper (Penetrator, Arthrex) through the inferior tissue. The suture is then advanced through the superior tissue, either with the Spectrum suture hook (Linvatec) or a spinal needle, and retrieved with the grasping instrument. In either case, the suture ends are retrieved through the anterior portal, after backing up the cannula, and secured using an arthroscopic sliding knot. This knot is tied blindly, extra-articularly over the anterior soft tissues. Alternatively, the sutures can be retrieved from within the subacromial space by viewing from within the space posteriorly. They can then be retrieved from a standard anterior portal and secured with an arthroscopic knot. Additional sutures may be added as needed. Again, care should be taken to position the arm in external rotation and adduction during suture placement and tensioning.

Capsular Laxity

Suture Plication

Excessive capsular laxity can be addressed by suture plication. Currently, this is the authors' method of choice for addressing pathologic glenohumeral capsular laxity with or without an associated Bankart lesion. The plication can be performed with either nonabsorbable or absorbable sutures. The technique involves either lateral to medial or inferior to superior shift of the capsule. This can be accomplished either using the pinch-tuck method, suturing capsule to capsule, or as a shift, plicating the capsule to the labrum.

The capsule is initially prepared by abrading it with a full-radius shaver. If the suction is turned off, unintentional capsular damage by the shaver will be minimized. Next, a suture passing device, such as a Spectrum suture hook, Suture Lasso (Arthrex), or similar device, is used to grasp the capsule. The capsule is then shifted the desired amount by penetrating another region of the capsule with the suture passing device. Sutures are then passed and tied arthroscopically, using standard techniques as described previously in this chapter. This effectively decreases capsular volume and decreases glenohumeral joint laxity.

Thermal Capsulorrhaphy

Thermal capsulorrhaphy has been used as an adjunct to tighten the capsule if persistent capsular laxity remains after the capsulolabral repair. Unfortunately, few published peer-reviewed studies advocating its routine use appear in the literature. Initial enthusiasm for this technique has been tempered because several series have documented unacceptably high failure rates[56,57] (DF D'Alessandro, JP Bradley, Orlando, FL, unpublished data, 2000; TJ Noonan, KK Briggs, RJ Hawkins, Miami Beach, FL, unpublished data, 2000; DF D'Alessandro, JP Bradley, PM Connor, personal communication, 2001). If thermal energy is used for a lax capsule, it should be applied after all anchors have been placed and all knots have been tied. Shrinking before suture placement increases the level of difficulty in assessing, approximating, and repairing the soft tissue to the glenoid rim. After suture repair, care should be taken to avoid thermal treatment near the suture line because of the risk of soft-tissue weakening and failure. Either a monopolar radiofrequency device or a bipolar radiofrequency device can be used. To date, no prospective, randomized comparisons of these devices with control groups have been conducted. Thus, the technique of thermal treatment of the capsule remains empiric. A grid-like or "cornrow" pattern is preferred because this theoretically maintains normal areas of the capsule between thermally treated areas, allowing viable cells to repopulate thermally modified areas. Results with this technique have been variable, with recurrence rates from 0 to 59%; in general, the results have been less favorable than those achieved with traditional open repair techniques. In light of this and the development of better techniques for suture plication, there is currently a trend away from thermal capsulorrhaphy and toward arthroscopic suture plication for excessive capsular laxity.

The notable exception is throwing athletes with internal impingement. Levitz and associates[58] found thermal capsular shrinkage useful as an adjunct to the standard surgical treatment of pathology in the overhead athlete's shoulder. They reported that it significantly improved the rate of return to competition. In treating the underlying capsular pathology that leads to rotational instability, data from this series support the adjunctive use of thermal capsulorrhaphy in this specific patient population. The authors stress that the postoperative rehabilitation of these athletes must be carefully monitored by both therapist and physician and that the rehabilitation is as important as the surgical treatment.

Postoperative Rehabilitation

Postoperative rehabilitation after arthroscopic repair is identical to that following open reconstruction. Sling immobilization is generally required for 4 to 6 weeks depending on the methods used and the instability pattern treated. Active and unrestricted range of motion of the hand, wrist, and elbow begins immediately following surgery. Similarly, deltoid isometrics and gentle pendulum exercises begin immediately. Some surgeons allow active, forward elevation restricted to 120° after the first 2 to 3 weeks, as experimental studies have shown that this places little load on the capsulolabral region. At this point, external rotation may be permitted to 30° to 40° as well, depending on the extent of repair. At 4 to 6 weeks, rotation limits are gradually extended; at 8 to 10 weeks, progressive resistive exercises begin. Return to sport occurs at 18 to 36 weeks.

Summary

Arthroscopic stabilization for anterior glenohumeral instability has developed rapidly over the past 20 years. Better understanding of the pathoanatomy associated with glenohumeral instability and advances in surgical technology and technique now make it possible to duplicate and perhaps even exceed the results of open stabilization techniques. The pathoanatomy of instability is quite complex and can involve both soft tissue and bony elements. Failure to recognize and address the pathoanatomy can result in poor results with high recurrence rates. Each element of the instability must be addressed surgically, whether through arthroscopic or open techniques.

A variety of arthroscopic techniques are now available to restore anterior glenohumeral stability. The principal goal is to repair the capsulolabral sleeve carefully with appropriate tension. The techniques described in this chapter allow a thorough evaluation of the patient with instability and present a variety of arthroscopic methods for treating the patholaxity. Direct repair of the capsule and labrum, plication of the capsule, and closure of the rotator interval can all be accomplished with the arthroscopic techniques described in this chapter. At this point, the use of thermal capsulorrhaphy as an adjunct remains unclear. In certain settings, it may prove useful to shrink the capsule and address residual capsular laxity that would otherwise lead to failure. Perhaps more predictably, variable degrees of capsular tightening can be performed using suture plication techniques. Fortunately, peer-reviewed studies on many of these techniques is forthcoming.

Unfortunately, there are no well-designed, randomized, prospective studies comparing arthroscopic stabilizations to control groups, although several recent uncontrolled, prospective studies confirm the efficacy of these techniques. The arthroscopic suture anchor techniques described in this chapter are preferable because they best restore the anatomy and most closely duplicate the traditional open Bankart repair. Patient selection is still critical to the ultimate success, as is appropriately addressing all the pathology at the time of surgery. Postoperative rehabilitation is not significantly different from that following traditional open techniques, and appropriate intervals for healing are needed. Obviously, premature return to activities that place stress on the reconstruction will result in early failure. Surgeons are encouraged to practice these techniques in a forum of continuing education before performing them in an operating room setting.

References

1. Cole B, Warner J: Anatomy, biomechanics, and pathophysiology of glenohumeral instability, in Iannotti J, Williams J, GR (eds): *Disorders of the Shoulder: Diagnosis and Management.* Philadelphia, PA, Lippincott Williams & Wilkins, 1999, pp 207-232.
2. Cooper D, Arnoczky S, O'Brien S, Warren RF, DiCarlo E, Allen AA: Anatomy, histology, and vascularity of the glenoid labrum: An anatomical study. *J Bone Joint Surg Am* 1992;74:46-52.
3. Cole BJ, Rodeo SA, O'Brien SJ, et al: The anatomy and histology of the rotator interval capsule of the shoulder. *Clin Orthop* 2001;390:129-137.
4. Neviaser TJ: The anterior labroligamentous periosteal sleeve avulsion lesion: A cause of anterior instability of the shoulder. *Arthroscopy* 1992;9:17-21.
5. Bigliani LU, Kurzweil PR, Schwartzbach CC, Wolfe IN, Flatow EL: Inferior capsular shift procedure for anterior-inferior shoulder instability in athletes. *Am J Sports Med* 1994;22:578-584.
6. Bigliani L, Pollock R, Soslowsky L, Flatow E, Pawluk R, Mow V: Tensile properties of the inferior glenohumeral ligament. *J Orthop Res* 1992;10:187-197.
7. Caspari R, Savoie F: Arthroscopic reconstruction of the shoulder: The Bankart repair, in McGinty J (ed): *Operative Arthroscopy*. New York, NY, Raven Press, 1991, pp 507-516.
8. Morgan CD, Burkhart SS, Palmeri M, Gillespie M: Type II SLAP lesions: Three subtypes and their relationship to superior instability and rotator cuff tears. *Arthroscopy* 1998;14:553-565.
9. Burkhart SS, Morgan CD, Kibler WB: Shoulder injuries in overhead athletes: The "dead arm" revisited. *Clin Sports Med* 2000;19:125-158.
10. Wolf EM: Arthroscopic capsulolabral repair using suture anchors. *Orthop Clin North Am* 1993;24:59-69.
11. Harryman DT II, Sidles JA, Harris SL, Matsen FA III: The role of the rotator interval capsule in passive motion and stability of the shoulder. *J Bone Joint Surg Am* 1992;74:53-66.
12. Rowe C, Sakellarides H: Factors related to recurrences of anterior dislocations of the shoulder. *Clin Orthop* 1961;20:40-48.
13. Burkhart SS, De Beer JF: Traumatic glenohumeral bone defects and their relationship to failure of arthroscopic Bankart repairs: Significance of the inverted-pear glenoid and the humeral engaging Hill-Sachs lesion. *Arthroscopy* 2000;16:677-694.
14. Burkhart SS, De Beer JF, Tehrany AM, Parten PM: Quantifying glenoid bone loss arthroscopically in shoulder instability. *Arthroscopy* 2002;18:488-491.
15. Rowe C, Patel D, Southmayd W: The Bankart procedure: A long-term end-result study. *J Bone Joint Surg Am* 1978;60:1-16.
16. Pagnani M, Dome D: Surgical treatment of traumatic anterior shoulder instability in American football players. *J Bone Joint Surg Am* 2002;84:711-715.
17. Magnusson L, Kartus J, Ejerhed L, Hultenheim I, Sernert N, Karlsson J: Revisiting the open Bankart experience: A four- to nine-year follow-up. *Am J Sports Med* 2002;30:778-782.
18. Matsen FA, Thomas SC, Rockwood CAJ: Glenohumeral instability, in Rockwood C, Matsen F (eds): *The Shoulder.* Philadelphia, PA, WB Saunders, 1990, pp 526-622.
19. Belzer J, Snyder J: Abstract: Arthroscopic capsulorrhaphy for traumatic anterior shoulder instability using suture anchors and nonabsorbable suture. *Proceedings from the Annual Meeting of the Arthroscopy Association of North America.* Rosemont, IL, Arthroscopy Association of North America, 1995, p 359.
20. Hoffman F, Reif G: Arthroscopic shoulder stabilization using Mitek anchors. *Knee Surg Sports Traumatol Arthrosc* 1995;3:50-54.

21. Guanche CA, Quick DC, Sodergren KM, Buss DD: Arthroscopic versus open reconstruction of the shoulder with isolated Bankart lesions. *Am J Sports Med* 1996;24:144-148.

22. Bacilla P, Field LD, Savoie FH III: Arthroscopic Bankart repair in a high demand patient population. *Arthroscopy* 1997;13:51-60.

23. Sisto DJ, Cook DL: Intraoperative decision making in the treatment of shoulder instability. *Arthroscopy* 1998;14:389-394.

24. Field L, Savoie F, Griffith P: A comparison of open and arthroscopic Bankart repair. *J Shoulder Elbow Surg* 1999;8:195.

25. Gartsman GM, Roddey TS, Hammerman SM: Arthroscopic treatment of anterior-inferior glenohumeral instability: Two to five-year follow-up. *J Bone Joint Surg Am* 2000;82:991-1003.

26. Cole BJ, Romeo AA: Arthroscopic shoulder stabilization with suture anchors: Technique, technology, and pitfalls. *Clin Orthop* 2001;390:17-30.

27. Mishra D, Fanton G: Two-year outcome of arthroscopic Bankart repair and electrothermal-assisted capsulorrhaphy for recurrent traumatic anterior shoulder instability. *Arthroscopy* 2001;17:844-849.

28. Kim SH, Ha KI, Kim SH: Bankart repair in traumatic anterior shoulder instability: open versus arthroscopic technique. *Arthroscopy* 2002;18:755-763.

29. Abrams J, Savoie F, Tauro J, Bradley J: Recent advances in the evaluation and treatment of shoulder instability: Anterior, posterior, multidirectional. *Arthroscopy* 2002;18:1-13.

30. Johnson L: Techniques of anterior glenohumeral ligament repair, in Johnson L (ed): *Arthroscopic Surgery: Principles and Practice*. St Louis, MO, CV Mosby, 1986, pp 1405-1420.

31. Morgan C, Bodenstab A: Arthroscopic Bankart suture repair: Technique and early results. *Arthroscopy* 1987;3:111-122.

32. Savoie FH III, Miller CD, Field LD: Arthroscopic reconstruction of traumatic anterior instability of the shoulder: The Caspari technique. *Arthroscopy* 1997;13:201-209.

33. Torchia ME, Caspari RB, Asselmeier MA, Beach WR, Gayari M: Arthroscopic transglenoid suture repair: 2 to 8 year results in 150 shoulders. *Arthroscopy* 1997;13:609-619.

34. Walch G, Boileau P, Levigne C, Mandrino A, Neyret P, Donell S: Arthroscopic stabilization for recurrent anterior shoulder dislocation: Result of 59 cases. *Arthroscopy* 1995;11:173-179.

35. Mologne T, Lapoint J, Morin W, Zilberfarb J, O'Brien J: Arthroscopic anterior labral reconstruction using a transglenoid suture technique. *Am J Sports Med* 1996;24:268-274.

36. Marcacci M, Zaffagnini S, Petitto A, Pia Neri M, Iacono F, Visani A: Arthroscopic management of recurrent anterior dislocation of the shoulder: Analysis of technical modifications on the Caspari procedure. *Arthroscopy* 1996;12:144-149.

37. Speer KP, Warren RF, Pagnani M, Warner JJ: An arthroscopic technique for anterior stabilization of the shoulder with a bioabsorbable tack. *J Bone Joint Surg Am* 1996;78:1801-1807.

38. Arciero RA, St Pierre P: Acute shoulder dislocation: Indications and techniques for operative management. *Clin Sports Med* 1995;14:937-953.

39. Arciero R, Taylor D, Snyder R, Uhorchak J: Arthroscopic bioabsorbable tack stabilization of initial anterior shoulder dislocations: A preliminary report. *Arthroscopy* 1995;11:410-417.

40. Resch H, Povacz P, Wambacher M, Sperner G, Golser K: Arthroscopic extra-articular Bankart repair for the treatment of recurrent anterior shoulder dislocation. *Arthroscopy* 1997;13:188-200.

41. Laurencin C, Stephens S, Warren R, Altchek D: Arthroscopic Bankart repair using a degradable tack: A followup study using optimized indications. *Clin Orthop* 1996;332:132-137.

42. Warner JJ, Miller MD, Marks P, Fu FH: Arthroscopic Bankart repair with the Suretac device: Part I. Clinical observations. *Arthroscopy* 1995;11:2-13.

43. Warner J, Pagnani M, Warren R, Cavanaugh J, Montgomery W: Arthroscopic Bankart repair utilizing a cannulated absorbable fixation device. *Orthop Trans* 1991;15:761-762.

44. Snyder S: *Shoulder Arthroscopy*. New York, NY, McGraw Hill, 1994, pp 179-214.

45. Geiger D, Hurley J, Tovey J, Rao J: Results of arthroscopic versus open Bankart suture repair. *Orthop Trans* 1993;17:973.

46. Steinbeck J, Jerosch J: Arthroscopic transglenoid stabilization versus open anchor suturing in traumatic anterior instability of the shoulder. *Am J Sports Med* 1998;26:373-378.

47. Cole BJ, Warner JJ: Arthroscopic versus open Bankart repair for traumatic anterior shoulder instability. *Clin Sports Med* 2000;1:19-48.

48. Karlsson J, Magnusson L, Ejerhed L, Hultenheim I, Lundin O, Kartus J: Comparison of open and arthroscopic stabilization for recurrent shoulder dislocation in patients with a Bankart lesion. *Am J Sports Med* 2001;29:538-542.

49. Sperber A, Hamburg P, Karlsson J, Sward L, Wredmark T: Comparison of an arthroscopic and an open procedure for posttraumatic instability of the shoulder: A prospective, randomized multicenter study. *J Shoulder Elbow Surg* 2001;10:105-108.

50. Speer K, Hannafin J, Altchek D, Warren R: An evaluation of the shoulder relocation test. *Am J Sports Med* 1994;22:177-183.

51. Green M, Christensen K: Magnetic resonance imaging of the glenoid labrum in anterior shoulder instability. *Am J Sports Med* 1994;22:493-498.

52. Iannotti JP, Zlatkin MB, Esterhai J, Kressel HY, Dalinka MK, Spindler KP: Magnetic resonance imaging of the shoulder: Sensitivity, specificity, and predictive value. *J Bone Joint Surg Am* 1991;73:17-29.

53. Kinnard P, Tricoire J, Levesque R, Bergeron D: Assessment of the unstable shoulder by computed arthrography: A preliminary report. *Am J Sports Med* 1983;11:157-159.

54. Singson RD, Feldman F, Bigliani L: CT arthrographic patterns in recurrent glenohumeral instability. *AJR Am J Roentgenol* 1987;149:749-753.

55. Altchek DW, Warren RF, Skyhar MJ, Ortiz G: T-plasty modification of the Bankart procedure for multidirectional instability of the anterior and inferior types. *J Bone Joint Surg Am* 1991;73:105-112.

56. Fitzgerald B, Watson B, Lapjoint J: The use of thermal capsulorrhaphy in the treatment of multidirectional instability. *J Shoulder Elbow Surg* 2002;11:108-113.

57. Anderson K, Warren RF, Altchek DW, Craig EV, O'Brien SJ: Risk factors for early failure after thermal capsulorrhaphy. *Am J Sports Med* 2002;30:103-107.

58. Levitz CL, Dugas J, Andrews JR: The use of arthroscopic thermal capsulorrhaphy to treat internal impingement in baseball players. *Arthroscopy* 2001;17:573-577.

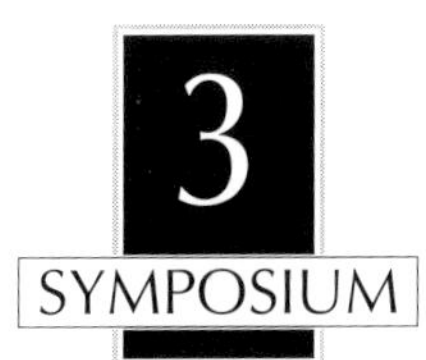

Arthroscopic Versus Open Treatment of Anterior Shoulder Instability

April Armstrong, MD
Dory Boyer, MD
Konstantinos Ditsios, MD
Ken Yamaguchi, MD

Abstract

Open repair is the accepted mainstay of treatment for anterior shoulder instability, and consistently good clinical results have been reported in the literature. With the development of newer arthroscopic imbrication techniques, however, arthroscopy may eventually provide equivalent long-term efficacy.

In the early 1900s, shoulder instability was first described as the "shearing off of the fibrous capsule of the joint from its attachment to the fibrocartilaginous glenoid ligament."[1,2] Since then, improved understanding of both the anatomy of normal glenohumeral stability and pathology of shoulder instability has changed the surgical treatment of this condition. Classically, unilateral (most often anterior) instability and multidirectional instability were thought to be distinct patterns. Unilateral instability was historically related to a traumatic injury. Treatment addressed associated Bankart lesions, and high recurrence rates were reported. Multidirectional instability, in contrast, was considered to have an atraumatic origin, was often bilateral, and had an instability pattern in more than one direction. Treatment of multidirectional instability addressed the pathology of capsular redundancy in the form of an anteroinferior capsular shift.

The current understanding of anterior shoulder instability is that it is actually a continuum of instability ranging from traumatic to atraumatic origins with varying degrees of laxity. Patients with traumatic anterior shoulder instability may or may not have a Bankart lesion but almost always have associated capsular laxity; disregarding associated capsular pathology can limit the efficacy of traditional Bankart repair. Patients with multidirectional instability may have predominant instability in one direction and therefore require more focused treatment.

Pathoanatomy

Because several anatomic structures around the shoulder provide stability, a clear understanding of shoulder anatomy as it relates to glenohumeral stability is crucial for treating patients with anterior shoulder instability. The ultimate goal of treatment should be restoration of normal anatomy around the shoulder to restore functional stability and minimize disability.

The bony articulations are more important for marginal congruency in the shoulder than they are in other joints. As evidence of this marginal congruency, Hill-Sachs lesions have been observed arthroscopically in 80% of patients with anterior shoulder dislocations[3] (Figure 1). When Hill-Sachs lesions cover over 30% of the articular surface of the humeral head, treatment in addition to capsular imbrication may be required.[4]

Capsuloligamentous structures supplement the bony and muscular anatomy, contributing to glenohumeral joint stability. The glenoid labrum deepens the articulation of the glenoid to improve joint congruity. It also anchors the capsular attachments via the superior glenohumeral ligament (SGHL), middle glenohumeral ligament (MGHL), and inferior glenohumeral ligament complex (IGHLC).

Biomechanical studies conducted to assess these ligaments demon-

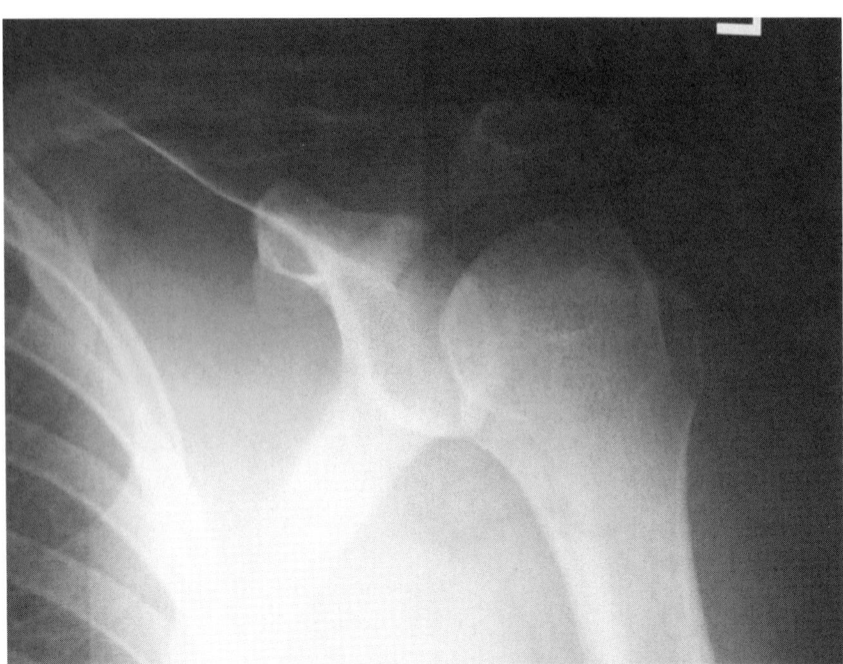

Figure 1 Radiograph of a Hill-Sachs lesion after an anterior shoulder dislocation.

strate variable tensional restraint depending on the position of the arm in space.[5,6] The SGHL acts as an inferior restraint when the arm is in an adducted position. The MGHL acts as an inferior restraint with the arm abducted less than 90°. The IGHLC acts as the primary inferior restraint with extension and external rotation and the arm in 90° abduction. The location of the capsular stabilizers has been shown to shift inferiorly as the arm is increasingly abducted, with the IGHLC most taut in the provocative position. In this position, the MGHL and SGHL rotate superiorly and are not taut.

Insufficiency of the inferior capsuloligamentous structures has been shown to disengage the chock-block effect of the anterior labrum and eliminate the inherent added stability afforded by the anterior labrum by a factor of 50%.[7] Lippitt and Matsen[8] demonstrated that concavity compression and anterior translatory resistance was decreased by 20% with the presence of a Bankart lesion. Other authors have shown similar diminished restraints correlating with decreased stability.[9]

It was once believed that this anteroinferior capsulolabral avulsion (Bankart lesion) was the "essential lesion" for anterior shoulder instability. Recent anatomic cadaveric studies have shown that transection of the anterior band of the IGHLC only slightly increased anterior translation of the shoulder,[10] and researchers have speculated that permanent change in the tensile properties of the IGHLC may be responsible for additional instability.[11] Moreover, Bigliani and associates[12] observed that stretching of the IGHLC was necessary for the recurrence of anterior shoulder dislocation.

Bigliani and associates[12] also demonstrated three failure sites for the inferior glenohumeral ligament: the glenoid insertion (40%), the ligament substance (35%), and the humeral insertion (25%) and observed plastic deformity no matter where failure occurred. Baker[13] confirmed these findings in vivo from arthroscopic examination of acute shoulder dislocations. These findings demonstrated the importance of addressing both the IGHLC as well as any labral avulsions at the time of repair. McMahon and associates[11] demonstrated that the tautness of the IGHLC can be recovered, and concluded that only a small capsular plication is necessary for adequate repair.

Treatment Goals

For both open and arthroscopic repair, many different implants and techniques have been used to stabilize the shoulder joint. Whatever the treatment method, the main goals of treatment should focus on repairing the labral detachment to restore the anterior bumper and addressing the associated capsular laxity.

Surgical options for open techniques include a classic Bankart procedure, capsular shift, or a combination of the two. Historically, arthroscopic techniques were used to address the labral avulsion (arthroscopic Bankart procedure) but were limited in their ability to imbricate a lax capsule.

The advantages of open stabilization include proven reliability, direct visualization of capsular tightening, and early motion; it generally requires less technical expertise than arthroscopy. A primary disadvantage of open stabilization is the required subscapularis takedown. It has also been suggested that patients undergoing open repair of anterior shoulder instability are at increased risk of losing motion, particularly external rotation, which is a concerning limitation for overhead athletes.[14,15] Although patients who undergo arthroscopic repair of anterior shoulder instability report consistently more external rotation than those who undergo open repair, there is little support for this outcome in the literature.

An analysis of 26 studies of open repair was conducted that included 1,399 shoulders (K Yamaguchi, MD, St. Louis, MO, unpublished data, 2002). Follow-up ranged from 22 to 180 months. Failure rates averaged 4.7% (range, 0% to 13.3%). Eighty-five percent to 98% of the patients returned to work, 79% returned to sports activity (range, 48% to 97%), and 56% of overhead athletes returned to throwing (range, 33% to 86%). In light of the increased reliability of this procedure and its ability to correct secondary pathologies of instability, open repair is the preferred method of treatment for patients with recurrent dislocations. Athletes who participate in contact sports that do not require the arms to be lifted overhead, especially those athletes with poor anterior tissue quality, are also likely to receive more benefit from an open procedure than arthroscopic repair.

Takedown of the subscapularis muscle is not required during arthroscopic repair of anterior shoulder instability. Other advantages over open repair include improved cosmesis, less perioperative morbidity, improved motion, and the potential for a shorter, easier operation. Additionally, direct inspection of the glenohumeral joint can allow other shoulder pathology to be addressed and thereby improve overall results.[7] Moreover, decreased surgical time, fewer complications in the perioperative period, shorter hospital stays, and reduced costs have been reported with arthroscopic versus open repair.[16,17] Disadvantages include a reported failure rate higher than that of open repair.

An analysis of the literature revealed 21 studies on arthroscopic repair that included 1,221 patients.[14,18-24] The overall average recurrence of instability for arthroscopic shoulder stabilization was 17.4%. These findings, however, may be misleading because early studies used various techniques that are now outdated, such as staple imbrication.[25] Because staple imbrication often resulted in problems with nonanatomic repair, staple migration, and painful subscapularis bursitis, it is no longer a favored technique. Similarly, transosseous suture imbrication of the capsule had promising early results, but longer follow-up showed that this technique was unreliable, and the risk of suprascapular nerve injury rendered it unacceptable by current standards. In addition, both staple imbrication and transosseous suture imbrication may have resulted in the creation of anterior labroligamentous periosteal sleeve avulsion lesions.[26]

More recently, Snyder and Strafford[27] described the use of suture anchors for fixation, and Karlsson and associates[14] reported a 15% recurrence rate with this technique compared to 10% with open techniques. The problems encountered using suture anchors include migration and breakage, and overall success rates for this technique have not yet been established. Initial success was achieved with a relatively simple procedure using cannulated bioabsorbable transfixation devices[28,29] to arthroscopically repair anterior shoulder instability, but a 6% incidence of synovitis and phagocytosis in the joint capsule was subsequently reported.[30] The recently introduced Suretac device (Smith-Nephew, Boston, MA) is limited in its ability to address associated joint laxity[31] and is unlikely to prove favorable for patients with multidirectional instability. The actual incidence of failure with this device is unknown, but it likely exceeds the failure rate of open repair.

Open and arthroscopic repair were compared in a recent prospective, randomized study that reported a recurrence rate of 12% and 23%, respectively.[19] Although these recurrence rates were higher than those reported in previous studies, a greater risk of redislocation was noted for patients in the arthroscopic group. Recently published data from Cole and associates[20] and Karlsson and associates[14] show similar results. Rook and associates,[32] offering a more optimistic assessment of using arthroscopy to repair anterior shoulder instability, reported satisfactory outcomes in 97% of patients who underwent treatment for Bankart lesions and 93% of those who underwent treatment for multidirectional instability.

Surgical expertise is required for both arthroscopic and open repair, and the existence of a learning curve to master these procedures must be understood. As surgeons continue to master arthroscopic techniques, the efficacy of arthroscopic treatment of shoulder instability is improving. Antoniou and associates[33] suggest that the successful outcomes of arthroscopic stabilization may be dependent on the efficacy of new capsular tightening techniques (Figure 2). Newer suture imbrication techniques used in the arthroscopic repair of shoulder instability that address associated capsular pathology in addition to labral pathology may result in recurrence rates comparable to those for open repair. Moreover, with the use of arthroscopic capsular tucks, the loss of external rotation may be better regulated than as classically seen with the use of open

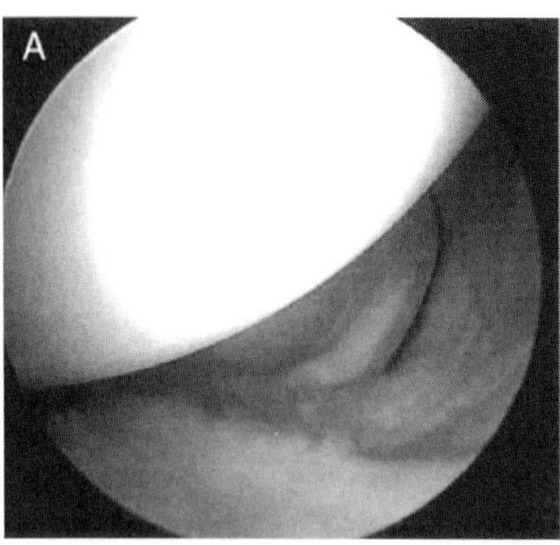

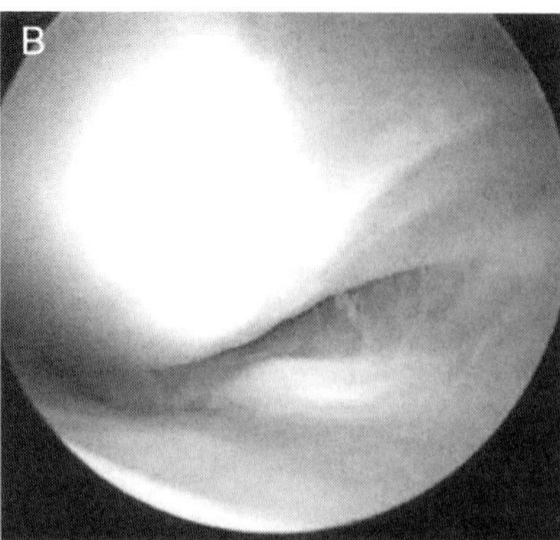

Figure 2 A, Anterior arthroscopic view of the shoulder showing an absorbable suture before tying for capsular imbrication. **B,** Arthroscopic view of the same shoulder following imbrication stitch. Note the marked decrease in joint volume after tying of the suture.

techniques. As a result, athletes with shoulder instability may obtain better outcomes without an open procedure.

It is important to understand that bias exists in the general literature regarding arthroscopic repair for shoulder instability because all of the published studies have been conducted by shoulder specialists. Therefore, the applicability of these results for surgeons with less technical experience and a poorer understanding of the anatomy and pathology of shoulder instability is questionable. An informed patient is also crucial to the success of arthroscopic surgery; the treatment must be highly individualized, and the patient must understand and be willing to accept the inherent risks. Age, mode of onset, and degree of future participation in sports activities are factors that must be considered when determining the appropriate method of fixation. Examination under anesthesia, a careful history and physical examination, and appropriate imaging modalities all play a part in choosing the correct procedure for each patient. That patients with less capsular laxity may have a better result with arthroscopic treatment than those with a significant laxity pattern should also be considered when determining the appropriate treatment. Postoperative rehabilitation should also be tailored individually and patients should be observed at weekly intervals for the first 6 to 8 weeks, with the goal of achieving full range of motion by 8 weeks. In patients with a posterior component to their instability, the shoulder should be immobilized in a gunslinger brace.

Summary

The understanding of the pathology of glenohumeral instability and improved open and arthroscopic techniques will continue to evolve and help in the treatment of anterior shoulder instability. Although open shoulder stabilization remains the gold standard for treatment of this condition, arthroscopic shoulder stabilization techniques are improving. With the development of newer arthroscopic imbrication techniques, the indications for using arthroscopic stabilization may begin to approach those for open stabilization.

References

1. Perthes G: Ueber operationen bei habitueller schutterluxation. *Deutsche Zeitschr Chir* 1906;85:199-227.
2. Bankart AS: Recurrent or habitual dislocation of the shoulder-joint. *BMJ* 1923;2:1132-1133.
3. Calandra JJ, Baker CL, Uribe J: The incidence of Hill-Sachs lesions in initial anterior shoulder dislocations. *Arthroscopy* 1989;5:254-257.
4. Connolly J, Regen E, Evans OB: The management of the painful, stiff shoulder. *Clin Orthop* 1972;84:97-103.
5. Turkel SJ, Panio MW, Marshall JL, Girgis FG: Stabilizing mechanisms preventing anterior dislocation of the glenohumeral joint. *J Bone Joint Surg Am* 1981;63:1208-1217.
6. Warner J, Caborn D, Berger R, Fu FH, Seel M: Dynamic capsuloligamentous anatomy of the glenohumeral joint. *J Shoulder Elbow Surg* 1993;2:115-133.
7. Cole BJ, Warner JJ: Arthroscopic versus open Bankart repair for traumatic anterior shoulder instability. *Clin Sports Med* 2000;19:19-48.
8. Lippitt S, Matsen F: Mechanisms of glenohumeral joint stability. *Clin Orthop* 1993;291:20-28.
9. Lazarus MD, Sidles JA, Harryman DT II, Matsen FA III: Effect of a chondral-labral defect on glenoid concavity and glenohumeral stability: A cadaveric model. *J Bone Joint Surg Am* 1996;78:94-102.
10. Speer KP, Deng X, Borrero S, Torzilli PA, Altchek DA, Warren RF: Biomechanical evaluation of a simulated Bankart lesion. *J Bone Joint Surg Am* 1994;76:1819-1826.
11. McMahon PJ, Dettling JR, Sandusky MD, Lee TQ: Deformation and strain characteristics along the length of the anterior band of the inferior glenohumeral ligament. *J Shoulder Elbow Surg* 2001;10:482-488.
12. Bigliani LU, Pollock RG, Soslowsky LJ, Flatow EL, Pawluk RJ, Mow VC: Tensile properties of the inferior glenohumeral ligament. *J Orthop Res* 1992;10:187-197.
13. Baker CL: Intraarticular pathology in acute, first-time anterior shoulder dislocation: An arthroscopic study. *Arthroscopy* 1994;10:478-479.
14. Karlsson J, Magnusson L, Ejerhed L, Hultenheim I, Lundin O, Kartus J: Comparison of open and arthroscopic stabilization for recurrent shoulder dislocation in patients with a Bankart lesion. *Am J Sports Med* 2001;29:538-542.
15. Kartus J, Ejerhed L, Funck E, Kohler K, Sernert N, Karlsson J: Arthroscopic and open shoulder stabilization using

absorbable implants: A clinical and radiographic comparison of two methods. *Knee Surg Sports Traumatol Arthrosc* 1998;6:181-188.

16. Green MR, Christensen KP: Arthroscopic versus open Bankart procedures: A comparison of early morbidity and complications. *Arthroscopy* 1993;9:371-374.
17. Barber FA, Click SD, Weideman CA: Arthroscopic or open Bankart procedures: What are the costs? *Arthroscopy* 1998;14:671-674.
18. Kim SH, Ha KI, Kim SH: Bankart repair in traumatic anterior shoulder instability: Open versus arthroscopic technique. *Arthroscopy* 2002;18:755-763.
19. Sperber A, Hamberg P, Karlsson J, Sward L, Wredmark T: Comparison of an arthroscopic and an open procedure for posttraumatic instability of the shoulder: A prospective, randomized multicenter study. *J Shoulder Elbow Surg* 2001;10:105-108.
20. Cole BJ, L'Insalata J, Irrgang J, Warner JJ: Comparison of arthroscopic and open anterior shoulder stabilization: A two to six-year follow-up study. *J Bone Joint Surg Am* 2000;82:1108-1114.
21. Gartsman GM, Roddey TS, Hammerman SM: Arthroscopic treatment of anterior-inferior glenohumeral instability: Two to five-year follow-up. *J Bone Joint Surg Am* 2000;82:991-1003.
22. Dora C, Gerber C: Shoulder function after arthroscopic anterior stabilization of the glenohumeral joint using an absorbable tac. *J Shoulder Elbow Surg* 2000;9:294-298.
23. O'Neill DB: Arthroscopic Bankart repair of anterior detachments of the glenoid labrum: A prospective study. *J Bone Joint Surg Am* 1999;81:1357-1366.
24. Treacy SH, Savoie FH III, Field LD: Arthroscopic treatment of multidirectional instability. *J Shoulder Elbow Surg* 1999;8:345-350.
25. Detrisac DA, Johnson LL: Arthroscopic shoulder capsulorrhaphy using metal staples. *Orthop Clin North Am* 1993;24:71-88.
26. Neviaser TJ: The anterior labroligamentous periosteal sleeve avulsion lesion: A cause of anterior instability of the shoulder. *Arthroscopy* 1993;9:17-21.
27. Snyder SJ, Strafford BB: Arthroscopic management of instability of the shoulder. *Orthopedics* 1993;16:993-1002.
28. Speer KP, Warren RF, Pagnani M, Warner JJ: An arthroscopic technique for anterior stabilization of the shoulder with a bioabsorbable tack. *J Bone Joint Surg Am* 1996;78:1801-1807.
29. Torchia ME, Caspari RB, Asselmeier MA, Beach WR, Gayari M: Arthroscopic transglenoid multiple suture repair: 2 to 8 year results in 150 shoulders. *Arthroscopy* 1997;13:609-619.
30. Edwards DJ, Hoy G, Saies AD: Adverse reactions to an absorbable shoulder fixation device. *J Shoulder Elbow Surg* 1994;3:230-233.
31. Cole BJ, Romeo AA, Warner JJ: Arthroscopic Bankart repair with the Suretac device for traumatic anterior shoulder instability in athletes. *Orthop Clin North Am* 2001;32:411-421.
32. Rook RT, Savoie FH III, Field LD: Arthroscopic treatment of instability attributable to capsular injury or laxity. *Clin Orthop* 2001;390:52-58.
33. Antoniou J, Duckworth DT, Harryman DT: Capsulolabral augmentation for the management of posteroinferior instability of the shoulder. *J Bone Joint Surg Am* 2000;82:1220-1230.

Superior Labral Anterior and Posterior Lesions and Internal Impingement in the Overhead Athlete

Laith M. Jazrawi, MD
George M. McCluskey III, MD
James R. Andrews, MD

Abstract

Superior labral lesions and internal impingement are believed to be the primary cause of shoulder pathology in the overhead athlete, particularly the baseball player. Increased shoulder external rotation can lead to repetitive impingement of the rotator cuff and superior labrum resulting in a superior labrum anterior and posterior lesion and partial articular-sided rotator cuff tearing. Although the etiology for this phenomenon remains controversial, the end result remains the same: pathology in the rotator cuff and superior labrum. Isolated treatment of the pathology alone, without addressing the capsular laxity, results in lower return to play rates. Addressing the capsular laxity arthroscopically at the same time as the intra-articular pathology is necessary to give these athletes the best chance to return to their prior competitive level. Although short-term results are promising, long-term follow-up is necessary to determine the ultimate usefulness of this treatment philosophy.

The understanding of throwing injuries in the overhead athlete has evolved over the past several decades. The pathologic shoulder in the overhead athlete was initially believed to be psychologically based.[1] After Neer's description of subacromial impingement syndrome in 1972, external impingement was thought to be the main culprit.[2] However, open acromioplasty in athletes with shoulder pain had a greater than 50% failure rate with only 22% of throwing athletes returning to their preinjury level of competitive throwing.[3] Kennedy and associates[4] also demonstrated poor long-term results with coracoacromial ligament division in swimmers.

With the advent of shoulder arthroscopy, Andrews and associates[5] were the first to report, in 1985, on superior labral lesions associated with the long head of the biceps brachii origin. They reported on the arthroscopic findings in a group of high-level throwing athletes with shoulder dysfunction. In addition to tears of the rotator cuff, they described changes in the anterosuperior labral tissue that included fraying, detachment, and, sometimes, partial tearing of the biceps tendon. They suggested the cause in these individuals was attrition secondary to repetitive tension overload on the rotator cuff and biceps anchor. Snyder and associates[6] later classified these injuries as superior labrum anterior and posterior lesions and coined the term SLAP lesion. They described these injuries of the superior labrum that begin posteriorly and extend anteriorly, stopping before or at the midglenoid notch and including the anchor of the biceps tendon to the labrum. The arthroscopic appearances of these lesions were classified into four distinct types. Three variations based on the original classification of Snyder and associates[6] were later described because only 62% of SLAP tears fit into Snyder's classification[7] (Fig. 1).

In 1989, Jobe and associates[8] suggested that instability in the shoulder of the overhead athlete could lead to the development of rotator cuff pathology and shoulder dysfunction. They postulated that repetitive throwing gradually stretches out the anterior capsule and allows the humeral head to migrate anterosuperiorly, causing external or subacromial impingement type symptoms (impingement-instability overlap).[9,10] In 1992, Walch and associates[11] were the first to present arthroscopic clinical evidence that partial, articular-sided rotator cuff tears were a direct consequence of what they termed internal impingement. Internal impingement is characterized by

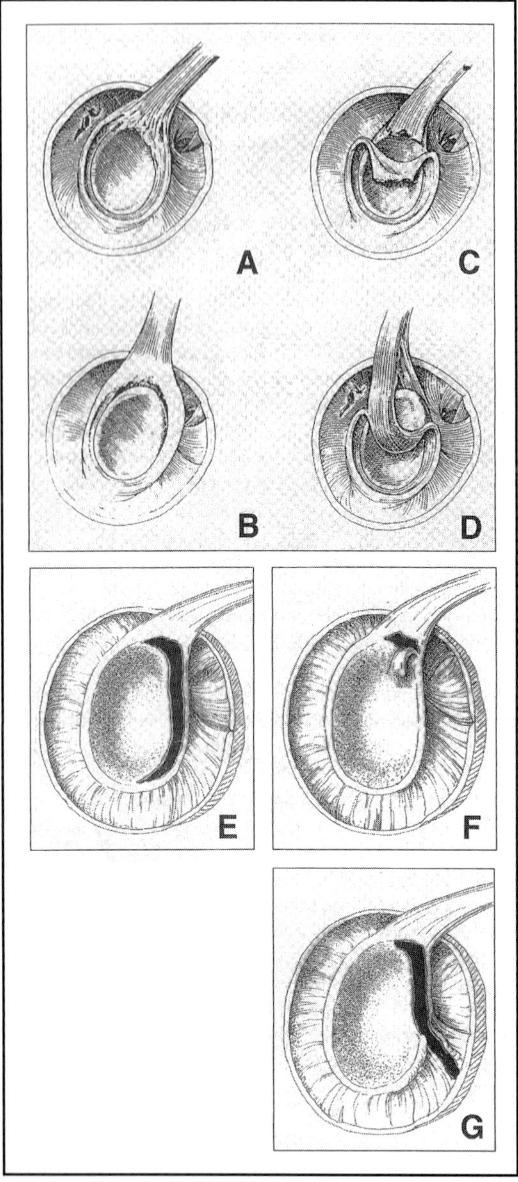

Fig. 1 A, Schematic representation of a type I SLAP lesion showing marked fraying of the superior labrum with degenerative appearance. **B,** Type II SLAP lesion demonstrating superior labral fraying and detachment of the superior biceps-labral anchor. **C,** Type III SLAP lesion demonstrating bucket handle tear of the superior labrum with displacement into the joint. **D,** Type IV SLAP lesion with bucket handle tear of the labrum and extension into biceps tendon. **E,** Type V SLAP lesion where anteroinferior labral lesion extends into superior biceps-labral complex. **F,** Type VI SLAP lesion is a type II SLAP lesion with an associated unstable flap tear of the superior labrum. **G,** Type VII SLAP lesion is superior biceps-labral detachment extending anteriorly to include middle glenohumeral ligament. (Reproduced with permission from Musgrave DS, Rodosky MW: SLAP lesions: Current concepts. *Am J Orthop* 2001;30:29-38.)

contact of the articular surface of the rotator cuff and the greater tuberosity with the posterior and superior glenoid rim and labrum in the extremes of shoulder abduction and external rotation. Jobe[12,13] expanded the concept of internal impingement by applying his observations to overhead athletes with injury to the rotator cuff, glenoid labrum, and glenoid bone as a result of internal impingement and coined the term posterosuperior glenoid impingement. He also believed that anterior microinstability aggravated the internal impingement phenomenon.

In 1998, Morgan and associates[14] expanded the classification by describing three subtypes of type II SLAP lesions: anterior, posterior, and combined anterior-posterior (Fig. 2). They noted that the posterior and combined anterior-posterior type II SLAP lesions were frequently observed in the overhead athlete. Type II SLAP lesions with a posterior component represented 62% of all SLAP lesions in their series and were three times more common in throwers than nonthrowers. They believe that these posterior type II SLAP lesions are mainly responsible for shoulder dysfunction in the overhead athlete.

Anatomy, Function, and Biomechanics

The glenoid labrum is a fibrocartilaginous ring around the bony glenoid rim, which not only deepens the socket, but also serves as the attachment site for the glenohumeral ligaments and biceps tendon.[15] It also adds to shoulder stability by increasing glenoid surface area.[16] The glenoid labrum is composed primarily of fibrous tissue with an occasional fibrocartilaginous transitional zone into the glenoid. Detrisac and Johnson[17] divided normal glenoid labrum into five types based primarily on which labrum quadrant remains unattached to the underlying glenoid (Fig. 3). Williams and associates[18] later simplified this into two types: (1) a peripheral attachment on the glenoid with a fibrocartilaginous transitional zone which, superiorly, at the biceps insertion, is meniscoid in appearance; and (2) a labrum secured to the glenoid both peripherally and centrally.

The long head of the biceps tendon arises from the posterosuperior labrum and the supraglenoid tubercle, which is 5 mm medial to the superior glenoid rim. Cadaveric dissections have shown that 40% to 60% of the time, the tendon arises from the supraglenoid tubercle and surrounding labrum. The remaining specimens arise from the labrum alone.[19] The biceps labral attachment has also been classified into four types depending on the location of its attachment on the superior glenoid: type 1, the labral attachment is entirely posterior (22%); type 2, most of the labral contribution is posterior, with some anterior component (33%); type 3, contribution is equal from both the anterior and posterior labrums (37%); and type 4, most of the contribution is anterior[19] (Fig. 4).

Branches of the suprascapular, posterior humeral circumflex, and circumflex scapular arteries supply the labrum via capsular and periosteal vessels rather than through the bone. Vascularity tends to be greater peripherally than centrally.[20] The superior labrum has been shown to receive the fewest collateral vessels, the number of which continues to decrease with age.[21] This may explain the limited ability for unrepaired SLAP lesions to heal.

Typically the inferior labrum, in contrast to the anterosuperior labrum, is a rounded fibrous structure that is continuous with the articular cartilage. Several normal anatomic variants of the anterior labrum have been described. Knowledge of these variants is necessary to avoid overconstraining the shoulder by repairing normal structures. These variants include variations in insertions of the middle glenohumeral ligament (MGL). The MGL normally appears as a sheet-like structure that drapes over the subscapularis tendon at a 45° angle. In 19% of shoulders, there is a thickening of the MGL with the appearance of a cord-like structure rather than a sheet-like structure.[21] The cord can be seen alone attaching to the superior glenoid where the biceps tendon attaches or it may be associated with a sublabral hole or foramen where there is a bare area on the glenoid labrum at about the 2 o'clock position (Fig. 5). This hole beneath the labrum is most commonly seen at the anterior labrum just below the biceps anchor from the 12 to 3 o'clock positions. No true labral detachment is present, with no evidence of trauma. No increased laxity is attributed to this condition, and the sublabral foramen should not be closed. The incidence of a sublabral foramen in shoulder arthroscopy is 12% and as high as 73% in MRI and cadaver studies.[19] When a cord-like MGL is associated with absence of labral tissue from the 12 to 3 o'clock positions, it is called a Buford complex[19] (Fig. 6). This variant is seen in approximately 1.5% of shoulders.

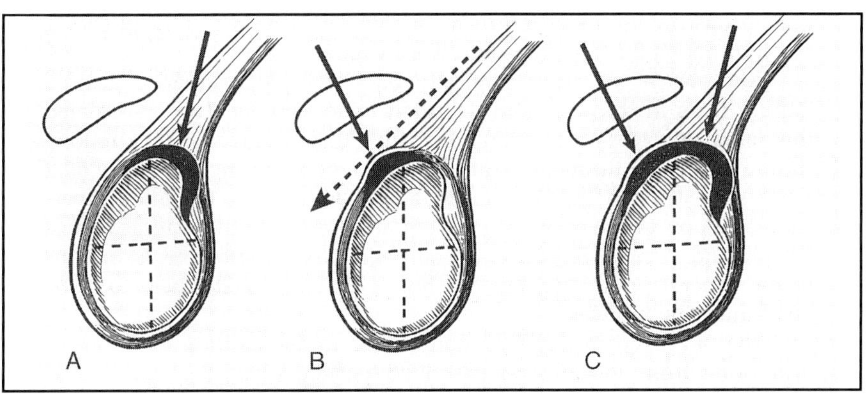

Fig. 2 Three subtypes of type II SLAP lesions. **A**, Anterior, **B**, posterior, **C**, combined anterior and posterior. (Reproduced with permission from Morgan CD, Burkhart SS, Palmeri M, et al: Type II SLAP lesions: Three subtypes and their relationship to superior instability and rotator cuff tears. *Arthroscopy* 1998;14:553-565.)

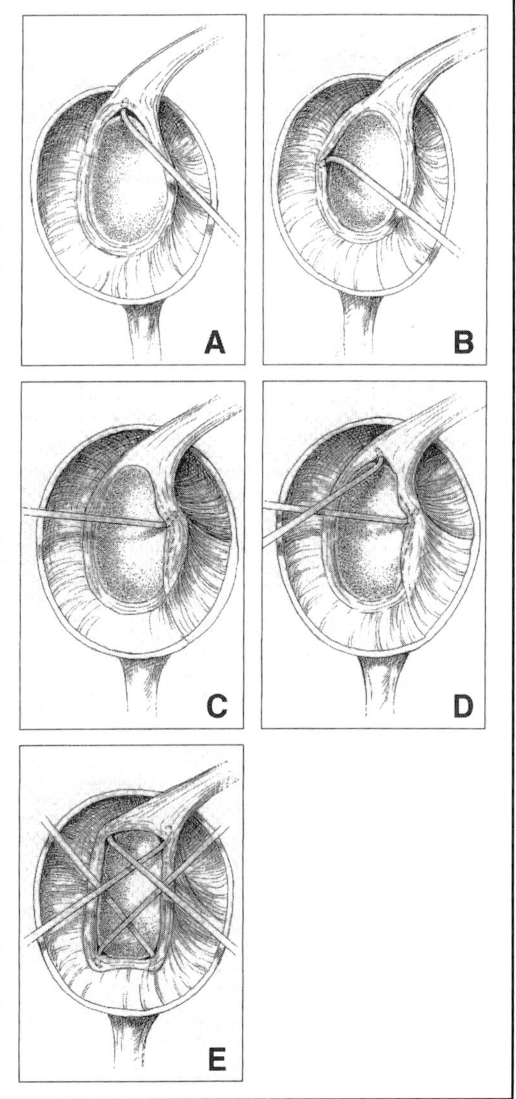

Fig. 3 A, Schematic representation of a type A (superior wedge) labrum in which the superior labrum is triangular in cross section and not attached to the glenoid centrally, allowing a probe to be placed under the superior central free edge. Posterior, inferior, and anterior portions of the labrum remain firmly attached to the glenoid centrally and peripherally. **B,** Type B (posterior wedge) labrum in which the posterior labrum is triangular in cross section and is not attached to the glenoid centrally. The rest of the labrum is attached to glenoid centrally and peripherally. **C,** Type C (anterior wedge) labrum in which the superior band of the IGHL is large and overlaps the relatively small anterior labrum. The rest of the labrum is firmly attached both centrally and peripherally. **D,** Type D (superior and anterior wedge) labrum. **E,** Type E (meniscal) labrum in which there is a central free edge around the entire glenoid. (Reproduced with permission from Musgrave DS, Rodosky MW: SLAP lesions: Current concepts. *Am J Orthop* 2001;30:29-38.)

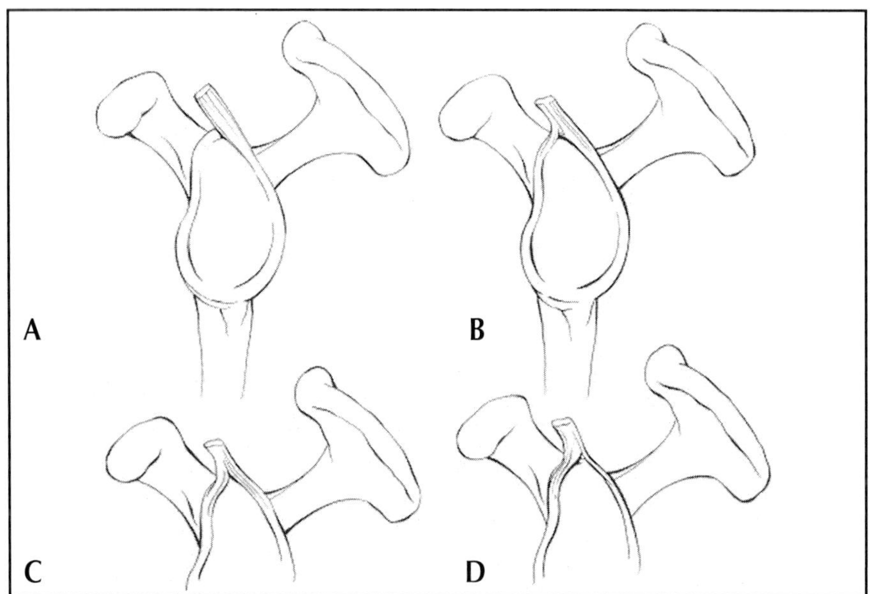

Fig. 4 Biceps contribution to superior labral contribution. **A,** Type 1. **B,** Type 2. **C,** Type 3. **D,** Type 4. (Reproduced with permission from Yamaguchi K, Binder R: Disorders of the biceps tendon, in Iannotti JP, Williams GR (eds): *Disorders of the Shoulder: Diagnosis and Management.* Philadelphia, PA, Lippincott-Williams & Wilkins, 1999, pp 159-190.)

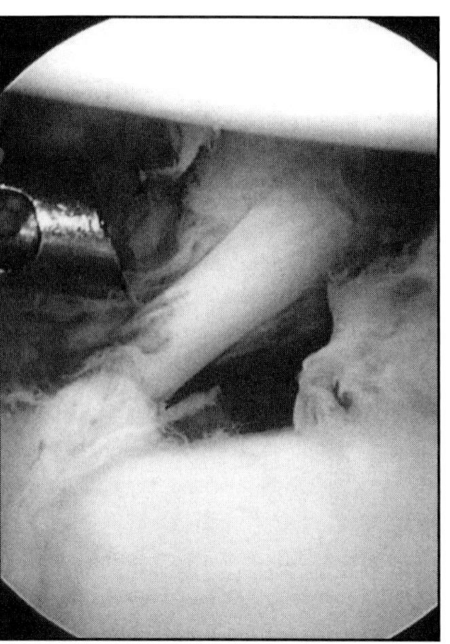

Fig. 6 Right shoulder arthroscopy in lateral decubitus position demonstrating Buford complex.

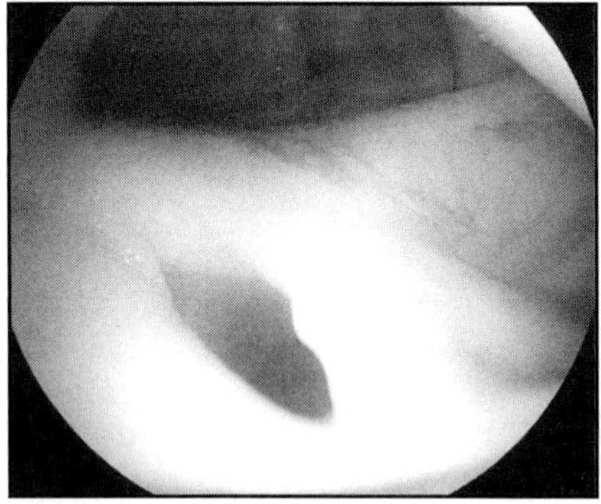

Fig. 5 Right shoulder arthroscopy in lateral decubitus position demonstrating sublabral foramen.

It has been shown that the biceps tendon functions biomechanically as a humeral head depressor, especially in the presence of a large rotator cuff tear, and as a secondary restraint to glenohumeral translation when the shoulder is placed into abduction and external rotation.[22,23] The presence of a SLAP lesion decreases the ability of the biceps to resist external rotation forces on the shoulder in the abducted, externally rotated, or cocked position.[23] Furthermore, lack of an intact superior labrum causes greater stress demand on the inferior glenohumeral ligament (IGHL), which theoretically could lead to damage of the IGHL and subsequent anterior instability.[23] These findings have been confirmed by others who demonstrated that loading of the long head of the biceps tendon resulted in decreases in anterior, posterior, and inferior glenohumeral translation.[24,25] The stabilizing effects of the biceps tendon become more pronounced with decreasing stability of the shoulder.[24] These effects have been confirmed clinically.[26]

Whereas the biomechanical data seem fairly conclusive in suggesting a stabilizing effect of the long head of the biceps brachii, the muscles' complete role in shoulder function has yet to be fully delineated. Electromyogram (EMG) data have been conflicting and inconclusive. However, pitchers with unstable shoulders have an increased EMG response in the biceps tendon when compared to those who were asymptomatic.[27]

Pathophysiology

Internal impingement is caused by the repeated extreme movements of glenohumeral abduction and external rotation seen in overhead throwers, which results in contact of the superior and posterior glenoid rim with the supraspinatus and infraspinatus muscles and posterior humeral head and greater tuberosity.[11] This contact results in partial articular-sided and undersurface rotator cuff tears, tearing of the posterosuperior labrum, and changes on the posterior humeral head including an expanded bare area and cyst formation[11,13] (Fig. 7). Internal impingement is considered to be physiologic and occurs normally when the shoulder is placed in the cocked, abducted, and externally rotated position.[11,28] Jobe[13] hypothesized that this normal phenomenon progressively worsens in overhead throwers because throwing causes gradual repetitive stretching of the anterior capsuloligamentous structures, resulting in anterior microinstability. The anterior instability is theorized to worsen the internal impingement, thereby increasing the degree of contact between the greater tuberosity, rotator cuff, and posterosuperior glenoid rim. This increase results in undersurface rotator cuff tears and superior labrum pathology. The successful treatment of pathologic internal impingement depends on dealing with this anterior microinstability, initially supporting the use of open anterocapsulolabral reconstruction (ACLR).[9] Initial reports with ACLR reported a 68% return to play at prior competitive levels for at least 1 year.[9] Further larger follow-up reports with modification of the procedure (horizontal instead of a T-capsulotomy) demonstrated improved return to play rates with 81% of patients returning to the same sport at the same level of competition.[29]

Burkhart and Morgan,[30] on the other hand, believe the torsional SLAP lesion rather than internal impingement is the main pathologic finding in the overhead athlete with shoulder dysfunction. Their explanation of shoulder pain in the overhead athlete is secondary to an acquired tight posteroinferior capsule and peel-back mechanism of the biceps labral anchor that results in posterosuperior glenohumeral instability and anteroinferior pseudolaxity. Treatment involves superior biceps stabilization and posteroinferior capsular flexibility (stretching or arthroscopic capsular release). They agree that the Jobe model of internal impingement properly describes posterosuperior glenoid impingement and anterior instability.[13] They disagree with the belief that the instability is secondary to progressive stretching of the middle and inferior glenohumeral ligaments and, thus, disagree with the proposed treatment using anterior stabilization procedures.

The Peel-Back Sign

The cocking position of throwing, maximum abduction and external rotation, causes the biceps tendon to assume a more vertical and posterior angle (Fig. 8).

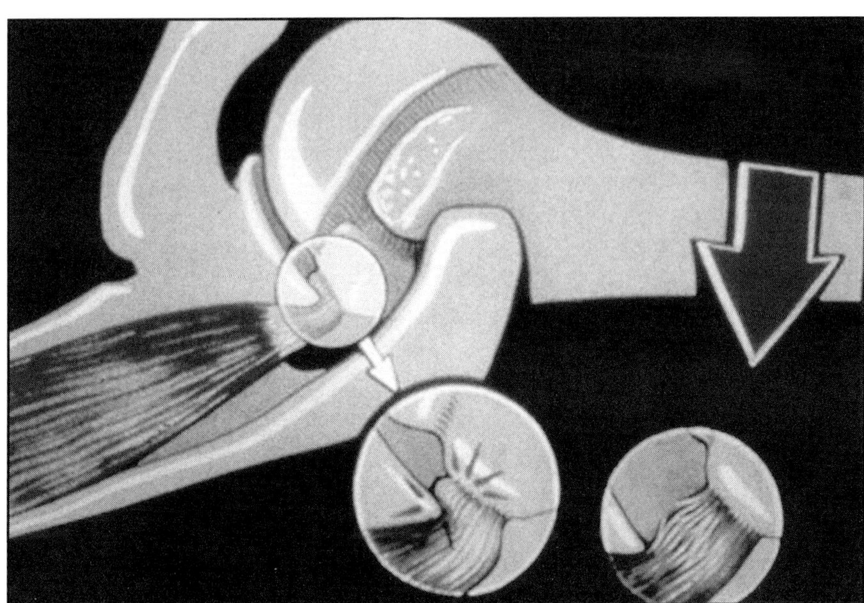

Fig. 7 Impingement of the articular surface of the rotator cuff tendon between the greater tuberosity and posterior glenoid rim characteristic of internal impingement. (Reproduced with permission from Walch G, Boileau P, Noel E, et al: Impingement of the deep surface of the supraspinatus tendon on the posterosuperior glenoid rim: An arthroscopic study. *J Shoulder Elbow Surg* 1992;1:238-245.)

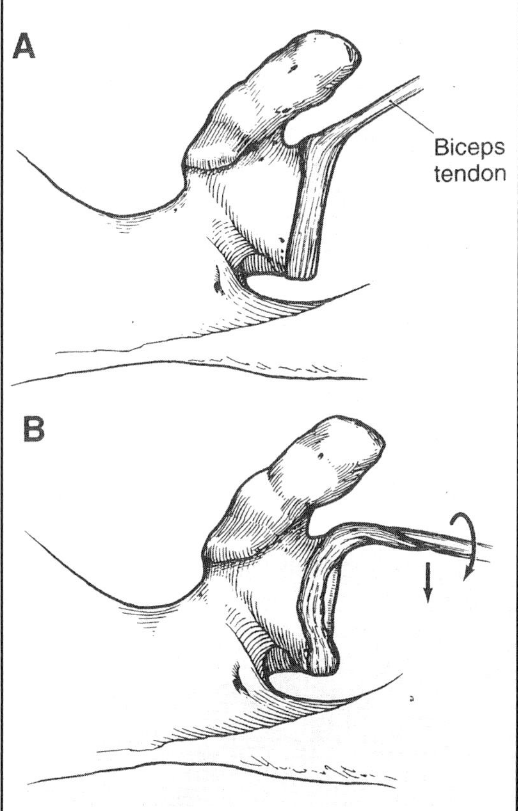

Fig. 8 A, Superior view of resting position of biceps anchor. **B,** With maximum abduction and external rotation the biceps anchor assumes a more vertical position with a torsional force transmitted to the posterosuperior labrum. (Reproduced with permission from Burkhart SS, Morgan CD: The peel-back mechanism: Its role in producing and extending posterior type II SLAP lesions and its effect on SLAP repair rehabilitation. *Arthroscopy* 1998;14: 637-640.)

The dynamic angle change produces a twist at the base of the biceps, transmitting a torsional force to the posterosuperior labrum. In normal shoulders, the intact biceps anchor resists this torsional force. In throwers with posterior and combined anterior and posterior type II SLAP lesions, the torsional force transmitted to the posterosuperior labrum is not effectively resisted, causing it to rotate medially over the corner of the glenoid onto the posterior scapular neck. The phenomenon was described by Burkhart and Morgan[30] and Morgan and associates[14] and called the peel-back sign. Surgical repair eliminates the peel-back sign by neutralizing the torsional force transmitted to the posterosuperior labrum.

Instability Versus Pseudolaxity

Inherent in the internal impingement concept supported by Walch and associates[11] and Jobe[13] is some type of subtle anterior instability with anterior capsular stretching, which results in pathologic internal impingement and ultimately shoulder dysfunction in the throwing athlete. Both Morgan and associates[14] and Burkhart and Morgan[30] also believe that these shoulders have some degree of instability, which they confirmed arthroscopically by the presence of a positive drive-through sign[31] in which the arthroscope can easily be driven with little resistance through the shoulder from superior to inferior between the humeral head and glenoid. While the clinical significance of this sign has been questioned recently, Burkhart and Morgan's surgical approach to the overhead throwing athlete is dictated by the presence of this arthroscopic drive-through sign.[32-35] If SLAP repair eliminates the drive-through sign, nothing further is done surgically. If the drive-through sign persists after SLAP repair, either thermal capsulorrhaphy or capsular suture plication to address the anterior instability is performed. Burkhart and Morgan believe the posterosuperior torsional SLAP lesion, rather than anterior capsular stretching, to be the main culprit of the instability, which is posterosuperior in direction.[30] This secondary posterosuperior instability is similar clinically to the instability caused by anteroinferior labral detachment. Although the humeral head cannot dislocate superiorly because of the acromion, repetitive superior translation or subluxation can lead to partial articular-sided rotator cuff damage. In Morgan and associates' study,[14] partial articular-sided rotator cuff tears associated with anterior type II SLAP lesions were all located within the anterior to mid portion of the rotator crescent. Partial articular-sided rotator cuff tears associated with posterior type II SLAP tears were all located in the posterior part of the rotator cuff crescent. Morgan and associates[14] believe these lesion-specific location rotator cuff tears, associated with type II SLAP subtypes, are consistent with the concept of superior instability as the main factor causing the cuff to tear from inside-out, with the tear location corresponding to the location of increased tensile force in the zones that are maximally stressed. When this laxity is present with type II SLAP lesions it is referred to as pseudolaxity.[14]

The concept of pseudolaxity is consistent with the circle concept in which the periarticular labral fibers of the glenoid act as a unit so that disruption of the fibers in one part of the labrum manifests itself as an apparent laxity on the opposite side.[14,36,37] Huber and Putz[38] postulated a periarticular fiber system consisting of the labrum, glenohumeral ligaments, and the biceps anchor. This system of parallel collagen fibers surrounding the circumference of the glenoid acts as a basket or a tension brace to provide hoop stresses at the periphery. The labrum thus acts as bumper in all directions to resist dislocation or subluxation of the humeral head. As a result, the end effect of the peel-back sign is laxity of the glenohumeral joint secondary to disruption of the superior labrum. This concept is further supported by Pagnani and associates[37] who demonstrated in a cadaver model that lesions of the superior labrum alone, destabilizing the biceps anchor, resulted in an increase in anteroposterior and superoinferior glenohumeral translation. Theoretically, repairing the posterosuperior labral fibers will restore the circle and eliminate the anteroinferior pseudolaxity.

Etiology and Mechanism of Injury

Arthroscopic and laboratory observations point to several possible etiologies for SLAP lesions. Patients who have superior labral pathology fall into two categories. The first consists of overhead athletes (eg, baseball players, tennis players, swimmers), most commonly baseball players, more specifically pitchers, with a history of repetitive overhead activity and no history of trauma. The second category consists of patients who have had an acute traumatic injury.[6] These injuries can be traction- or compression-related. Traction injuries result from a sudden pull on the arm, which can be in an inferior direction (eg, losing hold of a heavy object such as a couch), an anterior direction (for example, water skiing), superior direction (for example, grabbing a railing while falling down stairs). Compression injuries result from a fall on an outstretched hand with the arm in slight forward flexion and abduction or a motor vehicle accident with the arms on the steering wheel with the elbows extended and force transmitted to the humerus. Finally, a direct blow to the shoulder could theoretically result in superior labral injury.

Andrews and associates[5] initially attributed SLAP lesions to tensile overload predominantly occurring during the deceleration phase of throwing in which electromyographic (EMG) studies have indicated that the biceps is active. Arthroscopic electrical stimulation of the long head of the biceps brachii caused the tendon to become taut and raised its origin at the superior labrum off the glenoid.[5] We believe these data explain only part of the etiology of SLAP lesions in the overhead athlete. Currently, we believe the cause of SLAP lesions in the overhead athlete is explained by the "weed-pull theory" (J Conway, MD, personal communication) in which abduction of the humerus brings the biceps tendon groove close to the superior glenoid rim and biceps tendon origin and external rotation of the humerus rotates the biceps tendon groove posterior to the biceps tendon origin. This is essentially the same as the peel-back sign espoused by Morgan and associates[14] and Burkhart and Morgan,[30] which we believe only partly explains the etiology of SLAP lesions. External rotation of the humerus causes strain in the anterior segment of the biceps and deformity in the posterior segment of the biceps tendon anchor. Internal rotation of the humerus relieves the stress but is accompanied by tension forces at the biceps anchor acting to decelerate the elbow.[5] This rapid, forceful, repetitious back-and-forth motion pulls the biceps tendon away from the glenoid rim. In a biomechanical study investigating the potential etiology of SLAP lesions, the lesions were reliably produced with traction on the long head of the biceps tendon with the shoulders inferiorly subluxated.[39] This study supports the theory that the deceleration phase of throwing may be partly responsible for SLAP lesions, which are exacerbated in individuals with preexisting laxity.[5]

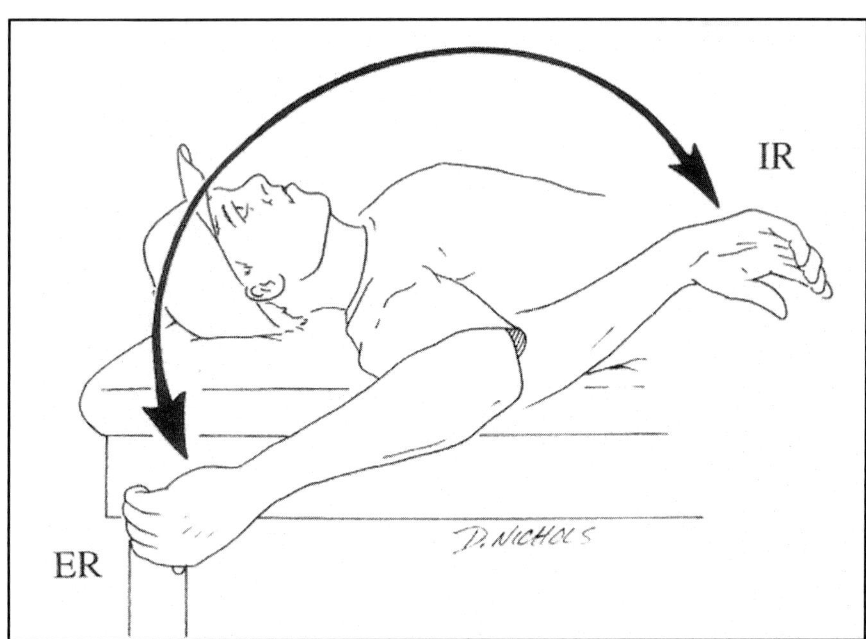

Fig. 9 The total arc of motion concept: external rotation + internal rotation = total motion. (Reproduced with permission from Wilk KE, Meister K, Andrews JR: Current concepts in the rehabilitation of the overhead throwing athlete. *Am J Sports Med* 2002;30:136-151.)

Morgan and associates[14] and Burkart and Morgan[30] believe the culprit is the peel-back sign caused by the cocking position of throwing (maximum abduction and external rotation). This phenomenon transmits a torsional force to the posterosuperior labrum, which is magnified by a tight posterior capsule. This torsional force causes the posterosuperior labrum and biceps anchor to rotate medially over the corner of the glenoid onto the scapular neck. These authors[14,30] also believe that a tight posterior capsule in the throwing shoulder, demonstrated by a lack of internal rotation greater than 40° compared with the nonthrowing shoulder, predisposes this select group to develop type II SLAP lesions by enhancing the peel-back sign. In the cocking position, the presence of a tight posterior capsule causes a posterosuperior shift of the glenohumeral fulcrum, or contact point between the glenoid and humerus. As the shoulder externally rotates around this new rotation point, there is increased contact of the rotator cuff and posterior glenoid labrum with increased torsional forces at the biceps anchor. They believe this force produces the type II SLAP lesion, which in turn magnifies the posterosuperior shift or instability problem, and that these lesions are not purely deceleration injuries.

The healthy throwing shoulder will have increased external rotation in abduction at the expense of internal rotation. The gains in external rotation are roughly equal to the loss of internal rotation maintaining a total 180° arc of motion, which is consistent with the total arc of motion concept demonstrated by Wilk and associates[40] (Fig. 9). Burkhart and Morgan[30] and Morgan and associates[14] believe that patients who develop SLAP lesions have an altered total arc of motion less than 180° with symptomatic decreases in internal rotation up to 40° to 60°, making these patients become more susceptible to SLAP lesions. The etiology for this altered arc of motion is believed to be multifactorial and may also be developmental, with alterations in glenoid and humeral head retroversion accounting for the changed range of motion.[28,41,42,43]

The humeral and glenoid retroversion may be protective against the development of internal impingement. The lack of spinback or retroversion of the proximal humerus may be related to age at onset of throwing, technique, level of play, length of play, or other factors. This concept is currently the focus of further studies at the American Sports Medicine Institute in Birmingham, Alabama.

Clinical Examination

It is important to obtain an accurate history. The athlete is often vague about the onset of shoulder pain and the inciting event. The throwing history should include the most recent activity and changes in level of performance (velocity, control, stamina, pain). Pain should be evaluated for location, quality, and duration of symptoms. The point in the throwing cycle at which symptoms are worse should be documented. Any recent changes in throwing mechanics or schedule should be noted. Any prior history of shoulder or elbow problems should be noted and previous upper extremity surgery documented.

The diagnosis of SLAP lesions can be difficult and challenging in that they can mimic rotator cuff pathology and glenohumeral instability. Definitive diagnosis can only be made with arthroscopy. Overhand throwing athletes with internal impingement with or without SLAP lesions typically complain of pain in the late cocking phase, which is often poorly localized but classically located posteriorly at the junction of infraspinatus/supraspinatus humeral head insertion. However, the pain is often vague and inconsistent.

Mechanical symptoms can be present and include catching, locking, popping, or grinding. Overhead athletes often complain that their arm goes "dead" when they try to throw hard. Rowe and Zairns[44] initially defined the dead arm syndrome in patients with recurrent transient anterior subluxation of the shoulder. More recently the syndrome has been defined as a pathologic condition in which the throwers are unable to throw with their preinjury velocity and control because of a combination of pain and subjective unease in the shoulder.[45] A variety of pathologic entities result in this clinical entity (ie, rotator cuff tendinitis, biceps tendinitis, posterior glenoid calcifications [Bennett's lesion], acromioclavicular pathology, and scapula dysfunction). Internal impingement with or without SLAP lesion in throwers is one of the more common causes of the dead arm syndrome.

Physical examination should begin with visual inspection. Overdevelopment of the dominant throwing arm is expected.[46] Scapular position and periscapular musculature should be examined. Functional abnormalities of the scapula are evaluated by observing from behind while the patient does a sitting lift-off test. Scapulothoracic motion is evaluated by active forward flexion of the glenohumeral joint and by a wall push-off test because scapula dysfunction can predispose to shoulder dysfunction.[45] With the patient seated, palpation should proceed from the sternoclavicular joint, along the clavicle and the acromioclavicular (AC) joint, and to the lateral acromion so that point tenderness can be detected. Proceeding from anterior to lateral to posterior, the examiner evaluates the anterior capsule, bicipital groove, coracoid, deltoid insertion, posterior capsule, and posterior soft tissue for tenderness. The shoulder is palpated for circumduction crepitus, which is frequently positive with subacromial disease. Cross-arm adduction is helpful to assess AC pathology. Speed's and Yergason's tests are used to assess pathology in the bicipital groove. Seated passive internal rotation is assessed by determining position of the thumb tip on the vertebral column. Rotator cuff strength is also assessed in a seated patient. External impingement is checked with Neer and Hawkins tests.[47,48]

At the American Sports Medicine Institute all shoulders are assessed for the presence of labral pathology using the active compression test as described by O'Brien and associates[49] and the clunk test described by Andrews and associates.[50,51] Numerous labral provocative tests are described in the literature and their accuracy and usefulness in detecting superior labral pathology is currently being investigated, including the anterior slide test (Kibler test), the crank test, the biceps load tests I and II, the Mimori test, the biceps tension test (Speed's test), and the Jobe relocation test (for posterior SLAP).[14,52-57] Morgan and associates[14] demonstrated that the Speed and O'Brien tests were useful in predicting anterior type II SLAP lesions, whereas the Jobe relocation test was more useful in predicting posterior SLAP lesions.

For the clunk test, the patient is placed supine with the affected shoulder maximally elevated. The examiner stands at the head of the bed, cephalad to the affected shoulder. The examiner places the hand nearest to the patient's head posterior to the humeral head and applies an anteriorly directed force. With the hand furthest from the patient, the examiner grasps the distal humerus, abducts it maximally, and applies gentle rotatory forces. Labral tears are trapped between the humeral head/greater tuberosity and glenoid rim, producing a palpable or audible clunk or reproduction of pain.

Stability is assessed initially with the patient seated. The Lachman test is performed, and glenohumeral translation is classified according to the scale proposed by Altchek and associates.[58] The sulcus sign is used to test for inferior laxity in a seated patient; it is graded according to the distance in centimeters the humeral head can be inferiorly subluxated from the acromion (1+, 1 cm; 2+, 2 cm; 3+, > 3 cm). The Lachman test is repeated with the patient supine because it is often difficult to assess in a seated patient, particularly one with a muscular athletic shoulder. The humerus is then abducted and externally rotated as the examiner anteriorly translates the humeral head. The subjective assessment of the end point of anterior translation is as important as the amount of translation. In the normal shoulder and the asymptomatic throwing shoulder, the anterior band of the glenohumeral ligament will become the most important static restraint in this position. To detect more subtle instability, we use the relocation test described by Kvitne and Jobe.[59] The test is performed with the patient supine and the arm positioned at 90° abduction and maximal shoulder external rotation. The test will recreate anterior pain or apprehension if subtle anterior instability is present, as opposed to the internal impingement test, which recreates posterior pain with maximum external rotation. The test is positive if the anterior pain is relieved when a posteriorly directed force is applied to the humeral head.

With the patient supine, passive forward elevation and passive external rotation and internal rotation at 0° and 90° of shoulder abduction are documented. High-level throwers often have increased passive external rotation and decreased internal rotation of the dominant shoulder.[40,60,61] While the patient is still supine, the test for internal impingement is performed with the arm abducted to 90° and maximally externally rotated. The test is positive if pain is elicited in the posterior aspect of the shoulder in the region of the infraspinatus.[62] The patient is then placed prone and the posterior cuff palpated. In this position, the posterior capsule and the adjacent soft tissue are assessed for palpation tenderness. Any pain in the region of the infraspinatus insertion is considered significant and may be the only clinical sign of a partial thickness tear associated with internal impingement.

Radiologic Evaluation

Radiologic evaluation of the overhead throwing athlete begins with plain radiographs. These include internal and external AP views, an axillary view, a Stryker notch view, and a supraspinatus outlet view. The AP views often reveal increased sclerosis at the base of the greater tuberosity of the throwing shoulder.[63] This sclerosis occurs secondary to the contact erosive areas on the greater tuberosity with the posterior glenoid rim, which occurs from repetitive maximal external rotation of the shoulder. The Stryker notch projection is helpful in demonstrating a thrower's exostosis at the posteroinferior glenoid as well as a Hill-Sachs lesion, which is pathognomonic for a previous anterior shoulder dislocation.[64,65] Other less common abnormalities, including AC joint arthrosis or osteophyte formation on the undersurface of the clavicle, can be seen on the AP shoulder or AC joint view. Both situations can predispose to external impingement and rotator cuff disease. Supraspinatus outlet views are helpful in determining acromial type. However, acromial spurs are uncommon in the overhead athlete. The axillary and West Point views are helpful in the diagnosis of osseous Bankart lesions. Although these studies are valuable to rule out concomitant pathology, plain radiographs are not usually helpful for the evaluation of the overhead athlete with internal impingement and superior labral pathology. However, a supraglenoid tubercle fracture seen on a shoulder AP view may be diagnostic of a SLAP lesion.[66]

Plain radiographs, while noninvasive and inexpensive, do not show soft-tissue pathology. Ultrasound, also noninvasive and inexpensive, has been shown in some centers to be useful for the identification of rotator cuff pathology.[67] However, it has not been proven to be useful in identifying labral pathology. The test is highly operator dependent, with the viewing area constrained by the bony anatomy. Because the acromial process cannot be penetrated, medial pathology at the joint line, such as labral defects, are not well visualized.[67]

Plain radiographs are followed with MRI for evaluation of the rotator cuff and labrum. CT arthrography has been used in the past; however, recent improvements in MRI resolution have limited its use. Double-contrast CT arthrography has a 90% sensitivity, 73% specificity, and 83% accuracy in detecting anterior labral defects.[68] Limitations include poor visualization of the posterior labrum, difficult evaluation of the labrum in the presence of a complete rotator cuff tear, difficulty identifying SLAP lesion types, and inability to diagnose partial rotator cuff tears.[69]

Magnetic resonance arthrography (MRA) of the shoulder has been used at the American Sports Medicine Institute since 1991. The intra-articular contrast improves diagnostic accuracy, especially in the presence of labral pathology. Although there is controversy in the literature regarding the use of intra-articular contrast to detect labral and rotator cuff pathology, its use should be based on the preference of the referring clinician and the radiologist performing the test. The highly magnetic contrast agent allows a short T1 time and yields images with low signal-to-noise ratio and spatial resolution. While intra-articular gadolinium is off-label and not approved by the Food and Drug Administration (FDA), the required dose is small compared with the FDA-approved intravenous dose, and to our knowledge no problems with its use have been reported.[51] MRI sensitivity in detecting labral lesions in general has been as high as 95%;[70] however, nonenhanced MRI is less sensitive in detecting superior labral lesion compared with middle and inferior labral tears.[71] Iannotti and associates[72] demonstrated nonenhanced MRI to have an 88% sensitivity, 93% specificity, 97% positive predictive value, and 87% negative predictive value in identifying labral pathology. However, it was not able to distinguish between SLAP lesions and other labral tears. Smith and associates[73] noted that nonenhanced MRI detected only 17% of SLAP lesions preoperatively, whereas Connell and associates,[74] reported that nonenhanced MRI can accurately diagnose superior labral lesions with a 86% sensitivity and 100% specificity. Monu and associates[75] reported 100% retrospective

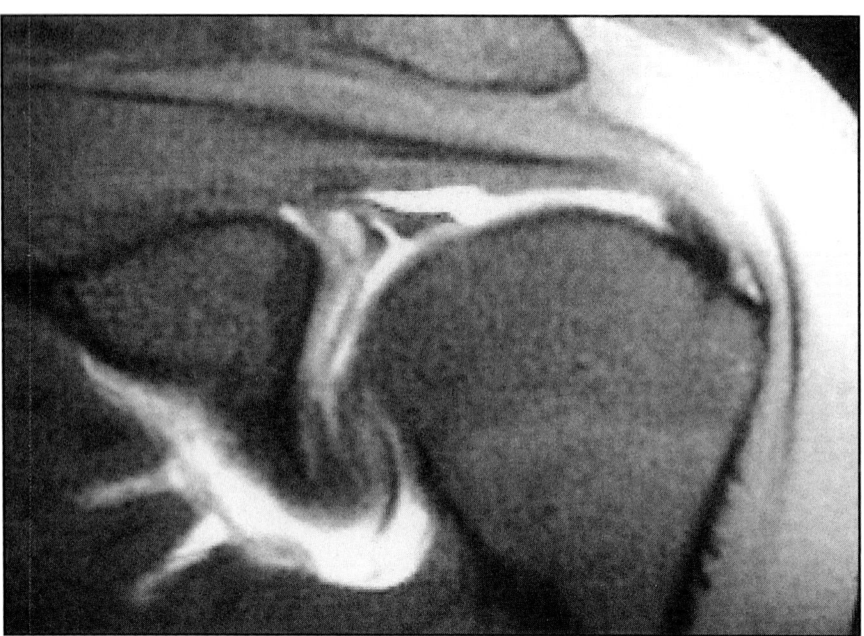

Fig. 10 Coronal oblique gadolinium-enhanced MRI scan of the left shoulder demonstrating increased signal in posterior labrum consistent with a type II SLAP lesion.

detection of arthroscopically confirmed SLAP lesions with nonenhanced MRI. However, our experience as well as that of others has not been as good.[51,70,71,76-80]

Flannigan and associates[70] reported that MRA detected all nine patients with surgically proven SLAP tears, while nonenhanced MRA detected only three (33%). Eleven of 14 surgically proven rotator cuff tears were detected by MRA (3 partial tears on the bursal surface were missed) while nonenhanced MRI detected 9 of the tears (three partial tears of the articular side of the tear as well as two complete tears were missed). These results suggest that MRA enhances the accuracy of MRI in the evaluation of the superior labrum as well as the rotator cuff. Chandnani and associates[81] reported 89% sensitivity, 88% specificity, and 89% accuracy of MRA in detecting SLAP lesions. Critics of comparative studies evaluating enhanced and unenhanced MRI claim that nonenhanced MRI protocols use relatively low resolution and standardized spin-echo techniques and that less than optimal MRI parameters can be faulted as the potential cause for the diminished accuracy in use of the traditional noncontrast techniques.[82] Proponents of nonenhanced MRI believe that simply using a high magnetic field strength with a dedicated shoulder coil is not adequate to impart sufficient diagnostic accuracy, and attention to pulse sequence parameters and pixel size is essential to provide accurate, reproducible results.[82]

At the American Sports Medicine Institute all overhead athletes with potential shoulder pathology have MRA of the shoulder. A dilute mixture of gadopentate dimeglumine (Magnevist, Berlex Laboratories, Wynne, NJ) and saline (1 mL gadopentate dimeglumine in 250 mL saline) is sterilely injected into the shoulder under fluoroscopic guidance. After injection of 15 to 20 mL the shoulder is taken through a passive range of motion (ROM). In investigations of the intra-articular use of gadolinium in animals there was no accumulation in synovium and cartilage, and there have been no adverse reports with clinical use.[83] Alternatives to intra-articular gadolinium include saline alone, which is inert and inexpensive but does not enhance T1-weighted images. However, sensitivities and specificities as high as 89% have been reported.[80]

Superior labral tears are best visualized on coronal oblique images as T- or Y- shaped areas of increased signal that extend to the labral surface (Fig. 10). Superior labral cysts are also highly suggestive of labral tears.[81] Other findings suggestive of superior labral pathology on MRA include (1) contrast material extending into the insertion of the long head of the biceps tendon or irregularity of the insertion or superior labrum displacement on oblique coronal images, (2) accumulation of contrast between the labrum and glenoid fossa on axial images and (3) contrast material extending into the insertion of the long head of the biceps tendon or irregularity of the insertion or superior labrum displacement on sagittal oblique images.[84] Distinguishing irregularity of the labral margin is important because it separates labral trauma from a sublabral foramen or other anatomic variants.[82] In addition, the displaced labrum commonly lies adjacent to hyperintense, frayed glenohumeral ligaments.[82]

MRI and MRA have been shown to accurately identify ganglion cysts involving the spinoglenoid notch, which have been associated with SLAP lesions.[85-88] EMG and nerve conduction velocity studies can also be used to identify suprascapular nerve compression. However, secondary to complex suprascapular nerve and spinoglenoid notch anatomy, these tests are often not sensitive enough to detect suprascapular nerve entrapment.[85,86]

Partial articular-sided rotator cuff tears, characteristic of internal impingement, are best seen on the coronal oblique MRA images as irregularity of the undersurface of the supraspinatus-infraspinatus. Contrast-enhanced MRI was shown by Karzel and Snyder[83] to improve the diagnostic accuracy of the detection of partial articular-sided rotator cuff tears. Others have also confirmed improved accuracy in the detection of partial rotator cuff tears with MRA.[70] More recently, Meister and associates[89] have shown, with arthroscopic confirmation, that MRA is greater than 90% sensitive in detecting partial-thickness tears of less than 25% of the cuff thickness.

Nonsurgical Treatment

Internal Impingement

Wilk and associates'[40] nonsurgical treatment protocol for internal impingement is summarized briefly here. The primary goal of the rehabilitation program for internal impingement (Table 1) is to enhance the athlete's dynamic stabilization abilities, thereby controlling anterior humeral head translation, which we believe is partially responsible for symptomatic internal impingement. Posterior rotator cuff muscle flexibility is encouraged as well. Aggressive stretching of the anterior and inferior glenohumeral structures is avoided, because it may increase anterior translation. Restoring dynamic stabilization is an essential goal to minimize the anterior translation of the humeral head during the late cocking and early acceleration phases of throwing. Exercise drills such as proprioceptive neuromuscular facilitation patterns with rhythmic stabilization are incorporated as well as stabilization drills performed at end-range external rotation.[90] Perturbation training to the shoulder joint is performed to enhance proprioception, dynamic stabilization, and neuromuscular control.

Once posterior flexibility is restored, glenohumeral strength ratios normalized, scapular muscular strength enhanced, and patient's symptoms diminished, an interval-throwing program with an increase in throwing intensity based on symptoms is initiated. During this phase, correction of throwing pathomechanics is critical to returning the athlete to asymptomatic and effective throwing.

SLAP Lesions

The nonsurgical treatment of SLAP lesions depends on lesion type. Most lesions in the overhead athlete are type II, which are not amenable to nonsurgical treatment. The rehabilitation program prior to surgical correction emphasizes restoration of ROM through stretching exercises within the patient's tolerance. A strengthening program should be performed in an attempt to prevent muscular atrophy. Strengthening exercises such as external rotation and internal rotation with the arm at the side or scapular plane, scapular strengthening, and deltoid exercises to 90° of abduction can be safely performed. Exercises such as shoulder press, bench press, and latissimus dorsi pull downs (behind the neck) are avoided because of increased stress to the superior labrum and anterior glenohumeral joint capsule.

Surgical Indications

One of the most challenging decisions facing clinicians who treat overhead athletes is whether or not surgical treatment is indicated, and when is the appropriate time for surgery. In the past, shoulder surgery in the throwing athlete may have been a career-ending event. We believe that previous poor surgical results in patients with internal impingement with or without SLAP lesions have resulted from the surgeon's inability to deal with the acquired laxity in the throwing shoulder and to repair labral pathology rather than using débridement.[58,59] Laxity, if recognized, was treated with an open capsular reconstruction, which initially had been associated with poor results in this population in part secondary to decreased postoperative external rotation in the surgically corrected shoulder.[9] Although the postoperative external rotation decreases were in most cases minimal, they were enough to prevent some from returning to their preinjury level of play. The greatest challenge in management of these patients with internal

Table 1
Rehabilitation for Internal Impingement: Phases and Goals

Phase One: Acute Phase	
Goals	Diminish pain and inflammation Normalize motion Retard muscular atrophy Reestablish dynamic stability Control functional stress and strain
Exercises and Modalities	Cryotherapy, ultrasound, electrical stimulation Flexibility and stretching for posterior shoulder muscles Rotator cuff strengthening (especially external rotators) Scapular muscles strengthening (especially retractors, protractors, depressors) Dynamic stabilization exercises (rhythmic stabilization) Closed kinetic chain exercises Proprioception training Abstain from throwing
Phase Two: Intermediate Phase	
Goals	Progress strengthening exercise Restore muscular balance (external rotation/internal rotation) Enhance dynamic stability Control flexibility and stretches
Exercises and Modalities	Continue stretching and flexibility Progress isotonic strengthening Complete shoulder program Throwers Ten program Rhythmic stabilization drills Initiate core strengthening program Initiate leg program
Phase Three: Advanced Strengthening Phase	
Goals	Aggressive strengthening Progress neuromuscular control Improve strength, power, and endurance Initiate light throwing activities
Exercises and Modalities	Flexibility and stretching Rhythmic stabilization drills Throwers Ten program Initiate plyometric program Initiate endurance drills Initiate short distance throwing program
Phase Four: Return to Activity Phase	
Goals	Progress to throwing program Return to competitive throwing Continue strengthening and flexibility drills

impingement with or without SLAP tears is attention to what Wilk and associates[40] refer to as the thrower's shoulder paradox. The paradox refers to the thrower's need to be able to obtain the extreme degree of external rotation seen in the late cocking phase, while maintaining stability in light of an almost certain degree of capsular laxity.[62]

We believe that internal impingement accounts for a significant percentage of partial-thickness articular-sided rotator cuff tears and posterosuperior labral tears in the overhead athlete. While successful results with rotator cuff débridement have been reported in athletes who participate in overhand athletics (ie, tennis, badminton), none were baseball throwers.[11,42] We agree with Meister[62] that this is because of the lower physical demands placed on the throwing shoulder of athletes who are not baseball pitchers, which makes these athletes more amenable to less aggressive treatment. Payne and associates[91] reported only a 25% to 50% return to sports with rotator cuff débridement alone in patients with associated instability. We believe that inability to address the occult instability in these throwing athletes led to poor results.

The treatment of occult instability in the throwing athlete continues to remain a major challenge today. The ability of these athletes to pitch has much to do with their ability to maintain excessive physiologic laxity, specifically, increased external rotation of the shoulder.[62] It is their ability to maintain a dynamic balance through muscular control in the face of static laxity that allows them to function efficiently and effectively as baseball throwers. When this fine balance is broken, either from partial articular-sided rotator cuff tearing, labral tearing, or internal impingement, the athlete has crossed over from physiologic to pathologic laxity.[62] The goal in treatment of these overhead athletes is to eliminate the pathologic laxity while maintaining motion.

Open procedures to address this instability have included ACLR popularized by Jobe and associates.[9] Only 68% of 25 patients returned to prior competitive levels for at least 1 year. In a more recent study in which they used ACLR with modifications (horizontal rather than a T-capsulotomy, suture anchors instead of bone tunnels) there was an 81% (33 of 36) return of players to their prior competitive levels.[92] However, additional studies using open capsulorrhaphy for reconstruction have had poorer results.[93-95]

Arthroscopic suture plication techniques to address the capsular laxity, particularly in the patient with multidirectional instability, have also been described.[96-104] Theoretically, these techniques are intended to be minimally invasive, curing the instability while maintaining motion. Although results are short term, they are encouraging. However, none of these studies has focused entirely on the overhead athlete.

Fair to good results at short-term follow-up deteriorated with time at longer term follow-up in the arthroscopic treatment of patients with internal impingement with or without SLAP lesions when standard arthroscopic techniques of débridement with or without labral repair were used.[58,105-108] Theoretically, débridement was believed to promote healing and acromioplasty was used to decrease bursal-sided impingement. We believe previous poor results were secondary to failure to address the pathophysiology of internal impingement, which is instability. The rarity of external impingement in this patient population explains the poor results with acromioplasty.[109]

The mechanism of injury to the rotator cuff in internal impingement is different from what occurs in the nonthrower or nonoverhead athlete. Overuse injuries in the nonthrower frequently have characteristics of external impingement with no glenohumeral laxity. Because of the different pathophysiology involved in the cuff damage in the baseball player or overhead athlete, acromioplasty should be avoided in this patient group. We tend to perform acromioplasty only when an overhead athlete has failed a previous surgical treatment aimed at addressing internal impingement and the associated instability.

Surgical Technique

If a true superior labral detachment is noted, arthroscopic repair is the procedure of choice. SLAP tears in the overhead athlete, if present, are almost entirely type II. These tears must be repaired if present. We initially identify whether the type II SLAP lesion has a predominant posterior or anterior component as described by Burkhart and Morgan[30] and Morgan and associates.[14] The SLAP lesion is repaired according to its location. Posterior lesions are treated with the use of suture anchors placed posteriorly followed by arthroscopic knot tying. Lesions with anterior extension are treated with an additional suture anchor placed through the anterior portal followed by arthroscopic knot tying. However, superior lesions with posterior extension are more difficult to repair through the anterior cannula because of the angle of insertion for the anchor or other fixation device used. Therefore, we routinely use a small bioabsorbable anchor placed through a posterolateral stab incision. This procedure produces the smallest possible defect in the rotator cuff without compromising the arthroscopic repair and fixation. Before placing any anchor or tack, the glenoid rim should be débrided down to bleeding bone. The fixation should be at the articular margin, not recessed on the glenoid neck. Fixation on the glenoid neck as opposed to the correct periarticular location may lead to instability and subsequent reinjury. The superior labrum should be carefully inspected before repair to ensure that the attachment is in fact detached. The normal superior labrum may be recessed or meniscoid with its fibers attaching medial to the articular surface. This condition should not be mistaken for a true labral tear.

We prefer not to use bioabsorbable tacks for labral repairs despite several positive reports,[110-115] secondary to fear of tack fragmentation and foreign body reaction.[116,117] We also fear that impingement of the head of the tack and the greater tuberosity of the humerus may occur in the late cocking phase of pitching. According to Burkhart and Parten,[35] the use of translabral tacks provides, at least visually, less effective resistance to the peel-back syndrome than suture anchors. With a suture anchor, the circumferential suture loop around the labrum develops tensile force in response to the peel-back torsional load, providing a peripherally placed opposing torque. On the other hand, tacks have a single point of contact on the labrum, by virtue of their design, and resist the torsional load by means of a flexural bending load on the shaft of the tack.[35] From a mechanical standpoint, this is a less effective and predictable way of resisting an applied torque. The only report in the literature on the use of suture anchors for SLAP repairs noted a 97% success rate (99 of 102)[30] compared with success rates of 71% to 88% with absorbable tacks.[110-115]

Our technique of addressing capsular laxity in the overhead athlete with internal impingement involves the use of thermal capsular shrinkage. We use a monopolar radiofrequency probe (Oratec, Menlo Park, CA) although several devices are currently available. The technique consists of slowly painting the shoulder capsule while initially viewing through the anterior portal. The anterior band of the IGHL is treated initially followed by the posterior band and then the rest of the posterior capsule. The probe is placed first at the glenoid side of the capsule working laterally to its insertion on the humerus. The probe is passed over the capsule until there is visible response of tissue shrinkage. We do not use a cannula for the probe because its use limits maneuverability. The arthroscope is then moved to the posterior portal. The cannula is initially maintained anteriorly so that the location of capsular penetration can be seen to avoid multiple penetrations of the capsule. Once this location is confirmed, the cannula is removed and the thermal probe inserted. The remaining portion of the anterior capsule and rotator interval from an inferior to superior direction and medial (glenoid) to lateral (humerus) direction are then treated with the thermal probe. We currently treat the capsule in a paintbrush rather than grid pattern despite reported benefits of a grid pattern.[118]

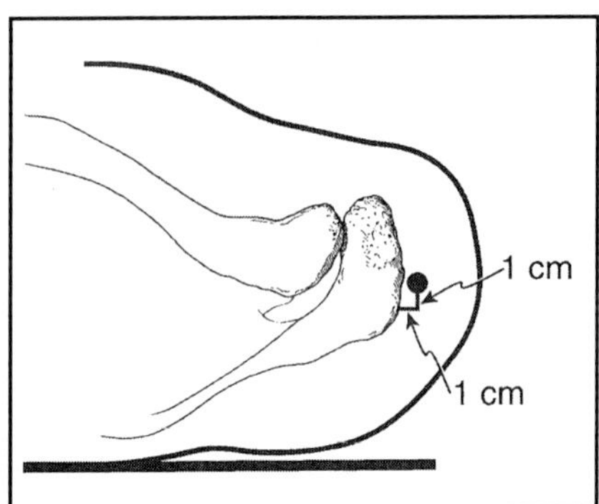

Fig. 11 Location of posterolateral portal for fixation of type II SLAP lesions with posterior extension. (Reproduced with permission from Morgan CD, Burkhart SS, Palmeri M, Gillespie M: SLAP lesions: Three subtypes and their relationships to superior instability and rotator cuff tears. *Arthroscopy* 1998;14:558-565.)

Preferred Technique

The patient is placed in the lateral decubitus position and the affected shoulder is placed in balance suspension traction of 10 to 15 lb at 35° to 45° of abduction and 10° to 15° of forward flexion. After creation of a standard posterior arthroscopy portal (3 cm inferior and 1 cm medial to the posterolateral acromial edge), a standard 4.0 mm, 30° arthroscope is inserted into the glenohumeral joint. The diagnosis of a SLAP lesion requires a thorough knowledge of normal arthroscopic anatomy because it can sometimes be difficult to differentiate a SLAP lesion from normal anatomic variants, including a sublabral hole and a Buford complex.[19] A blunt trochar is placed through an anterior portal in the rotator interval and the biceps anchor is evaluated. Acute lesions are easy to diagnose because there is hemorrhage in the area of the avulsed labrum. Acute lesions are rarely seen in the overhead athlete because SLAP lesions in ballplayers are usually chronic conditions. Granulation tissue beneath the biceps labral anchor may also be seen in chronic SLAP lesions. The key difference is that in the normal shoulder, articular cartilage extends to the labral attachment.[119] Arthroscopic findings suggestive of a type II SLAP lesion include the presence of a space between the edge of the glenoid articular cartilage and the attachment of the biceps anchor, a sublabral sulcus greater than 5 mm in depth, and arching of the biceps-labral complex greater than 3 to 4 mm away from the glenoid when traction is applied to the biceps tendon.[119]

The evaluation of the rotator cuff begins with use of the posterior portal to look for tearing. Complete tears are rare in the overhead athlete. The overhead athlete with internal impingement classically displays partial-thickness tearing of the posterior rotator cuff at the junction of the supraspinatus and infraspinatus. The tear is inspected with an arthroscopic trochar or probe to determine its thickness. It is often difficult to quantify the thickness of the tear. Because the rotator cuff inserts over a 15-mm base from medial to lateral the percentage of tearing present can be quantified. Partial-thickness tears greater than 75% of the thickness of the rotator cuff tendon are taken down and repaired through a mini-open incision.

The type II SLAP lesion is evaluated and categorized as one of the subtypes (posterior, anterior, or combined). Posterior SLAP lesions are repaired through

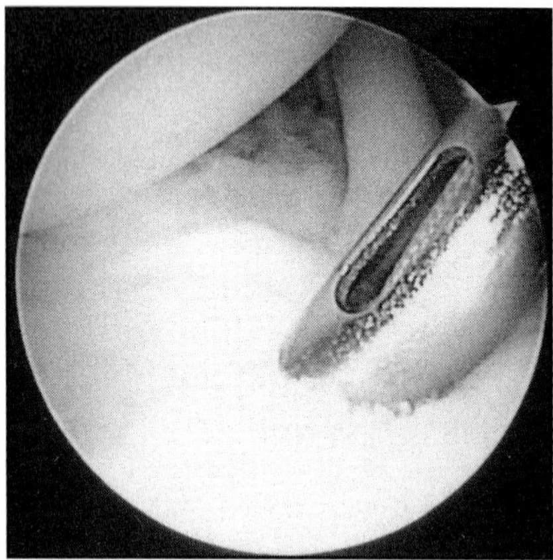

Fig. 12 Repair of type II SLAP lesion with insertion of cannula and suture anchor through posterolateral portal.

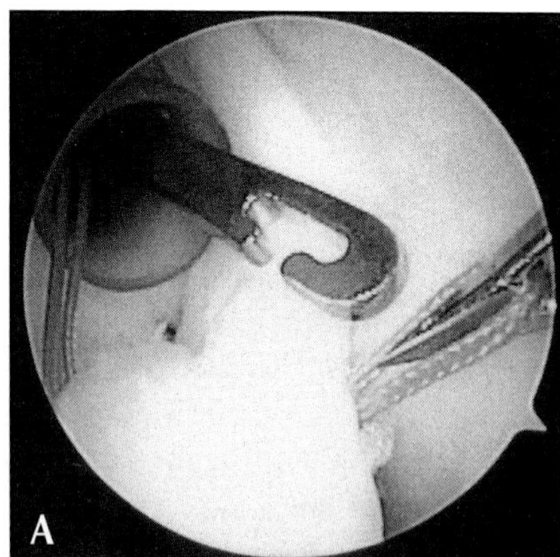

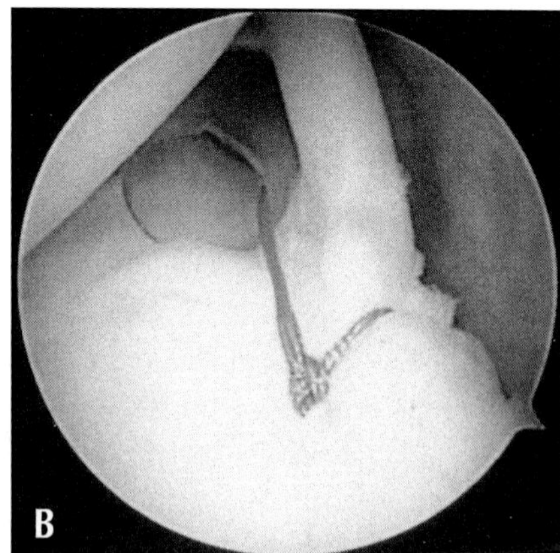

Fig. 13 A, Repair of type II SLAP lesion with birdbeak suture grasper placed through posterolateral portal to grasp suture from anterior portal after piercing posterior labrum. **B**, Repair of type II SLAP lesion with posterior extension of SLAP tied down from anterior cannula.

a posterolateral portal (Fig. 11). This portal is located 1 cm lateral and 1 cm anterior to the posterolateral acromion; it allows an adequate angle of approach for suture anchor placement into the posterosuperior glenoid. Prior to creation of the posterolateral portal, we use a motorized shaver through the anterior portal to prepare the bony bed beneath the detached labrum to the bleeding base while carefully avoiding removal of excessive bone.

For creation of the posterolateral portal, needle localization with an 18-gauge spinal needle is performed initially to determine the proper angle of insertion, followed by insertion of a suture anchor, such as the 3.0-mm Bio-FASTak (Arthrex, Naples, FL). The use of this biodegradable poly-lactic acid anchor avoids insertion of a large cannula, which can damage the rotator cuff tendon at this posterolateral location. A small diameter, 3.5-mm Spear guide (Arthrex, Naples, FL) insertion guide for the Bio-FASTak suture anchor is inserted on the posterosuperior glenoid margin at a 45° angle. This step is followed by insertion through the Spear guide of a pointed trochar punch that is impacted into the bone with a mallet to create a pilot hole. A bone tap is then placed through the Spear guide followed by insertion of the anchor (Fig. 12).

Sutures are then retrieved through the anterior portal. At this point a variety of tissue-penetrating devices can be used that allow the retrieval of either a suture relay device or a looped suture for suture passage through tissue or the deployment of a hooked device to grasp the suture limb. We prefer to use the 45° Ideal Suture Grasper (Mitek, Westwood, MA) or 45° angled Birdbeak (Arthrex, Naples, FL) to penetrate the biceps anchor from the posterolateral portal (Fig. 13, *A*). After this is complete, both sutures are retrieved using a crochet hook and brought through the anterior portal and tied through the anterior cannula (Fig. 13, *B*). Two half-hitches in the same direction, a reversal of the half-hitch, and two reversals of the post and direction of the half-hitch for a total of 5 throws are used. It is critical that the first two half-hitches are thrown in the same direction to allow sliding of the knot.

Although a variety of arthroscopic sliding knots have been described, we have not had difficulty with firmly seating the knots with simple half-hitches. A standard single hole arthroscopic knot pusher is used to seat the half-hitches The security of the knot is tested with a probe placed through the anterior working portal, and the anterior extent of the tear is evaluated. If it still remains unstable after insertion of the posterior anchor, an additional anchor is placed just anterior to the biceps root attachment securing the SLAP tear (Fig. 14). For these combined anterior and posterior type II SLAP lesions, placement of anchors should be anterior and posterior to the biceps root rather than within the body of the biceps.[14] This placement may result in biceps fiber injury within the body of the biceps tendon substance.

We have not had difficulty inserting the anterior suture anchor through an anterior rotator interval portal. A Bio-FASTak suture anchor or, alternatively, the 2.8-mm ROC suture anchor (Mitek, Westwood, MA) can then be inserted. The insertion of the ROC anchor requires insertion of an 8.0-mm drill guide, which may be damaging to the rotator cuff tendon if used through the posterolateral portal. However, the anterior portal is created through the rotator interval, preventing damage to the cuff tendon, followed by securing the anterior extension of the SLAP lesion. Alternatively, Morgan and associates[14] described use of an anterosuperior portal, which is located 1 cm lateral to the anterolateral acromion. If this portal is used, a large cannula should be avoided because this portal may partially traverse through the supraspinatus tendon. The 3.0-mm Bio-FASTak suture anchor can be used through this portal to limit damage to the rotator cuff tendon. However, we have not found it necessary to use this portal and have been able to adequately insert suture anchors into the anterior superior glenoid through a portal located in the superior aspect of the rotator interval.

Alternatively, Getelman and Snyder[119] recommend use of a "suture sling" repair, which avoids use of the posterolateral portal. The standard anterosuperior and midglenoid anterior portals traversing through the rotator interval are used. A suture anchor that is double loaded with a No. 2 braided permanent suture is inserted via the anterosuperior portal at the 12 o'clock position. A variety of suture passing and retrieval systems can then be used to place one limb of the suture anterior to the biceps anchor and the other limb posterior to the biceps anchor. This procedure avoids both the need for multiple suture anchor placement and the need for additional posterior portal placement. However, type II SLAP lesions with posterior extension may be difficult to adequately secure with this one-anchor technique; they require the use of an additional suture anchor placed through the posterolateral portal.

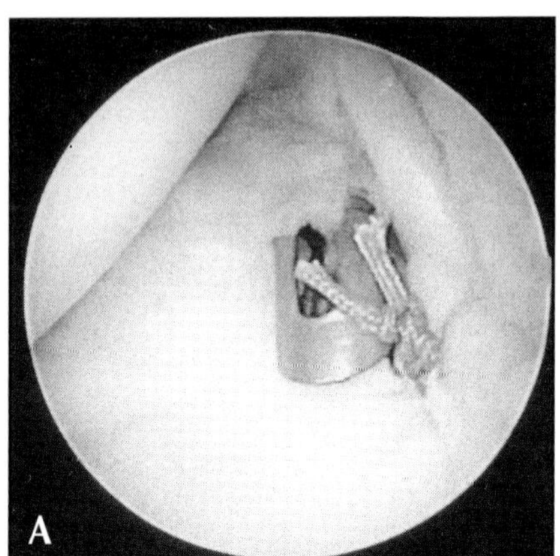

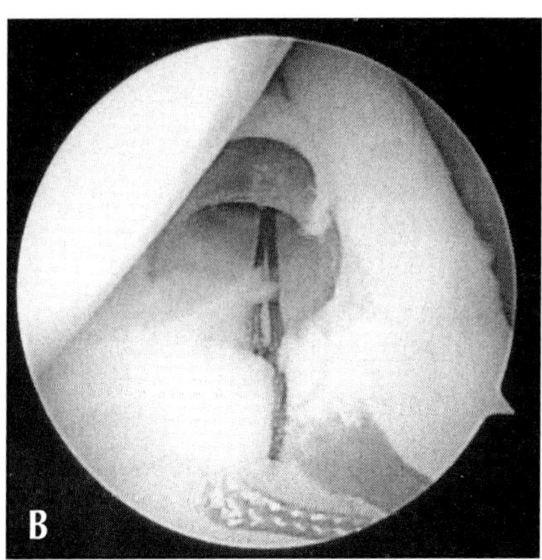

Fig. 14 A, Anterior extension of type II SLAP lesion repaired with the drill guide placed through the rotator interval. **B,** Anterior extension of type II SLAP lesion secured after a suture was passed through the labrum.

Results

Superior labrum surgical results are strongly influenced by stability of the shoulder. In unstable shoulders, the prognosis for labral resection and biceps anchor stabilization remains poor unless concomitant anterior or multidirectional instability is corrected. Ogilvie-Harris and Wiley[107] reported that arthroscopic labrum resection yielded poor results in unstable shoulders. Glasgow and associates[108] similarly reported poor results in patients with SLAP tears and associated instability, with 75% poor and fair results when SLAP débridement alone was performed in shoulders with evidence of glenohumeral instability.

Cordasco and associates[105] demonstrated that labral débridement alone for superior labral lesions afforded 78% excellent results at 1-year follow-up, which declined to 63% at 2-year follow-up. Full return to sports was only 52% initially, declining to 44% at 2 years. They concluded that an isolated labral tear without concomitant mechanical derangement is uncommon and that most superior labral tearing results from instability. Although none of the patients had a history of clinically evident instability, 70% had evidence of instability on examination under anesthesia.[105] When treating SLAP lesions in the overhead athlete, a careful assessment of glenohumeral instability must be performed. Others have also had poor experience with simple débridement of type II SLAP lesions.[120]

Yoneda and associates[121] used a 5.5-mm staple inserted arthroscopically to treat 10 athletes with type II SLAP lesions. Staples were removed at 3 to 6 months, and all lesions appeared healed. Field and Savoie[122] fixed 15 type II SLAP tears and 5 type IV with transosseous suture fixation. At 12- to 42-month follow-up, all of 20 patients had a good or excellent result. All athletes were able to return to their previous sport with no limitation. Resch and associates[123] reported their experience with stabilizing 14 SLAP tears. In six they used a cannulated screw and washer construct and in eight they used the Suretac (Smith & Nephew, Inc, Dyonics, Memphis, TN) absorbable polyglyconate tack. At 18-month follow-up, eight patients (57%) were able to return to preinjury level of competition. An additional four patients were débrided alone, and only one (25%) improved.

Stetson and associates[124] identified type II SLAP tears in 55% of their 140 cases. However, most of the patients were not overhead athletes. At an average follow-up of 3.2 years, 79% of patients with SLAP tears had good or excellent results on the University of California at Los Angeles shoulder rating score. Their results included 19 of 61 patients with type II lesions that were treated with only glenoid abrasion, which is associated with higher failure rates. In addition, several of the type II lesions were also treated with bioabsorbable tacks, which in their series, were noted to have higher failure rates compared with standard suture anchors. They concluded that, with their current treatment protocol of suture anchor technique, long-term good and excellent results can be expected to exceed 85% to

90%.

Most rotator cuff tears in the overhead throwing athlete occur secondary to internal impingement. In the nonathletic population, débridement alone has a success rate from 80% to 90%.[125-128] In Andrews and associates[5] original series, 76% of 73 baseball pitchers treated with rotator cuff and labral débridement had an excellent result. However, average follow-up was only 13 months. Payne and associates[91] reported on rotator cuff débridement in overhead athletes with longer follow-up (minimum, 2 years). In 43 athletes with associated instability, only 25% to 50% returned to their preinjury level of activity. Riand and associates[42] reported on 104 patients with the diagnosis of internal impingement. Rotator cuff débridement alone was successful in 80% of the patients. However, none were baseball players. Although the successful treatment of internal impingement with rotator cuff débridement alone has been reported, none of the overhead athletes in these series (ie, badminton, European handball) were baseball players.[11,42] The lower physical demands placed on the shoulder of the athlete who does not play baseball makes them more amenable to less aggressive treatment.[62] Therefore, Andrews began using thermal-assisted capsular shrinkage (TACS) in 1997 to address the instability associated with internal impingement in baseball players. A retrospective study investigating the treatment of internal impingement in baseball players with TACS was then conducted.[129]

In the non-TACS group, 41 of 51 throwers (80%) returned to competition at a mean time of 7.2 months. At 30-month follow-up, only 34 (67%) were still competing, and only 31 (61%) were competing at their preinjury level of competition. In the TACS group, 30 of 31 throwers (97%) returned to competition at a mean of 8.4 months. Twenty-eight (90%) were still competing 30 months after surgery, and 27 (87%) were still competing at their preinjury level of competition. When comparing return to play at 30 months after surgery, the use of TACS was associated with a statistically significant increase in rate of return to play compared to the non-TACS group ($P = 0.01$).

Phase 2 Study Results

Of the 12 players who underwent arthroscopic SLAP repair without TACS, five (42%) were competing at 27 months. Of the 11 players who had TACS in addition to a SLAP repair, 10 (91%) were competing at 27 months.

The results of these studies clearly demonstrate that addressing the capsular laxity at the time of surgery (in our case with TACS) led to an increased rate of return to play in baseball throwers with internal impingement and SLAP lesions. As the interval from surgery increased, the overall percentage of players who were able to return to play at the same or higher level tended to increase. The results also demonstrated that presence of a SLAP lesion negatively affected the overall results and increased the time necessary to return to competition.

Morgan and associates[14] reported on 102 type II SLAP lesions (53 in overhead throwers) without associated anterior instability who underwent isolated SLAP repair. They demonstrated arthroscopically that repair of the SLAP lesion eliminated the peel-back sign and the drive-through sign. At 1-year follow-up, 87% of 53 throwers returned to their preinjury level of play. Of the 53 throwers, 44 were baseball pitchers, 84% of whom returned to their preinjury levels of activity or better. The remaining seven pitchers who did not reach their preinjury levels of pitching had associated undersurface rotator cuff tears. The authors documented that all throwers in their study had marked internal rotation deficits caused by a tight posteroinferior capsule.[14] The authors implicated the contracture of the posteroinferior capsule as ultimately responsible in causing the SLAP lesions.

Results from one recent study of 41 high school and college baseball players with SLAP lesions were reported (GM McCluskey III, MD, personal communication, 2002). Forty-one players were separated into three groups: (1) 22 players with cuff débridement and SLAP repair; (2) 16 players with cuff débridement, SLAP repair, and thermal shrinkage; and (3) 5 players with cuff repair, SLAP repair, and thermal shrinkage. Rate of return to sport at previous level for the three groups was: (1) 64%, (2) 71%, and (3) 40%. Players who had instability addressed with thermal shrinkage had a higher return to play rate, and players undergoing rotator cuff repair had the lowest return to play rates.

Postoperative Management

The first 6 weeks after surgery are spent regaining ROM along with dynamic stability. The second 6 weeks are used to regain strength and proprioception, along with initiating plyometric exercise. By 3 to 4 months, the interval throwing program is initiated. If thermal shrinkage alone is performed, return to competition can be expected by 7.5 months. If labral repair is performed in addition to the shrinkage the average return time is 11.2 months[128] (Tables 2 and 3).

Summary

The treatment and management of the overhead throwing athlete is complex. Many factors enter into the decision regarding the nature and timing of appropriate intervention. Because of the nature of the mechanical aspects of the throwing motion, increased external rotation (over-rotation) is often necessary to throw at a highly competitive level. The increased motion is associated with acquired increased glenohumeral laxity, which by itself is generally not problematic. However, in the overhead athlete the increased external rotation can lead to

Table 2
Thermal-Assisted Anterior Capsulorrhaphy (For Acquired Laxity)

Phase 1 Protection Phase (Day 1 to Week 6)	
Goals	Allow soft-tissue healing Diminish pain and inflammation Initiate protected motion Retard muscular atrophy
Weeks 0 to 2	Sling use for 7 to 10 days Sleep in sling/brace for 14 days
Exercises	Hand gripping exercises Elbow and wrist ROM exercises AROM cervical spine Passive and AAROM exercises Elevation to 75° to 90° (flexion to 70°, week 1; flexion to 90°, week 2) IR in scapular plane (45° by 2 weeks) ER in scapular plane (25° by 2 weeks) No aggressive stretching Rope and pulley (flexion) AAROM Cryotherapy to control pain (before and after treatment) Submaximal isometrics (ER, IR, Abd, Flex, Ext) Rhythmic stabilization exercises at 7 days Proprioception and neuromuscular control drills
Weeks 3 to 4	ROM exercises (AAROM, PROM, AROM) Elevation to 125° to 135° IR, in scapular plane, full motion ER, in scapular plane, 45° by week 4 At week 4, begin ER/IR at 90° abduction ER at 90° abduction to 45° to 50° No aggressive stretching Strengthening Exercises Active ROM program (begin at week 3) Initiate light isotonic program (use 1 lb at week 4) ER/IR exercise tubing (0° abduction) Continue dynamic stabilization drills Scapular strengthening exercises Biceps/triceps strengthening Proprioceptive neuromuscular facilitation flex/ext manual resistance (limited ROM) Emphasize ER strengthening and scapular musculature Continue use of cryotherapy and modalities to control pain
Weeks 5 to 6	Continue all exercise listed above Progress ROM to the following: Elevation to 160° by week 6 ER at 90° abduction (75° to 80°) by 6 weeks IR at 90°abduction (60° to 65°) by 6 weeks Initiate Throwers Ten strengthening program Continue emphasis on ER and scapular muscles
Phase II Intermediate Phase (Week 7 to 12)	
Goals	Restore full ROM (week 8) Restore functional ROM (week 10 to 11) Normalize arthrokinematics Improve dynamic stability, muscular strength
Weeks 7 to 8	Progress ROM to the following Elevation to 180° ER at 90° abduction to 90° to 100° by week 8 IR at 90° abduction to 60° to 65° by week 8 Continue stretching program May become more aggressive with ROM progression and stretching May perform joint mobilization techniques Strengthening Exercises Continue Throwers Ten Program Continue manual resistance, dynamic stabilization drills Rhythmic stabilization drills Initiate plyometrics (two-handed drills)
Weeks 9 to 12	Progress ROM to the overhead athlete's demands Gradual progression from weeks 9 to 12 Continue stretching into ER ER at 90° abduction to 110° to 115° by weeks 10 to 12 Continue stretching program for posterior structures (IR, horizontal adduction) Strengthening exercises Progress isotonic program Continue Throwers Ten Program May initiate more aggressive strengthening Push ups Bench press (do not allow arm below body) Lateral pull downs (in front of body) Single hand plyometrics throwing (initiate 14 to 18 days following the introduction of two hand plyos) Plyoball wall drills
Phase III Advanced Activity and Strengthening Phase (Weeks 12 to 20)	
Goals	Improve strength, power, and endurance Enhance neuromuscular control Functional activities
Criteria to Enter Phase III	Full ROM No pain or tenderness Muscular strength 80% of contralateral side
Weeks 12 to 16	Continue all stretching exercises Self capsular stretches, AROM, passive stretching Continue all strengthening exercises Throwers Ten Program Progress isotonics Plyometrics Two-hand drills progress to one-hand drills Throwing into plyoback 1 lb ball (week 13) Neuromuscular control/dynamic stabilization drills
Weeks 16 to 22	Initiate interval sport program (throwing, tennis, swimming, etc) week 16 Progress all exercises listed above May resume normal training program Continue specific strengthening exercises Progress interval program (throwing program to phase II) weeks 22 to 23
Week 22	Progress to Phase II interval throwing program or sport specific training Continue isotonic strengthening Continue flexibility and ROM Continue plyometrics
Phase IV Return to Activity Phase (Week 26)	
Goals	Gradual return to unrestricted activities Maintain static and dynamic stability of shoulder joint
Criteria to Enter Phase IV	Full functional ROM No pain or tenderness Satisfactory muscular strength (isokinetic test) Satisfactory clinical examination
Exercises	Continue maintenance for ROM (stretching) Continue strengthening exercises (Throwers Ten) Gradual return to competition Progress throwing program to game situation—months 6 to 7

ROM = assisted range of motion; AAROM = active-assisted range of motion; ER = external rotation; IR = internal rotation; Abd = abduction; Flex = flexion; Ext = extension; PROM = passive range of motion; ROM = range of motion

Table 3
Arthroscopic SLAP Lesion Repair (Type II) With Thermal Capsular Shrinkage

Phase I Immediate Postoperative Phase "Restrictive Motion" (Day 1 to Week 6)

Goals
- Protect the anatomic repair
- Prevent negative effects of immobilization
- Promote dynamic stability
- Diminish pain and inflammation

Weeks 0 to 2
- Sling for 4 weeks
- Sleep in immobilizer for 4 weeks
- Elbow/hand ROM
- Hand gripping exercises
- Passive and gentle active assistive ROM exercises
  - Flexion to 60° (week 2: Flexion to 75°)
  - Elevation in scapular plane to 60°
  - ER/IR with arm in scapular plane
  - ER to 10° to 15°
  - IR to 45°
- No active ER or extension or abduction
- Submaximal isometrics for shoulder musculature
- No isolated biceps contractions
- Cryotherapy, modalities as indicated

Weeks 3 to 4
- Discontinue use of sling at 4 weeks
- Sleep in immobilizer until week 4
- Continue gentle ROM exercises (PROM and AAROM)
  - Flexion to 90°
  - Abduction to 75° to 80°
  - ER in scapular plane and 35° abd to 25° to 30°
  - IR in scapular plane and 35° abd to 55° to 60°
- Note: Rate of progression based on evaluation of the patient
  - No active ER, extension or elevation
  - Initiate rhythmic stabilization drills
  - Initiate proprioception training
  - Tubing ER/IR at 0° abduction
  - Continue isometrics
  - Continue use of cryotherapy

Weeks 5 to 6
- Gradually improve ROM
  - Elevation to 145°
  - ER at 45° abduction: 45° to 50°
  - ER at 45° abduction: 55° to 60°
  - At 6 weeks begin light and gradual ER to 90° abduction—progress to 30° to 40° ER
- May initiate stretching exercise
- May initiate light (easy) ROM at 90° abduction
- Continue tubing ER/IR (arm at side)
- PNF manual resistance
- Initiate active shoulder abduction (without resistance)
- Initiate "full can" exercise (weight of arm)
- Initiate prone rowing, prone horizontal abduction
- No biceps strengthening

Phase II - Intermediate Phase Moderate Protection Phase (Weeks 7 to 14)

Goals
- Gradually restore full ROM (week 10)
- Preserve the integrity of the surgical repair
- Restore muscular strength and balance

Weeks 7 to 9
- Gradually progress ROM:
  - Flexion to 180°
  - ER at 90° abduction: 90° to 95°
  - IR at 90° abduction: 70° to 75°
- Continue to progress isotonic strengthening program
- Continue PNF strengthening
- Initiate Throwers Ten program

Weeks 10 to 12
- May initiate slightly more aggressive strengthening
- Progress ER to throwers motion
  - ER at 90° abduction: 110° to 115° in throwers (weeks 10 to 12)
- Progress isotonic strengthening exercises
- Continue all stretching exercises
- Progress ROM to functional demands (ie, overhead athlete)
- Continue all strengthening exercises

Phase III Minimal Protection Phase (Week 14 to 20)

Goals
- Establish and maintain full ROM
- Improve muscular strength, power, and endurance
- Gradually initiate functional activities

Criteria to Enter Phase III
- Full nonpainful ROM
- Satisfactory stability
- Muscular strength (good grade or better)
- No pain or tenderness

Weeks 14 to 16
- Continue all stretching exercises (capsular stretches)
- Maintain throwers motion (especially ER)
- Continue all strengthening exercises:
  - Throwers Ten program or fundamental exercises
  - PNF manual resistance
  - Endurance training
  - Initiate light plyometric program
  - Restricted sport activities (light swimming, half golf swings)

Weeks 16 to 20
- Continue all exercises listed above
- Continue all stretching
- Continue Throwers Ten Program
- Continue plyometric program
- Initiate interval sport program (throwing, etc)
  - See interval throwing program

Phase IV Advanced Strengthening Phase (Weeks 20 to 26)

Goals
- Enhanced muscular strength, power, and endurance
- Progress functional activities
- Maintain shoulder mobility

Criteria to Enter Phase IV
- Full nonpainful ROM
- Satisfactory static stability
- Muscular strength 75% to 80% of contralateral side
- No pain or tenderness

Weeks 20 to 26
- Continue flexibility exercises
- Continue isotonic strengthening program
- PNF manual resistance patterns
- Plyometric strengthening
- Progress interval sport programs

Phase V Return to Activity Phase (Months 6 to 9)

Goals
- Gradual return to sport activities
- Maintain strength, mobility, and stability

Criteria to Enter Phase V
- Full functional ROM
- Muscular performance isokinetic (fulfills criteria)
- Satisfactory shoulder stability
- No pain or tenderness

Exercises
- Gradually progress sport activities to unrestrictive participation
- Continue stretching and strengthening program

ROM = range of motion; ER = external rotation; IR = internal rotation; PNF =proprioceptive neuromuscular facilitation repetitive impingement of the rotator cuff and superior labrum resulting in a SLAP lesion and partial articular-sided rotator cuff tearing. Although the etiology for this phenomenon remains controversial, the end result remains the same: pathology in the rotator cuff and superior labrum. Isolated treatment of the pathology alone without addressing the capsular laxity often results in lower return to play rates. Addressing the capsular laxity arthroscopically at the same time as the intra-articular pathology is necessary to give these athletes the best chance to return to their prior competitive level. Although short-term results are promising, long-term follow-up is necessary to determine the ultimate usefulness of this treatment philosophy.

References

1. Rowe CR, Pierce DS, Clark DG: Voluntary dislocation of the shoulder. *J Bone Joint Surg Am* 1973;55:445-460.
2. Neer CS II: Anterior acromioplasty for chronic impingement syndrome of the shoulder. *J Bone Joint Surg Am* 1972;54:41-50.
3. Tibone JE, Jobe FW, Kerlan RF, et al: Shoulder impingement syndrome in athletes treaterd by anterior acromioplasty. *Clin Orthop* 1985;188:134-140.
4. Kennedy JC, Hawkins RJ, Krusoff WJ: Orthopaedic manifestations of swimming. *Am J Sports Med* 1978;6:309-322.
5. Andrews JR, Carson WG, McLoed WD: Glenoid labrum tears related to the long head of the biceps. *Am J Sports Med* 1985;13:337-340.
6. Snyder SJ, Karzel RP, Del Pizzo W, et al: SLAP lesions of the shoulder. *Arthroscopy* 1990;6: 274-279.
7. Maffet MW, Gartsmann GM, Moseley B: Superior labrum-biceps tendon complex lesions of the shoulder. *Am J Sports Med* 1995;23:93-98.
8. Jobe F, Kivitne R, Giangarra C: Shoulder pain in the overhand or throwing athlete: The relationship of anterior instability and rotator cuff impingement. *Orthop Rev* 1989;18:963-975.
9. Jobe FW, Giangarra CE, Kvitne RS, Glousman RE: Anterior capsulolabral reconstruction of the shoulder in athletes in overhand sports. *Am J Sports Med* 1991;19:428-434.
10. Jobe FW, Tibone JE, Jobe CM, et al: The shoulder in sports, in Rockwood CA Jr, Matsen FA III (eds): *The Shoulder*. Philadelphia, PA, WB Saunders, 1990, pp 963-967.
11. Walch G, Boileau P, Noel E, et al: Impingement of the deep surface of the supraspinatus tendon on the posterosuperior glenoid rim: An arthroscopic study. *J Shoulder Elbow Surg* 1992;1:238-245.
12. Jobe CM: Posterior superior glenoid impingement: Expanded spectrum. *Arthroscopy* 1995;11:530-537.
13. Jobe CM: Superior glenoid impingement: Current concepts. *Clin Orthop* 1996;330: 98-107.
14. Morgan CD, Burkhart SS, Palmeri M, et al: Type II SLAP lesions: Three subtypes and their relationship to superior instability and rotator cuff tears. *Arthroscopy* 1998;14:553-565.
15. Howell S, Galinat B: The glenoid-labral socket. *Clin Orthop* 1989;243:122-125.
16. Soslowsky LJ, Flatow EL, Bigliani LU, Mow VC: Articular geometry of the glenohumeral joint. *Clin Orthop* 1992;285:181-190.
17. Detrisac DA, Johnson LL: Glenoid labrum, in *Arthroscopic Shoulder Anatomy: Pathologic and Surgical Implications*. Thorofare, NJ, SLACK, 1986, pp 71-89.
18. Williams MM, Karzel RP, Snyder SJ: Labral disorders, in Hawkins RJ, Misamore GW (eds): *Shoulder Injuries in the Athlete: Surgical Repair and Rehabilitation*. New York, NY, Churchill Livingstone,1996, pp 291-305.
19. Vangsness CT, Jorgenson SS, Watson T, Johnson DL: The origin of the long head of the biceps from the scapula and glenoid labrum: An anatomic study of 100 shoulders. *J Bone Joint Surg Br* 1994;76:951-954.
20. Cooper DE, Arnoczky SP, O'Brien SJ, Warren RF, DiCarlo E, Allen AA: Anatomy, histology, and vascularity of the glenoid labrum. *J Bone Joint Surg Am* 1992;74:46-52.
21. Prodromos CC, Ferry JA, Schiller AL, Zarins B: Histological studies of the glenoid labrum from fetal life to old age. *J Bone Joint Surg Am* 1990;72:1344-1348.
22. Kumar VP, Satku K, Balasubramaniam P: The role of the long head of the biceps brachii in stabilization of the head of the humerus. *Clin Orthop* 1989;244:172-175.
23. Flatow EL, Raimondo RA, Kelkar R, et al: Active and passive restraints against superior humeral translation: The contributions of the rotator cuff, the biceps tendon, and the coracoacromial arch. Presented at the annual meeting of the American Society of Shoulder and Elbow Surgeons, 1996.
24. Itoi E, Kuechle DK, Newman SR, Morrey BF, An K-N: Stabilizing function of the biceps in stable and unstable shoulders. *J Bone Joint Surg Br* 1993;75:564-550.
25. Pagnani MJ, Deng XH, Warren RF, Torzilli PA, O'Brien SJ: Role of the long head of the biceps brachii in glenohumeral stability:a biomechanical study in cadavera. *J Shoulder Elbow Surg* 1996;5255-5262.
26. Warner JJP, McMahon PJ: The role of the long head of the biceps brachii in superior stability of the glenohumeral joint. *J Bone Joint Surg Am* 1995;77:336-372.
27. Jobe FW, Moynes DR, Tibone JE, Perry J: An EMG analysis of the shoulder in pitching: A second report. *Am J Sports Med* 1984;12: 218-220.
28. Halbrecht JL, Tirman P, Atkin D: Internal impingement of the shoulder: Comparison of findings between the throwing and non-throwing shoulders of college baseball players. *Arthroscopy* 1999;15:253-258.
29. Montgomery WH III, Jobe FW: Functional outcomes in athletes after modified anterior capsulolabral reconstruction. *Am J Sports Med* 1994;22:352-358.
30. Burkhart SS, Morgan CD: The peel-back mechanism: It's role in producing and extending posterior type II SLAP lesions and its effect on SLAP repair rehabilitation. *Arthroscopy* 1998;14:637-640.
31. Pagnani MJ, Warren RF: Arthroscopic shoulder stabilization. *Oper Tech Sports Med* 1993;1: 276-284.
32. McFarland EG, Neira CA, Gutierrez MI, Cosgarea AJ, Magee M: Clinical significance of the arthroscopic drive-through sign in shoulder surgery. *Arthroscopy* 2001;17:38-43.
33. Pagnani MJ, Warren RF, Altchek DW, Wickiewicz TL, Anderson AF: Arthroscopic shoulder stabilization using transglenoid sutures. *Am J Sports Med* 1996;24:459-467.
34. Peterson CA, Altchek DW, Warren RF: Operative arthroscopy, in Rockwood CA, Matsen FA (eds): *The Shoulder*, ed 2. Philadelphia, PA, WB Saunders, 1998.
35. Burkhart SS, Parten PM: Dead arm syndrome: Torsional SLAP lesions versus internal impingement. *Tech Shoulder Elbow Surg* 2001;2:74-84.
36. O'Brien SJ, Warren RF: Anterior shoulder instability. *Orthop Clin North Am* 1987;18: 395-408.
37. Pagnani MJ, Deng XH, Warren RF, et al: Effects of lesions of the superior portion of the glenoid labrum on glenohumeral translation. *J Bone Joint Surg Am* 1995;77:1003-1010.
38. Huber WP, Putz RV: The periarticular fiber system (PAFS) of the shoulder joint. *Arthroscopy* 1997;13:680-691.
39. Bey MJ, Elders GJ, Huston LJ, Kuhn JE, Blaiser RB, Soslowsky LJ: The mechanism of creation of superior labrum, anterior, and posterior lesions in a dynamic biomechanical model of the shoulder: The role of inferior subluxation. *J Shoulder Elbow Surg* 1998;7: 397-401.
40. Wilk KE, Meister K, Andrews JR: Current concepts in the rehabilitation of the overhead throwing athlete. *Am J Sports Med* 2002;30: 136-151.
41. Crockett HC, Gross LB, Wilk KE, Schwartz ML, et al: Osseous adaptation and range of motion at the glenohumeral joint in professional baseball pitchers. *Am J Sports Med* 2002;30:20-31.
42. Riand N, Levigne C, Renaud E, et al: Results of derotational humeral osteotomy in posterosuperior glenoid impingement. *Am J Sports Med* 1998;26:453-459.

43. Pieper H: Humeral torsion in the throwing arm of handball players. *Am J Sports Med* 1998;26:247-253.

44. Rowe CR, Zarins B: Recurrent transient subluxation of the shoulder. *J Bone Joint Surg Am* 1981;63:863-872.

45. Burkhart SS, Morgan CD, Kibler WB: Shoulder injuries in overhead athletes: The dead arm revisited. *Clin Sports Med* 2000;19:125-157.

46. King JW, Brelsford HJ, Tullos HS: Analysis of the pitching arm of the professional baseball. *Clin Orthop* 1969;67:116-123.

47. Neer CS, Welsh RP: The shoulder in sports. *Orthop Clin North Am* 1977;8:583-591.

48. Hawkins RJ, Kennedy JC: Impingement syndrome in athletes. *Am J Sports Med* 1980;8: 151-158.

49. O'Brien SJ, Pagnani MJ, Fealy S, McGlynn SR, Wilson JB: The active compression test: A new and effective test for diagnosing labral tears and acromioclavicular joint abnormality. *Am J Sports Med* 1998;26:610-613.

50. Andrews JR, Gidumal RH: Shoulder arthroscopy in the throwing athlete: Perspectives and prognosis. *Clin Sports Med* 1984;6:565-571.

51. Andrews JR, Fairbanks JH, Wilk KE, Flesig GS, Schwartz ML: Labral tears in throwing sports, in Garrett WE, Speer KP, Kirkendall DT (eds): *Principles and Practice of Orthopaedic Sports Medicine*. Philadelphia, PA, Lippincott-Williams & Wilkins, 2000, pp 457-477.

52. Kim SH, Ha KI, Ahn JH, Kim SH, Choi HJ: Biceps load test II: A clinical test for SLAP lesions of the shoulder. *Arthroscopy* 2001;17: 160-164.

53. Bennett WF: Specificity of the Speed's test: Arthroscopic technique for evaluating the biceps tendon at the level of the bicipital groove. *Arthroscopy* 14:789-796.

54. Mimori K, Muneta T, Nakagawa T, Shinomiya K: A new pain provocation test for superior labral tears of the shoulder. *Am J Sports Med* 1999;27:137-142.

55. Kibler WB: Specificity and sensitivity of the anterior slide test in throwing athletes with superior glenoid labral tears. *Arthroscopy* 1995;11:296-300.

56. Liu SH, Henry MH, Nuccion SL: A prospective evaluation of a new physical examination in predicting glenoid labral tears. *Am J Sports Med* 1995;24:721-725.

57. Kim SH, Ha KI, Han KY: Biceps load test: A clinical test for superior labrum anterior and posterior lesions in shoulders with recurrent anterior dislocations. *Am J Sports Med* 1999;27:300-303.

58. Altchek DW, Warren RF, Wickiewicz TL, et al: Arthroscopic labral debridement: A three year follow-up study. *Am J Sports Med* 1992;20: 702-706.

59. Kvitne RS, Jobe FW: The diagnosis and treatment of anterior instability in the throwing athlete. *Clin Orthop* 1993;291:107-123.

60. Brown LP, Niehues SL, Harrah A, et al: Upper extremity range of motion and isokinetic strength of the internal and external shoulder rotators in major league baseball players. *Am J Sports Med* 1988:16:577-585.

61. Johnson L: Patterns of shoulder flexibility among college players. *J Athletic Training* 1992;27:44-49.

62. Meister K: Injuries to the shoulder in the throwing athlete: Part Two. Evaluation and treatment. *Am J Sports Med* 2000;28:587-601.

63. Wohlwend J, van Holsbeeck H, Craig J, et al: The association between irregular greater tuberosities and rotator cuff tears: A monographic study. *AJR Am J Roentgenol* 1998;171:229-233.

64. Meister K, Andrews JR, Batts J, et al: Symptomatic thrower's exostosis: Arthroscopic evaluation and treatment. *Am J Sports Med* 1999;23:638-642.

65. Bennett GE: Shoulder and elbow lesions of the professional baseball pitcher. *JAMA* 1959;117:510-514.

66. Iannotti JP, Wang ED: Avulsion fracture of the supraglenoid tubercle: A variation of the SLAP lesion. *J Shoulder Elbow Surg* 1992;1:26-30.

67. Middleton WD, Reinus WR, Totty WG, Melson GL, Murphy WA: Ultrasonographic evaluation of the rotator cuff and biceps tendon. *J Bone Joint Surg Am* 1986;68:440-50.

68. Callaghan JJ, McNeish LM, Dehaven JP, et al: A prospective comparison study of double contrast computed tomography arthrography and arthroscopy of the shoulder. *Am J Sports Med* 1998;16:13-19.

69. Hunter JC, Blatz DJ, Escobedo EM: SLAP lesions of the glenoid labrum: CT arthrographic and arthroscopic correlation. *Radiology* 1992;184:513-518.

70. Flannigan B, Kursunoglu-Brahme S, Snyder S, Karzel R, Del Pizzo W, Resnick D: MR arthrography of the shoulder: Comparison with conventional MR imaging. *AJR Am J Roentgenol* 1990;155:829-832.

71. Legan JM, Burkhard TK, Gaft WB, et al: Tears of the glenoid labrum: MR imaging of 88 cases arthroscopically confirmed cases. *Radiology* 1992;183:35-37.

72. Iannotti JP, Zlatkin MB, Esterhai JL, et al: Magnetic resonance imaging of the shoulder: Sensitivity, specificity and predictive value. *J Bone Joint Surg Am* 1991;73:17-29.

73. Smith AM, McCauley TR, Jokl P: SLAP lesions of the glenoid labrum diagnosed with MR imaging. *Skeletal Radiol* 1993;22:507-510.

74. Connell DA, Potter HG, Wickiewicz TL, et al: Noncontrast magnetic resonance imaging of superior labral lesions: 102 cases confirmed at arthroscopic surgery. *Am J Sports Med* 1999;27:208-213.

75. Monu JU, Pope TL, Chabon SJ, Vanarthos WJ: MR diagnosis of superior labral anterior posterior (SLAP) injuries of the glenoid labrum: Value of routine imaging without intraartricular injection of contrast material. *AJR Am J Roentgenol* 1994;163:1425-1429.

76. Chandnani VP, Yeager TD, DeBerardino TD, et al: Glenoid labral tears: Prospective evaluation with MR imaging, MR arthrography, and CT arthrography. *AJR Am J Roentgenol* 1993;161:1229-1235.

77. Hodler J, Kursunoglu-Brahme S, Flannigan B, et al: Injuries of the superior portion of the glenoid labrum involving the insertion of the biceps tendon: MR imaging in 9 cases. *AJR Am J Roentgenol* 1992;159:565-568.

78. Smith DK, Chopp TM, Aufdemorte TB, et al: Sublabral recess of the superior glenoid labrum: Study of cadavers with conventional nonenhanced MR imaging, MR arthrography, anatomic dissection, and limited histologic examination. *Radiology* 1996;201:251-256.

79. Palmer WE, Caslowitz PL: Anterior shoulder instability: Diagnostic criteria determined from prospective analysis of 121 MR arthrograms. *Radiology* 1995;197:819-825.

80. Tirman PFJ, Stauffer AE, Crues JV III, et al: Saline magnetic resonance arthrography in the evaluation of glenohumeral instability. *Arthroscopy* 1993;9:550-559.

81. Chandnani VP, Gagliardi JA, Murnane TG, et al: Glenohumeral ligaments and shoulder capsular mechanism: Evaluation with MR arthrography. *Radiology* 1995;196:27-32.

82. Potter HG: Magnetic resonance imaging of the unstable shoulder. *Tech Shoulder Elbow Surg* 2000;1:25-38.

83. Karzel RP, Snyder SJ: Magnetic resonance arthrography of the shoulder: A new technique of shoulder imaging. *Clin Sports Med* 1993;12:123-126.

84. Beltran J, Rosenberg ZS, Chandnani VP, et al: Glenohumeral instability: Evaluation with MR arthrography. *Radiographics* 1997;17:657-673.

85. Moore TP, Fritts HM, Quick DC, Buss DD: Suprascapular nerve entrapment caused by spinoglenoid cyst compression. *J Shoulder Elbow Surg* 1997;6:455-462.

86. Fritz RC, Helms CA, Steinbach LS, Genant HK: Suprascapular nerve entrapment: Evaluation with MR imaging. *Radiology* 1992;182:437-444.

87. Catalano JB, Fenlin JM Jr: Ganglion cysts about the shoulder girdle in the absence of suprascapular nerve entrapment. *J Shoulder Elbow Surg* 1994;3:34-41.

88. Tirman PFJ, Feller JF, Janzen DL, Peterfy CG, Bergman AG: Association of glenoid labral cysts with labral tears and glenohumeral instability: Radiologic findings and clinical significance. *Radiology* 1994;190:653-658.

89. Meister K, Walczak S, Fontenot W, et al: Abstract: Evaluation of partial undersurface tears of the rotator cuff in the overhand athlete: MRI arthrography versus arthroscopy. *Arthroscopy* 1999;14:451.

90. Wilk KE, Andrews JR, Arrigo CA, et al: The strength characteristics of internal and external rotator muscles in professional baseball pitchers. *Am J Sports Med* 1993;21:61-66.

91. Payne LZ, Altchek DW, Craig EV, et al: Arthroscopic treatment of partial rotator cuff

tears in young athletes: A preliminary report. *Am J Sports Med* 1997;25:299-305.

92. Montgomery WH III, Jobe FW: Functional outcomes in athletes after modified anterior capsulolabral reconstruction. *Am J Sports Med* 1994;22:352-358.

93. Altchek DW, Warren RF, Wickiewicz TL, et al: T-plasty modification of the Bankart procedure for multidirectional instability of the anterior and inferior types. *J Bone Joint Surg Am* 1991;73:105-112.

94. Bigliani LU, Kurzweil PR, Schwartzbach CC, et al: Inferior capsular shift procedure for anterior-inferior shoulder instability in athletes. *Am J Sports Med* 1994;22:578-584.

95. Warner JP, Johnson D, Miller M, et al: Technique for selecting capsular tightness in repair of anterior-inferior shoulder instability. *J Shoulder Elbow Surg* 1995;4:352-364.

96. Capsari RB, Savoie FH: Arthroscopic reconstruction of the shoulder, in McGinty JB, Caspari RB, Jackson RW, et al (eds): *Operative Arthroscopy*. New York, NY, Raven Press, 1991, pp 507-515.

97. McIntyre LF: Arthroscopic capsulorrhaphy for multidirectional instability. *Oper Tech Sports Med* 1997;5:233-237.

98. Tauro JC, Carter FM II: Arthroscopic capsular advancement for anterior and anterior-inferior shoulder instability: A preliminary report. *Arthroscopy* 1994;10:513-517.

99. Wichman MT, Snyder SJ: Arthroscopic capsular plication for multidirectional instability of the shoulder. *Oper Tech Sports Med* 1997;5: 238-243.

100. Duncan R, Savoie FH: Arthroscopic inferior capsular shift for multidirectional instability of the shoulder: A preliminary report. *Arthroscopy* 1993;9:24-27.

101. McIntyre LF, Capsari RB, Savoie FH: The arthroscopic treatment of posterior shoulder instability: Two-year results of a multiple suture technique. *Arthroscopy* 1997;13:426-432.

102. Savoie FH, Field LD: Thermal versus suture treatment of capsular laxity. *Clin Sports Med* 2000;19:63-75.

103. Snyder SJ, Stafford BB: Arthroscopic management of instability of the shoulder. *Orthopedics* 1993;16:993-1002.

104. Rook RT, Savoie FH, Field LD: Arthroscopic treatment of instability attributable to capsular injury or laxity. *Clin Orthop* 2001;390:52-58.

105. Cordasco FA, Steinmann S, Flatow EL, et al: Arthroscopic treatment of glenoid labral tears. *Am J Sports Med* 1993;21:425-430.

106. Martin DR, Garth WP: Results of arthroscopic debridement of glenoid labral tears. *Am J Sports Med* 1995;23:447-451.

107. Ogilvie-Harris DJ, Wiley AM: Arthroscopic surgery of the shoulder: A general appraisal. *J Bone Joint Surg Br* 1986;68:201-207.

108. Glasgow SG, Bruce RA, Yacobucci GN, Torg JS: Arthroscopic resection of glenoid labral tears in the athlete: A report of 29 cases. *Arthroscopy* 1992;8:48-54.

109. Tibone JE, Jobe FW, Kerlan RK, et al: Shoulder impingement syndrome in athletes treated by subacromial decompression. *Clin Orthop* 1985;198:134-140.

110. Resch H, Gloser K, Thoeni H, Sperner G: Arthroscopic repair of superior glenoid labral detachment (the SLAP lesion). *J Shoulder Elbow Surg* 1993; 2:147-155.

111. Pagnani MJ, Speer KP, Altchek DW, Warren RF, Dines DM: Arthroscopic fixation of superior labral lesions using a biodegradable implant: A preliminary report. *Arthroscopy* 1995;11: 194-198.

112. Segmuller HE, Hayes MG, Saies AD: Arthroscopic repair of glenolabral injuries with an absorbable fixation device. *J Shoulder Elbow Surg* 1997;6:383-392.

113. Warner JJP, Kann S, Marks P: Arthroscopic repair of combined bankart and superior labral detachment anterior and posterior lesions: Technique and preliminary results. *Arthroscopy* 1994;10:383-391.

114. Berg EE, Ciullo JV: The SLAP lesion: A cause for failure after distal clavicle resection. *Arthroscopy* 1997;13:85-89.

115. Samani JE, Martson SB, Buss DD: Arthroscopic stabilization of type 2 SLAP lesions using an absorbable tack. *Arthroscopy* 2001;17:19-24.

116. Snyder SJ, Banas MP, Karzel RP: An analysis of 140 injuries to the superior glenoid labrum. *J Shoulder Elbow Surg* 1995;4:243-248.

117. Burkart A, Imhoff AB, Roscher E: Foreign-body reaction to the bioabsorbable suretac device. *Arthroscopy* 2000;16:91-95.

118. Medvecky MJ, Ong BC, Rokito AS, Sherman OH: Thermal capsular shrinkage: Basic science and clinical application. *Arthroscopy* 2001;17:624-635.

119. Getelman MH, Snyder SJ: Arthroscopic management of SLAP lesions and biceps tendon injuries, in Chow JCY (ed): *Advanced Arthroscopy*. New York, NY, Springer-Verlag, 2001.

120. Mileski RA, Snyder SJ: Superior labral lesions in shoulder: Pathoanatomy and surgical management. *J Am Acad Orthop Surg* 1998;6: 121-131.

121. Yoneda M, Hirooka A, Saito S, Yamamoto T, Ochi T, Shino K: Arthroscopic stapling for detached superior glenoid labrum. *J Bone Joint Surg Br* 1991;73:746-750.

122. Field LD, Savoie FH III: Arthroscopic suture repair of superior labral detachment lesions of the shoulder. *Am J Sports Med* 1993;21:783-790.

123. Resch H, Golser K, Thoeni H, Sperner G: Arthroscopic repair of superior glenoid labral detachment (the SLAP lesion). *J Shoulder Elbow Surg* 1993;2:147-155.

124. Stetson WB, Karzel RP, Banas MP, et al: Long-term clinical follow-up of 140 consecutive patients with injury to superior labrum. *Arthroscopy* 1997;13:376-377.

125. Budoff JE, Nirschl RP, Guidi EJ: Debridement of partial thickness tears of the rotator cuff without acromioplasty: Long term follow-up and review of the literature. *J Bone Joint Surg Am* 1998;80:733-748.

126. Gartsman GM, Milne JC: Articular surface partial thickness rotator cuff tears. *J Shoulder Elbow Surg* 1995;4:409-415.

127. Snyder SJ, Pachelli AF, Del Pizzo W, et al: Partial thickness rotator cuff tears: Results of arthroscopic treatment. *Arthroscopy* 1991;7:1-7.

128. Wright SA, Cofield RH: Management of partial-thickness rotator cuff tears. *J Shoulder Elbow Surg* 1996;5:458-466.

129. Levitz CL, Dugas J, Andrews JR: The use of arthroscopic thermal capsulorraphy to treat internal impingement in baseball players. *Arthroscopy* 2001;17:53-577.

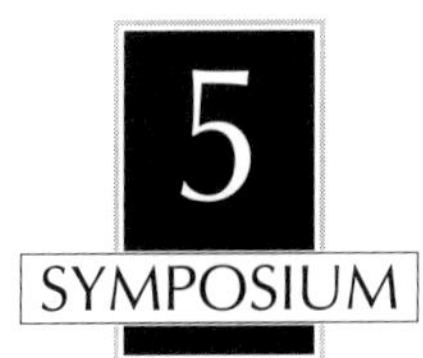

Multidirectional Instability: Surgical Decision Making

Ian K.Y. Lo, MD, FRCSC
Julie Y. Bishop, MD
Anthony Miniaci, MD
Evan L. Flatow, MD

Abstract

Although previous authors have described multidirectional instability of the shoulder, it was not until 1980 that Neer and associates solidified the current understanding and treatment of inferior and multidirectional instability. They emphasized the importance of differentiating this condition from the more common unidirectional instabilities and introduced the concept of an inferior capsular shift to globally tension the capsule anteriorly, inferiorly, and posteriorly, while thickening and reinforcing it on the side of greatest instability (ie, anterior or posterior). Since the time of this initial description, the diagnosis and treatment of multidirectional instability has been fraught with difficulty and confusion. More recently, the advent of shoulder arthroscopy has blazed the trail for minimally invasive techniques to correct multidirectional instability, including arthroscopic thermal capsulorrhaphy and suture plication. However, despite strong opinions regarding these surgical techniques, when comparing open approaches to arthroscopic techniques for the treatment of multidirectional instability, long-term outcomes of arthroscopic techniques have yet to replicate those of open surgery.

Multidirectional instability may be defined as symptomatic glenohumeral instability in more than one direction: anterior, inferior, and posterior.[1-4] Although this definition may at first appear straightforward, several areas of confusion have pervaded the orthopaedic literature that have compounded the complexities of treating this challenging condition.

First, there is a common misconception that multidirectional instability is limited to young, sedentary patients with bilateral symptoms and signs and is classically acquired in an atraumatic fashion. In reality, many patients with multidirectional instability are often athletic and may have acquired their disease through repetitive microtrauma (eg, butterfly swimming and gymnastics). In these patients, an evaluation of other joints usually does not reveal generalized ligamentous laxity.

Second, classic anterior unidirectional instability actually involves dislocation of the humeral head anteriorly and inferiorly. However, this is not the same as bidirectional instability (ie, anterior and inferior instability) and should be differentiated from such. In patients with instability both anteriorly and inferiorly, inferior instability may be demonstrated by a sulcus sign with the arm in adduction and inferior sag of the humerus with the arm in abduction.

Third, not all loose shoulders are symptomatic; thus, it is imperative that the surgeon be convinced that the instability is symptomatic before considering repair. Furthermore, there may be elements of asymptomatic laxity and symptomatic instability in the same shoulder (eg, symptomatic anterior instability with "normal" inferior and posterior laxity).[5-7] Therefore, the entire spectrum of multidirectional instability may include patients with primary unidirectional instability, bidirectional instability, and patients with unidirectional or bidirectional instability but multidirectional laxity. However, patients with classic multidirectional instability have symp-

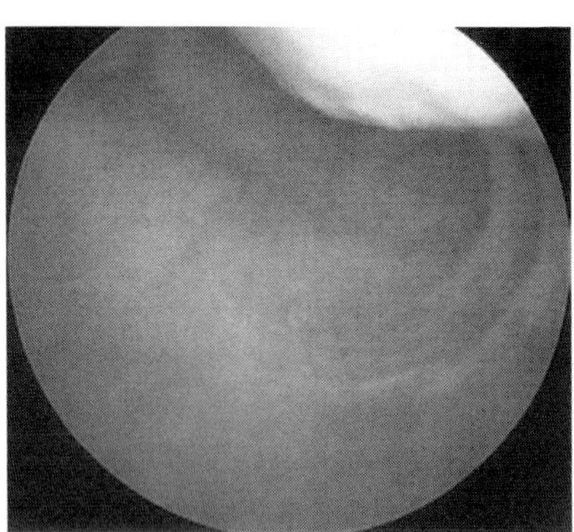

Figure 1 Arthroscopic view through a posterior portal demonstrates a capacious inferior recess characteristic of patients with multidirectional instability.

tomatic instability in at least two directions that is characterized pathologically by a grossly patulous and redundant capsule (Figure 1).

Finally, a small subset of patients with multidirectional instability can dislocate their shoulders at will or on command (ie, voluntary dislocators). In many instances, this ability is related to the position of the arm (ie, posterior dislocation with the arm raised in forward elevation and slight adduction). In these patients, this maneuver can be done, but the patient is reluctant to do so and usually avoids this position. These patients usually do not have a psychiatric disorder and may be amenable to surgical correction. However, some voluntary dislocators, who may have accompanying psychiatric disorders, can use asymmetric muscle pull to dislocate their shoulders or even statically dislocate their joints to great dramatic effect. Another group includes habitual dislocators who have developed improper muscle firing patterns and produce dislocations by asymmetric muscle pull. These patients are usually best treated with skillful neglect and muscular retraining.

Nonsurgical Management

Rehabilitation of the muscles that stabilize the humerus is the mainstay of treatment of classic multidirectional instability. This is not only important in nonsurgical management but is essential in protecting the capsule repair postoperatively.[2] Rehabilitation is focused on strengthening the deltoid and rotator cuff muscles with the arm below the shoulder[8,9] as well as strengthening the scapulothoracic stabilizing muscles. Therapy is aimed at improving muscle tone and coordination and improving the patient's functional adaptation. Occasionally, patients with multidirectional instability may develop secondary impingement. In these patients, a subacromial steroid injection may provide sufficient pain relief to allow participation in a rehabilitation program. Furthermore, a brief course of nonsteroidal anti-inflammatory medication may also benefit patients with baseline shoulder pain.

Open Surgical Treatment

The procedure for open surgical treatment of multidirectional instability has been outlined in the literature.[1,2] This procedure is designed to reduce the capsular volume on all sides by thickening and overlapping the capsule on the side of greatest instability and tensioning the capsule inferiorly and on the opposite side. This procedure can usually be performed from one surgical approach, either anterior or posterior. Although some authors have routinely performed all procedures using an anterior approach,[10] others have preferred to approach the shoulder from the side of greatest instability because this side will be best reinforced and strengthened by the overlapping of capsular flaps and the scarring of surgery.[11-14] Shoulders that dislocate both anteriorly and posteriorly equally are probably easiest to approach from the anterior side. **(DVD-51.1)**

Because the capsule is funnel-shaped (ie, wider laterally than medially), a humeral-based shift is performed by making a horizontal T incision between the middle and the inferior glenohumeral ligaments, thereby creating a superior flap (containing the superior and middle glenohumeral ligaments) and an inferior flap (containing all three parts of the inferior glenohumeral ligament) (Figure 2). Shifting the capsule on the humeral side reduces capsular volume where the capsular circumference is the largest and avoids the axillary nerve medially. Although the primary goal of this shift is to reduce the inferior capsular laxity in a north-south direction, a complete release of the capsule is required (ie, the posterior capsule must be released off the humerus) to provide sufficient capsular mobility to obtain an effective shift. A finger placed in the inferior pouch can help assess the size of the inferior pouch and how much redundant capsule must be released from the humerus before repair. Following release and mobilization of the capsule, the axillary pouch should be obliterated and can be evaluated by placing a finger inferiorly in the axillary pouch and pulling on the inferior flap in a superior direction (Figure 3).

In addition to a capsular shift, a closure of the rotator interval is performed. Neer[12] believed that this area was enlarged in patients with multidirectional instability and described closing it and drawing the superior flap tight inferiorly so that the middle glenohumeral ligament could act as a sling against inferior subluxation.[2] Recent biomechanical studies have supported this principle;

both the inferior capsule and rotator interval have been shown to be important stabilizers to inferior subluxation of the arm.[15-18]

All concomitant pathologies (eg, loose bodies and labral tears) are treated, and the capsule is repaired with the arm in approximately 25° of external rotation and 20° of abduction. This is modified based on the patient's particular needs and pathology. The inferior flap is shifted superiorly and repaired first while the superior flap is shifted inferiorly and repaired (Figure 4).

In 1980, Neer and Foster[2] reported the preliminary results of using an inferior capsular shift to treat 36 patients with multidirectional instability of the shoulder. Only one patient demonstrated recurrent subluxation at early follow-up. More recently, several authors have reported on the successful treatment of multidirectional instability using an inferior capsular shift procedure.[1-14,19-25] In 1992, Cooper and Brems[10] reported on 43 shoulders in 38 patients following an inferior capsular shift. An anterior surgical incision was used for all patients, and all had a minimum 2-year follow-up. Overall, 89% of the patients were satisfied with no recurrent instability and 11% of patients developed recurrent symptomatic instability. These failures generally occurred less than 2 years following surgery.

In 2000, Pollock and associates[13] reported on 49 shoulders following inferior capsular shift. At a mean 61-month follow-up, 94% of patients had good or excellent results and 96% of patients remained stable. Of the 36 athletes who underwent this procedure, 86% were able to return to sports, but only 69% were able to return to their premorbid level of athletic activity. These results collectively emphasize that excellent clinical results may be obtained with careful patient selection and the use of meticulous surgical technique in this difficult patient population.

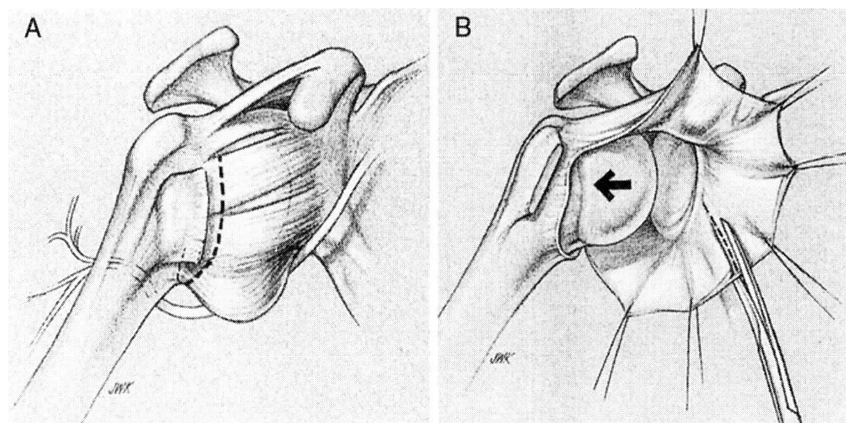

Figure 2 Capsular incision during open inferior capsular shift. **A,** The capsular incision (*dotted line*) is made 5 mm medial to the lateral cuff of the subscapularis tendon while the arm is maintained in external rotation and adduction to avoid injury to the axillary nerve. **B,** The capsule is incised horizontally (*dotted line*) in a T fashion between the middle and inferior glenohumeral ligaments. The bone of the humerus lateral to the articular margin is freshened to facilitate healing (*arrow*). (Reproduced with permission from Yamaguchi K, Flatow EL: Management of multidirectional instability. *Clin Sports Med* 1995;14:885-902.)

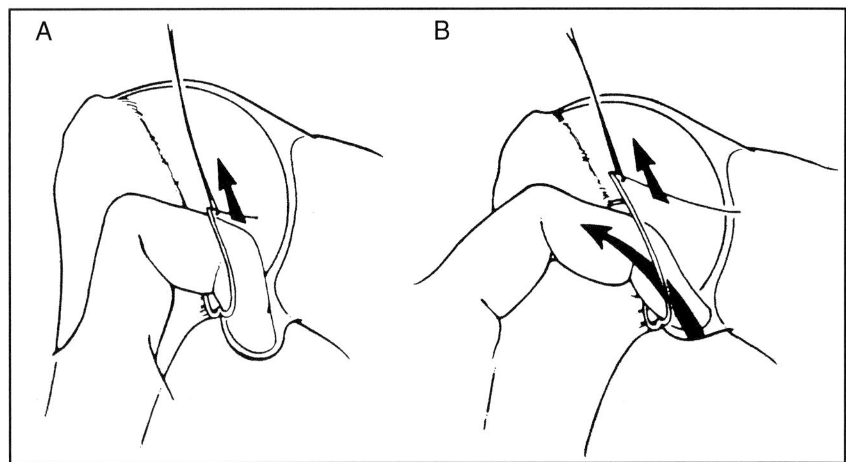

Figure 3 A and **B,** The dissection proceeds inferiorly, until pulling up on the capsular traction sutures (*short arrows*) extrudes the surgeon's index finger (*long arrow*) from the redundant inferior pouch. (Reproduced with permission from Pollock RG, Owens JM, Flatow EL, Bigliani LU: Operative results of the inferior capsular shift procedure for multidirectional instability of the shoulder. *J Bone Joint Surg Am* 2000;82:919-928.)

Problems and Complications

Technical Considerations Although open surgical treatment can lead to excellent results in expert hands, several surgical considerations are important in minimizing potential complications during an open inferior capsular shift. In particular, the temptation to shift the capsule from an east-west (ie, medial to lateral) direction must be avoided. This is

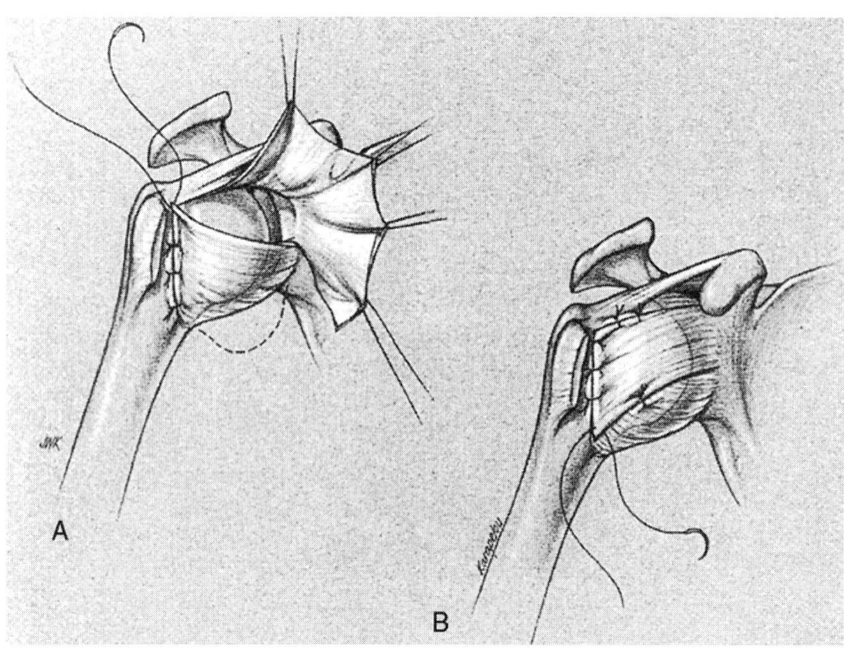

Figure 4 A, The capsular shift begins as the inferior flap of the capsule is shifted superiorly and repaired to the lateral cuff of capsule. **B,** After the repair of the superior cleft (ie, the capsular portion of the rotator interval), the superior capsular flap is then shifted inferiorly and repaired. (Reproduced with permission from Yamaguchi K, Flatow EL: Management of multidirectional instability. *Clin Sports Med* 1995;14:885-902.)

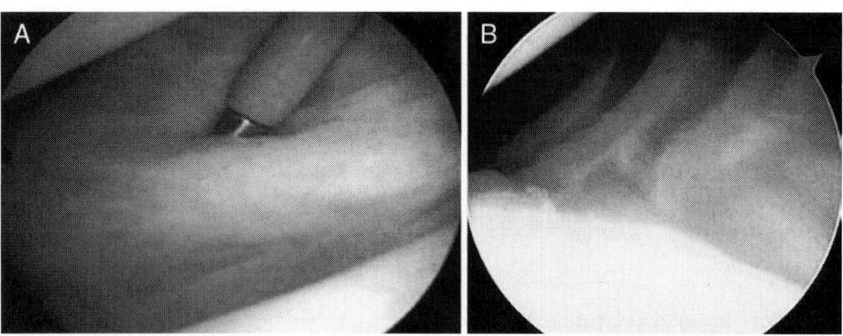

Figure 5 Arthroscopic views of right shoulder during thermal capsulorrhaphy. **A,** The thermal probe is introduced through an anterior portal, and the anterior band of the inferior glenohumeral ligament and anterior inferior capsule are shrunk. **B,** The thermal probe is used in a stripe fashion to maintain an interval of viable tissue between the thermally treated tissues and minimize the potential for capsular necrosis. (Courtesy of J.J.P. Warner, MD.)

commonly a result of inadequate mobilization of the capsule inferiorly and posteriorly. An east-west capsular shift inadvertently shortens the glenohumeral ligaments, limits external rotation, and does not reduce the patulous inferior capsule. Furthermore, an east-west tightening can exacerbate symptomatic instability. Patients with true multidirectional instability who undergo anterior capsular tightening may develop symptomatic posterior instability or may develop a flask deformity of the capsule. In a flask deformity, patients develop a superior east-west capsular constriction, which limits external rotation and exacerbates inferior instability. Adherence to these surgical principles and careful postoperative immobilization and rehabilitation can lead to excellent results following open surgical treatment.

Arthroscopic Thermal Capsulorrhaphy

Arthroscopic techniques, particularly the thermal modification of the capsule, have gained wide popularity in the treatment of multidirectional instability and capsular laxity. Because these techniques are relatively easy to use, they have become popular despite a lack of scientific evidence of their effectiveness. The most popular techniques include the use of either laser or radiofrequency energy. Although laser techniques are more expensive and require specialized training and equipment, both laser and radiofrequency energy work by transferring energy from the probe tip or laser into the tissue (Figure 5). The resultant heat that is generated by movement of molecules causes collagen shrinkage and depends on many factors, including time, temperature, and tissue quality.[26] The critical temperature for collagen shrinkage in ligamentous or capsular tissue is between 65°C and 75°C and depends on the time of exposure and the collagen cross-linkage of the tissue. Importantly, cell death begins at 45°C, and when local tissue reaches 55°C to 60°C, all the cells in that area within the tissue have died and the tissue is essentially dead.

Although several in vitro studies have demonstrated the effectiveness of thermal techniques in shrinking collagenous tissue, time-zero in vitro mechanical data may have little correlation with the eventual mechanical properties of the tissue.[26-34] Studies have reported a degradation of mechanical properties after thermal treatment that is slowly reconstituted with time.[26-34] However, these techniques are not easy to apply because it is difficult to predict a patient's biologic response to injury. The biologic response following thermal injury is variable and is characterized by a fibroplasia and angiogenesis. Hayashi and associates[35] have reported that biopsy specimens of some patients even 1 year following thermal treatment demonstrate a persistent synovial, cellular, and vascular reaction. Clinically, some patients may demonstrate continued inferior instability, whereas others may be extraordinarily stiff. Furthermore, complications including nerve injury[36,37] or capsular necrosis[26,38] (Figure 6) can leave patients worse off and permanently disabled. Although newer techniques (eg, thermal treatment applied in a stripe or grid pattern) may improve outcomes, they do not allow surgeons to accurately titrate the amount of thermal modification necessary during arthroscopic surgery to provide a stable joint postoperatively.

The clinical results of thermal capsulorrhaphy for multidirectional instability are variable. Some researchers have reported success rates approaching 100%,[39-41] whereas others have reported lower success rates[42-47] and 40% to 60% failure rates.[36,48] As stated previously, some of the variability may in part be related to the diagnosis and spectrum of disease of multidirectional instability.

In 2003, Joseph and associates[48] reported on 25 shoulders in 21 patients who underwent laser capsulorrhaphy to treat multidirectional instability. Patients were subclassified as having congenital/inherited multidirectional instability (ie, generalized ligamentous laxity, atraumatic onset, symptoms caused by activities of daily living, and younger age), acquired multidirectional instability (ie, history of repetitive microtrauma, isolated laxity to the shoulder girdle, less severe laxity, and symptoms caused by sports activity), or posttraumatic multidirectional instability (ie, traumatic event and pain being the most significant component). Overall, 40% of shoulders experienced recurrent instability postoperatively at a mean follow-up of 32 months; moreover, the incidence of recurrence varied according to the subclassification of multidirectional instability, although not significantly. Patients with congenital/inherited multidirectional instability had a 60% recurrence rate, patients with repetitive microtrauma had a 17% recurrence rate, and patients with posttraumatic multidirectional instability had a 33% recurrence rate.

Miniaci and associates[49] also reported the results of patients treated with thermal capsulorrhaphy for multidirectional instability. At 2-year follow-up of 19 patients, 9 had failed surgical outcomes, 5 demonstrated significant restrictions in motion, and 4 had axillary nerve irritation or injury. Of the patients with failed surgical outcomes requiring revision, one third demonstrated capsular deficiency that complicated revision surgery. Collectively, these results should caution against the widespread use of thermal capsulorrhaphy in the treatment of true multidirectional instability.

The most effective use of thermal energy may be to augment or enhance suture reconstructions (eg, Bankart repairs and suture capsulorrhaphy).[40,50,51] However, its use in the treatment of multidirectional instability has yet to be determined, and some researchers now consider multidirectional instability as a risk factor for the failure of thermal capsulorrhaphy.[47,52] As an isolated treatment, thermal capsulorrhaphy may be indicated only in patients with subtle instability patterns (ie, anterior inferior subluxation or microinstability), particularly in throwing athletes.[53,54] Although there may be a place for thermal treatment in shoulder surgery, additional studies are necessary to determine the appropriate indications.

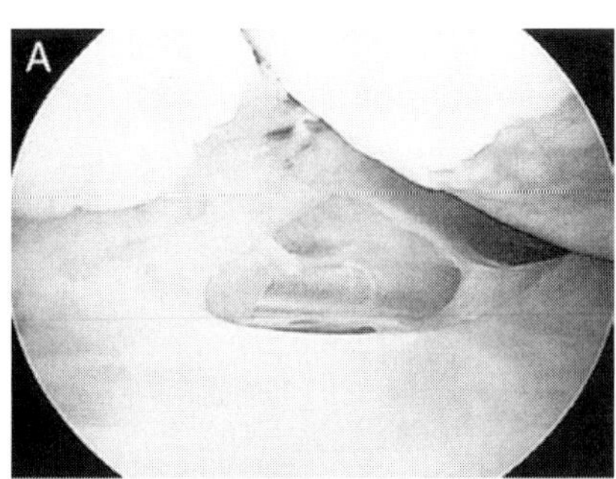

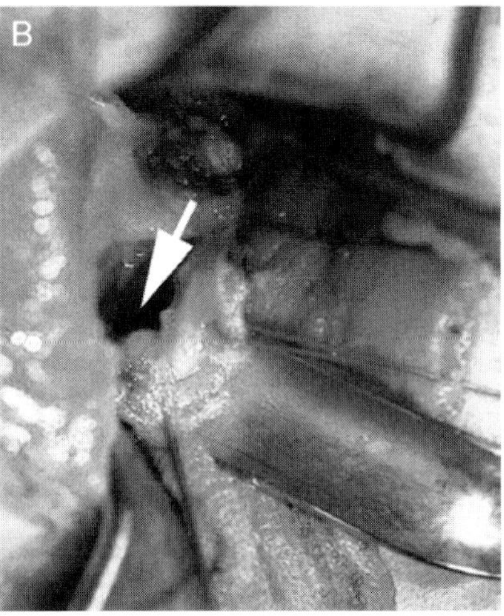

Figure 6 **A,** Arthroscopic view demonstrating capsular necrosis and deficiency after thermal capsulorrhaphy. (Courtesy of J. Bradley, MD.) **B,** Photograph of open capsular reconstruction after thermal capsulorrhaphy demonstrates a hole in the inferior capsule (*arrow*).

Arthroscopic Capsular Shift

Recently, arthroscopic capsular shift procedures have been used to treat

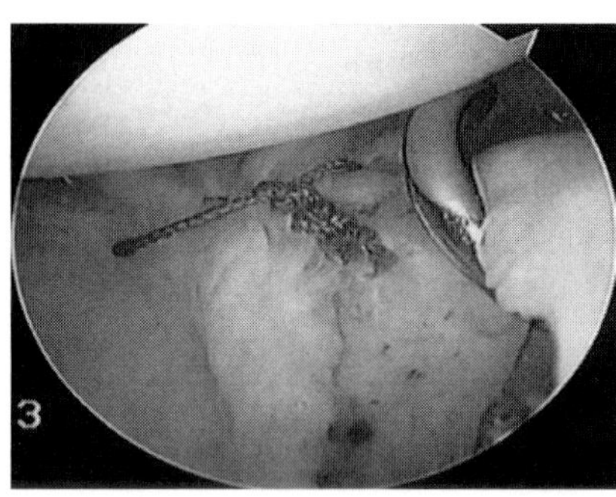

Figure 7 Arthroscopic view of a left shoulder through an anterosuperolateral portal demonstrates plication of the anterior capsule to the labrum.

multidirectional instability.[55-60] These arthroscopic techniques are based on the same principles as an open inferior capsular shift; however, because arthroscopic capsular shift is generally glenoid based, the potential amount of mechanical capsular shift achieved is less than that achieved with a traditional open humeral based shift.[61] **(DVD- 51.2)** Although capsular plication can effectively decrease capsular volume, open surgery does afford the advantages of thickening and overlapping of tissues and allows mobilization of the external surface of the capsule to allow a more effective shift.

By using capsular tucks and other techniques, the capsular volume may be reduced arthroscopically by plicating the capsule to the labrum (Figure 7). In patients with a deficient labrum, a suture anchor may be used to plicate the capsule and reconstruct the labrum. Care must be taken to shift the capsule more superiorly than medially to avoid restricting range of motion. The addition of an interval closure can further improve inferior stability.

Several authors have recently reported the results of using arthroscopic capsular shift for the treatment of multidirectional instability.[55-60] In general, they report 88% to 95% good to excellent results, with approximately 85% of patients able to return to sports activity.[55-60] Although these early results appear promising, concern has been raised regarding the ability of soft-tissue capsular tucks to heal, and many of these surgeries were performed in patients with subtle instability.

Summary

The treatment of multidirectional instability continues to progress toward the use of minimally invasive techniques, with the ultimate goals being maximizing outcomes and minimizing morbidity. In patients with multidirectional instability who primarily report pain and minimal instability symptoms, an arthroscopic capsular shift may be the ideal treatment. Patients with pain commonly demonstrate other pathologic conditions (eg, labral tears), which may be concomitantly treated and may contribute to glenohumeral laxity. Although thermal augmentation has not definitively demonstrated any clear benefit, thermal capsulorrhaphy may be used to address subtle capsular laxity in the throwing athlete. However, in patients with true dislocations or instability in multiple directions, particularly if generalized ligamentous laxity can be demonstrated, open surgery remains a good option. Although arthroscopic capsular shift may be used to treat these patients, an open inferior capsular shift can provide a larger shift, and for many surgeons open repair is still the gold standard for the treatment of classic multidirectional instability.

References

1. Neer CS II: Involuntary inferior and multidirectional instability of the shoulder: Etiology: Recognition and treatment. *Instr Course Lect* 1985;34:232-238.
2. Neer CS II, Foster CR: Inferior capsular shift for involuntary inferior and multidirectional instability of the shoulder: A preliminary report. *J Bone Joint Surg Am* 1980;62:897-908.
3. Cordasco FA, Pollock RG, Flatow EL, Bigliani LU: Management of multidirectional instability. *Oper Tech Sports Med* 1993;1:293-300.
4. Ozaki J: Glenohumeral movement of the involuntary inferior and multidirectional instability. *Clin Orthop* 1989;238:107-111.
5. Fu FH, Burkhead WZ Jr, Flatow EL, et al: Controversies in reconstruction of the unstable shoulder: Mobility versus instability. Part I. *Contemp Orthop* 1993;26:301-322.
6. Fu FH, Burkhead WZ Jr, Flatow EL, et al: Controversies in reconstruction of the unstable shoulder: Mobility versus instability. Part II. *Contemp Orthop* 1993;26:407-427.
7. Mok DW, Fogg AJ, Hokan R, Bayley JI: The diagnostic value of arthroscopy in glenohumeral instability. *J Bone Joint Surg Br* 1990;72:698-700.
8. Burkhead WZ Jr, Rockwood CA Jr: Treatment of instability of the shoulder with an exercise program. *J Bone Joint Surg Am* 1992;74:890-896.
9. An YH, Friedman RJ: Multidirectional instability of the glenohumeral joint. *Orthop Clin North Am* 2000;31:275-285.
10. Cooper RA, Brems JJ: The inferior capsular-shift procedure for multidirectional instability of the shoulder. *J Bone Joint Surg Am* 1992;74:1516-1521.
11. Bigliani LU: Anterior and posterior capsular shift for multidirectional instability. *Tech Orthop* 1989;3:36-45.
12. Neer CS II: *Shoulder Reconstruction*. Philadelphia, PA, WB Saunders, 1990, pp 273-341.
13. Pollock RG, Owens JM, Flatow EL, Bigliani LU: Operative results of the inferior capsular shift procedure for multidirectional instability of the shoulder. *J Bone Joint Surg Am* 2000;82:919-928.
14. Yamaguchi K, Flatow EL: Management of multidirectional instability. *Clin Sports Med* 1995;14:885-902.
15. Warner JJ, Deng XH, Warren RF, Torzilli PA: Static capsuloligamentous restraints to superior-inferior translation of the glenohumeral joint. *Am J Sports Med* 1992;20:675-685.

16. Motzkin NE, Itoi E, Morrey BF, An KN: Contribution of capsuloligamentous structures to passive static inferior glenohumeral stability. *Clin Biomech (Bristol, Avon)* 1998;13:54-61.

17. Soslowsky LJ, Malicky DM, Blasier RB: Active and passive factors in inferior glenohumeral stabilization: A biomechanical model. *J Shoulder Elbow Surg* 1997;6:371-379.

18. Harryman DT II, Sidles JA, Harris SL, Matsen FA III: The role of the rotator interval capsule in passive motion and stability of the shoulder. *J Bone Joint Surg Am* 1992;74:53-66.

19. Altchek DW, Warren RF, Skyhar MJ, Ortiz G: T-plasty modification of the Bankart procedure for multidirectional instability of the anterior and inferior types. *J Bone Joint Surg Am* 1991;73:105-112.

20. Lebar RD, Alexander AH: Multidirectional shoulder instability: Clinical results of inferior capsular shift in an active-duty population. *Am J Sports Med* 1992;20:193-198.

21. Mallon WJ, Speer KP: Multidirectional instability: Current concepts. *J Shoulder Elbow Surg* 1995;4:54-64.

22. Hamada K, Fukuda H, Nakajima T, Yamada N: The inferior capsular shift operation for instability of the shoulder: Long-term results in 34 shoulders. *J Bone Joint Surg Br* 1999;81:218-225.

23. Bak K, Spring BJ, Henderson JP: Inferior capsular shift procedure in athletes with multidirectional instability based on isolated capsular and ligamentous redundancy. *Am J Sports Med* 2000;28:466-471.

24. van Tankeren E, De Waal Malefijt MC, van Loon CJ: Open capsular shift for multi directional shoulder instability. *Arch Orthop Trauma Surg* 2002;122:447-450.

25. Choi CH, Ogilvie-Harris DJ: Inferior capsular shift operation for multidirectional instability of the shoulder in players of contact sports. *Br J Sports Med* 2002;36:290-294.

26. Barber FA, Uribe JW, Weber SC: Current applications for arthroscopic thermal surgery. *Arthroscopy* 2002;18(suppl 1): 40-50.

27. Arnoczky SP, Aksan A: Thermal modification of connective tissues: Basic science considerations and clinical implications. *J Am Acad Orthop Surg* 2000;8:305-313.

28. Schaefer SL, Ciarelli MJ, Arnoczky SP, Ross HE: Tissue shrinkage with the holmium:yttrium aluminum garnet laser: A postoperative assessment of tissue length, stiffness, and structure. *Am J Sports Med* 1997;25:841-848.

29. Schulz MM, Lee TQ, Sandusky MD, Tibone JE, McMahon PJ: The healing effects on the biomechanical properties of joint capsular tissue treated with Ho:YAG laser: An in vivo rabbit study. *Arthroscopy* 2001;17:342-347.

30. Medvecky MJ, Ong BC, Rokito AS, Sherman OH: Thermal capsular shrinkage: Basic science and clinical applications. *Arthroscopy* 2001;17:624-635.

31. Khan AM, Fanton GS: Electrothermal assisted shoulder capsulorrhaphy: Monopolar. *Clin Sports Med* 2002,21:599-618.

32. Wallace AL, Hollinshead RM, Frank CB: Creep behavior of a rabbit model of ligament laxity after electrothermal shrinkage in vivo. *Am J Sports Med* 2002;30:98-102.

33. Wallace AL, Hollinshead RM, Frank CB: Electrothermal shrinkage reduces laxity but alters creep behavior in a lapine ligament model. *J Shoulder Elbow Surg* 2001;10:1-6.

34. Wallace AL, Hollinshead RM, Frank CB: The scientific basis of thermal capsular shrinkage. *J Shoulder Elbow Surg* 2000;9:354-360.

35. Hayashi K, Massa KL, Thabit G III, et al: Histologic evaluation of the glenohumeral joint capsule after the laser-assisted capsular shift procedure for glenohumeral instability. *Am J Sports Med* 1999;27:162-167.

36. D'Alessandro DF, Bradley JP, Fleischli JF, Connor PM: Prospective evaluation of electrothermal arthroscopic capsulorrhaphy (ETAC) for shoulder instability: Indications, techniques, and preliminary results. *J Shoulder Elbow Surg* 1999;8:663.

37. Greis PE, Burks RT, Schickendantz MS, Sandmeier R: Axillary nerve injury after thermal capsular shrinkage of the shoulder. *J Shoulder Elbow Surg* 2001;10:231-235.

38. Abrams JS: Thermal capsulorrhaphy for instability of the shoulder: Concerns and applications of the heat probe. *Instr Course Lect* 2001;50:29-36.

39. Ceballos C, Zvijac JE, Uribe JW, Hechtman KS: Arthroscopic thermal capsulorrhaphy in multidirectional glenohumeral instability. *Arthroscopy* 2000;16:428.

40. Savoie FH III, Field LD: Thermal versus suture treatment of symptomatic capsular laxity. *Clin Sports Med* 2000;19:63-75.

41. Lyons TR, Griffith PL, Savoie RH III, Field LD: Laser-assisted capsulorrhaphy for multidirectional instability of the shoulder. *Arthroscopy* 2001;17:25-30.

42. Frostick SP, Sinopidis C, Al Maskari S, Gibson J, Kemp GJ, Richmond JC: Arthroscopic capsular shrinkage of the shoulder for the treatment of patients with multidirectional instability: Minimum 2-year follow-up. *Arthroscopy* 2003;19:227-233.

43. Giffin JR, Annunziata CC, Bradley JP: Thermal capsulorrhaphy for instability of the shoulder: Multidirectional and posterior instabilities. *Instr Course Lect* 2001;50:23-28.

44. Levy O, Wilson M, Williams H, et al: Thermal capsular shrinkage for shoulder instability: Mid-term longitudinal outcome study. *J Bone Joint Surg Br* 2001;83:640-645.

45. Favorito PJ, Langenderfer MA, Colosimo AJ, Heidt RS Jr, Carlonas RL: Arthroscopic laser-assisted capsular shift in the treatment of patients with multidirectional shoulder instability. *Am J Sports Med* 2002;30:322-328.

46. Fitzgerald BT, Watson BT, Lapoint JM: The use of thermal capsulorrhaphy in the treatment of multidirectional instability. *J Shoulder Elbow Surg* 2002;11:108-113.

47. Fanton GS, Khan AM: Monopolar radiofrequency energy for arthroscopic treatment of shoulder instability in the athlete. *Orthop Clin North Am* 2001;32:511-523.

48. Joseph TA, Williams JS Jr, Brems JJ: Laser capsulorrhaphy for multidirectional instability of the shoulder: An outcomes study and proposed classification system. *Am J Sports Med* 2003;31:26-35.

49. Miniaci A, McBirnie JL, Miniaci SL: Thermal capsulorrhaphy for the treatment of multi-directional shoulder instability. *68th Annual Meeting Proceedings*. Rosemont, IL, American Academy of Orthopaedic Surgeons, 2001, p 617.

50. Mishra DK, Fanton GS: Two-year outcome of arthroscopic Bankart repair and electrothermal-assisted capsulorrhaphy for recurrent traumatic

anterior shoulder instability. *Arthroscopy* 2001;17:844-849.

51. Hawkins RJ, Karas SG: Arthroscopic stabilization plus thermal capsulorrhaphy for anterior instability with and without Bankart lesions: The role of rehabilitation and immobilization. *Instr Course Lect* 2001;50:13-15.

52. Anderson K, Warren RF, Altcheck DW, Craig EV, O'Brien SJ: Risk factors for early failure after thermal capsulorrhaphy. *Am J Sports Med* 2002;30:103-107.

53. Andrews JR, Dugas JR: Diagnosis and treatment of shoulder injuries in the throwing athlete: The role of thermal-assisted capsular shrinkage. *Instr Course Lect* 2001;50:17-21.

54. Dugas JR, Andrews JR: Thermal capsular shrinkage in the throwing athlete. *Clin Sports Med* 2002;21:771-776.

55. Gartsman GM, Roddey TS, Hammerman SM: Arthroscopic treatment of multidirectional glenohumeral instability: 2- to 5-year follow-up. *Arthroscopy* 2001;17:236-243.

56. Duncan R, Savoie FH III: Arthroscopic inferior capsular shift for multidirectional instability of the shoulder: A preliminary report. *Arthroscopy* 1993;9:24-27.

57. McIntyre LF, Caspari RB, Savoie FH III: The arthroscopic treatment of multidirectional instability: Two-year results of a multiple suture technique. *Arthroscopy* 1997;13:418-425.

58. McIntyre LF, Caspari RB, Savoie FH: The arthroscopic treatment of anterior and multidirectional shoulder instability. *Instr Course Lect* 1996;45:47-56.

59. Treacy SH, Savoie FH III, Field LD: Arthroscopic treatment of multidirectional instability. *J Shoulder Elbow Surg* 1999;8:345-350.

60. Rook RT, Savoie FH III, Field LD: Arthroscopic treatment of instability attributable to capsular injury or laxity. *Clin Orthop* 2001;390:52-58.

61. Deutsch A, Barber JE, Davy DT, Victoroff BN: Anterior-inferior capsular shift of the shoulder: A biomechanical comparison of glenoid-based versus humeral-based shift strategies. *J Shoulder Elbow Surg* 2001;10:340-352.

Arthroscopic Stabilization in Posterior or Multidirectional Instability of the Shoulder

Michael H. Metcalf, MD
Felix H. Savoie III, MD
Larry D. Field, MD

Abstract

The diagnosis and treatment of posterior or multidirectional instability of the shoulder can be difficult. Normal laxity must be differentiated from pathologic instability. Once clinically diagnosed, there are several likely factors that contribute to pathologic instability. Although many patients with posterior or multidirectional instability of the shoulder respond well to nonsurgical treatment, when surgical intervention is required, the success rate has not been as favorable as that for repairing isolated anterior instability of the shoulder.

Despite advances in surgical procedures for stabilization of the shoulder, the results for the surgical management of recurrent posterior or multidirectional instability (MDI) remain inferior to those used to treat anterior instability.[1,2] Several surgical techniques have been developed to treat posterior instability or MDI, the majority of which involve manipulating soft tissue to increase glenohumeral stability (posteroinferior capsular shift,[3,4] posterior Bankart repair,[5,6] posterior staple capsulorrhaphy,[7-9] posterior capsular plication and infraspinatus advancement,[10-13] transposition of subscapularis,[14,15] biceps tendon transfer,[16,17] and fascia lata reconstruction[12]), and some include modifications of the effective shape of the glenoid fossa (extracapsular bone blocks,[6,18,19] intra-articular bone blocks,[20] and posteroinferior glenoplasty[21,22]).

The fact that many techniques have been developed to treat a relatively rare condition suggests the presence of a multifactorial etiology, which has been shown to include the use of capsular restraints, widening of the rotator interval, labral shape and tears, glenoid shape and version, dynamic pull of the rotator cuff, intra-articular negative pressure, and collagen laxity.[23-32] With multiple factors involved, and a combination of those factors often responsible for the instability, it is therefore unlikely that a single procedure will reproducibly result in shoulder stability for every patient. Optimal treatment then would involve defining which factors may be causing instability and addressing as many of those factors as possible, a therapeutic modality for which arthroscopic approaches may be better suited than traditional open techniques.

Diagnosis

Multidirectional Instability

The diagnosis of MDI relies heavily on a complete patient history. The acronym AMBRI (which refers to those who are Atraumatic, Multidirectional, Bilateral, treated with Rehabilitation, and, when rehabilitation is unsuccessful, are subsequently treated with open Inferior capsular shift and Interval closure) has been used to describe classic MDI. Although many patients with MDI may be classified as being "bone loose" (having generalized ligamentous laxity), some athletes have an acquired deformity from repetitive microtrauma and overuse of the upper extremities, which fatigues the dynamic stabilizers. Still others experience traumatic episodes that cause underlying instability to become symptomatic. Pain is often the presenting symptom and is usually associated with activities that put inferior traction on the shoulder, such as carrying a suitcase with the affected arm.

Physical examination includes evaluation for generalized ligamentous laxity. It is important to differentiate laxity from instability—the latter implies apprehension with re-creation of symptoms. A sulcus sign greater than 2 cm is usually pathognomonic for MDI, but pain and the reproduction of feeling of instability should also be present for diagnosis. Load and shift tests, standard anterior instability tests (apprehension, relocation, and augmentation), posterior evaluation with apprehension signs, and the jerk test are equally important in confirming the diagnosis. Muscle strength testing should be done and range of motion assessed.

Radiographs typically are normal but may reveal a flattened glenoid fossa, excessive retroversion, and even Hill-Sachs or reverse Hill-Sachs lesions. MRI studies often are normal but may reveal labral tears, capsular avulsion, or a wide rotator interval.

Examination under anesthesia is an important part of surgical treatment, but its role in diagnostic evaluation is unclear. For patients with suspected MDI of the shoulder, both shoulders must be compared; the same maneuvers used for clinical evaluation may exaggerate the degree of instability in the patient under anesthesia.

Posterior Instability

Because pure posterior instability is rare compared with anterior instability or MDI, the diagnosis of this condition is often delayed. Trauma is the underlying etiology in approximately 50% of patients. Athletes who participate in activities such as football and weight lifting and in sports requiring the arm to be lifted overhead are at greater risk for traumatic injury. Many patients with posterior instability actually have MDI but are symptomatic primarily in the posterior direction, and pain is a more common presenting symptom than instability.

Physical examination for patients with suspected posterior instability of the shoulder is similar to that for patients with suspected MDI, but evaluation of the posterior glenoid rim with both palpation and load and shift tests is particularly important. The jerk test position of flexion, adduction, and internal rotation has been described.

Radiographic evaluation must include careful assessment of the glenoid on the axillary view. Because glenoid abnormalities may contribute to failure of soft-tissue repairs, making surgical correction necessary, a CT scan is sometimes needed if the glenoid version is unclear. Patients who have actually dislocated the shoulder may have a reverse Hill-Sachs lesion on the humeral head.

Nonsurgical Treatment

Multidirectional Instability

Burkhead and Rockwood[33] have demonstrated that a persistent exercise program results in satisfactory results in 90% of patients with MDI of the shoulder. Most authors suggest waiting a minimum of 6 months before considering a surgical procedure. Rehabilitative exercises strengthen the entire shoulder complex, including the rotator cuff, large external muscles, and scapular stabilizers. Activity modification and patient education are also necessary components of a comprehensive rehabilitation program.

Posterior Instability

Although rehabilitation is the initial treatment of choice for patients with posterior instability of the shoulder, the success rate of physical therapy has not been as convincingly established as it has for MDI. Rehabilitative exercises should emphasize strengthening of the entire shoulder complex, and activities should be modified to avoid positions placing the shoulder at risk for injury.

Arthroscopic Treatment

Arthroscopic stabilization of posterior instability or MDI requires a familiarity with anterior stabilization techniques. The surgeon and assistants must be comfortable with anchor placement, intra-articular stitching, suture management, and arthroscopic knot tying. A thorough knowledge of relevant arthroscopic anatomy is also necessary in order to address all factors that may be causing the instability. **(DVD-3.1)**

Examination under anesthesia should be done prior to positioning the patient so that the opposite extremity can be compared. As noted earlier, apparent laxity will increase when the patient is under a general anesthetic.

When positioning the patients, the lateral position allows better access to both anterior and posterior aspects of the shoulder, but the beach chair position may also be used. With the patient in the lateral position, access to the anterior portals is improved by rolling the shoulders back 30° while keeping the pelvis vertical. This position also places the glenoid perpendicular to the floor, which can improve orientation. The patient is then secured with the assistance of a beanbag and straps, and the arm is suspended via single or double traction.

Diagnostic arthroscopy is performed via the posterior portal. Care should be taken to establish the portal so that the arthroscope can be inserted parallel to the glenoid. The anterior portal is created after confirming the appropriate position with a spinal needle. A probe is used to inspect the biceps root and the entire labrum for evidence of tearing. Criteria for traumatic lesions include separation and fraying of the labrum with corresponding chondromalacia of the glenoid cartilage. The rotator interval and capsular insertions should also be evaluated. Patients with MDI will typically have increased glenohumeral joint space, defined by the "drive-through" sign (ie, the arthroscope can easily be passed from anterior to posterior), a large inferior capsular pouch, and a widened rotator interval. The rotator cuff should then be evaluated for partial-thickness or complete tears. The arthroscope is replaced in the anterior portal to completely visualize the posterior structures.

In a recent series of patients, the following lesions have been noted: superior labrum anterior and posterior tears, superior labrum anterior cuff tears, anterior Bankart lesions, posterior Bankart lesions, widened rotator intervals, partial-thickness and full-thickness rotator cuff tears, Hill-Sachs lesions (standard and reverse), humeral avulsions of capsule, and excessive inferior glenoid recesses. All such lesions must be identified and corrected to maximize the outcome.

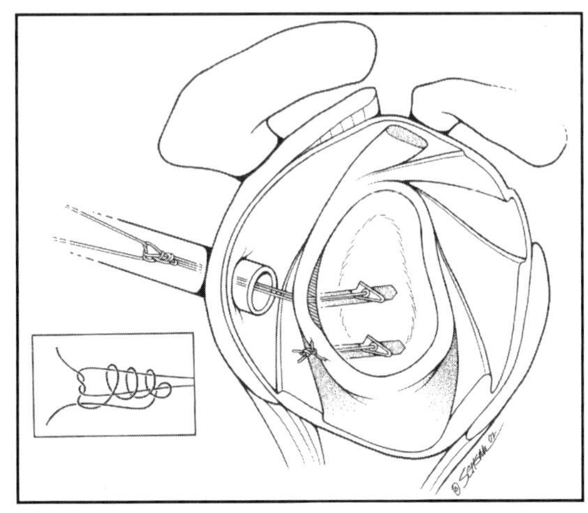

Fig. 1 Posterior Bankart lesion repair with anchors and No. 2 Ethibond suture. Inset, diagram of an arthroscopic modified Roeder knot.

Labral Lesions

Labral lesions can be stabilized with arthroscopic anchors and arthroscopic knots. The lesion is carefully elevated from the glenoid neck and extended to allow shifting of the capsule. The bone is débrided and decorticated to provide a bleeding bed. Anchors are used to allow tissue to be placed on the glenoid rim, not on the neck. Tissue is gathered with a Caspari suture punch, suture hooks, or a retrograde suture retriever and shifted superiorly to the anchor. Horizontal mattress sutures allow for the creation of a larger bumper. Nonabsorbable braided sutures provide better knot stability, resulting in less concern with potential synovitis (Fig. 1).

A bioabsorbable tissue tack can be used for lesions involving the posteroinferior glenohumeral ligament or the anterosuperior quadrant. The capsular tissue is then abraded, the glenoid decorticated, and a pilot hole drilled at the articular margin of the glenoid. The capsuloligamentous complex is subsequently speared with a wire, shifted superiorly, and inserted into the hole. The tack is then tapped into position (Fig. 2).

Stabilization of the biceps root is important in the surgical repair of superior labrum anterior and posterior tears. Although several techniques have been described, including the use of suture anchors and arthroscopic knots[34] and bioabsorbable tacks,[35] the authors prefer using arthroscopic anchors and nonabsorbable braided suture.

Rotator Interval Widening

Rotator interval closure is imperative for the successful repair of widened rotator intervals. A rasp or soft-tissue shaver is used to débride the capsule to promote a bleeding response. A thin-walled spinal needle will allow passage of a No. 2 braided suture. The spinal needle is passed approximately 1 cm medial to the humeral insertion and anterior to the anterior edge of the supraspinatus. The suture is passed superior to the biceps tendon to avoid capturing the tendon in the closure. A suture grasper is brought through the anterior portal and placed through the subscapularis through the capsule anterior and posterior to the subscapularis. This end of the suture is retrieved through the anterior cannula that has been allowed to back out superficial to the subscapularis. A suture hook is used to retrieve the suture end passed through the supraspinatus tendon from the subacromial space. An arthroscopic knot is then tied and tensioned to close the interval (Figs. 3 and 4).

Excessive Capsular Tissue

Redundant tissue can be managed with thermal shrinkage or with arthroscopic capsular shift. Arthroscopic knots generally provide more reproducible results. Typically, there is no labral tear and the redundant tissue is shifted and gathered onto the glenoid rim to enhance the existing labrum and deepen the effective glenoid dish. The area of the capsule that is to be shifted is lightly débrided to provide bleeding. An assortment of curved suture needles will allow the gathering of tissue and the shifting of the capsule onto the glenoid. Monofilament suture is used in combination with the arthroscopic suture needles and tied with arthroscopic knots. Alternatively, braided suture can be used in combination with a Crawford spinal needle and suture grasper (Figs. 5 and 6).

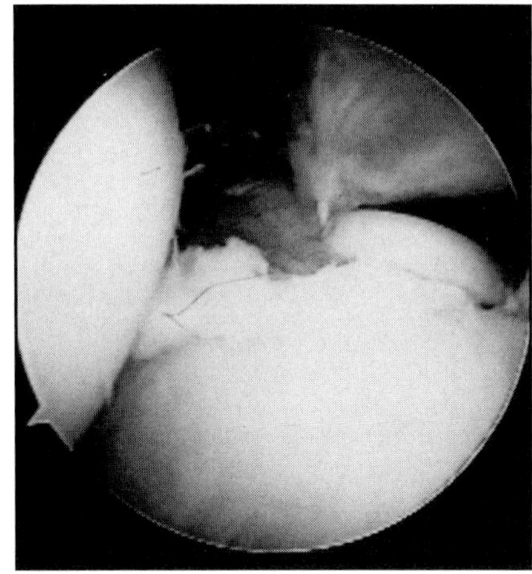

Fig. 2 Repair of posterior capsulolabral lesion with a bioabsorbable tack.

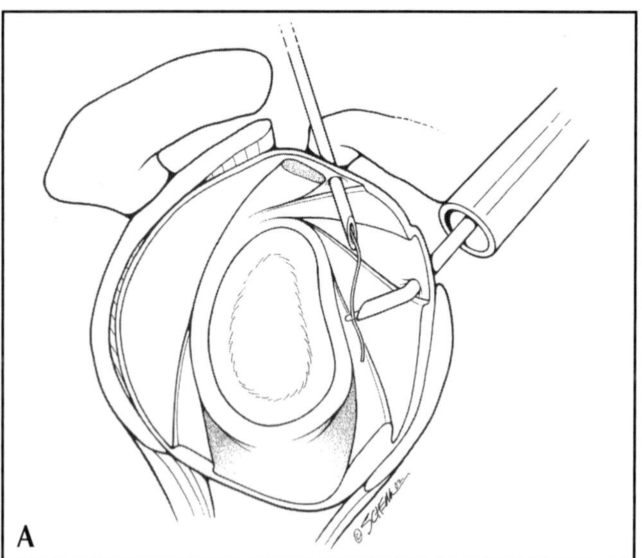

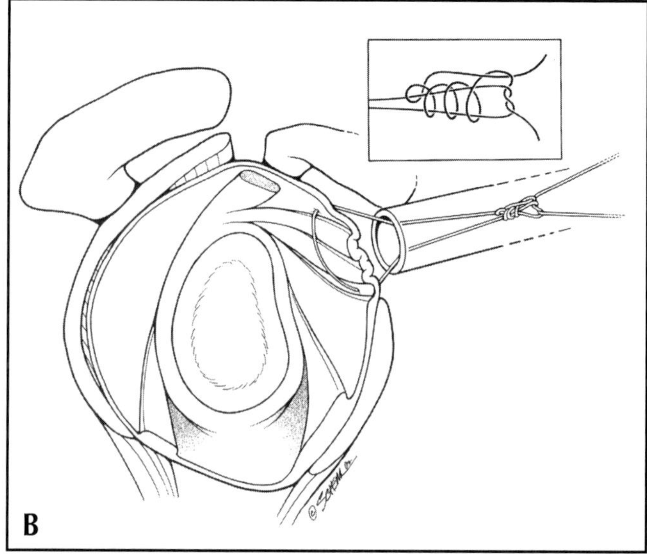

Fig. 3 Technique for arthroscopic closure of widened rotator interval. **A,** No. 2 Ethibond suture is placed via a Crawford spinal needle, and a suture grasper is advanced through the capsule at the inferior border and used to grasp the suture. **B,** The superior suture is retrieved from the subacromial space, and the interval is closed via arthroscopic knot tying.

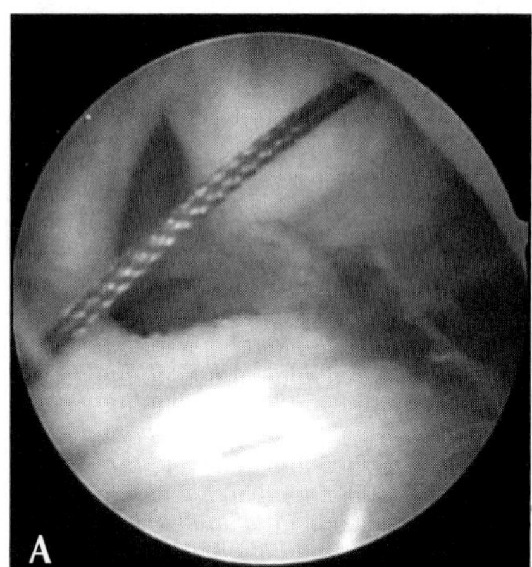

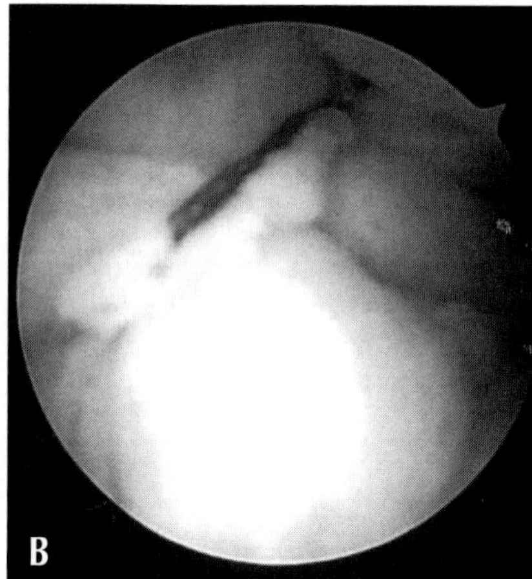

Fig. 4 Arthroscopic view of **(A)** widened interval prior to closure and **(B)** closure of interval.

Thermal capsulorrhaphy is performed with a temperature-specific thermal device. The amount of shrinkage is dependent on the total amount of heat absorbed by the tissue and is a component of both the temperature of the probe and the timing of the probe's placement on the tissue. Several studies have advocated using a grid pattern,[36] in which adjacent areas of tissue are spared thermal treatment. The treated area can be supplemented by placing a protective "lasso" monofilament absorbable suture. Rotator interval closure is typically needed as well because thermal capsulorrhaphy alone is not sufficient to treat a widened rotator interval.

Rehabilitation

Successful postoperative rehabilitation requires immobilization in a sling that provides approximately 30° of abduction. The sling should be worn full-time for 3 to 6 weeks, depending on the type of repair performed and the degree of patient compliance. The patient should perform active external rotation exercises with the arm adducted and scapular stabilization exercises for the next 3 weeks. At 6 weeks, more aggressive range-of-motion and strengthening exercises are started. Resistive exercises are initiated between 8 and 12 weeks, and sport-specific exercises typically begin 12 to 16 weeks after surgery. Exercise is continued until the operated side has symmetrical range of motion and the same level of strength as the opposite shoulder.

Rehabilitation must be patient specific and take into account patient factors (collagen quality, dependability, and future demand on shoulder) and surgical factors (quality of repair). Rehabilitative progression should be more gradual with a nonathletic social dislocator with hyperlaxity.

Clinical Results

Arthroscopic Capsular Shift and Labral Repair

Duncan and Savoie[37] reported on 10 consecutive patients with involuntary MDI

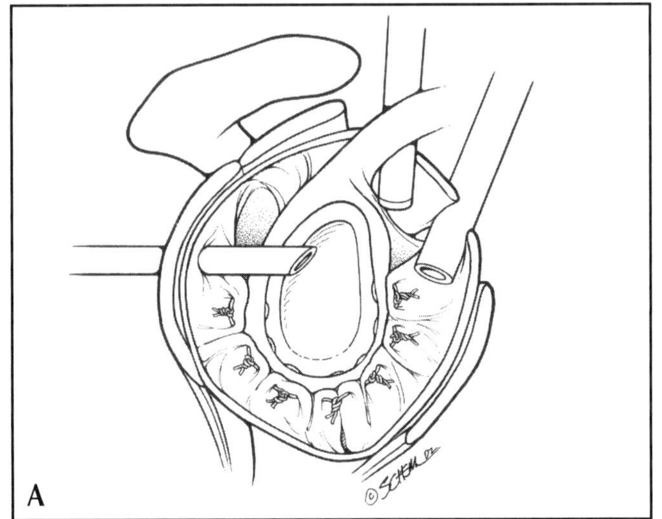
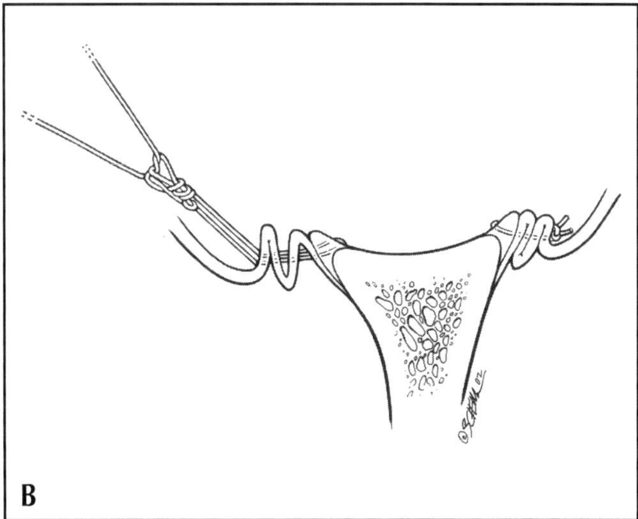

Fig. 5 Arthroscopic capsular shift. Horizontal mattress sutures **(A)** are placed in areas of redundant capsule **(B)**.

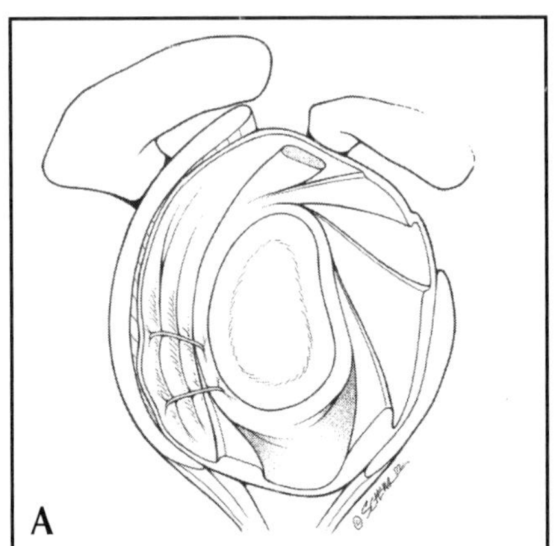
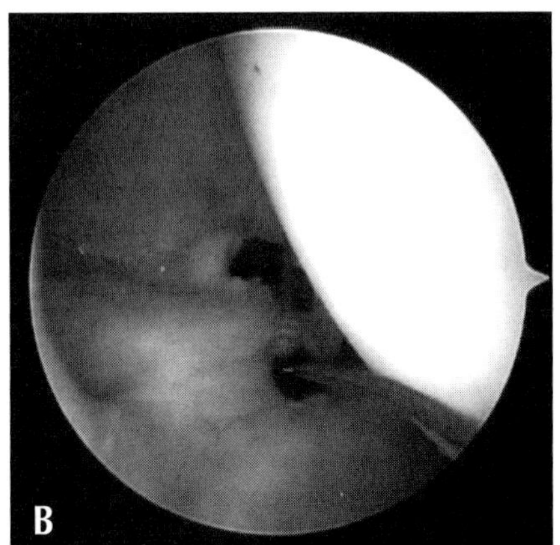
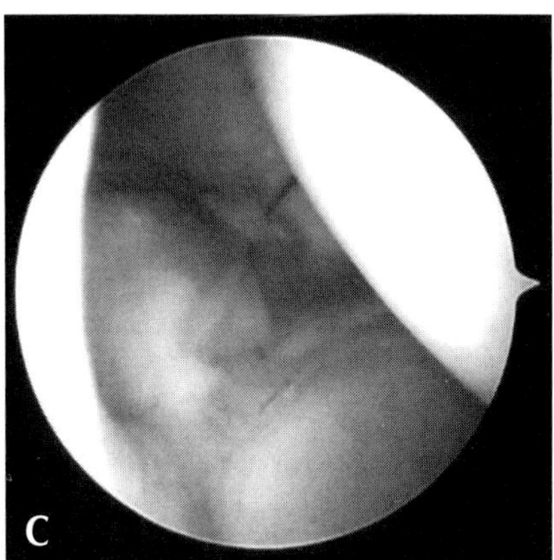

Fig. 6 Capsular shift performed for posterior instability **(A)**. The inferior recess decreases in size with tightening of the suture **(B** and **C)**.

treated with arthroscopic inferior capsular shift. The mean Bankart score was 90 for these patients and all had satisfactory results according to the Neer classification system.[37]

Treacy and associates[38] reported on 25 patients a mean of 60 months after arthroscopic capsular shift. The mean Bankart score was 95 for these patients. Three patients experienced postoperative instability. All but one patient regained full symmetric range of motion after 60 months. Twenty-one patients (88%) achieved satisfactory results according to the Neer classification system.

McIntyre and associates[39] reported on 19 patients at 34 months after undergoing arthroscopic capsular shift for MDI of the shoulder. The mean postoperative Bankart score was 91 out of a possible 100, with 13 patients achieving excellent results, 5 achieving good results, and 1 achieving fair results. Although none of the 19 patients were elite throwers, all but one of them returned to their previous levels of athletic performance. One patient had recurrent anterior subluxations, which were treated with a second arthroscopic capsular shift procedure with good results. The patient rated as fair had no improvement in her pain after surgery.

McIntryre and associates[40] reported on 20 patients who were treated with an arthroscopic posterior capsular shift for symptomatic posterior shoulder instability. Mean follow-up was 31 months. Twelve of the 20 patients had posterior Bankart lesions and 10 had anterior Hill-Sachs lesions. The average postoperative Bankart score was 83 out of a possible 100, with 15 patients achieving excellent results, 2 achieving good results, 1 achieving fair results, and 3 achieving poor results. Among these patients, there were two recurrent dislocations and three subluxations, resulting in an overall recurrence rate of 25%.

Wolf and Eakin[41] reported on 14 patients with recurrent posterior shoulder instability who underwent posterior capsular plication with or without suture anchors. Mean follow-up was 33 months. Twelve patients had excellent results and two had fair results. Nine of 10 patients who participated in recreational or competitive athletics reported a full return to their preinjury level of function in their respective sports. There was one recurrence of posterior shoulder instability, which was remedied with a second arthroscopic posterior capsular reconstruction. All 14 patients were satisfied with the results of their surgery.

Antoniou and associates[42] reported on 41 patients with posteroinferior instability of the shoulder who were treated with an arthroscopic shift of the posteroinferior aspect of the capsule to the adjacent labrum. These patients were observed for a mean of 28 months. Eighty-five percent had improved stability of the shoulder, and the findings on all physical examinations had improved significantly. Sixty-eight percent had a perception of residual stiffness despite having increased flexibility on examination.

Gartsman and associates[43] reported on a group of 47 patients with MDI 35 months after surgery. At final follow-up, 44 of 47 patients (94%) had good to excellent surgical results. One patient experienced persistent instability and underwent a second surgical procedure. Another patient noted a loss of strength during sports, and two other patients had pain that limited throwing ability. Twenty-two of 26 patients (85%) returned to their desired levels of athletic activity following the operations. In another study, Gartsman and associates[44] reported on bidirectional instability in 54 patients with a mean follow-up of 34 months. At final evaluation, 91% of patients had good to excellent results. Forty patients returned to sports activities, but 10 (25%) of them participated at a reduced level of activity.

Rotator Interval Closure

Field and associates[45] reported on 15 patients in whom history and examination were consistent with MDI. At the time of open stabilization, however, only a hole in the rotator interval was found. This interval widening was closed without any additional capsular shift. At a mean follow-up of 40 months, all patients achieved good or excellent results according to American Shoulder and Elbow Surgeons criteria.

Arthroscopic Thermal Capsulorrhaphy

Lyons and associates[46] reported that 26 of 27 shoulders (96%) remained stable and asymptomatic for a minimum of 2 years after surgery. Of 14 athletes in the study group, 12 (86%) returned to their previous levels of sports participation.

Thabit[47] reported on 41 patients who were treated with laser-assisted capsulorrhaphy. All competitive athletes returned to sports activities. Younger patients generally had better results than older patients.

Savoie and Field[48] compared 30 patients who were treated with a combination of thermal capsulorrhaphy and rotator interval closure with patients who were treated with either inferior shift or placation. No difference between these two groups of patients was reported.

Levy and associates[49] performed laser-assisted capsular shrinkage on 56 patients (61 shoulders), and 34 patients (38 shoulders) were treated with radiofrequency capsular shrinkage. In the laser-assisted group, 59% of patients considered their shoulders to be "much better" or "better," but there was a failure rate of 36.1%. For the radiofrequency group, 76.3% of patients considered their shoulders to be "much better" or "better," but there was a failure rate of 23.7%.

Levitz and associates[50] compared two groups of baseball players with internal impingement. One group underwent thermal capsulorrhaphy in addition to traditional treatment of labral repair and either débridement or repair of rotator cuff pathology, and the other group underwent traditional treatment alone. Those who underwent traditional treatment and thermal capsulorrhaphy returned to competition in 8.4 months compared with 7.2 months for those who underwent traditional treatment alone. However, 93% of those who underwent traditional treatment and thermal capsulorrhaphy eventually were able to return to competition compared with only 80% of those who underwent traditional treatment alone. At 30 months after surgery, 90% of those who underwent traditional treatment and thermal capsulorrhaphy returned to competition compared with only 67% of those who underwent traditional treatment alone.

Summary

Posterior instability and MDI of the shoulder can be difficult to treat because multiple etiologies often occur among patients and multiple coexisting factors occur in individual patients. For patients in whom rehabilitation is unsuccessful, arthroscopic evaluation is warranted. Careful arthroscopic examination helps to identify the underlying pathology, which can then be addressed with the appropriate arthroscopic techniques. The ability to identify and repair multiple coexisting factors that contribute to instability gives arthroscopic surgical techniques an advantage over traditional open techniques.

References

1. Hawkins RJ, Belle RM: Posterior instability of the shoulder. *Instr Course Lect* 1989;28:211-215.
2. Rowe CR: Prognosis in dislocations of the shoulder. *J Bone Joint Surg Am* 1956;38:957-977.
3. Bigliani LU, Pollock RG, McIlveen SJ, Endrizzi DP, Flatow EL: Shift of the posteroinferior aspect of the capsule for recurrent posterior glenohumeral instability. *J Bone Joint Surg Am* 1995;77:1011-1020.
4. Neer CS II, Foster CR: Inferior capsular shift for involuntary inferior and multidirectional instability of the shoulder: A preliminary report. *J Bone Joint Surg Am* 1980;62:897-908.

5. Rowe CR, Yee LB: A posterior approach to the shoulder joint. *J Bone Joint Surg Am* 1944;26:580-584.
6. Hindenach JC: Recurrent posterior dislocation of the shoulder. *J Bone Joint Surg Am* 1947;29:582-586.
7. Matsen FA III: Letter: Capsulorrhaphy with a staple for recurrent posterior subluxation of the shoulder. *J Bone Joint Surg Am* 1991;73:950.
8. Tibone JE, Prietto C, Jobe FW, et al: Staple capsulorrhaphy for recurrent posterior shoulder dislocation. *Am J Sports Med* 1981;9:135-139.
9. Tibone J, Ting A: Capsulorrhaphy with a staple for recurrent posterior subluxation of the shoulder. *J Bone Joint Surg Am* 1990;72:999-1002.
10. Greenhill BJ: Abstract: Persistent posterior shoulder dislocation: Its diagnosis and its treatment by posterior Putti-Platt repair. *J Bone Joint Surg Br* 1972;54:763.
11. Hawkins RJ, Koppert G, Johnston G: Recurrent posterior instability (subluxation) of the shoulder. *J Bone Joint Surg Am* 1984;66:169-174.
12. Norwood LA, Terry GC: Shoulder posterior subluxation. *Am J Sports Med* 1984;12:25-30.
13. Severin E: Anterior and posterior recurrent dislocation of the shoulder: The Putti-Platt operation. *Acta Orthop Scand* 1954;23:14-22.
14. Hawkins RJ, McCormack RG: Posterior shoulder instability. *Orthopedics* 1988;11:101-107.
15. McLaughlin HL: Posterior dislocation of the shoulder. *J Bone Joint Surg Am* 1952;34:584-590.
16. Boyd HB, Sisk TD: Recurrent posterior dislocation of the shoulder. *J Bone Joint Surg Am* 1972;54:779-786.
17. Nobel W: Posterior traumatic dislocation of the shoulder. *J Bone Joint Surg Am* 1962;44:523-538.
18. Fried A: Habitual posterior dislocation of the shoulder-joint: A report on 5 operated cases. *Acta Orthop Scand* 1949;18:329-345.
19. Schwartz E, Warren RF, O'Brien SJ, Fronek J: Posterior shoulder instability. *Orthop Clin North Am* 1987;18:409-419.
20. Mowery CA, Garfin SR, Booth RE, Rothman RH: Recurrent posterior dislocation of the shoulder: Treatment using a bone block. *J Bone Joint Surg Am* 1985;67:777-781.
21. Kretzler HH Jr, Blue AR: Abstract: Recurrent posterior dislocation of the shoulder in cerebral palsy. *J Bone Joint Surg Am* 1966;48:1221.
22. Scott DJ Jr: Treatment of recurrent posterior dislocations of the shoulder by glenoplasty: Report of three cases. *J Bone Joint Surg Am* 1967;49:471-476.
23. Andrews JR, Carson WG Jr, McLeod WD: Glenoid labrum tears related to the long head of the biceps. *Am J Sports Med* 1985;13:337-341.
24. Bankart ASB: The pathology and treatment of recurrent dislocation of the shoulder-joint. *Br J Surg* 1938;26:23-29.
25. Harryman DT II, Sidles JA, Clark JM, McQuade KJ, Gibb TD, Matsen FA III: Translation of the humeral head on the glenoid with passive glenohumeral motion. *J Bone Joint Surg Am* 1990;72:1334-1343.
26. Helmig P, Sojbjerg JO, Kjaersgaard-Andersen P, Nielsen S, Ovesen J: Distal humeral migration as a component of multidirectional shoulder instability: An anatomical study in autopsy specimens. *Clin Orthop* 1990;252:139-143.
27. Matsen FA III, Lippitt SB, Sidles JA, Harryman DT II (eds): *Practical Evaluation and Management of the Shoulder*. Philadelphia, PA, WB Saunders, 1994, pp 19-109.
28. Matsen FA III, Harryman DT II, Sidles JA: Mechanics of glenohumeral instability. *Clin Sports Med* 1991;10:783-788.
29. Bowen MK, Warren RF: Ligamentous control of shoulder stability based on selective cutting and static translation experiments. *Clin Sports Med* 1991;10:757-782.
30. Harryman DT II, Sidles JA, Harris SL, Matsen FA III: Laxity of the normal glenohumeral joint: A quantitative in vivo assessment. *J Shoulder Elbow Surg* 1992;1:66-76.
31. Howell SM, Galinat BJ: The glenoid-labral socket: A constrained articular surface. *Clin Orthop* 1989;243:122-125.
32. Lippitt SB, Vanderhooft JE, Harris SL, et al: Glenohumeral stability from concavity-compression: A quantitative analysis. *J Shoulder Elbow Surg* 1993;2:27-35.
33. Burkhead WZ Jr, Rockwood CA Jr: Treatment of instability of the shoulder with an exercise program. *J Bone Joint Surg Am* 1992;74:890-896.
34. Snyder SJ, Karzel RP, Del Pizzo W, Ferkel RD, Friedman MJ: SLAP lesions of the shoulder. *Arthroscopy* 1990;6:274-279.
35. Warner JJ, Cann S, Marko P: Arthroscopic repair of combined Bankart and superior labral detachment anterior and posterior lesions: Technique and results. *Arthroscopy* 1992;10:383-391.
36. Gerber A, Warner JJ: Thermal capsulorrhaphy to treat shoulder instability. *Clin Orthop* 2002;400:105-116.
37. Duncan R, Savoie FH III: Arthroscopic inferior capsular shift for multidirectional instability of the shoulder: A preliminary report. *Arthroscopy* 1993;9:24-27.
38. Treacy SH, Savoie FH III, Field LD: Arthroscopic treatment of multidirectional instability. *J Shoulder Elbow Surg* 1999;8:345-350.
39. McIntyre LF, Caspari RB, Savoie FH III: The arthroscopic treatment of multidirectional shoulder instability: Two-year results of a multiple suture technique. *Arthroscopy* 1997;13:418-425.
40. McIntyre LF, Caspari RB, Savoie FH III: The arthroscopic treatment of posterior shoulder instability: Two-year results of a multiple suture technique. *Arthroscopy* 1997;13:426-432.
41. Wolf EM, Eakin CL: Arthroscopic capsular plication for posterior shoulder instability. *Arthroscopy* 1998;14:153-163.
42. Antoniou J, Duckworth DT, Harryman DT II: Capsulolabral augmentation for the management of posteroinferior instability of the shoulder. *J Bone Joint Surg Am* 2000;82:1220-1230.
43. Gartsman GM, Roddey TS, Hammerman SM: Arthroscopic treatment of multidirectional glenohumeral instability: 2- to 5-year follow-up. *Arthroscopy* 2001;17:236-243.
44. Gartsman GM, Roddey TS, Hammerman SM: Arthroscopic treatment of bidirectional glenohumeral instability: Two- to five-year follow-up. *J Shoulder Elbow Surg* 2001;10:28-36.
45. Field LD, Warren RF, O'Brien SJ, Altchek DW, Wickiewicz TL: Isolated closure of rotator interval defects for shoulder instability. *Am J Sports Med* 1995;23:557-563.
46. Lyons TR, Griffith PL, Savoie FH III, Field LD: Laser-assisted capsulorrhaphy for multidirectional instability of the shoulder. *Arthroscopy* 2001;17:25-30.
47. Thabit G III: The arthroscopically assisted holmium:YAG laser surgery in the shoulder. *Oper Tech Sports Med* 1998;6:131-138.
48. Savoie FH III, Field LD: Thermal versus suture treatment of symptomatic capsular laxity. *Clin Sports Med* 2000;19:63-75.
49. Levy O, Wilson M, Williams H, et al: Thermal capsular shrinkage for shoulder instability: Midterm longitudinal outcome study. *J Bone Joint Surg Br* 2001;83:640-645.
50. Levitz CL, Dugas J, Andrews JR: The use of arthroscopic thermal capsulorrhaphy to treat internal impingement in baseball players. *Arthroscopy* 2001;17:573-577.

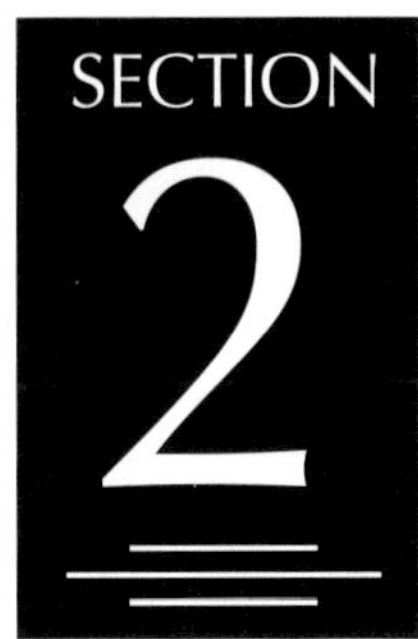

Rotator Cuff Injuries

Rotator Cuff Injuries

Dramatic advances in the basic science and clinical applications of shoulder surgery have occurred over the past 15 years, especially in our understanding of rotator cuff pathology. The prevalence of rotator cuff disorders increases with advancing age, and with the increased longevity of our population, orthopaedic surgeons are treating an increasing number of patients with these maladies. Advances in the clinical and radiographic diagnosis of these disorders also have resulted in increasing numbers of patients with rotator cuff pathology who may be relatively asymptomatic. Finally, because our patient population stays more physically active with advancing age, they expect to return to an active lifestyle. Thus, we can expect that the number of patients seeking treatment for rotator cuff problems will continue to rise.

The articles in this section not only serve as an excellent review of the state of knowledge of rotator cuff repairs, arthroscopic acromioplasty, and tendon transfers about the shoulder, but they also offer specific technical advice. Each article contains specific information and illustrations demonstrating how the experts perform these operations, which markedly enhances our understanding about on whom and when to perform such procedures, offers pearls for the surgeon, and supplies the rationale for the technical aspects of the treatment.

This compendium of articles also serves as an excellent introduction for residents and fellows regarding the state of the art of rotator cuff surgery. For practicing orthopaedic surgeons, this comprehensive review, coupled with the technical advice from thought leaders in the management of rotator cuff pathology, will advance their clinical acumen and enhance their surgical armamentarium. For those who specialize in shoulder surgery, these articles provide insight for those who wish to hone their surgical techniques.

The first article, authored by Blaine and associates, is principally a technique paper on open rotator cuff repair. The article begins with a brief introduction of the preoperative evaluation, highlighting the critical information that must be obtained and reviewed. The four distinct facets of open repair, namely the surgical approach, subacromial decompression, cuff mobilization and repair, and postoperative rehabilitation, are each systematically addressed, with essentially no stone left unturned. Well-positioned illustrations and the rationale for each step are supported by current literature. The sections on the mobilization of the rotator cuff and pearls in the management of both massive cuff tears and chronic cuff tears with retraction are expertly discussed. The quality of this article exceeds that of other technique articles because it includes a comprehensive review of the literature for each step in open rotator cuff repair, thereby addressing more than the "how" of each step by providing solid evidence about their approach.

The role of tendon transfers is expertly discussed by Dr. Warner in the second article. I consider this article the definitive review of the indications for tendon transfers with its comprehensive review of the germane literature on the topic. The discussion of pathoanatomy and pathomechanics is one of the best I've seen and truly sets his article above all others on the subject. He provides a comprehensive and rational explanation of the clinical problem, the underlying principles regarding tendon transfers, appropriate patient selection, and indications for a functional transfer in the shoulder. Even though tendon transfers are not commonly performed for posterior cuff deficiency, pectoralis major transfers are becoming more common for subscapularis deficiency, a condition that may be disabling for patients. What follows is a detailed guide that clearly delineates each step of pectoralis and latissimus transfers, illustrating not only how it is performed but also why each step is important. Specific details of postoperative rehabilitation are highlighted as well. These should be discussed with the physical therapist involved in the postoperative care in an effort to optimize outcomes.

Dr. Ken Yamaguchi provides a comprehensive review of mini-open rotator cuff repairs in the third article. He describes the evolution of this technique, citing the key articles that served as the impetus for moving to this technique for certain tears in lieu of formal open rotator cuff repair techniques. He clearly supports this trend. Critical steps in rotator cuff repair are detailed and then augmented with an explanation of how each step is accomplished using the mini-open technique. Thoughtful charts highlighting the critical differences among the various techniques (ie, formal open, mini-open, arthroscopic-assisted, and fully arthroscopic) add insight to both the surgical aspects and postoperative course for these procedures. The article concludes with a review of the pertinent literature regarding outcomes of mini-open repairs and highlights articles comparing mini-open to formal open techniques.

The fourth article is the most complete comparison of the above techniques in the literature and offers great insight into the advantages and disadvantages of the transition from open and mini-open techniques to a fully arthroscopic repair. Yamaguchi and associates dissect each step of the transition and provide invaluable, detailed guidelines and rationale as to when, why, and how to make the transition. What is critically important is the well-conceived gradual transition, which should serve as a model for those surgeons interested in making such a transition. The authors also have compiled a detailed list of pearls that assist with visualization during arthroscopic repairs, many of which are invaluable and not easily found in other articles. It is clear that there is great interest in this transition as arthroscopic techniques have dramatically improved, there is less blood loss, and patients typically report less postoperative discomfort. The long-term results of these techniques are still being investigated, but the current literature seems to support that intermediate-term results are as good as those with mini-open techniques.

The final article in the section describes the use of arthroscopic acromioplasty in treatment of impingement syndrome. Izquierdo and associates describe how the techniques for treating impingement syndrome have evolved to current arthroscopic methods, and landmark articles are succinctly reviewed. They clearly document that patients treated with arthroscopy have fewer complications and a shorter recovery period. A comprehensive review of the etiology follows, with a discussion of the newer theories on the etiology of impingement, including dynamic issues. Radiographic and physical findings are reviewed, with emphasis on new techniques of diagnosis. Finally, a detailed surgical methodology is presented, highlighting the critical components.

The treatment of rotator cuff tears has significantly changed over the past 15 years. With greater appreciation of the intrinsic causes of rotator cuff tears, we have turned our attention to surgical outcomes and failures. Now that we know more about the degenerative changes that accompany chronic tears and the profound effects on the musculotendinous unit, we can better appreciate why certain chronic tears may have diminished healing potential. These realizations have revolutionized our approach to both clinical and radiographic evaluation of patients. As a result, we have modified the indications for rotator cuff surgery, recognizing that tendon transfers will have an expanded role in the future. Finally, the healing potential of the tendon may be age related, and as such, strategies to enhance healing potential have evolved.

This collection of articles summarizes important advances in the treatment of rotator cuff pathology. From the discussion on the technique of open repairs to the transition through mini-open repairs to fully arthroscopic techniques, these articles serve as a roadmap to the future. Advanced techniques, including tendon transfers, complete our understanding of where we have been and where we are headed.

Laurence D. Higgins, MD
Division of Orthopaedic Surgery
Duke University Medical Center
Durham, North Carolina

Technique of Open Rotator Cuff Repair

Theodore A. Blaine, MD
Michael Q. Freehill, MD
Louis U. Bigliani, MD

Introduction

Rotator cuff repair is a common surgical procedure first described by Codman in 1911.[1,2] Since his initial series reporting 67% satisfactory results, several other authors have made modifications to open rotator cuff repair techniques. McLaughlin[3-5] described the pathogenesis of rotator cuff tears and emphasized surgical principles in achieving a tension-free repair. Further modifications in technique, including the use of anterior acromioplasty, cuff mobilization, and transosseous sutures were later proposed by Neer. With current surgical techniques, good to excellent results in both functional improvement (70% to 95%) and pain relief (85% to 100%) have recently been reported.[6-20]

However, the repair of large and massive tears remains a technical challenge. There is a higher incidence of postoperative failure that is related to a number of factors. The quality of remaining tissue may be poor,[8] and significant tendon retraction, bursal scarring, and adhesions to adjacent structures often accompany massive tears.[3,8,21-27] In many instances, the evolution of mobilization techniques has allowed for reconstruction of these large defects. In addition, local tendon transposition, tendon transfers, and tissue grafting with autograft, allograft, and synthetic material have all been described as potential options in repairing or augmenting the cuff repair.[3,8,21,24,25,28-32] Overall, satisfactory results have been attained more often in studies using mobilization or transposition of existing rotator cuff tissue.[5,8] This chapter will describe the technical aspects and considerations for open repair of large and massive rotator cuff tears.

Preoperative Evaluation

Patients with large or massive rotator cuff tears frequently complain of pain. Symptoms are often chronic in nature with a nocturnal component interrupting normal sleep. The use of narcotic analgesics is common in these patients. Physical examination may reveal significant weakness in forward elevation and external rotation, accompanied by atrophy of the spinati muscles. Patients will present with a wide discrepancy between active and passive range of motion. Patients with large tears have a positive lag sign, which indicates weakness of external rotation. A positive drop sign—inability to maintain neutral rotation with the arm at the side—usually indicates a tear of the infraspinatus and teres minor. Often patients with massive tears cannot actively elevate the arm above 90° of elevation. Patients with painless weakness require an expanded differential diagnosis. It is important that neurologic lesions, including cervical radiculopathy, brachial neuritis, suprascapular neuropathy, or syringomyelia, be considered in the diagnosis. A majority of patients will have signs and symptoms of subacromial impingement as this is often a contributing factor to full-thickness rotator cuff tears.

Routine radiographic evaluation should include supraspinatus outlet, axillary, and anteroposterior views in neutral, internal, and external rotation (Fig. 1). This evaluation allows determination of acromial morphology, the presence of an acromial spur, and an estimation of the acromiohumeral interval.[31] Patients with large or massive tears have a decreased acromiohumeral distance. In our series of massive tears, the average acromiohumeral interval was 7.1 mm. Early signs of cuff tear arthropathy must be considered in patients with superior migration of the humeral head, superior glenoid wear, and erosion into the acromioclavicular joint.[34]

Additional imaging studies may be necessary in the patient who has not responded to nonsurgical treatment. Arthrography, ultrasonography, and MRI can confirm the presence of a large or massive tear. MRI is the preferred modality because information regarding tear size, tear location, and tissue quality can be more clearly elucidated[35] (Fig. 2). It is important to perform MRI studies in the scapular plane to evaluate the infraspinatus attachment as more proximal cuts to determine muscle atrophy. Axillary images are needed to evaluate the subscapularis tendon and subluxation, dislocation, or rupture of the long head of the biceps.

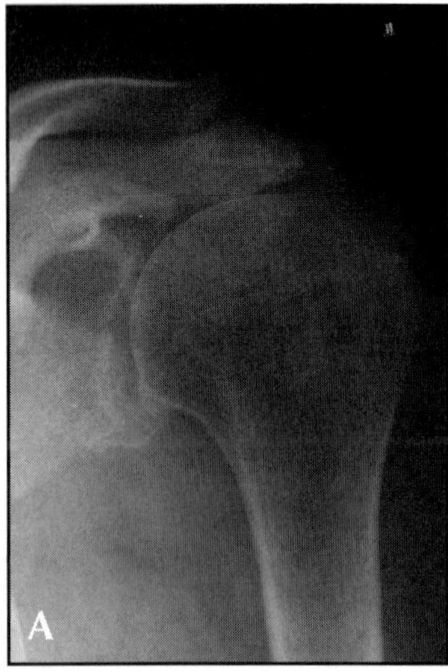
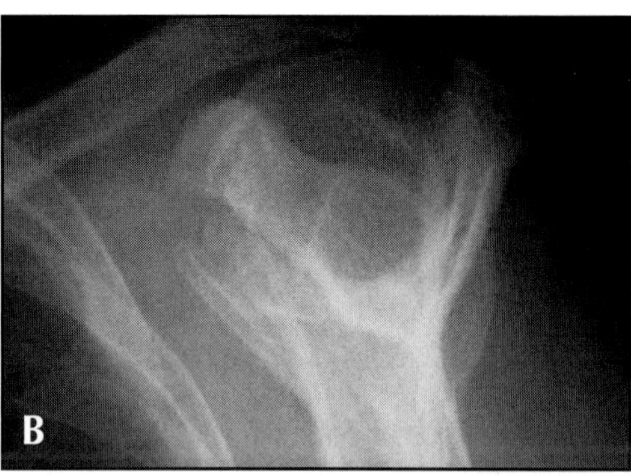

Fig. 1 A, Anteroposterior and **B,** lateral radiographs of a patient with a massive rotator cuff tear. There is proximal humeral migration and a decreased acromiohumeral interval.

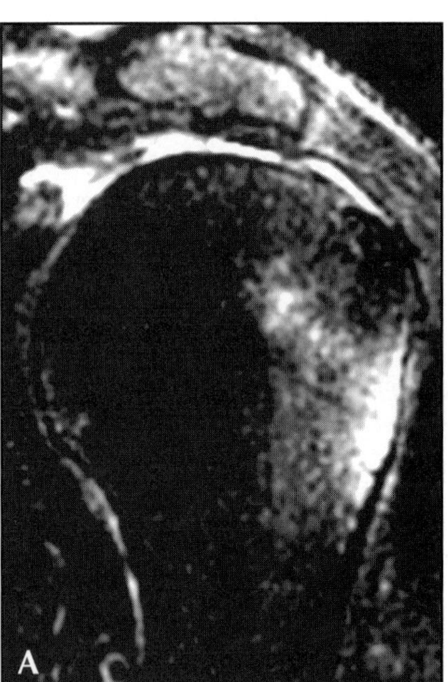
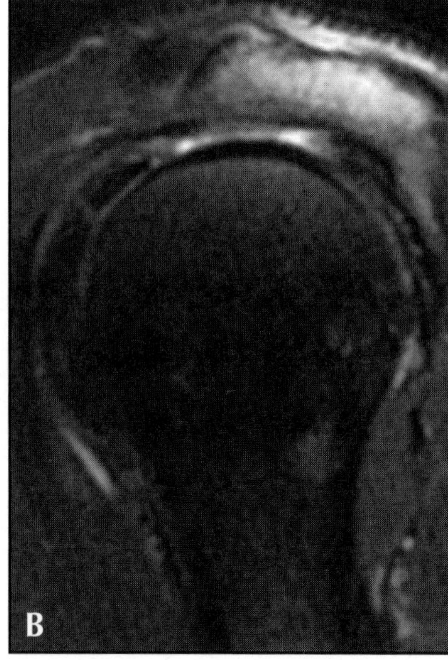

Fig. 2 A, Coronal oblique and **B,** sagittal oblique MRI studies in a patient with a massive rotator cuff tear.

Surgical Technique

Excellent results have been reported with the use of arthroscopic or combined approaches (mini-open) in the treatment of small and medium tears.[36-38] Large and massive tears, however, are managed more appropriately with open techniques. The technique of open repair has four distinct facets: the surgical approach, the decompression, the mobilization and repair, and the postoperative rehabilitation program. At our institution we have attained excellent intraoperative anesthesia and postoperative pain relief with interscalene regional anesthesia, which lasts between 8 and 9 hours.[39] This method has increased patient satisfaction and decreased postoperative pain, thus decreasing narcotic usage.

Approach

The patient is placed on the operating table in a supine position. An interscalene regional block is performed by the anesthesia team, and the patient is then placed in a modified beach chair position with the torso angled approximately 60° from the horizontal plane. The head is placed in a beach chair adapter or McConnell headrest with the neck in neutral position, which allows access to the superior and posterior aspects of the shoulder. The arm is draped free to permit full rotation, elevation, and rotation. Osseous landmarks are identified prior to incision. Antibiotics (first-generation cephalosporin or vancomycin for penicillin-allergic patients) are administered before skin incision is performed. The approach is initiated on the anterosuperior aspect of the shoulder with a 10- to 12-cm incision within Langer's lines. This approach promotes improved cosmesis with diminished potential for hypertrophic scar formation. The incision extends from the lateral aspect of the anterior acromion toward the lateral tip of the coracoid. This extensile incision allows for access to the acromioclavicular joint, the superior aspect of the subscapularis, and the posterior rotator cuff. The subcutaneous layer is divided, and needle-tip electrocautery is used to expose the superficial deltoid fascial layer. It is imperative to keep the fascial layer intact while creating full-thickness subcutaneous flaps. This allows for anatomic reconstruction of the deltoid split after cuff repair. Mobilization of the flaps is performed to allow exposure of the acromioclavicular joint, the anterolateral acromion, and the lateral deltoid in preparation for the deltoid split.

Kessel and Watson[40] initially described a transacromial or acromial-splitting approach for exposure of the rotator cuff. More recently, this approach has been advocated as an option in the management of massive tears involving the posterior cuff.[41] Satisfactory results were reported in 70% of the patients despite a 24% fibrous union rate. Complete detachment of the deltoid origin and modifications have been described as a method of obtaining unimpeded access to the rotator cuff.[42] Theoretically, these techniques can increase the possibility of deltoid origin disruption or symptomatic nonunion and should be avoided.[41,43,44] With modifications that consist of osseous detachment of the deltoid muscle, good results have been reported in 89%, and there are no complications related to deltoid function.[45] We prefer an approach that involves a deltoid split performed with electrocautery beginning 5 mm anterior to the acromioclavicular joint and extending past the anterolateral acromion. A strong, healthy cuff of tissue remains, allowing for excellent tissue reapproximation and preservation of the deltoid origin. The deltoid split is extended slightly posterior within a raphe of the middle deltoid for a distance of 3 to 4 cm past the tip of the lateral acromion, which safely avoids the axillary nerve (Fig. 3). The split is centered over the greater tuberosity to allow for improved visualization of the posterior cuff with internal rotation. Stay suture placement at the distal end of the split is performed to prevent propagation that may injure the axillary nerve. The superficial lateral bursal tissue is excised to improve visualization. The lateral aspect of the coracoacromial ligament is identified. The ligament should be removed in a subperiosteal fashion with electrocautery from the undersurface of the acromion and acromioclavicular joint and tagged so that it can be repaired back to the acromion in a more medial position after cuff repair (Fig. 4). This may aid in maintaining the "buffering" function of the coracoacromial arch and prevent anterosuperior humeral head subluxation in patients who have compromised rotator cuff function.[46,47] Exposure of the ligament and acromion can be facilitated by placing a wide, flat retractor (Darrach) inferior to the acromion, allowing the humeral head to be levered inferiorly. The entire rotator cuff can be visualized with simple maneuvering of the humerus in flexion, extension, and rotation.

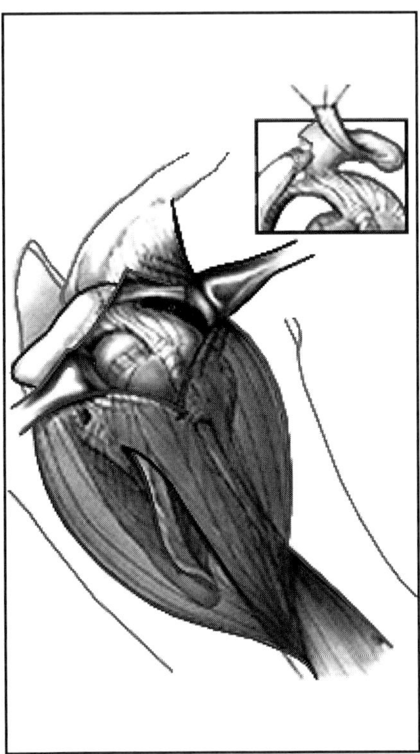

Fig. 3 Deltoid split for a distance of 3 to 4 cm. The coracoacromial ligament is preserved. (Reproduced with permission from Bigliani LU: Rotator cuff repair, in Bigliani LU, Flatow EL, Pollock RA, Post MP (eds): *The Shoulder: Operative Technique*. Baltimore, MD, Williams & Wilkins, 1998, pp 133-135.)

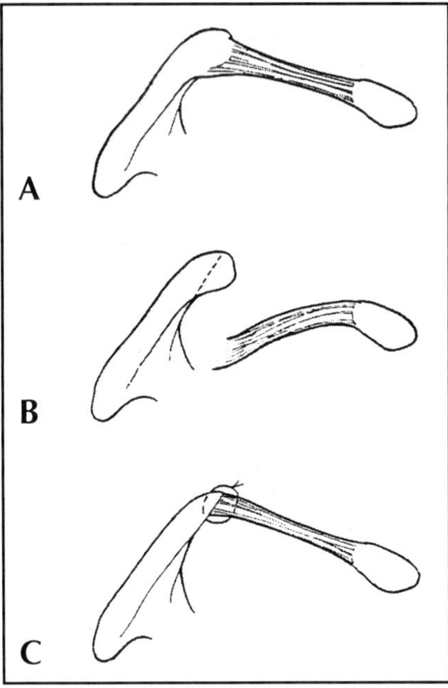

Fig. 4 Repair of the coracoacromial ligament. (Reproduced with permission from Bigliani LU: Rotator cuff repair, in Bigliani LU, Flatow EL, Pollock RA, Post MP (eds): *The Shoulder: Operative Technique*. Baltimore, MD, Williams & Wilkins, 1998, pp 133-135.)

Decompression

The etiology of subacromial impingement can involve three elements: the anterolateral coracoacromial ligament, the anteroinferior acromion, and the acromioclavicular joint.[17,18] A decompression usually includes a coracoacromial ligament release as well as an anterior acromioplasty. If the acromioclavicular joint is symptomatic, then a modified or complete acromioclavicular joint arthroplasty is indicated. Meticulous elevation of the deltoid origin is performed to expose the anterior aspect of the acromion, and adherent cuff and bursal tissue is cleared from the inferior aspect of the acromion. Prior to performing the acromioplasty, the thickness of the acromion and the presence of a spur should be assessed. A thin, sharp, beveled osteotome is then used to perform the acromioplasty, keeping the bevel directed superiorly to avoid excessive bone removal or fracture (Fig. 5). The osteotomized region should consist of the full acromial width, leaving a smooth contour on the anteroinferior acromion. A double-action ronguer, rasp, or burr can also be used when performing a modified acromioplasty. A complete acromioclavicular arthroplasty or distal clavicle resection is reserved for patients who

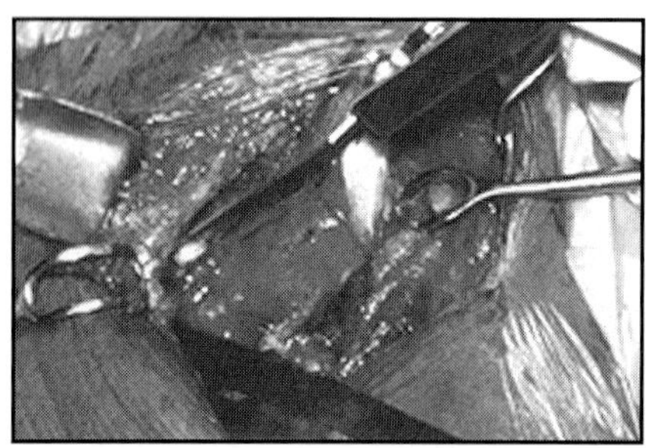

Fig. 5 A conservative acromioplasty is performed with a sharp, beveled osteotome. Prior to performing the procedure, the acromion is palpated to assess its thickness.

exhibit associated tenderness and pain with cross-body adduction during clinical examination. The resection should allow for preservation of the superior acromioclavicular ligaments, thereby maintaining anterior-posterior stability of the joint. If patients do not have tenderness but have inferior osteophytes extending inferiorly from the acromioclavicular joint, then a modified acromioclavicular arthroplasty where just the undersurface of the joint is resected should be performed.

Also, lateral or radical acromioplasty should be avoided because these procedures are often deforming in nature.[48] Radical acromionectomy weakens the deltoid by removing the fulcrum provided by the acromion. As a result, the middle deltoid can become permanently contracted. Subsequently, these patients frequently present with associated functional deficits and diminished range of motion.[49] In addition, these aggressive techniques have demonstrated an increased incidence of postoperative complications, including sinus tract formation and deltoid origin disruption.[50,51] Moreover, revision surgery becomes technically demanding with a greater opportunity for an unsatisfactory outcome.[52-56]

Bursal Resection

The subacromial bursa is bordered superiorly by the acromion and coracoacromial ligament, medially by the coracoid process, laterally by the deltoid muscle, and inferiorly by the rotator cuff tendons and the greater tuberosity.[57] The role of bursal resection in rotator cuff surgery is controversial. Many surgeons believe that the bursa is important in the healing process that leads to repair of a degenerated rotator cuff tendon.[58-60] Others routinely resect the subacromial bursa, primarily to obtain better exposure to the rotator cuff.[61] Recent studies have identified an increase in inflammatory mediators, afferent nerve endings and their products in inflamed subacromial bursa.[62-66] Often with full-thickness rotator cuff tears the bursa is thickened, inflamed, or fibrotic; therefore, resection of the bursa can reduce the pain and inflammation produced by this reactive bursal membrane. For bursal resection, the superficial inflamed and fibrotic tissue overlying the rotator cuff is grasped with a straight Adson clamp and extensive resection is performed using Mayo or Metzenbaum scissors. The distal end of the bursa may be a considerable distance from the edge of the acromion. Care should be taken to avoid resection of the rotator cuff tendons, which often are tightly adhered to the fibrotic bursal tissue. The thick fibrotic bursa will lead to the edge of rotator cuff tendon that can be differentiated by identifying the capsule on the deep articular side of the cuff.

Assessment of Tear

After subacromial decompression and bursal resection, the size of the tendon defect is determined by several parameters. The width of the tear at its insertion to the greater tuberosity can be measured as well as its greatest diameter in any direction. Small tears are less than 1 cm in width; medium tears are 1 to 3 cm; large tears 3 to 5 cm, and massive tears greater than 5 cm in width.[67] The tear can also be characterized by the number of tendons involved. Large and massive tears typically involve two or more tendons. This technique of classification, however, may be unreliable because of confluence of the tendons at their insertion into the greater tuberosity.[68]

The presence of associated pathology should also be noted. In a review of 200 shoulder arthroscopies for patients with full-thickness tears, 60.5% had associated intra-articular pathology, including 15% biceps tendon lesions. However, only three of these (1.5%) were considered major lesions that required surgical intervention.[69] A low incidence of biceps tendon pathology in association with rotator cuff tears was noted, with only 33 subluxations or dislocations at a tertiary referral center over a 9-year period. If a biceps tear is present, a subscapularis tear should be suspected. Some authors have argued that the biceps tendon has a humeral head depressing function and should be preserved in patients with massive rotator cuff tears.[70] These recommendations have been questioned by a more recent study examining biceps activity using electromyography, where biceps activity remained low (1.6%-4.4% maximum muscle contraction), even in the setting of a rotator cuff tear.[71] We recommend biceps tenodesis in conjunction with rotator cuff repair if greater than 50% of the biceps tendon is involved or significant dislocation is present. We do not advocate biceps transection, posterior transposition, tenodesis of the distal part, or using the proximal part as a substitute for a deficient rotator cuff. On rare occasions the biceps can be sutured in situ into the cuff repair to achieve continuity.

Cuff Mobilization

The first step in cuff mobilization is to identify the leading edge of the torn rotator cuff tendons anteriorly, superiorly, and posteriorly. It is helpful to tag the edges of the tendons with nonabsorbable sutures. The Gerber retractor may be used for better visualization during cuff mobilization. The rotator

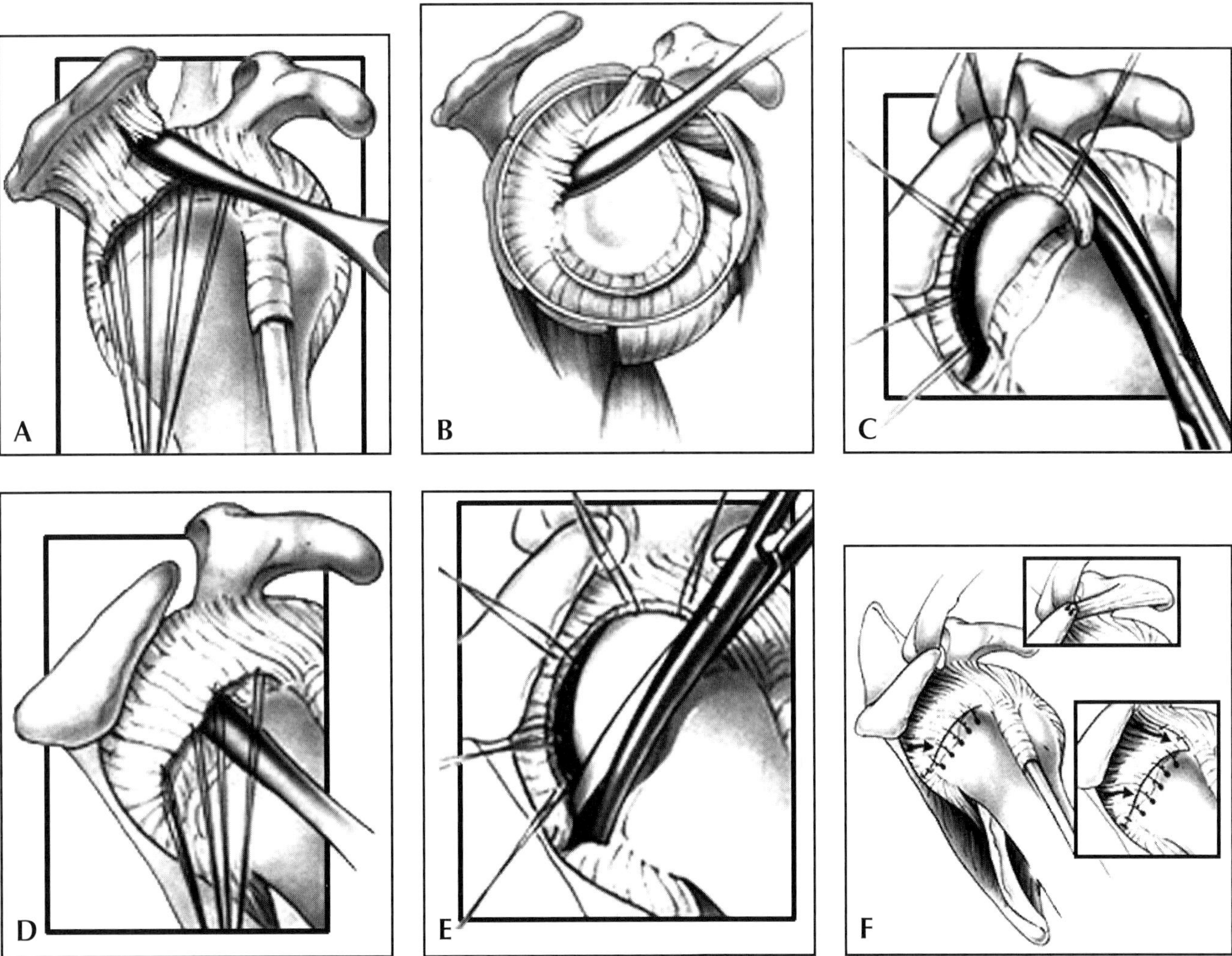

Fig. 6 Cuff mobilization. **A**, The adherent rotator cuff is elevated from the undersurface of the acromion. **B,** The rotator cuff is released from the glenoid rim with an elevator. **C**, Interval slide. The rotator interval and coracohumeral ligament are incised to the coracoid base. **D** and **E,** The tendon is mobilized posteriorly using blunt and sharp dissection. **F**, The rotator cuff is mobilized to the tuberosity. Simple transosseous sutures secure a tension-free repair. (Reproduced with permission from Bigliani LU: Rotator cuff repair, in Bigliani LU, Flatow EL, Pollock RA, Post MP (eds): *The Shoulder: Operative Technique*. Baltimore, MD, Williams & Wilkins, 1998, pp 133-135.)

cuff is released from any subacromial adhesions by sweeping a periosteal elevator in the subacromial space (Fig. 6, *A*). Sharp dissection may be performed when needed with Mayo scissors, and dissection is continued around anteriorly over the subscapularis tendon and beneath the coracoid. Often the leading edge of the torn rotator cuff is stuck up under the acromion or more laterally under the origin of the deltoid muscle as it leaves the acromion. The edge of tendon is closely adherent and gives an impression that there is no rotator cuff tissue. However, soft tissue can be palpated and with sharp dissection the leading edge of tendon can be liberated and then mobilized. Posterolateral adhesions between the rotator cuff and deltoid in the lateral gutter should also be addressed.[72]

Dissection is then performed on the articular side of the remaining rotator cuff tendons to free any attachments to the glenoid rim (Fig. 6, *B*). This is accomplished with a combination of both blunt and sharp dissection. Blunt dissection should be performed initially and if sharp dissection is required, great care should be taken with posterior dissection to avoid injury to the suprascapular nerve.[73] In a previous study on dissection of the suprascapular nerve in 90 cadavers, the suprascapular nerve was on average between 2.5 and 3 cm medial to the glenoid rim.[74] Therefore, a relative safe zone for dissection in the posterosuperior aspect of the glenoid is within 2 cm of the glenoid rim. A Gerber retractor may be used during posterior cuff mobilization to improve visualization. This retractor increases the acromiohumeral distance by depressing the humeral head.

Often, the coracohumeral ligament and the anteromedial portion of the supraspinatus tendon is retracted and scarred down to the base of the coracoid. In this case, an interval slide—a complete longitudinal release of the rotator interval and coracohumeral ligament to the superior aspect of the coracoid—may be performed (Fig. 6, *C*). In an anatomic study of the coracohumeral ligament and its insertions present in 55 cadavers, 14 (25%) inserted into the supraspinatus tendon, and 16 (29%) had a secondary slip of insertion to the subscapularis tendon in addition to the usual insertion in the rotator interval.[75] We have found that release of the coracohumeral ligament from its origin at the base of the coracoid allows an additional excursion of the supraspinatus tendon of 1 to 1.5 cm. This technique has also obviated the need for subscapularis transfer in most cases. The coracohumeral ligament is released at its origin from the coracoid process using Mayo scissors and electrocautery. Dissection should not be performed medial to the coracoid because of the risk of injury to the musculocutaneous nerve and axillary vessels.

Often, there is differential retraction of the rotator cuff tendons.[76] If the supraspinatus is retracted more medially than the subscapularis, dividing the rotator interval can free the supraspinatus from its contracture to the subscapularis, allowing advancement to its insertion at the tuberosity. Differential retraction can also occur posteriorly between the supraspinatus and infraspinatus tendons. A similar interval release can be performed between these tendons to allow supraspinatus advancement. This can also be performed by both sharp and blunt dissection (Fig. 6, *D* and *E*). We prefer spreading gently with scissors rather than cutting with a knife when visualization is less than optimal. An alternative technique of supraspinatus advancement has previously been described by Debyre and others which involves elevating the muscle from its scapular origin.[25,26] This technique should be avoided as it will significantly weaken the muscle and tendon.

Subscapularis tendon transfer has also been advocated in cases of massive tears.[24] We have performed transfer of the upper one third of the tendon in severe cases but have been dissatisfied with the results. In 1994, Burkhart and associates[77] demonstrated that this transfer may lead to superior migration of the humeral head by destabilizing force couples. We prefer partial repair over transfer of the subscapularis tendon, as even partial transfer of an intact subscapularis may further destabilize the shoulder and adversely affect active motion.

The mobility of the remaining cuff tendons must be assessed following release. To achieve satisfactory repair, the tendons should extend past the anatomic neck of the humerus with the arm in a functional position. In the beach chair position, the arm is in relative extension, which puts great stress across the rotator cuff. Placing the arm in the functional position of approximately 10° to 15° of forward flexion, abduction, and internal rotation will facilitate repair. If interval slides have been performed as described, tendons should be repaired first to the tuberosity, followed by interval closure with nonabsorbable sutures.

Preparation of Tendon and Bone

Once the tendon has been mobilized adequately and traction sutures placed in the tendon ends, attention is turned to performing a tension-free tendon to bone repair. Débridement of the tendon edges to healthy bleeding tissue has been proposed by several authors.[78] More recent studies using laser Doppler flowmetry in patients with rotator cuff tears have demonstrated that the tendon edges are well vascularized.[79] Furthermore, Uhthoff and associates[80] have demonstrated healthy granulation tissue present over the tendon edges indicating a neovascular response. We believe that maximum tendon length should be maintained and therefore do not recommend routine débridement of the tendon edges.

Once the rotator cuff tendons have been successfully mobilized to reach the greater tuberosity of the humerus, the bone must be prepared for tendon insertion. We do not recommend making a bony trough because this will increase the distance of tendon excursion and may create a sharp edge of bone over which the tendon has to pass. It is important to have bleeding bone adjacent to the anatomic neck of the humerus to promote healing from tendon to bone. However, recent studies have demonstrated that the healing of rotator cuff tendons to cortical bone is comparable to healing in a cancellous bony trough.[81] Therefore, we perform only minimal débridement of the cortical bone on the superficial aspect of the greater tuberosity using a scalpel blade, rongeur, or burr. The tendon should be advanced to the proximal aspect of the greater tuberosity past the anatomic neck.

Sutures and Suture Anchors

McLaughlin[4] emphasized in his early work that the primary concern in rotator cuff repair is to obtain tension-free apposition of tendon to bone. Because the humeral head is spherical, there is obligatory rotation with movement; and preliminary data reveal that stress and strain occur in oblique directions and not in a straight line. Therefore, despite the importance placed on the concept of suture and suture anchor pullout strength, it is important to emphasize that minimal tissue tension in all directions is critical to successful rotator cuff repair. Great care should be taken to ensure that excessive stress is not placed on the repair until adequate healing has occurred.

Multiple studies have been performed to determine the strength of transosseous versus suture anchors in rotator cuff repair. A transosseous suture technique is preferred, unless the bone stock is insufficient to provide a reasonable bone tunnel. Studies have shown that suture pullout strength is increased by placing the transosseous sutures in the hard bone distal to the tuberosity and by using a wide bridge of bone.[82] A 1- to 1.5-cm bridge is preferred between the medial and lateral drill holes with the lateral hole exiting in the hard cortical bone distal to the tip of the tuberosity. Holes are connected and enlarged using a small curette to allow passage of nonabsorbable sutures with a medium-sized Mayo needle. Simple sutures are used, because the mechanical strength of mattress sutures have been demonstrated to be inferior.[83] Other investigators have also recommended augmenting the insertion site with a plastic or metal button.[82,84,85] Suture fixation with transosseous bone tunnels has been found to be adequate in most cases.

Once the bone tunnels are made, 0 to #1 braided nylon sutures are passed through the holes. A larger caliber of suture is not necessary, as failure is typically noted at the knot of the suture or at the bony insertion.[83] Larger sutures may also promote excess scar formation or direct impingement of the knot underneath the acromion. Sutures are then passed through the tendon, grasping at least 1 cm of tissue. Because of the concern that Mason Allen sutures do not slide or allow slack and may lead to suture breakage, we typically use simple sutures for repair. However, in compromised tendon tissue, a modified Mason Allen stitch may be used for better grasping power.[86] The Mason-Allen stitch is a locking stitch where the transverse suture limb is placed perpendicular to the tendon fibers in the tendon edge. The vertical limb of the suture then loops behind the transverse limb, allowing the suture to grasp both the tendon and the transverse suture limb for improved holding power. Although any locking suture configuration may be used to improve grasping power in the compromised tendon (such as the Krackow or Bunnell stitch), the Mason-Allen stitch has been found to be the simplest and most effective when it is required. The arm is then held in 10° to 15° of flexion and 10° of abduction with slight internal rotation while the sutures are tied. The anterior and posterior tendon to bone stitches are tied first and then the middle sutures. It is important to tie the knots on top of the tendon to create superior compression. The knot can also be advanced distally over the tuberosity to avoid impingement. The longitudinal component of the tear may then be closed side to side, followed by the lateral portion of the rotator interval (Fig. 6, *E*).

Multiple studies have examined the pullout strength of suture anchors and compared them to the transosseous technique. One study has demonstrated improved anchor strength over transosseous sutures, although the transosseous technique for this study used only an 8 mm bony bridge and horizontal mattress sutures, which have been shown to be inadequate in other studies.[87] A second study comparing four different suture anchors with the transosseous technique found comparable results in all techniques, with the exception of one anchor that was found to be inferior.[88] The transosseous technique is preferred because it is both less expensive and does not pose the risk of hardware migration that suture anchors present.[89] We are not opposed to the use of suture anchors, however, especially as newer bioabsorbable anchors that do not have the risks of retained hardware become available.

Deficient Rotator Cuff

Many procedures have also been proposed to augment a deficient rotator cuff. Although rotator cuff débridement alone for "irreparable tears"[90] caused by the disastrous complication of anterosuperior humeral head migration is not advised,[91] the routine use of allografts or synthetic grafts in this setting is not advocated.[29,30] Instead, partial repair of the rotator cuff has been used successfully. Burkhart and associates[22] initially described this technique in 14 patients with "irreparable" rotator cuff tears, with the goal of restoring force couples and converting the defect to a "functional cuff tear." Complete coverage of the defect was not essential, and average residual defect size measured 2.9 cm^2. With this technique, forward elevation improved from 59.6° preoperatively to 150.4° postoperatively, and only one patient had a poor result according to the UCLA score. We have had success using a modification of this partial repair technique, leaving the posterolateral aspect of the head uncovered.

If a partial repair is not adequate, transfer of either the latissimus dorsi or teres major in cases of posterior cuff deficiency or pectoralis major transfer in the absence of a subscapularis tendon has been performed.[32] With the tendon mobilization techniques described here as well as partial repair proposed by Burkhart, we have seldom had to use tendon transfer procedures.

As mentioned previously, in large to massive tears, the coracoacromial ligament is reattached in a more medial position to provide improved anterosuperior stability.[46,47] Firm reattachment is performed with 0 or No. 1 nonabsorbable sutures with transosseous sutures placed through the acromion.

Deltoid Reattachment and Closure

Deltoid reattachment is a critical component of rotator cuff repair. In a study of 31 patients undergoing surgical treatment for failed rotator cuff repair, poor results were associated with previous lateral acromionectomy or deltoid detachment.[52] In another study, there was a 48% incidence of prior deltoid detachment or lateral acromionectomy in those patients

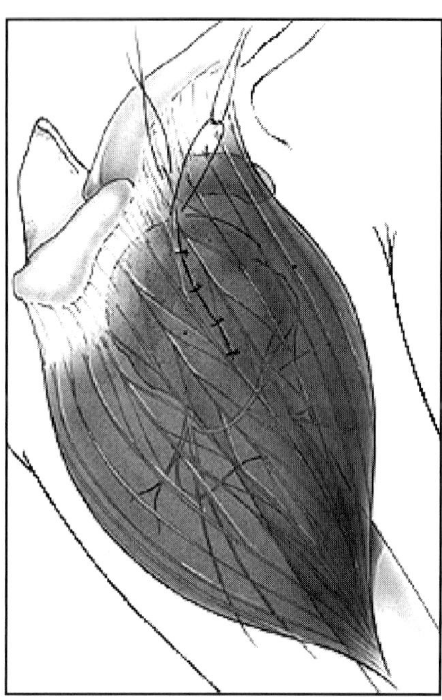

Fig. 7 Meticulous deltoid repair to the cuff of tissue at the anterior acromial edge using nonabsorbable sutures is shown.

presenting for a second rotator cuff repair.[55] For deltoid reapproximation, we repair the longitudinal deltoid split with nonabsorbable sutures in a simple fashion. The anterior portion of the deltoid fascia is then reapproximated to the cuff or soft tissue origin on the acromion with 0 or No. 1 nonabsorbable sutures (Fig. 7). Drill holes through bone are used only if the deltoid tissue is adequate to hold the sutures. Absorbable sutures are then placed in the subcutaneous tissue, followed by a running subcuticular monocryl stitch for the skin closure.

Rehabilitation

The rehabilitation begins with passive-assisted range of motion exercises on the first postoperative day. Patients with large or massive tears undergo a modified Neer phase I protocol for 6 weeks that includes pendulum exercises, passive-assisted forward elevation to 140°, and passive-assisted external rotation (while supine) to 30°. Pulley exercises are avoided for the first 6 weeks in order to protect the cuff repair. Strengthening with isometric exercises is also initiated at 6 weeks, accompanied by active-assisted range of motion. Use of weights is avoided for at least 3 months in the rehabilitation period to avoid re-tear of the cuff. Early use of weights has been reported to cause cuff failure.[19,43] However, resistance exercises with light weights (1 to 3 lb) can be initiated at 12 weeks, progressing to dynamic strengthening exercises at 6 to 8 months. Patients should be aware that full return of strength may take as long as 12 to 18 months.[8]

Results

With these techniques, long-term results for repair of large and massive rotator cuff tears have been excellent. In a 7-year average follow-up study of 61 patients who underwent repair of massive rotator cuff tears, 85% excellent or satisfactory results were achieved by Neer's criteria.[8] Ninety-two percent of patients had adequate pain relief and the ability to raise the arm above the horizontal position. Only two re-tears occurred, and these were secondary to significant trauma. In a more recent study at the New York Orthopaedic Hospital of 231 shoulder massive rotator cuff tears there were 90% satisfactory results with primary rotator cuff repair. Function was improved postoperatively, with average active forward elevation 160°, external rotation 55°, and internal rotation to T-9. This represented an average improvement of 46° elevation, 22° external rotation, and internal rotation of two vertebral levels. External rotation power was improved from an average of 3.1 to 4.7. Satisfactory results were slightly less (76.5%) in patients with four-tendon involvement. These results support the role of open primary rotator cuff repair for patients with large to massive rotator cuff tears.

Summary

With current surgical techniques, open rotator cuff repair can provide significant functional improvement and pain relief in the majority of patients. Important principles include performing anterior acromioplasty, bursal resection, rotator cuff mobilization, tension-free repair to the greater tuberosity with nonabsorbable sutures, and meticulous deltoid repair. In massive rotator cuff tears, the coracoacromial ligament should be repaired to prevent anterosuperior instability, and partial repair of the rotator cuff is recommended over performing transfer procedures. Postoperative rehabilitation requires the patient to avoid active exercises for 6 weeks and weights for 3 months. With these techniques, 85% to 90% satisfactory results can be expected.

References

1. Codman EA: Complete rupture of the supraspinatus tendon: Operative treatment with report of two successful cases. *Boston Med Surg J* 1911;164:708-710.
2. Codman EA (ed): *The Shoulder: Rupture of the Supraspinatus Tendon and Other Lesions In or About the Subacromial Bursa*. Boston, MA, Thomas Todd, 1934.
3. McLaughlin HL: Lesions of the musculotendinous cuff of the shoulder: I. The exposure and treatment of tears with retraction. *J Bone Joint Surg Am* 1944;26:31-51.
4. McLaughlin HL: Repair of major cuff ruptures. *Surg Clin North Am* 1963;43:1535-1540.
5. McLaughlin HL, Asherman EG: Lesions of the musculotendinous cuff of the shoulder: IV. Some observations based upon the results of surgical repair. *J Bone Joint Surg Am* 1951;33:76-86.
6. Cofield RH: Rotator cuff disease of the shoulder. *J Bone Joint Surg Am* 1985;67:974-979.
7. Ellman H, Hanker G, Bayer M: Repair of the rotator cuff: End-result study of factors influencing reconstruction. *J Bone Joint Surg Am* 1986;68:1136-1144.
8. Bigliani LU, Cordasco FA, McIlveen SJ, et al: Operative treatment of massive cuff tears: Long term results. *J Shoulder Elbow Surg* 1992;1:120-130.
9. Rokito AS, Cuomo F, Gallagher MA, Zuckerman JD: Long-term functional outcome of repair of large and massive chronic tears of the rotator cuff. *J Bone Joint Surg Am* 1999;81:991-997.

10. Gupta R, Leggin BG, Iannotti JP: Results of surgical repair of full-thickness tears of the rotator cuff. *Orthop Clin North Am* 1997;28: 241-248.

11. Iannotti JP, Bernot MP, Kuhlman JR; Kelley MJ; Williams GR: Postoperative assessment of shoulder function: A prospective study of full-thickness rotator cuff tears. *J Shoulder Elbow Surg* 1996;5:449-457.

12. Iannotti JP: Full-thickness rotator cuff tears: Factors affecting surgical outcome. *J Am Acad Orthop Surg* 1994;2:87-95.

13. Worland RL, Arredondo J, Angles F, Lopez-Jimenez F: Repair of massive rotator cuff tears in patients older than 70 years. *J Shoulder Elbow Surg* 1999;8:26-30.

14. Adamson GJ, Tibone JE: Ten-year assessment of primary rotator cuff repairs. *J Shoulder Elbow Surg* 1993;2:57-63.

15. Bassett RW, Cofield RH: Acute tears of the rotator cuff: The timing of surgical repair. *Clin Orthop* 1983;175:18-24.

16. Misamore GW, Ziegler DW, Rushton JL II: Repair of the rotator cuff: A comparison of results in two populations of patients. *J Bone Joint Surg Am* 1995;77:1335-1339.

17. Neer CS II: Impingement lesions. *Clin Orthop* 1983;173:70-77.

18. Neer CS II, Flatow EL, Lech O: Tears of the rotator cuff: Long-term results of anterior acromioplasty and repair. *Orthop Trans* 1988;12:673-674.

19. Packer NP, Calvert PT, Bayley JI, Kessel L: Operative treatment of chronic ruptures of the rotator cuff of the shoulder. *J Bone Joint Surg Br* 1983;65:171-175.

20. Pollock RG, Black AD, Self EB, Flatow EL, Bigliani LU: Abstract: Surgical management of rotator cuff disease. *J Shoulder Elbow Surg* 1996;5:S37.

21. Bateman JE: The diagnosis and treatment of ruptures of the rotator cuff. *Surg Clin North Am* 1963;43:1523-1530.

22. Burkhart SS, Nottage WM, Ogilvie-Harris DJ, Kohn HS, Pachelli A: Partial repair of irreparable rotator cuff tears. *Arthroscopy* 1994;10: 363-370.

23. Bush LF: The torn shoulder capsule. *J Bone Joint Surg Am* 1975;57:256-259.

24. Cofield RH: Subscapular muscle transoposition for repair of chronic rotator cuff tears. *Surg Gynecol Obstet* 1982;154:667-672.

25. Debyre J, Patte D, Elmelik E: Repair of ruptures of the rotator cuff of the shoulder: With a note on advancement of the supraspinatus muscle. *J Bone Joint Surg Br* 1965;47:36-42.

26. Ha'eri GB, Wiley AM: Advancement of the surpraspinatus muscle in the repair of ruptures of the rotator cuff. *J Bone Joint Surg Am* 1981;63:232-238.

27. Neviaser JS: Ruptures of the rotator cuff of the shoulder: New concepts in the diagnosis and operative treatment of chronic ruptures. *Arch Surg* 1971;102:483-485.

28. Neviaser RJ, Neviaser TJ: Transfer of subscapularis and teres minor for massive defects of the rotator cuff, in Bayley I, Kessel L (eds): *Shoulder Surgery*. Berlin, Germany, Springer-Verlag, 1982, pp 60-63.

29. Neviaser JS, Neviaser RJ, Neviaser TJ: The repair of chronic massive ruptures of the rotator cuff of the shoulder by use of a freeze-dried rotator cuff. *J Bone Joint Surg Am* 1978;60: 681-684.

30. Ozaki J, Fujimoto S, Masuhara K, Tamai S, Yoshimoto S: Reconstruction of chronic massive rotator cuff tears with synthetic materials. *Clin Orthop* 1986;202:173-183.

31. Karas SE, Giachello TL: Subscapularis transfer for reconstruction of massive tears of the rotator cuff. *J Bone Joint Surg Am* 1996;78:239-245.

32. Gerber C, Vinh TS, Hertel R, Hess CW: Latissimus dorsi transfer for the treatment of massive tears of the rotator cuff: A preliminary report. *Clin Orthop* 1988;232:51-61.

33. Weiner DS, Macnab I: Superior migration of the humeral head: A radiological aid in the diagnosis of the rotator cuff. *J Bone Joint Surg Br* 1970;52:524-527.

34. Neer CS II, Craig EV, Fukuda H: Cuff-tear arthropathy. *J Bone Joint Surg Am* 1983;65: 1232-1244.

35. Tirman PF, Steinbach LS, Belzer JP, Bost FW: A practical approach to imaging of the shoulder with emphasis on MR imaging. *Orthop Clin North Am* 1997;28:483-515.

36. Gartsman GM, Hammerman SM: Full-thickness tears: Arthroscopic repair. *Orthop Clin North Am* 1997;28:83-98.

37. Weber SC: Abstract: All arthroscopic versus mini-open repair in the management of complete tears of the rotator cuff. *Arthroscopy* 1997; 13:398.

38. Pollock RG, Flatow EL: The rotator cuff: Full-thickness tears: Mini-open repair. *Orthop Clin North Am* 1997;28:169-177.

39. Brown AR, Weiss R, Greenberg C, Flatow EL, Bigliani LU: Interscalene block for shoulder arthroscopy: Comparison with general anesthesia. *Arthroscopy* 1993;9:295-300.

40. Kessel L, Watson M: The painful arc syndrome: Clinical classification as a guide to management. *J Bone Joint Surg Br* 1977;59:166-172.

41. Paulos LE, Meislin RJ, Drawbert J: The acrominon- splitting approach for large and massive rotator cuff tears. *Am J Sports Med* 1994;22:306-312.

42. Cubbins WR, Callahan JJ, Scuderi CS: The reduction of old or irreducible dislocations of the shoulder joint. *Surg Gynecol Obstet* 1934;58:129-135.

43. Neviaser RJ, Neviaser TJ: Reoperation for failed rotator cuff repair: Analysis of fifty cases. *J Shoulder Elbow Surg* 1992;1:283-286.

44. Sher SJ, Iannotti JP, Warner JJ, Groff Y, Williams GR: Surgical treatment of postoperative deltoid origin disruption. *Clin Orthop* 1997;343:93-98.

45. Habernek H, Weinstabl R, Schabus R, Schmid L: A new approach to the subacromial space: Technique and 2-year results in 28 rotator-cuff repair cases. *Acta Orthop Scand* 1993;64:92-94.

46. Flatow EL, Weinstein DM, Duralde XA, Compito CA, Pollock RG, Bigliani LU: Abstract: Coracoacromial ligament preservation in rotator cuff surgery. *J Shoulder Elbow Surg* 1994;3:S73.

47. Flatow EL, Connor PM, Levine WN, Arroyo JS, Pollock RG, Bigliani LU: Abstract: Coracoacromial arch reconstruction for antero-superior subluxation after failed rotator cuff surgery: A preliminary report. *J Shoulder Elbow Surg* 1997;6:228.

48. Neer CS II, Marberry TA: On the disadvantages of radical acromionectomy. *J Bone Joint Surg Am* 1981;63:416-419.

49. Bigliani LU, Steinmann S, Flatow EL, et al: Complications, in Iannotti JP (ed): *Rotator Cuff Disorders: Evaluation and Treatment*. Park Ridge, IL, American Academy of Orthopaedic Surgeons, 1991, pp 63-74.

50. Hammond G: Complete acromionectomy in the treatment of chronic tendinitis of the shoulder: A follow-up of ninety operations on eighty-seven patients. *J Bone Joint Surg Am* 1971;53:173-180.

51. Groh GI, Simoni M, Rolla P, Rockwood CA: Loss of the deltoid after shoulder operations: An operative disaster. *J Shoulder Elbow Surg* 1994;3:243-253.

52. Bigliani LU, Cordasco FA, McIlveen SJ, Musso ES: Operative treatment of failed repairs of the rotator cuff. *J Bone Joint Surg Am* 1992;74: 1505-1515.

53. Wolfgang GL: Surgical repair of tears of the rotator cuff of the shoulder: Factors influencing the result. *J Bone Joint Surg Am* 1974;56: 14-26.

54. Cordasco FA, Bigliani LU: The treatment of failed rotator cuff repairs. *Instr Course Lect* 1998; 47:77-86.

55. DeOrio JK, Cofield RH: Results of a second attempt at surgical repair of a failed initial rotator-cuff repair. *J Bone Joint Surg Am* 1984;66:563-567.

56. Neviaser RJ: Evaluation and management of failed rotator cuff repairs. *Orthop Clin North Am* 1997;28:215-224.

57. Strizak AM, Danzig L, Jackson DW, Resnick D, Staple T: Subacromial bursography: An anatomical and clinical study. *J Bone Joint Surg Am* 1982;64:196-201.

58. Rahme H, Nordgren H, Hamberg H, Westerberg CE: The subacromial bursa and the impingement syndrome: A clinical and histological study of 30 cases. *Acta Orthop Scand* 1993;64:485-488.

59. Ishii H, Brunet JA, Welsh RP, Uhthoff HK: 'Bursal reactions' in rotator cuff tearing, the impingement syndrome, and calcifying tendinitis. *J Shoulder Elbow Surg* 1997;6:131-136.

60. Uhthoff HK, Sarkar K: Surgical repair of rotator cuff ruptures: The importance of the subacromial bursa. *J Bone Joint Surg Br* 1991;73:399-401.

61. Gerber C: Massive rotator cuff tears, in Iannotti JP, Williams GR Jr (eds): *Disorders of the Shoulder: Diagnosis and Management.* Philadelphia, PA, Lippincott-Williams & Wilkins, 1999, pp 57-92.

62. Soifer TB, Levy H, Soifer FM, Kleinbart F, Vigorita V, Bryk E: Neurohistology of the subacromial space. *Arthroscopy* 1996;12:182-186.

63. Gotoh M, Hamada K, Yamakawa H, Inoue A, Fukuda H: Increased substance P in subacromial bursa and shoulder pain in rotator cuff diseases. *J Orthop Res* 1998;16:618-621.

64. Gotoh M, Hamada K, Yamakawa H, et al: Increased interleukin-1 beta production in the synovium of glenohumeral joints with anterior instability. *J Orthop Res* 1999;17:392-397.

65. Rodeo SA, Hannafin JA, Tom J, Warren RF, Wickiewicz TL: Immunolocalization of cytokines and their receptors in adhesive capsulitis of the shoulder. *J Orthop Res* 1997,15:427-436.

66. Stone D, Green C, Rao U, et al: Cytokine-induced tendinitis: A preliminary study in rabbits. *J Orthop Res* 1999;17:168-177.

67. Post M, Silver R, Singh M: Rotator cuff tear: Diagnosis and treatment. *Clin Orthop* 1983;173: 78-91.

68. Clark JM, Harryman DT II: Tendons, ligaments, and capsule of the rotator cuff: Gross and microscopic anatomy. *J Bone Joint Surg Am* 1992;74:713-725.

69. Gartsman GM, Taverna E: The incidence of glenohueral joint abnormalities associated with full-thickness, reparable rotator cuff tears. *Arthroscopy*. 1997;13:450-455.

70. Kumar VP, Satka K, Balasubralmaniam P: The role of the long head of biceps brachii in the stabilization of the head of the humerus. *Clin Orthop* 1989;244:172-175.

71. Yamaguchi K, Riew KD, Galatz LM, Syme JA, Neviaser RJ: Biceps activity during shoulder motion: An electromyographic analysis. *Clin Orthop* 1997;336:122-129.

72. Cordasco FA, Bigliani LU: The rotator cuff: Large and massive tears: Technique of open repair. *Orthop Clin North Am* 1997;28:179-193.

73. Warner JP, Krushell RJ, Masquelet A, Gerber C: Anatomy and relationships of the suprascapular nerve: Anatomical constraints to mobilization of the supraspinatus and infraspinatus muscles in the management of massive rotator-cuff tears. *J Bone Joint Surg Am* 1992;74:36-45.

74. Bigliani LU, Dalsey RM, McCann PD, April EW: An anatomical study of the suprascapular nerve. *Arthroscopy* 1990;6:301-305.

75. Neer CS II, Satterlee CC, Dalsey RM, Flatow EL: The anatomy and potential effects of contracture of the coracohumeral ligament. *Clin Orthop* 1992;280:182-185.

76. Codd TP, Flatow EL: Anterior acromioplasty, tendon mobilization, and direct repair of massive rotator cuff tears, in Burkhead WZ Jr (ed): *Rotator Cuff Disorders.* Baltimore, MD, Williams & Wilkins, 1996, pp 323-334.

77. Burkart SS, Nottage WM, Ogilvie-Harris DJ, Kohn HS, Pachelli A: Partial repair of irreparable rotator cuff tears. *Arthroscopy* 1994;10: 363-370.

78. Rathbun JB, Macnab I: The microvascular pattern of the rotator cuff. *J Bone Joint Surg Br* 1970;52:540-553.

79. Swiontkowski MF, Iannotti JP, Boulas HJ, Esterhai JL: Intraoperative assessment of rotator cuff vascularity using Laser Doppler Flowmetry, in Post M, Morrey BF, Hawkins RJ (eds): *Surgery of the Shoulder.* St. Louis, MO, Mosby-Year Book, 1990; pp 208-212.

80. Uhthoff HK, Sarkar K, Lohr J: Repair in rotator cuff tendons, in Post M, Morrey BF, Hawkins RJ (eds): *Surgery of the Shoulder.* St. Louis, MO, Mosby-Year Book, 1990, pp 216-219.

81. St Pierre P, Olson EJ, Elliott JJ, O'Hair KC, McKinney LA, Ryan J: Tendon-healing to cortical bone compared with healing to a cancellous trough: A biomechanical and histological evaluation in goats. *J Bone Joint Surg Am* 1995;77:1858-1866.

82. Caldwell GL, Warner JP, Miller MD, Boardman D, Towers J, Debski R: Strength of fixation with transosseous sutures in rotator cuff repair. *J Bone Joint Surg Am* 1997;79: 1064-1068.

83. Burkhart SS, Fischer SP, Nottage WM, et al: Tissue fixation security in transosseous rotator cuff repairs: A mechanical comparison of simple versus mattress sutures. *Arthroscopy* 1996; 12:704-708.

84. Burkhart SS, Johnson TC, Wirth MA, Athanasiou KA: Cyclic loading of transosseous rotator cuff repairs: Tension overload as a possible cause of failure. *Arthroscopy* 1997;13: 172-176.

85. Sward L, Hughes JS, Amis A, Wallace WA: The strength of surgical repairs of the rotator cuff: A biomechanical study on cadavers. *J Bone Joint Surg Br* 1992;74:585-588.

86. Gerber C, Schneeberger AG, Beck M, Schlegel U: Mechanical strength of repairs of the rotator cuff. *J Bone Joint Surg* Br 1994;76:371-380.

87. Reed SC, Glossop N, Ogilvie-Harris DJ: Full-thickness rotator cuff tears: A biomechanical comparison of suture versus bone anchor techniques. *Am J Sports Med* 1996;24:46-48.

88. Craft DV, Moseley JB, Cawley PW, Noble PC: Fixation strength of rotator cuff repairs with suture anchors and the transosseous suture technique. *J Shoulder Elbow Surg* 1996;5:32-40.

89. Zuckerman JD, Matsen FA III: Complications about the glenohumeral joint related to the use of screws and staples. *J Bone Joint Surg Am* 1984;66:175-180.

90. Rockwood CA Jr, Williams GR Jr, Burkhead WZ Jr: Debridement of degenerative, irreparable lesions of the rotator cuff. *J Bone Joint Surg Am* 1995;77:857-866.

91. Wiley AM: Superior humeral dislocation: A complication following decompression and debridement for rotator cuff tears. *Clin Orthop* 1991;263:135-141.

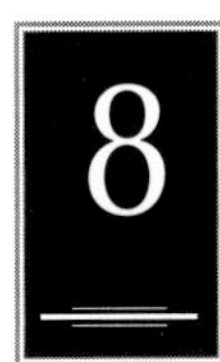

Management of Massive Irreparable Rotator Cuff Tears: The Role of Tendon Transfer

Jon J.P. Warner, MD

The Problem

Most rotator cuff tears can be repaired by conventional methods. Even in the case of massive tears, repair or reconstruction is usually feasible and the outcome is usually good.[1,2] While there is no universal agreement on the definition, in North America Cofield's[3] definition of a massive tear as one with a diameter of 5 cm or greater is used. Furthermore, there appear to be two distinct patterns of tears, each with a different epidemiology, mechanism of injury, associated disability, and prognosis.[4] The more common, posterosuperior configuration involves the supraspinatus and the infraspinatus, and the less common, anterosuperior configuration involves the subscapularis and the supraspinatus.

Massive posterosuperior rotator cuff tears are not common. Even in clinical practices limited to the treatment of shoulder problems, less than one third of all rotator cuff tears are massive. Neer[5] reported that, of 340 rotator cuff tears operated on over a 13-year period, 145 were massive. Bigliani and associates[2] described 61 massive rotator cuff tears requiring surgery over a 6-year period. Ellman and associates[6] reported that 9 of 54 rotator cuff repairs involved a massive tear. Harryman and associates[7] reported that 28 of 105 surgically-treated tears were massive. Of 407 rotator cuff tears that I repaired surgically over a period of 6 years, 146 were massive posterosuperior lesions (unpublished data).

Massive anterosuperior rotator cuff tears are even less common. A recent European study included 88 combined subscapularis and supraspinatus tendon tears from seven centers; 24 such tears were reported in a series of 301 tears that were repaired over a 5-year period.[4] Of 105 tears reported on by Harryman and associates,[7] 22 involved the subscapularis as well as the supraspinatus. Of the 407 rotator cuff tears that I repaired surgically during a period of 6 years, 19 were combined supraspinatus and subscapularis tears (unpublished data).

Although most tears that involve two or more tendons can be repaired with good results, in some patients the size of the defect and the quality of the tendon tissue preclude secure repair to bone.[7-9] As these tears are, by definition, massive, not all can be repaired. An irreparable tear is one in which the quality of the tendon tissue is so poor that direct tendon-to-bone repair is not possible. In such cases, alternative surgical techniques are considered. Both open and arthroscopic débridement have been suggested; however, while some authors have thought that this provides good pain relief and function, strength is not restored.[10-12] Furthermore, the durability of this pain relief has been questioned.[13] In general, this technique is best suited for elderly patients whose predominant symptom is pain. Tendon allografts and synthetic fabrics have also been used in such patients but without reproducible results.[14,15]

Both local tendon transposition and distant tendon transfer have been proposed to manage irreparable rotator cuff tears in patients who have both pain and weakness. The former has included use of a portion of the subscapularis and the teres minor to cover a large superior defect of the rotator cuff.[16-18] While some surgeons have reported success with these methods, the results have not been reproducible by others. In Europe, anterior deltoid transposition has also been suggested for the reconstruction of irreparable tears of the cuff;[19-21] however, this technique has not gained favor in North America.

Historically, extrinsic tendon transfer about the shoulder has been proposed for the management of paralysis.[22-25] Transfer of the trapezius tendon was once recommended for the management of massive rotator cuff tears;[26] however, the results of this technique were not reproducible. Several authors[27,28] have suggested that the teres major may be a reasonable substitute for an infraspinatus muscle with an irreparable lesion; however, clinically it has been found that this tendon is too short and bulky for transfer.[9] In 1988, Gerber and associates[9] documented the anatomic potential and clinical effectiveness of latissimus dorsi tendon transfer for the management of the functional deficit associated with a massive irreparable posterosuperior rotator cuff tear. Gerber's[29] long-term follow-up study of this series, reported in 1992, added to the enthusiasm for this method. Others[30,31] have reported similarly successful outcomes with this approach.[4] This is currently the favored method for the reconstruction of irreparable massive posterosuperior rotator cuff tears.

The principal problem with management of irreparable anterosuperior tears is the subscapularis component of the tear. This is the most important muscle-tendon unit for both function and stability of the glenohumeral joint.[32-36] Although subscapularis rupture has been well recognized as a complication of anterior dislocation, it has only recently been appreciated that disruption of this structure without instability can lead to severe pain and weakness.[33,34,37-40] While Gerber and associates[33,34] highlighted the physical findings that allow the detection of subscapularis rupture and the technical steps necessary for repair, little has been written about the management of an irreparable subscapularis tendon tear. Recent anecdotal experience and one published report[32] have suggested that transfer of the pectoralis major may be a method for the management of chronic irreparable subscapularis deficiency. No other type of tendon transfer has proved useful in this situation.

Preoperative Considerations

All considerations with regard to treatment must be placed in the context of the individual patient's disability and expectations for pain relief and functional recovery. Concomitant medical problems must also be considered, as they have a bearing on the patient's potential for recovery and for postoperative compliance with therapy.

Pathoanatomy and Pathomechanics

The functional contribution of a muscle to the rotation of a joint is determined by multiplying its physiologic cross-sectional area by its leverage. Physiologic cross-sectional area is an expression of a muscle's force potential.[41] The leverage of a muscle is determined by drawing a perpendicular line from the muscle's line of action to the center of rotation of the joint.[42] If this analysis is applied to the rotator cuff muscles, it is clear that the supraspinatus makes a small (14%) contribution to the overall moment arm for abduction of the shoulder,[41,42] whereas the infraspinatus and teres minor contribute 32% and the subscapularis contributes 52%.[41] Thus, the anterior and posterior components of the rotator cuff are of primary importance in determining the rotation of this joint.

The excursion of the rotator cuff tendons is also relatively small (range, 0.5 to 4.0 cm) during scapular abduction. In comparison, the deltoid muscle has an excursion of 6.5 cm during abduction.[35] The rotator cuff muscles are thus critical stabilizers of the humeral head, providing a fixed fulcrum for rotation powered by the deltoid during abduction.[35] Disruption of the supraspinatus in combination with either the infraspinatus or the subscapularis can result in loss of the fulcrum for the rotation that is necessary for full abduction.[36,43-45]

The role of the long head of the biceps remains a matter of some debate. While some authors[46-48] have provided evidence for its action as a humeral head depressor, others[49,50] have suggested that it does not play an important biomechanical role in the setting of a massive rotator cuff tear.

Clinical[10,12] and experimental[36,37] work has demonstrated that, in some patients who have a massive rotator cuff tear, shoulder function remains good. In these patients, the tear involves the entire supraspinatus and, while it may extend into the subscapularis or the infraspinatus, it does not disrupt these tendons inferior to the equator of the humeral head. Thus, the remaining anterior and posterior aspects of the rotator cuff can exert sufficient force to maintain a fixed fulcrum for rotation of the humeral head in the glenoid. Extension of the tear inferior to the equator results in biomechanical decompensation with loss of containment of the humeral head.[9,29,36,37] Paradoxically, some patients with a smaller rotator cuff tear may have very poor function while others with a larger tear may maintain good function. The fact that tear size does not always correlate with function is reflected in the literature in terms of the disparity among treatment outcomes.[2,3,10,12] Several surgeons have suggested that this disparity between tear size and function can be explained by the degree of atrophy and fatty degeneration of the muscles of the rotator cuff[34,51] (Fig. 1).

Another important factor that must be considered is the integrity of the coracoacromial arch. This structure may act as a stabilizer against unchecked anterosuperior movement of the humeral head in the setting of a tendon tear involving the supraspinatus and at least one other tendon.[52,53] Thus, it is now commonly recommended that the arch be preserved in the surgical management of such patients.

Because massive rotator cuff tears are found in a heterogeneous population of patients, it remains difficult to select the optimal form of treatment. The determination that a rotator cuff tear is irreparable can be made prior to surgery. Currently, it is possible to identify individuals who have poor quality tissue and a large tear that preclude successful primary tendon repair. Factors that predict these findings include profound weakness of external rotation, superior displacement of the humeral head, and MRI imaging showing not only atrophy but also fatty replacement of the muscles of the rotator cuff. An anteroposterior radiograph that shows an acromiohumeral interval of less than 5 mm usually means that the tear involves at least two tendons of the rotator cuff. Hersche and Gerber[54] demonstrated that the duration of the tendon tear is associated with the stiffness of the muscle-tendon unit at the time of surgery. I have found that the degree of fatty replacement of the muscle seen on a preoperative MRI study predicts the quality and stiffness of the tendon tissue as well. Therefore, primary repair or local reconstruction of the torn rotator cuff tendon is not recommended for patients with this combination of findings.

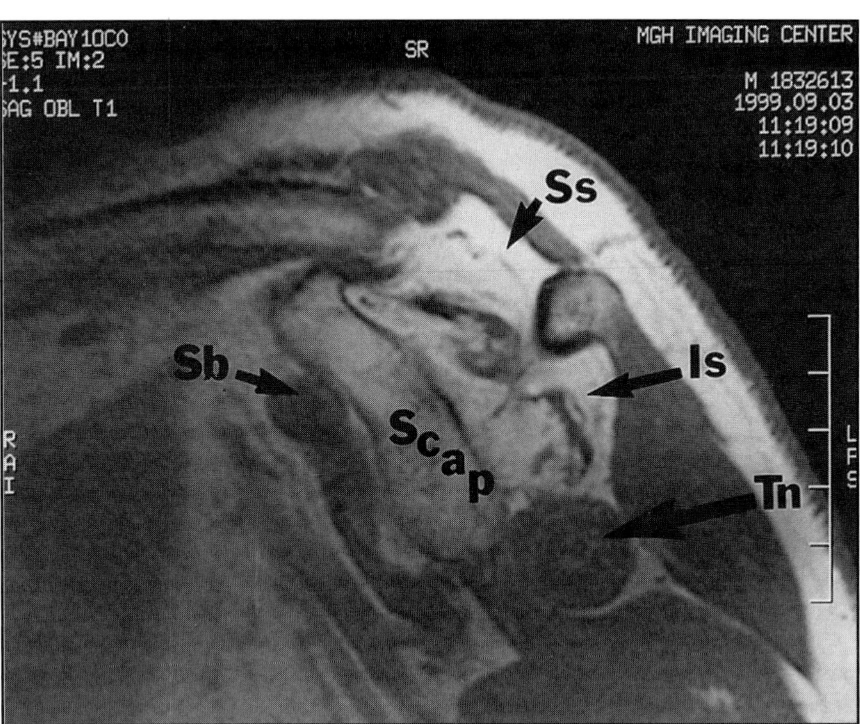

Fig. 1 Oblique sagittal plane MRI study of a left shoulder with a chronic massive tear involving the supraspinatus (Ss) and the infraspinatus (Is). These muscles are atrophic and have a signal characterized as fat. The teres minor (Tn) and the subscapularis (Sb) are not torn and do not demonstrate fatty replacement. Scap = scapula.

Indications for Tendon Transfer

The clinical experience of several authors provides some guidelines for the appropriate selection of patients for tendon transfer for the reconstruction of an irreparable tear.[9,29-31] In general, it is appropriate to consider tendon transfer for patients who have a painful rotator cuff tear that is associated with poor function and in whom there is a low probability that primary reconstruction will be successful.

For patients who have had failure of a prior tendon repair, the indications for tendon transfer are less clear; a number of factors may mitigate against successful improvement of function in this situation.[29,30] These factors include disruption of the coracoacromial arch, deltoid deficiency, stiffness, and nerve injury. In addition, with an irreparable tear of the supraspinatus and infraspinatus, disruption of the subscapularis is a relative contraindication for latissimus dorsi tendon transfer.[9] This is due to disruption of the anterior component of the anteroposterior force couple of the rotator cuff.

The Mechanical Basis of Tendon Transfer for Reconstruction of the Rotator Cuff

The anatomic and biomechanical basis of muscle transfer has been previously published.[55] The relative length of a muscle and its line of action relative to the center of rotation of the joint determine its usefulness as a transfer to restore motion. The rotator cuff muscles have a relatively short amplitude compared with extrinsic shoulder muscles such as the deltoid, pectoralis major, and latissimus dorsi. For the most part, the important function of the rotator cuff that needs to be restored is its action as an external and internal rotator of the humeral head. Thus, the function of the infraspinatus or subscapularis is of primary concern. The subscapularis has an amplitude of 7.3 cm and is the strongest of the rotator cuff muscles.[55] It acts as a powerful internal rotator, but it also maintains the stability of the humeral head by pulling it both downward and posteriorly during abduction of the arm. It acts in synergy with the infraspinatus both to abduct the shoulder and to provide centering of the humeral head in the glenoid.

Comparison of the orientation of the subscapularis with that of other muscles about the shoulder reveals that there are no tendons available for optimal restoration of function if the subscapularis cannot be repaired. Use of the trapezius and the pectoralis major has been proposed.[32] Clinical experience with the trapezius has not been reported in the peer-reviewed literature, to my knowledge, but its line of action seems unfavorable as a substitute for subscapularis function. The pectoralis major has a favorable amplitude (14.4 cm for the clavicular head and 18.8 cm for the sternal head), but its line of action is anterior to the normal orientation of the subscapularis as it originates from the chest wall and thus it cannot pull the humeral head backward.[32,55] Several surgeons have suggested that this line of action can be improved if the pectoralis major is transferred underneath the conjoined tendon and to the lesser tuberosity; however, I am aware of no published reports of this technique.

Transfer of the trapezius[26] or the lateral head of the deltoid[19,21] has been proposed for use in the management of supraspinatus tendon insufficiency; however, neither technique has been shown to

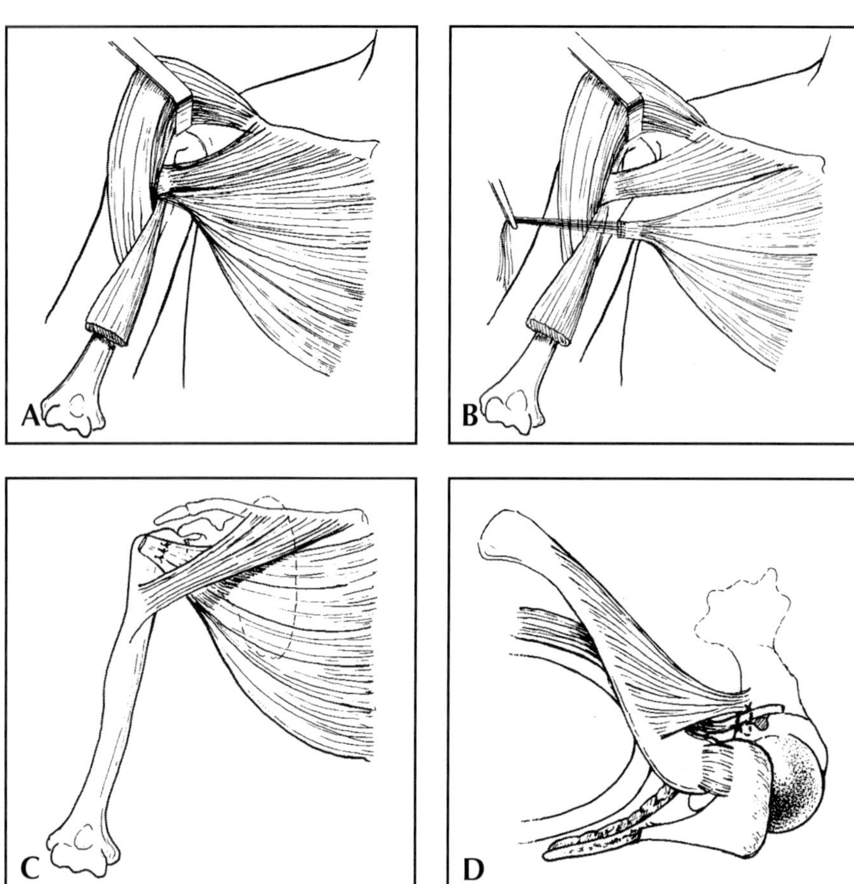

Fig. 2 Drawings showing the surgical technique for the pectoralis major tendon transfer. **A**, The superior and inferior borders of the pectoralis major are exposed. **B**, The sternal portion is dissected, with preservation of the clavicular portion. **C**, The sternal portion is transferred underneath the clavicular portion and is repaired into the lesser tuberosity. **D**, The sternal head of the pectoralis passes underneath the clavicular head, which acts as a pulley, keeping the line of pull of the sternal head closer to the line of the subscapularis tendon.

be effective when there is an irreparable infraspinatus or subscapularis tear.

Disruption of the infraspinatus is always associated with a supraspinatus tear. The combination, which is irreparable, is very disabling for some patients because they lose not only abduction but also external rotation, which prevents movement of the hand to the mouth or to the top of the head. The two muscles that have been proposed as best suited to restore external rotation and abduction are the teres major and the latissimus dorsi. The maximum potential amplitude of the infraspinatus is 8.6 cm, that of the latissimus dorsi is 34 cm, and that of the teres major is 15 cm. Each of these muscles has sufficient strength to be effective as a transferred muscle. While the teres major appears to qualify as a good substitute on the basis of its line of action, it has a rather bulky short tendon, and experimental study has demonstrated that it may not reach superior to the posterior portion of the greater tuberosity when it is transferred underneath the acromion.[28] The latissimus dorsi has been shown to have sufficient excursion to be transferred over the humeral head; however, this muscle crosses both the scapulothoracic and the glenohumeral articulation, and its function is completely different from that of the muscle for which it is acting as a substitute. It normally functions as a powerful adductor and extends the humerus.

My personal preference is to use a modified pectoralis major transfer for reconstruction of an irreparable subscapularis tendon tear and to use a latissimus dorsi transfer for reconstruction of an irreparable infraspinatus tear.

Split Pectoralis Major Transfer for Reconstruction of an Irreparable Subscapularis Tear

The technical steps for the mobilization and repair of the subscapularis were described by Gerber and associates.[9] It is important to attempt to mobilize the subscapularis tendon because even a partial repair may be of some advantage. It is sometimes possible to repair the inferior portion of the tendon while the superior one half remains irreparable. The pectoralis major can then be used to augment the function of the deficient portion.

Wirth and Rockwood[32] described use of the superior portion of the pectoralis major for reconstruction. With their technique, this portion is released from the humerus and transferred lateral to the bicipital groove with the arm in internal rotation. My approach modifies this technique for several reasons. First, the sternal portion of the pectoralis is identified and used for the transfer because this component has sufficient strength and amplitude to act effectively as a transfer. Second, transfer of this component of the pectoralis underneath the remaining clavicular portion of the tendon brings its line of action closer to that of the subscapularis muscle (Fig. 2).

Surgical Technique An extended deltopectoral approach is used. The deltopectoral groove is identified, and the dissection proceeds through this interval to the level of the clavipectoral fascia. The interval underneath the conjoined tendon is developed by both blunt and sharp dissection. There is usually a thin layer of tissue overlying the humeral head; this is not the subscapularis but rather scar tissue in continuity with the subscapularis tendon that has retracted medially deep to the conjoined tendon. This layer is detached along the lesser tuberosity from superior to inferior. Often, a few remaining muscle fibers of the subscapularis attached inferiorly to the lesser tuberosity are visible. A humeral head retractor is then inserted into the joint to displace the humeral head posteriorly, improving exposure for mobilization of the scarred subscapularis tendon. A long, thin retractor is then placed underneath the conjoined tendon, and the axillary nerve and the circumflex vessels are identified. The circumflex vessels are mobilized and then controlled with suture ligature, and the axillary nerve is mobilized and a vessel loupe is placed underneath it. Dissection then frees the inferior scar of the subscapularis while protecting the axillary nerve. Sutures are placed through the scarred edge of the subscapularis so that it can be manipulated to allow for release of adhesions. Sharp dissection releases the contracted subscapularis from the labrum, and the muscle is then mobilized from its fossa. Finally, the scarred coracohumeral ligament is released from the base of the coracoid process. When there is fatty replacement of the muscle, the muscle-tendon unit feels stiff. Usually, the entire subscapularis tendon cannot be repaired to the lesser tuberosity, but in some cases its inferior portion can be reattached to the lesser tuberosity with use of a transosseous repair technique.[4,34]

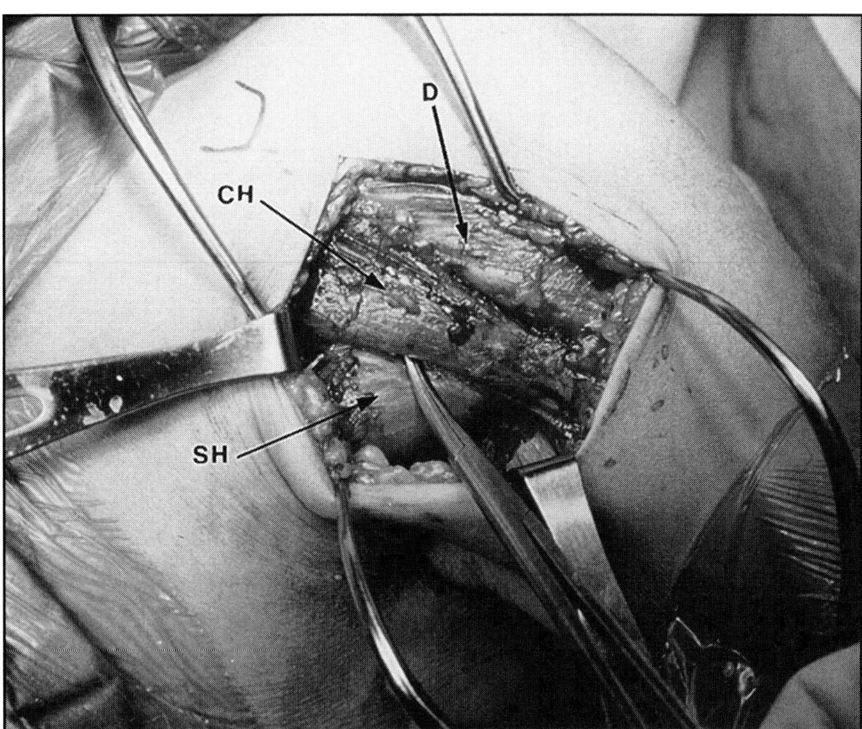

Fig. 3 Photograph showing the interval between the sternal head (SH) and the clavicular head (CH) of the pectoralis major. The sternal head passes posterior to the clavicular head as it approaches its insertion on the humerus. D = deltoid.

The pectoralis major is then exposed, and the dissection is continued medially on its superficial surface. Knowledge of the anatomy of the tendon insertion is important for harvesting the sternal head of the muscle. The sternal portion originates from the inferior part of the sternum and the fifth and sixth ribs. Its tendon courses superiorly underneath that of the clavicular head, so that it twists 180° and inserts superiorly on the humerus. The interval between the two heads and the orientation of the tendon usually can be clearly identified (Fig. 3). This interval is then developed bluntly just medial to the muscle-tendon junction, and a large clamp is placed underneath the sternal portion of the muscle. The clamp is replaced with a Penrose drain. The dissection then proceeds distally, with separation of the two components of the tendon and detachment of the sternal portion from the humerus. Nonabsorbable No. 2 braided sutures are placed in the tendon end. The muscle split between the two heads is extended about 3 to 4 cm medially in order to facilitate transfer of the sternal head underneath the clavicular head. After decortication of the area of the lesser tuberosity and the bicipital groove, the tendon is repaired to bone with use of either bone anchors or a transosseous repair technique. This is done with the arm in neutral rotation and the pectoralis pulled superiorly to the top of the lesser tuberosity. The incision is then closed in layers, and the arm is placed in a shoulder immobilizer.

Postoperative care consists of immobilization in a sling for 4 weeks, during which time passive flexion is performed below the horizontal and passive external rotation is limited to about 30°. After 4 weeks, active assisted motion is commenced. Strengthening exercises are delayed for 4 months.

Results Experience with transfer of the pectoralis major for the reconstruction of irreparable subscapularis tears is limited. Wirth and Rockwood[32] reported on 13 patients with an irreparable subscapularis tendon tear who had had failure of a capsular repair for the treatment of instability. Seven of these patients had transfer of the pectoralis major only, five had transfer of both the pectoralis major and the pectoralis minor, and one had transfer of the pectoralis minor only. Ten patients had a satisfactory outcome, and three had failure of the

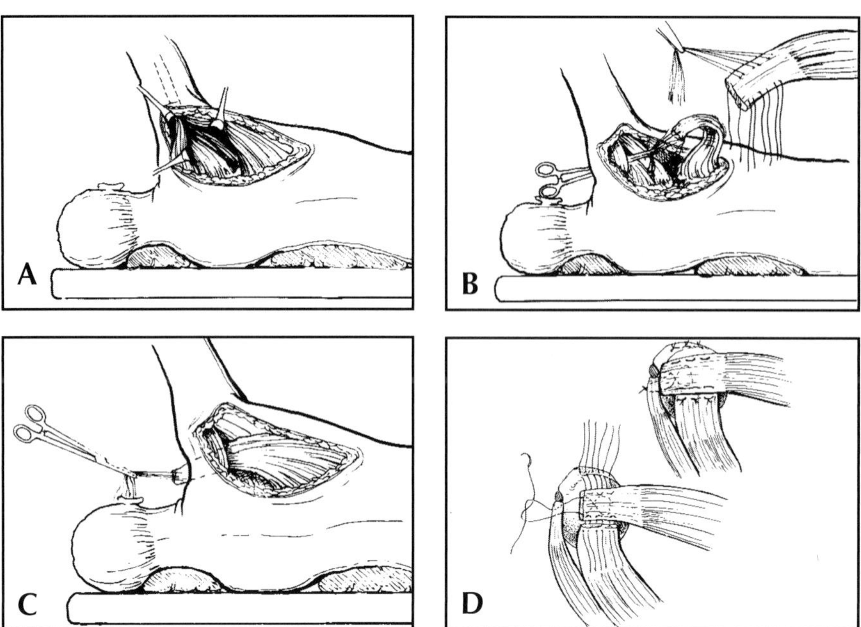

Fig. 4 Drawings showing the surgical technique for the latissimus dorsi tendon transfer. **A,** The patient is placed in the lateral decubitus position, and an accessory posterior incision is made in order to identify and harvest the latissimus dorsi tendon. **B,** The tendon is detached from the humerus and then dissected retrograde to the neurovascular pedicle. The tendon is freed from its fascial connections to the chest wall. Sutures are then placed in the tendon prior to its transfer underneath the acromion. **C,** The tendon is transferred underneath the deltoid and the acromion. **D,** With the shoulder abducted and in external rotation, the tendon is secured to the remnant of the rotator cuff tendons medially, to the greater tuberosity laterally, and to the subscapularis anteriorly.

procedure. All of the patients with a satisfactory outcome had resolution of the instability as well as a marked reduction in pain. Two patients had restoration of a normal lift-off test.[32] (This test measures the ability to lift the internally rotated arm off of the lower back, and it indicates normal terminal internal rotation performed by the subscapularis.)

My experience with split pectoralis major transfer has included 10 patients over the past 4 years. In five patients, the procedure was done after failure of prior rotator cuff surgery; in three, it was done after failure of surgery for the treatment of instability; and in two, it was done in the setting of instability after hemiarthroplasty. All patients had pain and the perception of instability when the arm was placed either overhead or behind the plane of the body. The results were graded according to pain relief, improved function, and resolution of instability. All patients thought that the shoulder was stable and indicated that the pain had decreased, although only six reported minimal or no pain. Functional gains were more limited, with only two patients indicating marked improvement and the ability to participate in sports such as golf and tennis. Three patients thought that they had much improvement, but they still had limited overhead use of the arm, and five had minimal functional improvement despite relief of pain and of the sense of apprehension. No patient had a normal lift-off test.

Latissimus Dorsi Transfer for Reconstruction of an Irreparable Posterosuperior Rotator Cuff Tear

The technique for transfer of the latissimus dorsi tendon to reconstruct posterosuperior rotator cuff tears has been described in detail previously.[4,9,29] Over the 8 years of my experience, it has been modified technically as described below.

Surgical Technique The patient is placed in the lateral decubitus position and is stabilized on a long beanbag, which is contoured to support the torso (Fig. 4, *A*). The entire arm and hemithorax are prepared with use of sterile technique and are draped. An anterosuperior incision is made in order to expose the rotator cuff tear. This incision begins on top of the shoulder, over the lateral one third of the acromion, and continues anteriorly about 1 cm lateral to the coracoid process. In all cases, an attempt is made to preserve the coracoacromial arch. This is done by splitting the deltoid from the lateral aspect of the acromion and elevating it subperiosteally off of the anterior aspect. The interval between the deltoid and the coracoacromial ligament is identified, so that the latter is not detached from the acromion. The lateral deltoid split also allows easier access to the posterior aspect of the rotator cuff, improving exposure for transfer of the tendon. The edges of the rotator cuff are then identified, and steps to mobilize the retracted tendon edges are performed. These steps include release of the coracohumeral ligament, extra-articular lysis of adhesions that may be tethering the tendons, and intra-articular release in the plane between the labrum and the tendon surface. This will increase tendon excursion only modestly, usually less than a centimeter. Braided nonabsorbable No. 2 sutures are then placed through the tendon edges.

The greater tuberosity is then prepared by abrading its surface and placing holes from the edge of the tuberosity to the lateral cortex of the humerus. Loops of braided No. 2 suture are placed through these holes so that sutures from the transferred tendon can be passed subsequently.

In order to harvest the latissimus dorsi tendon, a separate posterior incision is

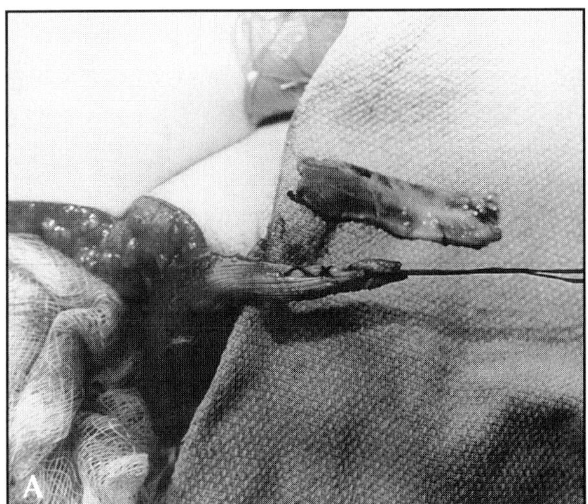

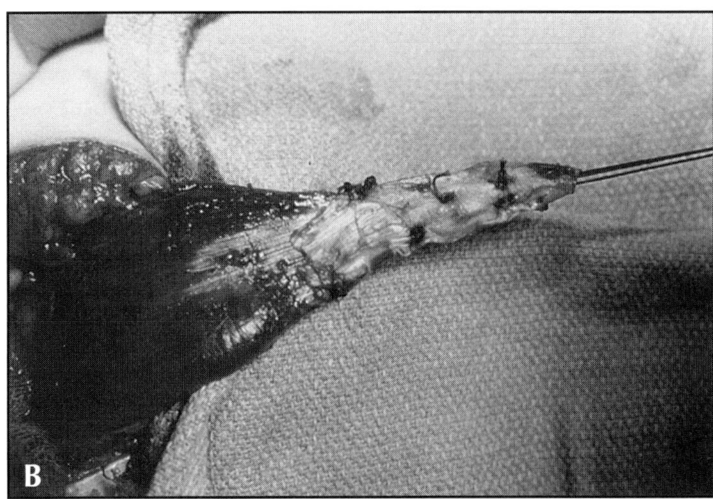

Fig. 5 A, The latissimus dorsi tendon is often small and thin. The fascia lata autograft that will be used to augment the tendon is shown in the background of the photograph. **B,** Photograph showing the latissimus dorsi tendon after the fascia lata autograft has been sewn over it to reinforce it prior to transfer.

made over the muscle belly and curved superiorly over the posterior aspect of the deltoid at the level of the joint line. The posterior aspect of the deltoid, the long head of the triceps, the teres major, and the latissimus dorsi muscles are identified. The latissimus dorsi is then dissected free from the teres major and the fascia of the chest wall. There are often substantial connections between the latissimus dorsi and the teres major, so dissection is easier if it begins at the level of the muscle and continues toward its insertion. The arm is positioned in flexion and internal rotation, which makes access to the tendon insertion easier. Long retractors are used to expose the tendon insertion while an assistant holds the arm in this position. Once the tendon has been detached from its insertion on the humerus, several No. 2 braided sutures are placed through the end of the tendon in order to maintain tension on it as it is dissected in a retrograde fashion (Fig. 4, *B*). The tendon is freed from fascial extensions to the chest wall, and the neurovascular pedicle is isolated and protected. The muscle-tendon unit has been sufficiently mobilized for transfer when the tendon end can reach superior to the posterior aspect of the acromion. Braided nonabsorbable No. 2 sutures are then placed through the tendon's lateral edge to be used to repair the tendon to the greater tuberosity once it has been transferred underneath the acromion.

The interval underneath the deltoid and the acromion is developed by both blunt and sharp dissection, and the tendon is then transferred with use of a curved clamp (Fig. 4, *C*). The arm is positioned in 45° of abduction in the scapular plane and 30° of external rotation and is held in that position with use of a special articulated arm-holder (McConnell Shoulder Holder; McConnell, Greenville, TX) until the transferred tendon is sutured in place. Use of the arm-holder seems to work better than having an assistant hold the arm, as it allows better exposure of the shoulder because of its thin profile. It also maintains the arm in a consistent position, whereas an assistant might become fatigued and allow the arm position to move during the tendon transfer and repair. At this stage, a lamina spreader placed between the greater tuberosity and the acromion may help with exposure for suturing of the tendon. The tendon is held in position over the greater tuberosity while it is sutured along its medial edge to the remaining cuff tendons and then to the subscapularis as well (Fig. 4, *D*). Finally, the sutures in the lateral edge of the tendon are transferred through the greater tuberosity with use of the loops of the previously placed suture.

Because the latissimus tendon is thin and I have noted late rupture of the graft in 20% to 30% of cases, the tendon is now routinely augmented with autogenous fascia lata (Fig. 5, *A*). A 2 × 4-cm strip of iliotibial band is harvested from the ipsilateral thigh and sewn over the tendon in order to reinforce it (Fig. 5, *B*).

Postoperative care is very important following this transfer. For the first 6 weeks, the patient continually wears an abduction brace that maintains the arm in 45° of abduction and 30° of external rotation in order to allow the tendon to heal without tension. Throughout this period, a therapist performs passive motion with the arm in abduction and external rotation, but internal rotation and adduction are not permitted. This motion ensures that the tendon graft does not adhere to the surrounding soft tissue and that the glenohumeral joint does not become stiff. After 6 weeks, the brace is removed and the patient is encouraged to perform activities of daily living.

The patient is then taught to initiate and maintain active contraction of the latissimus dorsi during flexion and external rotation of the arm. This is not the normal phase of activity for this musculotendinous unit, so a concerted effort must be made to retrain the muscle. This is achieved in two ways. With the first method, the arm is positioned in the midrange of abduction and the patient is asked to adduct the shoulder toward the midline, which causes the latissimus dorsi to contract. As the latissimus dorsi contracts, the arm is guided into flexion and the patient is coached to maintain this contraction in order to facilitate flexion. Gradually, the patient acquires the ability to maintain contraction of the latissimus dorsi. Similarly, the patient is asked to maintain contraction as the arm is moved into external rotation.

The second method for retraining the latissimus dorsi is with use of biofeedback. A small biofeedback unit with cutaneous electrode pads is applied over the muscle belly of the latissimus dorsi. This unit provides audible feedback (a higher pitch indicates more muscle activity) and visual feedback (red to green indicates more muscle activity). The patient tries to maintain contraction of the latissimus dorsi during flexion and external rotation and is gradually able to do so through biofeedback. Overall, it may take between 6 and 12 months for complete training of the transferred muscle.

Results Gerber and associates[9] originally reported good-to-excellent short-term results in four patients who were followed for more than 1 year after a latissimus dorsi transfer. Gerber[29] subsequently evaluated 16 patients who had been followed for an average of 33 months after such a transfer. He reported an excellent subjective result in eight patients, a good result in five, a fair result in two, and a poor result in one. The average improvement in flexion was 53°. Aoki and associates[31] reported on 12 shoulders at an average of 36 months after a latissimus dorsi transfer. The subjective improvement was rated as excellent in four shoulders, good in four, fair in one, and poor in three. The average improvement in flexion was 36°. Miniaci and MacLeod[30] reported on 17 patients who had undergone a latissimus dorsi transfer for revision of a failed rotator cuff repair. At an average of 51 months postoperatively, 14 of the 17 patients had marked relief of pain and increased function. My experience has been more varied. Of 407 rotator cuff repairs performed by my colleagues and myself over 6 years, 22 were latissimus dorsi tendon transfers (unpublished data). Of these 22 transfers, 6 were done to reconstruct an irreparable rotator cuff tear that had not been treated with prior surgery and 16 were performed after failure of a prior repair of a rotator cuff tear. When the results were analyzed according to these two groups, the outcomes were quite different. Of the 16 patients who had had a revision, only 8 reported a satisfactory outcome, and the average gain in flexion was 44°. Negative prognostic factors included a prior deltoid injury, associated stiffness, and poor tendon quality of the remaining rotator cuff. In contrast, a satisfactory outcome was achieved in five of the six patients who had had the latissimus dorsi transfer as a primary procedure, and the average gain in flexion was 60°. Late rupture of the transferred tendon was thought to have occurred in about 20% to 30% of the patients on the basis of the inability of the examiner to palpate contraction of the muscle and on the basis of a decrease in shoulder function. While others have not reported this problem, to my knowledge, I believe that it was due to the relatively small size of the latissimus tendon and the good early results in some patients, which led to increased activity before adequate healing was obtained. This has led me to augment these tendon transfers with autogenous iliotibial band. In the past year, four such procedures have been performed, and none have led to a late rupture at the time of this writing.

Summary

The inability to repair a rotator cuff tear is not uncommon, and in practices devoted to the management of shoulder injuries up to 30% of rotator cuff tears may be irreparable. The anterior and posterior components of the rotator cuff are the most important deficient areas. In the case of an irreparable subscapularis tendon tear, pain relief and stability appear to be reliably achieved by a split pectoralis major transfer; however, functional improvement is less certain because the biomechanics associated with this tendon transfer do not appear to be optimal. In the case of an irreparable posterosuperior rotator cuff tear, a latissimus dorsi tendon transfer reliably restores flexion and relieves pain; however, its use after failure of prior rotator cuff surgery makes the outcome less predictable. Both anterior and posterior reconstructions with tendon transfer require precise surgical technique and patient compliance with postoperative rehabilitation.

References

1. Rokito AS, Cuomo F, Gallagher MA, Zuckerman JD: Long-term functional outcome of repair of large and massive chronic tears of the rotator cuff. *J Bone Joint Surg Am* 1999;81:991–997.
2. Bigliani LU, Cordasco FA, McIlveen SJ, Musso ES: Operative repairs of massive rotator cuff tears: Long-term results. *J Shoulder Elbow Surg* 1992;1:120–130.
3. Cofield RH: Rotator cuff disease of the shoulder. *J Bone Joint Surg Am* 1985;67:974–979.
4. Warner JJP, Gerber C: Treatment of massive rotator cuff tears: Posterior-superior and anterior-superior, in Iannotti JP (ed): *The Rotator Cuff: Current Concepts and Complex Problems.* Rosemont, IL, American Academy of Orthopaedic Surgeons, 1998, pp 59–94.
5. Neer CS II (ed): *Shoulder Reconstruction.* Philadelphia, PA, WB Saunders, 1990, pp 41–142.
6. Ellman H, Hanker G, Bayer M: Repair of the rotator cuff: End-result study of factors influencing reconstruction. *J Bone Joint Surg Am* 1986;68:1136–1144.

7. Harryman DT II, Mack LA, Wang KY, Jackins SE, Richardson ML, Matsen FA III: Repairs of the rotator cuff: Correlation of functional results with integrity of the cuff. *J Bone Joint Surg Am* 1991;73:982–989.

8. Gazielly DF, Gleyze P, Montagnon C: Functional and anatomical results after rotator cuff repair. *Clin Orthop* 1994;304:43–53.

9. Gerber C, Vinh TS, Hertel R, Hess CW: Latissimus dorsi transfer for the treatment of massive tears of the rotator cuff: A preliminary report. *Clin Orthop* 1988;232:51–61.

10. Rockwood CA Jr, Williams GR Jr, Burkhead WZ Jr: Debridement of degenerative, irreparable lesions of the rotator cuff. *J Bone Joint Surg Am* 1995;77:857–866.

11. Apoil A, Dautry P, Moinet P, Koechlin P: The syndrome "rupture of the cap of the rotations of the scapula:" A propos of 70 cases. *Rev Chir Orthop Reparatrice Appar Mot* 1977:63(suppl 2): 145–149.

12. Burkhart SS: Arthroscopic debridement and decompression for selected rotator cuff tears. Clinical results, pathomechanics, and patient selection based on biomechanical parameters. *Orthop Clin North Am* 1993;24:111–123.

13. Melillo AS, Savoie FH III, Field LD: Massive rotator cuff tears: Debridement versus repair. *Orthop Clin North Am* 1997;28:117–124.

14. Neviaser JS, Neviaser RJ, Neviaser TJ: The repair of chronic massive ruptures of the rotator cuff of the shoulder by use of freeze-dried rotator cuff. *J Bone Joint Surg Am* 1978;60:681–684.

15. Ozaki J, Fujimoto S, Masuhara K, Tamai S, Yoshimoto S: Reconstruction of chronic massive rotator cuff tears with synthetic materials. *Clin Orthop* 1986;202:173–183.

16. Cofield RH: Subscapular muscle transposition for repair of chronic rotator cuff tears. *Surg Gynecol Obstet* 1982;154:667–672.

17. Debeyre J, Patte D, Elmelik E: Repairs of ruptures of the rotator cuff of the shoulder: With a note on advancement of the supraspinatus muscle. *J Bone Joint Surg Br* 1965;47:36–42.

18. Neviaser RJ, Neviaser TJ: Transfer of subscapularis and teres minor for massive defects of the rotator cuff, in Bayley I, Kessel L (eds): *Shoulder Surgery*. Berlin, Germany, Springer-Verlag, 1982, pp 60–63.

19. Apoil A, Augereau B: Deltoid flap repair of large losses of substance of the shoulder rotator cuff. *Chirurgie* 1985;111:287–290.

20. Dierickx C, Vanhoof H: Massive rotator cuff tears treated by a deltoid muscular inlay flap. *Acta Orthop Belg* 1994:60:94–100.

21. Gazielly DF: Deltoid muscular flap transfer for massive defects of the rotator cuff, in Burkhead WZ Jr (ed): *Rotator Cuff Disorders*. Baltimore, MD, Williams & Wilkins, 1996, pp 356–367.

22. L'Episcopo JB: Tendon transplantation in obstetrical paralysis. *Am J Surg* 1934; 25:122–125.

23. Covey DC, Riordan DC, Milstead ME, Albright JA: Modification of the L'Episcopo procedure for brachial plexus birth palsies. *J Bone Joint Surg Br* 1992;74:897–901.

24. Hoffer MM, Wickenden R, Roper B: Brachial plexus birth palsies: Results of tendon transfers to the rotator cuff. *J Bone Joint Surg Am* 1978;60:691–695.

25. Phipps GJ, Hoffer MM: Latissimus dorsi and teres major transfer to rotator cuff for Erb's palsy. *J Shoulder Elbow Surg* 1995;4:124–129.

26. Mikasa M: Trapezius transfer for global tear of the rotator cuff, in Bateman JE, Welsh RP (eds): *Surgery of the Shoulder*. Philadelphia, PA, BC Decker, 1984, pp 196–199.

27. Combes JM, Mansat M: Lambeau de muscle grand rond dans les ruptures massives de la coiffe des rotateurs: Etude experimentale, in Bonnel F, Blotman F, Mansat M (eds): *L'epaule: L'epaule Degenerative, l'epaule Traumatique, l'epaule du Sportif*. Paris, France, Springer, 1993, pp 318–330.

28. Wang AA, Strauch RJ, Flatow EL, Bigliani LU, Rosenwasser MP: The teres major muscle: An anatomic study of its use as a tendon transfer *J Shoulder Elbow Surg* 1999; 8:334–338.

29. Gerber C: Latissimus dorsi transfer for the treatment of irreparable tears of the rotator cuff. *Clin Orthop* 1992;275:152–160.

30. Miniaci A, MacLeod M: Transfer of the latissimus dorsi muscle after failed repair of a massive tear of the rotator cuff: A two to five-year review. *J Bone Joint Surg Am* 1999:81:1120–1127.

31. Aoki M, Okamura K, Fukushima S, Takahashi T, Ogino T: Transfer of latissimus dorsi for irreparable rotator-cuff tears. *J Bone Joint Surg Br* 1996;78:761–766.

32. Wirth MA, Rockwood CA Jr: Operative treatment of irreparable rupture of the subscapularis. *J Bone Joint Surg Am* 1997:79:722–731.

33. Gerber C, Krushell RJ: Isolated rupture of the tendon of the subscapularis muscle: Clinical features in 16 cases. *J Bone Joint Surg Br* 1991;73:389–394.

34. Gerber C, Hersche O, Farron A: Isolated rupture of the subscapularis tendon. *J Bone Joint Surg Am* 1996;78:1015–1023.

35. McMahon PJ, Debski RE, Thompson WO, Warner JJ, Fu FH, Woo SL: Shoulder muscle forces and tendon excursions during glenohumeral abduction in the scapular plane. *J Shoulder Elbow Surg* 1995;4:199–208.

36. Thompson WO, Debski RE, Boardman ND III, at al: A biomechanical analysis of rotator cuff deficiency in a cadaveric model. *Am J Sports Med* 1996;24:286–292.

37. Burkhart SS: Reconciling the paradox of rotator cuff repair versus debridement: A unified biomechanical rationale for the treatment of rotator cuff tears. *Arthroscopy* 1994;10:4–19.

38. DePalma AF, Cooke AJ, Prabhakar M: The role of the subscapularis in recurrent anterior dislocations of the shoulder. *Clin Orthop* 1967;54:35–49.

39. Neviaser RJ, Neviaser TJ, Neviaser JS: Concurrent rupture of the rotator cuff and anterior dislocation of the shoulder in the older patient. *J Bone Joint Surg Am* 1988;70:1308–1311.

40. Turkel SJ, Panio MW, Marshall JL, Girgis FG: Stabilizing mechanisms preventing anterior dislocation of the glenohumeral joint. *J Bone Joint Surg Am* 1981;63:1208–1217.

41. Keating JF, Waterworth P, Shaw-Dunn J, Crossan J: The relative strengths of the rotator cuff muscles: A cadaver study. *J Bone Joint Surg Br* 1993;75:137–140.

42. Bassett RW, Browne AO, Morrey BF, An KN: Glenohumeral muscle force and moment mechanics in a position of shoulder instability. *J Biomech* 1990;23:405–415.

43. Bernageau J: Roentgenographic assessment of the rotator cuff. *Clin Orthop* 1990;254:87–91.

44. LeClerq R: Diagnostic de la rupture du sous-epineoux. *Rev Rheum* 1950;10:510–515.

45. Weiner DS, Macnab I: Superior migration of the humeral head: A radiological aid in the diagnosis of tears of the rotator cuff. *J Bone Joint Surg Br* 1970;52:524–527.

46. Itoi E, Kuechle DK, Newman SR, Morrey BF, An KN: Stabilising function of the biceps in stable and unstable shoulders. *J Bone Joint Surg Br* 1993;75:546–550.

47. Kumar VP, Satku K, Balasubramaniam P: The role of the long head of biceps brachii in the stabilization of the head of the humerus. *Clin Orthop* 1989:244:172–175.

48. Warner JJ, McMahon PJ: The role of the long head of the biceps brachii in superior stability of the glenohumeral joint. *J Bone Joint Surg Am* 1995;77:366–372.

49. Yamaguchi K, Riew KD, Galatz LM, Syme JA, Neviaser RJ: Biceps activity during shoulder motion: An electromyographic analysis. *Clin Orthop* 1997;336:122–129.

50. Walch G, Boileau P, Noel E, Liotard JP, Dejour H: Surgical treatment of painful shoulders caused by lesions of the rotator cuff and biceps, treatment as a function of lesions: Reflections on the Neer's concept. *Rev Rhum Mal Osteoartic* 1991;58:247–257.

51. Goutallier D, Postel JM, Bernageau J, Lavau L, Voisin MC: Fatty muscle degeneration in cuff ruptures: Pre- and postoperative evaluation by CT scan. *Clin Orthop* 1994;304:78–83.

52. Arntz CT, Matsen FA III, Jackins S: Surgical management of complex irreparable rotator cuff deficiency. *J Arthroplasty* 1991;6:363–370.

53. Flatow EL, Raimondo RA, Kelkar R, et al: Abstract: Active and passive restraints against superior humeral translation: The contribution of the rotator cuff, the biceps tendon and the coracoacromial arch. *Orthop Trans* 1996:20:121.

54. Hersche O, Gerber C: Passive tension in the supraspinatus musculotendinous unit after long-standing rupture of its tendon: A preliminary report. *J Shoulder Elbow Surg* 1998;7:393–396.

55. Gerber C, Hersche O: Tendon transfers for the treatment of irreparable rotator cuff defects. *Orthop Clin North Am* 1997;28:195–203.

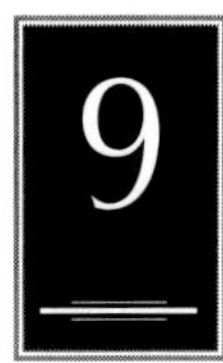

Mini-Open Rotator Cuff Repair: An Updated Perspective

Ken Yamaguchi, MD

Introduction

Once regarded as a "cutting edge" procedure performed only by a select few arthroscopists, the mini-open or arthroscopically assisted rotator cuff repair has quickly become a popular procedure and for many the standard of care for rotator cuff repair.[1-8] In just 5 to 10 years, the mini-open repair has gained acceptance comparable to formal open repair and ironically now lies as a "sensible" middle ground between the traditional formal open repair and the unproven, newer complete arthroscopic rotator cuff repair techniques.[9,10] From several standpoints, the mini-open or arthroscopically assisted approach to rotator cuff repair combines many of the advantages of the former open repair and complete arthroscopic repair while avoiding many of the disadvantages. As complete arthroscopic rotator cuff repair becomes a more viable option, mini-open repair represents an excellent transitional procedure in which a surgeon can become experienced in many of the arthroscopic-specific techniques such as release, tendon mobilization, suture and suture anchor placement necessary in order to perform complete arthroscopic repairs. This chapter will review some of the relevant history regarding the mini-open repair, the relationship to the formal open and arthroscopic repair alternatives, specifics of surgical technique, and the overall results reported with mini-open repair. Additionally, a rationale for the use of the mini-open repair technique for rotator cuff tears of all sizes and as a transition procedure toward complete arthroscopic repair, if desirable, will be described.

Table 1
Fundamentals of rotator cuff repair

Glenohumeral inspection
Anterior-inferior acromioplasty
Release of the coracoacromial ligament
Complete release/mobilization of any fixed contracted tendons around the following structures:
Glenoid labrum
Superficial bursa
Coracoid base (coracohumeral ligament)
Rotator interval
Posterior interval (scapular spine)
Tendon grasping suture placement
Secure bone fixation
Minimize deltoid surgical insult/meticulous repair
Early restoration of passive motion and surgeon-directed rehabilitation

Historical Considerations

The advent of shoulder arthroscopy has had an important impact on the evolution of rotator cuff treatment. Since the initial description of arthroscopic subacromial decompression by Ellman and Kay[11] only a short time ago, there has been a significant trend toward more minimally invasive surgery to accomplish the same results seen previously with the formal open repair. It is important, however, to review formal open repairs as the gold standard or benchmark when reviewing results with arthroscopic treatment. Many of the fundamental principles required in the successful outcome from formal open repair (Table 1) are applicable to achieving good outcome from the mini-open or complete arthroscopic repairs.

The surgical experience with formal open repair of the rotator cuff as presented in the peer-reviewed literature has been extensive.[12-26] Codman[27,28] reported on his experience with rotator cuff repair first described as early as 1911 in which he noted 20 of 31 patients with successful results after repair of full-thickness tears. In 1972, Neer[29] reported results on rotator cuff repair employing routine anterior acromioplasty. He reported 19 of 20 satisfactory results and highlighted four important principles for open rotator cuff surgery: (1) anterior-inferior acromioplasty or reshaping rather than acromionectomy; (2) meticulous repair of the deltoid origin and avoidance of those procedures that may place this area at risk for injury; (3) releasing, mobilizing, and repairing the torn rotator cuff tendons; (4) early restoration of passive motion through surgeon-directed and individualized rehabilitation. These principles have been generally accepted and have led to relatively uniform open treatment of full-thickness rotator cuff tears. Not surprisingly, many subsequent large series of rotator cuff repairs have shown similarly good results. In a series of 100 consecutive rotator cuff repairs with a mean follow-up of 4.2 years, Hawkins and and associates[18] showed that 86% had no or slight pain and average postoperative improvement in abduction of 44°. In a later series of 245 shoulders, Neer and associates[22] reported a 92% excellent or satisfactory rating. Multiple later series have shown similar results for either small or massive repairs.[12-17,20,21,24-26] A common denominator for the articles referred to above has been the adherence to strict surgical principles of deltoid preservation, anterior-inferior acromioplasty, cuff mobilization, and then repair.

Despite a track record of a high percentage of good or excellent results, the formal open repair was associated with some disadvantages. The open repair required some form of anterior deltoid takedown combined with a lateral deltoid split; if associated with a long, difficult procedure, open repair could also be associated with some traction injury. Although the surgical injury imparted to the deltoid has generally been reported to repair and heal in a predictable fashion, experienced shoulder surgeons report a 0.5% incidence of deltoid avulsion.[19,30-32] The incidence reported by less experienced shoulder surgeons may be substantially higher. Loss of the integrity of the anterior deltoid origin is a serious and devastating complication for which there are no satisfying surgical alternatives.[30,32-33] In the context of a rotator cuff tear, results following loss of anterior deltoid function were almost uniformly poor.

Fortunately, deltoid-related complications from formal open approaches appear to be rare. However, a formal open approach has two additional disadvantages related to surgical insult to the deltoid during the rotator cuff repair. The deltoid takedown and repair usually requires a period of protection in order to avoid any inadvertent avulsion. This may preclude accelerated rehabilitation in terms of active-assisted or active motion in smaller rotator cuff tears. Additionally, although not formally qualified, the open repair appears to be associated with more perioperative pain than mini-open or complete arthroscopic alternatives.[1,6,8,34-36] The increased pain may be related to the transdeltoid approach required for formal open repair. This pain can hinder early rehabilitation and early motion as well. Finally, formal open repair, while highly successful over the long term, has been associated with significant recovery times.[24,25] It is generally considered to require 18 months for full recovery to take place. These recovery times appear to be longer than those required for mini-open or complete arthroscopic approaches and again may be related to surgical insult to the deltoid.

In order to avoid anterior deltoid detachment, Levy and associates,[3] in a preliminary report, and then Paulos and Kody[6] in a long-term follow-up study first described the arthroscopically enhanced "mini approach" to rotator cuff repair in 1994. The authors described a technique performed in the lateral decubitus position in which an arthroscopic decompression was first performed followed by an open rotator cuff repair through a lateral deltoid split. As the anterior-inferior acromioplasty had been performed in an arthroscopic fashion, an anterior deltoid detachment was no longer necessary. The rotator cuff repair technique at this point was essentially the same as a complete open repair. All releases were performed in an open fashion and then a combination of transosseous sutures and suture anchors used to secure bone-tendon fixation. Paulos and Kody reported 88% good and excellent results at average follow-up of 48 months.[6] In their opinion, the technique resulted in less perioperative morbidity and, because the deltoid muscle was not detached, more safe initiation of rehabilitation exercises. Conceptionally, the strategy of arthroscopic decompression and then lateral deltoid split has been appealing and several subsequent studies have shown comparable good and excellent results.

Although the results reported thus far have been encouraging, mini-open repair generally is not advised for all rotator cuff tears.[7] For those who rely on open rotator cuff releases and mobilization, the small lateral approach is generally insufficient for repairs of large or massive size tears. For this reason, small, easily mobilized tears are the best indication for the originally described mini-open repair[4,7,9,10] However, with increasing experience in arthroscopic mobilization and tagging of rotator cuff tears, large or massive tears are becoming more easily amenable to repair through mini-open lateral deltoid-splitting approaches.

Strategy and Indications for Surgery

In general, there have been two strategies for surgical technique when using the mini-open repair. The more established method has been arthroscopic decompression followed by a standard open repair through a lateral deltoid split. This technique was initially described by Paulos and Kody.[6] An alternative strategy uses more extensive arthroscopic assistance. In this case, an arthroscopic decompression is performed as in the previous scenario, but in addition an extensive rotator cuff mobilization is performed during the arthroscopic portion procedure. Afterward, arthroscopic tagging sutures or stay sutures are placed and perhaps preparation of the greater tuberosity, débridement of the rotator cuff tendon, and placement of suture anchors are all done arthroscopically. The small lateral deltoid split is then performed in order to place tendon gripping sutures on the previously mobilized

Table 2
Comparison of mini-open surgical techniques

	Inspection	Decompression	Releases	Placement of Tagging Sutures	Tendon Gripping Stitches	Bone-Tendon Fixation
Arthroscopically-assisted open repair	Arthroscopic	Arthroscopic	Open	Open	Open	Open
Mini-open assisted arthroscopic repair	Arthroscopic	Arthroscopic	Arthroscopic	Arthroscopic	Open	Open

cuff and then to fixate the cuff to bone using the surgeon's preferred method, whether it be suture anchors or transosseous sutures.

The two strategies of mini-open repair are fundamentally different in the manner in which arthroscopic assistance is used (Table 2). In the more established method, arthroscopic surgery is used simply to perform a decompression and plays a small role in the actual performance of the rotator cuff repair. This method can be referred to by the traditional designation of an arthroscopically assisted open repair technique. In the second strategy, the decompression and rotator cuff repair are primarily performed arthroscopically and a small portal-extension approach is performed simply to obtain secure tendon to bone fixation of a previously mobilized cuff. This surgical strategy can be referred to as a mini-open assisted arthroscopic rotator cuff repair. In the first case, the emphasis is on open repair techniques; in the second, the emphasis is on arthroscopic repair. Because a lateral open deltoid-splitting approach is used in both strategies, the term mini-open repair can be applicable to both. However, the surgical techniques are distinctly different and associated with different advantages and disadvantages (Table 3).

Table 3
Comparison of rotator cuff repair techniques

	Formal Open	Arthroscopically Assisted Open Repair	Mini-Open Assisted Arthroscopic Repair	Complete Arthroscopic Repair
Glenohumeral evaluation	No	Yes	Yes	Yes
Limited mobilization	Yes	Yes	Yes	Yes
Extensive mobilization	Yes	No	Yes	Yes
Limited deltoid surgical insult	No	No/Yes	Yes	Yes
Tendon-gripping stitches (Mason-Allen)	Yes	Yes	Yes	No
Transosseous sutures	Yes	Yes	Yes	No
Suture anchors	Yes	Yes	Yes	Yes
Early passive motion	Yes	Yes	Yes	Yes
Early active assisted motion	No/Yes	Yes	Yes	Yes
Early active motion (small tears)	No	Yes	Yes	Yes

For the more established arthroscopically assisted open repair technique, less arthroscopic experience or expertise is required. For those surgeons with less experience in performing shoulder arthroscopy, the technique is less technically demanding and more readily performed. However, this technique is directly limited by the size of the lateral deltoid split. When using a smaller approach for larger or massive rotator cuff tears that are chronic in nature, performing all necessary surgical releases can be difficult, if not impossible, through a limited transdeltoid opening. If a large or massive rotator cuff repair is attempted in this fashion, the surgeon is essentially "squeezing" a large operation through a small opening. Although a formal anterior deltoid takedown is not performed in a classic mini-open approach, attempting to repair a large tear can still lead to significant deltoid injury from surgical traction. This may help explain why some surgeons have reported increased episodes of frozen shoulder and even deltoid injury following mini-open repair.

In contrast, a mini-open assisted arthroscopic repair should not be limited by the size of the lateral deltoid split. All rotator cuff preparation is done in an arthroscopic fashion including débridement of cuff edges, extensive releases, cuff mobilization, tuberosity preparation, and even suture anchor placement if desired. Because the rotator cuff has been previously mobilized and tagged, the tendon edges can be delivered directly to the small opening for placement of tendon gripping sutures and then fixation to bone. Because a majority of the surgery has been performed arthroscopically, the

Table 4
Progression toward minimally invasive rotator cuff repair

Formal open repair
↓
Arthroscopically assisted open repair (Arthroscopic decompression followed by lateral open repair)
↓
Mini-open assisted arthroscopic repair (Arthroscopic decompression, arthroscopic rotator cuff preparation followed by mini-open exposure for bone-tendon fixation)
↓
Complete arthroscopic repair

time requirement and exposure for the deltoid splitting portion should be reduced and deltoid injury minimized.

The technique, however, is associated with some significant disadvantages. A large amount of arthroscopic experience around the shoulder is probably a prerequisite for most surgeons in order to obtain expertise in performing all the necessary surgical releases and suture placement. The technique also relies heavily on uncompromising visualization of the rotator cuff and surrounding structures. Without this, the surgeon can be easily misled during rotator cuff preparation. However, as technically demanding as the arthroscopic portion of this procedure can be, it is still significantly easier from a technical standpoint than complete arthroscopic repair (Table 4). Additionally, in comparison to complete arthroscopic repair, more secure bone to tendon fixation is probably possible, because tendon-gripping Mason-Allen sutures and bone augmentation can be used.[37,38]

Surgical Technique

Basic Setup

Open and arthroscopic shoulder surgery at my institution is performed with the patient under interscalene block regional anesthesia and supplemental laryngeal masked general anesthesia (LMA). The interscalene block regional anesthesia has been a reliable and safe method for obtaining intraoperative and postoperative pain relief.[39] The intraoperative pain relief obtained with the block significantly reduces the general anesthetic requirements for the LMA. Laryngeal mask anesthesia is performed in addition to the interscalene block to obtain a more reliable, responsive control of systolic blood pressure, which is essential for the more complex arthroscopic techniques. The patient is placed in a semisitting, upright beach chair position with the back elevated to approximately 70° to 80°. A shoulder arthroscopic positioning device is often helpful. In my institution, a universal locking head and arm holder is used. Once the patient is positioned on the table with the medial aspect of the scapula in line with the lateral aspect of the table, 20 mL of 0.25% bupivacaine hydrochloride containing epinephrine is injected into the subacromial space. Early injection of the bupivacaine hydrochloride with epinephrine prior to prepping and draping of the patient allows for enhanced vascular constriction from the epinephrine. This step can significantly decrease surgical bleeding and improve visualization. Once the shoulder is prepped and draped, all bony landmarks are carefully outlined with a marking pen to help facilitate accurate portal placement.

Accurate portal placement is especially important when instituting advanced arthroscopic techniques about the shoulder. The posterior portal is generally drawn approximately 1 to 2 cm inferior to the posterior edge of the acromion and 2 cm medial to the posterior lateral corner. This portal is generally drawn slightly more superior than the usual posterior portal for arthroscopy in order to obtain a better line of sight to the subacromial bursa for arthroscopic repair. The anterior portal is positioned just lateral to the palpable coracoid tip. The lateral portal is generally placed 1 cm posterior and 3 cm inferior to the anterior lateral corner of the acromion. The exact placement of this portal is determined by needle localization during arthroscopy.

The arthroscope is first placed in the glenohumeral joint through the posterior portal. A standard glenohumeral inspection is performed. Of particular importance, the biceps tendon should be visualized carefully. Often the pathology in the biceps tendon is in the intertubercular groove portion and not readily seen on initial inspection of the intra-articular portion. A hook should be used to pull the tendon into the joint and ensure there are no structural difficulties with the tendon laterally. In those situations in which there is structural pathology to the tendon; such as a partial tear, atrophy, or chronic enlargement, either biceps tenodesis or tenotomy is preferred as the treatment of choice.[40] In those situations in which the tendon either looks normal or inflamed, surgical treatment for the biceps is not recommended. Next, the rotator cuff tear should be visualized and the tear location and size qualified. This will give an idea as to where the appropriate lateral portal placement should be. Finally, the subscapularis should be carefully visualized and its integrity verified.

Rotator cuff mobilization starts with an intra-articular release. This should be performed with the arthroscope in the posterior portal and a hook multipolar cautery device in the anterior portal. Normally a pouch is present superior to the glenoid labrum between the undersurface of the rotator cuff and the superior or posterior-superior portion of the lateral glenoid neck. A hook probe should be placed in this location to determine if the rotator cuff is scarred to the superior labrum. The release is performed by taking the hook cautery and sharply releasing adhesions between the undersurface of the cuff and the superior glenoid labrum starting from anterior and progressing toward posterior (Fig. 1). The multipolar cautery is oriented away from the suprascapular nerve, which is medial. A circumferential release around the posterior, anterior-superior and posterior-superior labrum can be accomplished all the way to the posterior portal. This release is probably the most important to obtain mobilization of the cuff. In addition, it is probably more readily performed arthroscopically than open, where access to the posterior glenoid and posterior-superior rim is difficult secondary to obstruction by the humeral head. Once this intra-articular release has been performed, the arthroscope is then withdrawn and attention placed to the subacromial space.

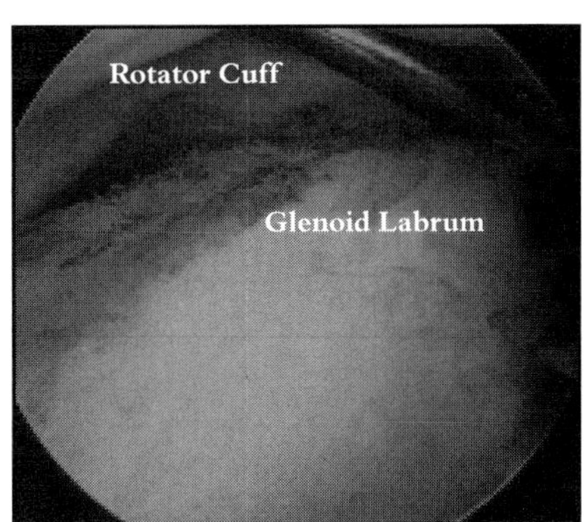

Fig. 1 Release of superior glenoid adhesions.

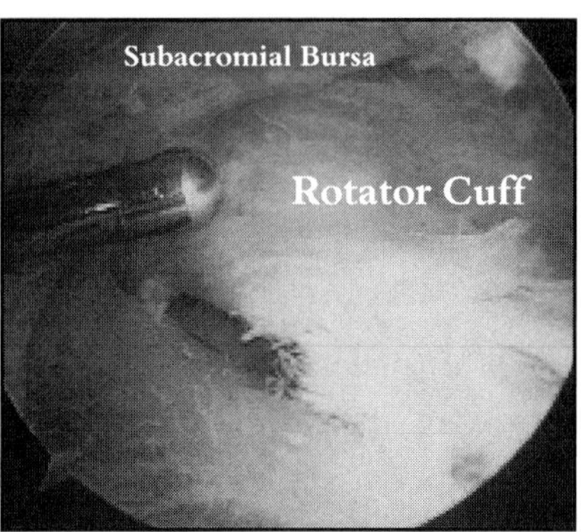

Fig. 2 Release of the superficial surface of the rotator cuff.

An arm holder is used in order to apply inline traction on the humerus. The arm is adducted, forward flexed, and slightly internally rotated. This opens up the subacromial space for good visualization. The arthroscope is then redirected into the subacromial space from posterior. Upon entrance into the subacromial bursa, a needle is used to localize the appropriate location for the lateral portal. The lateral portal location should allow a parallel orientation of the burr to the undersurface of the acromion, and it should also be centered over the middle of the rotator cuff tear. In general, this portal is located 1 cm posterior to the anterior-lateral corner of the acromion and 3 cm interior. The portal is made in the direction of Langer's skin lines in a horizontal fashion.

A subacromial bursectomy is then performed, initially starting out with the full radius resector and usually followed by a multipolar electrocautery device. Care should be taken to visualize the cuff first to make sure that bursa, and not rotator cuff, is being débrided. The anteriormost portions of the bursa are débrided first and the débridement also includes the undersurface of the acromion, which is excavated of soft tissues from the anterior-inferior edge and posteriorly. The arthroscope is then generally switched to the lateral portal and the cautery device placed posterior (Fig. 2). The cautery device is then swept from lateral toward medial and then from anterior toward posterior, again excavating bursa off of the rotator cuff all the way medial to the base of the acromion. Generally, a complete removal of bursa from the underlying rotator cuff can be achieved in this fashion. Because the arthroscope is placed laterally, visualization can be obtained all the way around the teres minor posteriorly and inferiorly. Excellent visualization of the subacromial space and the undersurface of the acromion should be obtained in this fashion. At this time, the scope is replaced into the posterior portal and a burr placed into the anterior portal and an anterior-inferior acromioplasty performed. The degree of acromioplasty performed and whether or not a coracoacromial ligament release is also added depends on the reparability[41] of the cuff tear and the size of the anterior-inferior spur if present. These are precautions to avoid anterior-superior instability.[33] At this point, the mini-open approach through a lateral deltoid split can be performed if the surgeon is not experienced with the more technically difficult arthroscopic procedures.

It should be noted that throughout the subacromial procedure, careful attention should be applied to blood pressure control. As a general rule, systolic blood pressure should not exceed 120 mm Hg. The pump pressure is generally placed at 40 mm Hg, but it can be raised to 60 mm Hg (as necessary to control bleeding). Elevated pump pressures, however, are associated with more rapid soft-tissue distention and edema, conditions that will eventually obscure visualization. Following decompression, an uncompromising visualization of the rotator cuff should be achieved (Fig. 3). The rotator cuff tear should be seen from its most anterior aspect all the way to its most posterior aspect. This is a prerequisite to performing further rotator cuff preparation arthroscopically.

At this point, an arthroscopic shaver is placed into the lateral portal and débridement performed of the greater tuberosity for later rotator cuff repair. The tuberosity is slightly decorticated and extraneous soft tissue removed. A formal bone

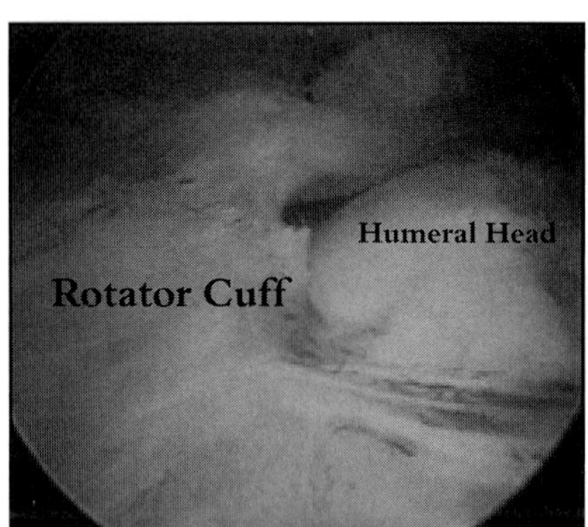

Fig. 3 Arthroscopic visualization of the rotator cuff.

trough is not performed and is contraindicated if a suture anchor is used. Next, the shaver is used to débride any of the torn cuff edge that appears to be nonviable or attenuated. Care should be taken here to do only a limited débridement.

At this point, stay suture placement is initiated. Several different alternative devices are available to achieve this. The Caspari suture punch (Linvatec, Largo, FL) is delivered through the lateral portal (Fig. 4). A place in the midportion of the rotator cuff tear is selected and the suture punch is used to grasp this location. The suture punch is then used to access the mobility of the rotator cuff tendon. For the majority of cases, a release of the rotator cuff from the superior glenoid labrum as well as a superficial bursa generally results in a significant mobilization of the rotator cuff tissue. In rare cases, when assessing the cuff with the suture punch, further releases may be necessary. If the releases are necessary, the suture punch is withdrawn and the arthroscope is placed to the lateral portal. A cautery device is then placed into the anterior portal and this is brought down into the base of the coracoid. At this point, a coracohumeral ligament release is performed right down to the base of the coracoid on the superficial surface. It should be noted that the base of the coracoid has already been débrided on the articular side during the circumferential glenoid release. The sharp débridement can be taken from the base of the coracoid all the way out laterally to the bicipital groove as a rotator interval release as necessary, although this option is rarely needed. Finally, if this release is not sufficient, a posterior interval release can be performed arthroscopically. The scope remains in the lateral portal and the electrocautery device is then switched back to the posterior portal. The base of the acromion and scapular spine can be visualized quite readily from the lateral portal and the cautery device is delivered to this location. The rotator cuff is then mobilized from the scapular spine and base of the acromion in a sharp fashion. Once these releases are performed, mobility of the cuff is reassessed by grasping the tissue with a Caspari suture punch.

After all of these releases are performed, it is a rare case in which the rotator cuff will not be reducible to the greater tuberosity. At this point, multiple shuttle-relay devices (Linvatec, Largo, FL) are delivered by the Caspari suture punch into the anterior, middle, and posterior portions of the rotator cuff tear. In general, these stay sutures are separated by 1 cm and the number required depends on the transverse dimension of the rotator cuff tear. Use of a shuttle-relay device, or alternatively, a No. 1 prolene doubled onto itself allows the surgeon to use these sutures both to control the rotator cuff into a reduced location and also to later pass either transosseous sutures or suture anchors into the cuff for bone fixation.

At this point the mini-open approach is initiated. The horizontal lateral incision is enlarged to a length of 3 to 4 cm (Fig. 5). The subcutaneous tissue is then undermined to expose underlying deltoid fascia. The deltoid is then split inline, with fibers incorporating the arthroscopic puncture site. This split is generally taken up to the acromion and distally about 3 to 4 cm. As the cuff has been previously mobilized and stay sutures already placed, a surprisingly small deltoid split is necessary at this time. Further bursectomy can be performed around the split site to improve visualization, but this is generally not necessary secondary to the extensive bursectomy previously performed with the electrocautery device. Rotating the arm allows different portions of the cuff to be visualized through the deltoid split.

Bone-tendon fixation is then performed at this time. If the tear is small and easily mobilized, then simple stitches placed through suture anchors, which are embedded in the superior lateral aspect of the greater tuberosity, are preferred. For large tears under some tension, Mason-Allen stitches in the cuff, once again placed through suture anchors in the superior lateral location on the greater tuberosity, are preferred.[37,42] Alternatively, transosseous fixation can be used; however, many studies have documented that suture anchors placed in the superior-lateral portion of the greater tuberosity to be at a strength equal to or greater than that of transosseous sutures.[42-44]

Results

The reported outcome from mini-open or arthroscopically assisted rotator cuff repair performed through a lateral deltoid-splitting approach has been generally good and comparable to long-term results seen in multiple open rotator cuff repair series.[1,3-8,41] First reported in 1990 as a preliminary report of 1-year follow-up on 25 patients treated with an arthroscopic subacromial decompression and then lateral deltoid-splitting open repair, Levy and associates[3] reported that 80% of the patients had good or excellent results according to the UCLA shoulder rating. Flynn and associates[45] reported a satisfactory outcome from mini-open repair performed in 10 recreational athletes who participated in overhead and nonthrowing sports. Accelerated reha-

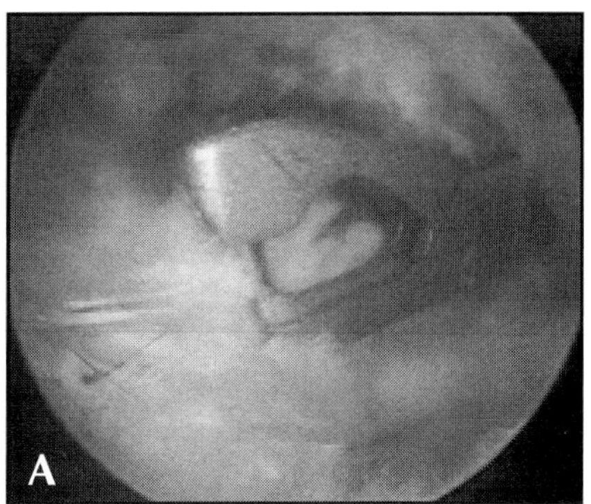

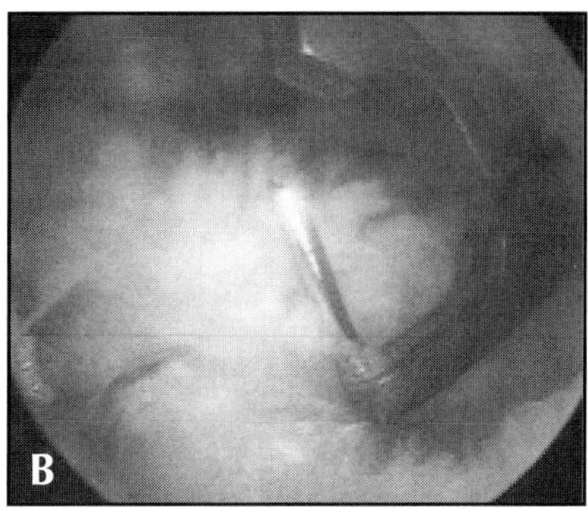

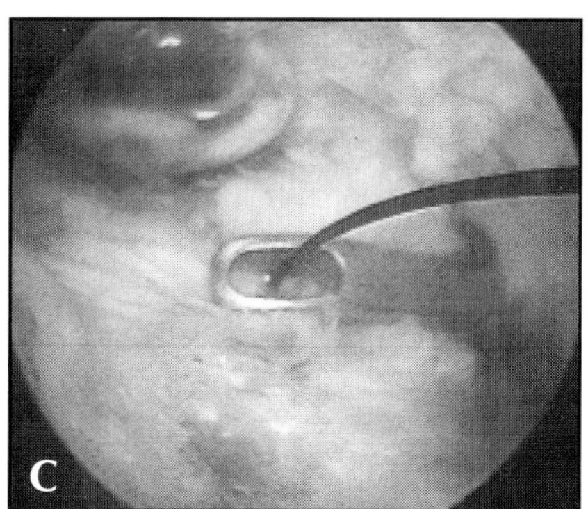

Fig. 4 The Caspari suture punch (Linvatec, Largo, FL) is helpful to insert stay sutures into the rotator cuff. **A** and **B**, This suture punch can be inserted from the lateral portal. **C**, A monofilament suture or a shuttle relay device is then inserted into the rotator cuff to pull traction into the lateral deltoid split.

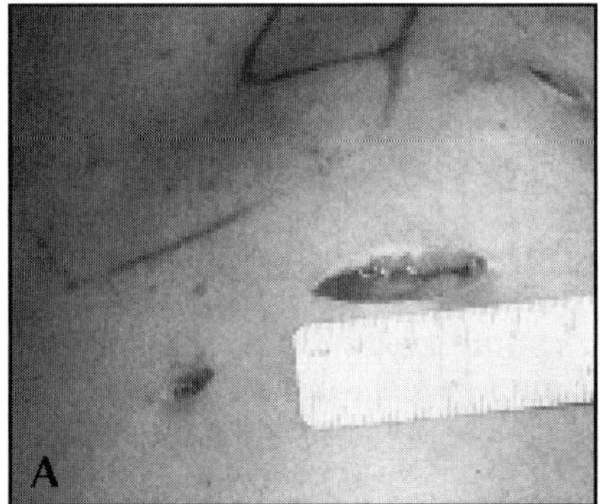

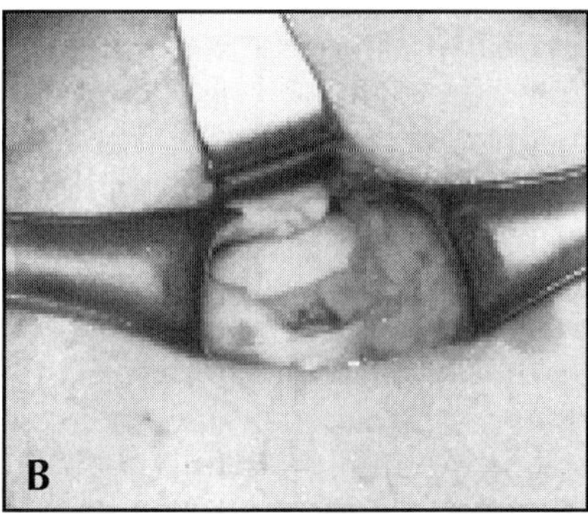

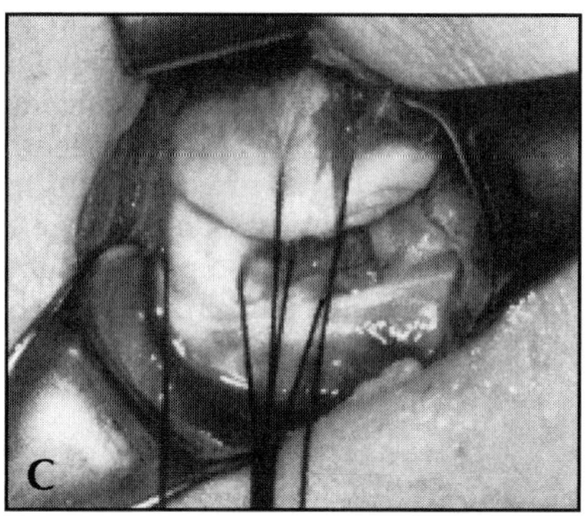

Fig. 5 The mini-open approach. **A**, The anterior-lateral portal is extended. This portal usually measures between 3 and 4 cm in length. Skin incisions within Langer's lines are preferred. **B**, Once subcutaneous dissection is performed, a deltoid split is made in line with the previous portal wound to expose the tear. **C**, Stay sutures are then placed. If arthroscopic preparation has been performed, the previously placed stay sutures can then be brought out through the portal to pull the rotator cuff into view. (Reproduced with permission from Bigliani LU: Rotator cuff repair, in Post M, Bigliani LU, Flatow EL, Pollack RG (eds): *The Shoulder: Operative Technique*. Baltimore, MD, Williams & Wilkins, 1998, pp 133-165.)

bilitation appeared to be present as all these patients returned to their sports within 9 months.

Paulos and Kody[6] presented the first long-term results in 18 patients with an average follow-up of 46 months. In this series, 88% had excellent or good results with the only two poor results seen in patients with pending worker's compensation cases. Pain and function were significantly improved. In another long-term study, Liu and Baker[4] reviewed 44 patients with full-thickness tears treated with an arthroscopically assisted approach. The average follow-up was 4.2 years and 84% of the patients had an excellent or good result. With this surgical technique, the authors correlated outcome to size of tear and showed less satisfactory results in large and massive tears. The authors also showed the procedure to be associated with a shortened hospital stay and more rapid rehabilitation, presumably from less soft-tissue damage. Blevins and associates[2] also reported on results of a large series of patients in which large rotator cuff tears were repaired in addition to the smaller or easily accessible tears. In this study, 83% of the patients achieved a good or excellent rating based on the Hospital for Special Surgery shoulder score. The authors concluded that the procedure was effective for larger rotator cuff tears, but it was more technically demanding. Warner and associates[7] reported on an average 4-year follow-up of 24 patients who were specifically selected for arthroscopically assisted rotator cuff repair. In this focused series, 17 patients underwent a transosseous arthroscopically assisted rotator cuff repair when intraoperative selection criteria showed an avulsion-type tear configuration with good tendon quality and absence of subscapularis tendon involvement. Using specific selection criteria, the authors showed that the arthroscopically assisted repair can achieve excellent results. Average American Shoulder and

Elbow Surgeons Function Index of 96 out of 100 was achieved, along with an 89 out of 100 activity of daily living score.

Two studies have sought to compare open and arthroscopically assisted rotator cuff repairs. Baker and Liu[1] compared open and arthroscopically assisted rotator cuff repairs in 37 patients. The open group had 80% good or excellent results compared with 85% for the arthroscopically assisted repair group. Of the patients who had an open repair, 88% were satisfied in comparison to 92% for the arthroscopically assisted repair group. The shoulder strength and functional outcome did not differ significantly between the two groups; however, the arthroscopically assisted repair group had shorter hospital stays and returned to their previous activity an average of 1 month earlier.

Weber and Schaefer[8] also compared mini-open and formal open repair in a retrospective series. The authors studied 69 patients who had open repair and 60 patients in a mini-open group with a minimum 2-year follow-up. The mini-open repair group was seen to require significantly less parenteral narcotics and had shorter hospital stays. The final outcome, however, was not significantly different between the two groups. The authors concluded that the primary advantage of a mini-open technique was to offer a significant decrease in perioperative morbidity without compromising long-term results.

Summary

The mini-open rotator cuff or arthroscopically assisted surgical procedure for repair of the rotator cuff has become a popular procedure with proven clinical results. The development of this procedure has followed a natural progression toward more minimally invasive means to accomplish rotator cuff repair. For many, it represents a middle ground between the traditional formal open repair and the newer complete arthroscopic rotator cuff repairs. As arthroscopic rotator cuff repair becomes more refined and accepted,[35,36,45-48] the mini-open repair can also represent an excellent transitional technique to someday accomplish the more technically difficult complete arthroscopic repair. Whether used as the definitive rotator cuff repair procedure or as a transitional procedure toward arthroscopic repair, the mini-open repair can be thought of as two different types of procedures, an arthroscopically assisted open repair in which the actual repair is performed in a primarily open fashion, or as a mini-open assisted arthroscopic repair in which most of the repair is performed arthroscopically and an open exposure provided just for bone-tendon fixation. With either strategy, the mini-open repair represents an excellent technique for treating full-thickness rotator cuff tears and offers many of the advantages of either formal or complete arthroscopic repair while minimizing many of the disadvantages.

References

1. Baker CL, Liu SH: Comparison of open and arthroscopically assisted rotator cuff repairs. *Am J Sports Med* 1995;23:99-104.
2. Blevins FT, Warren RF, Cavo C, et al: Arthroscopic assisted rotator cuff repair: Results using a mini-open deltoid splitting approach. *Arthroscopy* 1996;12:50-59.
3. Levy HJ, Uribe JW, Delaney LG: Arthroscopic assisted rotator cuff repair: Preliminary results. *Arthroscopy* 1990;6:55-60.
4. Liu SH, Baker CL: Arthroscopically assisted rotator cuff repair: Correlation of functional results with integrity of the cuff. *Arthroscopy* 1994;10:54-60.
5. Liu SH: Arthroscopically-assisted rotator-cuff repair. *J Bone Joint Surg Br* 1994;76:592-595.
6. Paulos LE, Kody MH: Arthroscopically enhanced "mini approach" to rotator cuff repair. *Am J Sports Med* 1994;22:19-25.
7. Warner JJ, Goitz RJ, Irrgang JJ, Groff YJ: Arthroscopic-assisted rotator cuff repair: Patient selection and treatment outcome. *J Shoulder Elbow Surg* 1997;6:463-472.
8. Weber SC, Schaefer R: Abstract: "Mini-open" versus traditional open repair in the management of small and moderate size tears of the rotator cuff. *Arthroscopy* 1993;9:365-366.
9. Pollock RG, Flatow EL: The rotator cuff: Full-thickness tears: Mini-open repair. *Orthop Clin North Am* 1997;28:169-77.
10. Yamaguchi K, Flatow EL: Arthroscopic evaluation and treatment of the rotator cuff. *Orthop Clin North Am* 1995;26:643-659.
11. Ellman H, Kay SP: Arthroscopic subacromial decompression for chronic impingement: Two- to five-year results. *J Bone Joint Surg Br* 1991;73:395-398.
12. Adamson GJ, Tibone JE: Ten-year assessment of primary rotator cuff repairs. *J Shoulder Elbow Surg* 1993;2:57-63.
13. Bigliani L, Cordasco F, McIlveen S, et al: Operative treatment of massive rotator cuff tears: Long-term results. *J Shoulder Elbow Surg* 1992;1:120-130.
14. Gazielly DF, Gleyze P, Montagnon C: Functional and anatomical results after rotator cuff repair. *Clin Orthop* 1994;304:43-53.
15. Grana WA, Teague B, King M, Reeves RB: An analysis of rotator cuff repair. *Am J Sports Med* 1994;22:585-588.
16. Gupta R, Leggin BG, Iannotti JP: Results of surgical repair of full-thickness tears of the rotator cuff. *Orthop Clin North Am* 1997;28:241-248.
17. Hattrup SJ: Rotator cuff repair: Relevance of patient age. *J Shoulder Elbow Surg* 1995; 4:95-100.
18. Hawkins RJ, Misamore GW, Hobeika PE: Surgery for full-thickness rotator-cuff tears. *J Bone Joint Surg Am* 1985;67:1349-1355.
19. Karas EH, Iannotti JP: Failed repair of the rotator cuff: Evaluation and treatment of complications. *Instr Course Lect* 1998;47:87-95.
20. Kronberg M, Wahlstrom P, Brostrom L-A: Shoulder function after surgical repair of rotator cuff tears. *J Shoulder Elbow Surg* 1997;6:125-130.
21. Kirschenbaum D, Coyle MP Jr, Leddy JP, Katsaros P, Tan F Jr, Cody RP: Shoulder strength with rotator cuff tears: Pre- and postoperative analysis. *Clin Orthop* 1993;288:174-178.
22. Neer CS II, Flatow EL, Lech O: Tears of the rotator cuff: Long term results of anterior acromioplasty and repair. *Orthop Trans* 1988;12:673-674.
23. Neer CS II (ed): *Shoulder Reconstruction.* Philadelphia, PA, WB Saunders, 1990, pp 41-142.
24. Rokito AS, Cuomo F, Gallagher MA, Zuckerman JD: Long-term functional outcome of repair of large and massive chronic tears of the rotator cuff. *J Bone Joint Surg Am* 1999;81:991-997.
25. Rokito AS, Zuckerman JD, Gallagher MA, Cuomo F: Strength after surgical repair of the rotator cuff. *J Shoulder Elbow Surg* 1996;5:12-17.
26. Romeo AA, Hang DW, Bach BR Jr, Shott S: Repair of full thickness rotator cuff tears: Gender, age, and other factors affecting outcome. *Clin Orthop* 1999;367:243-255.
27. Codman EA (ed): *The Shoulder: Rupture of the*

Supraspinatus Tendon and Other Lesions In or About the Subacromial Bursa. Boston, MA, Thomas Todd, 1934.

28. Codman EA: Complete rupture of the supraspinatus tendon: Operative treatment with report of two successful cases. *Boston Med Surg J* 1911;164:708-710.
29. Neer CS II: Anterior acromioplasty for the chronic impingement syndrome in the shoulder: A preliminary report. *J Bone Joint Surg Am* 1972;54:41-50.
30. Mansat P, Cofield RH, Kersten TE, Rowland CM: Complications of rotator cuff repair. *Orthop Clin North Am* 1997;28:205-213.
31. Mormino MA, Gross RM, McCarthy JA: Captured shoulder: A complication of rotator cuff surgery. *Arthroscopy* 1996;12:457-461.
32. Yamaguchi K: Complications of rotator cuff repair. *Tech Orthop* 1997;12:33-41.
33. Wiley AM: Superior humeral dislocation: A complication following decompression and débridement for rotator cuff tears. *Clin Orthop* 1991;263:135-141.
34. Gartsman GM: Arthroscopic management of rotator cuff disease. *J Am Acad Orthop Surg* 1998;6:259-266.
35. Gartsman GM, Brinker MR, Khan M: Early effectiveness of arthroscopic repair for full-thickness tears of the rotator cuff: An outcome analysis. *J Bone Joint Surg Am* 1998;80:33-40.
36. Gartsman GM, Hammerman SM: Full-thickness tears: Arthroscopic repair. *Orthop Clin North Am* 1997;28:83-98.
37. Gerber C, Schneeberger AG, Beck M, Schlegel U: Mechanical strength of repairs of the rotator cuff. *J Bone Joint Surg Br* 1994;76:371-380.
38. Gerber C, Schneeberger AG, Perren SM, Nyffeler RW: Experimental rotator cuff repair: A preliminary study. *J Bone Joint Surg Am* 1999;81:1281-1290.
39. Brown AR, Weiss R, Greenberg C, Flatow EL, Bigliani LU: Interscalene block for shoulder arthroscopy: Comparison with general anesthesia. *Arthroscopy* 1993;9:295-300.
40. Sethi N, Wright R, Yamaguchi K: Disorders of the long head of the biceps tendon. *J Shoulder Elbow Surg* 1999;8:644-654.
41. Gartsman GM: Arthroscopic assessment of rotator cuff tear reparability. *Arthroscopy* 1996;12:546-549.
42. Burkhart SS, Diaz Pagan JL, Wirth MA, Athanasiou KA: Cyclic loading of anchor-based rotator cuff repairs: Confirmation of the tension overload phenomenon and comparison of suture anchor fixation with transosseous fixation. *Arthroscopy* 1997;13:720-724.
43. Reed SC, Glossop N, Ogilvie-Harris DJ: Full-thickness rotator cuff tears: A biomechanical comparison of suture versus bone anchor techniques. *Am J Sports Med* 1996;24:46-48.
44. Barber FA, Cawley P, Prudich JF: Suture anchor failure strength: An in vivo study. *Arthroscopy* 1993;9:647-652.
45. Flynn L, Flood S, Clifford S, et al: Arthroscopically assisted rotator cuff repair with the Mitek anchor. *Am J Arthroscopy* 1991;1:15-18.
46. Snyder SJ: Technique of arthroscopic rotator cuff repair using implantable 4-mm Revo suture anchors, suture Shuttle Relays, and no. 2 nonabsorbable mattress sutures. *Orthop Clin North Am* 1997;28:267-275.
47. Stollsteimer GT, Savoie FH III: Arthroscopic rotator cuff repair: Current indications, limitations, techniques, and results. *Instr Course Lect* 1998;47:59-65.
48. Tauro JC: Arthroscopic rotator cuff repair: Analysis of technique and results at 2- and 3-year follow-up. *Arthroscopy* 1998;14:45-51.

Transitioning to Arthroscopic Rotator Cuff Repair: The Pros and Cons

Ken Yamaguchi, MD
William N. Levine, MD
Guido Marra, MD
Leesa M. Galatz, MD
Steven Klepps, MD
Evan L. Flatow, MD

Abstract

There has been much recent enthusiasm regarding complete arthroscopic rotator cuff repair, and it is becoming apparent that, for many, this newer technique may be a preferable alternative to the more traditional mini-open rotator cuff repair. Several short-term studies have demonstrated that complete arthroscopic repair has excellent results comparable with those of mini-open repair, which is also an excellent technique. The choice of which procedure may be better for an individual patient or surgeon can be based on a variety of considerations, including the patient's expectations, the pathoanatomy of the cuff, and the surgical experience of the surgeon. The relative merits and disadvantages of arthroscopic rotator cuff repair are discussed on the basis of those considerations. When a surgeon is deciding which procedure to perform, it is important that the basic principles of rotator cuff repair not be compromised and that he or she perform the procedure that is most reproducible given his or her level of experience; however, for those who are now utilizing mini-open repair, arthroscopic repair may have important advantages and may be worth pursuing in the future. If a surgeon chooses to obtain the skills necessary to perform a complete arthroscopic repair, performance of the mini-open procedure offers an excellent opportunity to make an orderly transition.

Although the best method for repair of full-thickness rotator cuff tears has been controversial, complete arthroscopic rotator cuff repair techniques have been evolving as a future alternative to traditional open and mini-open repairs.[1-13] Early reported experience has been promising, and the technique has become increasingly popular among experienced shoulder surgeons as a preferred means to obtain repair of the rotator cuff. In experienced hands, the technique appears to offer less pain and morbidity as well as quicker recovery than do alternative techniques such as open or mini-open repair. In this chapter, we review the advantages of arthroscopic rotator cuff repair in comparison with the more established mini-open repair. Both techniques will be reviewed for their merits and disadvantages. Additionally, there will be a discussion of how the mini-open technique can be used to gradually transition to an all-arthroscopic technique.[1,3,11]

Historical Perspective

Rotator cuff tears have long been recognized as a disabling problem of the upper extremity that can be treated effectively with surgical repair. Codman[14] reportedly performed the first open rotator cuff repair in 1911. Over the next three decades, surgical treatment of rotator cuff tears became increasingly popular, with many different techniques being described;[15-20] however, the results were variable, and a high percentage of unsatisfactory results was reported in some series.[15,21,22]

Neer[23] reported the results of anterior acromioplasty in combination with cuff mobilization and repair in 1972. The surgical fundamentals emphasized in that report substantially improved the reliability of the outcomes of repairs of rotator cuff tears. The fundamentals include (1) preservation or meticulous repair of the deltoid origin, (2) adequate decompression of the subacromial space by resection of any anteroinferior osteophytes, (3) surgical releases as necessary to obtain freely mobile muscle-tendon units,

(4) secure fixation of the tendon to the greater tuberosity, and (5) closely supervised rehabilitation including early passive motion within a protected range.

It is important to remember the fundamentals of surgical treatment that have proved successful in open rotator cuff repair when considering new minimally invasive techniques. It is likely that the results of arthroscopically assisted or completely arthroscopic procedures will be best if those fundamentals are preserved.

Arthroscopic Treatment Options

The use of arthroscopy in the shoulder has expanded dramatically since its introduction in 1980. As surgeons have become increasingly comfortable with use of the arthroscope in the shoulder, the indications for shoulder arthroscopy have increased. Ellman's seminal 1987 article describing a technique for arthroscopic subacromial decompression led to further interest in the use of the arthroscope as an alternative to open rotator cuff repairs.[24]

At this time, there are two primary methods of arthroscopically assisted repair of the rotator cuff: the mini-open rotator cuff repair, initially described by Levy and associates[25] in a preliminary study and then validated by Paulos and Kody,[26] and the complete arthroscopic rotator cuff repair, popularized by Gartsman and associates.[3] The traditional mini-open approach can be further subdivided into two different types,[27-29] reflecting the increasing use of the arthroscope to accomplish many of the surgical procedures used in a traditional open repair. In the first type of mini-open repair, the arthroscope is used primarily to obtain a decompression; the remainder of the procedure is done through an open approach. In the second type of mini-open repair, the operation is performed primarily arthroscopically: the arthroscope is used to carry out the decompression, release adhesions, and place tagging sutures. A mini-open approach is then performed at the end of the procedure in order to obtain suture management and tendon-to-bone fixation. The expanded options for arthroscopically assisted rotator cuff repair thus can be classified as follows: (1) Arthroscopically assisted open repair, which consists of arthroscopic subacromial decompression followed by open repair of the rotator cuff through a lateral deltoid-splitting approach. (2) Mini-open arthroscopically assisted repair, which includes arthroscopic subacromial decompression, release of adhesions, placement of tagging sutures, and débridement of the tendon edges followed by a mini-open deltoid-splitting approach to obtain suture management and bone-tendon fixation. (3) Complete arthroscopic repair, in which subacromial decompression, release of adhesions, and bone-tendon fixation are all carried out in an arthroscopic fashion.[27-29]

Each of these treatment options has inherent advantages and disadvantages. Additionally, all have common advantages in comparison with traditional open techniques. Understanding the relative merits of these different procedures can help to determine which technique is most appropriate for each individual surgeon and patient so that a good clinical result can be obtained.

Advantages Common to Mini-Open and Complete Arthroscopic Repair

Deltoid Preservation

When the anterior acromioplasty is performed arthroscopically, the deltoid muscle does not have to be detached from the acromion, thus preserving the deltoid muscle origin during repair of the torn tendons. This is a major advantage over traditional open approaches. Deltoid detachment following rotator cuff repair is a devastating, albeit rare, complication.[30-33] Preservation of the deltoid origin, therefore, is an extremely attractive option. In addition, the postoperative rehabilitation of the shoulder can be less restricted if it is not necessary to wait for the deltoid to heal to the acromion.

Arthroscopic Evaluation and Treatment of the Glenohumeral Joint

An important potential advantage of arthroscopic treatment over traditional open repair is an improved ability to diagnose and treat lesions within the glenohumeral joint. Miller and Savoie[34] found a 76% prevalence of intra-articular pathologic disorders in patients undergoing mini-open rotator cuff repair and concluded that glenohumeral arthroscopy was useful. However, they did not comment on the importance of the documented lesions, which made it difficult to interpret the results of their study. In a recent study of patients who had undergone arthroscopic rotator cuff repair, Gartsman and associates[1] showed that the treatment of intra-articular lesions can affect outcome. In that study, patients with a major intra-articular lesion had a preoperative University of California at Los Angeles score of 10.9 points compared with 23.7 points for patients without an intra-articular lesion. Postoperatively, the scores were 29.9 and 31.2 points, respectively ($P = 0.23$). Thus, despite the fact that the group with a major intra-articular lesion had more severe preoperative disease, treatment of the lesions led to outcomes that were similar to those in patients without such a lesion.

Advantages Associated With Complete Arthroscopic Repair

Mobilization and Release of the Rotator Cuff

Arthroscopic mobilization and release of the rotator cuff has generally been considered an advantage of complete arthroscopic repair over mini-open repair. More recently, a modern approach to mini-open repair has included arthroscopic releases. However, this advantage is still primarily associated with the complete arthroscopic repair, and surgeons who are capable of performing arthroscopic releases can generally advance to complete arthroscopic repair in very little time. If arthroscopic lysis of adhesions is performed, the fundamental principles of open rotator cuff repair can be preserved with both arthroscopic and mini-open repairs.

Decreased Surgical Insult to the Deltoid

While the original technique of mini-open repair substantially decreased deltoid injury compared with that associated with formal open techniques, the complete arthroscopic repair represents an additional opportunity to decrease the surgical insult to the deltoid. Although there is only a small difference in the size of the lateral skin incision (3.5 cm compared with 1.5 cm), the amount of surgery and retraction performed through the opening differs substantially between the complete arthroscopic and mini-open repairs. In the mini-open repair, the lateral deltoid split is generally followed by the placement of self-retaining retractors or other devices to obtain visualization. This retraction, performed for any amount of time, can lead to substantial injury to the deltoid muscle. This consideration is especially relevant to surgeons who perform traditional mini-open techniques with open surgical release of the cuff through a limited lateral approach. The increased rate of postoperative stiffness seen after traditional mini-open repairs may in fact be due to this injury to the deltoid.[35] These concerns are decreased with more modern techniques of mini-open repair in which the releases and cuff mobilization are performed arthroscopically.

In contrast to the mini-open repair involving the lateral deltoid split, the arthroscopic repair requires a small incision for insertion of a 9- to 10-mm cannula. No retraction is applied to the deltoid during the course of the surgery, and the only insult to the deltoid occurs during the insertion of the cannula.

Decreased Immediate Postoperative Pain and Better Rehabilitation

There is very little available information with which to compare mini-open and complete arthroscopic techniques. However, two recent presentations[9,11] indicated that complete arthroscopic repair is associated with a better early range of motion and a decreased requirement for overnight hospitalization. These two advantages reflect the fact that complete arthroscopic repair appears to be associated with less perioperative pain than is mini-open repair. These findings are not surprising considering the decreased surgical insult to the deltoid associated with arthroscopic repair. Comparative prospective studies are needed to substantiate this potential advantage.

Decreased Postoperative Stiffness

Although we are not aware of any reports in the literature on the topic, several presentations at national meetings have suggested that the prevalence of adhesive capsulitis is higher after mini-open rotator cuff repair than it is after traditional open rotator cuff repair. In his series of patients treated with mini-open rotator cuff repair, Nicholson[35] found that 6 of 54 patients (11%) required an arthroscopic release to treat stiffness and that 2 additional patients had stiffness with a functional impact. Williams and associates[36] also reported that a high percentage of patients (about 20%) had substantial stiffness following mini-open rotator cuff repair.

It is possible that the stiffness reported in those series reflects the procedure in its infancy: namely, an arthroscopic decompression without an attempt to release adhesions and mobilize the tendons arthroscopically. It is possible to injure the deltoid tendon when releases are performed through the mini-open incision.

Limitations in the Size of the Rotator Cuff Tear Amenable to Mini-Open Repair

There is a major limitation to the size or chronicity of a tear that can be treated with a traditional mini-open repair in which the cuff is released and mobilized through the deltoid approach. Open release and mobilization of a chronically retracted cuff may require a prolonged period of traction on the deltoid. In effect, the surgeon would be attempting to "squeeze" a large repair through a small approach. As stated earlier, these limitations are reduced with more advanced mini-open techniques in which arthroscopic releases are performed.

Disadvantages of Complete Arthroscopic Repair

Bone-Tendon Fixation

Fixation in transosseous tunnels has traditionally been the method of choice for rotator cuff repair. Suture anchors were originally designed for use in the glenoid in Bankart reconstructions. The original designs of these anchors were ill-suited for use in the osteoporotic proximal part of the humerus, leading to many anecdotal reports of failed repairs secondary to anchor problems.[37,38] Major advances in the design of suture anchors over the last decade eliminated some of the early concerns about anchor failure. The modern improvements in suture anchor fixation are pertinent to complete arthroscopic repairs as they are limited primarily to simple suture grasping of the tendon and suture anchor fixation to bone. The use of transfixation devices has also been suggested; however, there are concerns that such fixation will not be stronger than that provided by sutures and may, in fact, be worse.

Whereas the fixation provided by suture anchors has been repeatedly shown to be as strong or stronger than that provided by traditional transosseous techniques,[39,40] the lack of a tendon-gripping suture on the rotator cuff may be a concern. Although it may not be intuitive, this disadvantage may be more pertinent for patients with good-quality, relatively healthy tendon tissue in whom consistent bone-to-tendon healing would be expected if the fixation can be sustained for 6 weeks or longer. In such cases, a lack of good mechanical fixation may lead to a failure of healing when otherwise healing would have been possible. The strength of fixation of healthy tendons to the greater tuberosity may be important.[2,41] Gerber and associates[41] studied the mechanical properties provided by several techniques of tendon-to-bone suture fixation. They found that the most commonly used technique—the simple stitch—provided mechanically poor results, whereas a new modification of the Mason-Allen suture technique improved the ultimate tensile strength nearly twofold.

In contrast, the healing of large, degenerative tears appears to be inconsistent at best, regardless of the fixation method or operative approach. More recently, Gerber and associates[2] updated their previous work by studying experimental rotator cuff repair in a sheep model. They again found that the modified Mason-Allen stitch was superior to simple sutures; however, both fixation methods had a large failure rate, and modifications of the rehabilitation protocol (to include protective immobilization and delayed mobilization) were found to be more important.[2]

To some, the fact that Mason-Allen stitches can be used with mini-open repairs is a potential advantage of those repairs over completely arthroscopic techniques, in which it has been technically difficult to use tendon-grasping sutures. It is important to note that the strength of initial fixation may not be as important as other considerations such as the biologic capacity for healing and the type of rehabilitation. At this time, the early results of arthroscopic repair seem to be equivalent to those of mini-open repair despite concerns about fixation strength.[1,11-13]

Technical Difficulty

Complete arthroscopic rotator cuff repair is widely considered to be a technically difficult procedure. It may be necessary to perform a relatively large number of these procedures to obtain the experience required to carry them out in a reliable fashion. For surgeons with less experience with arthroscopic surgery of the shoulder, the mini-open repair is a more familiar technique with less complexity. The lateral deltoid split and open repair of the rotator cuff that are performed with the more established mini-open technique are only slightly different from the procedures done in a traditional open repair. The technical difficulties associated with performing an arthroscopic decompression first are relatively minor compared with those associated with performing a complete arthroscopic repair. Thus, for surgeons who are less experienced with these types of surgical procedures, the mini-open repair offers a real advantage in that it is less difficult.

However, although complete arthroscopic rotator cuff repair may be a more technically difficult procedure than a mini-open repair, it should not preclude a surgeon from eventually transitioning to this method if it is deemed to be superior. With a proper transition strategy, those with less experience with arthroscopic surgery can still achieve the skills necessary to do a complete arthroscopic repair. Of course, the transition period for those with less experience may be longer than that for those with more experience.

Indications for Complete Arthroscopic Repair

The pros and cons of transitioning from a mini-open to a complete arthroscopic rotator cuff repair should be considered carefully when an orthopaedic surgeon is deciding which procedure is best. Ideally, the choice between mini-open and arthroscopic tendon repair should depend on the preoperative surgical expectations of the patient (for example, how much he or she values a minimally invasive approach), the mechanical properties of the torn cuff (for example, where simple sutures will hold the tendon edge), the surgical experience of the surgeon (currently perhaps a dominant factor), and the reported outcomes obtained with the various types of procedures (still preliminary). Furthermore, while it is usually stated that the choice of technique should not change the indications for surgery, it is not only likely but also probably appropriate that as the morbidity of the surgery decreases more patients will proceed with a repair. In comparison with the situation 20 years ago, when surgery involved general anesthesia, several days of hospitalization, and a large incision with extensive muscular dissection, the risk-benefit profile is now more in favor of surgical treatment for refractory pain.

Patient Factors

Although most patients would prefer a small incision or decreased surgical morbidity, patient preference should not distract the treating surgeon from performing the most appropriate procedure to achieve a good result. Other patient factors are probably more important when the surgeon considers the indications for an arthroscopic repair. These include the chief symptom—that is, whether it is pain or loss of strength and function. While some surgeons may think that open repair is best for all patients and others have a similar conviction about arthroscopic repair, many believe that arthroscopic repair yields a somewhat weaker mechanical construct. Thus, many surgeons will offer arthroscopic repair to patients with reasonable function who are primarily seeking pain relief and will reserve open or mini-open repair for patients who are concerned about loss of strength and may require a more solid repair. The former group might include young patients with a small tear. A patient with a repairable tear and little muscle atrophy who is seeking strength more than pain relief may want the most mechanically secure repair, such as that provided by the mini-open procedure. In contrast, an elderly patient with a very large defect and rotator cuff muscle atrophy in whom deltoid preservation and reduced morbidity are of paramount importance may benefit more from the less invasive arthroscopic repair.

Pathoanatomic Factors

The most important pathoanatomic factors are tissue quality, tear size, tendon mobility, and status of the articular surfaces. In most cases, these can be adequately evaluated by arthroscopic means.[12]

Tendon quality may be decreased by the chronicity of the tear, previous surgery, repeated injections, chronic steroid use, rheumatoid arthritis, or other conditions, with an increased risk of suture pull-out.[3,4,13] Mason-Allen sutures may be better at distributing the force onto the suture rather than the tendon and may have a role in such cases.[41] Although these sutures can be placed arthroscopically, doing so is difficult. As stated above, this is a controversial consideration and may be most relevant to younger patients with a smaller tear and a good potential for healing.

The condition of the bone is also an important factor.[13] The bone should hold bone anchors adequately. Advanced age, a long-standing tear, metabolic disease, and compromised function all negatively influence bone density. If bone anchors cannot be placed, then an open technique involving use of bone tunnels may be more appropriate, but this is controversial. Several studies have shown that bone anchors provide stronger fixation than do bone tunnels in cadaveric specimens.[39,40] At this time, osteoporotic bone per se is not a contraindication to arthroscopic repair.

Initially, arthroscopic repair was described for small to medium tears (< 5 mm) with less than 2 cm of retraction.[13,42] Some believe that if the tendon cannot be advanced without excess tension, then arthroscopic repair should be abandoned in favor of open repair.[1,13,43] However, this approach has been vigorously debated because of the increasing ability to achieve equal or perhaps better mobilization with arthroscopic techniques.[27,44] As arthroscopic methods have improved in terms of mobilization and suture placement, the indications have been modified to include larger tears.[5,43] Furthermore, techniques such as side-to-side repair, margin convergence, and partial repair have been developed to assist with the treatment of massive tears.[5] Currently, the size of the tear has become irrelevant to many surgeons when they determine arthroscopic repairability.

Surgeon Factors

Surgeons must offer patients techniques with which they feel comfortable and with which they have adequate experience and skill. A well-performed open repair is far better than a poorly performed arthroscopic one. Frank discussions with patients regarding relative surgical experience and expected results may help them to choose an approach. Many patients prefer the operation to be performed with the method most familiar to a trusted orthopaedist to being part of a difficult learning process. Although the technical difficulty associated with an arthroscopic repair may be intimidating to less-experienced surgeons, the learning curve can be controlled with an appropriate transition strategy. Hence, a transition to arthroscopic repair may still be a reasonable goal for even less-experienced surgeons if they believe that a well-performed arthroscopic repair is better than a well-performed mini-open repair.

Results of Arthroscopic Repair

The proper indications for arthroscopic rotator cuff repair should be developed on the basis of data. Multiple short-term studies have revealed a substantial improvement in function, decrease in pain, and improvement in satisfaction for patients who have undergone arthroscopic rotator cuff repair. The level of success has been similar to that achieved with use of the mini-open technique[1,5-9,13,45] (Table 1). Even though these studies were mostly retrospective reviews or scientific presentations, and we do not yet have the benefit of randomized, prospective studies, it is important to review the early studies as we continue to assess and modify our techniques.

As is typical of retrospective reviews, these studies have several weaknesses and are difficult to interpret. For instance, in some of the early reports, arthroscopic repairs were reserved for small, nonretracted tears, while open techniques were used for large or massive tears.[11,13] In the study by Stollsteimer and Savoie,[13] of 891 rotator cuff repairs performed during the study period, 48 were performed arthroscopically and 843 were performed with an open technique. By selecting patients with simpler tears for arthroscopic repair, Stollsteimer and Savoie created and subsequently compared two different patient populations. Despite such limitations, these studies have documented positive outcomes in several different patient populations, leading to the increasing popularity of arthroscopic rotator cuff repairs. Subsequent studies have shown that any size of tear can be repaired arthroscopically without compromising the result.[1,9,13] In those studies, comparison of patient populations with small (< 1 cm), medium (1 to 3 cm), and large (> 3 cm) tears revealed no differences in University of California at Los Angeles or American Shoulder and Elbow Surgeon scores. Also, no difference in outcome was noted among patients of different ages, suggesting that the arthroscopic repair is equally effective in all age groups.[13]

The only studies of which we are aware that have directly compared mini-

Table 1
Results of Arthroscopic Rotator Cuff Repairs Reported in the Literature

				Score (points)						
				UCLA*		Pain		Constant		
Author	Year of Study	No. of Patients	Duration of Follow-up (mo)	Pre-operative	Post-operative	Pre-operative	Post-operative	Pre-operative	Post-operative	Success Rate (%)
Tauro[7]	1998	53	24	17	41/45	2.3	8.4			92
Stollsteimer and Savoie[13]	1998	48	34		33					
Gartsman et al[1]	1998	73	30	12.4	31.1	1.4	7.6	41.7	83.6	90
Burkhart[5]	2000	24	38	15.1	32.3					96
Hoffmann et al[6]	2000	45	34					46	91	
Gleyze et al[45]	2000	87	25			4.05	12.3	49.7	83.5	95
Wolf[8]	2000	96	74		32.3					
Nottage and Severud[9]	2001	35	38		32.6					91
Weber[11]	2001	126	36		32.3					92

*UCLA = University of California at Los Angeles

open and arthroscopic techniques by the same surgeon and in the same patient populations have shown the results of the two methods to be similar.[9,11] In Weber's[11] study, 95% of the arthroscopic repairs were done on an outpatient basis, whereas only 28% of the mini-open repairs were. Although these two studies have contributed to our confidence in performing these repairs, the ideal study, which would include random selection and prospective and blind evaluation of patients, has not yet been done.

Most of the early studies on arthroscopic rotator cuff repair have focused on clinical outcome. Little has been done to evaluate the integrity of the rotator cuff with either imaging or arthroscopic techniques. Although a fairly high prevalence of incomplete healing has been reported after mini-open repairs, patients still had a good clinical outcome; however, patients in whom the repaired rotator cuff remained intact had better strength.[30,46-49] The two studies in which imaging was used to evaluate arthroscopic rotator cuff repairs postoperatively both revealed a substantial rate of incomplete healing.[10,46] Ball and associates[10] performed ultrasound for 20 consecutive patients who had had an arthroscopic repair of a massive, chronic tear and, despite excellent clinical results, found disruption in 90%.

Complications of Arthroscopic Repair

Complications have been rarely reported after arthroscopic rotator cuff repair,[9,11,13,50] and some believe that the rate of complications is lower than that after open repair after these procedures.[3,27] Weber[11] reported three loose anchors that led to a reoperation, Nottage and Severud[9] reported one sinus tract infection, and Grondel and associates[50] reported two superficial infections. Although to our knowledge stiffness has not been reported after arthroscopic repairs, in some studies stiffness developed in 10% to 20% of patients treated with the mini-open technique.[9,28,35] In both the study by Nicholson and Duckworth[35] and that by Nottage and Severud,[9] the stiffness required surgical manipulation or release.

Technique of Arthroscopic Repair

The arthroscope is placed into the glenohumeral joint through the posterior portal, and an anterior working portal is established. The glenohumeral joint is systematically examined. The articular surfaces of the glenoid and humerus must be carefully assessed for chondral damage, which is graded when present.[51] Articular defects are not uncommon in patients who have rotator cuff lesions.[52] Attention is then turned to the biceps tendon and the superior aspect of the glenoid labrum. Fraying and degeneration of the superior aspect of the labrum is seen frequently and is of uncertain importance. The stability of the biceps insertion is tested with a probe. The long head of the biceps is drawn into the glenohumeral joint and inspected.[53] The rotator cuff is inspected with the arm in the abducted position. Internal and external rotation of the arm allows inspection of the entire rotator cuff. The supraspinatus insertion is at the articular margin, whereas there is an intervening bare area between the articular margin and the infraspinatus and teres minor. When the tendon edge is frayed, débridement to normal tissue is performed to evaluate the extent of the tendon injury. If there is any question about whether the tear is full-thickness, a colored suture placed in the area in question is used to localize the area on the bursal surface.

A retracted tear of the rotator cuff is often associated with adhesions of the articular side of the cuff to the glenoid.

These are released with the use of electrocautery or arthroscopic basket forceps (Fig. 1). When there is substantial retraction of the anterior aspect of the supraspinatus, the rotator interval can also be released under direct visualization.

Bursal Arthroscopy

The arthroscopic sheath is redirected into the subacromial bursa through the posterior portal. The sheath is used to lyse adhesions from the undersurface of the acromion and the lateral part of the deltoid. The lateral working portal is established under direct visualization. It should be positioned to allow the motorized shaver to move freely under the acromion. If the portal is positioned too close to the acromion, resection of the anteromedial aspect of the acromion will be difficult. The portal incision is placed parallel to the Langer lines for cosmetic reasons. The bursa veil is resected with a motorized shaver or an electrocautery device. Arthroscopic evaluation of the subacromial space includes assessment of the coracoacromial ligament for wear and the bursal side of the rotator cuff. If a suture marker was placed through the rotator cuff, it should be located, and the rotator cuff should be inspected for wear and thickness.

A motorized shaver is used to remove the periosteum on the undersurface of the acromion. The coracoacromial ligament is released from the lateral and anterior aspects of the acromion. It should be noted that the coracoacromial ligament is usually composed of an anterolateral band and a posteromedial band. The anterolateral band extends posteriorly on the acromial undersurface and beyond the anterolateral corner of the acromion.[54] An incomplete release of this portion of the ligament can result in clinical failure of an arthroscopic acromioplasty.

After exposure of the anterior aspect of the acromion, bone is removed by gently sweeping the motorized burr from anterior to posterior while moving it from lateral to medial. All osseous prominences are removed so that the remaining anterior third of the acromion is relatively flat. The acromioplasty is then viewed through the lateral portal to ensure that it is complete. Any final contouring is performed through the posterior portal.

Bursal Preparation for Arthroscopic Rotator Cuff Repair

With the advanced mini-open arthroscopic rotator cuff repair technique, the bursal resection is more extensive and is performed to facilitate visualization and mobilization of the torn tendons. Bursal resection is initially performed from the lateral portal, with removal of the bursa from the lateral aspect of the subacromial space to completely visualize the greater tuberosity. Resection then proceeds medially toward the acromioclavicular joint. Care must be taken to avoid injury to the muscle when the bursa over the supraspinatus is resected. The arthroscope is then switched to the lateral portal, and resection of the bursa is completed from the posterior portal. A rotator interval release can be completed by excising the tissue back to the base of the coracoid, which divides the coracohumeral ligament. The arthroscope is then switched back to the posterior portal, and an acromioplasty is performed as previously described. It should be noted that, at this point, all of the traditionally open releases have now been performed arthroscopically. These include release of adhesions on the deep surface between the glenoid labrum and the rotator cuff as well as adhesions superficial to the cuff between the acromion, subtrapezial fat, and scapular spine. If needed, a rotator interval release, including division of the coracohumeral ligament, can also be performed arthroscopically.

Next, the edge of the tear is débrided with use of arthroscopic basket forceps and a motorized shaver. The greater tuberosity is cleared of soft tissue and is lightly decorticated. Several traction sutures are then passed through the rotator cuff. This can be done with various commercially available suture-passing devices. The sutures are passed through the lateral portal, and the mobility of the rotator cuff is evaluated.

A 10-mm clear cannula vent is then placed through the anterolateral portal.

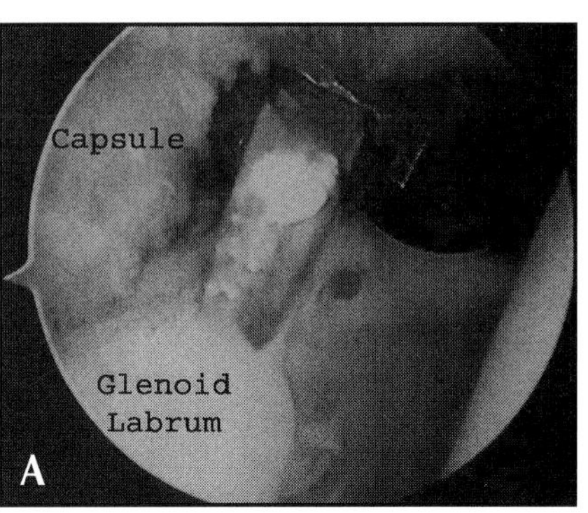

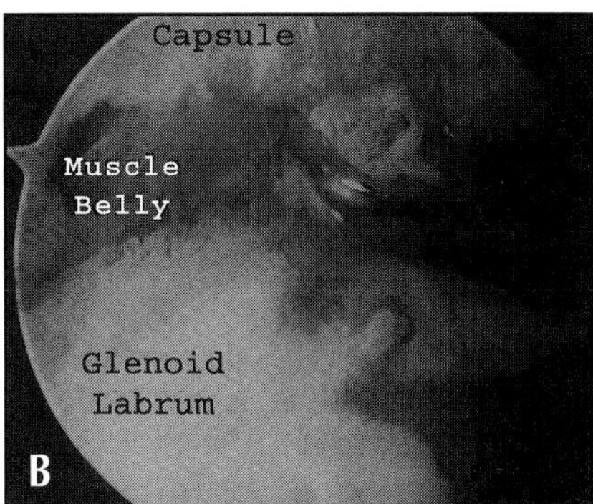

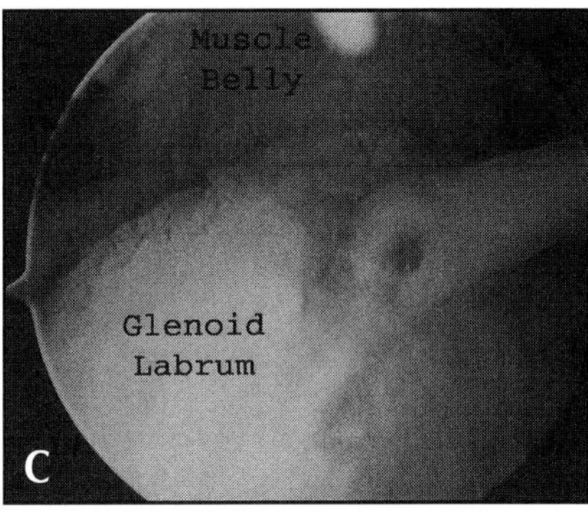

Fig. 1 Capsular release of adhesions of the articular side of the rotator cuff to the glenoid rim is performed with the use of electrocautery or arthroscopic basket forceps. **A,** Basket forceps removing capsular tissue at the edge of the glenoid labrum. **B,** View of the capsule and overlying muscle. **C,** Completed release.

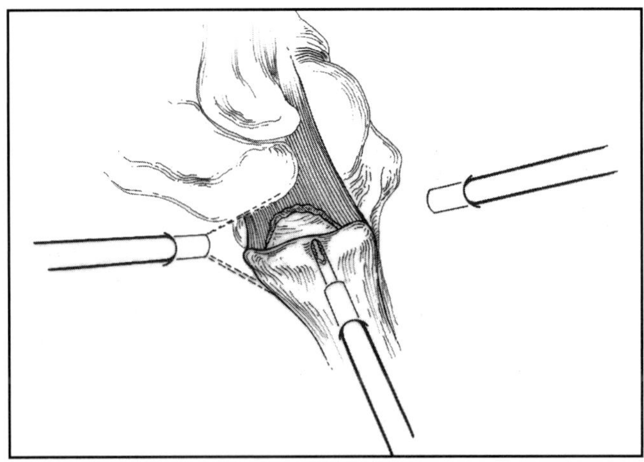

Fig. 2 The edge of the rotator cuff and the greater tuberosity are débrided with a shaver inserted through the anterolateral portal. A limited débridement of the greater tuberosity is performed in order to maintain bone integrity and thus ensure adequate suture anchor fixation.

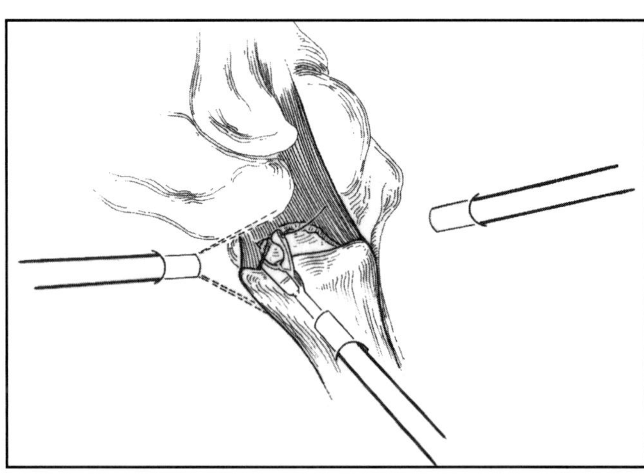

Fig. 3 A suture punch or a similar suture-passing device is inserted through the anterolateral portal and is used to pass a suture shuttle through the edge of the rotator cuff tear.

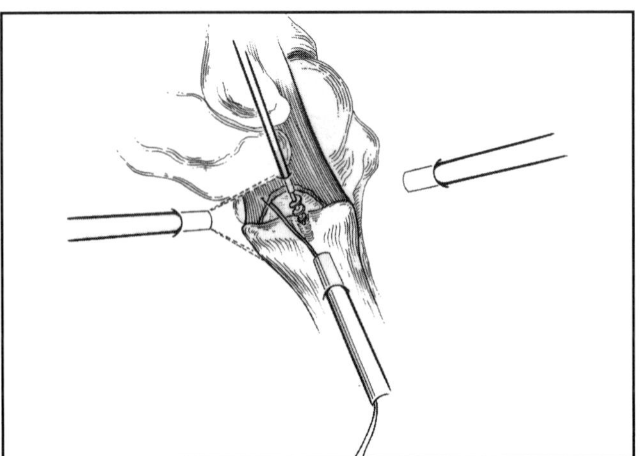

Fig. 4 A superior accessory portal is made proximal to the anterolateral working portal, just lateral to the acromion, in order to drill a bone hole and insert the suture anchor. The purpose of this superior accessory portal is to ensure that the anchor is inserted at the proper orientation into the greater tuberosity.

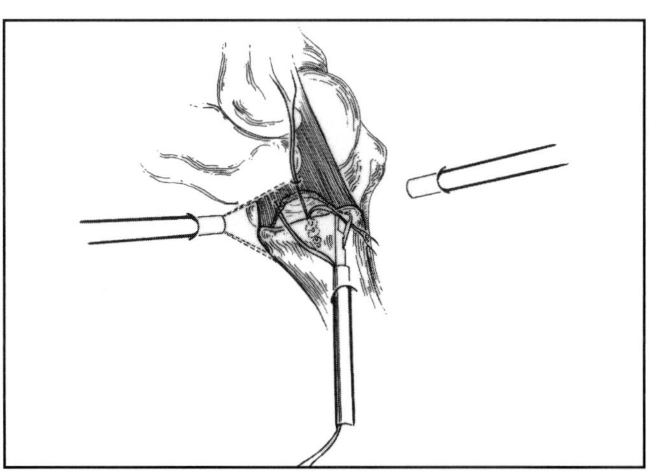

Fig. 5 A suture grasper is used to bring the sutures from the suture anchor out of the anterolateral cannula. The suture shuttle and anchor sutures are now both passed through the lateral cannula.

This cannula helps to facilitate passage of instruments and sutures in and out of the subacromial space while protecting the deltoid. The edge of the rotator cuff and the insertion site on the greater tuberosity are débrided with a shaver (Fig. 2). In order to ensure adequate bone for secure anchor fixation, a limited débridement is performed on the greater tuberosity. A Caspari Suture Punch (Linvatec, Largo, FL) or a similar suture-passing device is inserted through the clear cannula and No. 0 Prolene (polypropylene) suture is inserted through the tendon in order to act as a suture shuttle (Fig. 3). Some manufacturers produce a specific suture shuttle. A superior accessory portal is made just lateral to the acromion, proximal to the working anterolateral portal (Fig. 4), to serve as an introduction site for the anchor. The superior position of this portal ensures that the anchor and the drill hole will be inserted into the greater tuberosity at the appropriate position and angle. After the hole is impacted into the greater tuberosity with an awl and the anchor is implanted in the bone, a suture grasper is used to bring the sutures out through the anterolateral clear cannula (Fig. 5). The suture shuttle is then used to shuttle one limb of the anchor suture into the inferior surface of the rotator cuff to exit the tendon along

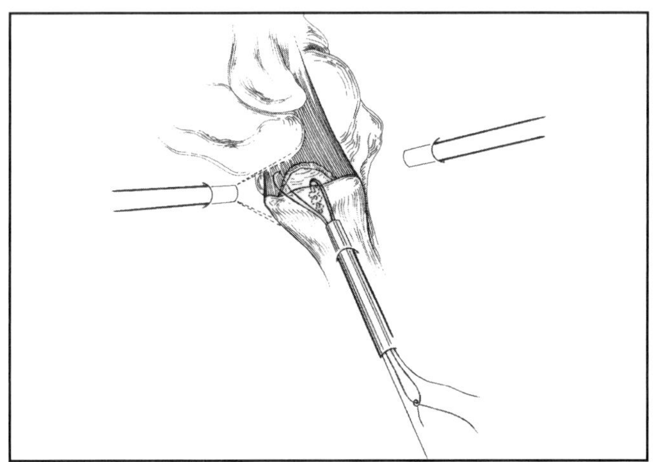

Fig. 6 The suture shuttle is then tied to one limb of the suture through the anchor. This limb is shuttled from the inferior to the superficial surface of the rotator cuff tear.

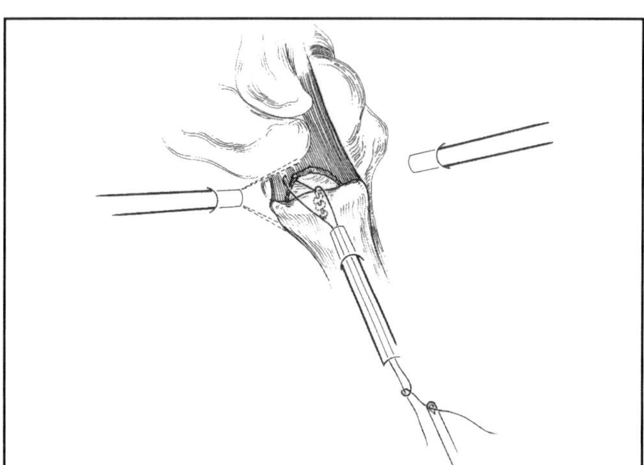

Fig. 7 A knot is tied with use of a knot-tying device, reducing the rotator cuff to the greater tuberosity.

its superficial surface (Fig. 6). Arthroscopic knot tying is then performed (Fig. 7). The limb of the suture exiting the tendon is used as the post. The surgeon should be familiar with various knot-tying techniques, including those for making sliding and nonsliding knots. The process is repeated sequentially with another suture and anchor. Passing each suture anchor separately after the preceding suture anchor has been tied and cut minimizes problems with suture management; it substantially decreases the complexity of the procedure and avoids problems of suture tangling. The disadvantage of this type of strategy, however, is that the final sutures can be difficult to pass underneath the rotator cuff as there is less and less room to insert a suture passer as the rotator cuff is secured to the bone. In general, it is helpful to work from anterior to posterior as this ensures anatomic reduction of the supraspinatus and improves visualization for the remainder of the procedure.

Alternatively, some surgeons prefer to place all anchors and sutures through the tendon before tying any knots. A smaller cannula is inserted through the anterior portal into the subacromial space. Sutures from the anchors can be "stored" in this cannula while subsequent anchors and sutures are being placed. Suture management is of paramount importance when this technique is used to keep sutures untangled and separated before knot tying.

Some L-shaped tears may require side-to-side sutures. In this situation, the suture-passing device is used to pass first one suture shuttle through one side of the tear and then another shuttle through the opposite side of the tear. An extra-long No. 2 suture is then passed first through one and subsequently through another side of the tendon, and the knot is tied over the top. If side-to-side sutures are necessary, it is often helpful to place them before anchoring the remaining tendon to the greater tuberosity. This decreases the size of the tear and makes subsequent mobilization of the remaining edge to the greater tuberosity easier. This technique, which has been termed "margin convergence," has become popular for obtaining arthroscopic repair of the rotator cuff. It was, however, rarely a starting point in traditional open repair. While margin convergence is appropriate for many tears with a substantial side-to-side or intrasubstance extension, it should not be substituted for traditional releases to obtain a reduction of the rotator cuff to the greater tuberosity. In most cases, margin convergence is not necessary to obtain an anatomic reduction of the rotator cuff to the greater tuberosity if complete releases have been performed.

There are several ways to increase the ease of repair: (1) Proper portal placement is necessary. Portals should be positioned to allow access to all necessary structures. One common mistake is to place the anterolateral working portal for the subacromial space too proximal and close to the acromion, so that instruments enter the subacromial space in a downward direction, making it difficult to reach the undersurface of the acromion and to place a subsequent superior accessory portal. (2) Establishing a second lateral portal posterior to the primary anterolateral working portal can be helpful when a tear is large and extends around the posterior aspect of the humeral head. It allows working instruments and anchors to be placed closer to the site of reattachment. (3) Effective suture management is extremely important. Until the surgeon becomes adept at suture management, it can be helpful to place one rotator cuff suture at a time and to tie it prior to placing the next suture.

This avoids the need to manage multiple sutures prior to arthroscopic knot tying. (4) Downward traction generally increases the working space available for the subacromial space. Even minimal traction can make a major difference in visualization. (5) It is critical that the intra-articular portion of the arthroscopy and the subacromial decompression be performed in a timely fashion, so that the majority of the time is left for the arthroscopic rotator cuff repair. When the intra-articular arthroscopy and decompression are performed quickly, soft-tissue edema is kept to a minimum during the repair. This substantially improves visualization. (6) As is true for any other procedure, adequate exposure is necessary for visualization during arthroscopic rotator cuff repair. Adequate exposure is obtained with thorough débridement of the bursa and complete lysis of adhesions between the bursa and the cuff.

Finally, several pitfalls can prevent the timely completion of a rotator cuff repair. The usual culprits include inadequate visualization, suture entanglement, problems with arthroscopic knot tying, and incomplete release of adhesions. **(DVD-8.1)**

Strategies for Making a Transition to Arthroscopic Rotator Cuff Repair

Making a direct transition from a traditional mini-open repair technique to a complete arthroscopic cuff repair can be very difficult for even the most skilled arthroscopic surgeon. This type of one-step jump in surgical technique may inappropriately subject the patient to complications associated with the surgeon's inexperience. However, an orderly transition strategy may help the surgeon to progress from the traditional mini-open repair to the arthroscopic repair. A logical plan for making this transition includes the use of the traditional mini-open repair as a starting point and then successively adding more arthroscopic procedures as the surgeon gains confidence and experience.

The strategy can start with the performance of an arthroscopic decompression of the subacromial space. While many surgeons are comfortable with carrying out a standard decompression, more visualization is required for a decompression performed in an arthroscopic repair. The surgeon should aim for more comprehensive removal of the subacromial bursa that allows for visualization of the entire space. During this resection, the surgeon should become adept at controlling bleeding. Visualization of the subacromial space should allow the surgeon to become comfortable with observing torn edges of the rotator cuff as well as the musculotendinous junction. Finally, an essential part of the decompression procedure for rotator cuff repair is the performance of bursal resection and decompression in a timely fashion. This allows the majority of the procedure time to be allocated to rotator cuff repair.

The next step in a transition to arthroscopic repair includes arthroscopic deep surface releases of the rotator cuff. First, a circumferential lysis of adhesions from the undersurface of the rotator cuff to the superior aspect of the glenoid labrum is completed. This is a relatively easy skill to obtain, as most surgeons are comfortable with performing glenohumeral arthroscopy. After the deep surface releases and an extensive subacromial bursectomy have been carried out, much of the rotator cuff should be freely mobile for repair. The final release, which can be difficult, involves mechanical or sharp débridement around the coracoid base, including the coracohumeral ligament.

Once a surgeon is able to perform the arthroscopic releases and decompression of the rotator cuff in a timely fashion, the next step is to place sutures in the rotator cuff. A variety of commercial suture punches are now available to accomplish this task. Initially, the surgeon may place only a couple of sutures, which can be used for control of the rotator cuff once a mini-open deltoid split is performed. Later, the suture tags can be used to "shuttle relay" a suture anchor loaded stitch.

The next step following suture placement is placement of suture anchors. The surgeon should become adept at placing the anchors in a relatively anatomic fashion lateral on the tuberosity with good visualization of the bone holes and uncovered bone. Finally, he or she must become skilled at arthroscopic knot-tying. This is a particularly important step, which usually requires repetition and experience. It is relatively easy to tie a poor arthroscopic knot and generally difficult to tie a good one.

As the surgeon works toward acquiring the necessary arthroscopic skills mentioned above, any procedure can be quickly changed to a mini-open technique if difficulties are encountered. Thus, the mini-open procedure offers the surgeon the opportunity to gradually transition to the complete arthroscopic rotator cuff repair in an orderly and individualized fashion.

Summary

The complete arthroscopic rotator cuff repair is an excellent procedure that can provide pain relief and restore function to patients with disorders of the rotator cuff. Most short-term studies have shown excellent results comparable with those of mini-open repair.[1,3,7,13] The choice of the best technique for an individual patient or surgeon can be based on a variety of considerations, including the patient's expectations, the pathoanatomy of the cuff, and the surgical experience of the surgeon. When deciding which procedure to pursue, the surgeon should make sure that the basic principles of rotator cuff repair are not compromised and should consider which would be the most reproducible procedure given his or her level of experience. If a surgeon chooses to obtain the experience necessary to perform a complete arthroscopic repair, the mini-open procedure provides an excellent opportunity to make an orderly transition.

References

1. Gartsman GM, Khan M, Hammerman SM: Arthroscopic repair of fullthickness tears of the rotator cuff. *J Bone Joint Surg Am* 1998;80: 832-840.
2. Gerber C, Schneeberger AG, Perren SM, Nyffeler RW: Experimental rotator cuff repair: A preliminary study. *J Bone Joint Surg Am* 1999;81:1281-1290.
3. Gartsman GM, Brinker MR, Khan M: Early effectiveness of arthroscopic repair for full-thickness tears of the rotator cuff: An outcome analysis. *J Bone Joint Surg Am* 1998;80:33-40.
4. Gartsman GM, Hammerman SM: Full-thickness tears: Arthroscopic repair. *Orthop Clin North Am* 1997;28:83-98.
5. Burkhart S: Arthroscopic repair of massive rotator cuff tears: Concept of margin convergence. *Tech Shoulder Elbow Surg* 2000;1:232-239.
6. Hoffmann F, Schiller M, Reif G: Arthroscopic rotator cuff reconstruction. *Orthopade* 2000;29:888-894.
7. Tauro JC: Arthroscopic rotator cuff repair: Analysis of technique and results at 2- and 3-year follow-up. *Arthroscopy* 1998;14:45-51.
8. Wolf E: All arthroscopic rotator cuff repair report. Presented at the Annual Shoulder Surgery Controversies Meeting, Costa Mesa, CA, 2000.
9. Nottage W, Severud E: A comparison of all arthroscopic vs. mini-open rotator cuff repair: Results at 45 months. Presented at the Summer Institute Meeting of the American Academy of Orthopaedic Surgeons, San Diego, CA, 2001.
10. Ball CM, Galatz LM, Teefey SA, Middleton WD, Yamaguchi K: Complete arthroscopic repair of large and massive rotator cuff tears: Correlation of functional outcome with repair integrity, in *69th Annual Meeting Proceedings*, AAOS, Rosemont, IL, 2002.
11. Weber S: Comparison of all arthroscopic and mini-open rotator cuff repairs. Presented at the Annual Meeting of the Arthroscopic Association of North America, Seattle, WA, 2001.
12. Gartsman GM: Arthroscopic assessment of rotator cuff tear reparability. *Arthroscopy* 1996;12: 546-549.
13. Stollsteimer GT, Savoie FH III: Arthroscopic rotator cuff repair: Current indications, limitations, techniques, and results. *Instr Course Lect* 1998;47:59-65.
14. Codman EA: Complete rupture of the supraspinatus tendon: Operative treatment with report of two successful cases. *Boston Med Surg J* 1911;164:708-710.
15. Bosworth DM: An analysis of twenty-eight consecutive cases of incapacitating shoulder lesions, radically explored and repaired. *J Bone Joint Surg* 1940;22:369-392.
16. McLaughlin HL: Lesions of the musculotendinous cuff of the shoulder: I. The exposure and treatment of tears with retraction. *J Bone Joint Surg* 1944;26:31-51.
17. McLaughlin HL: Repair of major cuff ruptures. *Surg Clin North Am* 1963;43:1535-1540.
18. McLaughlin HL, Asherman EG: Lesions of the musculotendinous cuff of the shoulder: IV. Some observations based upon the results of surgical repair. *J Bone Joint Surg Am* 1951;33: 76-86.
19. Watson M: Major ruptures of the rotator cuff: The results of surgical repair in 89 patients. *J Bone Joint Surg Br* 1985;67:618-624.
20. Wolfgang GL: Surgical repair of tears of the rotator cuff of the shoulder: Factors influencing the result. *J Bone Joint Surg Am* 1974;56:14-26.
21. Codman EA: Rupture of the supraspinatus—1834 to 1934. *J Bone Joint Surg Am* 1937;19: 643-652.
22. Codman EA: The shoulder: Rupture of the supraspinatus tendon and other lesions in or about the subacromial bursa, in *The Shoulder*. Boston, MA, Thomas Todd, 1934.
23. Neer CS II: Anterior acromioplasty for the chronic impingement syndrome in the shoulder: A preliminary report. *J Bone Joint Surg Am* 1972;54:41-50.
24. Ellman H: Arthroscopic subacromial decompression: Analysis of one- to three-year results. *Arthroscopy* 1987;3:173-181.
25. Levy HJ, Uribe JW, Delaney LG: Arthroscopic assisted rotator cuff repair: preliminary results. *Arthroscopy* 1990;6:55-60.
26. Paulos LE, Kody MH: Arthroscopically enhanced "miniapproach" to rotator cuff repair. *Am J Sports Med* 1994;22:19-25.
27. Yamaguchi K: Mini-open rotator cuff repair: An updated perspective. *Instr Course Lect* 2001;50:53-61.
28. Yamaguchi K, Ball CM, Galatz LM: Arthroscopic rotator cuff repair: transition from mini-open to all-arthroscopic. *Clin Orthop* 2001;390:83-94.
29. Yamaguchi K: Mini-open rotator cuff repair. An updated perspective. *Instr Couse Lect* 2001;50: 53-61.
30. Bigliani LU, Cordasco FA, McIlveen SJ, Musso ES: Operative treatment of failed repairs of the rotator cuff. *J Bone Joint Surg Am* 1992;74: 1505-1515.
31. DeOrio JK, Cofield RH: Results of a second attempt at surgical repair of a failed initial rotator-cuff repair. *J Bone Joint Surg Am* 1984;66: 563-567.
32. Neer CS II, Marberry TA: On the disadvantages of radical acromionectomy. *J Bone Joint Surg Am* 1981;63:416-419.
33. Neviaser RJ, Neviaser TJ: Reoperation for failed rotator cuff repair: analysis of fifty cases. *J Shoulder Elbow Surg* 1992;1:283-286.
34. Miller C, Savoie FH: Glenohumeral abnormalities associated with full-thickness tears of the rotator cuff. *Orthop Rev* 1994;23:159-162.
35. Nicholson G, Duckworth M: Mini-open rotator cuff repair for supraspinatus tears. Presented at the Second Biennial Shoulder and Elbow Meeting, Miami Beach, FL, 2000.
36. Williams GR, Ianotti JP, Luchetti W, Ferron A: Mini vs open repair of isolated supraspinatus tears. *J Shoulder Elbow Surg* 1998;7:310.
37. Carpenter JE, Fish DN, Huston LJ, Goldstein SA. Pull-out strength of five suture anchors. *Arthroscopy* 1993;9:109-113.
38. Barber FA, Cawley P, Prudich JF. Suture anchor failure strength—an in vivo study. Arthroscopy 1993;9:647-652.
39. Hecker AT, Shea M, Hayhurst JO, Myers ER, Meeks LW, Hayes WC: Pull-out strength of suture anchors for rotator cuff and Bankart lesion repairs. *Am J Sports Med* 1993;21:874-879.
40. Reed SC, Glossop N, Ogilvie-Harris DJ: Full-thickness rotator cuff tears: A biomechanical comparison of suture versus bone anchor techniques. *Am J Sports Med* 1996;24:46-8.
41. Gerber C, Schneeberger AG, Beck M, Schlegel U: Mechanical strength of repairs of the rotator cuff. *J Bone Joint Surg Br* 1994;76:371-380.
42. Baker CL, Liu SH: Comparison of open and arthroscopically assisted rotator cuff repairs. *Am J Sports Med* 1995;23:99-104.
43. Gartsman GM: Massive, irreparable tears of the rotator cuff: Results of operative debridement and subacromial decompression. *J Bone Joint Surg Am* 1997;79:715-721.
44. Tauro JC: Arthroscopic "interval slide" in the repair of large rotator cuff tears. Arthroscopy 1999;15:527-530.
45. Gleyze P, Thomazeau H, Flurin P, Lafosse L, Gazielly DF, Allard M: Arthroscopic rotator cuff repair: A multicentric retrospective study of 87 cases with anatomical assessment. *Rev Chir Reparatrice Appar Mot* 2000;86:566-574.
46. Cohen B, Nicholson G, Romeo A: Arthroscopic rotator cuff repair: Is miniopen just of historical interest? *Curr Opin Orthop* 2001;12:331-336.
47. Burkhart SS, Diaz Pagan JL, Wirth MA, Athanasiou KA: Cyclic loading of anchor-based rotator cuff repairs: Confirmation of the tension overload phenomenon and comparison of suture anchor fixation with transosseous fixation. *Arthroscopy* 1997;13:720-724.
48. Harryman DT II, Mack LA, Wang KY, Jackins SE, Richardson ML, Matsen FA III: Repairs of the rotator cuff: Correlation of functional results with integrity of the cuff. *J Bone Joint Surg Am* 1991;73:982-989.
49. Kirschenbaum D, Coyle MP Jr, Leddy JP, Katsaros P, Tan F Jr, Cody RP: Shoulder strength with rotator cuff tears: Pre- and post-operative analysis. *Clin Orthop* 1993;288: 174-178.
50. Grondel RJ, Savoie FH III, Field LD: Rotator cuff repairs in patients 62 years of age or older. *J Shoulder Elbow Surg* 2001;10:97-99.

51. Outerbridge RE: The etiology of chondromalacia patellae. *J Bone Joint Surg Br* 1961;43:752-757.

52. Weinstein DM, Bucchieri JS, Pollock RG, Flatow EL, Bigliani LU: Arthroscopic debridement of the shoulder for osteoarthritis. *Arthroscopy* 2000;16:471-476.

53. Sethi N, Wright R, Yamaguchi K: Disorders of the long head of the biceps tendon. *J Shoulder Elbow Surg* 1999;8:644-654.

54. Soslowsky LJ, An CH, Johnston SP, Carpenter JE: Geometric and mechanical properties of the coracoacromial ligament and their relationship to rotator cuff disease. *Clin Orthop* 1994;304:10-17.

Arthroscopic Acromioplasty: History, Rationale, and Technique

Rolando Izquierdo, MD
Walter G. Stanwood, MD
Louis U. Bigliani, MD

Abstract

Subacromial impingement or supraspinatus syndrome has been known to exist in some form since the early 1900s. Several early studies have discussed subacromial impingement or supraspinatus syndrome. Arthroscopic acromioplasty has evolved as a useful surgical treatment. Pertinent physical examination and radiographic evaluation findings must be identified. In order for the surgery to be successful, it is important to understand the rationale for treatment of impingement syndrome and the technical aspects of arthroscopic acromioplasty.

Meyer[1] proposed that tears in the rotator cuff occurred because of attrition secondary to friction with the undersurface of the acromion. Corresponding lesions on the greater tuberosity and the undersurface of the acromion were identified. Codman[2] described the critical zone in the supraspinatus tendon where most degenerative changes occur, which is located 1 cm medial to the insertion of the supraspinatus tendon on the greater tuberosity. Watson-Jones[3] discussed the excision of the acromion for supraspinatus tendinitis and later published his surgical techniques and results. Other studies[4,5] on complete acromionectomy were reported, with satisfactory results. However, there was significant controversy during the 1960s regarding treatment options for supraspinatus syndrome and subacromial bursitis with regard to the amount and location of acromial bone resection.

History

In 1972, Neer[6] was the first to coin the term "impingement syndrome." In an anatomic study of 100 dissected scapulae, Neer observed evidence of impingement in 11 scapulae. He found a characteristic ridge of proliferative spurs and excrescences on the undersurface of the anterior acromion, which he attributed to repetitive impingement of the rotator cuff and humeral head with traction on the coracoacromial ligament. He described impingement as a compression of the supraspinatus tendon against the anterior edge of the acromion, the coracoacromial ligament, and, occasionally, a prominent acromioclavicular joint. He also described a commonly occurring acromial spur within the coracoacromial ligament (Figure 1). Neer believed that impingement syndrome was chronic and repetitive, characterized by microtrauma causing a progressive inflammatory process and a subsequent degenerative process within the rotator cuff tendon. Because of these findings, Neer recommended an anterior acromioplasty with removal of the anterior edge and undersurface of the acromion, the attached coracoacromial ligament, as well as resection of overhanging osteophytes at the acromioclavicular joint when indicated. Neer believed that this procedure would relieve impingement while preserving the osseous architecture of the acromion and the insertion of the deltoid, preventing cosmetic deformity, and preserving deltoid function.

In 1981, Neer and Marberry[7] studied 30 consecutive patients who had previous radical acromionectomies at other institutions. All had poor results: 27 had persistent pain, all had marked weakness of the

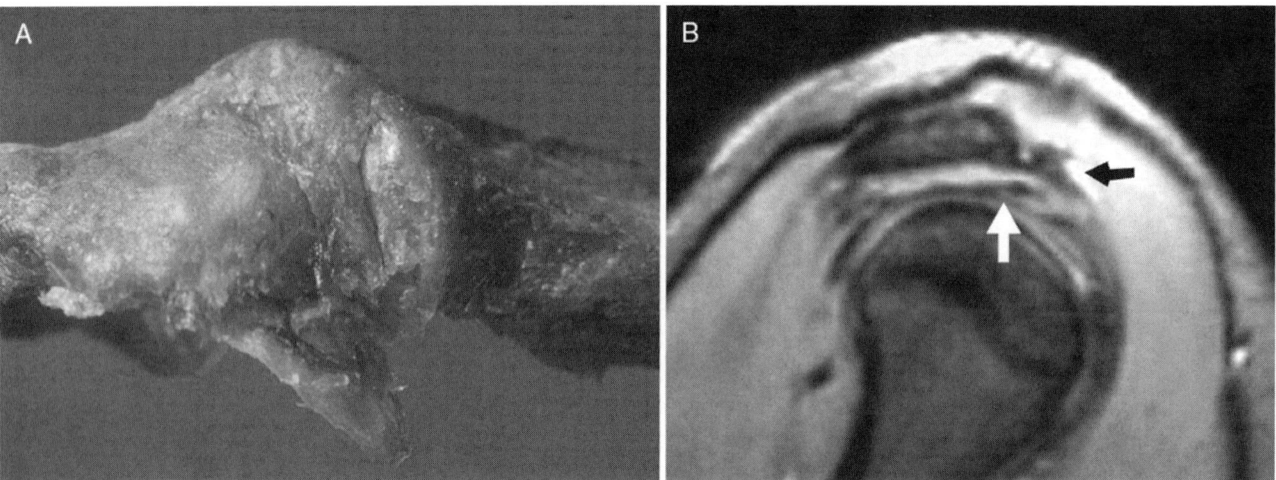

Figure 1 **A**, Cadaveric specimen showing the characteristic calcification within the coracoacromial ligament. **B**, Sagittal oblique MRI depicts a calcified ligament (black arrow) and an area of bursitis above the rotator cuff (white arrow).

shoulder, and none could raise the arm above the horizontal position. Eight patients had serious wound complications, and none was satisfied with the appearance of the shoulder. Neer and Marberry concluded that radical acromionectomy weakened the deltoid by removing its lever arm and by encouraging retraction of the deltoid origin. The retracted middle section of the deltoid became adherent to either the rotator cuff or the humerus and became fibrotic and permanently shortened. This combination of altered anatomy and fibrotic changes of the deltoid made reconstruction of the deltoid mechanism very difficult. Again, Neer stressed the importance of performing only an anterior acromioplasty and removal of the coracoacromial ligament in treating patients with refractory impingement.

Many different surgical procedures[4,5,8] were used to treat impingement syndrome with variable success before the advent of the anterior acromioplasty as described by Neer.[6] This procedure has gained widespread acceptance with reproducible, excellent long-term results ranging from 80% to 90% in most series.[6,9-12] In 1985, Ellman[13] described an arthroscopic alternative for decompression of the subacromial space, and his preliminary results were comparable to the results of open procedures. The 1- to 3-year results for Ellman's initial 50 cases of arthroscopic subacromial decompression were published in 1987.[14] Eighty-eight percent of the patient results were rated satisfactory (excellent or good), and 12% were rated unsatisfactory (fair or poor). Subsequent reports have described comparable results.[15-20] Speer and associates[21] reported good or excellent results in 88% of patients with intact rotator cuffs who underwent arthroscopic acromioplasty. Similarly, Gartsman[22] reported 88% satisfactory results in patients without cuff tears and 83% satisfactory results with associated partial thickness cuff tears.

Although this arthroscopic technique was initially embraced as a technically feasible and reproducible procedure with consistently good results, following the initial description by Ellman,[13] a great deal of skepticism arose regarding the technical difficulties and adequacy of acromial resection when compared with the original open procedure as described by Neer.[6] In response to this, Gartsman and associates[23] published results from a cadaveric study in which the predictability of the bone resection in the arthroscopic technique was found to be equal to that of the open technique. Prospective randomized trials have also validated the efficacy of arthroscopic acromioplasty. For example, Sachs and associates[24] reported on 41 patients randomized into open or arthroscopic treatment groups. They found that patients in the arthroscopic treatment group regained flexion and strength more rapidly than did those in the open treatment group, had shorter hospitalizations, required less narcotics for pain relief, and returned more quickly to work and activities of daily living. In both groups, full recovery took at least 1 year for most patients, and more than 90% of patients achieved a satisfactory result at 1 year. More recently, Spangehl and associates[25] performed a prospective, randomized, controlled clinical trial to determine if arthroscopic acromioplasty was equivalent or superior to open acromioplasty. Sixty-two patients with a minimum follow-up of 12 months (mean, 25 months) were prospectively randomized to have either arthroscopic or open acromioplasty. No significant differences in visual analog scale scores for postoperative improvement, patient satisfaction, UCLA shoulder scores, or strength were reported. Overall, 67% of patients had good or excellent results. This increased to 87% when unsettled compensation claims were excluded. Open acromioplasty was found to be equivalent to arthroscopic acromioplasty in terms of UCLA scores and patient satisfaction.

A comparison of both techniques reveals several advantages of arthroscopic acromioplasty. Open acromioplasty requires detachment of the anterior deltoid and protection of the deltoid during the early rehabilitation period. Arthroscopic acromioplasty preserves the deltoid origin and allows safe participation in an active rehabilitation regimen in the early postoperative period. Lindh and Norlin[26] performed a prospective study and reported that both methods resulted in adequate subacromial decompression and bone resection. However, the arthroscopic method required less operating time and resulted in earlier restoration of active motion and return to work. Arthroscopy also allows direct visualization of the glenohumeral joint, which may help identify other unrecognized problems, such as osteoarthritis, subtle instability, labral tears, biceps tendon lesions, and undersurface rotator cuff tears.

Etiology and Associated Anatomy

Subacromial bursitis, rotator cuff tendinitis, and rotator cuff tears are common problems in the shoulder and may result in pain, weakness, and difficulties with activities of daily living.[27,28] Many factors have been implicated in the development of impingement and subsequent rotator cuff pathology, including extrinsic tendon injury from compression against an abnormal coracoacromial arch,[6,29-32] abutment on the glenoid rim, tendon and bursal swelling in a confined space,[33,34] altered glenohumeral kinematics,[35,36] intrinsic injury from tendinitis,[34] and calcific tendinitis and altered vascularity.[37] Subacromial impingement is considered a component in a spectrum of rotator cuff pathology that probably begins with tendinitis and ends in a full-thickness tear. Therefore, if subacromial impingement is identified during the treatment of a rotator cuff injury, it is reasonable to consider subacromial decompression.

Neer[6] first proposed that variations in acromial slope and morphology were clinically important. Stimulated by Neer's initial observations, Bigliani and associates[31] reviewed 140 shoulders in 71 cadavers and described three basic types of acromial morphology. Type I is flat and occurred in 17% of the specimens, type II is curved and occurred in 43%, and type III is hooked and occurred in 40%. Bilateral occurrence of similar shapes was noted in 58% of the cadaveric specimens. Thirty-three percent of the inspected specimens had full-thickness rotator cuff tears, 73% were associated with type III acromial morphology, and 24% were associated with type II. Morrison and Bigliani[38] followed their initial cadaveric study with a clinical review of 200 modified scapular lateral radiographs. They found that 80% of patients with full-thickness cuff tears had type III acromial morphology, and the remainder had type II morphology. In 1990, Gartsman[22] reviewed his results for arthroscopic acromioplasty and identified an additional type of acromial morphology associated with impingement (a type I acromial morphology with an increased angle of inclination that subsequently narrows the subacromial space).

Flatow and associates[39] performed contact studies on the subacromial space of cadaveric specimens and found that contact was centered on the supraspinatus insertion where rotator cuff tears generally initiate. The acromial undersurface and rotator cuff tendons are in closest proximity between 60° and 120° of elevation, and contact was consistently more pronounced for type III acromions. These data correlate well with the findings and theories described by Neer[6] and Bigliani and associates.[31,38]

The volume within the subacromial space may be decreased by other causes, including hypertrophy and calcification of the coracoacromial ligament, osteophytes of the acromioclavicular joint, greater tuberosity fracture malunion, calcific tendinitis, and inflammatory bursitis. All of these processes must be considered and addressed at the time of surgery because they decrease the overall volume of the subacromial space and may lead to rotator cuff degeneration and tearing. Occasionally, the volume of the subacromial space is compromised only by the tight embrace of the coracoacromial ligament (Figure 2). This is seen most frequently in young, overhead athletes with impingement syndrome who have no radiographic or arthroscopic evidence of an acromial spur. However, upon arthroscopic inspection, signs of attritional wear on both the surface of the coracoacromial ligament and the bursal surface of the rotator cuff may be apparent. In these patients, treatment with

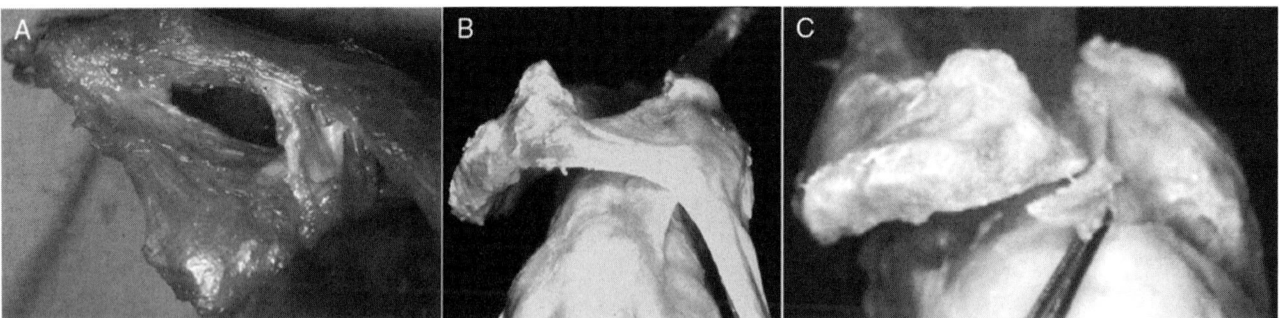

Figure 2 **A**, AP photograph of the anterolateral and posteromedial bands of the coracoacromial ligament. **B**, Arthroscopic outlet view of the shoulder and the coracoacromial arch. **C**, Arthroscopic view of the broad attachment of the coracoacromial ligament on the undersurface of the acromion.

a soft-tissue decompression without acromioplasty may be sufficient.

Dynamic impingement occurs as a result of the imbalance between the weakened rotator cuff and normal deltoid, causing abnormal superior migration of the humeral head during arm elevation. Deutsch and associates[40] found that patients with normal shoulders evaluated radiographically did not show a significant change in position of the humeral head with arm elevation. In contrast, those with stage II impingement had significant superior displacement of the center of the humeral head with arm elevation ($P < 0.05$), and patients with rotator cuff tears demonstrated a significant rise in displacement during the first 40° of abduction ($P < 0.05$). The average position of the humeral head in the two pathologic patient groups was superior to the average head position in the normal patient group ($P < 0.05$). This dynamic process gives credence to the role of rehabilitation of the shoulder musculature in patients with impingement syndrome. Theoretically, successful strengthening of the rotator cuff and scapular stabilizers should restore the ability of the rotator cuff to center the humeral head in the glenoid during arm elevation.

Physical Examination

Recent advances in diagnostic imaging and arthroscopic techniques have helped confirm the diagnosis of subacromial impingement, but the mainstay in the evaluation of the painful shoulder is a thorough history and physical examination. The patient's chief complaint should direct the surgeon to an initial differential diagnosis. Impingement syndrome is typically characterized by anterosuperior shoulder pain during overhead activities. The pain may awaken the patient from sleep or make it difficult to lie on the affected side. Pain may radiate down the lateral side of the arm toward the deltoid insertion because the subacromial bursa extends distally beneath the deltoid muscle. A careful assessment of motion and motor muscle strength should be performed during the evaluation of subacromial impingement and rotator cuff injury. However, most patients with impingement do not report a loss of motion unless an associated adhesive capsulitis is present, which is more frequently seen in diabetic populations. Shoulder motion should be compared with that of the opposite side, with documentation of forward flexion, external rotation at the side, external rotation at 90° of abduction, and internal rotation. An examination of the neck should also be performed to rule out abnormalities of the cervical spine, such as radiculitis and degenerative disease that may cause symptoms in the shoulder.[41,42] Subacromial impingement and cervical radiculopathy may exist simultaneously; therefore, it is imperative to clearly document the presence of both entities.

Several specific tests may be helpful in making the diagnosis of impingement syndrome. Neer[28] described the impingement sign elicited by passively elevating the arm in the scapular plane while stabilizing the scapula. Pain is usually present in the arc between 70° and 120°. Hawkins and Kennedy[43] modified this test by internally rotating the arm at 90° of forward flexion. Both impingement maneuvers are based on the concept of impingement of the greater tuberosity and cuff on the undersurface of the anterior acromion and the coracoacromial ligament.

Neer's impingement test can also be useful in the diagnosis of impingement. After sterile injection of 10 mL of lidocaine into the subacromial space, the test for the impingement sign is repeated. When the pathology is confined to the subacromial space, the injection typically eliminates the pain. Abnormalities of the acromioclavicular joint should be identified by direct palpation of the joint, internal rotation of the extended arm, and adduction of the arm across the chest. However, these maneuvers also may cause impingement in the subacromial space and therefore may not be specific for the identification of pathology in the acromioclavicular joint. Selective injections into both the acromioclavicular joint and subacromial bursa are helpful in identifying the source of symptoms. Stability assessment is performed for those patients in whom the relative contributions of instability and rotator cuff pathology are uncertain.

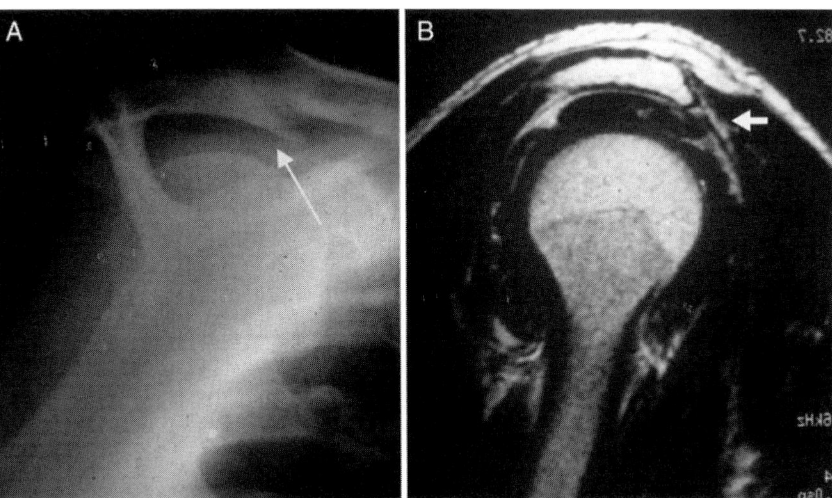

Figure 3 **A**, Radiographic outlet view showing a type III acromion (arrow). **B**, Sagittal oblique MRI showing the corresponding acromial morphology and coracoacromial ligament (arrow).

Radiographic Evaluation

Routine radiographs are also helpful in the evaluation of subacromial impingement. AP radiographs may show subchondral cysts or sclerosis of the greater tuberosity, with corresponding areas of sclerosis or spur formation on the anterior edge of the acromion. AP radiographs may also help identify other sources of pain, such as osteoarthritis of the glenohumeral or acromioclavicular joints, calcific tendinitis, and glenohumeral instability. An axillary radiograph may be needed to confirm the diagnosis of an unfused acromial epiphysis. The subacromial space, however, is not well visualized on AP radiographs because of the superimposition of the scapular spine and body. The supraspinatus outlet view, which is a lateral radiograph made in the plane of the scapula with the x-ray beam directed 10° caudally, is widely used in the diagnosis of subacromial impingement.[44] However, the findings may be difficult to reproduce consistently because of thoracic kyphosis or superimposition of adjacent osseous structures, such as the clavicle, ribs, or scapular body.

If the history, physical examination, and radiographs are consistent with subacromial impingement without rotator cuff pathology, additional imaging studies may not be needed. However, if a tear of the rotator cuff is suspected, additional imaging studies may be indicated. The use of MRI has increased the ability to diagnose partial tears and small full-thickness tears, but differentiating these lesions from rotator cuff tendinitis remains difficult. MRI can also be helpful in evaluating the acromioclavicular joint, unfused acromial epiphysis, and lateral acromial morphology. The sagittal oblique images from a typical MRI evaluation may be comparable to the supraspinatus outlet view (Figure 3). These images allow evaluation of the acromial morphology, coracoacromial ligament, and acromioclavicular joint. Coronal views allow evaluation of the rotator cuff, especially the supraspinatus and infraspinatus, and the acromioclavicular joint. The axial views allow visualization of the subscapularis, teres minor, and long head of the biceps, as well as an os acromiale when present.

Surgical Technique

Surgical intervention is considered only after patients have failed to respond to at least 3 months of physical therapy, nonsteroidal anti-inflammatory medications, and subacromial corticosteroid injections. Arthroscopic procedures are performed using an interscalene block with intravenous sedation, thereby avoiding the morbidity and potential complications associated with general anesthesia.[45] The beach-chair position with the arm draped free is preferred because the arm can be rotated throughout the procedure. The lateral decubitus position is also an option. Regardless of the position chosen, it is important to have full access to the anterior, lateral, and posterior aspects of the shoulder. The superficial osseous landmarks (the coracoid; the anterior, lateral, and posterior aspects of the acromion; and the acromioclavicular joint) are outlined with a sterile marking pen. Before the start of the procedure, 10 to 15 mL of

0.25% bupivacaine with epinephrine is injected into the subacromial space to distend the subacromial bursa, provide hemostasis, and help provide anesthesia into the early postoperative period.

The first step in arthroscopy is examination of the glenohumeral joint. A standard arthroscopy portal is made in the posterior aspect of the shoulder 2 cm inferior and medial to the posterolateral tip of the acromion. If pathology warrants, an anterior portal is made by placing a spinal needle just lateral and superior to the coracoid. The needle is visualized arthroscopically as it enters the joint in the triangle between the biceps and subscapularis tendons. Any inflamed synovium should be débrided and labral pathology addressed as indicated.[46,47] Attention is then turned to the undersurface of the rotator cuff, which can be visualized with gentle external rotation and abduction of the arm.

Before the advent of arthroscopy, excision and repair of partial-thickness rotator cuff tears seemed logical and added little morbidity to the open procedure. However, patients with partial-thickness tears that are less than 50% of the thickness of the tendon are currently treated with arthroscopic débridement and subacromial decompression.[22,48-50] This débridement can be performed with a 4.5-mm full-radius resector. However, if the partial tear is greater than 50% of the tendon thickness, then mini-open or arthroscopic repair is indicated after the arthroscopic decompression.

During subacromial arthroscopy, an additional anterolateral portal located approximately 2 cm lateral to the anterolateral tip of the acromion is made as the working portal. The 4.5-mm full-radius resector is placed through the anterolateral portal, and the thick bursa and undersurface of the coracoacromial ligament are débrided. This is done in a fanning-type fashion starting from the lateral aspect of the coracoacromial ligament and progressing to its medial aspect near the coracoid. In addition, the rotator cuff tendon can be inspected for a full-thickness tear and arthroscopically débrided before performing a mini-open repair.

The coracoacromial ligament is an important part of the coracoacromial arch and often extends inferior and lateral to the leading edge of the bony acromion. It has a broad insertion on the entire anterior undersurface, extending from the medial to the lateral side. Therefore, it may be the initial and primary source of subacromial impingement leading to disability, especially in overhead athletes. In patients who do not have a prominent acromion, it may be the only source of impingement. Adequate removal of the coracoacromial ligament is an important step in arthroscopic acromioplasty. Removal enhances visualization of the acromion so that a more accurate determination can be made concerning the bony prominence of the anterior acromion and spur formation.

Technically, the coracoacromial ligament is sequentially removed using electrocautery from the undersurface of the acromion by starting laterally and extending medially. The undersurface of the acromion is then exposed. The full-radius resector is then used to débride the soft tissue from the entire undersurface of the acromion so that the deltoid insertion into the acromion can be seen. Inserting an 18-gauge needle on the palpable, anterolateral edge of the acromion may aid in the arthroscopic identification of the lateral margin of the acromion. The acromioclavicular joint can also be seen using the established portals and preoperatively resected if it is symptomatic. A 6.0-mm longitudinally tapered burr is preferred for the acromioplasty rather than a round burr. The thickness and morphology of the acromion[31] and the size of the bone spur will dictate the amount of bone removal in each patient. Approximately 2 to 3 mm of bone is removed from the undersurface of the anteroinferior acromion. Simply changing the acromial morphology from type II or III to type I is advocated. It is critical not to remove an excessive amount of bone, and the level of the acromioclavicular joint and the white fibers of the deltoid origin can be used as landmarks to assess the depth of resection. The amount of bone removed is not as important as the way in which it is removed. A smooth acromial undersurface establishes a smooth transition to the deltoid insertion. No residual bone spurs or coracoacromial ligament attachment should be left on the anterolateral aspect of the acromion. The arthroscope may be switched to the anterolateral portal or anterior portal to better assess this area for any residual bone. After decompression, the arthroscopic instruments are removed and portals are closed with absorbable suture and sterile bandage strips. The patient is then placed in a bulky dressing and sling. Postoperative exercises are generally started within the first 48 hours, when the patient's pain has decreased.

Summary

Arthroscopic acromioplasty is useful for the treatment of subacromial impingement and has been associated with a high incidence of satisfactory results. However, to consistently achieve satisfactory results, certain conditions must be met. First, there must be an accurate diagnosis of subacromial impingement. Second, the pertinent anatomy and pathology must be identified. Third, the proper surgical techniques must be used, which include adequate bursectomy, removal of the coracoacromial ligament, and changing the acromial morphology with minimal bone resection.

References

1. Meyer AW: The minuter anatomy of attrition lesions. *J Bone Joint Surg* 1931;13:341-360.
2. Codman EA (ed): *The Shoulder: Rupture of the Supraspinatus Tendon and Other Lesions in or About the Subacromial Bursa.* Boston, MA, Thomas Todd, 1934.
3. Watson-Jones R (ed): *Fractures and Joint Injuries*, ed 3. Edinburgh, Scotland, ES Livingstone, 1943, p 418.
4. Armstrong JR: Excision of the acromion in the treatment of the supraspinatus syndrome: Report of ninety-five excisions. *J Bone Joint Surg Br* 1949;31:436-442.
5. Hammond G: Complete acromionectomy in the treatment of chronic tendinitis of the shoulder. *J Bone Joint Surg Am* 1962;44:494-504.
6. Neer CS II: Anterior acromioplasty for the chronic impingement syndrome in the shoulder: a preliminary report. *J Bone Joint Surg Am* 1972;54:41-50.
7. Neer CS II, Marberry TA: On the disadvantages of radical acromionectomy. *J Bone Joint Surg Am* 1981;63:416-419.
8. Hammond G: Complete acromionectomy in the treatment of chronic tendinitis of the shoulder: A follow-up of ninety operations on eighty-seven patients. *J Bone Joint Surg Am* 1971;53:173-180.
9. Bigliani LU, D'Alessandro DF, Duralde XA, McIlveen SJ: Anterior acromioplasty for subacromial impingement in patients younger than 40 years of age. *Clin Orthop* 1989;246:111-116.
10. Ha'eri GB, Wiley AM: Shoulder impingement syndrome: Results of operative release. *Clin Orthop* 1982;168:128-132.
11. Hawkins RJ, Brock RM, Abrams JS, Hobeika P: Acromioplasty for impingement with an intact rotator cuff. *J Bone Joint Surg Br* 1988;70:795-797.
12. Post M, Cohen J: Impingement syndrome: A review of late stage II and early stage III lesions. *Clin Orthop* 1986;207:126-132.
13. Ellman H: Arthroscopic subacromial decompression: A preliminary report. *Orthop Trans* 1985;9:49.
14. Ellman H: Arthroscopic subacromial decompression: Analysis of one- to three-year results. *Arthroscopy* 1987;3:173-181.
15. Paulos LE, Franklin JL: Arthroscopic shoulder decompression development and application: A five year experience. *Am J Sports Med* 1990;18:235-244.
16. Roye RP, Grana WA, Yates CK: Arthroscopic subacromial decompression: Two- to seven-year follow-up. *Arthroscopy* 1995;11:301-306.
17. Ryu RK: Arthroscopic subacromial decompression: A clinical review. *Arthroscopy* 1992;8:141-147.
18. Esch JC, Ozerkis LR, Helgager JA, Kane N, Lilliott N: Arthroscopic subacromial decompression: Results according to the degree of rotator cuff tear. *Arthroscopy* 1988;4:241-249.
19. Esch JC: Arthroscopic subacromial decompression and postoperative management. *Orthop Clin North Am* 1993;24:161-171.
20. Altchek DW, Warren RF, Wickiewicz TL, Skyhar MJ, Ortiz G, Schwartz E: Arthroscopic acromioplasty: Technique and results. *J Bone Joint Surg Am* 1990;72:1198-1207.
21. Speer KP, Lohnes J, Garrett WE Jr: Arthroscopic subacromial decompression: Results in advanced impingement syndrome. *Arthroscopy* 1991;7:291-296.
22. Gartsman GM: Arthroscopic acromioplasty for lesions of the rotator cuff. *J Bone Joint Surg Am* 1990;72:169-180.
23. Gartsman GM, Blair ME Jr, Noble PC, Bennett JB, Tullos HS: Arthroscopic subacromial decompression: An anatomical study. *Am J Sports Med* 1988;16:48-50.
24. Sachs RA, Stone ML, Devine S: Open vs. arthroscopic acromioplasty: A prospective, randomized study. *Arthroscopy* 1994;10:248-254.
25. Spangehl MJ, Hawkins RH, McCormack RG, Loomer RL: Arthroscopic versus open acromioplasty: A prospective, randomized, blinded study. *J Shoulder Elbow Surg* 2002;11:101-107.
26. Lindh M, Norlin R: Arthroscopic subacromial decompression versus open acromioplasty: A two-year follow-up study. *Clin Orthop* 1993;290:174-176.
27. Cofield RH: Rotator cuff disease of the shoulder. *J Bone Joint Surg Am* 1985;67:974-979.
28. Neer CS II: Impingement lesions. *Clin Orthop* 1983;173:70-77.
29. Soslowsky LJ, An CH, Johnston SP, Carpenter JE: Geometric and mechanical properties of the coracoacromial ligament and their relationship to rotator cuff disease. *Clin Orthop* 1994;304:10-17.
30. Nicholson GP, Goodman DA, Flatow EL, Bigliani LU: The acromion: Morphologic condition and age-related changes. A study of 420 scapulas. *J Shoulder Elbow Surg* 1996;5:1-11.
31. Bigliani LU, Morrison DS, April EW: The morphology of the acromion and its relationship to rotator cuff tears. *Orthop Trans* 1986;10:228.
32. Bigliani LU, Ticker JB, Flatow EL, Soslowsky LJ, Mow VC: The relationship of acromial architecture to rotator cuff disease. *Clin Sports Med* 1991;10:823-838.
33. Fukuda H, Hamada K, Nakajima T, Tomonaga A: Pathology and pathogenesis of the intratendinous tearing of the rotator cuff viewed from en bloc histologic sections. *Clin Orthop* 1994;304:60-67.
34. Uhthoff HK, Hammond DI, Sarkar K, Hooper GJ, Papoff WJ: The role of the coracoacromial ligament in the impingement syndrome: A clinical, radiological and histological study. *Int Orthop* 1988;12:97-104.
35. Jobe FW, Bradley JP: Rotator cuff injuries in baseball: Prevention and rehabilitation. *Sports Med* 1988;6:378-387.
36. Jobe FW, Kvitne RS, Giangarra CE: Shoulder pain in the overhand or throwing athlete: The relationship of anterior instability and rotator cuff impingement. *Orthop Rev* 1989;18:963-975.
37. Rathbun JB, Macnab I: The microvascular pattern of the rotator cuff. *J Bone Joint Surg Br* 1970;52:540-553.
38. Morrison DS, Bigliani LU: Roentgenographic analysis of acromial morphology and its relationship to rotator cuff tears. *Orthop Trans* 1987;11:439.
39. Flatow EL, Soslowsky LJ, Ticker JB, et al: Excursion of the rotator cuff under the acromion: Patterns of subacromial contact. *Am J Sports Med* 1994;22:779-788.
40. Deutsch A, Altchek DW, Schwartz E,

Otis JC, Warren RF: Radiologic measurement of superior displacement of the humeral head in the impingement syndrome. *J Shoulder Elbow Surg* 1996;5:186-193.

41. McCann PD, Bigliani LU: Shoulder pain in tennis players. *Sports Med* 1994;17:53-64.
42. Hawkins RJ, Hobeika PE: Impingement syndrome in the athletic shoulder. *Clin Sports Med* 1983;2:391-405.
43. Hawkins RJ, Kennedy JC: Impingement syndrome in athletes. *Am J Sports Med* 1980;8:151-158.
44. Neer CS II, Poppen NK: Supraspinatus outlet. *Orthop Trans* 1987;11:234.
45. Brown AR, Weiss R, Greenberg C, Flatow EL, Bigliani LU: Interscalene block for shoulder arthroscopy: Comparison with general anesthesia. *Arthroscopy* 1993;9:295-300.
46. Cordasco FA, Steinmann S, Flatow EL, Bigliani LU: Arthroscopic treatment of glenoid labral tears. *Am J Sports Med* 1993;21:425-431.
47. Flatow EL, Cordasco FA, Bigliani LU: Arthroscopic resection of the outer end of the clavicle from a superior approach: A critical, quantitative, radiographic assessment of bone removal. *Arthroscopy* 1992;8: 55-64.
48. Andrews JR, Broussard TS, Carson WG: Arthroscopy of the shoulder in the management of partial tears of the rotator cuff: A preliminary report. *Arthroscopy* 1985;1:117-122.
49. Ellman H: Diagnosis and treatment of incomplete rotator cuff tears. *Clin Orthop* 1990;254:64-74.
50. Olsewski JM, Depew AD: Arthroscopic subacromial decompression and rotator cuff debridement for stage II and stage III impingement. *Arthroscopy* 1994;10:61-68.

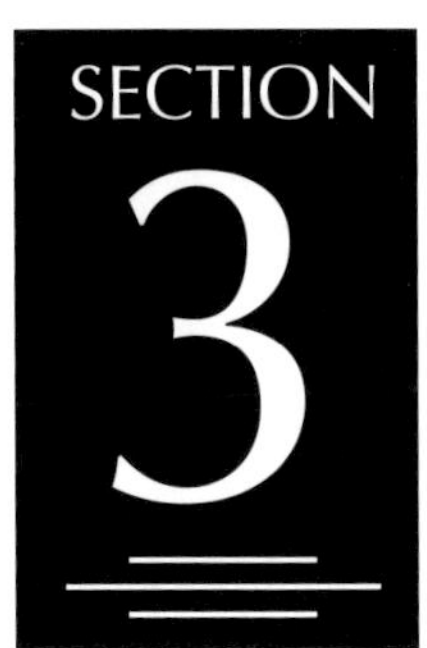

Degenerative Diseases About the Shoulder

Degenerative Diseases About the Shoulder

The six articles that make up this section cover the breadth and depth of management of degenerative disease of the shoulder, focusing on state-of-the art treatment of shoulder arthritis.

The first article in this section by Shapiro and Zuckerman clearly explains the relevant bony anatomy and soft-tissue pathology associated with glenohumeral arthritis. The principal causes of glenohumeral arthritis, including infection, rheumatoid arthritis, osteoarthritis, osteonecrosis, dislocation arthropathy, rotator cuff arthropathy, crystalline arthropathy, hemophiliac arthropathy, neuropathic arthropathy, septic arthritis, and posttraumatic arthritis, are reviewed. Overall, this article is an excellent, clear, and concise introduction to the section.

Hayes and Flatow review treatment alternatives for young patients with shoulder arthritis, including pharmacologic treatment, arthroscopic methods, osteotomies, and allograft resurfacing of the glenoid. Indications for hemiarthroplasty versus total shoulder arthroplasty and a comparison of expected durability in each case are presented. Modern surgical technique also is detailed, with emphasis on soft-tissue releases and the best cement technique in glenoid fixation. Finally, results and complications are clearly outlined. This article is one of the few publications that focuses on this difficult population of patients who demand both pain relief and excellent shoulder function.

Brems' article on complications of shoulder arthroplasty provides a detailed account of all potential complications and reasons for failure. He summarizes the available literature on this topic and provides one of the most comprehensive presentations on this subject that I have ever read. Acute and chronic infection and their care are presented, as is an extensive discussion of glenoid and humeral component loosening.

In the fourth article, Dutta and associates point out that the long-term glenoid aseptic loosening rates of 4% to 11% represent a major reason for late failure of shoulder arthroplasty. They also describe indications for placement of a glenoid component, as well as alternative methods such as biologic resurfacing, discuss management of glenoid deformities and deficiencies, and present ongoing controversies such as keeled versus pegged glenoid and metal-backed versus all-polyethylene glenoid components.

In a follow-up lecture presented 2 years later, Baumgarten and associates review the controversy between hemiarthroplasty and total shoulder arthroplasty in greater detail, and it points out the excellent long-term results with total shoulder arthroplasty. The authors carefully distinguish between radiolucent lines and clinical loosening of the glenoid and provide evidence that few patients with radiolucent lines actually develop clinical loosening of the glenoid component. Finally, guidelines for management of eccentric glenoid erosion are presented.

The final article in this section, by Pearl and associates, is a "must read" for all surgeons who perform state-of-the-art shoulder arthroplasty. It provides an excellent overview of the evolution of component design, which has great implications for restoration of anatomy and component durability and presents, in detail, the most recent three-dimensional anatomic studies on which all current third-generation shoulder arthroplasty designs are based. The importance of restoring anatomic geometry of the proximal humerus in terms of version, offset, and head height is stressed. Controversies between hemiarthroplasty and total shoulder arthroplasty, as well as alternative allograft resurfacing of the glenoid, are presented in detail. Finally, indications for the new technique of reverse shoulder arthroplasty are summarized.

Jon J.P. Warner, MD
Chief, The Harvard Shoulder Service
Professor of Orthopaedic Surgery
Harvard Medical School
Boston, Massachusetts

Glenohumeral Arthroplasty: Indications and Preoperative Considerations

Joel Shapiro, MD
Joseph D. Zuckerman, MD

Introduction

The use of prosthetic replacements for advanced glenohumeral arthritis has become commonplace in orthopaedic surgery. The development of proximal humeral replacement in the 1950s and early 1960s led to total shoulder replacement in the late 1970s and 1980s.[1-7] The results of shoulder arthroplasty have been gratifying, both in terms of pain relief and improvement in function.[8-17] The indications for glenohumeral arthroplasty in the treatment of glenohumeral arthritis are examined in this chapter. Each of the different types of glenohumeral arthritis is described, particularly with respect to the clinical disease and radiographic manifestations. In addition, important preoperative considerations essential for surgical planning are outlined.

Indications

The general indications for prosthetic replacement of the glenohumeral joint are similar to those for other joint arthroplasties. The appropriate candidate has severe shoulder pain with significantly restricted range of motion and compromised activities of daily living. Radiographs usually show advanced glenohumeral arthritis. The patient also should have undergone a program of unsuccessful nonsurgical management (rest, physical therapy, anti-inflammatory medications) before being considered for surgical management.

Several important factors that apply to the various types of arthritides to varying degrees must be recognized and then carefully considered in planning glenohumeral arthroplasty, including bony anatomy, soft-tissue status, associated degenerative conditions of the extremities, and infection. Appropriate measures to increase the chances for a successful surgical result may then be initiated.

Bony Anatomy

Radiographs of the involved shoulder provide the basis for an evaluation of the bony anatomy. The bony structures should be evaluated for quantity, quality, and deformity. Bone quantity refers to the degree of bone loss that may be present as a result of inflammatory, traumatic, or degenerative processes. This can apply to both the humeral head and the glenoid. In addition, bone loss may be asymmetric, particularly involving the glenoid. Bone quality refers to the structure of the available bone. With extensive osteoporotic changes, the bone can be expected to be soft and easily deformed or fractured during the surgical procedure. In some cases, radiographs will show the available bone to be significantly sclerotic, which can also be problematic. Bone deformity is especially important in posttraumatic situations because the tuberosities may be malunited. This is particularly true in the greater tuberosity, which may be displaced superiorly or posteriorly and medially. After proximal humeral fractures, the humeral head may heal in a rotated or angulated position. Similarly, significant deformity of the proximal portion of the humeral shaft may interfere with the ability to insert the stem of the humeral prosthesis.

Evaluation of these aspects of the bony anatomy requires a complete radiographic assessment: standard plain radiographic views, including AP with internal and external rotation of the proximal humerus, scapular Y, and an axillary view.[18] CT scanning of the glenohumeral joint is particularly useful for evaluating the degree of bone loss as well as bone deformity. This is essential preoperative information.

Soft Tissues

The condition of the soft tissues about the shoulder is an equally important preoperative consideration. The range of motion that can be obtained postoperatively, and hence the degree of improvement of shoulder function, depends in large measure on intact, functioning soft tissues. The most important aspects of the soft tissues are the deltoid and rotator cuff muscles. After trau-

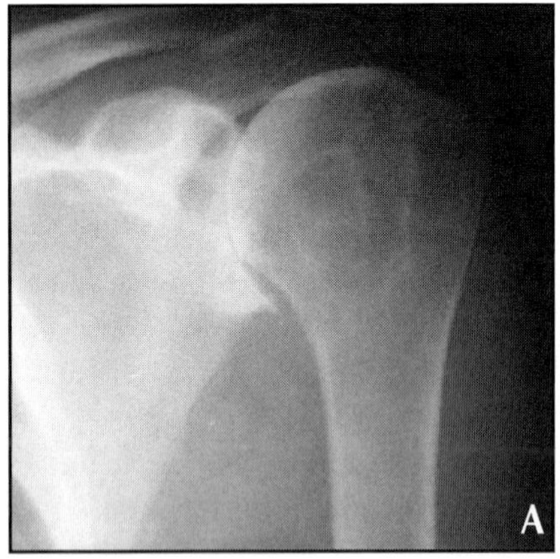

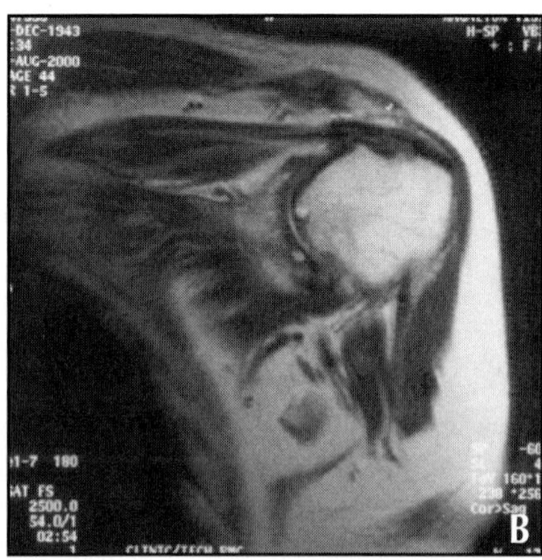

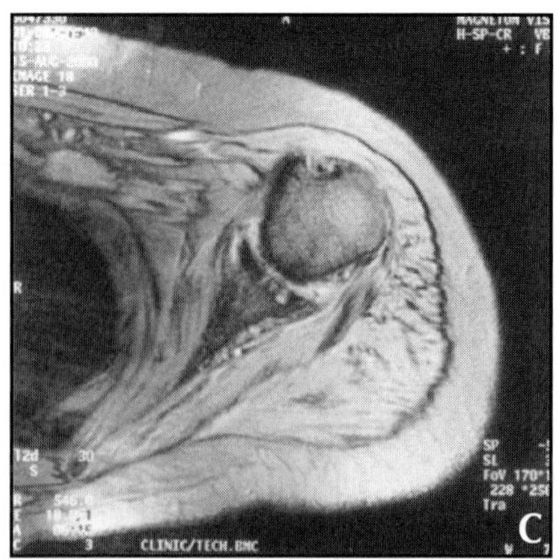

Fig. 1 Inflammatory arthritis in a 57-year-old woman with rheumatoid arthritis and severe shoulder pain despite maximal medical management. AP radiographic (**A**) and coronal (**B**) and axial (**C**) MRI views of early rheumatoid arthritis demonstrating lack of osteophytes, symmetric loss of joint space, and subchondral cysts with minimal loss of glenoid bone stock. Note the attenuated but intact rotator cuff.

ma or previous surgery, the deltoid may be significantly scarred and adherent to the underlying tissues. Previous surgery also carries the risk of deltoid muscle detachment with distal displacement, which is a very difficult problem to overcome.

Involvement of the rotator cuff is frequently present in inflammatory arthritis but much less so in osteoarthritis. Assessment of the rotator cuff integrity preoperatively is valuable because of the positive correlation between rotator cuff status and a successful surgical result. Displaced tuberosities imply scarring and contracture of the rotator cuff, which will require intraoperative release.

Possible denervation of the deltoid and the rotator cuff muscles also must be evaluated preoperatively. Injuries to the axillary nerve or suprascapular nerve that compromise the function of these muscles will affect the indications for surgical management. Electrodiagnostic studies are helpful in any situation in which the status of these muscles is in question.

Associated Conditions

Associated degenerative problems of the affected upper extremity also must be carefully considered. In patients with polyarticular inflammatory arthritis, ipsilateral involvement of the elbow, wrist, and hand may be present, requiring careful staging of the surgical procedures.[19] In some cases, completing hand and wrist reconstructions before proceeding to shoulder reconstruction may be necessary.

Associated degenerative problems of the lower extremity also must be carefully considered. A patient with advanced glenohumeral arthritis who is also in need of total hip or total knee replacement should completely recover from the lower extremity procedure before undergoing the shoulder procedure. The use of assistive walking devices early after a shoulder arthroplasty may compromise the result and lead to complications. Generally, waiting a minimum of 6 to 9 months after shoulder arthroplasty before allowing the use of assistive devices for ambulation is recommended. Whenever possible, completing lower extremity reconstructions before performing shoulder arthroplasty is preferable.

Infection

Infection is an important preoperative consideration for any patient undergoing arthroplasty. Patients who have had previous surgery may have low-grade indolent infections that contribute to the degenerative problem. This should be considered and appropriate tests ordered preoperatively, including aspiration arthrogram and a technetium Tc 99m bone scan combined with either a gallium Ga 67 nitrate or indium In 111 scan. Such tests should also be performed for any destructive type of arthritis or in any case in which a septic process is considered in the differential diagnosis.

If all preoperative testing is negative for infection, intraoperative use of frozen sections also may be helpful in identifying any septic process. Patients with a history of septic process many years previously may be considered candidates for shoulder arthroplasty, but only after a complete preoperative evaluation. In any case, before shoulder arthroplasty is undertaken, any distant site of infection must be eradicated, including periodontal problems, urinary tract infections, and such seemingly innocuous problems as an infected ingrown toenail. Hematogenous spread of the infection to the prosthesis is a significant risk in these situations.

Glenohumeral Arthritides

Several glenohumeral arthritides have been described. Knowledge of their clinical and radiographic characteristics is an important component of preoperative planning for shoulder arthroplasty.

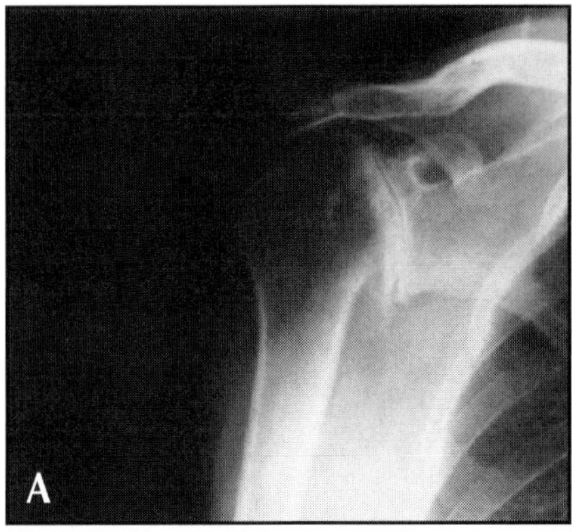

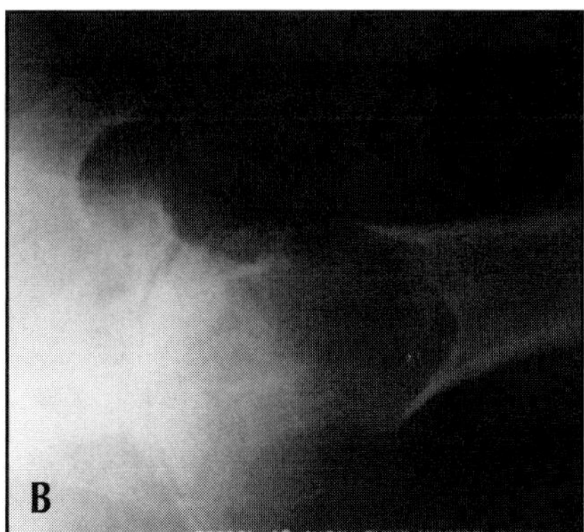

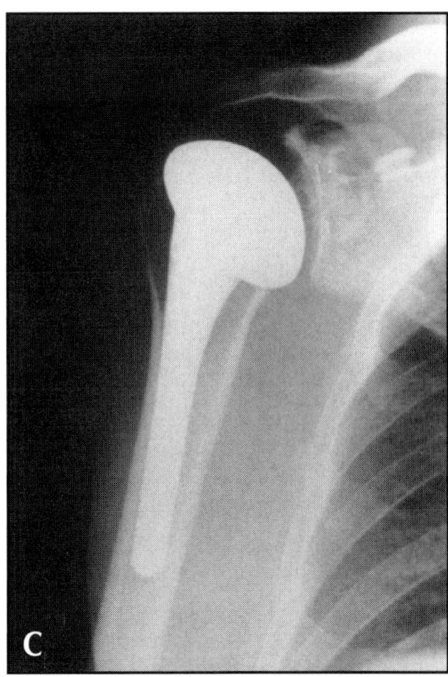

Fig. 2 Osteoarthritis in a 68-year-old man with a long clinical history of worsening shoulder pain with crepitation and progressive loss of range of motion. AP (**A**) and axillary (**B**) radiographic views of advanced osteoarthritis demonstrating large osteophyte formation, subchondral cysts and sclerosis, and posterior glenoid wear with posterior humeral head subluxation. **C,** AP radiographic view of osteoarthritis after total shoulder arthroplasty with anatomic reconstruction.

Rheumatoid Arthritis

Patients with advanced rheumatoid arthritis of the glenohumeral joint are generally younger than 65 years of age and likely to be female, reflecting the epidemiologic characteristics of the disease itself (Fig. 1). These patients also tend to have polyarticular disease with involvement not only of multiple joints of the ipsilateral and/or contralateral upper extremities but also of the lower extremities. Recognizing such multiple involvements is another key aspect in planning the time of shoulder arthroplasty.[20] Patients also may have systemic manifestations, including hematologic, vascular, and renal problems, which must be evaluated carefully before surgery. Also, the presence of instability of the cervical spine, particularly at the C1-C2 level, must be evaluated before administering general anesthetic.

The condition and function of the rotator cuff muscle is another important consideration. Shoulders with advanced rheumatoid arthritis have an extremely high incidence of rotator cuff pathology. Up to 75% of rotator cuffs will be abnormal, and 20% to 35% will have full-thickness tears.[21-25] Generalized atrophy of the muscles about the shoulder often is found as a result of a long period of disuse. The periarticular inflammatory nature of the disease also results in significant soft-tissue contracture. Radiographs often show extensive osteoporosis, which may progress to extensive erosions of the humeral head as well as the glenoid. Glenoid erosion may be extreme, with medialization beyond the base of the coracoid process. The acromioclavicular joint also may show erosive changes because it is a synovial joint.[26] The degree of erosion and the resultant bone loss must be evaluated carefully before surgery because this will impact the choice between hemiarthroplasty and total shoulder replacement.[27,28]

Osteoarthritis

Patients with advanced osteoarthritis of the glenohumeral joint generally are older than 65 years of age and more commonly male than female. Osteoarthritis often presents as a monoarticular problem, although many patients can have one or two major joints involved. The rotator cuff muscle is much less frequently involved than it is in patients with rheumatoid arthritis; in osteoarthritis, the rotator cuff is almost invariably intact, with only 5% of patients having full-thickness rotator cuff tears.[14] Anterior capsular contracture is commonly encountered, resulting in a significant loss of external rotation.

Radiographically, the bone of the humeral head and glenoid appears sclerotic, with extensive osteophyte formation (Fig. 2). The humeral head is generally flattened and enlarged. Flattening of the glenoid is also present, often with asymmetric wear, usually resulting in posterior glenoid erosion. Although bone loss generally is not a problem, osteoarthritic patients may have a history of impingement-type symptoms with anterior acromial osteophytes. This extensive osteophyte formation makes it necessary to carefully identify the normal bony anatomy at the time of shoulder arthroplasty.[29]

Osteonecrosis

Osteonecrosis of the humeral head generally is encountered in patients younger than 65 years of age who present with an underlying medical problem. Predisposing

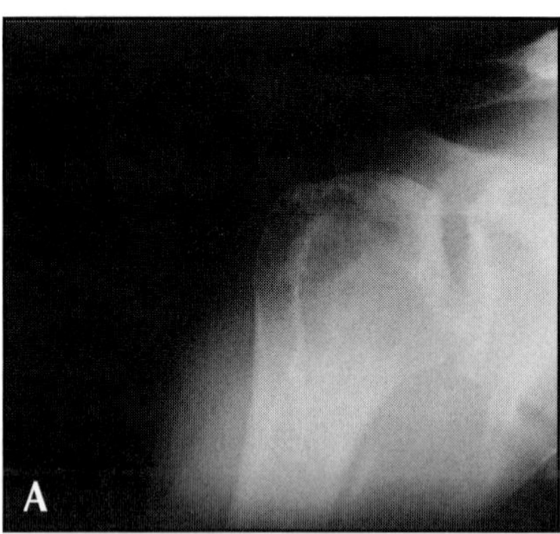

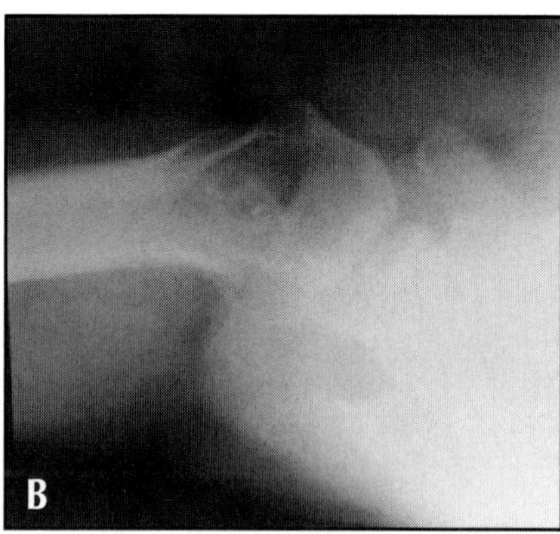

Fig. 3 Osteonecrosis in a 34-year-old patient with steroid-dependent asthma and a 4-month history of shoulder pain of insidious onset. AP (**A**) and axillary (**B**) radiographic views of early osteonecrosis demonstrating pattern of localized collapse of the humeral head without significant glenoid involvement.

conditions include the use of exogenous steroids, systemic lupus erythematosus, alcohol abuse, and sickle cell anemia.[30,31] Osteonecrosis differs from the other conditions discussed here in that nonsurgical management is often successful in limiting symptoms and maintaining function.[32] When such treatment is unsuccessful, surgical management consisting of either proximal humeral replacement or total shoulder arthroplasty may be indicated.

The early stages of osteonecrosis often do not manifest radiographically. The first radiographic sign may be sclerosis of the humeral head, but even this can be difficult to recognize. The appearance of the crescent sign heralds the onset of humeral head collapse. Although initially the collapse may be limited to a relatively small area (Fig. 3), over time it often progresses to extensive humeral head collapse. Early in the process the soft tissues are spared, but as secondary degenerative arthritis develops, soft-tissue contracture becomes common. As the humeral head deforms, joint incongruity results in secondary degenerative changes of the glenoid (Fig. 4), often producing a picture more typical of osteoarthritis.

Dislocation Arthropathy

Arthritis of dislocations is generally encountered in patients younger than 50 years of age and is more common in men. Most of these patients have undergone previous surgery for recurrent instability.[33] Many of these procedures used staples or screws about the shoulder that, because of malposition or migration, resulted in articular cartilage injury.[34] In some cases, an anterior repair was excessively tight, resulting in fixed posterior subluxation and eventual degenerative arthritis. By far the most common etiology is when a "standard" surgical procedure is performed to remedy what are thought to be recurrent unidirectional dislocations but actually is multidirectional instability.

In general, dislocation arthropathy is characterized by a significant amount of soft-tissue scarring from the previous surgery. The anterior structures generally are tight and, as noted, fixed posterior subluxation may be present. The possibility of neurologic injury from the previous surgery should be considered carefully; the anatomy may be significantly abnormal, particularly if the coracoid process has been transferred (for example, via a Bristow procedure). In addition, any soft-tissue repair about the anterior aspect of the shoulder may result in displacement of neurovascular structures. Dissection must be performed carefully to avoid injury to these structures. The axillary nerve is particularly at risk because of its proximity to the inferior aspect of the joint capsule. Other special considerations include the possible need for a deltoidplasty, glenoid bone deficiency, and the threat of postoperative instability of components.

Rotator Cuff Arthropathy

Cuff tear arthropathy represents the end stage of rotator cuff disease. It is an uncommon entity, usually encountered in patients of either sex older than age 70 years; many have had previous rotator cuff surgery (Fig. 5).

On physical examination, there often is a significant amount of swelling about the shoulder as well as extensive atrophy of the rotator cuff muscles. Fluid accumulation within the subacromial bursa results in the classic "fluid sign." These patients have a massive tear of the rotator cuff with probable involvement of all four tendons. The loss of integrity of the glenohumeral joint results in upward migration of the humeral head, often leading to secondary erosive changes of the underside of the acromion and the acromioclavicular joint (Fig. 6). Later stages are characterized by humeral head collapse as well as significant glenoid erosion. The absence of the rotator cuff results in significant instability via the posterior mechanism, and often the humeral head is subluxated anterosuperiorly.

Total shoulder arthroplasty for cuff tear arthropathy is one of the most challenging procedures in orthopaedic surgery. The absence of the rotator cuff and the degree of bony erosions make reconstruction difficult. Postoperative expectations generally fall into the "limited goals" category in which pain relief is the goal; significant improvement in motion or overhead function usually is not possible.[35]

Crystalline Arthropathy

Crystalline arthropathy (Fig. 7) may represent gout, pseudogout, or hydroxyapatite (Milwaukee shoulder) disease. There has

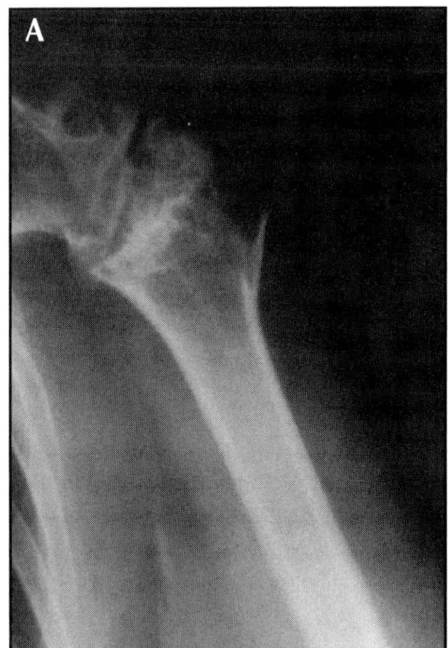
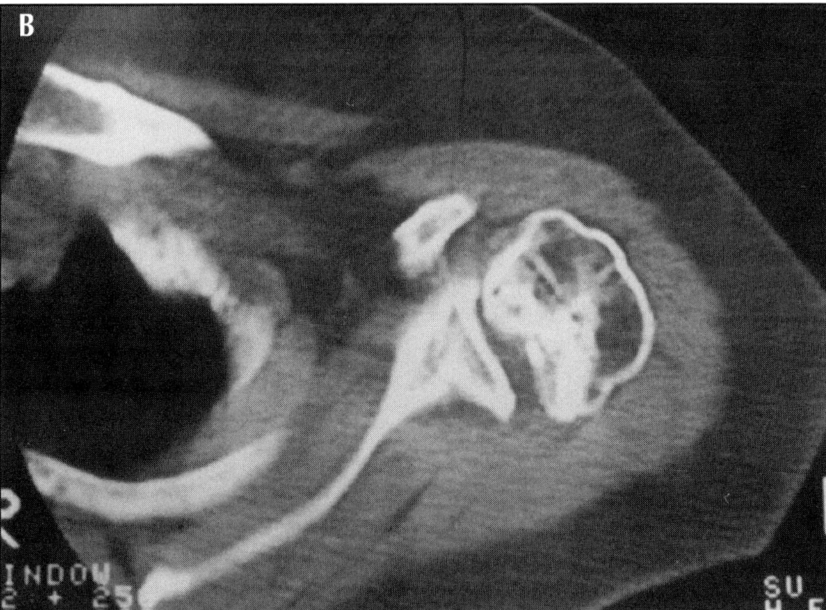

Fig. 4 Osteonecrosis in a 44-year-old man with an 8-year history of shoulder pain that has worsened over a 6-month period. Late osteonecrosis is shown. AP (**A**) and CT (**B**) axillary views demonstrate severe collapse and glenoid wear.

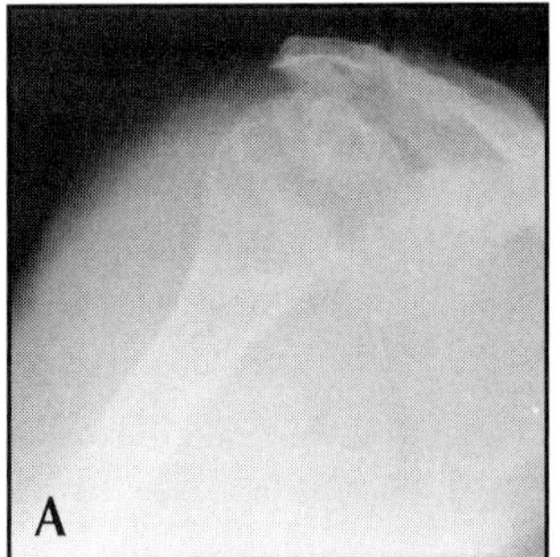
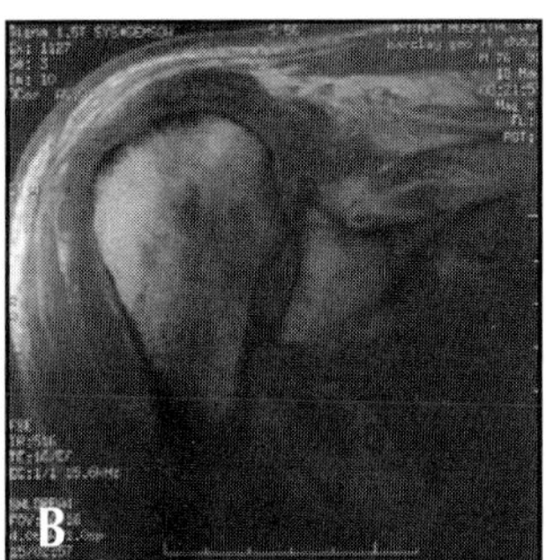
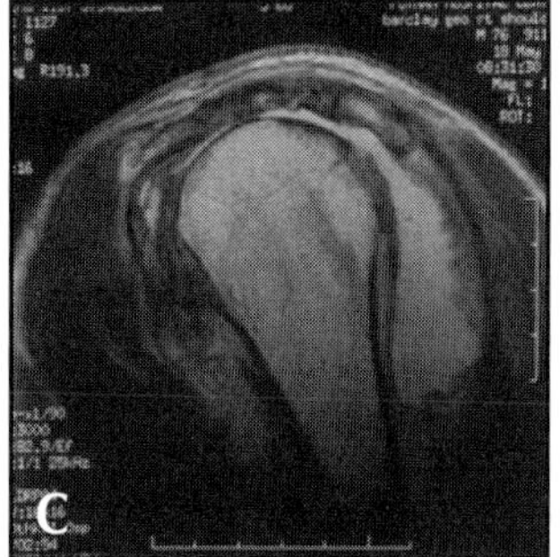
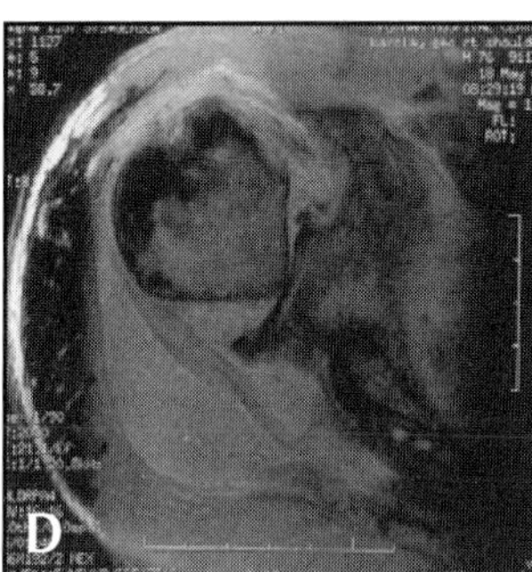

Fig. 5 Rotator cuff arthropathy in a 76-year-old man with a history of massive rotator cuff tear previously treated with débridement, the patient has progressive shoulder pain and dysfunction. AP radiographic (**A**) and MRI coronal (**B**), sagittal (**C**), and axial (**D**) views demonstrate severe superior migration of the humeral head, massive rotator cuff defect, and extreme secondary degenerative changes.

been some disagreement as to whether Milwaukee shoulder (Fig. 8) and rotator cuff arthropathy represent the same or different disease entities. Certain characteristics are common in both, but it is difficult to determine whether these represent the same entity. In general, crystalline arthropathy of the shoulder is uncommon. It is generally found in patients older than 70 years of age, with men more commonly involved than women. The degree of bony involvement as well as soft-tissue involvement is variable, ranging from the appearance of a mild inflammatory arthritis to one of extensive soft-tissue and bone destruction. These patients are candidates for total shoulder arthroplasty. When bony erosions and soft-tissue deterioration are extensive, reconstruction becomes more problematic.

Hemophiliac Arthropathy

Hemophiliac arthropathy generally is encountered in patients with factor VIII and factor IX deficiency and von Willebrand's disease. Because of the sex-linked nature of factor VIII deficiency, men are much more commonly involved. Hemophiliac arthropathy is a type of inflammatory arthropathy. This is essentially a synovial disease, with progressive deterioration of articular cartilage followed by bony erosions and soft-tissue deterioration over time. Thus, the appearance of hemophiliac arthropathy can be similar to that of rheumatoid arthritis. These patients are candidates for total shoulder arthroplasty. Careful consideration must be given, however, to intra-

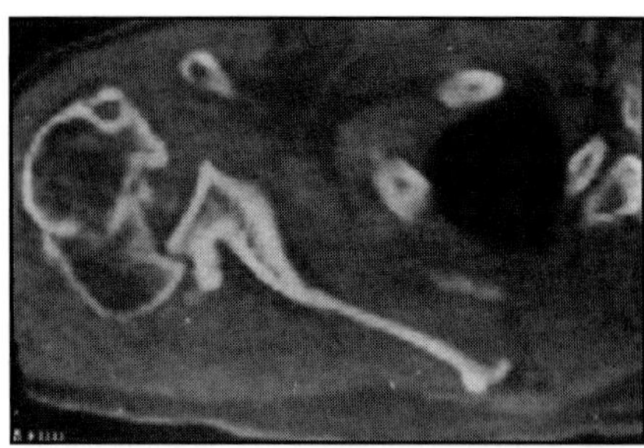

Fig. 6 Posttraumatic arthritis in a 39-year-old man who refused treatment at the time of his original injury. Six months later, he presented for treatment of a stiff, painful shoulder. This axial CT view demonstrates the previous fracture dislocation with resultant chronic dislocation and malunion of the humeral head.

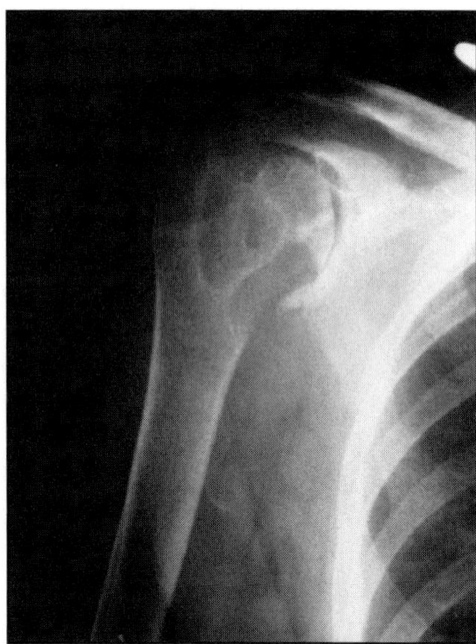

Fig. 7 AP radiographic view of crystalline arthropathy in a 51-year-old man with long-standing gout and recurrent episodes of pain in multiple joints. Note the cystic changes in the humeral head and severe glenoid wear, similar to inflammatory arthritis.

operative bleeding and the need for transfusions and factor replacement. In addition, the fact that a high percentage of hemophiliacs are positive for human immunodeficiency virus requires the surgeon to use extreme caution in performing this procedure.

Neuropathic Arthropathy

Neuropathic arthropathy is an uncommon diagnosis, generally encountered in the patient older than 70 years of age who presents with marked derangement of the glenohumeral joint, as evidenced by bone destruction and fragmentation, but generally with relatively minimal pain (Fig. 9). The most common etiologies include syringomyelia, tabes dorsalis, and diabetes mellitus. Neuropathic shoulders usually exhibit significant swelling and marked deformity. Radiographs show extensive bone destruction and fragmentation, as well as new bone formation. There often is a classic histologic appearance of bone shards embedded within inflamed synovial tissue. Because the process of bone destruction can be expected to continue, total shoulder arthroplasty should not be considered for patients with neuropathic arthropathy. Other contraindications to total shoulder arthroplasty include septic arthritis, paralysis of both the rotator cuff and deltoid muscles, and patient inability to perform postoperative rehabilitation.

Septic Arthritis

Acute septic arthritis (Fig. 10) with joint destruction should be easily recognized and appropriate treatment instituted. Difficulty arises in the diagnosis of patients with inactive or quiescent sepsis; this should be suspected in patients with factors predisposing to septic arthritis, including exogenous steroid use, diabetes mellitus, and in patients undergoing chemotherapy and intravenous drug use, or who have undergone previous intra-articular injections or previous surgery. If ancient sepsis is suspected, the preoperative workup should include a bone scan, indium In 111 scan, and aspiration arthrogram. Total shoulder arthroplasty is contraindicated in a patient with septic arthritis. If shoulder arthroplasty is considered in a patient with a history of joint infection, a frozen section should be performed at the time of surgery. Any histologic evidence of active infection is an indication for either resection arthroplasty or arthrodesis.

Posttraumatic Arthritis

Patients with posttraumatic arthritis can present a very complicated clinical picture (Fig. 6). Of variable age and not predominantly male or female, these patients have sustained previous proximal humeral fractures and also may have undergone previous surgery. Radiographic characteristics of posttraumatic arthritis usually include significant malunion involving both the tuberosities and the articular segment. There may be malalignment of the shaft with respect to the proximal humerus. The bone usually is sclerotic, and significant collapse of the humeral head may be present when there is associated osteonecrosis. Asymmetric glenoid erosion, particularly involving the posterior aspect, is often present.

A subcategory of posttraumatic arthritis involves chronic dislocations and fracture-dislocations of the proximal humerus. These generally represent misdiagnoses, often the result of an unrecognized seizure disorder. Such fixed anterior and posterior dislocations, often with associated fracture, result in significant distortion of the bony and soft-tissue anatomy. Retracted tuberosities result in scarring of the rotator cuff, which may pose significant difficulties in mobilization. Bony deformity, including malunion and nonunion, also may be problematic, particularly when there is significant osteoporosis of the fragments. There may be associated nerve injuries involving the axillary nerve, the suprascapular nerve, or the cords of the brachial plexus, which should be evaluated before considering surgical management. In general, surgical treatment of chronic fracture–dislocations of the proximal humerus represents one of the most challenging reconstructive problems of shoulder surgery.[36-39]

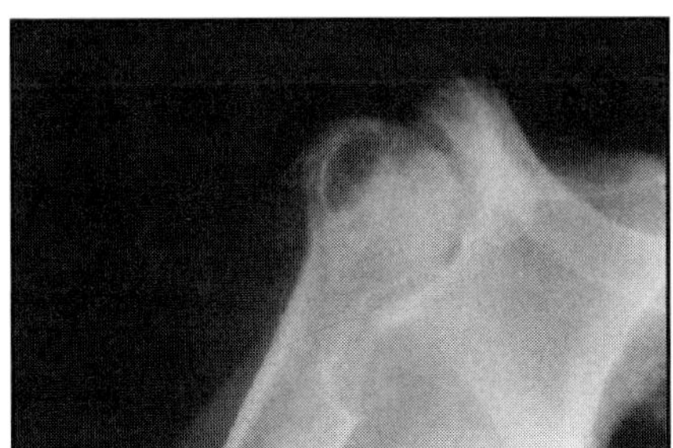

Fig. 8 AP radiographic view of Milwaukee shoulder in a 43-year-old man who has had severe shoulder pain for 1 year, demonstrating extreme erosive changes along the humeral neck and glenoid.

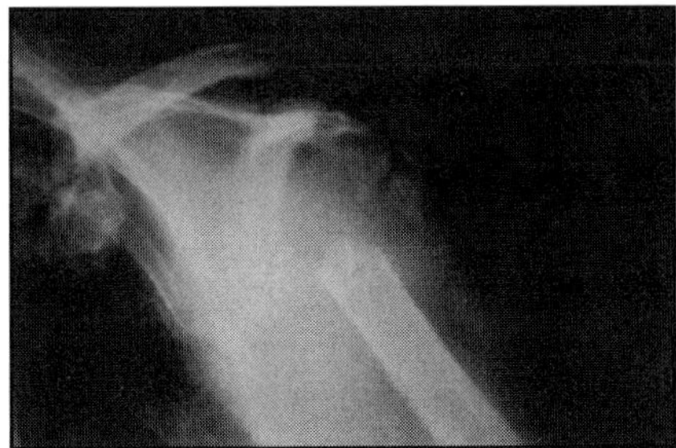

Fig. 9 AP radiographic view of neuropathic arthropathy in a 26-year-old woman with known cervical syringomyelia. She presented with progressively worsening shoulder function but minimal discomfort. Note the complete destruction and resorption of the humeral head, with massive glenoid bone loss.

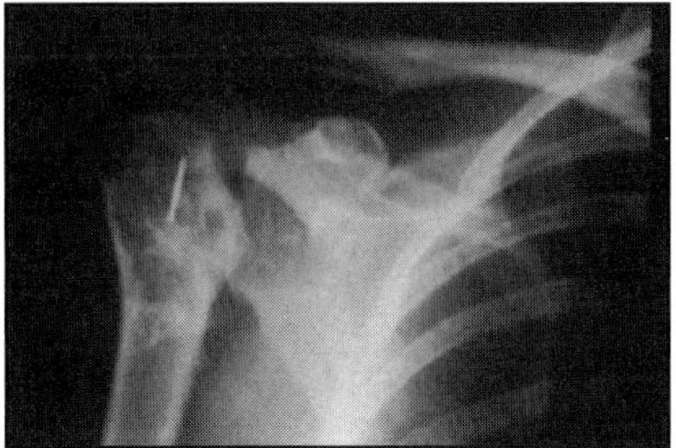

Fig. 10 AP radiographic view of a previously septic shoulder with a history of osteomyelitis, complicating the previous internal fixation of a fracture in a 49-year-old woman. Note the old hardware, which was buried within the humeral head.

Summary

The indications for glenohumeral arthroplasty are severe pain and restricted range of motion associated with radiographic evidence of advanced glenohumeral arthritis. Nonsurgical management consisting of rest, physical therapy, and anti-inflammatory medication should be tried before considering surgical management. It is important that each patient be evaluated on the basis of the clinical disease and radiographic characteristics of the underlying diagnosis. Preoperative considerations should include a careful assessment of bone quality and quantity and associated deformity. Evaluation of the soft tissues, particularly the rotator cuff and deltoid muscles, is essential because the success of total shoulder arthroplasty depends greatly on the integrity of these structures. Associated upper and lower extremity degenerative arthritis should be evaluated and carefully considered, particularly with respect to the timing of surgical management. Careful consideration of these factors is invaluable in obtaining successful outcomes of total shoulder arthroplasty.

References

1. Stone KD, Grabowski JJ, Cofield RH, Morrey BF, An KN: Stress analyses of glenoid components in total shoulder arthroplasty. *J Shoulder Elbow Surg* 1999;8:151-158.
2. Anglin C, Wyss UP, Pichora DR: Mechanical testing of shoulder prostheses and recommendations for glenoid design. *J Shoulder Elbow Surg* 2000;9:323-331.
3. Ehnes DL, Stone JJ, Cofield RH, An KN: Analysis of the shoulder implant. *Biomed Sci Instrum* 2000;36:129-134.
4. Sait S, Scott WA: Early results of isoelastic hemiarthroplasty in chronic shoulder arthritis. *Orthopedics* 2000;23:467-469.
5. Walch G, Boileau P: Prosthetic adaptability: A new concept for shoulder arthroplasty. *J Shoulder Elbow Surg* 1999;8:443-451.
6. Arredondo J, Worland RL: Bipolar shoulder arthroplasty in patients with osteoarthritis: Short-term clinical results and evaluation of birotational head motion. *J Shoulder Elbow Surg* 1999;8:425-429.
7. Vitale MG, Krant JJ, Gelijns AC, et al: Geographic variations in the rates of operative procedures involving the shoulder, including total shoulder replacement, humeral head replacement, and rotator cuff repair. *J Bone Joint Surg Am* 1999;81:763-772.
8. Cofield RH: Total shoulder arthroplasty with the Neer prosthesis. *J Bone Joint Surg Am* 1984;66:899-906.
9. Sperling JW, Cofield RH, Rowland CM: Neer hemiarthroplasty and Neer total shoulder arthroplasty in patients fifty years old or less: Long-term results. *J Bone Joint Surg Am* 1998;80:464-473.
10. Kelly IG, Foster RS, Fisher WD: Neer total shoulder replacement in rheumatoid arthritis. *J Bone Joint Surg Br* 1987;69:723-726.
11. McCoy SR, Warren RF, Bade HA III, Ranawat CS, Inglis AE: Total shoulder arthroplasty in rheumatoid arthritis. *J Arthroplasty* 1989;4: 105-113.
12. Neer CS II: Replacement arthroplasty for glenohumeral osteoarthritis. *J Bone Joint Surg Am* 1974;56:1-13.
13. Neer CS II, Watson KC, Stanton FJ: Recent experience in total shoulder replacement. *J Bone Joint Surg Am* 1982;64:319-337.
14. Gartsman GM, Roddey TS, Hammerman SM: Shoulder arthroplasty with or without resurfacing of the glenoid in patients who have osteoarthritis. *J Bone Joint Surg Am* 2000;82:26-34.
15. Thomas BJ, Amstutz HC, Cracchiolo A: Shoulder arthroplasty for rheumatoid arthritis. *Clin Orthop* 1991;265:125-128.
16. Barrett WP, Thornhill TS, Thomas WH, Gebhart EM, Sledge CB: Nonconstrained total shoulder arthroplasty in patients with polyarticular rheumatoid arthritis. *J Arthroplasty* 1989;4:91-96.
17. Kuhn JE, Blasier RB: Assessment of outcome in shoulder arthroplasty. *Orthop Clin North Am* 1998;29:549-563.
18. Cuomo F, Checroun A: Avoiding pitfalls and complications in total shoulder arthroplasty. *Orthop Clin North Am* 1998;29:507-518.
19. Gill DR, Cofield RH, Morrey BF: Ipsilateral total shoulder and elbow arthroplasties in patients who have rheumatoid arthritis. *J Bone Joint Surg Am* 1999;81:1128-1137.
20. Figgie HE III, Inglis AE, Goldberg VM, Ranawat CS, Figgie MP, Wile JM: An analysis of factors affecting the long-term results of total shoulder arthroplasty in inflammatory arthritis. *J Arthroplasty* 1988;3:123-130.
21. Arntz CT, Jackins S, Matsen FA III: Prosthetic replacement of the shoulder for the treatment of defects in the rotator cuff and the surface of the glenohumeral joint. *J Bone Joint Surg Am* 1993;75:485-491.
22. Zeman CA, Arcand MA, Cantrell JS, Skedros JG, Burkhead WZ Jr: The rotator cuff-deficient arthritic shoulder: Diagnosis and surgical management. *J Am Acad Orthop Surg* 1998;6: 337-348.
23. Franklin JL, Barrett WP, Jackins SE, Matsen FA III: Glenoid loosening in total shoulder arthroplasty: Association with rotator cuff deficiency. *J Arthroplasty* 1988;3:39-46.
24. Sneppen O, Fruensgaard S, Johannsen HV, Olsen BS, Sojbjerg JO, Andersen NH: Total shoulder replacement in rheumatoid arthritis:

Proximal migration and loosening. *J Shoulder Elbow Surg* 1996;5:47-52.

25. Rozing PM, Brand R: Rotator cuff repair during shoulder arthroplasty in rheumatoid arthritis. *J Arthroplasty* 1998;13:311-319.

26. Lehtinen JT, Kaarela K, Belt EA, Kautiainen HJ, Kauppi MJ, Lehto MU: Relation of glenohumeral and acromioclavicular joint destruction in rheumatoid shoulder: A 15 year follow up study. *Ann Rheum Dis* 2000;59:158-160.

27. Alund M, Hoe-Hansen C, Tillander B, Heden BA, Norlin R: Outcome after cup hemiarthroplasty in the rheumatoid shoulder: A retrospective evaluation of 39 patients followed for 2-6 years. *Acta Orthop Scand* 2000;71:180-184.

28. Sojbjerg JO, Frich LH, Johannsen HV, Sneppen O: Late results of total shoulder replacement in patients with rheumatoid arthritis. *Clin Orthop* 1999;366:39-45.

29. Walch G, Boulahia A, Boileau P, Kempf JF: Primary glenohumeral osteoarthritis: Clinical and radiographic classification: The Aequalis Group. *Acta Orthop Belg* 1998;64(suppl 2): 46-52.

30. Hattrup SJ, Cofield RH: Osteonecrosis of the humeral head: Results of replacement. *J Shoulder Elbow Surg* 2000;9:177-182.

31. Mont MA, Payman RK, Laporte DM, Petri M, Jones LC, Hungerford DS: Atraumatic osteonecrosis of the humeral head. *J Rheumatol* 2000;27:1766-1773.

32. Hattrup SJ, Cofield RH: Osteonecrosis of the humeral head: Relationship of disease stage, extent, and cause to natural history. *J Shoulder Elbow Surg* 1999;8:559-564.

33. Neer CS II: Arthritis of dislocations, in Neer CS II (ed): *Shoulder Reconstruction*. Philadelphia, PA, WB Saunders, 1990, pp 208-212.

34. Zuckerman JD, Matsen FA III: Complications about the glenohumeral joint related to the use of scews and staples. *J Bone Joint Surg Am* 1984;66:175-180.

35. Nwakama AC, Cofield RH, Kavanagh BF, Loehr JF: Semiconstrained total shoulder arthroplasty for glenohumeral arthritis and massive rotator cuff tearing. *J Shoulder Elbow Surg* 2000;9:302-307.

36. Bosch U, Skutek M, Fremerey RW, Tscherne H: Outcome after primary and secondary hemiarthroplasty in elderly patients with fractures of the proximal humerus. *J Shoulder Elbow Surg* 1998;7:479-484.

37. Wiater JM, Flatow EL: Posttraumatic arthritis. *Orthop Clin North Am* 2000;31:63-76.

38. Dines DM, Warren RF, Altchek DW, Moeckel B: Post-traumatic changes of the proximal humerus: Malunion, nonunion, and osteonecrosis: Treatment with modular hemiarthroplasty or total shoulder arthroplasty. *J Shoulder Elbow Surg* 1993;2:11-21.

39. Norris TR, Green A, McGuigan FX: Late prosthetic shoulder arthroplasty for displaced proximal humerus fractures. *J Shoulder Elbow Surg* 1995;4:271-280.

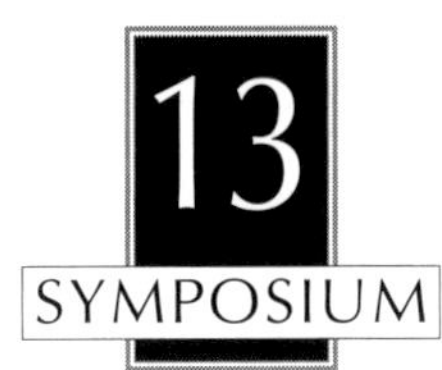

Total Shoulder Arthroplasty in the Young Patient

Patrick R.L. Hayes, MD
Evan L. Flatow, MD

Introduction

Neer ushered in the era of modern shoulder arthroplasty in 1953, reporting on his first anatomic humeral head prosthesis.[1] In 1955 he described using his redesigned vitallium, anatomic humeral head prosthesis (the Neer I) in patients with four-part fractures, fracture-dislocations, and osteonecrosis (ON).[2,3] He then expanded the indications for humeral head replacement to include degenerative glenohumeral arthritis.[4] In the 1970s several authors reported on the implantation of a polyethylene glenoid component with which the humeral prosthesis articulated.[4-7] The Neer II prostheses was designed to articulate with any of Neer's glenoid components.[4] Since then, many other shoulder prostheses have been developed. To date the most reliable long-term results in shoulder arthroplasty with respect to pain relief, restoration of function, and longevity of the prosthesis appear to occur with unconstrained prostheses of anatomic design.[4,8-19]

As success with shoulder arthroplasty has grown and orthopaedists have become more familiar and adept with the technique, the indications for shoulder arthroplasty have expanded. In young patients with severe proximal humerus fractures; ON; posttraumatic, inflammatory, and degenerative arthritides; humeral replacement and total shoulder arthroplasty remain viable options.[20-23] It is critical, however, to remember the limits of the technique, to remain clear on the indications and contraindications, and to accurately educate patients on the risks, benefits, alternatives, and expected outcomes of shoulder arthroplasty in the young patient.

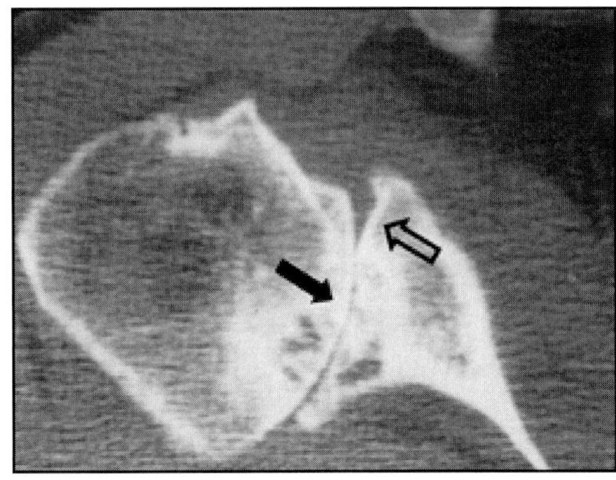

Fig. 1 CT scan showing eccentric posterior glenoid wear in this patient with OA. Version is easily seen on CT. The hollow arrow shows native glenoid contour; the solid arrow shows posterior eroded contour.

Alternatives

Shoulder arthroplasty remains the optimal procedure for pain relief and restoration of function in most shoulders with severe articular disease.[20-23] In more moderate cases the pathology may not warrant such definitive intervention, and in some settings prosthetic replacement is contraindicated. It is important to be familiar with conservative and other surgical options in treating glenohumeral pathology.[24]

Etiology of the arthritis plays an important part in a patient's natural history and prognosis after arthroplasty. The shoulder joint is an uncommon site of primary osteoarthritis (OA). Radiographic signs of OA in the shoulder include large inferior osteophytes, sclerosis, subchondral cysts, and posterior erosion of the glenoid (Fig. 1). An OA presentation in young patients often is the result of trauma[24] or of prior instability repairs. Humeral trauma or surgery that alters shoulder biomechanics and results in humeral roughness or eccentric loading of the glenoid eventually can progress to glenoid degeneration.[22,23,25] Radiographic findings do not necessarily correlate with symptoms.

In rheumatoid arthritis (RA), the glenohumeral joint is commonly involved

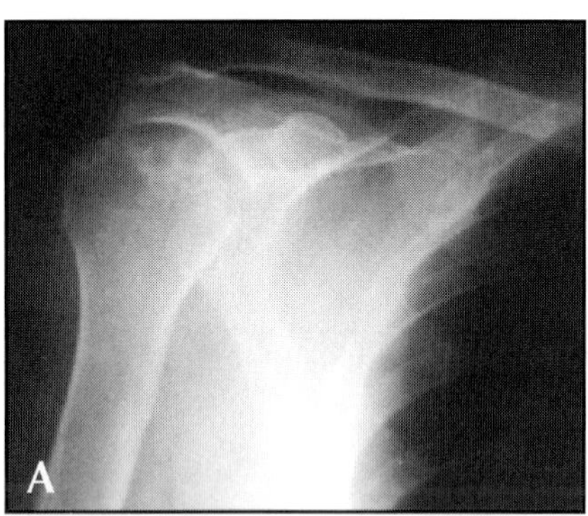

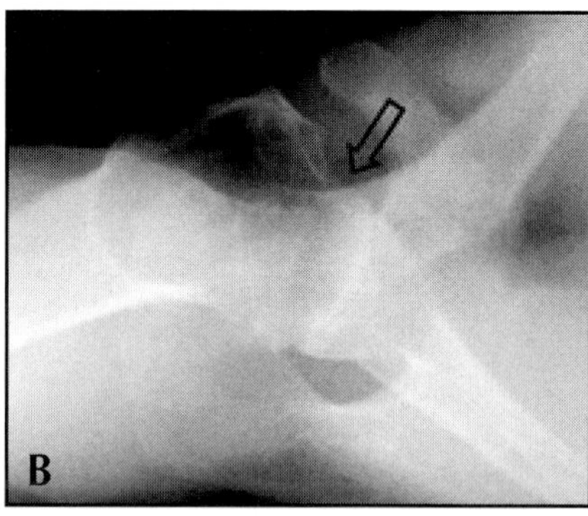

Fig. 2 Radiographs from a patient with glenohumeral RA. **A,** AP view. Note the subchondral erosions, relative osteopenia, and absence of osteophytes. **B,** Axillary view. Note central glenoid erosion, relative osteopenia, periarticular erosions, and lack of osteophytes. The arrow points to anterior periarticular erosion.

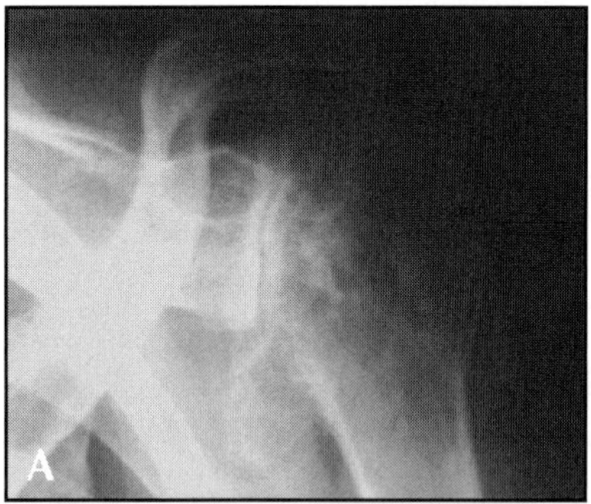

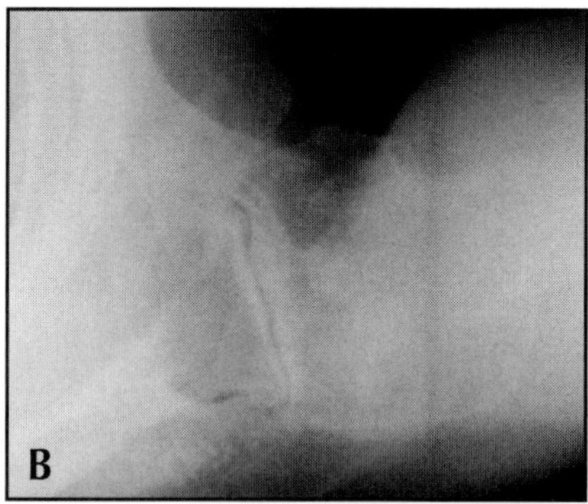

Fig. 3 Radiograph from a patient with Cruess stage V idiopathic ON. **A,** AP view. Note joint space narrowing, huge inferior humeral osteophyte, and humeral head collapse. The dotted line marks the native cortex and underscores the size of the humeral osteophyte. **B,** Axillary view. Flattened humeral head caused like changes on the glenoid.

and is usually part of a polyarthropathy[26] (Fig. 2). Symptomatic RA of the shoulder typically occurs in women between 35 and 55 years of age who have positive rheumatoid factor.[24] Loss of motion, fatigue, and muscle weakness occur. Rotator cuff tears occur in approximately 25% of these patients.[24]

ON can occur in patients with trauma, steroid use, alcoholism, sickle-cell disease, hemophilia, a history of decompression sickness, lipid storage diseases, or lupus erythematosus.[23,27,28] Often the cause is unknown. Disease progression was staged by Cruess as follows: preradiographic stage (I), humeral head involvement (II), subchondral humeral head fracture (crescent sign, III), humeral head collapse (IV), and glenoid involvement (V) (Fig. 3). The later stages of ON are typically more symptomatic, are more likely to progress, and most often require prosthetic replacement.[27]

Degenerative glenohumeral arthritis can occur after stabilization surgery for instability.[29,30] This arthritis may result from postsurgical, iatrogenic subluxations; persistent multidirectional instability; inadequate or inappropriate surgery; or as a complication of hardware, and it is often multifactorial in nature[30] (Fig. 4). In Bigliani and associates' series,[29] symptomatic arthritis came to prosthetic replacement an average of 16 years after the initial stabilization procedure.

Nonsurgical Treatment

Patient education about natural history and prognosis can ensure that the patients understand what to expect and how they can influence their disease process. Understanding what is in store allows them to make realistic job and recreational choices, participate in strength and motion preserving exercises, and avoid detrimental activities.

Physical therapy can especially benefit patients who are stiff and weak prior to the onset of end-stage arthritis. Motion and strength can be restored or at least maintained. End-stage arthritis with stiffness secondary to joint incongruity actually may be exacerbated with aggressive stretching exercises. Preferential strengthening of muscles that specifically resist instability may be beneficial in patients with a component of instability.[31] Cold therapy is useful in reducing inflammation and calming down shoulders after stretching and strengthening. Heat can help alleviate chronic pain and facilitate gaining joint motion. Ultrasound works to increase tissue temperature and blood flow to a depth of 5 cm.[24,32] Occupational therapy can provide strategies and assistive devices to patients with glenohumeral arthritis who struggle with daily functional limitations.

Local anesthetic injections can be valuable in determining the pain generators about a painful shoulder.[33-35] Steroid injections can efficaciously alleviate symptoms in the shoulder with RA, although the value of steroid injections is less clear in OA.[24,36,37] Nonsteroidal anti-inflammatory drugs (NSAIDs) also can be very effective in treating inflammatory glenohumeral arthritis. In OA it is not clear that NSAIDs are any better than acetaminophen.[38]

Surgical Alternatives

Arthroscopic débridement for degenerative arthritis of the knee has been used with reasonable success in the appropriate setting.[39] The indications for débridement of degenerative arthritis of the glenohumeral joint are not as clear. Often degenerative lesions of the glenohumeral joint are found incidentally during diagnostic arthroscopy.[40,41]

Results of arthroscopic débridement appear to depend on the extent of the degenerative changes found.[42] One series looked at arthroscopic débridement of OA of the shoulder in 54 patients with 3 years' follow-up. If mild changes were present, two thirds did well; if severe changes were seen, only one third were doing well at follow-up. Those who had débridement of degenerative labral tears did well.

Abrasion arthroplasty has been suggested in the shoulder, but its benefit remains to be proven.[24,43] In ON, abrasion of small lesions on the humeral head with removal of loose bodies may be helpful.[44] In a study by Weinstein and associates,[45] 27 patients were followed for an average of 30 months after arthroscopic débridement of degenerative arthritis of the shoulder. Loose bodies were removed, degenerative labral tissue and cartilage were débrided, and subacromial bursectomy was performed. Patients experienced significant gains in function and pain relief, with 78% satisfactory results. The authors concluded that arthroscopic débridement is a useful procedure in patients with mild glenohumeral OA. The addition of bursectomy in this series may have increased the success compared with results seen in other series.[24]

The efficacy of subacromial decompression (SAD) in the presence of glenohumeral arthritis has been established by two other series. Simpson and Kelley[46] performed SAD, bursectomy, and glenohumeral débridement in 24 patients with RA and advanced glenohumeral involvement. Nineteen of 22 patients at 30-months follow-up had good pain relief and significantly improved range of motion. Ellowitz and associates[47] looked at 21 patients who had OA with grade IV chondral changes in the glenohumeral joint. They performed SAD and reported uniformly good results. Given these results, Skedros and associates[24] could not recommend glenohumeral débridement as an isolated procedure in glenohumeral arthritis, and urged consideration of SAD and bursectomy as part of the débridement.

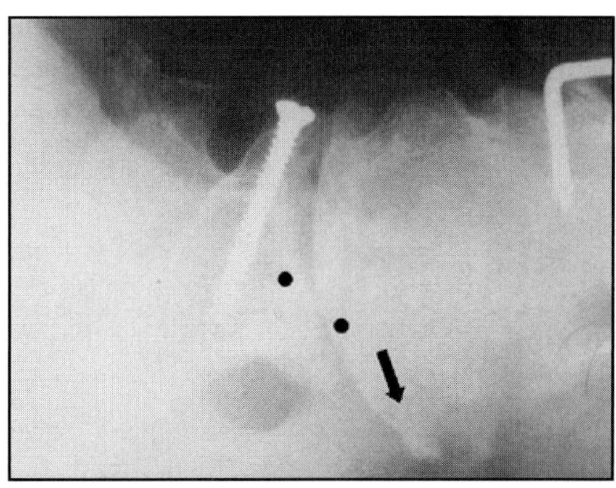

Fig. 4 Axillary view from a 32-year-old patient with painful arthritis of the glenohumeral joint following multiple procedures for instability, including a coracoid transfer and a Putti-Platt procedure, performed approximately 10 years earlier. Dots show the center of the glenoid and the humerus. The arrow underscores the fixed posterior subluxation that contributed to the arthrosis.

Capsular release has a role in the stiff, painful shoulder with mild arthritic changes. Hawkins and Angelo[48] reported arthritis in 10 patients who had previously undergone Putti-Platt capsulorrhaphies for anterior instability. Four patients were taken to surgery, all received open capsular releases to restore external rotation, and two received humeral head replacements. Ogilvie-Harris and Wiley[42] arthroscopically débrided 14 frozen shoulders with associated OA. If more than 20° of motion were lost, an arthroscopic capsular release was performed. Brems[30] reviewed arthritis of dislocation and found a large number of patients who developed arthritis in the setting of instability had had previous reconstructive procedures. Common factors contributing to the development of arthritis included failure to diagnose direction or degree of instability, inadequate or nonanatomic surgical reconstruction, prominent hardware, surgery on the wrong side of the joint, and inappropriate use of arthroscopic techniques. Brems[30] advocated soft-tissue rebalancing and prosthetic replacement in these patients if the cartilage surfaces were destroyed. Ideally, humeral head replacement without glenoid resurfacing could be performed if the surgery was performed before severe glenoid involvement.

Surgical synovectomy can give good local pain relief and improve motion in inflammatory arthropathies about the shoulder.[24] The synovectomy can be performed arthroscopically.[49] Done early in the disease process, it can slow disease progression. The procedure may have to be repeated in tenacious inflammatory arthropathies. The best overall symptomatic relief is obtained when the shoulder is the most symptomatic of the joints involved. It was found on 6-year follow-up of open shoulder synovectomies, that 75% of late stage RA patients were satisfied, 70% had improvements in swelling and motion, and 50% had lasting reduction in pain.[24]

Addressing comorbidities in mild or moderate arthritis can give significant relief and buy time before glenohumeral replacement, if the comorbidities are the dominant pain generators. Diagnostic injections can help identify portions of pain from symptomatic acromiocalvicular joints or subacromial bursae. According to Pollock,[50] cuff repair and humeral head replacement is the treatment of choice in severely painful shoulders with RA that have rotator cuff tears. If the cuff appears

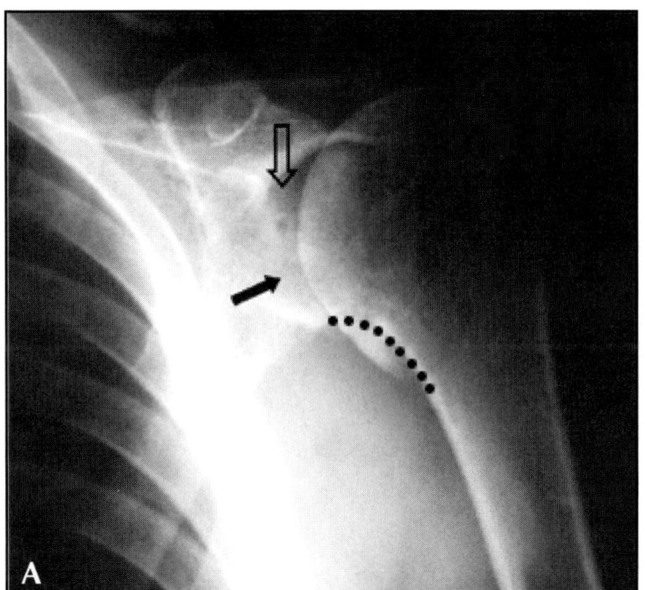

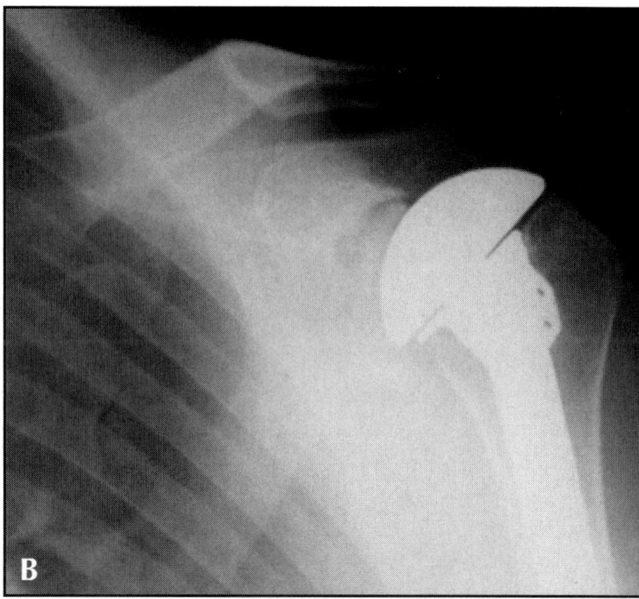

Fig. 5 Radiograph from a 35-year-old patient with painful glenohumeral arthritis and stiffness after multiple instability reconstructions performed during his late teens and early 20s. **A**, Dotted line outlines native cortex and shows size of inferior osteophyte. The solid arrow points to change in contour of humeral head from flattening; the hollow arrow points to nonmetallic anchor hole from prior repair for instability. **B**, AP view of hemiarthroplasty with biologic resurfacing of glenoid with reflected capsule.

to be dysfunctional and unable to center the glenoid even after repair, the glenoid should not be replaced.[51,52] Skedros and associates[24] recommended cuff repair without replacement in symptomatic tears if the arthritis is minor.

Benjamin and associates[53,54] described periarticular osteotomies for symptomatic treatment of glenohumeral arthritis. This is rarely done in the United States. The theory is that the osteotomies reduce subchondral venous congestion and bring new blood flow to the area with healing. The procedure has not been reported by other surgeons in peer reviewed journals.[24]

Osteotomies through the humerus have been described to correct abnormal glenohumeral biomechanics and reduce instability.[55] Theoretically this may prevent development of arthritis from fixed or recurrent instability. As pointed out by Brems,[30] most arthritis in the setting of instability usually occurs as the result of an unbalanced joint after previous surgery attempting to address the instability.[30] Glenoid osteotomies have been suggested to reduce increased glenoid retroversion and posterior instability.[56,57] In a patient with marked glenoid retroversion and instability, a scapular neck osteotomy may correct the abnormal biomechanics and avoid posterior glenoid wear. True glenoid hypoplasia is uncommon, and only a small percentage of these patients develop degenerative arthritis. If this arthritis occurs, most patients can be managed with a program of physical therapy.[58] If bone stock is inadequate, glenoid replacement should not be performed.

Most surgeons are reluctant to offer prosthetic replacement to young, active, high-demand patients, for fear of loosening and eventual failure. Alternative techniques have been developed which débride, resect, reshape, or fuse the articular surfaces. Humeral head resection results in significant loss of strength and motion because the fulcrum for the shoulder is lost.[23] In the era of arthroplasty, fusion is reserved for salvage efforts. Indications may include combined deltoid and rotator cuff dysfunction, irreparable rotator cuff tears with painful cuff tear arthropathy, paralytic disorders in infancy, joint destroying infections, failed arthroplasty, recurrent dislocations uncontrolled by other procedures, painful arthritis in patients who require power but not motion, and resections after tumors.[59] Fusion significantly limits the ability to place the hand in space and often transfers the stresses and pain to the periscapular muscles.

Interposition arthroplasty has been reported on both sides of the joint. The techniques described include reducing in size, then resurfacing the humeral head with a biologic membrane, and smoothing or flattening the glenoid and covering it with biologic tissue as well. The main indication appears to be in the young patient with end-stage RA who has an intact rotator cuff and is capable of following the postoperative regimen. Loss of cuff integrity and large destructive cysts in the humeral head are contraindica-

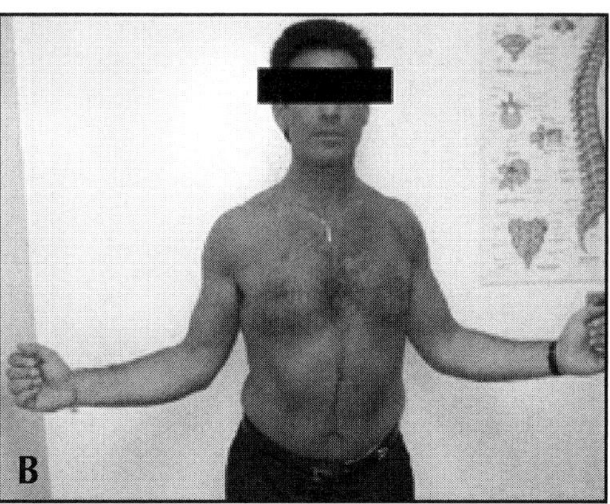

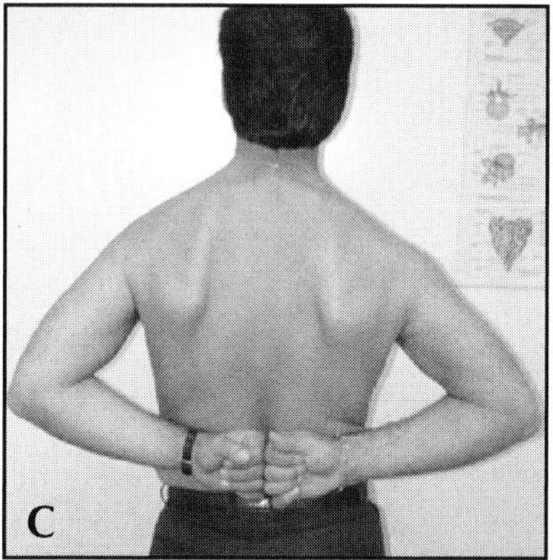

Fig. 6 Photographs of a patient who had infectious arthritis 1 year after left humeral head replacement with fascial arthroplasty. **A**, Maximum forward flexion compared with the normal side. **B**, Maximum external rotation. **C**, Maximum internal rotation. The patient is able to play golf and lift light weights.

tions. Burkhead and Hutton[60] reported on early results of biologic resurfacing of the glenoid with humeral head replacement in the young patient with glenohumeral arthritis. Excellent results were obtained in five of six patients at a minimum of 2 years' follow-up, with excellent pain relief and significant gains in motion (Figs. 5 and 6).

Indications and Contraindications

Shoulder arthroplasty is performed in many young patients with painful conditions of the glenohumeral joint, whose symptoms are refractory to conservative measures and less definitive procedures. The most common diagnoses in the young shoulder arthroplasty patient include trauma, posttraumatic arthritis, arthritis after reconstruction of instability, inflammatory arthritis, and ON of the humeral head.

Humeral head replacement (HHR) is offered to patients with severe pain and dysfunction of the shoulder resulting from destruction of the humeral head. HHRs work best in patients with functioning deltoid and rotator cuff muscles and a balanced soft-tissue envelope that centers the humeral head on the glenoid.[50-52] Soft tissues may have to be balanced or repaired, and the glenoid may have to be smoothed at surgery to achieve this.[23] In Levine and associates' series,[61] HHRs were most successful in the patients with OA who had concentric glenoid wear. Poorer results, with less forward elevation and external rotation, were seen in patients with increased posterior wear and were attributed to a less stable fulcrum for the humeral head. Rodosky and Bigliani[62] believed that patients with OA and eccentric glenoid wear do better with glenoid resurfacing. This belief is a relative indication to be weighed against the relative contraindication of resurfacing a glenoid in a young person.

HHR may be offered in the setting of prior infection (Fig. 7). The infection must have been quiescent for over 12 months, with laboratory tests and cultures negative for signs of active infection. Smith and Matsen[63] recommend a noncemented HHR. The glenoid is not replaced, and the patient is warned the humeral component will have to be removed if the infection recurs.

Nerve or muscle damage causing muscle imbalance and subluxation of the glenohumeral joint is another contraindication to glenoid replacement. Severe rotator cuff dysfunction can allow superior migration of the humerus and eccentric loading of the glenoid component, which increases the risk of early glenoid loosening,[64] the so-called "rocking horse" glenoid. Deltoid dysfunction could cause fixed inferior subluxation or dislocation of the humeral prosthesis.

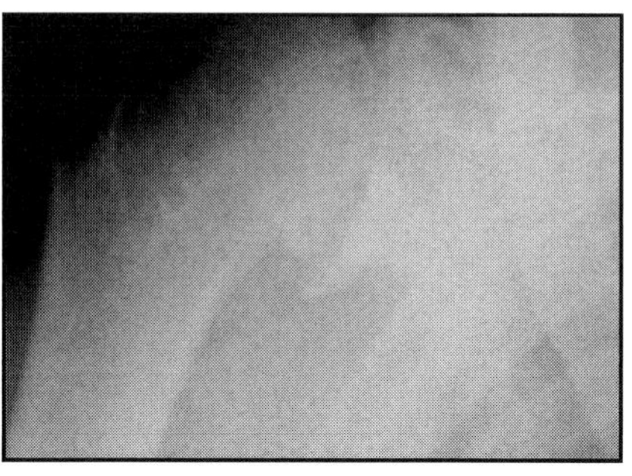

Fig. 7 AP view of postinfectious arthritis in a patient with prior hematogenous *Staphylococcus* infection. Note the erosive appearance and absence of osteophytes.

Caution is warranted in neuropathic arthropathy of the shoulder.[65] Central lesions such as syringomyelia and metabolic processes such as diabetes and chronic alcoholism can cause neuropathic arthropathy. The same lack of sensation that led to the joint destruction can loosen any prosthesis that is inserted. The neuropathy may progress and cause loss of rotator cuff or deltoid function. Arthroplasty is not recommended.

Glenoid replacement generally is avoided in the young, active patient for fear of loosening. In a series of patients

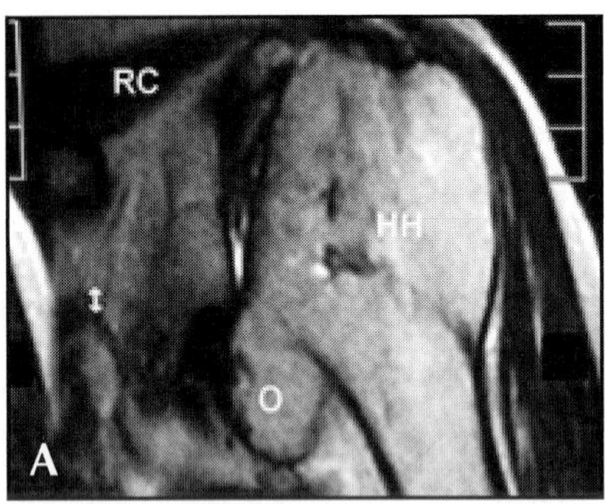

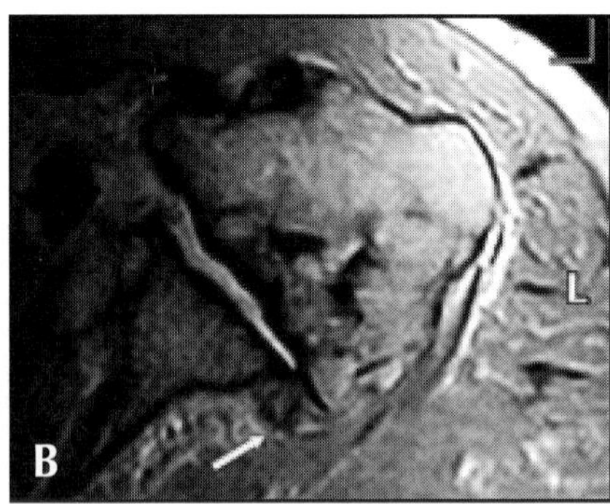

Fig. 8 A, Sagittal oblique MRI study of the patient in Figure 3. RC = rotator cuff, HH = humeral head, O = osteophyte. Cuff looks intact but thinned. **B,** Axial MRI study. Note how clear version is on this image. The arrow points to a posterior osteophyte that overhangs the posterior glenoid, which made dislocation of the glenohumeral joint impossible without extensive releases.

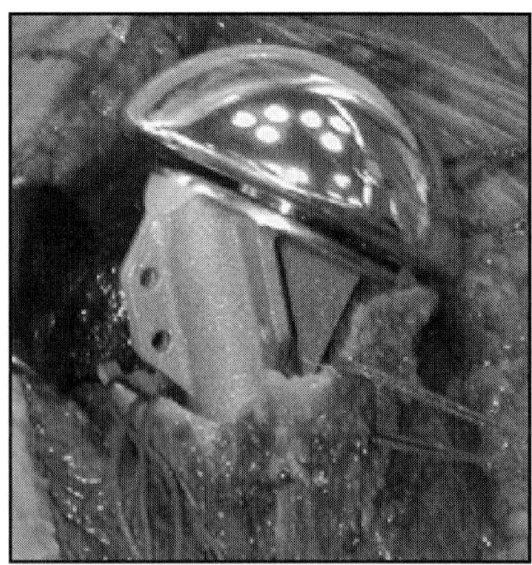

Fig. 9 HHR in a four-part fracture. Sutures are used to reattach tuberosities. Cement is always used to afford rotational stability. The stem may need to be cemented superior to the shaft fracture to obtain appropriate tension in myofascial sleeve.

younger than 50 years of age,[66] complete radiolucent lines around the glenoid were seen in 59% of 34 total shoulder arthroplasties (TSAs) at a mean follow-up of 12.3 years. Torchia and associates[19] reported the presence of radiolucent lines at the bone-cement interface of glenoid components in 84% of their patients followed an average of 12 years. By radiographic signs, 44% were definitely loose, and looseness was associated with pain. Biologic resurfacing should be considered if glenoid involvement is present in the young patient (Fig. 5). Revising a loose glenoid is technically demanding and may not be possible because of bone loss (2 of 9 in a small series).[67] Recurrent loosening after revision can occur (two of seven). Given these data, we recommend attempting humeral replacement and biologic resurfacing in the young, active patient with destruction on both sides of the joint (Fig. 6).

If the nonreplaced glenoid becomes symptomatic, resurfacing the glenoid can be undertaken as a later procedure with reasonable success. Sperling and Cofield[25] reported on 22 revisions of painful humeral replacements to TSAs. Revisions were performed an average of 4.4 years after their humeral replacements. Most patients had marked pain relief and increased motion after revision. This further reinforces a staged approach in the young patient, performing HHR and possibly biologic resurfacing, then addressing the glenoid later if it becomes symptomatic.

Glenoid resurfacing is avoided in patients with nonfunctioning deltoids or rotator cuffs,[23,50,51] a history of infection, inadequate bone stock to support a glenoid, very tight shoulders despite releases, and patients who cannot comply with the postoperative restrictions.

Preoperative Planning

Preoperative imaging studies are critical in planning for TSA. Standard plain films obtained include a true anteroposterior (AP) view in slight external rotation and a good quality axillary view. The AP will show superior migration suspicious for rotator cuff dysfunction. This view will also show joint space narrowing and humeral and glenoid osteophytes (Fig. 3, *A*). The axillary delineates the version of the glenoid and any rim erosions present (Fig. 3, *B*). If bony anatomy or glenoid involvement remains in question, a CT scan or MRI study can provide additional information about the glenoid (Figs. 1 and 8). MRI will show the condition of the rotator cuff. Electromyograms and nerve conduction studies may be necessary to evaluate or document preoperatively the patient's neural status.

In fracture cases, the goals of the procedure include preserving vascularity of the fracture fragments, getting the fracture to heal, and restoring appropriate tension in the soft-tissue envelope to restore function of the deltoid and rotator cuff postoperatively.[23,68,69] With significant comminution or bone loss, radiographs of the opposite, normal humerus with radiographic markers to correct for magnification may be helpful in planning where to seat the cemented humeral prosthesis. Traction radiographs or a CT scan can help define the fracture lines and the size and orientation of the fragments. Bone graft can be obtained from the discarded humeral head if this is available. Heavy suture or wire may be used to repair tuberosity fragments to each other and to the humeral stem (Fig. 9).

In tumor cases imaging studies including MRI and bone scintigraphy can delineate the extent of the tumor including skip lesions. Bulk allografts and custom prostheses may be needed; these must be planned for preoperatively.

Technique

Meticulous handling of the soft tissues is critical to successful TSA. The patient is met in the holding area before receiving anesthesia, and the surgical site and plan are confirmed. Usually, regional anesthesia is administered with interscalene block without general anesthesia. The patient is placed in the beach chair position over the edge of the table so that the extremity to be operated on can be adducted and extended in a vertical position without hitting the side of the table. Two folded towels are placed under the medial border of the scapula to support the glenoid. A headrest is used, and the head is taped in place.

The patient is prepped and draped. Bony landmarks, old scars, and the proposed incision are drawn on the skin. A medium-sized antimicrobial incise drape is placed over the surgical site, enveloping the shoulder.

The skin incision is made through dermis from superiomedial to the coracoid, crossing the coracoid, down toward the anterior aspect of the deltoid insertion on the upper arm. Needle tip electrocaudery is used to divide fat down to the fascia, which is left on the muscles. Medial and lateral skin flaps are raised to allow palpation of the anterior clavicle, the coracoid, and the insertion of the deltoid. A fatty triangle will open up at the superior edge of the deltopectoral interval. Near its insertion the deltoid will curve away from the pertoralis, opening up the interval. **(CD-10.1)**

The cephalic vein is identified and preferentially taken medially to avoid trauma to the vein during preparation of the humerus. The vein is unroofed, and any branches are cauterized or ligated. Branches reliably occur superiorly in the fat triangle near the coracoid, periodically along the lateral and deep aspects of the vein, and along the superior border of the pectoralis, right next to the deltoid tendon insertion.

Sweeping a finger in the interval further develops the deltopectoral interval. Any adhesions should be divided with electrocautery. The clavipectoral fascia is divided lateral to the strap muscle fibers lateral to the conjoined tendon. If the deltoid is still adherent, it is freed from underlying tissue as well. Bursa is resected for exposure. The axillary nerve can be located by sweeping a finger under the strap muscles, over the front of the subscapularis. The tug test[70] will reliably help identify the course of the axillary nerve in index procedures without scarring from previous trauma. The spaces under the acromion and deltoid must be fully developed. Retractors are placed under the deltoid and the strap muscles. For additional exposure, the anterior free edge of the coracoacromial ligament can be resected. The superior centimeter of the pectoralis can be divided as well. This usually is not repaired.

At this point, different surgical techniques are used to handle a variety of clinical situations. In fracture cases, technique depends on the fracture configuration. In old fractures, great care must be taken to incise scar, meticulously developing the planes described above. The axillary nerve must carefully be identified and freed from scar. The patient is not paralyzed, and electrocautery is used for the dissection. Nerve stimulation from the cautery warns the surgeon of the nerve's proximity.

With acute three- and four-part fractures,[68,69,71-73] the soft-tissue attachments to the tuberosities are preserved. The biceps is followed into the glenoid, and the rotator interval is opened. The tuberosity fragments are mobilized, preserving their cuff attachments, and the humeral head is removed. Sutures placed through the bone-tendon junction of each tuberosity piece can assist the surgeon in mobilizing these fragments from each other and enveloping adhesions. Any cartilage remaining on the tuberosities is removed. The humeral shaft is prepared for a cemented humeral stem. Version for the humeral component is selected, using the forearm as a goniometer. Less version may be selected for locked posterior dislocations. Drill holes and suture or wires are placed in the shaft before cementing the stem. Cement must be used in fracture cases to afford rotational stability because the proximal fins of the prosthesis do not engage the distal humeral shaft. The humerus is cemented above the fractured shaft the appropriate amount to restore height and soft-tissue tension (Fig. 9). If little comminution is present, the bony fragments can assist in assessing this length. Preoperative measurements and intraoperative soft-tissue tension must also be considered. The tuberosity fragments are repaired to the shaft and to the stem with wire or heavy suture. Cancellous bone may have to be removed from the tuberosities to allow them to fit around the cemented humeral stem.

In surgical neck fractures that go on to nonunions,[72] the inferior part of the humeral head often undergoes significant erosion. Prosthetic hemiarthroplasty can simultaneously bridge the nonunion and replace the eroded humeral head. An attempt can be made to approach the humeral head osteotomy through the rotator interval to preserve subscapularis insertion and blood supply to the proximal fragment. The subscapularis and capsule may have to be taken down in the usual fashion if this soft-tissue sparing approach is not successful or if releases are needed to regain motion. The subscapularis insertion can be taken with bone to facilitate healing. The prosthesis skewers the proximal humerus if there is adequate bone, preserving a ring of metaphysis proximally. Otherwise a horseshoe of metaphyseal bone is fashioned to fit around the proximal stem. The humeral prosthesis is cemented in the shaft in the correct position, with the appropriate amount of tension in the deltoid to

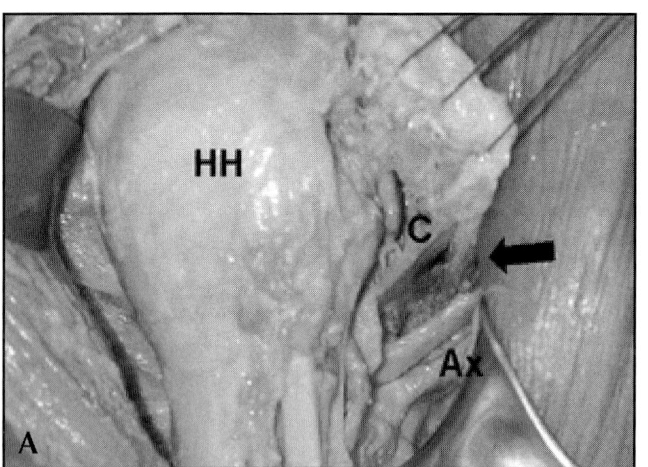

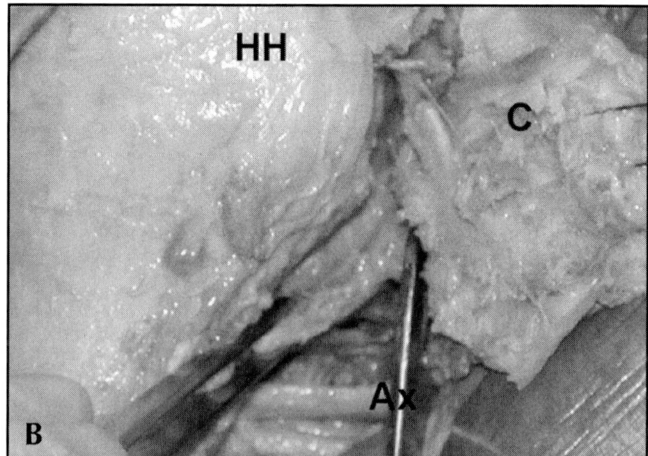

Fig. 10 A, Exposure in a cadaver after subscapularis release, just before dividing the capsule off the posterior aspect of the subscapularis. The anterior labrum can be left to deepen the socket in hemiarthroplasties. The capsule can be harvested off the subscapularis and reflected over the freshened glenoid surface for biologic resurfacing. In TSA, the anterior capsule and labrum are excised. HH = humeral head, C = capsule, Ax = axillary nerve. The arrow points to the subscapularis muscle anterior to the capsule. **B,** Cadaveric dissection showing standard anterior capsulectomy to release medial tethering effect on the subscapularis.

restore function. The nonunion site is bone grafted and can be reinforced with wire or heavy suture.

For chronic malunions of the proximal humerus, the different fragments may have collapsed on each other and coalesced into an amorphous ball. To replace the humeral head, the tuberosity fragments may have to be osteotomized off the shaft and each other. Reconstruction proceeds as in a three- or four-part fracture after the tuberosity fragments have been mobilized. Length may be considerably more difficult to judge than in the acute setting.

In inflammatory and degenerative arthritis, the circumflex vessels are ligated routinely. The subscapularis and capsule are divided together a centimeter medial and parallel to the biceps. If loss of external rotation is present preoperatively, completely freeing the subscapularis usually restores much of this motion. In cases of severe internal rotation contracture, z-lengthening of the subscapularis with a laterally based flap of capsule has been described.[23] For moderate contractures, the tendon of the subscapularis can be taken down adjacent to the bicipital groove and repaired to the humeral osteotomy site. This effectively lengthens the subscapularis, especially at its inferior aspect. We have rarely found these measures to be necessary, and in our hands the subscapularis is routinely repaired to its anatomic insertion at the end of the surgical procedure.

The capsule is stripped off the humerus past the 6 o'clock position. Medial to the biceps, inferior to the subscapularis, the soft tissue on the inframedial neck of the humerus is dissected subperiosteally. It is critical during dissection in this area to know at all times exactly where the nerve lies and to protect it. The subscapularis is freed from soft-tissue attachments in the rotator interval, at the inferiomedial base of the coracoid, and along its inferior border. The rotator interval tissue overlying the biceps as it enters the glenohumeral joint is released, effectively releasing the coracohumeral ligament.

The humeral head is dislocated, the glenoid is inspected, and a decision is made regarding the glenoid. If the glenoid is mildly involved and a biologic resurfacing is appropriate (given the patient's age and degree of glenoid involvement), the anterior capsular flap can be used to resurface it. The capsule must be harvested off the undersurface of the subscapularis to create a medially based flap. Care is taken to preserve length of the capsular flap so that it can reach the posterior and superior edges of the glenoid. The glenoid is reamed to a bleeding surface. The capsular flap is then sewn to the glenoid peripherally through the labrum and anchored centrally with suture anchors (Fig. 10).

If the glenoid is to be replaced, we proceed with our standard TSA technique. The capsule is excised from the posterior surface of the subscapularis to remove its medially tethering effect on the tendon. By pulling on the traction sutures placed along its cut edge, excursion of the subscapularis is tested. If more excursion is needed, the superior, rolled edge of the subscapularis is "recessed" with an oblique cut. This step can give an additional 7 to 10 mm excursion, in our experience. In stiff shoulders it is important to release the anterior edge of the supraspinatus from the superior base of the coracoid.

In intact proximal humerii, the canal of the humerus is found with a small, sharp hand reamer. The humerus is reamed by hand until cortical contact is obtained for noncemented humerii. If cement is used, the stem 1 to 2 mm under the diameter that was reamed is selected. The humeral cutting guide is placed on the final reamer and prongs that insert in the guide show the surgeon where 20° and 40° of retroversion fall in relation to the forearm. The forearm is used as a goniometer to select version for the cut. Metal fingers on the guide can help assess where the cut will be in relation to the cuff. The cut is made and the head fragment is used to assist in selection of prosthetic head size. The trial broach is inserted. Prostheses with a thin proximal body preserve proximal bone stock, and humeral fracture during broach insertion is less of a problem. The lateral fin of the prosthesis should fall on average 12 mm behind the biceps groove. The proximal plate of the prosthesis can be recessed into cancellous bone by using a special reamer. A trial head with variable offset is placed on the broach. Using the prosthetic head as a template, osteophytes are removed around the proximal humerus to make the bone even with the prosthesis. If the glenoid is replaced, the head must have the same radius of curvature as the glenoid component. If only the humerus is replaced, the head that is selected should match the size and the curvature of the head removed and the native glenoid.

If the glenoid is to be replaced, the trial head is removed and a Fukuda retractor is placed behind the posterior glenoid. The broach in the humerus partially protects the humerus from crushing during retraction, although some injury to the anterior metaphysis can still occur. A two-pronged retractor is placed medially on the anterior glenoid neck to hold back the subscapularis and strap muscles. Protecting the axillary nerve from damage, the inferior capsule is resected near the glenoid to facilitate further exposure. Overhanging soft tissue and labrum are resected, and any remaining cartilage on the glenoid is scraped away. These tissues are preserved in hemiarthroplasty to deepen the articulating socket for the HHR.

In OA, erosions occur posteriorly or centrally (Fig. 1). In arthritis following instability procedures, erosions occur opposite the side of the capsular reefing, if the capsule was overtightened (Fig. 4). If there is rim erosion on one side of the glenoid, a burr may be used to even the surface, prior to reaming. Care must be taken not to remove so much bone that the prosthesis cannot be inserted or supported. The glenoid size is selected from trials, choosing the biggest size that allows no overhang of the glenoid component. Reamers are used to smooth the glenoid surface. Straight reamers are preferred because these are easier to control, but adequate glenoid exposure is essential. For cemented glenoids, keel or peg fixation have been used. We prefer peg fixation in small glenoids. Prosthetic designs with anterior and posterior pegs can force the surgeon to place peg holes in thin areas, causing fracture or perforation of the rim.

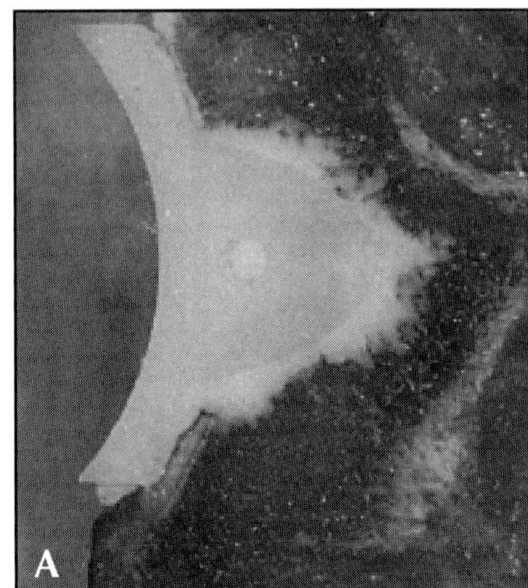

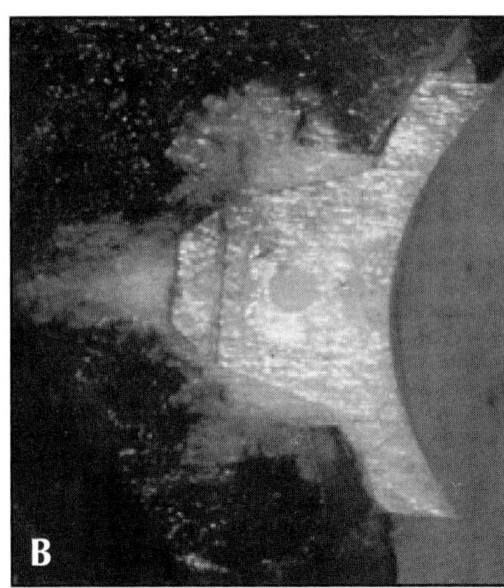

Fig. 11 Cadaveric specimen. **A,** Cut in coronal plane after cementing the glenoid with standard finger packing technique. **B,** Cut in coronal plane after cementing the glenoid with third-generation technique: serial pressurization of "wet" cement with special pressurization tools and sponges.

Trial reduction of the glenoid is performed to ensure the glenoid fits well, there is no rocking of the prosthesis against the glenoid, there is good rim coverage circumferentially, and there is no soft-tissue interposition. Third-generation cement technique is used while cementing the glenoid. The cancellous bone in the vault is prepared with pulsatile lavage, with thrombin-soaked gel foam, and finally with peroxide-soaked sponges. The cement is injected in the holes using a Tumey syringe. The cement is injected and pressurized a total of four times in rapid succession using special cement pressurizing instruments, then the prosthesis is inserted. These techniques have been shown to increase depth of penetration of cement into the bony glenoid in cadaver studies by 50% (Fig. 11). The glenoid prosthesis is held in place until the cement cures.

The proximal humerus is again exposed, and the broach is removed. The humeral canal is prepared for cementing similarly to the glenoid. A cement restrictor is placed 1 to 2 cm distal to the length of the stem. Sutures are placed through the proximal humerus prior to cementing to repair the subscapularis to bone. The humeral stem is cemented in place without excessive pressurization to avoid cement extrusion in the humerus. Care is taken to orient the stem in the appropriate position, and it is held securely in place until the cement cures. The humerus can also be inserted without cement. There is some controversy over which technique is best in the young patient.

Final trial reduction is performed. Care is taken to select a head size that allows 50% translation of the humeral head posteriorly and allows the hand to reach the opposite axilla. The top of the HHR should be superior to the greater tuberosity to avoid impingement. The neck of the proximal humerus is again inspected, and final contouring of the metaphysis is performed to create a smooth contour from neck to prosthetic head. The subscapularis is repaired anatomically with sutures through bone. Drains may be placed if needed. The deltopectoral interval is loosely approximated, and the superficial layers are closed meticulously.

Postoperative Course

Any drains are removed the first or second postoperative day. The arm is placed in a Velpeau dressing with a pillow under the elbow to protect the subscapularis repair while the interscalene block remains in effect. Starting the day after surgery, the patient is switched to a sling and is seen by a therapist twice a day. Neer Phase I exercises are begun postoperative day 1, including pendulum exercises, passive external rotation with a stick to 45°, and passive forward flexion to 140°, using a door pulley. These limits may need to be modified if the subscapularis is tight after repair or the tissue quality is poor. The patient is allowed to remove the sling for sponge bathing and exercises and is discharged from the hospital usually after 2 days. At 2 weeks additional assisted motion in all planes and isometrics are added except for resisted internal rotation and passive external rotation past 45°. At 6 weeks assisted motion in all planes is allowed and light resistive exercises are added in all planes. At 12 weeks more resistance and terminal stretching are added.

Results

Results in general from TSA are excellent. In Torchia and associates' series,[19] 113 TSA patients operated on between 1975 and 1981 were reviewed. Survivorship at 10 and 15 years was 93% and 87%, respectively. At a mean of 12.2 years' follow-up, relief of moderate or severe pain was achieved in 83%. Significant gains in motion were achieved, although gains in elevation were related to the condition of the rotator cuff.

Results in TSA can be markedly influenced by the underlying pathology. In OA early outcome data show substantial and statistically significant improvement in pain, motion, function, and general health by 6 months after surgery, and these remain stable, at least, with short-term follow-up.[17] Long-term follow-up studies are currently sparse in the literature for OA. In 1996 Wirth and Rockwood[74] surveyed the literature and found only four series with an average of more than 4 years' follow-up that included patients with OA.[74] OA in the young patient is rare, and arthritis of the glenohumeral joint in the young patient is usually secondary to trauma, prior instability repairs, ON, or inflammatory arthropathy.

Hemiarthroplasty for fractures has had less successful results. Zyto and associates[75] reviewed 27 hemiarthroplasty patients for fractures at an average of 39 months' follow-up. Most of their patients were older (median age 71 years). The median Constant score was 51 for three-part and 46 for four-part fractures. Median flexion was 70°, and 9 of the 27 patients still had moderate or severe pain. Movin and associates[76] looked at 29 patients, average age 71 years, at an average of 3 years after surgery. They also found significant persistent disability with pain, limited motion, and difficulty with activities of daily living. Goldman and associates[77] reported similar results in their series of 26 patients, average age 67 years, at 30 months' follow-up. Seventy-three percent of their population reported no or only slight pain. They concluded hemiarthroplasty was reliable for pain relief but much less predictable in restoring function, in three- and four-part proximal humerus fractures.

Bigliani[73] reviewed the literature with respect to hemiarthroplasty for proximal humerus fractures. Seventy-seven percent of 355 patients had excellent or satisfactory results. Achieving a relatively painless shoulder is reliable, with most studies reporting greater than 90% satisfactory pain relief. Return of active motion and function was more variable. Bigliani[73] reported expected forward flexion after hemiarthroplasty for proximal humerus fractures ranged from 90° to 120°. Factors cited as contributing to compromised motion and function included age, gender, motivation, fracture type, and timing of surgery. Adherence to technical details including restoration of humeral length and version, reconstruction and healing of the tuberosities, and soft-tissue tensioning are important. An extended supervised rehabilitation is also necessary in maximizing a patient's functional result. In 1994, Compito and associates[78] reported that unsatisfactory results in this type of patient were associated with tuberosity detachment, prosthetic loosening, inadequate or noncompliant rehabilitation, preoperative nerve injury, humeral malposition, dislocation, deep infection, and ectopic bone formation.

Arthritis following instability repairs is the most common cause of arthritis in patients younger than 40 years according to Brems.[30] In Samilson and Prieto's[79] series of 74 patients without prior surgery, older patients at first dislocation were at higher risk for developing arthritis. No correlation was found between the number of dislocations, the severity of initial trauma, and the presence of a Hill-Sachs lesion or a glenoid rim fracture and the development of arthritis. In surgical patients, the main risk factor for development of arthritis after instability repair is creation of an unbalanced joint, causing subluxation in the opposite direction and rim loading. Other surgical factors include failure to diagnose direction or degree of instability, inadequate or nonanatomic surgical reconstruction, prominent hardware, surgery on the wrong side of the joint, and inappropriate use of arthroscopic techniques. Arthroplasty after instability repair occurred an average of 16 years after the index procedure in Bigliani and associates' series.[29] Brems[30] reported that the average age of his patients was 38. He argued against fusion or chielectomy in these patients and for shoulder arthroplasty despite their young age, advocating glenoid replacement as well if the cartilage was destroyed. Releasing contractures and balancing the soft tissues, with particular attention to version of the components is critical. No long-term data after arthroplasty on this particular group are available.

In ON, the results of arthroplasty are often obscured by reporting results in mixed series with more common diagnoses. In 1998 Hattrup[80] gleaned 64 cases of shoulder arthroplasy for ON of the humeral head from the literature. Generally excellent results for pain relief and range of motion can be expected. Rutherford and Cofield[81] reported on 17 shoulders with 2 to 6.5 years' follow-up after shoulder arthroplasty for ON. Eleven had hemiarthroplasties and 6 had TSAs. Active abduction averaged 161° in the hemiarthroplasties and 150° in the total shoulder replacements. Differences between steroid-induced and posttraumatic ON have been reported by several authors. Tanner and Cofield[82] noted that reconstruction in the posttraumatic shoulder can be complicated by scarring, stiffness, cuff damage, nerve injury, and bony deformity. In nontraumatic causes of ON, scarring and stiffness are not present until the last stages of the disease. Hattrup[80] concluded pain relief and motion are generally excellent in ON. Results are superior in steroid-induced ON compared to posttraumatic ON.

Generally good and excellent results for shoulder arthroplasty can be expected in the patient with RA. Neer and associates[8] in a mixed series reported results in 43 patients with RA who received TSAs with a minimum of 2 years' follow-up. Twenty-eight were excellent, 12 were satisfactory, and 3 were unsatisfactory. Fourteen had rotator cuff tears that were repaired at surgery. All patients had excellent pain relief. The three failures were unable to actively elevate the arm past 90°. Cofield[13] reported on 29 arthroplasty patients with RA in a larger series of mixed diagnoses. The rotator cuff was normal in 5 and thinned in 17 patients. Pain relief was generally good or excellent. Postoperative abduction and external rotation averaged 103° and 35°, respectively. Stewert and Kelly[83] looked at 37 TSAs in patients with RA at 7 to 13 years' follow-up. Seventy-eight percent were pain free or had only slight discomfort. Abduction and external rotation postoperatively averaged 75° and 38°, respectively. In most series TSA is highly successful for pain relief in patients with RA. Significant gains in motion and function can also be obtained, even though postoperative elevation on average is 90°.[84]

Younger patients with arthroplasty may not fare as well as the older patient. Sperling and associates[66] reviewed 74 Neer hemiarthroplasties and 34 Neer TSAs in patients younger than 50 years of age with a mean of 12.3 years' follow-up. Both techniques resulted in significant long-term pain relief and significant gains in active abduction and external rotation with no statistically significant difference between the two groups. Results were graded according to a modified system of Neer and of Cofield. Thirty-five of 74 hemiarthroplasties and 17 of 34 TSAs had an unsatisfactory result according to the rating system. Caution was emphasized in offering shoulder arthroplasty to patients younger than age 50 years.[66]

Complications

TSA yields good or excellent results in over 90% of patients in midrange follow-up (< 10 years).[85] Despite these excellent results, Cofield and Edgerton[14] put the overall rate of complications in shoulder arthroplasty at 14% in their review. Complications can be related to one or more of the following: patient selection, underlying diagnoses (patient factors), surgical technique, rehabilitation, and natural history of the underlying diagnoses and shoulder arthroplasty.

Strict adherence to appropriate indications for TSA and hemiarthroplasty will limit a surgeon's postoperative complications. Replacing the glenoid in a rotator cuff deficient shoulder or performing arthroplasty in an unreliable patient with unrealistic expectations dooms the patient and the surgeon to increased complications.

Results from various diagnoses differ and were discussed above. OA most reliably fares well after TSA. RA has less reliable pain relief and restoration of function.[84] Arthroplasty for fracture[78] and for posttraumatic ON[80] typically gives the patient significant motion and pain relief but can fail to provide full active motion or function as discussed previously.

Cuomo and Checroun[85] reported instability occurs after shoulder arthroplasty in 0 to 22% of patients. Post and Pollock[23] put it at 1% to 2%. Appropriate version of the glenoid and humeral components are critical. Total combined retroversion of the glenoid and humeral components should average 35° to 45°. The largest glenoid that the bony glenoid can circumferentially support should be inserted. With a fixed radius of curvature, this will increase the wall height of the glenoid circumferentially, increasing stability.[85,86]

Anterior instability can be caused by excessive anteversion of either component, loss of subscapularis or anterior deltoid function, and excessive posterior capsular tightness.[85] Subscapularis rupture can lead to anterior instability postoperatively. Poor tendon repair, inadequate mobilization, poor tissue quality, oversized components, and inappropriate therapy can put the subscapularis at risk. Circumferential release of the subscapularis and, occasionally, lengthening are required to restore functional external rotation without placing excessive stress on the subscapularis repair.

Posterior instability typically is caused by excessive overall retroversion. Preoperative studies are obtained to assess glenoid version and posterior wear. The anterior high side can be smoothed with a burr and the glenoid reamed to lessen the glenoid retroversion.[23,87] Rarely bone grafting may be used to correct posterior deficiency[88] but severe bone loss will prevent glenoid resurfacing. Humeral retroversion can be decreased, but not too much, to avoid anterior instability. Intraoperative rotator cuff and capsular detachment can occur during the humeral osteotomy and contribute to instability. This cut should be made under direct vision. Newer humeral cutting guides are available in some systems. If these structures are detached they should be repaired to bone intraoperatively.

Placing the HHR too low in the humerus effectively lengthens the deltoid and leads to inferior instability.[23,85] The top of the head should rise about 5 mm above the tuberosity to avoid postoperative impingement. In cases with proximal bone loss the prosthesis may have to be cemented superior to the shaft fracture. Inferior instability can also be caused by axillary nerve palsy. Superior instability results from cuff dysfunction and overpull of the deltoid. Small rotator cuff tears should be repaired at the time of surgery. If the rotator cuff is likely not to center the head in the glenoid, the glenoid should not be replaced.[64] After releases and placement of components, the HHR should subluxate 50% on the glenoid, and the subscapularis should come to the humerus easily. Ideally the shoulder should externally rotate to 40° without excess tension on the subscapularis after repair. Treating the deltoid and rotator cuff with care, repairing the subscapularis securely, and taking care with soft-tissue balancing and version are critical in avoiding postoperative instability.

Postoperative rotator cuff tears occur from 1% to 13% of TSAs.[85] Degenerative changes in the cuff can progress years after arthroplasty. Progressive superior migration of the head may occur[23] as the deltoid overpowers the dysfunctional rotator cuff. Pain and dysfunction may result. Reoperation to repair a rotator cuff tear is best accomplished in acute traumatic tears with a sudden loss of function.

Nerve injury after shoulder arthroplasty rarely is reported.[23,85] Most represent traction neurapraxias and can be treated expectantly.[89] Lynch and associates[89] reported on 18 neurologic deficits after arthroplasty; 11 good and 5 fair recoveries were reported at 1 year. Traction on the brachial plexus in adduction, exernal rotation, and extension was postulated as the mechanism of injury. Careful attention to protecting the nerves and supporting the elbow during humeral preparation to take tension off the plexus is recommended. Nerves can be damaged by extruded cement. Care must be taken to avoid cortical perforations. Blunt-tipped humeral reamers are available to minimize these perforations. Excessive cement pressurization in fragile, osteoporotic bone can cause fractures and cement extrusion. Nerves can be damaged by crush or stretch from retractors. Care must be taken in placing and holding retractors to avoid crushing or stretching nerves. Serial electromyogram/nerve conduction studies can document nerve recovery. Failure of a dense, isolated peripheral nerve palsy to show improvement after 3 months may be reason to explore the nerve.

Infection is reported to occur in from 0.3% to 0.5%.[14,23] It is higher in immunocompromised patients and in patients who have had previous surgeries on the shoulder. Remote sites of potential bacteremia (teeth, bladder) need to be evaluated and treated preoperatively to minimize postoperative risk of infection. Routine preoperative antibiotics are given. Postoperative prophylactic antibiotics are given as recommended by the American Heart Association before dental, urologic and other procedures likely to cause transient bacteremia.[16] Any signs of infection postoperatively must be evaluated aggressively.

Intraoperative fractures are uncommon but do occur, especially in fragile osteoporotic or rheumatoid bone.[23] Humeral fractures during dislocation can be avoided by complete soft-tissue releases and gentle dislocation with adduction and external rotation. In end-stage ON or a locked posterior dislocation, the humeral head can hang up on the posterior glenoid rim and make dislocation particularly difficult (Fig. 8, *B*). Translating the head away from the glenoid to disengage the humeral head from the posterior rim before external rotation can ease dislocation.[85] Humeral fractures also can occur during broach or prosthesis insertion if the lateral fin contacts cortical bone, and the proximal body of the component is a large wedge. Thinner proximal body humeral components are available. Removing cortical bone behind the lateral fin with a thin rongeur before seating the broach is recommended.[85] In very weak bone it is recommended to avoid excessive pressurization, which can fracture the humerus.

On the glenoid side eccentric drilling can cause perforation of cortical bone on the scapular neck. It can be difficult determining the center of the glenoid. In OA, osteophytes typically occur posteriorly and inferiorly, which can lead the surgeon to placing the center hole too low and too posterior. Preoperative imaging studies and palpating the scapular neck intraoperatively can help the surgeon orient on the glenoid. A provisional shallow centering hole can be placed for reaming. This hole can be deepened after reaming, once the surgeon is satisfied the centering hole is appropriate. Perforations should be bone grafted or dammed prior to cementing. Glenoid fractures can occur during broaching or placement of a keeled prosthesis if the glenoid is small and the slot is narrow or not properly excavated. We use a pegged glenoid in small bony glenoids and use a keeled component in larger glenoids.

Humeral prostheses can be fixed with cement or press fit. Several authors assert uncemented humerii do as well as cemented stems. Advocates cite bone preservation and ease of surgery as reasons for using uncemented techniques. In the series by Sperling and associates[66] looking at shoulder arthroplasties in patients younger than age 50 years with an average follow-up of 12.3 years, radiolucent lines were present around the humeral prosthesis in 24% of the hemiarthroplasties and 53% of the TSAs. If humeral loosening occurred, which was rare before 10 years, it occurred in uncemented humerii.[66] Torchia and associates[19] reported humeral components shifted position in 49% of their press-fit components and in none of the cemented stems. Humeral component loosening was not associated with pain. It is unclear whether noncemented techniques result in bone preservation during later humeral revisions in the young patient, as asserted by proponents of this technique.

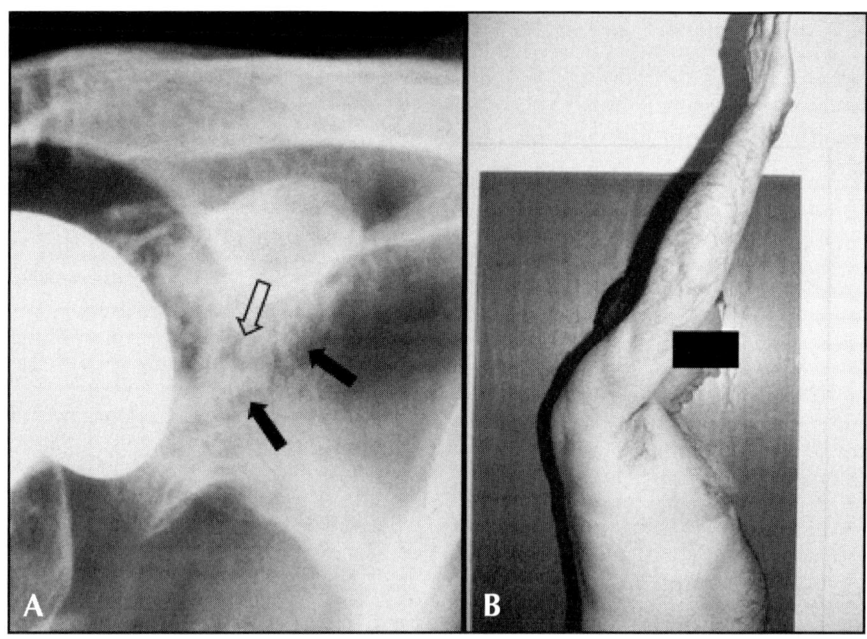

Fig. 12 Nineteen-year follow-up with evidence on left of glenoid loosening. **A,** Solid arrows point out wide radiolucent line at the bone-cement interface. The hollow arrow points to the prosthesis-cement interface. **B,** Patient has good function. He does not desire revision for current level of symptoms.

Glenoid loosening is the main problem with long-term survivorship in TSA, particularly in the young patient. A radiolucent line around the glenoid component was seen in 59% of the TSAs in Sperling and Cofield's series.[25] Erosion of the glenoid was present in 68% of the hemiarthroplasties. Torchia and associates[19] reported definite glenoid loosening was present in 44% of their patients, and glenoid loosening was associated with pain. In our experience, however, the ache associated with loosening is often not enough, in the patient's opinion, to warrant a revision surgery (Fig. 12).

Survivorship analysis for shoulder arthroplasty was conducted by Sperling and associates[66] in patients younger than age 50 years. Estimated survival of the hemiarthroplasties was 92% at 5 years, 83% at 10 years, and 73% at 15 years. Risk of revision was higher for hemiarthroplasties performed after trauma than for RA. Estimated survival for TSA was 97% at 5 and at 10 years, and 84% at 15 years. The risk of revision for TSA increased if a rotator cuff tear was present at the time of the surgery.[66]

Complications in shoulder arthroplasty may be minimized by appropriate patient selection; a thorough understanding of the anatomy, biomechanics, and underlying complications of particular disease states; meticulous attention to soft-tissue balancing, bony preparation, and component placement; and adherence to an appropriate, surgeon-directed rehabilitation program.

Discussion

In the young patient with glenohumeral arthritis, shoulder arthroplasty can generally result in excellent pain relief and significant gains in active motion. Care must be taken to exhaust measures short of arthroplasty in the young, active patient with a long life expectancy, given the finite survivorship of prosthetic components in patients younger than 50 years of age.

Careful preoperative studies help select and plan the appropriate procedure. History, physical examination, radiographic studies, and diagnostic injections can isolate the pain generators about the shoulder, including or excluding the acromioclavicular joint, subacromial bursa, glenohumeral joint, and sites outside the shoulder such as the cervical spine.

Nonsurgical means must be fully used to restore comfort and function, including activity modification; stretching and strengthening; ice, heat, and other physical modalities; pharmaceutical agents; and judicious use of steroid injections. Smaller procedures, such as débridement arthroscopy, subacromial decompression, distal clavicle resection, rotator cuff repair, and capsular releases may play a role, depending on the clinical setting.

Knowing the condition of the rotator cuff, deltoid, and neurovascular status about the shoulder is vital in planning shoulder arthroplasty. If any doubt exists, appropriate preoperative studies such as MRI or electromyography are ordered. We avoid glenoid replacement in the young patient, favoring biologic resurfacing in moderately involved glenoids. Glenoids are not replaced in patients with previous infections, nonfunctioning deltoids or rotator cuffs, tight shoulders despite releases, or in patients in whom it is known that there will be noncompliance with postoperative restrictions.

Results of shoulder arthroplasty are significantly influenced by the underlying pathogenesis, degree of arthrosis, and any concomitant comorbidities (like rotator cuff tears). Patients with OA typically fare very well with pain relief and restoration of function, although pure OA requiring shoulder arthroplasty in patients younger than age 40 years is very rare. Arthoplasty after fractures reliably relieves pain and results in significant gains of motion, but restoration of function and full active motion is less predictable. In ON, results are typically excellent in steroid-induced and other nontraumatic causes of ON. Prosthetic replacement of traumatic ON can be technically more difficult and results are not as good as in the atraumatic setting. In RA longevity of prostheses is statistically better than in the posttraumatic setting. Pain relief is excellent but restoration of function depends to a large degree on the condition of the rotator cuff.

Shoulder arthroplasty has a unique set of foibles in the young patient. Subtle nuances in pathogenesis (such as arthritis of dislocation) and unique clinical considerations (such as return to the work force and patient longevity) are seen that are not encountered in the older patient. Prosthetic survivorship is much more an issue in the young. Limitations of current techniques influence surgical decisions (such as whether to replace the glenoid or offer biologic resurfacing). Understanding the unique pathogenesis, surgical alternatives, technical considerations, and clinical results with arthroplasty in the young patient can help the shoulder surgeon choose wisely in offering surgical solutions to his young patients with glenohumeral arthritis.

References

1. Neer CS, Brown TH Jr, McLaughlin HL: Fracture of the neck of the humerus with dislocation of the head fragment. *Am J Surg* 1953;85:252-258.
2. Neer CS II: Articular replacement for the humeral head. *J Bone Joint Surg Am* 1955;37:215-228.
3. Neer CS II: Indications for replacement of the proximal humeral articulation. *Am J Surg* 1955;89:901-907.
4. Neer CS II: Replacement arthroplasty for glenohumeral osteoarthritis. *J Bone Joint Surg Am* 1974;56:1-13.
5. Post M, Jablon M, Miller H, Singh M: Constrained total shoulder joint replacement: A critical review. *Clin Orthop* 1979;144:135-150.
6. Hughes M, Neer CS II: Glenohumeral joint replacement and postoperative rehabilitation. *Phys Ther* 1975;55:850-858.
7. Paradis DK, Ferlic DC: Shoulder arthroplasty in rheumatoid arthritis. *Phys Ther* 1975;55:157-159.
8. Neer CS II, Watson KC, Stanton FJ: Recent experience in total shoulder replacement. *J Bone Joint Surg Am* 1982;64:319-337.
9. Neer CS II, Kirby RM: Revision of humeral head and total shoulder arthroplasties. *Clin Orthop* 1982;170:189-195.
10. Neer CS II: Unconstrained shoulder arthroplasty. *Instr Course Lect* 1985;34:278-286.
11. Figgie HE III, Inglis AE, Goldberg VM, Ranawat CS, Figgie MP, Wile JM: An analysis of factors affecting the long-term results of total shoulder arthroplasty in inflammatory arthritis. *J Arthroplasty* 1988;3:123-130.
12. Post M, Jablon M: Constrained total shoulder arthroplasty: Long-term follow-up observations. *Clin Orthop* 1983;173:109-116.
13. Cofield RH: Total shoulder arthroplasty with the Neer prosthesis. *J Bone Joint Surg Am* 1984;66:899-906.
14. Cofield RH, Edgerton BC: Total shoulder arthroplasty: Complications and revision surgery. *Instr Course Lect* 1990;39:449-462.
15. Fenlin JM Jr, Ramsey ML, Allardyce TJ, Frieman BG: Modular total shoulder replacement: Design rationale, indications, and results. *Clin Orthop* 1994;307:37-46.
16. Wirth MA, Rockwood CA Jr: Complications of shoulder arthroplasty. *Clin Orthop* 1994;307:47-69.
17. Matsen FA III: Early effectiveness of shoulder arthroplasty for patients who have primary glenohumeral degenerative joint disease. *J Bone Joint Surg Am* 1996;78:260-264.
18. Cofield RH: Uncemented total shoulder arthroplasty: A review. *Clin Orthop* 1994;307:86-93.
19. Torchia ME, Cofield RH, Settergren CR: Total shoulder arthroplasty with the Neer prosthesis: Long-term results. *J Shoulder Elbow Surg* 1997;6:495-505.
20. Neer CS II (ed): *Shoulder Reconstruction.* Philadelphia, PA, WB Saunders, 1990.
21. Friedman RJ (ed): Total shoulder arthroplasty. *Orthop Clin North Am* 1998;29.
22. Matsen FA III, Rockwood CA Jr, Wirth MA, Lippitt SB: Glenohumeral arthritis and its management, in Rockwood CA Jr, Matsen FA III, Wirth MA, Harryman DT II (eds): *The Shoulder*, ed 2. Philadelphia, PA, WB Saunders, 1998, vol 2, pp 840-964.
23. Post M, Pollock RG: Operative treatment of degenerative and arthritic diseases of the glenohumeral joint, in Post M, Flatow EL, Bigliani

LU, Pollock RG (eds): *The Shoulder: Operative Technique*. Baltimore, MD, Williams & Wilkins, 1998, pp 73-131.

24. Skedros JG, O'Rourke PJ, Zimmerman JM, Burkhead WZ Jr: Alternatives to replacement arthroplasty for glenohumeral arthritis, in Iannotti JP, Williams GR Jr (eds): *Disorders of the Shoulder: Diagnosis and Management*. Philadelphia, PA, Lippincott-Williams & Wilkins, 1999, pp 485-499.
25. Sperling JW, Cofield RH: Revision total shoulder arthroplasty for the treatment of glenoid arthrosis. *J Bone Joint Surg Am* 1998;80:860-867.
26. Barrett WP, Thornhill TS, Thomas WH, Gebhart EM, Sledge CB: Nonconstrained total shoulder arthroplasty in patients with polyarticular rheumatoid arthritis. *J Arthroplasty* 1989;4:91-96.
27. Hattrup SJ, Cofield RH: Osteonecrosis of the humeral head: Relationship of disease stage, extent, and cause to natural history. *J Shoulder Elbow Surg* 1999;8:559-564.
28. Cruess RL: Experience with steroid-induced avascular necrosis of the shoulder and etiologic considerations regarding osteonecrosis of the hip. *Clin Orthop* 1978;130:86-93.
29. Bigliani LU, Weinstein DM, Glasgow MT, Pollock RG, Flatow EL: Glenohumeral arthroplasty for arthritis after instability surgery. *J Shoulder Elbow Surg* 1995;4:87-94.
30. Brems JJ: Arthritis of dislocation. *Orthop Clin North Am* 1998;29:453-466.
31. Hurley JA, Anderson TE, Dear W, Andrish JT, Bergfeld JA, Weiker GG: Posterior shoulder instability: Surgical versus conservative results with evaluation of glenoid version. *Am J Sports Med* 1992;20:396-400.
32. Lehmann JF, Warren CG, Scham SM: Therapeutic heat and cold. *Clin Orthop* 1974;99:207-245.
33. Neer CS II: Impingement lesions. *Clin Orthop* 1983;173:70-77.
34. Rowe CR: Injection technique for the shoulder and elbow. *Orthop Clin North Am* 1988;19:773-777.
35. Kerlan RK, Glousman RE: Injections and techniques in athletic medicine. *Clin Sports Med* 1989;8:541-560.
36. Hollingworth GR, Ellis RM, Hattersley TS: Comparison of injection techniques for shoulder pain: Results of a double blind, randomised study. *Br Med J* 1983;287:1339-1341.
37. Blair B, Rokito AS, Cuomo F, Jarolem K, Zuckerman JD: Efficacy of injections of corticosteroids for subacromial impingement syndrome. *J Bone Joint Surg Am* 1996;78: 1685-1689.
38. Dieppe P: Drug treatment of osteoarthritis. *J Bone Joint Surg Br* 1993;75:673-674.
39. Jackson RW: Arthroscopic surgery. *J Bone Joint Surg Am* 1983;65:416-420.
40. Ellman H, Harris E, Kay SP: Early degenerative joint disease simulating impingement syndrome: Arthroscopic findings. *Arthroscopy* 1992;8:482-487.
41. Ellman H: Shoulder arthroscopy: Current indications and techniques. *Orthopedics* 1988;11:45-51.
42. Ogilvie-Harris DJ, Wiley AM: Arthroscopic surgery of the shoulder: A general appraisal. *J Bone Joint Surg Br* 1986;68:201-207.
43. Johnson LL: Arthroscopic abrasion arthroplasty historical and pathologic perspective: Present status. *Arthroscopy* 1986;2:54-69.
44. Hayes JM: Arthroscopic treatment of steroid-induced osteonecrosis of the humeral head. *Arthroscopy* 1989;5:218-221.
45. Weinstein DM, Bucchieri JS, Pollock RG, Flatow EL, Bigliani LU: Abstract: Arthroscopic debridement of the shoulder for osteoarthritis. *Arthroscopy* 1993;9:366.
46. Simpson NS, Kelly IG: Extra-glenohumeral joint shoulder surgery in rheumatoid arthritis: The role of bursectomy, acromioplasty, and distal clavicle excision. *J Shoulder Elbow Surg* 1994;3:66-69.
47. Ellowitz AS, Rosas R, Rodosky MW, Buss DD: Abstract: The benefit of arthroscopic subacromial decompression for impingement in patients found to have unsuspected glenohumeral osteoarthritis. *64th Annual Meeting Proceedings*. Rosemont, IL American Academy of Orthopaedic Surgeons, 1997, p 206.
48. Hawkins RJ, Angelo RL: Glenohumeral osteoarthrosis: A late complication of the Putti-Platt repair. *J Bone Joint Surg Am* 1990;72:1193-1197.
49. Caspari: Shoulder arthroscopy: A review of the current state of the art. *Contemp Orthop* 1982;4:523-530.
50. Pollock RG: Prosthetic replacement in rotator cuff-deficient shoulders. *J Shoulder Elbow Surg* 1992;1:173-186.
51. Flatow EL: Prosthetic replacement in the rotator cuff deficient shoulder in, Vastamäki M, Jalovaara P (eds): *Surgery of the Shoulder*. Amsterdam, The Netherlands, Elsevier, 1995, pp 335-345.
52. Codd TP, Pollock RG, Flatow EL: Prosthetic replacement in the rotator cuff-deficient shoulder. *Tech Orthop* 1993;8:174-183.
53. Benjamin A: Double osteotomy of the shoulder. *Scand J Rheumatol* 1974;3:65.
54. Benjamin A, Hirschowitz D, Arden GP: The treatment of arthritis of the shoulder joint by double osteotomy. *Int Orthop* 1979;3:211-216.
55. Kronberg M, Brostrom LA: Rotation osteotomy of the proximal humerus to stabilise the shoulder: Five years' experience. *J Bone Joint Surg Br* 1995;77:924-927.
56. Hawkins RH: Glenoid osteotomy for recurrent posterior subluxation of the shoulder: Assessment by computed axial tomography. *J Shoulder Elbow Surg* 1996;5:393-400.
57. Johnston GH, Hawkins RJ, Haddad R, Fowler PJ: A complication of posterior glenoid osteotomy for recurrent posterior shoulder instability. *Clin Orthop* 1984;187:147-149.
58. Wirth MA, Lyons FR, Rockwood CA Jr: Hypoplasia of the glenoid: A review of sixteen patients. *J Bone Joint Surg Am* 1993;75:1175-1184.
59. Gonzalez-Diaz R, Rodriguez-Merchan EC, Gilbert MS: The role of shoulder fusion in the era of arthroplasty. *Int Orthop* 1997;21:204-209.
60. Burkhead WZ Jr, Hutton KS: Biologic resurfacing of the glenoid with hemiarthroplasty of the shoulder. *J Shoulder Elbow Surg* 1995;4:263-270.
61. Levine WN, Djurasovic M, Glasson JM, Pollock RG, Flatow EL, Bigliani LU: Hemiarthroplasty for glenohumeral osteoarthritis: Results correlated to degree of glenoid wear. *J Shoulder Elbow Surg* 1997;6:449-454.
62. Rodosky MW, Bigliani LU: Indications for glenoid resurfacing in shoulder arthroplasty. *J Shoulder Elbow Surg* 1996;5:231-248.
63. Smith KL, Matsen FA III: Total shoulder arthroplasty versus hemiarthroplasty: Current trends. *Orthop Clin North Am* 1998;29:491-506.
64. Franklin JL, Barrett WP, Jackins SE, Matsen FA III: Glenoid loosening in total shoulder arthroplasty: Association with rotator cuff deficiency. *J Arthroplasty* 1988;3:39-46.
65. Hatzis N, Kaar TK, Wirth MA, Toro F, Rockwood CA Jr: Neuropathic arthropathy of the shoulder. *J Bone Joint Surg Am* 1998;80:1314-1319.
66. Sperling JW, Cofield RH, Rowland CM: Neer hemiarthroplasty and Neer total shoulder arthroplasty in patients fifty years old or less: Long-term results. *J Bone Joint Surg Am* 1998;80:464-473.
67. Hawkins RJ, Greis PE, Bonutti PM: Treatment of symptomatic glenoid loosening following unconstrained shoulder arthroplasty. *Orthopedics* 1999;22:229-234.
68. Fischer RA, Nicholson GP, McIlveen SJ, McCann PD, Flatow EL, Bigliani LU: Primary humeral head replacement for severely displaced proximal humerus fractures. *Orthop Trans* 1993;16:779.
69. Levine WN, Connor PM, Yamaguchi K, et al: Humeral head replacement for proximal humeral fractures. *Orthopedics* 1998;21:68-73.
70. Flatow EL, Bigliani LU: Tips of the trade: Locating and protecting the axillary nerve in shoulder surgery: The tug test. *Orthop Rev* 1992;21:503-505.
71. Connor PM, Flatow EL: Complications of internal fixation of proximal humeral fractures. *Instr Course Lect* 1997;46:25-37.
72. Duralde XA, Flatow EL, Pollock RG, Nicholson GP, Self EB, Bigliani LU: Operative treatment of nonunions of the surgical neck of the humerus. *J Shoulder Elbow Surg* 1996;5:169-180.

73. Bigliani LU: Proximal humerus fractures, in Post M, Flatow EL, Bigliani LU, Pollock RG (eds): *The Shoulder: Operative Technique.* Baltimore, MD, Williams & Wilkins, 1998, pp 43-71.

74. Wirth MA, Rockwood CA Jr: Complications of total shoulder-replacement arthroplasty. *J Bone Joint Surg Am* 1996;78:603-616.

75. Zyto K, Wallace WA, Frostick SP, Preston BJ: Outcome after hemiarthroplasty for three- and four-part fractures of the proximal humerus. *J Shoulder Elbow Surg* 1998;7:85-89.

76. Movin T, Sjoden GO, Ahrengart L: Poor function after shoulder replacement in fracture patients: A retrospective evaluation of 29 patients followed for 2-12 years. *Acta Orthop Scand* 1998;69:392-396.

77. Goldman RT, Koval KJ, Cuomo F, Gallagher MA, Zuckerman JD: Functional outcome after humeral head replacement for acute three- and four-part proximal humeral fractures. *J Shoulder Elbow Surg* 1995;4:81-86.

78. Compito CA, Self EB, Bigliani LU: Arthroplasty and acute shoulder trauma: Reasons for success and failure. *Clin Orthop* 1994;307:27-36.

79. Samilson RL, Prieto V: Dislocation arthropathy of the shoulder. *J Bone Joint Surg Am* 1983;65:456-460.

80. Hattrup SJ: Indications, technique, and results of shoulder arthroplasty in osteonecrosis. *Orthop Clin North Am* 1998;29:445-451.

81. Rutherford CS, Cofield RH: Osteonecrosis of the shoulder. *Orthop Trans* 1987;11:239.

82. Tanner MW, Cofield RH: Prosthetic arthroplasty for fractures and fracture-dislocations of the proximal humerus. *Clin Orthop* 1983;179:116-128.

83. Stewart MP, Kelly IG: Total shoulder replacement in rheumatoid disease: 7- to 13-year follow-up of 37 joints. *J Bone Joint Surg Br* 1997;79:68-72.

84. Waldman BJ, Figgie MP: Indications, technique, and results of total shoulder arthroplasty in rheumatoid arthritis. *Orthop Clin North Am* 1998;29:435-444.

85. Cuomo F, Checroun A: Avoiding pitfalls and complications in total shoulder arthroplasty. *Orthop Clin North Am* 1998;29:507-518.

86. Iannotti JP, Williams GR: Total shoulder arthroplasty: Factors influencing prosthetic design. *Orthop Clin North Am* 1998;29:377-391.

87. Ibarra C, Dines DM, McLaughlin JA: Glenoid replacement in total shoulder arthroplasty. *Orthop Clin North Am* 1998;29:403-413.

88. Neer CS II, Morrison DS: Glenoid bone-grafting in total shoulder arthroplasty. *J Bone Joint Surg Am* 1988;70:1154-1162.

89. Lynch NM, Cofield RH, Silbert PL, Hermann RC: Neurologic complications after total shoulder arthroplasty. *J Shoulder Elbow Surg* 1996;5:53-61.

Reference to Video

Flatow E, Yassamin H: Intraoperative video. New York, NY, Mt. Sinai Hospital, 2000.

Complications of Shoulder Arthroplasty: Infections, Instability, and Loosening

John J. Brems, MD

Introduction

The number of total shoulder replacements has increased significantly in the past decade: in the early 1990s, fewer than 10,000 shoulder arthroplasties were performed annually; in 1999, nearly 17,500 patients underwent either a humeral head replacement alone or a total shoulder replacement including humeral and glenoid components (unpublished data, 1999). The pain relief and improvements in patient function and activities of daily living resulting from successful shoulder arthroplasties paralleled, if not exceeded, those achieved with joint replacements of both hip and knee. In addition, the duration of implant survival is very good. Torchia and associates[1] reviewed 113 shoulder arthroplasties in long-term follow-up and found that Kaplan-Meier analysis yielded a probability of implant survival of 93% at 10 years and 87% at 15 years.

The potential complications associated with lower extremity joint replacement, including joint infection, joint instability, and component loosening also exist for shoulder replacement. The complications and their incidence rates are remarkably similar. Only because many fewer shoulders are replaced than hips and knees is the total number of complications lower.

Joint Infection

The shoulder joint enjoys a rich blood supply because of its proximity to the heart and because atherosclerotic vessel disease is uncommon in the subclavian and axillary arteries. With the abundant muscle enveloping a "deep" joint, infection after shoulder arthroplasty remains rare. However, when infection does develop, the consequences can be severe.

Infection of joint arthroplasty is either an acute, perioperative (intraoperative) event or a late event associated with hematologic or lymphatic contamination. The diagnosis, biology, bacterial agents, and treatment are usually very different for each, although both acute and late infections demand immediate attention to maximize chances for a functional limb after successful treatment. Because the soft-tissue sleeve is so much at risk of destruction with any inflammatory condition about the shoulder, an immediate and accurate diagnosis combined with definitive treatment is mandatory.

In anticipation of joint replacement surgery, preoperative assessment of risk factors for infection should be considered. Diabetes, malnutrition, systemic steroids, immunosuppressive agents, chemotherapy, and radiation are factors known to be associated with increased risk of infection.[2] Each must be addressed to minimize its impact on potential infection. Ensuring proper insulin-administration regimens to achieve steady-state blood glucose levels, maintaining proper caloric intake and establishing the proper nitrogen balance in nutrition, and ensuring the judicious use of systemic steroids may diminish the inherent risks of infection.

Acute Infection

Clinical Presentation Although the use of laminar flow operating suites and the judicious use of perioperative intravenous antibiotics have diminished the risk of this complication, the incidence of acute postoperative infection associated with shoulder arthroplasty is approximately 0.5%.[3-5] An infection is generally considered to be acute when it occurs within 4 to 6 weeks of the surgical procedure. Most infections that occur from intraoperative inoculation become clinically apparent within 3 to 12 days. Although the more virulent gram-negative organisms may not become clinically apparent as rapidly as the much more common gram-positive organisms, gram-negative bacteria can destroy much more soft tissue before a diagnosis is made.

Increasing pain is often the first symptom of an infectious process because most patients who undergo shoulder arthroplasty note significant improvement in their pain immediately after surgery. There are few other early clues. Radiographic studies, unless they show gas, offer little in establishing a diagnosis. With increasing incisional erythema, localized edema, and wound drainage, the diagnosis is not challenging, but more often than not, there are no local signs of sepsis, and laboratory analysis is of limited value in the acute postoperative period because acute-phase reactants have been elevated by the surgery itself. The clinical suspicion should mandate an aspiration for culture. The presence of drainage is sometimes considered to be a synovial leak through an incompetent cuff, but any presence of drainage should be considered an infection and an indication for immediate surgical exploration. Persistent wound drainage after 48 hours from the procedure demands extreme vigilance and concern for an infectious process.

Treatment Despite the few reports[6] of treating acute septic joint arthroplasties with intravenous antibiotics alone, most surgeons recommend open joint irrigation and débridement at the very least. With any evidence of chronicity, even by a few days, removal of prosthetic devices should be considered mandatory. Concomitant placement of an antibiotic-impregnated cement spacer is an option in an acute infection.[5] At the time of débridement, an attempt should be made to reapproximate cuff tendons to their physiologic length using monofilament sutures. Some surgeons recommend primary prosthetic exchange in acute gram-positive infections, but the more conservative approach is to perform a two-stage reimplantation after 6 weeks of appropriate intravenous antibiotics.[3,7-9]

Before reimplantation, laboratory analysis of erythrocyte sedimentation rate, C-reactive protein level, and other acute-phase reactants should approach baseline level or at least show a dramatic change toward that direction. If the rotator cuff tissue has been significantly destroyed and digested as a result of the infectious process, resection arthroplasty is likely the better choice, with subsequent reconstruction considerations to be made later when the infection is well controlled. I treat all infections after shoulder arthroplasty with removal of the components and cement interfaces, combined with implantation of a tobramycin-impregnated polymethylmethacrylate spacer for 6 weeks. At the time of spacer retrieval, consideration is given to prosthetic reimplantation only when there is a functional myofascial sleeve construct of the deltoid muscle and rotator cuff.

Chronic (Late) Infection

Clinical Presentation Late infections, those occurring many weeks to years after the joint replacement, are thought to be spread by the hematogenous or lymphatic routes. The usual portals of entry for these types of infections are associated with the oropharyngeal tract, the genitourinary tract, the gastrointestinal tract, and skin breaks. Pathogens that normally populate these biologic tissues presumably travel to the shoulder joint via direct blood and lymph pathways. The pharynx can contribute both gram-positive and gram-negative organisms, including aerobes and anaerobes. Oral tooth decay is not an uncommon source of gram-negative sepsis. Coliform bacteria populate the gastrointestinal and genitourinary tracts and can be spread by hematogenous routes. The skin harbors both *Staphylococcus epidermidis* and the more virulent *Staphylococcus aureus*. When hematogenous spread from some remote location is suspected, identification of the primary source must be undertaken as part of the evaluation and treatment of the shoulder infection.

Similar to acute infections, the most common symptom in a patient with a late infection is increasing pain, even when the arm is at rest. Joint motion and general use of the arm become increasingly painful. Night pain, described often as toothache-like, becomes typical. The shoulder displays more characteristic features of infection with increasing erythema, swelling, and warmth. Patients often have a low-grade fewer and will occasionally be frankly febrile, depending on the primary source of infection and the degree of joint involvement. The patient may have associated symptoms of pharyngitis or urinary tract infection or exhibit an identifiable skin lesion. Gastrointestinal sources of infection are more subtle and may require more sophisticated investigation.

Laboratory analysis in late infections is more classic, with elevations in white blood cell lines, including neutrophils and lymphocytes. Erythrocyte sedimentation rates are significantly elevated; C-reactive protein, fibrinogen, and glycoprotein levels also are increased. Urinalysis may show white cell casts and other chemical abnormalities, depending on the nature of the infectious agent.

Radiographic Findings Unlike acute infections, for which radiographs rarely offer insight, radiography in a patient with a late or chronic infection may be valuable. Except in the most severe of infections with gas-producing organisms, gas is rarely seen in shoulder infections. Rather, there is characteristic osteopenia of the humerus and glenoid. Bone cement interfaces may be widened, suggesting clear radiographic component loosening. The subacromial-humeral distance and glenohumeral distance often are subtly increased as a result of either fluid in the joint or soft-tissue edema of the cuff muscles. Long-standing low-grade infections may demonstrate frank erosions of the periarticular bone of the humerus and glenoid, similar to that seen in rheumatoid arthritis. Recently developed MRI scanning with pulse sequences that allow soft-tissue interpretation in the presence of the metal prosthesis may in time provide a more accurate diagnosis in patients with a painful prosthetic joint (J Sperling, MD, P Hollis, MD, E Craig, MD, Austin, TX, unpublished data, 2000).

Treatment Options The consensus concerning the management of late, deep infections after shoulder arthroplasty is that the prosthesis and all cement must be removed,[3,8] combined with radical soft-tissue débridement, drainage, and the use of long-term intravenous and oral antibiotics. Although empiric, 6 weeks of intravenous antibiotics followed by up to 3 months of oral antibiotics is considered standard. With such a complex array of antibiotics available, the expertise of an infectious diseases specialist should be relied on in the treatment of joint infections after arthroplasty.

Although a two-stage reimplantation would be the ideal, the soft-tissue sleeve usually is so severely deficient that even with reimplantation after the appropriate period of antibiotics, functional use is minimal, and continued low-level pain seems to be typical. By comparison, in the five patients I have treated with resection arthroplasty, pain relief has been very predictable, with only one patient requiring occasional narcotics. The degree of functional recovery after resection arthroplasty depends largely on patient personality and motiva-tion. Four of my five patients have active elevation against gravity of more than 140° and can effortlessly reach into an overhead kitchen cabinet. Resection arthroplasty followed by a well-structured, supine, eccentric deltoid muscle–strengthening program can result in a remarkably functional, minimally painful limb and can be considered the treatment of choice for late shoulder joint infections with significant soft-tissue (rotator cuff) loss. Attempting to reimplant a prosthesis in the face of a scarred bed without definable cuff tissue is a most challeng-ing exercise. Even when not evident on radiographs, abundant scar tissue, capsular contractures, and unrecognizable tissue planes will result in a painful, stiff limb that is severely functionally compromised. Some authors have reported successful reimplantation, but success depends on a functional myofascial sleeve.[4,7,10]

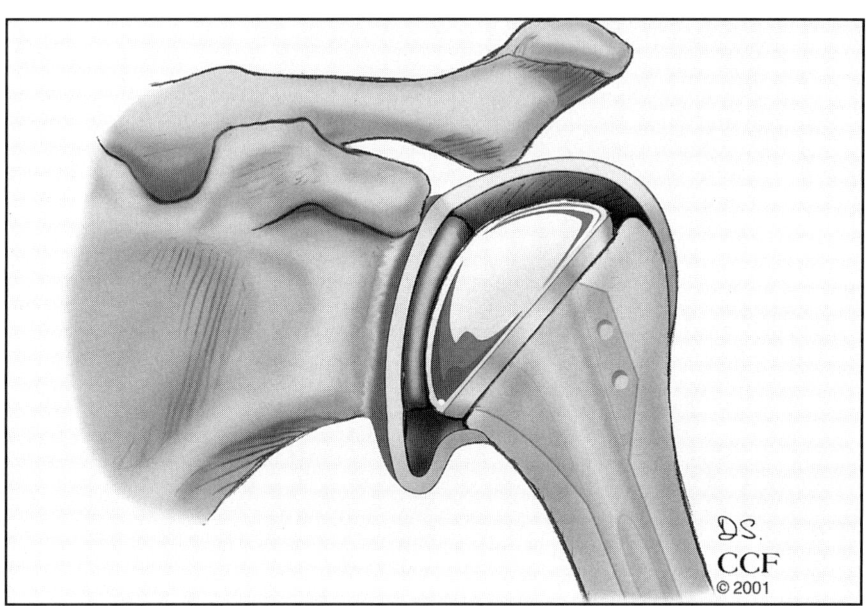

Fig. 1 The lateral offset (distance between the coracoid base and the humerus) must be respected and established at the time of joint replacement (©2001 Cleveland Clinic Foundation).

Joint Instability

In 1998, Cuomo and Checroun[11] reported that joint instability after arthroplasty represented 38% of all total shoulder replacement complications, with a frequency of occurrence ranging from 0 to 22%.[2,11,12] Determination of joint stability is a dynamic process that relies largely on surgeon experience. Precise soft-tissue balancing and proper prosthetic positioning are critical to restore both rotational and translational components of normal shoulder kinematics.[2,4,12-15] Neer and associates[16] stated that shoulder arthroplasty must be considered a soft-tissue procedure and that the version of the implanted components must confer the joint stability: the soft tissues are designed to move the joint, not provide stability of the joint. Improper version of the components will lead to excessive nonphysiologic forces both across and through the joint, resulting in a high incidence of instability and component loosening.

The pathology necessitating shoulder arthroplasty must be understood preoperatively because the procedure must address each component of the pathology during the reconstruction. Anterior instability is more commonly related to humeral version errors in the face of chronic incompetence and shortening of the subscapularis muscle. Posterior instability usually is caused by glenoid erosion and is a bony concern. Inferior instability appears to be iatrogenic in its etiology and results from the surgeon attempting to overstabilize the joint by overstuffing it. Since the advent of modular prostheses, there have been many more overstuffed joints resulting in poor outcome than there have been undersized joints resulting in instability.

Anterior Instability

Anterior instability after shoulder arthroplasty is primarily the result of excessive

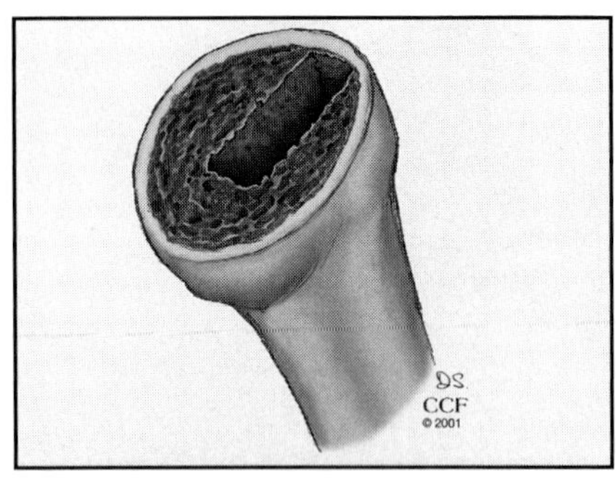

Fig. 2 The anatomic axis of the humerus is not centered on the anatomic neck. Most often, there is more bone posteriorly than anteriorly, resulting in posterior offset (©2001 Cleveland Clinic Foundation).

anteversion of the humeral component relative to the glenoid component. As discussed above, when the humeral and glenoid version are appropriate, anterior instability should be a rare event. Associated factors that aggravate the tendency for anterior instability include anterior deltoid muscle weakness and atrophy, coracoacromial arch incompetence, increased lateral offset of the joint, and incorrect humeral head offset with respect to the anatomic humeral axis. Complete subscapularis muscle incompetence or its absence may lead to weakness and functional deficits but should not lead to anterior instability of the reconstructed arthroplasty.

Deltoid muscle problems should be precluded by preserving the deltoid origin and respecting the axillary nerve during the initial dissection. Contemporary surgical approaches should use the anatomic, internervous plane defined by the deltopectoral interval. Delicate retraction of the deltoid muscle superolaterally allows very adequate exposure but may require ligation of the cephalic vein. The older concept that the coracoacromial ligament is a vestigial structure must be abandoned; even in a patient with healthy, robust rotator cuff tissue, I rarely resect or incise the coracoacromial ligament during shoulder arthroplasty. In rheumatoid patients and patients with rotator cuff–tear arthropathy, preservation of this ligament is of paramount concern. It clearly provides superior and anterior stability to the glenohumeral joint.

The surgeon must respect the concept of lateral offset, that is, the relationship of the humerus to the coracoid (Fig. 1). This simply means putting the joint line where it anatomically belongs while reestablishing the anatomically correct muscle lengths of the rotator cuff and deltoid muscle simultaneously. Glenoid components nearly always move the joint line lateral to its anatomic location with respect to the scapula. The polyethylene adds "thickness" and moves the joint line laterally. If the humeral head is not correspondingly smaller, the subscapularis muscle becomes functionally lengthened and thus is at risk for rupture as the arm is exercised into external rotation. Proper humeral retroversion can obviate this concern. The newest shoulder replacement systems offer the surgeon the ability to compensate for humeral head offset with respect to the anatomic humeral axis. Typically there is more bone posteriorly at the anatomic neck of the humerus with respect to the intramedullary canal (Fig. 2). If the implanted head is malpositioned, external rotation of the limb applies increased force to the subscapularis tendon, which may tear it. Furthermore, with correspondingly less articulating surface posteriorly, as the arm externally rotates, it may dislocate anteriorly. Again, proper version of the humeral component should preclude this iatrogenic problem.

Often the pathophysiology of arthritis results in long-standing internal rotation contractures and considerable loss of subscapularis tendon length. Intraoperative assessment of subscapularis and anterior capsular contracture is critically important to preserve anterior stability. Paradoxically, if the anterior capsule is not released and if the subscapularis tendon is not lengthened, the patient is at higher risk for anterior dislocation of the new joint. As the patient attempts to externally rotate (a particularly important motion for functional satisfaction), he or she will either tear these tight structures or translate the shoulder anteriorly to the point of dislocation. Because of the risk of significant postoperative loss of external rotation, anterior capsular release and subscapularis tendon advancement must be considered. Either Z-lengthening of the subscapularis tendon or advancement of the tendon to the osteotomy site is required (Fig. 3).

Posterior Instability

The most common cause of posterior shoulder instability after arthroplasty is overall combined excessive retroversion of both the glenoid and humeral components. Classic osseous pathology in osteoarthritis of the shoulder results in significant posterior wear or erosion of the glenoid. Preoperative axillary views or CT scans will define the extent of the posterior glenoid wear (Fig. 4). Because the surgical approach is anterior, it is often very difficult to treat extensive glenoid posterior bone loss.[17] Not infrequently, glenoid resurfacing is precluded because of severe malversion of the native glenoid. In some circumstances, the anterior aspect of the glenoid can be reamed and lowered to effectively change the orientation of the glenoid. Experience has shown that this may be effective when posterior wear and bone loss are minimal. However, only a small amount of anterior glenoid can be reamed away because the subchondral plate must be preserved, and not much bone is left to ream. Alternatively, bone grafting to the poster-ior glenoid may be considered, but this is technically very difficult, usually requires a second, simultaneous posterior approach, and adds to the lateral offset problem.

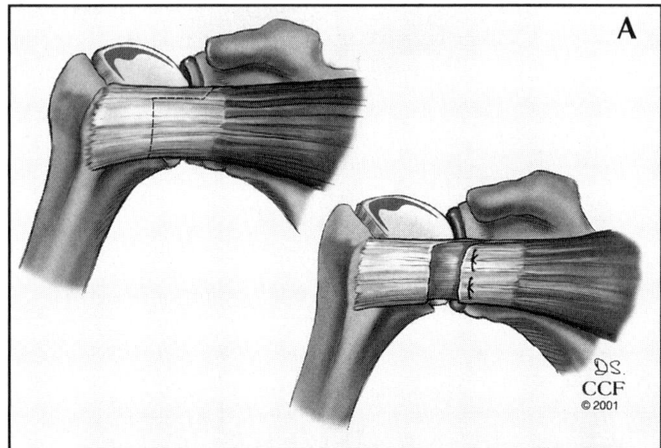

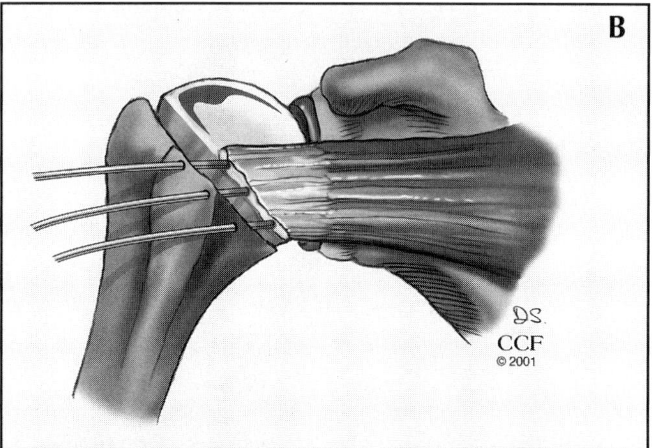

Fig. 3 When external rotation is compromised by long-standing internal rotation contractures, lengthening of the subscapularis is required. Two techniques are available. **A,** The subscapularis is lengthened by a coronal plane tenotomy. **B,** The medial advancement of the tendon to the osteotomy site is shown (©2001 Cleveland Clinic Foundation).

Manufacturers have designed a variety of posterior augmented glenoid components, but they are difficult to seat properly, and few surgeons have much experience in their use. More often than not, therefore, the surgeon performs humeral head replacement only.

When there is uncorrectable glenoid retroversion, the humeral osteotomy and reconstruction must have compensatory relative anteversion (less retroversion). If the surgeon proceeds with the textbook "recommendation" of 40° humeral retroversion, the shoulder arthroplasty will be posteriorly unstable, and as soon as the patient internally rotates the shoulder, it will dislocate. In the face of severe posterior glenoid wear, the humeral osteotomy may be in 0° retroversion or neutral (90° to the transepicondylar axis) (Fig. 5). One can always increase the retroversion intraoperatively as the specific osseous pathology dictates. Therefore, if preoperative axillary radiographs indicate posterior glenoid bone loss, the initial humeral osteotomy should be made more toward neutral and adjusted as necessary after full intraoperative consideration is given to the status of the glenoid.

With long-standing posterior subluxation and displacement of the arthritic joint, the posterior capsule and soft tissues my be overstretched, resulting in increased posterior volume, into which the new shoulder arthroplasty may translate or dislocate. If the version and size of the implanted components are ideal and if the midpoint of the humeral head can be translated posterior to the posterior glenoid rim with the arm in neutral rotation, then the posterior soft tissues must be imbricated to decrease the posterior volume of the joint (Fig. 6).

Another less common cause of posterior instability after joint arthroplasty is undersizing the surface area of the glenoid replacement. Because of the technically difficult surgical approach to the posteriorly worn glenoid, expedience may lead to the placement of a glenoid smaller than is appropriate because it is the only one that will fit into the tight surgical field. With a diminished anteroposterior dimension on which the humeral head must articulate, instability will occur even with optimal version and optimized soft-tissue balance. Consequently, appropriate glenoid sizing is equally important and may require more extensive surgical exposure.

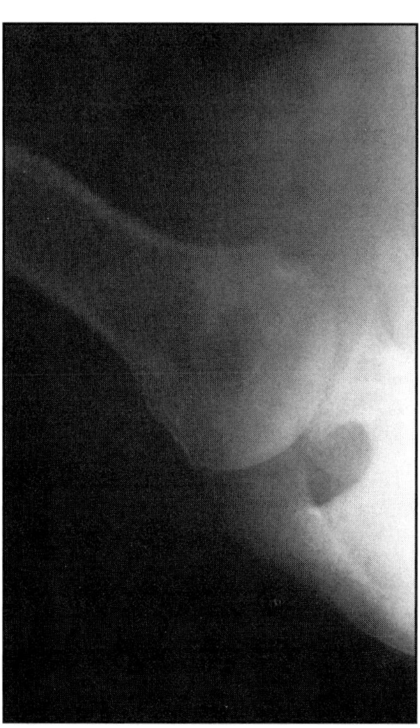

Fig. 4 Radiograph demonstrating the classic posterior wear of the humerus on the glenoid seen in osteoarthritis. A CT scan may better demonstrate the extent of posterior bone loss.

Inferior Instability

Inferior instability after shoulder replacement is caused by placing the humeral component too low within the

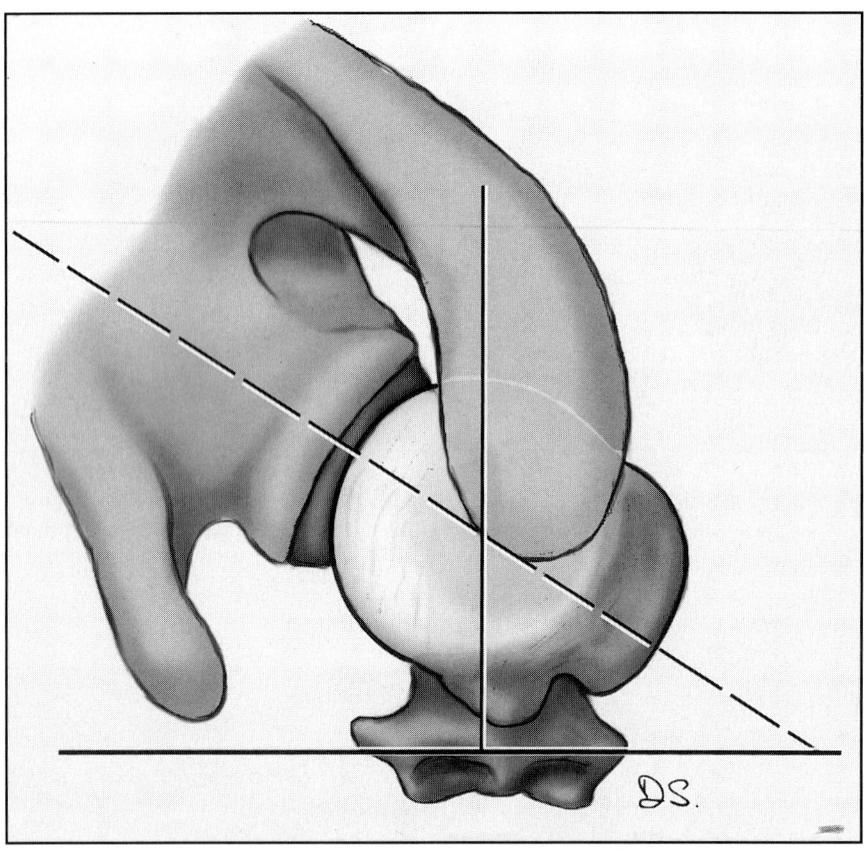

Fig. 5 The humeral osteotomy must compensate for the degree of glenoid retroversion. In severe cases of posterior glenoid loss, to enhance stability of the joint, the humeral osteotomy must be anteverted as shown (©2001 Cleveland Clinic Foundation).

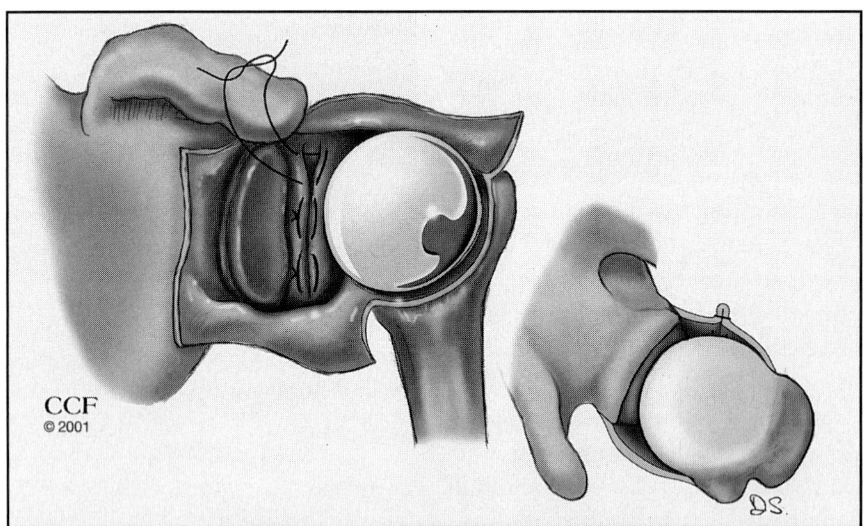

Fig. 6 When posterior soft-tissue laxity is present, the posterior capsule may be imbricated to restore posterior stability, especially when the arm is placed in internal rotation (©2001 Cleveland Clinic Foundation).

humeral canal.[4] In addition, it is possible with the modular systems to have the prosthetic humeral stem at the appropriate level but have the same functional and anatomic situation occur if the head size itself is too small. In simple terms, the humeral prosthesis merely functions as a spacer for the deltoid muscle. Furthermore, the deltoid force vector, on initiation of contraction when the arm is at the side, is directed superiorly. It has the effect of pulling the humerus in a cephalad direction. If a fulcrum cannot be effectively established through the cuff muscles, then the patient will not be able to elevate the arm. When the humeral component is situated too low, the arm will piston only in a superior-inferior direction. Another complication associated with an inferiorly placed humeral prosthesis is impingement syndrome occurring between the now proud tuberosity and the acromion (Fig. 7).

The most appropriate method to ensure proper humeral height is to keep the osteotomy at all times above the tip of the greater tuberosity. During trial reduction of the joint with the prosthetic components, as an inferior force is placed on the arm with the arm held in neutral rotation, the superior aspect of the head should not be displaced inferior to the midpoint of the glenoid (Fig. 8). It is equally important that the shoulder not be overstuffed in an effort to avoid inferior instability. It is not critical in the shoulder that the prosthesis sit firmly on the osteotomized neck. If the neck cut is too low, it is far better to cement the prosthesis proud to ensure proper myofascial sleeve tension of the deltoid muscle and rotator cuff. With acute fractures, malunions, and other pathologic processes, the proximal humeral anatomy may be so distorted as to be unrecognizable. It then becomes most important to preserve tuberosities, when possible, and to reestablish the correct deltoid muscle length-tension relationship by cementing the humeral component at the required height.

Shoulder Component Loosening

Glenoid Component Loosening

Nearly all published series that review total shoulder arthroplasties discuss glenoid loosening and glenoid lucent lines.[1,3-5,10,11,16,18-26] Symptomatic or clinically relevant humeral component loosening and subsidence are distinctly rare and occur in a very small proportion of shoulder arthroplasties compared with the frequency of glenoid component loosening.[27,28] Notwithstanding the relatively high incidence of radiographic lucent lines around glenoid components, clinically symptomatic loosening remains uncommon. Cofield summarized the complications of total shoulder arthroplasty from 29 separate series involving 1,459 shoulders.[3,29] Although only 2% of glenoid components were clinically loose at 3 years, the various studies documented radiographically loose glenoid components of from 30% to 90% at 3 years. Torchia and associates[1] reported a 5.6% glenoid revision rate at 12 years. But other findings have suggested that the incidence of lucent lines was most directly related to surgical technique.[27,30] Indeed, many of the identifiable factors associated with glenoid loosening are under the surgeon's control.

Several features unique to the glenoid result in the high incidence of loosening.[31,32] Although the shoulder is not burdened with the jackhammer-like loading associated with weight bearing on knees and hips, it is subjected to significant loads during normal activities that subject it to considerable physiologic forces. Biomechanical studies have determined that merely elevating the arm away from the side generates compressive forces across the glenohumeral joint equal to one half body weight.[33,34] When any mass or weight is placed in the hand and subsequently elevated, very considerable forces are created across the joint. Because of the physical and mechanical principles associated with lever arms and short fulcrums, very large forces are placed on the shoulder during normal daily

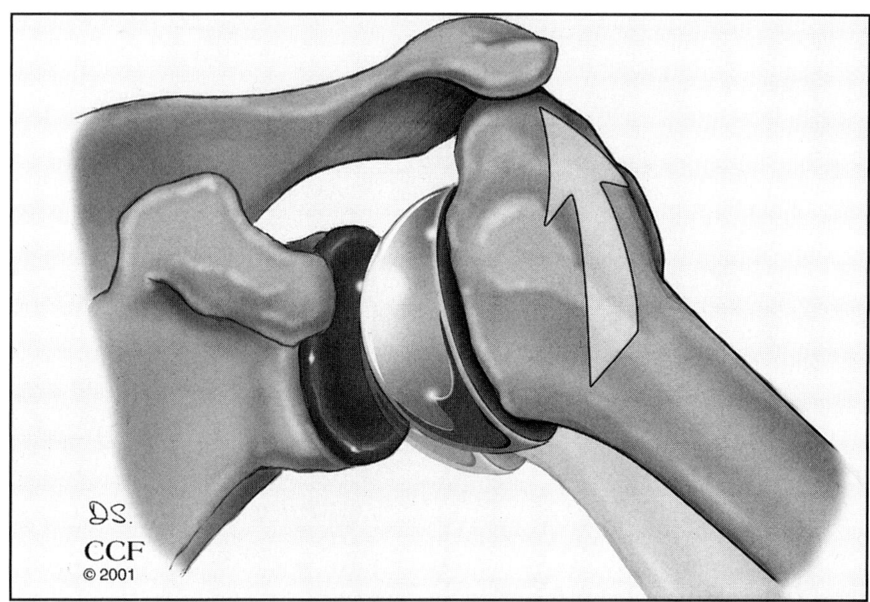

Fig. 7 When the humeral component is placed too inferiorly, the greater tuberosity becomes "proud" and may impinge on the acromion during elevation of the arm (©2001 Cleveland Clinic Foundation).

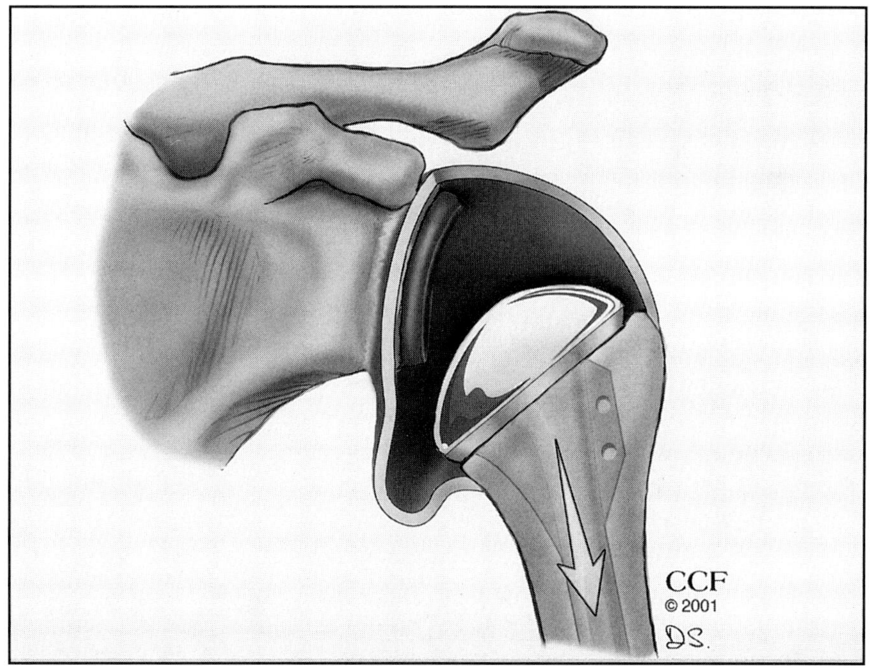

Fig. 8 During trial reduction, when an inferiorly directed force is placed on the limb, the superior aspect of the humeral component should not displace below the midpoint of the glenoid component (©2001 Cleveland Clinic Foundation).

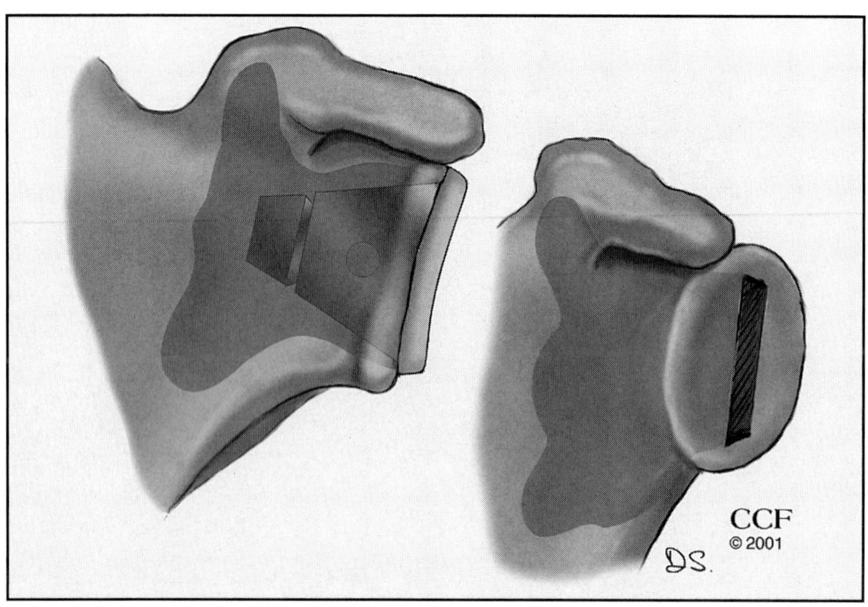

Fig. 9 When using cemented components, glenoid fixation is enhanced by placing cement into the base of the coracoid process.

recreational and occupational activities.[34] The surgeon thus will realize the importance of congruence between the native glenoid and the component.

Reeves and associates[35] found that the contact between the humerus and glenoid moves across the joint in many directions as a function of arm position and muscle activity. The humerus has three planes of motion across the glenoid, including rolling, sliding, and translation. True axial loading through the center of the glenoid rarely occurs because most forces in normal activity involve nonaxial and asymmetric forces. The resultant force is off center or eccentric and results in rim loading of the prosthesis.[14,36] If there is poor congruence between the glenoid subchondral bone and the back side of the glenoid component, micromotion, fretting, cold flow, and eventual failure will result from the repetitive eccentric loading of the component.[37]

As noted, the surgeon has great influence on the incidence of glenoid fixation failure. Although a host of total shoulder systems are available, principles of glenoid preparation remain constant. Surgical dissections that afford maximal exposure are critical: capsular releases and appropriate retraction benefit surgical exposure of the glenoid. As previously discussed, patients with osteoarthritis often present with a significantly retroverted glenoid, which makes preparation difficult and occasionally impossible; whenever possible, however, concentric reaming of the surface of the retroverted glenoid should be done in anticipation of resurfacing. Adequate glenoid bone stock seems an obvious prerequisite for satisfactory glenoid resurfacing,[38] yet despite adequate volume of bone, the surgeon must recognize the quality of the bone into which the glenoid component is fixed.[30] Inflammatory arthritides typically result in significant osteopenia or osteoporosis, leaving poor cancellous and cortical bone support. In cases of extremely poor bone, it may be more prudent to perform a humeral head replacement only.

Fixation may be enhanced by preparing an additional cement vault in the base of the coracoid process (Fig. 9). By developing this location for cement fixation, a noncoplanar construct of methylmethacrylate is created. Meticulous preparation of the vault is critically important before placing the cement.[39] Hemostasis is difficult yet mandatory because the bone bed of the glenoid vault must be meticulously clean, dry, and free from blood. There are several techniques to accomplish this, including pulsatile lavage and drying with hydrogen peroxide, thrombin, topical absorbable hemostatic fabric, or sterile absorbable gelatin sponge. Adherence to these proven principles of glenoid resurfacing should result in a very low incidence of glenoid loosening and very few radiographic lucent lines.

Clinical Presentation The patient with a loose glenoid usually has enjoyed a period of pain-free function of the arm. Deep, toothache-like pain associated with motion of the extremity is of gradual onset and not always related to a loose glenoid; the pain often relates to rotator cuff disease. The presence of night pain as part of the constellation of symptoms is more likely associated with a cuff tear than a loose glenoid. Only very rarely does catastrophic failure of the implant occur in which it dislodges from the native glenoid vault, causing mechanical locking of the joint.

The examination of the painful arthroplasty should concentrate on assessing passive and active motion differences. The pain of a loose glenoid is independent of active or passive motion of the joint, although the pain usually is more intense during active elevation because asymmetric compressive forces increase. When the examining physician loads the humerus axially while it is in 90° of abduction, the pain of a loose component increases significantly. Although the pain generated by a loose component may make the patient appear to be weak, isometric testing of both elevation and external rotation in the face of a rotator cuff tear reveals a distinctly different degree of weakness. Rotator cuff tears demonstrate much more weakness than that caused by pain alone.

Radiographic Assessment Plain radiographs will demonstrate a lucent line of at least 2 mm around the entire bone-cement interface of the implant. Because of the obliquity of the glenoid, three radiographic views to evaluate the bone-cement interface are recommended. The 40° posterior oblique view with the humerus in both internal and external rotation and an axillary view provide the best opportunity for analysis.[1,40] As Kelleher and associates[41] have noted, the three-dimensional nature of the construct may result in a high incidence of false-negative findings from plain radiographs alone. They recommend the use of fluoroscopy to better evaluate the painful arthroplasty in the search for a loose component.

Arthrography and digital subtraction arthrography remain useful tools in the radiologic assessment of the painful shoulder replacement when loosening is not evident on plain films. Newer pulse sequences that make MRI scanning possible in the presence of the metal humeral component may yet offer another technique to evaluate component loosening.[9]

Treatment of Loose Glenoid When a loose glenoid component is diagnosed early, although not necessarily immediately, revision should be considered. Particulate polyethylene debris, although microscopic, can have devastating effects on the local tissues, especially bone, as seen in lower extremity component wear. Osteolysis does occur in the upper extremity, but because the debris load generally is much less than that which occurs in the lower extremities, the rate of osteolysis and severe bone loss is considerably slower. Nevertheless, for patient comfort and satisfaction, and to preserve bone stock, early revision should be considered.

When sufficient bone stock remains at the time of revision, a thorough clean-out of the glenoid vault, including all soft tissue, scar, and cement, may be followed by reimplantation. Ideally, the surgeon would try to understand the mode of failure and correct whatever factors remain within his or her control. Assuring a congruent mating of the component to the native glenoid bone remains a critically important consideration. Meticulous cement technique preceded by thorough cleansing and drying of the vault is of paramount importance.

Not infrequently, at the time of revision the glenoid vault has had such significant bone loss that predictable stability of the implant is elusive. In this case, removal of the implant, cement, membrane, and scar is followed by grafting of the defect with allograft. Interposition arthroplasty in this circumstance may be an alternative to reimplantation in the face of precarious fixation.[42] Often, the more difficult issue is the presence of a cemented monoblock prosthesis, such as the original Neer fixed head-stem device. Its presence makes reimplantation particularly difficult because exposure of the glenoid is precluded by the humeral head. The amount of potential humeral destruction must be weighed against the relatively minimal problems of removing the glenoid component alone. If the humeral component can be retrieved, offering adequate exposure for glenoid revision, then there is no need to remove the cement mantle in the face of aseptic loosening. A smaller-diameter humeral component can be cemented over the retained cement within the humeral canal.

Humeral Component Loosening

Humeral component loosening is considered a very rare event and often is not included in a description or listing of complications associated with shoulder arthroplasty,[5,10,21,31,43] perhaps because the forces across the shoulder that occur with a completely nonconstrained joint result in only minimal bone-implant bone-cement interface stresses. The humerus is neither impact loaded nor rotationally constrained unless inappropriate components have been implanted. Even when the first generation of humeral components were press-fit, clinical loosening was a rare event (although with longer follow-up, radiographic evidence of loosening increased).

"Plastic disease," in which particulate wear debris results in characteristic osteolysis along the humeral stem, has been infrequently reported.[44] This is thought to be macrophage-induced osteolysis rather than primary mechanical loosening.[45-47] As discussed above, identification of this phenomenon may warrant earlier glenoid revision.

Whatever technique is used to treat humeral component loosening, immediate axial and rotational stability of the implant is of paramount importance. With osteoarthritic bone, which is usually robust, cement is rarely necessary. By contrast, in rheumatoid patients, bone quality is usually more precarious and often compromised by degenerative cysts. In this situation, cement is the wiser choice for immediate fixation. Patients with osteonecrosis who require humeral replacement are usually younger; consequently, methylmethacrylate should be used with caution in these patients. Fortunately, most of the dead bone in these situations occurs well within the confines of the excised humeral head, and the remaining metaphyseal bone is well vascularized, viable, and predictably able to support an uncemented implant. In the rare circumstance in which the avascular bone extends into the osteotomy site at the humeral neck, cement should be considered because the noncompliant dead bone will not provide adequate stability for the implant. Furthermore, adjacent dead bone obviously will not grow into the interstices of the porous metal surface, and subsequent loosening predictably will follow.

Clinical Presentation A patient with humeral component loosening will complain of activity-related pain radiating down the anterior aspect of the brachium. Biceps-related pain is remarkably similar and thus must be seriously considered in the differential diagnosis. As with glenoid loosening, there is almost always a history of a long, pain-free interval preceding the insidious onset of a low-intensity, aching pain radiating down the arm. The symptoms are aggravated by activity and generally absent at rest. There are no specific or reliable physical examination maneuvers that characteristically reproduce the pain of a loose humeral component. Clinical suspicion and radiographic confirmation must suffice.

Radiographic Findings As with the glenoid, plain radiographs will nearly always document a loose humeral component. The typical lucency will be apparent around the implant at the bone-implant interface. Frequently there is a scalloped appearance to the medullary bone, especially with osteolysis based on particulate debris. If there is humeral subsidence, evidence of the original humeral component placement will be apparent by noting the relationship of the tuberosities to the present subsided position. Distally, the prosthesis tip may demonstrate the windshield wiper phenomenon (distal toggle) characteristic of stem instability and micromotion.

In the rare circumstances in which plain radiographs fail to demonstrate humeral loosening that is suggested clinically, an arthrogram may be more defining. Because late loosening can be caused by infection, an aspirate should be sent for culture at the time of the arthrogram. In addition, just as MRI scanning noninvasively diagnoses glenoid loosening, the same technique may be refined and applied to the analysis of humeral component loosening.[9]

Treatment Options Humeral component loosening is usually sufficiently disabling to warrant revision surgery. The principles of revision surgery should be followed: meticulous dissection through anatomic tissue planes, retrieval of the loose prosthesis, removal of cement and fibrous tissue membrane, thorough preparation of the bone bed, and recementing of the new component using pressurized cement techniques. The humeral component should be positioned at the proper height and in the proper version to minimize the chance of postoperative instability. Unless the humeral component loosening is the result of sepsis, resection arthroplasty is rarely an option for the management of a loose humeral prosthesis.

References

1. Torchia ME, Cofield RH, Settergren CR: Total shoulder arthroplasty with the Neer prosthesis: Long-term results. *J Shoulder Elbow Surg* 1997; 6:495-505.
2. Wirth MA, Rockwood CA Jr: Complications of shoulder arthroplasty. *Clin Orthop* 1994;307: 47-69.
3. Cofield RH, Edgerton BC: Total shoulder arthroplasty: Complications and revision surgery. *Instr Course Lect* 1990;39:449-462.
4. Miller SR, Bigliani LU: Complications of total shoulder replacement, in Bigliani LU (ed): *Complications of Shoulder Surgery*. Baltimore, MD, Williams and Wilkins, 1993, pp 59-72.
5. Ramsey ML, Fenlin JM Jr: Use of an antibiotic-impregnated bone cement block in the revision of an infected shoulder arthroplasty: *J Shoulder Elbow Surg* 1996;5:479-482.
6. Marsh PK, Cotler JM: Management of an aerobic infection in a prosthetic knee with long-term antibiotics alone: A case report. *Clin Orthop* 1981;155:133-135.
7. Amstutz HC, Thomas BJ, Kabo JM, Jinnah RH, Dorey FJ: The DANA total shoulder arthroplasty. *J Bone Joint Surg Am* 1988;70:1174-1182.
8. Goss TP: Shoulder infections, in Bigliani LU (ed): *Complications of Shoulder Surgery*. Baltimore, MD, Williams and Wilkins, 1993, pp 202-213.
9. Soghikian GW, Neviaser RJ: Complications of humeral head replacement, in Bigliani LU (ed): *Complications of Shoulder Surgery*. Baltimore, MD, Williams and Wilkins, 1993, pp 81-92.
10. Bade HA III, Warren RF, Ranawat CS, Inglis AE: Long-term results of Neer total shoulder replacement, in Bateman JE, Welsh RP (eds): *Surgery of the Shoulder*. Philadelphia, PA, BC Decker, 1984, pp 294-302.
11. Cuomo F, Checroun A: Avoiding pitfalls and complications in total shoulder arthroplasty. *Clin Orthop North Am* 1998;29:507-518.
12. Karduna AR, Williams GR, Williams JL, Iannotti JP: Joint stability after total shoulder arthroplasty in a cadaver model. *J Shoulder Elbow Surg* 1997;6:506-511.
13. Friedman RJ: Glenohumeral translation after total shoulder arthroplasty. *J Shoulder Elbow Surg* 1992;1:312-316.
14. Harryman DT II, Sidles JA, Clark JM, McQuade KJ, Gibb TD, Matsen FA III: Translation of the humeral head on the glenoid with passive glenohumeral motion. *J Bone Joint Surg Am* 1990;72:1334-1343.
15. Moeckel BH, Altchek DW, Warren RF, Wickiewicz TL, Dines DM: Instability of the shoulder after arthroplasty. *J Bone Joint Surg Am* 1993;75:492-497.
16. Neer CS II, Watson KC, Stanton FJ: Recent experience in total shoulder replacement. *J Bone Joint Surg Am* 1982;64:319-337.
17. Neer CS II, Morrison DS: Glenoid bone-grafting in total shoulder arthroplasty. *J Bone Joint Surg Am* 1988;70:1154-1162.
18. Barrett WP, Franklin JL, Jackins SE, Wyss CR, Matsen FA III: Total shoulder arthroplasty. *J Bone Joint Surg Am* 1987;69:865-872.
19. Bell SN, Gschwend N: Clinical experience with total shoulder arthroplasty and hemi-arthroplasty of the shoulder using the Neer prosthesis. *Int Orthop* 1986;10:217-222.
20. Brenner BC, Ferlic DC, Clayton ML, Dennis DA: Survivorship of unconstrained total shoulder arthroplasty. *J Bone Joint Surg Am* 1989; 71:1289-1296.
21. Cofield RH: Total shoulder arthroplasty with the Neer prosthesis. *J Bone Joint Surg Am* 1984; 66:899-906.
22. Franklin JL, Barrett WP, Jackins SE, Matsen FA III: Glenoid loosening in total shoulder arthroplasty. *J Arthroplasty* 1988;3:39-46.
23. Hawkins RJ, Bell RH, Jallay B: Total shoulder arthroplasty. *Clin Orthop* 1989;242:188-194.
24. Neer CS II: Replacement arthroplasty for glenohumeral osteoarthritis. *J Bone Joint Surg Am* 1974;56:1-13.
25. Reckling FW, Asher MA, Dillon WL: A longitudinal study of the radiolucent line at the bone-cement interface following total joint-replacement procedures. *J Bone Joint Surg Am* 1977;59:355-358.
26. Wilde AH, Borden LS, Brems JJ: Experience with the Neer total shoulder replacement, in Bateman JE, Welsh RP (eds): *Surgery of the Shoulder*. BC Decker, Philadelphia, PA, 1984, pp 224-228.

27. Brems JJ: The glenoid component in total shoulder arthroplasty. *J Shoulder Elbow Surg* 1993;2:47-52.

28. Rodosky MW, Bigliani LU: Indications for glenoid resurfacing in shoulder arthroplasty. *J Shoulder Elbow Surg* 1996;5:231-248.

29. Cofield RH: Unconstrained total shoulder prostheses. *Clin Orthop* 1983;173:97-108.

30. Brems JJ, Wilde AH, Borden LS, Boumphrey FRS: Glenoid lucent lines. *Orthop Trans* 1986;10:231.

31. Frich LH, Odgaard A, Dalstra M: Glenoid bone architecture. *J Shoulder Elbow Surg* 1998; 7:356-361.

32. Friedman RJ, LaBerge M, Dooley RL, O'Hara AL: Finite element modeling of the glenoid component: Effect of design parameters on stress distribution. *J Shoulder Elbow Surg* 1992; 1:261-270.

33. Howell SM, Galinat BJ, Renzi AJ, Marone PJ: Normal and abnormal mechanics of the glenohumeral joint in the horizontal plane. *J Bone Joint Surg Am* 1988;70:227-232.

34. Poppen NK, Walker PS: Forces at the glenohumeral joint in abduction. *Clin Orthop* 1978;135:165-170.

35. Reeves BF, Jobbinis B, Dowson D, et al: A total shoulder endoprosthesis. *Engineering in Medicine* 1982;1:64-67.

36. Stone KD, Grabowski JJ, Cofield RH, Morrey BF; An KN: Stress analyses of glenoid components in total shoulder arthroplasty. *J Shoulder Elbow Surg* 1999;8:151-158.

37. Collins D, Tencer A, Sidles J, Matsen F III: Edge displacement and deformation of glenoid components in response to eccentric loading: The effect of preparation of the glenoid bone. *J Bone Joint Surg Am* 1992;74:501-507.

38. Frich LH, Jensen NC, Odgaard A, Pedersen CM, Sojbjerg JO, Dalstra M: Bone strength and material properties of the glenoid. *J Shoulder Elbow Surg* 1997;6:97-104.

39. Norris BL, Lachiewicz PF: Modern cement technique and the survivorship of total shoulder arthroplasty. *Clin Orthop* 1996;328:76-85.

40. Feldman F: The radiology of total shoulder prostheses. *Semin Roentgenol* 1986;21:47-65.

41. Kelleher IM, Cofield RH, Becker DA, Beabout JW: Fluoroscopically positioned radiographs of total shoulder arthroplasty. *J Shoulder Elbow Surg* 1992;1:306-311.

42. Burkhead WZ Jr, Hutton KS: Biologic resurfacing of the glenoid with hemiarthroplasty of the shoulder. *J Shoulder Elbow Surg* 1995;4: 263-270.

43. Cofield RH: The shoulder III: Glenohumeral arthritis and bad cuff disease. *60th Annual Meeting Proceedings*. Rosemont, IL, American Academy of Orthopaedic Surgeons, 1993, pp 397.

44. Klimkiewicz JJ, Iannotti JP, Rubash HE, Shanbhag AS: Aseptic loosening of the humeral component in total shoulder arthroplasty. *J Shoulder Elbow Surg* 1998;7:422-426.

45. Haynes DR, Rogers SD, Hay S, Pearcy MJ, Howie DW: The difference in toxicity and release of bone-resorbing mediators induced by titanium and cobalt-chromium-alloy wear particles. *J Bone Joint Surg Am* 1993;75:825-834.

46. Kim KJ, Chiba J, Rubash HE: In-vivo and in-vitro analysis of membranes from hip prostheses inserted without cement. *J Bone Joint Surg Am* 1994;76:172-180.

47. Shanbhag AS, Jacobs JJ, Black J, Galante JO, Glant TT: Human monocyte response to particulate biomaterials generated in-vivo and in-vitro. *J Orthop Res* 1995;13:792-801.

Glenoid Resurfacing in Shoulder Arthroplasty

Anil K. Dutta, MD
Gary Matthys, MD
Wayne Z. Burkhead, MD

Introduction

The current success of total shoulder arthroplasty is due, at least in part, to the emergence of successful techniques for glenoid resurfacing.[1-6] However, the most common cause of long-term failure of total shoulder arthroplasty remains the glenoid component. Aseptic loosening rates of 4% to 11% have been reported.[7-10] Rotator cuff deficiencies and anatomic limitations in specific patients may allow for arthroplasty but lead to premature glenoid failure.[11] When symptomatic glenoid loosening does occur, revision is further complicated by glenoid bone deficiency, often precluding reimplantation of a new component.[12] These complexities have engendered interest in glenoid-resurfacing alternatives and possible new implant options to solve this still frequent surgical dilemma in shoulder arthroplasty.

Indications

The decision to resurface the glenoid is based on many variables. In general, glenoid prosthetic resurfacing can be considered in patients with intact or repairable rotator cuffs, osteoarthritis, rheumatoid arthritis, arthritis with eccentric glenoid wear, or biconcave glenoid. Glenoid prosthetic resurfacing should not be considered in patients with irreparable rotator cuffs, fractures, stage III or IV osteonecrosis, concentric (not biconcave) glenoid, or severe glenoid bone deficiency.[13-16] Glenoid resurfacing is strongly recommended for men older than age 60 years with an intact rotator cuff and eccentric glenoid wear.

Exposure

Obtaining maximum glenoid exposure is critical to successful glenoid resurfacing. The decision to resurface the glenoid with a prosthesis is predicated on the ability to prepare the bone surface for implantation. Only with proper exposure can instrumentation be used effectively and bone defects be adequately treated. The quality of surgical technique has been shown to directly affect the immediate postoperative radiographic appearance of glenoid fixation.[8]

Positioning

The patient is placed in the beach chair position with a folded towel behind the scapula. An armrest behind the humerus is optional; it must be removed to allow extension of the arm during humeral preparation. The head is supported on a McConnell (McConnell Orthopedic Manufacturing, Greenville, TX) or Mayfield (Ohio Medical Instrument, Cincinnati, OH) headrest.

The incision begins at the anterior edge of the clavicle superiorly and bisects the coracoid process. Distally, the incision is extended to the insertion of the deltoid muscle anteriorly (just lateral to the muscle belly of the biceps). The deltopectoral interval is developed to identify the cephalic vein, which is mobilized medially, with the pectoralis major muscle. Care is taken to ligate branches of the vein, which may retract if not secured. A self-retaining retractor is placed between the deltoid and pectoralis major muscles. The superior one fourth of the pectoralis major insertion is released. The deltoid insertion can be partially released and tagged for later repair to prevent excessive tearing of the muscle, but this is not routinely necessary. For revision surgeries or chronic dislocations, takedown of the anterior deltoid from the acromion and clavicle may be required.

The clavipectoral fascia is incised lateral to the conjoined tendon. The coracoacromial ligament can be released off the coracoid for increased exposure but must be repaired if an irreparable cuff tear exists. The conjoined tendon is then retracted medially. The tendon can be released partially or totally off the coracoid to ease retraction, but care must be taken to protect the musculocutaneous nerve, which enters the coracobrachialis muscle 3 to 8 cm distal to the coracoid. If the conjoined tendon is taken down, the assistant must be careful not to pull too hard on the brachial plexus with the retractor.

The subscapularis tendon is identified, and the bursa overlying the tendon is removed. The axillary nerve position is noted (3 to 5 mm medial to the musculotendinous junction). The anterior

Table 1
Guidelines for Release of the Subscapularis Tendon

Subscapularis Tendon Release	Preoperative Range of Motion
Release 1.5 cm medial to insertion	Passive external rotation ≥ 20°
Release subperiosteally, reattach medially	Passive external rotation > -20° and < 20°
Subscapularis Z-lengthening	Passive external rotation ≤ -20°

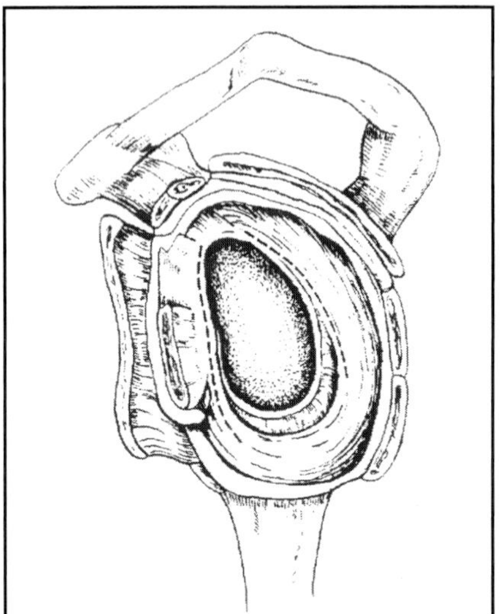

Fig. 1 Exposure and placement of capsulotomy.

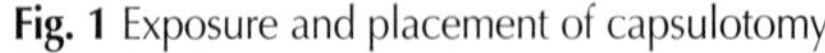

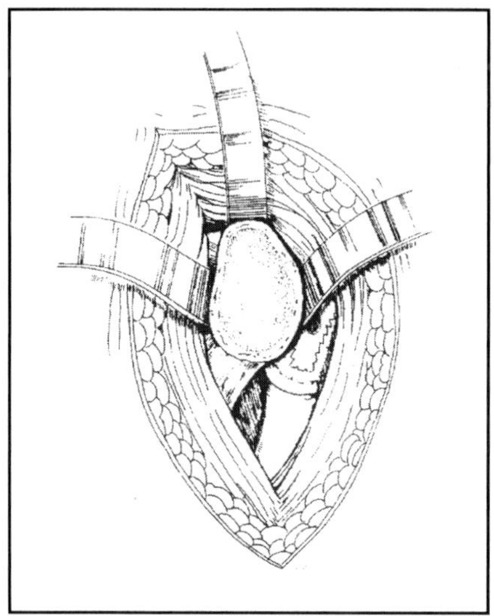

Fig. 2 Ideal placement of glenoid retractor.

humeral circumflex vessels are ligated at the inferior one third of the tendon. The treatment of the subscapularis tendon depends on the preoperative range of motion. Regardless of how the tendon is taken down, it is important to dissect subperiosteally just medial to the biceps down to the superior edge of the latissimus dorsi muscle. Guidelines for subscapularis release[17] are listed in Table 1.

The subscapularis tendon is released through the rotator interval superiorly. A biceps tenotomy can be done at this time, if needed. The conjoined tendon is released off the superficial surface; the inferior release is subperiosteal. The axillary nerve is protected with external rotation and flexion of the arm and by a retractor placed beneath the capsule. Before dislocation, an anterior glenoid capsulotomy is made from the 12 o'clock to 7 o'clock positions inferiorly (Fig. 1).

After dislocation, the humeral head is resected and marginal osteophytes are excised. Removal of the entire head superior to the capsule in the anteroposterior plane maximizes glenoid exposure. A position of 20° flexion and 30° abduction and slight internal rotation relaxes the posterior capsule after the humeral head resection and allows the humeral head to be retracted posteriorly. Glenoid retractors are placed. Behind the glenoid rim, a Fukuda or ring retractor is used to retract the humerus posteriorly.

Once the retractors are in place, the arm is positioned in increased external rotation, maintaining 30° of abduction and 20° of flexion. This arm position maximizes working exposure of the glenoid. A blunt Homan retractor is placed along the anterior rim. The superior capsule, biceps, and supraspinatus muscles are retracted with a Darrach retractor above. Correct placement of the retractors provides adequate exposure for inspection and preparation (Fig. 2).

Glenoid Prosthetic Resurfacing

The technique for glenoid prosthetic resurfacing is individualized for each model of prosthesis and depends on the resurfacing option chosen (such as conforming, nonconforming, or biologic resurfacing). Understanding important anatomic considerations and the technical aspects of preparation directly affects the quality of fixation and longevity and the function of the glenoid component.

Glenoid Version

Preparation of the glenoid begins after adequate exposure is assured. The glenoid center point is a useful landmark to identify initially. The index finger is used to palpate the anterior glenoid rim. The tip of the index finger should be placed on the point in the sulcus between the upper and lower crura of the scapula, past the glenoid neck. A drill guide is then used to drill a pilot hole from the center of the glenoid face to the point indicated by the index finger (Fig. 3). This centering point allows reconstruction of the native glenoid version. It is important to make sure the posterior retractor does not translate the drill guide anteriorly when creating this pilot hole.

A posterior capsular release off the posterior rim of the glenoid may be necessary to retract the humerus fully and allow proper centering of the drill on the glenoid. (Posterior release is avoided if there was posterior subluxation of the humeral head preoperatively.) The glenoid normally faces 5° to 10° superiorly.[18] Generally, the component should match this, although the surgeon may wish to reorient the glenoid to face more inferiorly in shoulders with poor restraints to superior migration of the humerus.

Glenoid Sizing

The back of the glenoid trial should precisely match the surface area of the native glenoid. If the component is too large, the periphery will be unsupported, leading to premature loosening and impingement in extremes of motion. Unrecognized glenoid osteophytes can lead to oversizing. The glenoid trial should seat without rocking on the glenoid face when tested.

Glenoid Preparation

Collins and associates[19] compared three techniques of in vitro preparation of the glenoid: (1) removal of the cartilage with a curette, (2) hand burring, and (3) spherical reaming with the radius of the reamer equal to the radius of the glenoid. The third technique was the best in reducing edge displacement and component deformation when stressed. Spherical reaming provides the most stable biomechanical configuration when implantation of a prosthetic component is possible (Fig. 4). When implantation of a component is not possible, the contour of the glenoid face after spherical reaming may provide an acceptable nonprosthetic glenoid arthroplasty.[20]

Preparation of the glenoid for a pegged component is done by following the individual specifications of the pegged implant. The peg holes are created and then checked with a curved hemostat. If perforation of the glenoid neck occurs, the hole is plugged with bone from the humeral head, and less or no cement is used for that peg; in addition, the penetrating peg holes are not pressurized. A double-pegged component allows a subchondral tunnel to be created and true pressurization into the glenoid vault to occur (Fig. 5).

Preparation for a keeled component is done with a hand burr (we recommend a dental burr). The landmark with the least bone for creation of the keel is the base of the coracoid process. The inferior landmark is the lateral margin of the scapula. Inferior osteophytes may lead to incorrectly lowering the component and should be excised. Once again, stability of the glenoid trial is digitally checked and irregularities addressed to correct any rocking of the component.

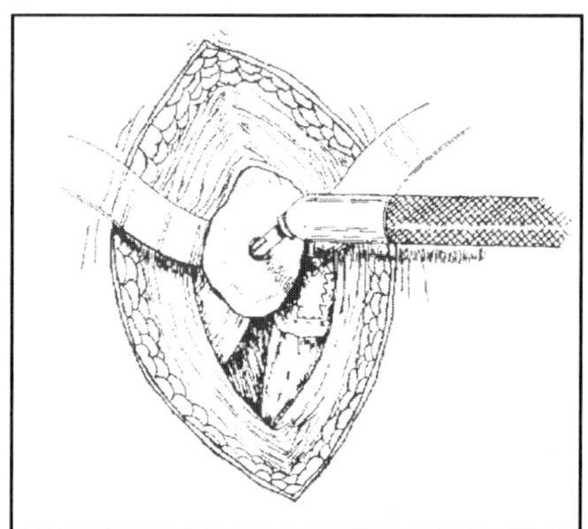

Fig. 3 Creation of glenoid center point.

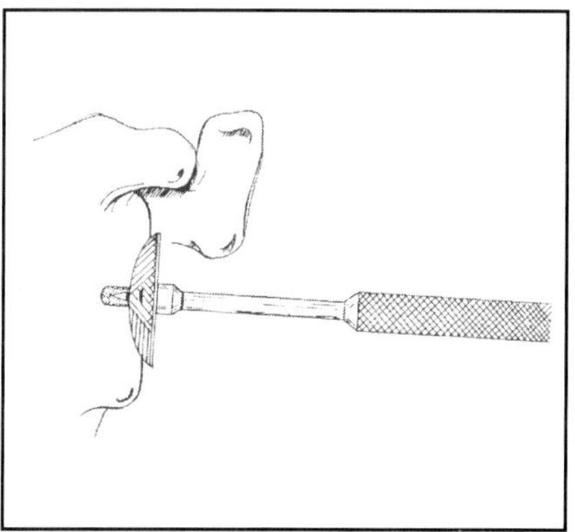

Fig. 4 Concentric reaming of the glenoid.

Cement technique is challenging in the confines of the glenoid cavity. Brems and associates[8] noted a 69% incidence of radiolucent lines immediately after cemented glenoid arthroplasty and also noted that the existence of these lines was related to surgeon practices intraoperatively. The standard cement technique for the keeled component is Neer's double-cement technique.[21] After creation of the keel slot, dry gauze or sterile absorbable gelatin sponge with thrombin is packed into the glenoid. Hydrogen peroxide is then used to bathe the bony surfaces. The gelatin sponge is removed and methylmethacrylate is applied in a liquid form with a syringe. The cement is then removed and allowed to become doughy before hand-packing the slot again. Cement is also placed on the back of the glenoid keel and the component is cemented into place. Placing cement on the back of the component (keeled or pegged) to make up for bone defects where it rests on the glenoid surface is not recommended because doing so may lead to cracking and loss of support. However, a relatively thin layer of cement will protect the bony surface from abrasion by the polyethylene and decrease polyethylene wear particles.[22]

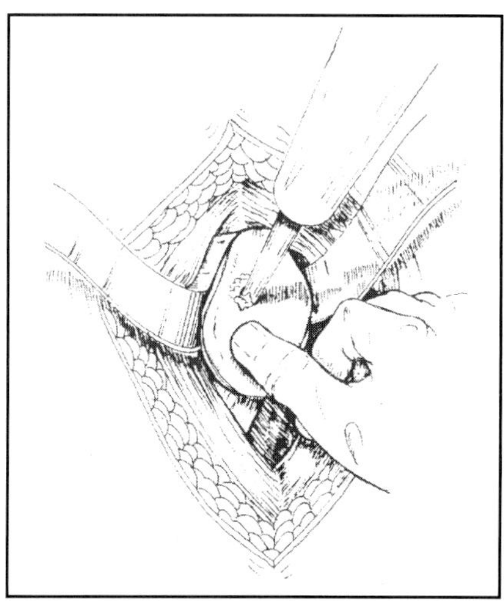

Fig. 5 Technique of glenoid cement pressurization.

Glenoid Bone Defects

Glenoid bone defects are common in primary arthroplasty and more so in revisions. Defects can be classified as mild, central (resorption or large cavity), peripheral, or segmental.[23-25] Central bone loss is most common in patients with rheumatoid arthritis. Cofield[12] recommends placing a centering hole and assessing the depth of the glenoid neck. A depth of less than 1 cm will probably not allow for adequate fixation and precludes placement of a prosthesis. Central cavities usually can be filled with local bone graft from the humeral head.

Peripheral defects are usually posterior in osteoarthritis. The reconstructive

Table 2
Management of Glenoid Bone Defects

Extent of Wear	Reconstructive Option
Minor wear (1-2 mm)	High side down
3-5 mm wear	High side down with increased retroversion
More than 5 mm wear	Bone graft fixed with screws or component augment

option is determined by the extent of wear (Table 2). One option is to place the component on the native surface, accepting the increased retroversion and compensating for it by anteverting the humeral component such that the sum of the two versions is roughly 30° to 40°. Alternatively, the high side can be burred down to match the low side. Bulk bone graft or augmented components can accommodate larger defects. However, both of these alternatives lead to higher complication rates.[12,26]

Glenoid Component Options

The various total shoulder designs can be grouped largely into three categories: constrained, semiconstrained, and nonconstrained.[27-29] Indications for the constrained and semiconstrained implants are few; the nonconstrained design is the standard in total shoulder arthroplasty. Nonconstrained designs can be further subdivided into conforming and nonconforming designs. In the conforming glenoid prosthesis, an exact match of the radius of curvature of the humerus is achieved. In the nonconforming design, the glenoid radius is mismatched to be slightly larger than the humerus radius of curvature.

The primary indications for a constrained design are shoulders with deficient rotator cuffs with superior migration of the humeral head. The Michael Reese prosthesis (Richards, Memphis, TN), a well-known constrained prosthesis designed by Post and Haskell,[28] is assembled in two components. The cavity has an internal diameter similar to that of the humeral head. The diameter of the peripheral cup is smaller, with metal-backed fixation into the glenoid. A self-locking metal ring first tightens around the humeral component and then around the glenoid. The four prerequisites for its use are (1) intact glenoid rim and neck, (2) strong anterior serratus and trapezius muscles, (3) no soft-tissue contracture that cannot be corrected, and (4) a strong deltoid muscle.[28]

Various constrained and semiconstrained prostheses have been used less frequently because good results have been reported with hemiarthroplasty alone in rotator cuff–deficient shoulders.[15] The constrained design has the highest rates of loosening (11.8%), dislocation (9.4%), and infection (2.9%).[12] The increased stresses placed on the glenoid component secondary to the higher degree of constraint lead to greater rates of aseptic loosening. Nonetheless, a constrained prosthesis may be indicated in selected patients with severe anterosuperior instability. A new constrained design, the Delta prosthesis, has shown promise in European trials but is not yet approved by the Food and Drug Administration for use in the United States.[30]

The principles of implantation of a nonconstrained glenoid prosthesis are based on reproducing key anatomy, obtaining initial fixation, and correcting bone defects. The options for glenoid implants are cemented polyethylene and metal-backed ingrowth components. The cemented polyethylene designs are divided into keeled or pegged fixation. Variations exist in keel design, although Neer's triangular keel is the gold standard. The DANA (designed after natural anatomy) hooded component (Howmedica, Rutherford, NJ) has an inferiorly directed keel, which may improve bending stability. The pegged components are differentiated by the number and size of the pegs.

Keeled Versus Pegged Components

The keeled design has shown excellent results in long-term studies of the Neer prosthesis,[12] and the keel remains the standard implant design for most total shoulder arthroplasties. Pegged glenoid components, however, may provide better fixation in higher quality bone, particularly in younger patients. Other advantages of pegs include the removal of less bone, which may allow for easier revision. Pegs also provide greater surface area for cement fixation and require less cement volume. The peg design also may offer another important variable: Giori and associates[31] have shown that multiple small pegs conserve bone stock and distribute stress more uniformly than do fewer large pegs (Figs. 6 and 7).

The keeled prostheses have greater ease of implantation and proven success. When the ability to implant a pegged component is precluded by the glenoid exposure, it may be necessary to convert to keeled preparation if instrumentation for proper peg hole creation cannot be properly placed on the glenoid surface. The potential for glenoid fracture is also greater with pegs. Lacaze and associates[32] tested in vitro pull-out strength and found a keel design with a round back to be superior to a keel design with a flat back, although both were stronger than pegged or cementless fixation. The ultimate decision to use pegged or keeled components may be affected by patient factors, however, and the surgeon should be able to adapt accordingly.

Metal-Backed Versus Polyethylene Components

The results of tissue-ingrowth glenoid components have been similar to those of cemented components in long-term studies. However, several concerns remain regarding cementless fixation. Metal increases the glenoid component thickness and lateralizes the joint line (Fig. 8); this may decrease the lever arm of the surrounding muscles. Metal backing also necessitates less polyethylene thickness, which can result in wear and polyethylene dissociation. Stress-shielding of bone may occur.[33] The larger keel and screws required may not be possible to use in smaller glenoids or where bone stock is limited. Screw osteolysis can serve as a source of early fixation failure. In contrast, Orr and associates[34] have shown that metal-backed components have improved stress transfer to bone and decreased polyethylene deformation. Wallace and associates[35] in a recent clinical study showed higher rates of early complications with metal-backed glenoids, but intermediate results are similar to those of cemented components. The in vitro study by Friedman and associates[36] suggests that polyethylene distributes stress more physiologically to bone. The stair-stepped keel design was found to be best.[36] Because improved longevity and function over cemented technique have not yet been elucidated to support ingrowth fixation, the cemented polyethylene glenoid (Fig. 9) remains the most common design in nonconstrained arthroplasty.

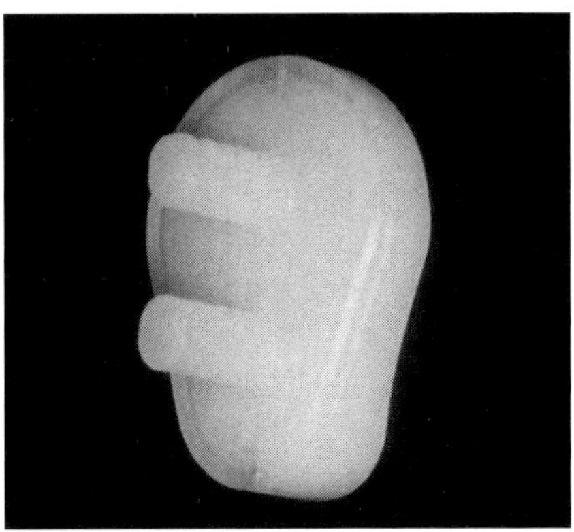
Fig. 6 Polyethylene pegged glenoid component.

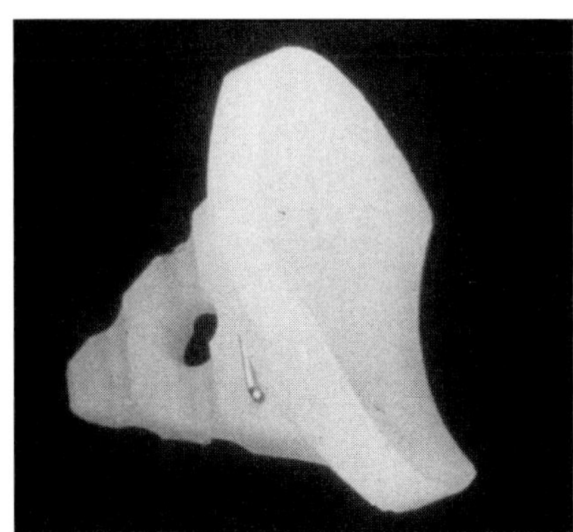
Fig. 7 Polyethylene keeled glenoid component.

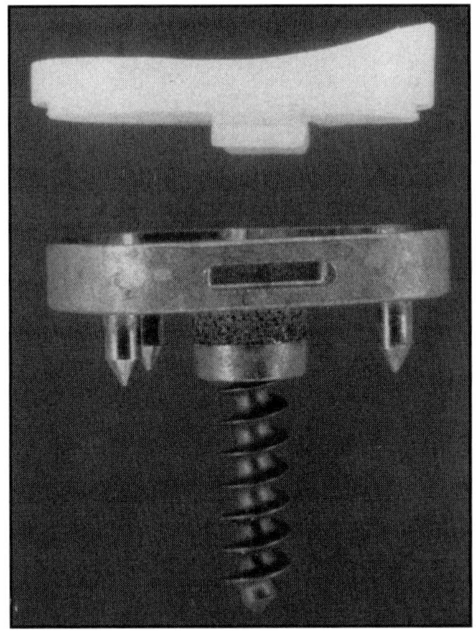
Fig. 8 Metal-backed glenoid component with screws for ingrowth fixation.

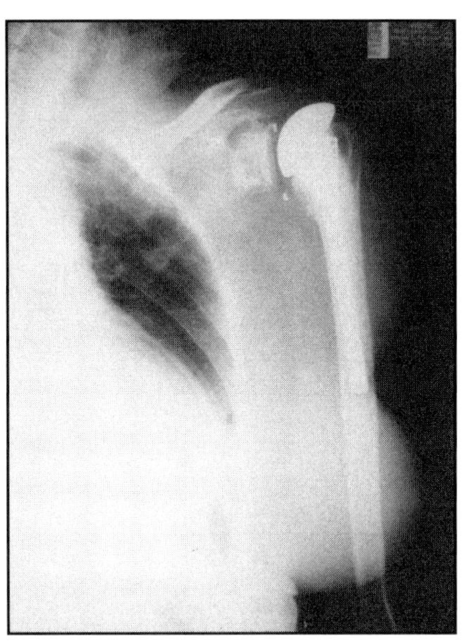
Fig. 9 Radiographic appearance of keeled cement fixation.

Conformity
The degree of conformity between the humeral head and the glenoid is determined by the radius of curvature of each. A perfectly congruent glenoid would match the humeral radius of curvature. This higher degree of conformity provides greater stability but, like the semiconstrained designs, increases glenoid stresses when the joint is loaded.[37] Mismatch of the radius of the glenoid, with a larger glenoid radius of curvature, will allow for some translation of the humeral head in the fossa.[38] However, the decreased conformity will lead to less contact area and increased linear contact stress. This may lead to increased polyethylene wear. The exact degree of mismatch to optimize results has yet to be determined, but the current recommendation of 4 mm to 6 mm of mismatch is optional.[39]

The curvature of the glenoid back is another design factor that is undergoing evaluation. Glenoid components can be flat-backed or curved-backed, regardless of whether the component is pegged or keeled. The flat-backed design may resist the rocking-horse phenomenon to some extent. The curved-backed or round-backed components were shown in the recent biomechanical study of Anglin and associates[40] and in the in vitro study by Lacaze and associates[32] to provide a greater degree of resistance to loosening with loading and pull-out stresses.

Alternatives

Hemiarthroplasty
When remaining bone stock is inadequate to support a prosthesis or the rota-

tor cuff is deficient, hemiarthroplasty with glenoidplasty of the remaining bone has been shown to have acceptable results for pain relief and motion.[15] In revision arthroplasty, the old component is removed and the remaining bone is reamed or shaped to conform to a hemiarthroplasty. Cofield[12] reported good results in eight of nine patients with loose glenoids treated with this technique.

Bone-grafting the remaining bone may allow for later reimplantation of a prosthesis.[12,41]

Biologic Resurfacing

Biologic resurfacing has been described by Burkhead and Hutton.[42] This technique was developed for younger, more active patients in whom concern for loosening of the glenoid precluded total shoulder arthroplasty. Fourteen patients were treated with hemiarthroplasty and biologic resurfacing. All patients had good results on follow-up.

Biologic resurfacing can be done with local capsule or autogenous fascia lata graft. After humeral osteotomy and removal of osteophytes, the glenoid surface is débrided, slightly increasing the anteversion in the process. If thick enough, the subscapularis-capsule complex is split in the coronal plane. The posterior leaf can then be draped over the glenoid and secured to the posterior labrum with suture or anchors. If inadequate capsule is present, a 2-in × 5-in segment of fascia is harvested from the thigh. After doubling the tissue upon itself, it is anchored to the center of the glenoid with a suture and to the anterior-posterior labrum with heavy suture, such as No. 1 cottony Dacron (Deknatel, Fall River, MA). More recently, one of us (W.Z.B.) has used Achilles tendon allograft to reduce graft morbidity and increase tissue availability. The long-term results of this procedure are yet to be elucidated.

Glenoidectomy

Wainwright[43] and Gariepy[44] have described the technique of glenoidectomy in patients with rheumatoid arthritis or cuff arthropathy. Glenoidectomy medializes the joint line and may allow closure of the cuff over a small humeral head implant. Pain relief is satisfactory with this procedure, and motion may be slightly increased.

References

1. Clayton MI, Ferlic DC, Jeffers PD: Prosthetic arthroplasties of the shoulder. *Clin Orthop* 1982;164:184-191.
2. Cofield RH: Total shoulder arthroplasty with the Neer prosthesis. *J Bone Joint Surg Am* 1984;66:899-906.
3. Neer CS II, Watson KC, Stanton FJ: Recent experience in total shoulder replacement. *J Bone Joint Surg Am* 1982;64:319-337.
4. Green A: Current concepts of shoulder arthroplasty. *Instr Course Lect* 1998;47:127-133.
5. Hawkins RJ, Bell RH, Jallay B: Total shoulder arthroplasty. *Clin Orthop* 1989;242:188-194.
6. Torchia ME, Cofield RH, Settergren CR: Total shoulder arthroplasty with the Neer prosthesis: Long-term results. *J Shoulder Elbow Surg* 1997;6:495-505.
7. Barrett WP, Franklin JL, Jackins SE, Wyss CR, Matsen FA III: Total shoulder arthroplasty. *J Bone Joint Surg Am* 1987;69:865-872.
8. Brems JJ, Wilde AH, Borden LS, Boumphrey FRS: Glenoid lucent lines. *Orthop Trans* 1986;10:231.
9. Brems J: The glenoid component in total shoulder arthroplasty. *J Shoulder Elbow Surg* 1993;2:47-54.
10. Brenner BC, Ferlic DC, Clayton ML, Dennis DA. Survivorship of unconstrained total shoulder arthroplasty. *J Bone Joint Surg Am* 1989;71:1289-1296.
11. Franklin JL, Barrett WP, Jackins SE, Matsen FA III: Glenoid loosening in total shoulder arthroplasty: Association with rotator cuff deficiency. *J Arthroplasty* 1988;3:39-46.
12. Cofield RH: Total shoulder arthroplasty: Complications and revision surgery. *Instr Course Lect* 1990;39:449-462.
13. Gartsman GM, Roddey TS, Hammerman SM: Shoulder arthroplasty with or without resurfacing of the glenoid in patients who have osteoarthritis. *J Bone Joint Surg Am* 2000;82:26-34.
14. Rodosky MW, Bigliani LU: Indication for glenoid resurfacing in shoulder arthroplasty. *J Shoulder Elbow Surg* 1996;5:231-248.
15. Boyd AD Jr, Thomas WH, Scott RD, Sledge CB, Thornhill TS: Total shoulder arthroplasty versus hemiarhroplasty: Indications for glenoid resurfacing. *J Arthroplasty* 1990;5:329-336.
16. Sperling JW, Cofield RH, Rowland CM: Neer hemiarthroplasty and Neer total shoulder arthroplasty in patients fifty years old or less: Long-term results. *J Bone Joint Surg Am* 1998;80:464-473.
17. Schenk T, Iannotti JP: Prosthetic arthroplasty for glenohumeral arthritis with an intact or repairable rotator cuff: Indications, techniques and results, in Iannotti JP, Williams GR Jr (eds): *Disorders of the Shoulder: Diagnosis and Management.* Philadelphia, PA, Lippincott Williams & Wilkins, 1999, pp 521-558.
18. Iannotti JP, Gabriel JP, Schneck SL, Evans BG, Misra S: The normal glenohumeral relationships: An anatomical study of one hundred and forty shoulders. *J Bone Joint Surg Am* 1992;74:491-500.
19. Collins D, Tenser A, Sidles J, Matsen F III: Edge displacement and deformation of glenoid components in response to eccentric loading: The effect of preparation of the glenoid bone. *J Bone Joint Surg Am* 1992;74:501-507.
20. Matsen FA III, Rockwood CA Jr, Wirth MA, Lippitt SB: Glenohumeral arthritis and its management, in Rockford CA Jr, Matsen FA III, Wirth MA, Harryman DT II (eds): *The Shoulder*, ed 2. Philadelphia, PA, WB Saunders, 1998, vol 2, pp 840-964.
21. Rockwood CA Jr: The technique of total shoulder arthroplasty. *Instr Course Lect* 1990;39:437-447.
22. Norris BL, Lachiewicz PF: Modern cement technique and the survivorship of total shoulder arthroplasty. *Clin Orthop* 1996;328:76-85.
23. Sperling JW, Cofield RH: Revision total shoulder arthroplasty for the treatment of glenoid arthritis. *J Bone Joint Surg Am* 1998;80:860-867.
24. Peterson SA, Hawkins RJ: Revision of failed total shoulder arthroplasty. *Orthop Clin North Am* 1998;29:519-533.
25. Steinmann SP, Cofield RH: Bone grafting for glenoid deficiency in total shoulder replacement. *J Shoulder Elbow Surg* 2000;9:361-367.
26. Neer CS II, Morrison DS: Glenoid bone-grafting in total shoulder arthroplasty. *J Bone Joint Surg Am* 1988;70:1154-1162.
27. Gristina AG, Webb LX, Carter RE, Romano RL: The monospherical total shoulder. *Orthop Trans* 1985;9:54-55.
28. Post M, Haskell SS, Jablon M: Total shoulder replacement with a constrained prosthesis. *J Bone Joint Surg Am* 1980;62:327-335.
29. Coughlin MJ, Morris JM, West WF: The semiconstrained total shoulder arthroplasty. *J Bone Joint Surg Am* 1979;61:574-581.
30. Grammont PM, Baulot E: Delta shoulder prosthesis for rotator cuff rupture. *Orthopedics* 1993;16:65-68.
31. Giori NJ, Beaupre GS, Carter DR: The influence of fixation peg design on the shear stability of prosthetic implants. *J Orthop Res* 1990;8:892-898.
32. Lacaze F, Kempf JF, Bonnomet F, Boutney P, Colin F: Primary fixation of glenoid implants: An in vitro study, in Walch G, Boileau P (eds): *Shoulder Arthroplasty*. Berlin, Germany, Springer-Verlag, 1999, pp 141-146.

33. Stone KD, Grabowski JJ, Cofield RH, Morrey BF, An KN: Stress analyses of glenoid components in total shoulder arthroplasty. *J Shoulder Elbow Surg* 1999;8:151-158.

34. Orr TE, Carter DR, Schurman DJ: Stress analyses of glenoid component designs. *Clin Orthop* 1988;232:217-224.

35. Wallace AL, Phillips RL, MacDougal GA, Walsh WR, Sonnabend DH: Resurfacing of the glenoid in total shoulder arthroplasty: A comparison, at a mean of five years, of prostheses inserted with and without cement. *J Bone Joint Surg Am* 1999;81:510-518.

36. Friedman RJ, LaBerge M, Dooley RL, O'Hara AL: Finite element modeling of the glenoid component: Effect of design parameters on stress distribution. *J Shoulder Elbow Surg* 1992;1:261-270.

37. Ballmer FT, Lippitt SB, Romeo AA, Matsen FA III: Total shoulder arthroplasty: Some considerations related to glenoid surface contact. *J Shoulder Elbow Surg* 1994;3:299-306.

38. Harryman DT II, Sidles JA, Clark JM; McQuade KJ, Gibb TD, Matsen FA III: Translation of the humeral head on the glenoid with passive glenohumeral motion. *J Bone Joint Surg Am* 1990;72:1334-1343.

39. Harryman DT, Sidles JA, Harris SL, Lippitt SB, Matsen FA III: The effect of articular conformity and the size of the humeral head component on laxity and motion after glenohumeral arthroplasty: A study in cadavera. *J Bone Joint Surg Am* 1995;77:555-563.

40. Anglin C, Wyss UP, Pichora DR: Mechanical testing of shoulder prostheses and recommendations for glenoid design. *J Shoulder Elbow Surg* 2000;9:323-331.

41. Hawkins RJ, Greis PE, Bonutti PM: Treatment of symptomatic glenoid loosening following unconstrained shoulder arthroplasty. *Orthopedics* 1999;22;229-234.

42. Burkhead WZ Jr, Hutton KS: Biologic resurfacing of the glenoid with hemiarthroplasty of the shoulder. *J Shoulder Elbow Surg* 1995;4:263-270.

43. Wainwright D: Abstract: Glenoidectomy: A method of treating the painful shoulder in severe rheumatoid arthritis. *Ann Rheum Dis* 1974;33:110.

44. Gariepy R: Abstract: Glenoidectomy in the repair of the rheumatoid shoulder. *J Bone Joint Surg Br* 1997;59:122.

Glenoid Resurfacing in Shoulder Arthroplasty: Indications and Contraindications

Keith M. Baumgarten, MD
Cyrus J. Lashgari, MD
Ken Yamaguchi, MD

Abstract

The indications for glenoid resurfacing are controversial. Advantages of glenoid resurfacing include decreased glenoid pain from metal-on-bone articulation, increased stability provided by the conforming glenoid component in the presence of asymmetric glenoid wear, and lateralization of the joint line providing for improved range of motion and strength. Proponents of hemiarthroplasty claim that function and pain relief are equivalent to glenoid resurfacing without the concomitant risk of glenoid loosening and loss of glenoid bone stock. In addition, hemiarthroplasty requires less surgical time and is less expensive than total shoulder arthroplasty.

Total shoulder arthroplasty has been shown to be superior to hemiarthroplasty with regard to pain relief, range of motion, and function. Resurfacing of the glenoid has been indicated in older patients with primary osteoarthritis. In addition, patients with rheumatoid arthritis generally have better improvement in pain and function when treated with total shoulder arthroplasty than with hemiarthroplasty.

Patients with severe rotator cuff disease, persistent instability, and lack of glenoid bone stock should be treated with hemiarthroplasty alone because glenoid resurfacing is associated with early loosening and failure. Patients with osteonecrosis isolated to the humeral head should be treated with hemiarthroplasty to preserve the native, congruent glenoid.

Treatment of glenohumeral disease was revolutionized in the 1970s when Neer[1] first reported successful results with resurfacing of the glenoid with a polyethylene component. Glenoid resurfacing with humeral head arthroplasty, known as total shoulder arthroplasty, has several theoretical advantages over humeral head hemiarthroplasty alone: first, resurfacing of the glenoid decreases glenoid-derived pain from a metal-on-bone articulation; second, increased stability is provided by the articulation between the prosthetic humeral head and the conforming glenoid component; third, the conforming glenoid component helps recenter the articulation when asymmetric wear is present; and fourth, the glenoid component lateralizes the wear-derived medialization of the joint line, anatomically tensions the rotator cuff and deltoid, and provides a better fulcrum for added range of motion and strength.

Despite these advantages, the indications for total shoulder replacement remain controversial. Advocates of hemiarthroplasty have described several theoretical advantages of the procedure. Hemiarthroplasties perform as well as total shoulder arthroplasties in improving motion and function and in providing pain relief. There is no concern for glenoid component failure in patients treated with humeral hemiarthroplasty, and there is no bone loss from the glenoid vault if revision surgery is necessary. Hemiarthroplasty is technically easier, requires less surgical time, and the total monetary cost is less than that for total shoulder arthroplasty. Finally, there may be a perception that only a minority of patients have glenoid-derived pain after hemiarthroplasty, and conversion to a total shoulder arthroplasty can relieve pain and dysfunction.

The previously mentioned considerations can be confusing and the issue of glenoid resurfacing in the treatment of glenohumeral disease has been a controversial one; however, a review of the literature has shown substantial support for glenoid resurfacing for the most common indications for glenohumeral arthroplasty.

Table 1
Classification of Glenoid Loosening

Classification	Description
Not loose	No radiolucent lines, or radiolucent lines limited to the flange; no change in position
Minimal risk of loosening	Incomplete line less than 2 mm and involving less than one third of the keel
Possibly loose	Incomplete line less than 2 mm that involves more than one third of the keel
Probably loose	Complete radiolucent line less than 1.5 mm Incomplete line greater than 2 mm involving more than one third of the keel
Definitely loose	Complete line greater than 1.5 mm or a shift in glenoid position

Total Shoulder Arthroplasty

Results of Total Shoulder Arthroplasty

Overall, the results of total shoulder arthroplasty have been very successful. Short-term survivorship was shown to be 97% at 5 years and 93% at 8 years with only 1 of 35 patients unsatisfied with the outcome.[2] Long-term follow-up of patients who had undergone total shoulder arthroplasty to treat a variety of glenohumeral diseases showed 93% survival at 10 years and 87% survival at 15 years.[3] Another long-term study showed a 75% survivorship at 11 years.[4] Eighty-three percent to 88% of patients had no or mild pain.[3-5] Neer showed a mean improvement of 77° of elevation and 51° of external rotation in patients with osteoarthritis and 57° of elevation and 60° of external rotation in patients with rheumatoid arthritis.[6]

The mean complication rate associated with total shoulder arthroplasty was 16%. Complications, listed in order of frequency, were component loosening, glenohumeral instability, rotator cuff tear, periprosthetic fracture, infection, implant failure, and deltoid dysfunction.[7] The symptomatic glenoid failure rate ranged from 0% to 12.5% of total shoulder arthroplasties.[8] Revision procedures due to glenoid loosening were necessary in only 5.6% of cases.[3]

Radiolucent Lines

Ever since the advent of cemented glenoid components, incomplete and complete radiolucent lines surrounding the glenoid have been observed on postoperative radiographs. The presence of these radiolucent lines are cause for concern; as a result, hemiarthroplasty has been advocated as a better treatment method for glenohumeral disease.

The reported incidence of partial or complete radiolucent lines on postoperative radiographs ranges from 26% to 100%.[8] Neer found that most lucent lines were present on immediate postoperative radiographs, and it was suggested that surgical technique might be responsible for these lines. One group noted that 69% of glenoid lucent lines were present on recovery room radiographs.[9] The presence of radiolucent lines was statistically correlated with methods of bone preparation. It was determined that the more meticulously the glenoid was prepared, the lower the incidence of radiolucent lines.[10] Modern cementing techniques, including pulsatile lavage, thorough drying, and pressurized cementing, were shown to decrease progressive radiolucencies and may improve implant survival.[2]

The presence of radiolucent lines on postoperative radiographs does not necessarily mean that the glenoid component is clinically loose. Radiographic lines isolated to the flange are not associated with glenoid loosening.[5] One system for assessing radiographic evidence of glenoid loosening classifies the glenoid into five categories as outlined in Table 1.[3] In addition, progression of radiolucencies causes concern for glenoid loosening. Progression of glenoid radiolucencies ranged from 0% to 36% of total shoulder arthroplasties in one literature review.[8]

The clinical significance of these radiolucent lines has been debated. Components that are deemed radiographically suspicious for loosening are not usually clinically relevant. In the 194 shoulders studied by Neer,[6] there were only two glenoids with radiographic evidence of loosening but no instances of clinical loosening. Another report described four asymptomatic patients with good function who had radiographic evidence of glenoid loosening including two glenoids that had a frank shift in position.[11] A study by Sperling and associates[12] showed no difference in pain, range of motion, or Neer results in patients who were at risk and who were not radiographically at risk for loosening. Despite these reference studies, there remains some concern about radiolucent lines; two retrospective reviews have shown a statistically significant correlation with glenoid loosening and pain.[3,13] One recent review showed that 58% of all total shoulder arthroplasties had radiolucent lines with 23% progressing over time.[13] The subgroup of patients without radiolucencies had more good and excellent results (86%) compared with the subgroup with glenoid radiolucencies (75%); however, of the 251 total shoulder arthroplasties done in the study, only 3 (1.2%) needed revisions for glenoid loosening: two cementless glenoids and one cemented glenoid.[13] In comparison, of 17 hemiarthroplasties followed in this same study, and 1 (5.9%) required a revision procedure for painful glenoid erosion. These authors noted that they did not use modern cementing techniques in this cohort and have therefore changed their practice in the hope of reducing the incidence of glenoid radiolucencies. Torchia and associates[3] also found that glenoid loosening was associated with pain. However, of the 44% of patients having radiographic evidence of loosening, only 5.6% of these patients needed revision surgery for symptomatic loosening . Thus, only a minority of patients with clinically evident loosening actually underwent revision surgery.

The relationship of radiolucent lines and glenoid loosening that is clinically relevant is still not clear. Very few patients with radiolucent lines develop clinically apparent loosening.[6,10,14,15] Even fewer patients require revision surgery for glenoid loosening.[3,13] Additionally, modern cementing techniques, not used in previous studies on glenoid longevity, should significantly reduce the incidence of radiolucencies around the glenoid.

Hemiarthroplasty

Results of Hemiarthroplasty

In 1974, Neer described the use of hemireplacement arthroplasty for the treatment of both primary and secondary osteoarthritis. Forty-eight shoulders were retrospectively reviewed after a mean follow-up of 6 years. Results were excellent in 20 shoulders, satisfactory in 20, and unsatisfactory in 6. According to Neer, total shoulder arthroplasty might correct the slow recovery in strength and continuing fatigability he noticed in his series of patients treated with hemiarthroplasty.[1] Zuckerman and Cofield[16] evaluated the efficacy of hemiarthroplasty in the treatment of osteoarthritis and rheumatoid arthritis in 83 shoulders with a mean follow-up of 39 months. They concluded that hemiarthroplasty can be successful in patients with glenohumeral arthritis, but the pain relief is not as great or as predictable as that for patients who have undergone total shoulder arthroplasty. Another retrospective review analyzed 31 shoulders with primary or secondary osteoarthritis treated with hemiarthroplasties.[17] Seventy-four percent of patients had good or excellent results. These results were inferior to the results of a study performed by the same investigators that found 97% good and excellent results in shoulders with osteoarthritis treated with total shoulder arthroplasty.[18] An additional finding of this study was that patients with asymmetric glenoids caused by wear had less successful results than patients with concentric glenoids after hemiarthroplasty. Pain relief was similar in both groups, but active external rotation and forward elevation was limited in patients with asymmetric glenoids.

Hemiarthroplasty Versus Total Shoulder Arthroplasty

Two studies have tried to compare the outcomes of hemiarthroplasty and total shoulder arthroplasty. The first study evaluated the use of hemiarthroplasty and total shoulder arthroplasty in a heterogeneous population. Boyd and associates[19] retrospectively reviewed 64 hemiarthroplasties compared with 146 total shoulder arthroplasties in patients with osteoarthritis, rheumatoid arthritis, osteonecrosis, and posttraumatic arthritis after a mean follow-up of 44 months. Treatment was determined individually on the basis of diagnosis, radiographs, preservation of cartilage, and available bone stock. There was no difference between shoulders treated with hemiarthroplasty and total shoulder arthroplasty regarding pain relief or range of motion. However, there was better pain relief, range of motion, and satisfaction in patients with rheumatoid arthritis treated with total shoulder arthroplasty than with hemiarthroplasty. These results did not meet statistical significance. The authors also reported that the hemiarthroplasty group tended to develop increased pain, subchondral sclerosis, and joint space narrowing over time. The findings of this study may be limited by treatment biases because the groups were not randomized.

Gartsman and associates[11] addressed the potential for treatment bias by performing a prospective, randomized trial that compared total shoulder arthroplasty with hemiarthroplasty in patients with primary osteoarthritis. Twenty-four shoulders were treated with hemiarthroplasty and 27 shoulders were treated with total shoulder arthroplasty with mean follow-ups of 34 months and 36 months, respectively. Patients who underwent total shoulder arthroplasty had a statistically significant better improvement in pain relief and internal rotation than those who underwent hemiarthroplasty. There was also a trend toward improved satisfaction, function, and strength, but these gains were not statistically significant with the small treatment sample used in this study. Fourteen of the 24 shoulders that underwent hemiarthroplasty also had progressive joint space narrowing postoperatively. Seven patients had increasing pain associated with loss of joint space, with three patients requiring a conversion to a total shoulder arthroplasty. None of the patients that initially had glenoid resurfacing required revision. Two important aspects of this study are worth emphasizing: (1) For the hemiarthroplasty group, 3 patients of 24 requiring revisions to a total shoulder arthroplasty represents a very significant failure rate in only short-term follow-up. (2) All patients, whether they received a hemiarthroplasty or total shoulder arthroplasty, were considered to have "concentric" glenoids. In other words, those patients with asymmetric wear of the glenoid were excluded from consideration. Hence, the study group most likely represented more earlier forms of osteoarthritis and was skewed to a population that was more likely to benefit from hemiarthroplasty alone.

Although the results from the Gartsman study favor total shoulder arthroplasty, they are not applicable to those patients with asymmetric wear in whom the difference between hemiarthroplasty and total shoulder arthroplasty is probably even more apparent. This is important, as patients with asymmetric wear of the glenoid are more likely to represent most of those people who require total shoulder arthroplasty.

Ease and Cost of Surgical Implantation

Opponents of total shoulder arthroplasty claim that it is associated with longer surgical times, more blood loss, and a higher monetary cost than hemiarthroplasty. Gartsman and associates[11] showed that the mean surgical time was 63 minutes for the hemiarthroplasty and 98 minutes for total shoulder arthroplasty. In addition, the mean intraoperative blood loss was 150 mL for hemiarthroplasty and 300 mL for total shoulder arthroplasty; however, no transfusions were needed for either group. As for the increased expense of glenoid resurfacing, the minimum increase for glenoid resurfacing was $1,177 more than a hemiarthroplasty. The 27 total shoulder arthroplasties cost $31,779 more than the 24 hemiarthroplasties done in this study. However, the total cost of the three revision operations necessary to convert a failed hemiarthroplasty to a total shoulder arthroplasty was $47,994.[11] No revisions were needed in the group receiving the total shoulder arthroplasties. Thus, the cost of hemiarthroplasty proved to be more than total shoulder arthroplasty when revision surgery was taken into account.

In addition to cost considerations, hemiarthroplasty is considered a less complex surgery than total shoulder arthroplasty because the glenoid does not have to be fully exposed. However, exposing the glenoid requires the same capsular releases necessary to provide adequate range of motion after a hemiarthroplasty. Thus, the most technically challenging aspect of a total shoulder arthroplasty is also necessary in a well-performed hemiarthroplasty. In any case, few surgeons would view the difference in cost or surgical difficulty as justification if an operation is considered inferior.

Conversion of a Hemiarthroplasty to a Total Shoulder Arthroplasty

The most common reason for reoperation after hemiarthroplasty is conversion to a total shoulder arthroplasty after the development of painful glenoid arthrosis. The prevalence of conversion of hemiarthroplasty to total shoulder arthroplasty ranges from 1.3% to 14%.[11,20,21] In patients who converted from hemiarthroplasty to a total shoulder arthroplasty, outcome was not promising; 39% had an unsatisfactory result according to the Neer rating system.[21] Although most patients had satisfactory pain relief, three patients required reoperations and five patients had limited range of motion, thereby defined as having an unsatisfactory result. Although the occurrence of painful glenoid arthrosis necessitating revision after hemiarthroplasty is rare, many of these conversions have unsatisfactory results. Therefore, a hemiarthroplasty must not be planned with the hopes of easily converting to a total shoulder arthroplasty if the initial procedure fails.

Indications for Glenoid Resurfacing

Resurfacing of the glenoid during shoulder arthroplasty has several advantages over humeral head arthroplasty alone. Resurfacing creates a smooth glenoid surface that decreases pain and progressive erosion of the unresurfaced glenoid. It provides a better fulcrum for added range of motion and strength, and it increases the inherent stability of the glenohumeral joint. Thus, total shoulder arthroplasty is generally indicated for most patients with primary osteoarthritis and rheumatoid arthritis with an intact glenoid and rotator cuff.

Osteoarthritis

Osteoarthritis affects both sides of the glenohumeral joint. The irregular glenoid surface, if left unresurfaced, is a potential pain generator when it articulates with a resurfaced humeral head. In contrast, total shoulder arthroplasty for primary osteoarthritis has reliably provided excellent pain relief and near-normal motion and function. In Neer's initial report on 39 total shoulder arthroplasties used to treat primary osteoarthritis, results were excellent in 36 shoulders and satisfactory in 3.[6] Eighty-eight percent of 67 shoulders (60 patients) had excellent results and 9% had good results in another study of intermediate follow-up.[18]

Posterior wear of the glenoid is often associated with glenohumeral osteoarthritis. Resurfacing of the glenoid creates a more anatomic version that decreases the risk of persistent posterior instability. In addition, glenoid resurfacing lateralizes the glenohumeral joint that has already been medialized by glenoid wear. This provides for a better lever arm for the deltoid and rotator cuff and improves range of motion and strength[20] (Figure 1). Rotator cuff disease is rare in patients with osteoarthritis, occurring in approximately 5% of patients. Thus, the risk for humeral head subluxation and asymmetric loading and glenoid loosening is less likely in patients with osteoarthritis. An important indication that favors glenoid resurfacing in glenohumeral osteoarthritis is that the patients afflicted by this disease are typically of more advanced age. The life expectancy of the glenoid component often outlasts the life expectancy of the patient. The risk of needing glenoid revision surgery is minimized with increasing age of the patient. In addition, older or elderly patients place less demand on their resurfaced glenoids, limiting the joint reactive forces that may cause loosening of the glenoid component.

Rheumatoid Arthritis

Several studies showed good short-term results of glenoid resurfacing in patients with rheumatoid arthritis. Approximately 90% of patients experienced substantial pain relief.[5,6,15,22] In one retrospective review, there was complete pain relief in 48% of total shoulder arthroplasties compared with 26% of hemiarthroplasties.[19] In addition, range of motion and patient satisfaction were improved in patients with glenoid resurfacing, although the improvements were not statistically significant. Total shoulder arthroplasty was also shown to be successful in patients with rheumatoid arthritis despite a high incidence of humeral head subluxation.[22] Kelly[23] determined that glenoid revision rates were only 5.6% in patients with rheumatoid arthritis after a mean 10-year follow-up. The high rate of glenoid survival despite humeral head luxation secondary to cuff disease suggests that glenoid resurfacing in patients with rheumatoid arthritis is acceptable even in the face of significant rotator cuff disease. The most probable reason for long-term survival despite rotator cuff dysfunction is the low activity levels of patients with rheumatoid arthritis. Generally, these patients have significant afflictions of other joints that severely limit the use of their extremities (Figure 2).

Contraindications to Glenoid Resurfacing

Several factors contribute to premature glenoid loosening and failure, including inadequate bone support for the glenoid component, rotator cuff disease, glenohumeral instability, trauma, and infection. Traumatic and infectious etiologies of failure cannot be anticipated. However, patients need to be evaluated for deficient bone stock, signs of instability, and rotator cuff disease before surgical intervention.

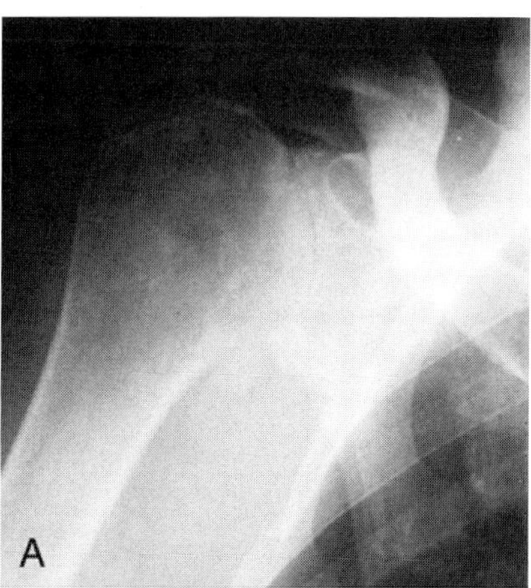

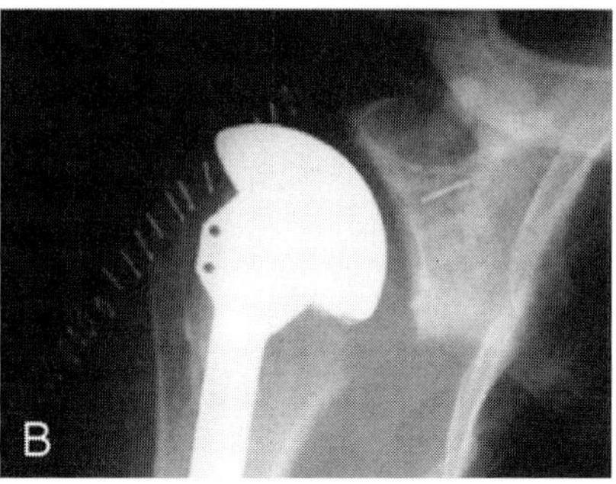

Figure 1 Total shoulder arthroplasty for osteoarthritis. **A,** The preoperative AP radiograph shows glenohumeral joint space narrowing and a prominent inferior osteophyte. **B,** The postoperative AP radiograph reveals a cemented keeled glenoid component without radiolucent lines. The humeral component has been inserted at the anatomic neck, recreating the normal proximal humerus anatomy.

Inadequate Bone Support of the Glenoid

In the normal glenoid, the volume of cancellous bone available for fixation is minimal. When disease further reduces the volume of bone, there is even less support for a glenoid component. Various disease states are known to destroy glenoid bone stock. Rheumatoid arthritis can cause large synovial cysts that destroy the cancellous bone needed for glenoid component fixation. Rheumatoid arthritis causes medial erosion of the glenoid, often diminishing the neck length to less than 1 cm.[10] Osteoarthritis may

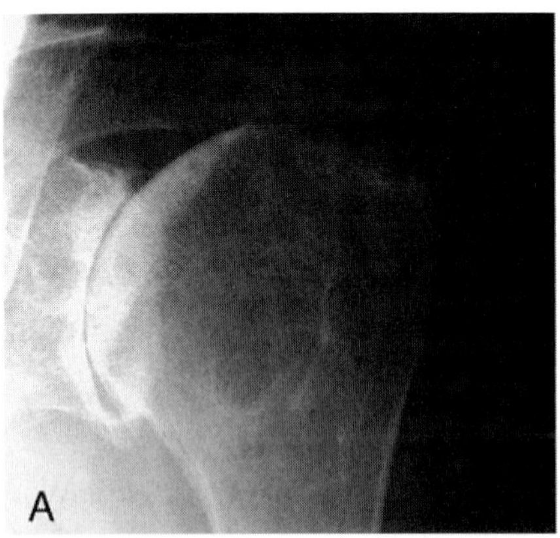

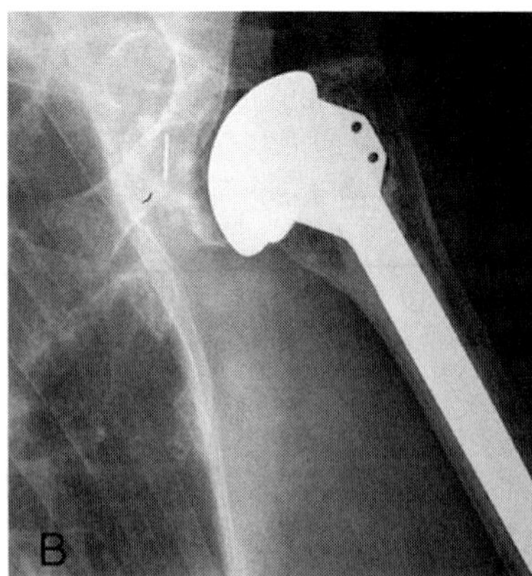

Figure 2 Total shoulder arthroplasty for rheumatoid arthritis. **A,** Preoperative AP radiograph. **B,** Postoperative AP radiograph of a cemented total shoulder. The rotator cuff was found to be thinned but intact at the time of surgery.

cause severe apparent retroversion of the glenoid due to posterior wear. This condition can lead to posterior instability that is associated with glenoid loosening.[3] Recurrent or chronic dislocations can cause anterior or posterior glenoid bone loss, further contributing to instability and the potential for glenoid component loosening. Mild peripheral glenoid loss can be treated with spherical reaming or by adjustment of the humeral version. When persistent, postreaming peripheral glenoid deficiencies are greater than 30% or an increase of persistent retroversion is greater than 15°, resurfacing should not be performed unless an ancillary procedure is done to restore bone stock or version.[24] Inadequate glenoid bone stock and a lack of congruent component contact are associated with an increased rate of component loosening. The use of methylmethacrylate to compensate for bone loss greater than 1 to 2 mm should be avoided. When the glenoid is supported by unconstrained cement, the cement may fragment, leading to glenoid loosening.

Severe Rotator Cuff Disease

The focus of treating glenohumeral arthritis in patients with rotator cuff disease is primarily to relieve pain. Functional status and active range of motion are unpredictable after shoulder arthroplasty in patients with rotator cuff disease.[25] These patients are often evaluated by the limited goals category of rehabilitation.[6] The goals of this rehabilitation program are very modest and include only painless use of the arm at the side. Patients with rotator cuff tears have less active range of motion compared with those without rotator cuff tears, and the extent of their range of motion is associated with the severity of the tear.[3,5,15]

Total shoulder arthroplasty initially was associated with successful results in the treatment of rotator cuff arthropathy in patients with a short follow-up period.[6,26] However, Franklin and associates[27] demonstrated in their retrospective series that rotator cuff arthropathy may have been associated with an increased rate of glenoid loosening and failure. The humeral head subluxated superiorly when the rotator cuff was torn and no longer maintained the congruent articulation of the humeral head and the glenoid. The subluxated humeral head caused an eccentric load on the glenoid component in total shoulder arthroplasty. This load promoted shifting of the glenoid into a more superior direction. Franklin and associates[27] termed this phenomenon "the rocking horse glenoid." Although the number of patients in this series was limited, the fundamental principles appeared sound and have generally been accepted as rotator cuff arthropathy has been associated with an increased need for revision surgery caused by glenoid loosening.[5]

Multiple series have shown improvement in both pain and range of motion in patients with rotator cuff arthropathy treated with humeral hemiarthroplasty.[28-32] In one series, 18 of 21 shoulders (86%) in 20 patients had no pain or mild pain and there was an average of 50° increase in forward flexion and a 19° increase in external rotation.[30] Hemiarthroplasty is more likely to be effective in the cuff tear population than in patients with osteoarthritis. These patients generally have much lower activity levels secondary to cuff dysfunction and have more glenoid conformity or less glenoid arthrosis. Humeral head arthroplasty provided pain relief and improvements in range of motion and function for rotator cuff arthropathy, although the results are significantly lower than those seen for total shoulder arthroplasties in osteoarthritis (Figure 3).

Instability

Total shoulder arthroplasty complicated by persistent instability and joint subluxation is associated with an increased incidence of radiographic loosening.[3] In a retrospective review of total shoulder arthroplasty, there was moderate or severe subluxation in 21 shoulders. Thirteen of these shoulders showed radiographic evidence of loosening that approached statistical significance ($P = 0.056$).

Rheumatoid Arthritis With a Grossly Deficient Rotator Cuff or Severe Glenoid Loss

Rheumatoid arthritis affects both the articular surfaces and the soft tissue surrounding the glenohumeral joint. The functionality of a nonconstrained shoulder arthroplasty in patients with rheumatoid arthritis is dependent on intact tendons, functioning muscles, and adequate bone stock. Rotator cuff failure has been reported to be as high as 50% in patients with rheumatoid arthritis.[33] If some cuff function or head coverage is obtainable, a glenoid resurfacing may still be effective if there is low activity level expectations. Of more concern, approximately 62% of patients with rheumatoid arthritis in another series had deficient glenoid bone stock.[22] Thus, these three factors must be accounted for when deciding whether to resurface the glenoid of a patient with rheumatoid arthritis.

Investigators have found high rates of glenoid loosening in some patients with rheumatoid arthritis treated with total shoulder arthroplasty. Fifty-five percent of shoulders with rheumatoid arthritis had proximal humeral migration and 40% had progressive glenoid loosening after a mean of 7.7 years.[33,34] Glenoid loosening was demonstrated in 25% of patients in another study.[23] The revision rates for glenoid loosening have remained low, between 5% and 8%.[23,24] The low revision rates most probably reflect the low activity demands in patients with rheumatoid arthritis.

Because of the varying degree of soft-tissue attenuation and glenoid loss in patients with rheumatoid arthritis, the decision to resurface the glenoid must be individualized for each patient. The key factors to analyze are the amount of bone stock available for the glenoid component, the quality of the rotator cuff, and the future ability of the rotator cuff to maintain the humeral head in a congruent relationship with the glenoid. If the rotator cuff is insufficient or there is substantial glenoid bone loss, a hemiarthroplasty may be better than a total shoulder arthroplasty.

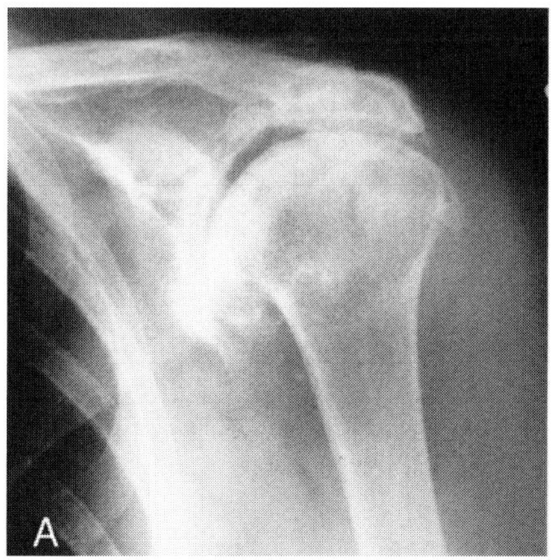

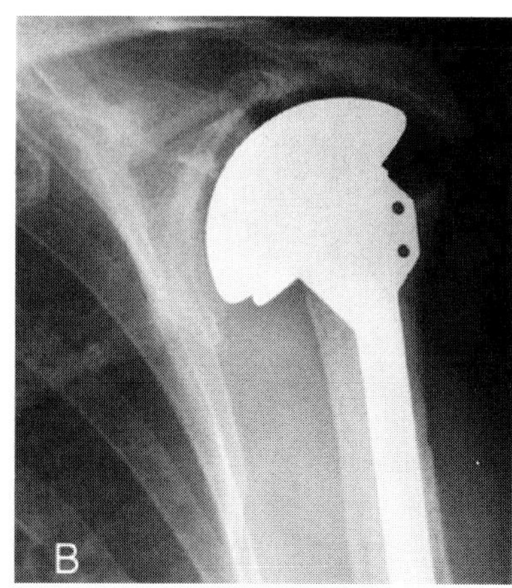

Figure 3 Hemiarthroplasty for rotator cuff arthropathy. **A,** Preoperative AP radiograph. Acetabularization of the acromion has occurred secondary to long-standing cuff deficiency. **B,** Postoperative AP radiograph. A cemented hemiarthroplasty was performed because of the irreparable rotator cuff.

Osteonecrosis of the Humeral Head

In a long-term follow-up of osteonecrotic shoulders treated with shoulder arthroplasty, there was little difference between humeral head replacement and total shoulder replacement.[35] Approximately 70 of 88 shoulders (80%) in 78 patients studied had subjective improvement. Glenoid loosening in the predominantly cemented glenoids was 38.3% at 10 years. A limitation of this study was that there was no stratification by stages of osteonecrosis to determine if there was glenoid articular destruction. Early stages of both primary and secondary osteonecrosis of the humeral head do not affect the articular surface of the glenoid. Thus, glenoid resurfacing is usually unnecessary in early stages of osteonecrosis (Figure 4). If the glenoid articular surface is damaged in the later stages of osteonecrosis by articulating with an incongruent humeral head, glenoid resurfacing should be considered to allow for a smooth, less painful articulation with the humeral prosthesis.

Controversial Issues in Glenoid Resurfacing

Young Patients

A theoretical concern in young patients is that they are more active and place greater demands on their shoulder arthroplasties, placing higher loads and joint reactive forces on their glenoid components than do older people who are more sedentary. This suggests that young patients are at higher risk for glenoid failure and revision surgery than their older counterparts. However, there was no statistically significant difference in outcome or survival of total shoulder arthroplasty and humeral hemiarthroplasty in patients younger than 50 years of age.[20] Both groups had a significant decrease in pain. Thirty-eight percent of the glenoid resurfacing group and 45% of the hemiarthroplasty group had unsatisfactory re-

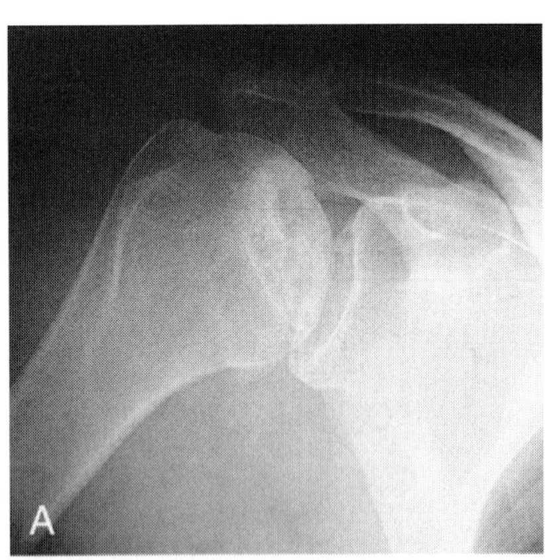

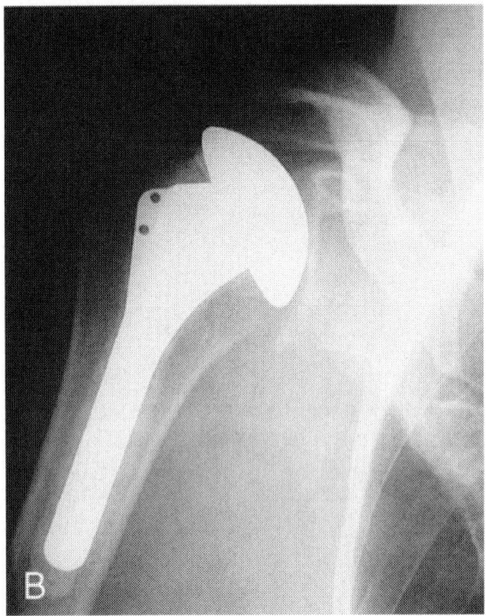

Figure 4 Hemiarthroplasty for osteonecrosis. **A,** Preoperative AP radiograph showing articular collapse of the humeral head. **B,** Postoperative AP radiograph. A cemented hemiarthroplasty was performed. The glenoid cartilage was found to be preserved at the time of surgery.

sults. These high rates of unsatisfactory results necessitate careful patient selection and the pursuit of alternate treatments when considering shoulder arthroplasty in the young patient. It may be that alternative forms of glenoid resurfacing such as the use of soft tissue could be preferable.

Biologic Resurfacing

Biologic resurfacing of the glenoid has been performed in a small number of patients. Younger patients with glenoid disease may benefit from biologic resurfacing because it is free of the complications associated with prosthetic glenoid resurfacing such as polyethylene wear, cement fragmentation, glenoid loosening and dissociation, and bone loss associated with glenoid revisions. In addition, it can be used in revision total shoulder arthroplasty when replacement of the glenoid component is contraindicated (WZ Burkhead Jr, MD, Orlando, FL, unpublished data presented at the American Shoulder and Elbow Surgeons annual meeting, 1995). The subscapularis-capsule complex and autogenous fascia lata graft was used to resurface the glenoid in six patients.[36] Pain relief and the Neer rating scale were excellent in five patients and satisfactory in one. Patients were able to return to heavy manual labor and sports activities.

The use of lateral meniscal allografts has been proposed as an alternative strategy in a series of six patients; all were satisfied with the procedure and had significant improvements in range of motion.[37] The use of meniscal allograft tissue has theoretical advantages for improved mechanical properties in comparison to capsular grafts. Another potential advantage of biologic resurfacing is that it does not preclude future procedures such as total shoulder arthroplasty or fusion. Additional studies with larger numbers of patients are necessary to determine the long-term success of biologic resurfacing.

Glenoid Revision Surgery

Revision of glenoid components as a result of loosening has been reported to be as high as 5.6%.[3] Cofield and Edgerton[38] showed that 89% of patients treated with glenoid removal at revision surgery had satisfactory pain relief. However, patient satisfaction and degree of external rotation were significantly higher in those who had glenoid resurfacing rather than glenoid component removal.[39] Replacement of the glenoid component is usually possible if central or peripheral bone loss is limited. When bone loss is severe, bone grafting can be considered.

Summary

Glenoid resurfacing is advocated to treat patients with an incongruent glenoid. Older patients with intact rotator cuffs and adequate bone stock are also good candidates for glenoid resurfacing because total shoulder arthroplasty has results that are superior to hemiarthroplasty in the treatment of osteoarthritis.

The risk of glenoid resurfacing is that the glenoid component can loosen, causing pain, decreased function, and the need for revision surgery. This risk has been realized in patients with glenohumeral subluxation (ie, instability and irreparable rotator cuff tears). Therefore, glenoid resurfacing is not recommended in patients with massive rotator cuff tears or persistent glenohumeral instability. Patients with significant glenoid bone loss cannot provide adequate subchondral bone for stable glenoid fixation, and glenoid resurfacing should be avoided in these patients. In addition, glenoid resurfacing should not be performed in patients with normal glenoids.

Glenoid resurfacing remains controversial in younger patients and patients with posttraumatic arthritis. Biologic resurfacing of the glenoid is a relatively new procedure that may aid in the treatment of patients with incongruent glenoids that are not eligible for a prosthetic component. Long-term studies are necessary to further delineate their efficacy in treating glenohumeral disease.

It is important to realize that the aforementioned indications and contraindications to glenoid resurfacing are not steadfast. However, they are guidelines to follow when treating individual patients with glenohumeral disease.

References

1. Neer CS II: Replacement arthroplasty for glenohumeral osteoarthritis. *J Bone Joint Surg Am* 1974;56:1-13.
2. Norris BL, Lachiewicz PF: Modern cement technique and the survivorship of total shoulder arthroplasty. *Clin Orthop* 1996;328:76-85.
3. Torchia ME, Cofield RH, Settergren CR: Total shoulder arthroplasty with the Neer prosthesis: Long-term results. *J Shoulder Elbow Surg* 1997;6:495-505.
4. Brenner BC, Ferlic DC, Clayton ML, Dennis DA: Survivorship of unconstrained total shoulder arthroplasty. *J Bone Joint Surg Am* 1989;71:1289-1296.
5. Barrett WP, Franklin JL, Jackins SE, Wysc CR, Matsen FA III: Total shoulder arthroplasty. *J Bone Joint Surg Am* 1987;69:865-872.
6. Neer CS II, Watson KC, Stanton FJ: Recent experience in total shoulder replacement. *J Bone Joint Surg Am* 1982;64:319-337.
7. Wirth MA, Rockwood CA Jr: Complications of shoulder arthroplasty. *Clin Orthop* 1994;307:47-69.
8. Rodosky MW, Bigliani LU: Indications for glenoid resurfacing in shoulder arthroplasty. *J Shoulder Elbow Surg* 1996;5:231-248.
9. Brems JJ, Wilde AH, Borden LS, Boumphrey RS: Glenoid lucent lines. *Orthop Trans* 1986;10:231.
10. Brems J: The glenoid component in total shoulder arthroplasty. *J Shoulder Elbow Surg* 1993;2:47-54.
11. Gartsman GM, Roddey TS, Hammerman SM: Shoulder arthroplasty with or without resurfacing of the glenoid in patients who have osteoarthritis. *J Bone Joint Surg Am* 2000;82:26-34.
12. Sperling JW, Cofield RH, O'Driscoll SW, Torchia ME, Rowland CM: Radiographic assessment of ingrowth total shoulder arthroplasty. *J Shoulder Elbow Surg* 2000;9:507-513.
13. Godeneche A, Boileau P, Favard L, et al: Prosthetic replacement in the treatment of osteoarthritis of the shoulder: Early results in 268 cases. *J Shoulder Elbow Surg* 2002;11:11-18.
14. Wallace AL, Phillips RL, MacDougal GA, Walsh WR, Sonnabend DH: Resurfacing of the glenoid in total shoulder arthroplasty: A comparison, at a mean of five years, of prostheses inserted with and without cement. *J Bone Joint Surg Am* 1999;81:510-518.
15. Cofield RH: Total shoulder arthroplasty with the Neer prosthesis. *J Bone Joint Surg Am* 1984;66:899-906.
16. Zuckerman JD, Cofield RH: Proximal humeral prosthetic replacement in glenohumeral arthritis. *Orthop Trans* 1986;10:231-232.
17. Levine WN, Djurasovic M, Glasson JM, Pollock RG, Flatow EL, Bigliani LU: Hemiarthroplasty for glenohumeral osteoarthritis: Results correlated to degree of glenoid wear. *J Shoulder Elbow Surg* 1997;6:449-454.
18. Pollock RG, Higgs GB, Codd TP, et al: Abstract: Total shoulder replacement for the treatment of primary glenohumeral osteoarthritis. *J Shoulder Elbow Surg* 1995;4:S12.
19. Boyd AD Jr, Thomas WH, Scott RD, Sledge CB, Thornhill TS: Total shoulder arthroplasty versus hemiarthroplasty: Indications for glenoid resurfacing. *J Arthroplasty* 1990;5:329-336.
20. Sperling JW, Cofield RH, Rowland CM: Neer hemiarthroplasty and Neer total shoulder arthroplasty in patients fifty years old or less: Long-term results. *J Bone Joint Surg Am* 1998;80:464-473.
21. Sperling JW, Cofield RH: Revision total shoulder arthroplasty for the treatment of glenoid arthrosis. *J Bone Joint Surg Am* 1998;80:860-867.
22. Kelly IG, Foster RS, Fisher WD: Neer total shoulder replacement in rheumatoid arthritis. *J Bone Joint Surg Br* 1987;69:723-726.
23. Kelly IG: Unconstrained shoulder arthroplasty in rheumatoid arthritis. *Clin Orthop* 1994;307:94-102.
24. Bell RH, Noble JS: The management of significant glenoid deficiency in total shoulder arthroplasty. *J Shoulder Elbow Surg* 2000;9:248-256.
25. Zeman CA, Arcand MA, Cantrell JS, Skedros JG, Burkhead WZ Jr: The rotator cuff-deficient arthritic shoulder: Diagnosis and surgical management. *J Am Acad Orthop Surg* 1998;6:337-348.
26. Pollock RG, Deliz ED, McIlveen SJ, et al: Prosthetic replacement in rotator cuff-deficient shoulders. *J Shoulder Elbow Surg* 1992;1:173-186.
27. Franklin JL, Barrett WP, Jackins SE, Matsen FA III: Glenoid loosening in total shoulder arthroplasty: Association with rotator cuff deficiency. *J Arthroplasty* 1988;3:39-46.
28. Field LD, Zubinski SJ, Dines DM, Warren RF, Altchek DW: Abstract: Hemiarthroplasty of the shoulder for rotator cuff arthropathy. *J Shoulder Elbow Surg* 1995;4:S62.
29. Poppen NK, Walker PS: Forces at the glenohumeral joint in abduction. *Clin Orthop* 1978;135:165-170.
30. Williams GR Jr, Rockwood CA Jr: Hemiarthroplasty in rotator cuff-deficient shoulders. *J Shoulder Elbow Surg* 1996;5:362-367.
31. Arntz CT, Matsen FA III, Jackins S: Surgical management of complex irreparable rotator cuff deficiency. *J Arthroplasty* 1991;6:363-370.
32. Williams GR: Glenohumeral acromio arthritis and severe cuff disease management with hemiarthroplasty. *Orthop Trans* 1992;16:743.
33. Sojbjerg JO, Frich LH, Johannsen HV, Sneppen O: Late results of total shoulder replacement in patients with rheumatoid arthritis. *Clin Orthop* 1999;366:39-45.
34. Sneppen O, Fruensgaard S, Johannsen HV, Olsen BS, Sojbjerg JO, Andersen NH: Total shoulder replacement in rheumatoid arthritis: Proximal migration and loosening. *J Shoulder Elbow Surg* 1996;5:47-52.
35. Hattrup SJ, Cofield RH: Osteonecrosis of the humeral head: Results of replacement. *J Shoulder Elbow Surg* 2000;9:177-182.
36. Burkhead WZ Jr, Hutton KS: Biologic resurfacing of the glenoid with hemiarthroplasty of the shoulder. *J Shoulder Elbow Surg* 1995;4:263-270.
37. Ball C, Galatz L, Yamaguchi K: Meniscal allograft interposition arthroplasty for the arthritic shoulder: Description of a new surgical technique. *Tech Shoulder Elbow Surg* 2001;2:247-254.
38. Cofield RH, Edgerton BC: Total shoulder arthroplasty: Complications and revision surgery. *Instr Course Lect* 1990;39:449-462.
39. Antuna SA, Sperling JW, Cofield RH, Rowland CM: Glenoid revision surgery after total shoulder arthroplasty. *J Shoulder Elbow Surg* 2001;10:217-224.

Decision Making in Contemporary Shoulder Arthroplasty

Michael L. Pearl, MD
Anthony A. Romeo, MD
Michael A. Wirth, MD
Ken Yamaguchi, MD
Gregory P. Nicholson, MD
R. Alexander Creighton, MD

Abstract

Clinical experience with humeral implants has evolved over the past decade, along with a better understanding of shoulder anatomy and function. There is no question that surgeons are getting better at restoring normal anatomic relationships than in preceding decades. Whether or not this impacts implant longevity will only be known with time and further follow-up. Even over the short term, it is difficult to ascertain whether new prosthetic designs have improved patient function as well as has been implied by the related biomechanical studies. Most surgeons with experience using old and new systems realize a greater sense of predictability in achieving their surgical goals when using more modern implants. Concerns over the durability of prosthetic systems with multiple moving parts and hand-tightened locking mechanisms have almost been forgotten in shoulder arthroplasty, but time will also reveal their importance. New glenoid designs have been less exciting, the major problem being one of developing appropriate materials. Polyethylene does not behave like normal cartilage, and its wear is constant and unforgiving. Surgeons now better understand how to reconstruct the normal glenoid position and achieve more secure early fixation than in the past, but this does not promise long-term durability and freedom from complications.

Instr Course Lect 2005;54:69-85.

Resurfacing arthroplasty of the glenohumeral joint is now well established as a means to restore comfort and function to the shoulder for many conditions that alter normal anatomy. Over the past decade, anatomic studies have added to the 50 years of clinical experience initiated by Neer that details the geometry of normal shoulder anatomy, particularly with respect to the proximal humerus. The prosthetic industry has been responsive to this new information, leading to the proliferation of new prosthetic designs. Although experience is not extensive with some of these new implants, many of the design features, such as an offset head, have already been recognized as useful by most orthopaedic surgeons. Other features, however, such as variable inclination angle, invite controversy.

The first 20 to 30 years of clinical experience with shoulder arthroplasty were based on the original Neer implant and then its successor, which was widely released in 1973. The Neer II implant is a single-piece (nonmodular) structure. It has only a few stem sizes and two head thicknesses, with the heads based on a 1-inch radius of curvature. The base of the head is inclined 50° relative to the axis of the stem. At the time of its introduction, relevant anatomic data were sparse and essentially nonexistent in the literature. The modular designs that followed were based on the clinical success of the Neer II implant and aimed to improve it with contemporary thinking on implant fixation and durability. These designs are exemplified by the Biomodular (Biomet, Warsaw, IN), Select (Intermedics Orthopaedics, Austin, TX), Global Shoulder (DePuy, Warsaw, IN), and Kirschner IIC Modular prostheses (Biomet) (Figure 1). Additional benefits of modularity were often discussed, including better fit in individual patients by mixing and matching various stem and head sizes. With each new prosthetic system, the number of stem and head sizes proliferated, as did the number of shoulder arthroplasties performed.

Rigorous study of shoulder anatomy in terms relevant to prosthetic geometry did not begin until the 1990s.[1-6] Not only did it become apparent that normal anatomy was aligned somewhat differ-

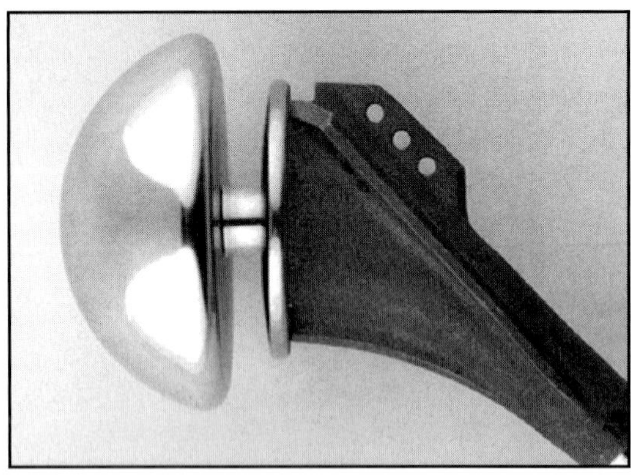

Figure 1 Photograph of a second-generation shoulder prosthesis. Note that the head is suspended from the collar by the taper locking mechanism and that there is one central position of the head for each head-stem combination.

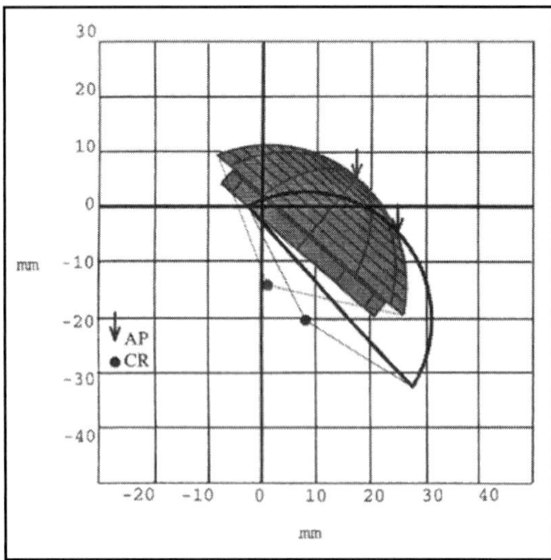

Figure 2 Two-dimensional plot showing typical mismatch between the position of prosthetic head (shaded) and the anatomic head (silhouette) as determined using a computer optimization algorithm. Note how for this prosthesis, the collar and locking mechanism accentuate the mismatch. AP, articulation point. CR, center of rotation. (Reproduced with permission from Pearl ML, Kurutz S: Geometric analysis of commonly used prosthetic systems for proximal humeral replacement. *J Bone Joint Surg Am* 1999;81:660-671.)

ently than common prosthetic devices, but it also became clear that normal anatomy was highly variable from individual to individual. In terms of replicating normal anatomy, the simple Neer II implant with its smooth stem offered some advantages over the larger modular designs, which were much more constrained with respect to their position in the canal. Most importantly, the Neer II implant placed the prosthetic head directly on the humeral osteotomy, whereas the modular systems propped it 4 to 5 mm above the osteotomy because of the prosthetic collar and the taper lock of the modular head (Figure 2). Ironically, these differences made it very difficult to restore normal anatomy using the more modern modular systems.[7,8]

Emphasis on anatomic humeral reconstruction initially came from Europe, where the Aequalis prosthesis (Tournier, Montbonnot, France) was developed. Other European designs followed, resulting in an explosion of implant options and design features in the 1990s. Concomitantly, independent anatomic studies validated many of the concerns raised by proponents of anatomic replacement.[1,4,5,7,8] Subsequent biomechanical studies further supported many of these conclusions.[9,10] New designs have continued to emerge from North America and Europe.

The questions that naturally arise are: How accurately must normal geometry be reproduced with a prosthetic head and how is this achieved surgically? (Figure 3) The first is a biomechanical question that has been well studied in cadaver models. Although it is difficult to show differences in clinical results with anatomic versus nonanatomic designs, the biomechanics of the shoulder are clearly altered in the laboratory when a prosthetic head is too thick, too thin, or shifted too far from its original position along the plane of the anatomic neck.[11,12] As a general guideline, using a head size that is within 4 mm of the original thickness and positioning it within the same range as the original should be the goal of prosthetic reconstruction. Having made this assertion, it is apparent that to achieve this goal, the surgeon must understand normal anatomy and the surgical techniques available to reconstruct it.

Normal Anatomy of the Proximal Humerus

Retroversion

Multiple studies have shown that the retroversion of the proximal humeral articular surface is markedly variable, not only among individuals but also between the left and right sides of the same individual.[2,13-15] Depending on the methodology used, retroversion ranged from 0 to 55°. Studies differ on the reference axes used to define retroversion. The proximal reference axis has been defined by the plane of the articular surface, a line connecting the center of rotation and the central point of the articular surface, or a line from the greater tuberosity to the central point of the articular surface. The distal reference axis has been defined by the trochlear axis, a line between the epicondyles, or the forearm itself. For any given individual, retroversion will measure differently, depending on which axes are used to make the measurement.

Head-Shaft Angle

The inclination of the proximal humeral articular surface relative to the shaft (head-shaft angle) is also variable, ranging from 30° to 55°, depending on the study

(Figure 4). Again, measurements vary, depending on methodology. The base of the articular surface can be approximated by a plane, but there is clearly room for interpretation in establishing this reference. Similarly, the proximal humeral canal is conical in shape, and defining its central axis is subject to variability.

Offset

The position of the proximal humeral articular surface relative to the shaft can be characterized by the distance of its center of rotation from the central axis of the canal, the humeral offset. In the coronal plane, this is the medial offset (Figure 4). In the transverse plane, this is the anteroposterior offset. Typically, the humeral head center is offset from the center of the canal in both the coronal and transverse planes. Medial offset ranges from 4 to 14 mm[2,4,15]; posterior offset ranges from –2 mm to 10 mm.[1,6]

Radius of Curvature and Head Height

The proximal humeral articular surface is variable in size as well as orientation. It is essentially spherical, particularly in its central portion, although some studies have found the radius of curvature greater in the coronal plane than in the sagittal plane.[16] Values for radius of curvature range from 20 mm to 30 mm, and it is typically smaller in women than in men. The thickness of the articular surface, head height, is equally variable but shows a striking proportionality to the radius of curvature. The ratio of the head height to radius of curvature is about 3/4, regardless of head size.[4] Importantly, this proportionality equates to a surface arc of the humeral articular surface of 150° (Figure 5).

Implant Considerations

Component design and surgical technique are inextricably intertwined. An implant is designed to fit in a certain manner, thereby endorsing a specific

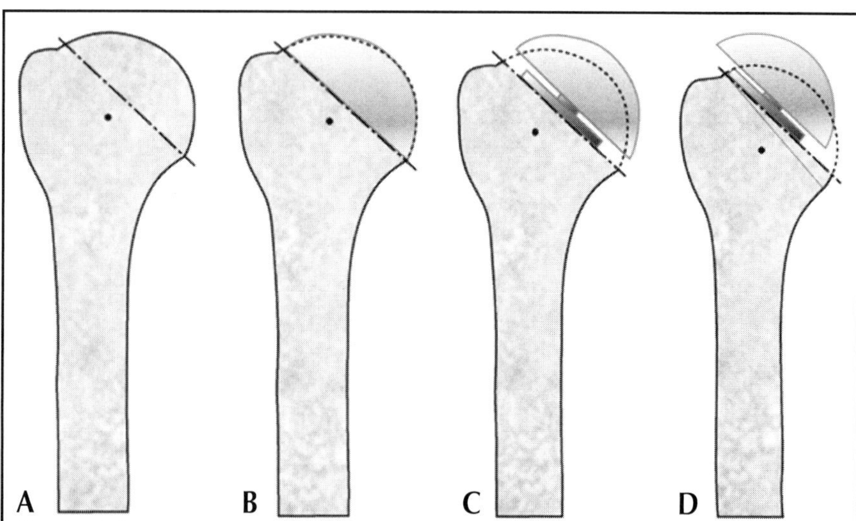

Figure 3 Schematic representation of a proximal humerus **(A)** replaced exactly with a prosthetic articular surface **(B)**, with a same size head suspended on collar and taper lock **(C)**, and malpositioning of the head that commonly occurs with second-generation prostheses **(D)**. (© Copyright ML Pearl, 2003.)

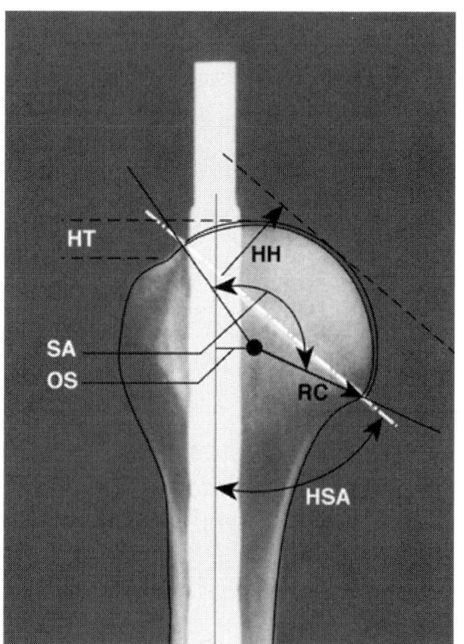

Figure 4 Radiograph marked to show the center of rotation (black dot), base of articular surface (dashed white line), center line of reamed canal (vertical black line), radius of curvature (RC), head height (HH), head to tuberosity height (HT), head-shaft angle (HSA), medial offset (OS), and surface arc (SA). (Reproduced with permission from Pearl ML, Volk AG: Coronal plane geometry of the proximal humerus relevant to prosthetic arthroplasty. *J Shoulder Elbow Surg* 1996;5:320-326.)

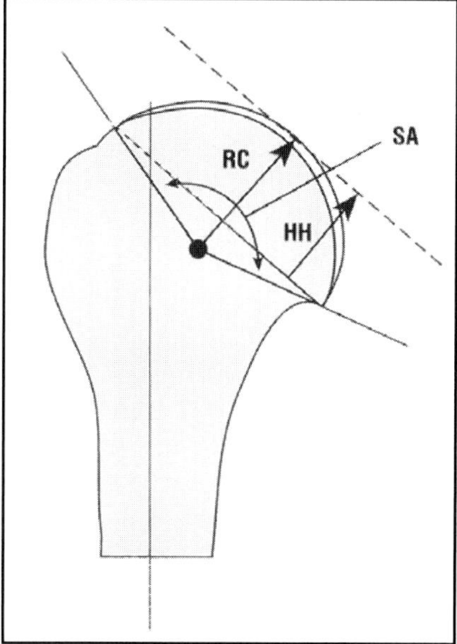

Figure 5 Schematic representation illustrating that the ratio of radius of curvature (RC) to head height (HH) is trigonometrically related to the surface arc (SA), a ratio of 3/4 equaling approximately 150°. SA = 180 – 360 arcsine[1-HH/RC]/Pi. (Reproduced with permission from Pearl ML, Volk AG: Coronal plane geometry of the proximal humerus relevant to prosthetic arthroplasty. *J Shoulder Elbow Surg* 1996;5:320-326.)

understanding of anatomy and function and the best means to restore it. This applies especially to shoulder arthroplasty over the past decade. An improved understanding of shoulder anatomy and mechanics has led to new implant design principles. Some principles have been universally adopted; others distinguish the prosthetic systems from each other. Accordingly, some elements of the surgical technique are consistent from system to system. Others are specific to the type of implant.

Humeral Head Size

The shape, size, and number of humeral heads incorporated into a prosthetic system clearly have an impact on the orthopaedic surgeon's ability to replicate normal anatomy. A greater selection of head sizes may offer greater flexibility than a limited supply, but may also add to the complexity of intraoperative decision making and lead to an unwieldy inventory of components. Without modularity between the head and stem, inventory issues are multiplied. With modularity, the biomechanical implications of suspending the head from the osteotomy because of a prosthetic collar and taper mechanism must be considered. With this proviso, the argument can be made that only anatomically sized heads are required. The counterargument is that the orthopaedic surgeon's surgical skills and the extent of the patient's joint destruction do not always allow for identical replication of anatomy. Nonetheless, modern anatomic findings caution against using head sizes that are markedly nonanatomic.

Anatomic replacement of the head size and position should produce the most accurate restoration of normal biomechanics. Increasing the humeral head thickness by 5 mm in vitro reduces the range of motion at the glenohumeral joint by 20° to 30° and results in obligate translations earlier in the range of motion.[11] It is not known, however, whether this concern applies in the context of significant glenoid bone loss where inevitable medialization of the glenohumeral joint line may slacken the overlying soft tissues. Decreasing the humeral head thickness by 5 mm may diminish the glenohumeral motion by a similar amount by reducing the surface arc available for differential motion between the humeral head and glenoid.[17] Smaller than average anatomic heads pose additional concerns of point loading of the glenoid because they alter normal glenohumeral translations and tuberosity impingement on the acromion and internally on the edge of the glenoid.[18] It is crucial that the head is not smaller than the prosthetic collar and does not allow the collar to grind on the glenoid at the end of the arc of motion. One in vivo clinical study found that smaller prosthetic heads within the anatomic range performed better than larger ones.[11]

Humeral Head Osteotomy

Humeral head size selection depends on multiple factors. The most important of these, other than the patient's original humeral head size, are the osteotomy performed by the surgeon and the inclination angle(s) of the prosthetic system. The prosthetic systems currently in use embody either of two philosophies or approaches to replacing the proximal humerus. Systems with variable inclination angles instruct the surgeon to resect the humeral head along the anatomic neck as best as possible and then provide either adjustable or variable prosthetic geometries to match the resultant inclination angle. When the anatomy allows for clear recognition of the anatomic neck, these prosthetic systems may allow for close replication of the anatomic head-shaft angle. In this context, the remaining reconstructive challenges for the surgeon are choosing the appropriate head size and putting it in the correct position.

Other prosthetic systems have a fixed inclination angle somewhere within the normal range and instruct the surgeon to make an osteotomy at this inclination, adjust the fit with additional preparation of the canal, and revise the osteotomy as necessary. For the fixed-angled systems, intramedullary guides can help achieve the provisional osteotomy and even relate it to the likely position of the prosthetic head. Surgeons using these systems develop techniques for altering prosthetic position, such as impaction bone grafting or cementing in a smaller component. The trial component often serves as a midsurgical cutting guide, allowing for revision of the first osteotomy. A wide array of head sizes that approximate the anatomic range also helps restore normal soft-tissue balance and reposition the center of rotation. It is important to realize that with either philosophy or approach, the osteotomy is an approximation of the anatomic inclination angle, and subsequent choices intraoperatively must still strive for a balanced, stable glenohumeral joint.

The osteotomy not only determines prosthetic inclination but also prosthetic version. Early descriptions of shoulder arthroplasty technique recommended an osteotomy at 30° to 45° of retroversion achieved by externally rotating the arm by this amount and cutting straight down. The known variability in anatomic retroversion challenges this recommendation in favor of individualizing the osteotomy for each patient so that it is more in line with the anatomic neck. This facilitates anatomic reconstruction of the humeral head and, most importantly, diminishes the likelihood that an errant cutting instrument violates the rotator cuff insertion (Figure 6).

Head-Stem Relationship

There are multiple indeterminate variables that result in the final position of the prosthetic body within the canal of the humerus. Different prosthetic systems have different stem lengths, some with flutes and others smooth, some in

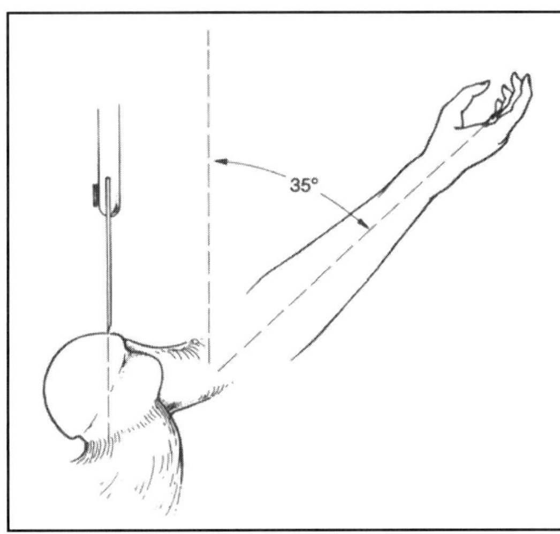

Figure 6 Schematic representation illustrating that a humeral head osteotomy with the arm in 30° to 40° of external rotation in a patient with significantly less retroversion (approximately 10°) not only makes anatomic reconstruction difficult but also runs the risk of detaching the rotator cuff insertion. (Reproduced with permission from Pearl ML, Volk AG: Retroversion of the proximal humerus in relationship to prosthetic replacement arthroplasty. *J Shoulder Elbow Surg* 1995;4: 286-289.)

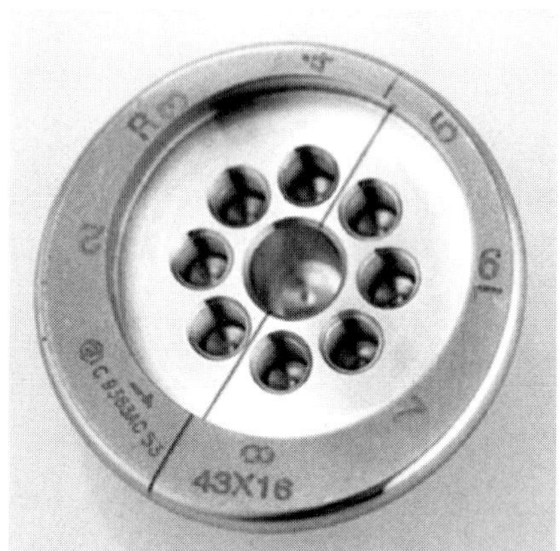

Figure 7 Photograph of the offset mechanism of the prosthetic head. For most contemporary prosthetic systems, the locking mechanism of the head is off center. Rotating the head around this off-center mechanism alters the offset accordingly.

1-mm increments and others in 2-mm increments, some cylindrical and others tapered. Prosthetic bodies have variable size, texture, fin placement, and shape. The metaphyseal region of the proximal humerus also differs among patients not only in morphology but also in the density of the bone. Altogether, these variables make the precise positioning of any given prosthetic system in any given patient unpredictable. The surgeon can influence prosthetic position to some extent; however, the goal of anatomic positioning of the prosthetic head is best served by the intraoperative flexibility afforded by an eccentric locking position of the Morse taper (Figure 7). This not only allows surgeons to make adjustments to the variable medial offset but to focus attention on the commonly encountered posterior offset.

As described, using a head that is too thin or thick has biomechanical consequences. The improper positioning of a humeral head of the correct size by over 4 mm also has untoward consequences.[10] Positioning the head too far superiorly puts additional tension on the overlying supraspinatus tendon and risks pinching it between the head and the acromion, which is an already vulnerable area of the shoulder. Positioning the head too far inferiorly may result in abutment of the greater tuberosity on the acromion or internal impingement on the rim of the glenoid. Positioning the head too far anterior or posterior similarly risks abutment of the uncovered humeral neck on the corresponding glenoid rim and excessive tension on the overlying subscapularis and posterior rotator cuff tendons, respectively.

Early prosthetic systems offered one centered position of the head for each head-stem combination. Over the past decade, most systems have offered heads that are offset by 3 to 4 mm, which allow surgeons to dial in the most suitable position for the head on the stem. Systems differ in whether they allow several discrete positions or free rotation around the taper. Some still have a centered head option. One of the most recently introduced systems (Epoca, Argomedical USA, Vista, CA) has a mechanism that allows for a range of eccentricities from 0 to several millimeters. Geometrically, more variability allows for better replication of the anatomy. How much variability is necessary and whether it is more useful in inclination, offset, or head sizes is not yet clear. These factors, however, distinguish the prosthetic systems from each other and their associated surgical technique.

A system that has variable inclination angles will instruct the surgeon to perform osteotomy of the head at the anatomic neck or the best approximation possible. The remaining challenge is then to position an anatomically sized head in the position of the original. This presupposes that the system offers enough control over offset and enough head sizes to make this possible. Proponents of these systems say that this is the only true way to completely replicate the original anatomy. Other systems offer a single or a few inclination angles that at first encounter may seem contrary to the variability found in normal anatomy. The counterargument is that the surgeon always approximates the anatomic neck anyway, especially when there has been extensive arthritic deformation of the anatomy; and if allowances are made for variable thickness in the prosthetic heads approximating the anatomic range, the normal geometry can be reconstructed around the prosthetic inclination angle (Figure 8).

Concerns and Issues Regarding Glenoid Resurfacing

It has been 30 years since Neer introduced glenoid resurfacing in shoulder replacement surgery by cementing a high-density polyethylene component

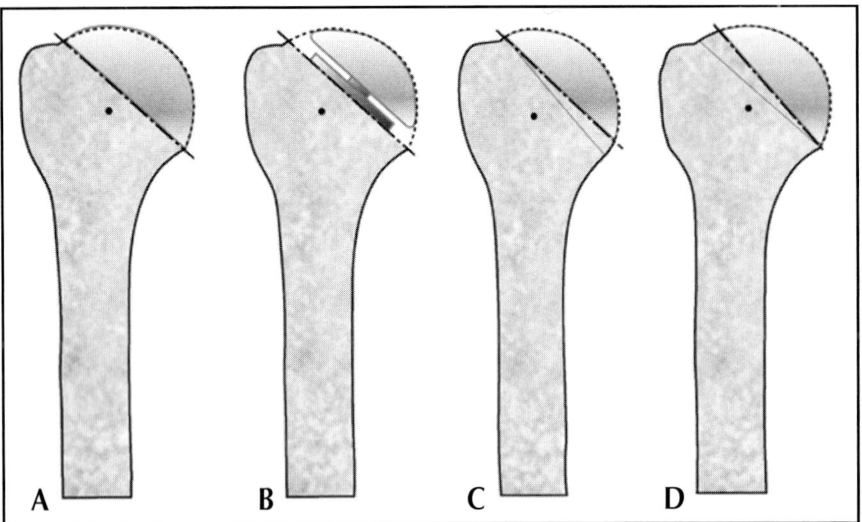

Figure 8 Schematic representation of a humeral head replaced exactly with a prosthetic articular surface **(A)**, with a smaller head suspended on collar and taper lock **(B)**, with a smaller prosthetic head placed on selective osteotomy that differs from (greater than) the inclination of the original anatomy **(C)**, and with a smaller prosthetic head placed on selective osteotomy that differs from (less than) the inclination of the original anatomy **(D)**. In all of these examples, the center of rotation is preserved as are the length-tension relationships of the overlying soft tissues. The differences in the articular surface arc and shapes of the prosthetic humeral heads may affect biomechanics, but this has not been well studied.

into the glenoid fossa.[19] The number of primary total shoulder arthroplasties performed annually is more than 10,000, and this number is increasing. Advances in total shoulder arthroplasty continue to evolve with knowledge gained from basic science and clinical research. The main objective for total shoulder arthroplasty is pain relief and improved shoulder function for everyday activities.[20-22] As the number of primary total shoulder arthroplasties increases, so does the potential for revision procedures. Although glenoid preparation and resurfacing techniques have improved, the glenoid is still the most common cause of long-term failure of total shoulder arthroplasties.[23] It is of the utmost importance to systematically evaluate the glenoid with preoperative imaging, adequate surgical exposure, and intraoperative confirmation of version and bone quality. Surgeons need to have several strategies to address the glenoid in a primary or revision setting as well as a thorough understanding of the anatomy of the glenoid, prosthetic options in the primary and revision setting, and alternatives to resurfacing.

Anatomy

The glenoid is shaped like a pear, with its superior AP diameter being smaller than its inferior AP diameter. This shape increases the arc of motion attainable and contributes to the shoulder joint having the greatest range of motion of any joint in the body. The superior AP diameter ranges from 18 to 30 mm, the inferior AP diameter from 21 to 35 mm, and the superoinferior diameter or height from 30 to 48 mm.[16] The inclination of the glenoid can vary considerably, with an average of 4.2° in the superior direction, but it can range from –7° to 20°. The version of the glenoid also is quite variable. The average glenoid version is 1.5° of retroversion, but with a range from 10.5° to 9.5° of anteversion.[24] In evaluating the osteoarthritic population, a CT study found the average version to be 11° of retroversion and the normal subject group to have an average version of 2° of anteversion.[25]

The shoulder is a conforming joint consistent with a sphere.[26] The surface area of the humeral head is roughly three times that of the glenoid, ranging from 11 to 19 mm and 4 to 6 mm, respectively. The small surface area of the glenoid does not enclose the humeral head, thereby contributing to the substantial motion of the joint. The cartilage thickness on average for the humeral head is 1.44 mm and 2.16 mm for the glenoid.[27] The glenoid has thicker articular cartilage at the periphery, and the opposite is true of the humeral head, which has thicker articular cartilage in the center. The radius of curvature of the humeral head ranges from 23 to 28 mm, and the glenoid ranges from 22 to 28 mm. The radius of curvature is within 2 mm in 88% of patients, and within 3 mm in 100% of patients, which contributes to the sphere concept of the glenohumeral joint. However, if the labrum of the glenoid is taken into account, then the radius of curvature of the glenoid exceeds that of the humeral head.[28]

Total shoulder arthroplasty has been modeled after normal anatomy.[29] The radius of curvature of new prosthetic glenoids is 2 to 6 mm larger than that of the humeral head in an attempt to recreate physiologic translation and allow for the correct balance of stability and function.[11,18,30] The goal of a prosthetic placement is 50% translation in the superior, anterior, and posterior directions.[28] One of the disadvantages of using a hemiarthroplasty or allograft replacement is that a standard size does not always match the radius of curvature of the natural glenoid.[31-33]

In deciding which type of glenoid prosthesis to use, the surgeon must first determine which patients are in need of glenoid resurfacing. Generally, a prosthesis should be used in patients with an intact or repairable rotator cuff as well as those with osteoarthritis (being aware of increased retroversion), rheumatoid arthritis (paying attention to the central defect, which is common), and arthritis with eccentric or biconcave wear. A surgeon should not place a glenoid prosthesis in patients with an irreparable rotator cuff tear, stage III or IV osteonecrosis, or severe bone deficiency. The shape and paucity of bone stock make fixation of the glenoid a perplexing dilemma.[34,35]

The importance of exposure to the glenoid cannot be overstated. This starts with the skin incision, which begins medial and superior to the coracoid, inferiorly around the axillary cleft, and laterally near the deltoid insertion. The use of proper retractors is necessary. The insertion of the pectoralis major can be released 50% to 80% to improve exposure. Identifying and tying off the anterior humeral circumflex vessels at the inferior border of the subscapularis will aid in hemostasis, thus improving exposure throughout the case. If external rotation of the arm is less than 10°, the subscapularis should be taken off its insertion, which improves external rotation by 20° to 30°. Otherwise, 1 cm of insertion should be left to repair at the completion of the case. After taking down the subscapularis and capsule, it is recommended that the release of the capsule be performed anteriorly and inferiorly to the 6 o'clock position to aid in exposure; the surgeon should always take care to be aware of the axillary nerve. After making the humeral head cut, appropriate retraction anteriorly, posteriorly, and superiorly is needed to expose the glenoid. Removal of the labrum and any osteophytes is necessary to appropriately size the glenoid. If the glenoid component is too large, then it will be unsupported; if it is too small, it will adversely affect stability. Both scenarios potentially increase the rate of wear and loosening.

After implantation of a glenoid prosthesis, the surgeon must observe the implant clinically and radiographically. The incidence of radiolucent lines ranges from 22% to 95% of patients; however, the significance of these lines remains controversial. Churchill and associates[24] found up to 69% of lucent lines are seen on immediate postoperative radiographs. Only 2.9% of the patients required revision for symptomatic loosening. These radiolucent lines remain a concern because of their significance in hip and knee arthroplasty. The radiolucent lines, however, can be influenced by imaging technique, surgical technique, duration of follow-up, and eccentric loading.[36,37] In another series, 55% of patients had radiographic evidence of radiolucent lines around the glenoid, but only 3% were revised. Collins and associates[38] reported that appropriate bone preparation with concentric reaming improves fit and enhances fixation. Visualization and meticulous hemostasis aid in this endeavor. Use of pulsatile lavage and hemostatic agents improve hemostasis and are required to get the best cement fixation possible. Improved cement techniques can lead to improved survivorship and a lower rate of component loosening.[39]

After the decision has been made to implant a glenoid prosthesis, the surgeon must then decide on the type of prosthesis. The main advantage of a metal-backed prosthesis is that it can achieve osseointegration with the potential for long-term survival. Preservation of bone stock and the modularity of metal-backed implants may also make revision surgery easier.[29] Another advantage is improved stress transfer to bone and decreased polyethylene deformation.[40] A metal-backed component may be better suited for rotator cuff-deficient shoulders displaying lower subchondral bone stresses under eccentric loading conditions. One study showed that when the trabecular bone under the glenoid was of good quality and quantity, the all-polyethylene components performed better.[41] There are disadvantages in using a metal-backed glenoid. A metal-backed prosthesis increases total glenoid thickness, which lateralizes the joint line and thereby decreases the lever arm of the shoulder. There is less polyethylene thickness, potentially resulting in increased wear. A metal-backed prosthesis has larger fixation, which requires more bone. It also can lead to stress shielding of bone and other potential areas of failure, including polyethylene dissociation and screw osteolysis. Despite these concerns, intermediate reports of using a metal-backed prosthesis are similar to cemented all-polyethylene components, but they did have increased rates of early failure.[42] An all-polyethylene component distributes stress more physiologically to bone, and until long-term clinical studies show improved result for the metal-backed prostheses, cemented all-polyethylene components remain the gold standard.[25,43]

The literature reports varying results in comparisons of keeled and pegged all-polyethylene components. The keeled prosthesis is easy to insert and has excellent long-term results.[44] A stair-stepped keeled design performed the best in distributing stress to bone most physiologically.[25] The pull-out strength was superior in a keeled round-backed prosthesis, compared with a flat-backed, pegged, or cementless prosthesis. Some studies suggest pegged components perform better.[45,46] They allow the surgeon to remove less bone, provide better fixation, and are potentially better for the younger patient population. Removing less bone allows for greater surface area for cement fixation and requires less cement volume, thereby distributing stress more uniformly throughout the glenoid.[45] One study reported that the pegged components had improved cement technique and better seating on the glenoid compared with the keeled prosthesis when evaluated using postoperative radiographs.[46] Surgeon experience also significantly affected cementing technique in this study. Because pegged components seem to better withstand shear stresses in a superoinferior direction, they are potentially better for patients with repairable rotator cuffs. On the other hand, keeled components are potentially better for patients with instability because they better withstand shear stresses anteroposteriorly.[29] Also, a component with a textured/waffled backing improves resistance to shear stresses. Until the results of longer clinical follow-up studies comparing keeled and pegged components are available, no definitive choice can be recommended. In some instances, the choice will be influenced by particular patient factors.

The incidence of revision surgeries for unconstrained total shoulder arthroplasty varies between 0 and 12.5% of patients, with glenoid loosening being the most common cause.[47,48] The reason for glenoid loosening is most often multifactorial, and treatment should be directed at those causes so the failure does not recur. Because several factors can cause glenoid failure, addressing instability, contracture, and rotator cuff failure will improve glenoid function and survival.[22,49] Glenoid failure is caused by loosening, polyethylene wear or dissociation, and component malposition. In a revision setting, the goal should be to resurface the glenoid when there is adequate bone stock. Satisfaction and pain relief have been reported to be improved in 86% of patients who underwent glenoid resurfacing compared with 66% of patients who did not undergo this procedure.[50] In removing the glenoid component and cement, the surgeon should preserve as much bone as possible. Replacement of a prosthesis is often possible in patients with mild or moderate bone loss. Concentric reaming and bone grafting may provide an adequate pedestal for reimplantation. The surgeon may also consider custom or augmented components. If the bone defects are severe or combined, reimplantation is often not possible. One study reported that only one of nine patients treated with removal of the glenoid component did not achieve satisfactory pain relief.[51] Other studies have found this approach to be satisfactory as well. Twelve of 18 patients (66%) reported satisfactory pain relief with component removal alone. The six patients who did not report satisfactory pain relief had significant glenoid arthritis.[50] Bone grafting of the deficient segment is a prudent option in this scenario because it may improve bone stock for later implantation if needed.

Alternatives

Hemiarthroplasty is useful when bone stock cannot support an implant or in patients with an irreparable rotator cuff. Hemiarthroplasty with a glenoplasty is also a reasonable option. Despite adequate success in most patients, development of painful glenoid arthrosis is the most common cause for revision of hemiarthroplasty. In a total shoulder arthroplasty revision setting, the old glenoid component is removed, and if one cannot be reimplanted, the glenoid should be reshaped. Bone grafting should be considered at this time, which may allow for later implantation of a glenoid component after bone incorporation, particularly if the patient still has a painful shoulder.[52,53]

Even though glenoid bone loss and altered version are common findings at surgery, they are most often addressed by altering the reaming direction. Alternatively, a bone graft procedure may be performed to improve bone quantity and version and allow for glenoid implantation.[49,53,54] In one series, 3.3% of patients undergoing total shoulder arthroplasty required bone grafting.[53] Neer and Morrison[49] reported on 19 patients, 16 of whom had excellent results, and the grafts incorporated with no loosening or shifting of position of the glenoid component. Steinmann and Cofield[53] reported on 28 patients, 23 of whom had satisfactory results, but radiographically more lucent lines were present than in the Neer and Morrison study. Hill and Norris[54] found that bone grafting restored version in 14 of 17 patients; however, only 50% had a satisfactory pain relief.[27] Because shoulder instability can be associated with glenoid failure, glenoid deficiency as well as the potential cause of this deficiency, instability, must be addressed. Although bone grafting is not done often, it should be considered when reaming in the opposite direction does not adequately correct version, when the patient has inadequate bone stock, and when excessive capsular laxity is present.

Biologic resurfacing for the glenoid was first described in 1995 in a younger patient population with osteoarthritis.[55] The goal was to improve pain relief and function above and beyond that which could be achieved by hemiarthroplasty alone. All patients had good results, but only six had greater than 2-year follow-up. All had substantial pain relief and improved forward elevation (average, 57°); external rotation (average, 45°); and internal rotation (average, six segments). The resurfacing was accomplished with local capsule or autogenous fascia lata graft. This technique may not only prove useful in the younger patients, but also in patients with severe bone loss who are undergoing primary arthroplasty or in a revision setting. At our institution, lateral meniscus allografts have been used in primary and revision settings. An allograft may be considered in a primary setting when the age and occupation of a patient indicate placement of a glenoid component. Also, in patients with significant bone loss in a primary setting that prevents glenoid placement, bone grafting and meniscal allograft may be considered. This scenario is more often encountered in a revision setting, and an allograft is useful when the glenoid bone quality is not sufficient to reimplant a glenoid prosthesis. The allograft meniscus is fixed through circumferential drill holes around the glenoid and sutured in place with nonabsorbable suture. This graft serves two functions. The first is to aid in conformity of the shoulder, which decreases pain and improves function. The second is to act as a barrier to the bone graft, which decreases stresses aiding incorporation of the graft. This graft incorporation will potentially allow for future placement of a glenoid prosthesis in this difficult patient population. The addition of the meniscal allograft may improve pain relief, aid in bone graft incorporation, and allow future implantation of a glenoid prosthesis if pain persists. Research is currently being conducted on this technique before routine use can be recommended.

Glenoidectomy should only be used as a salvage procedure after all other options have been exhausted. This procedure is potentially useful in patients with rheumatoid arthritis or in those with severe rotator cuff arthropathy. A glenoidectomy medializes the joint line, which improves the lever arm and potentially decreases tension to allow for rotator cuff repair. Pain relief is possible with glenoidectomy, but motion will be lost.[56]

Total shoulder arthroplasty has a proven track record of success in the correct patient population. Survivorship of total shoulder arthroplasties ranges from 88% to 97% at 5-year follow-up and 71% to 88% at 10-year follow-up.[39,42] The glenoid, however, remains a perplexing topic. The importance of an appropriate preoperative evaluation including detailed medical history, thorough physical examination, and appropriate radiographs and imaging studies cannot be overemphasized. Decisions regarding anatomic variations and associated pathology must be made by the surgeon on a patient-by-patient basis to maximize outcomes. The surgeon also needs to be familiar with the appropriate exposure, various implants, fixation options, and long-term function of the implants to make the best choice possible for a particular patient. Glenoid implantation can result in improved pain relief and function in a patient population with erosion of articular cartilage, adequate bone stock, and intact rotator cuff. In certain circumstances, not resurfacing the glenoid may be warranted, but the surgeon should be aware that the patient may still have discomfort related to glenoid arthrosis. Initial reports regarding the interposition of the glenoid side with a lateral meniscal allograft in a primary or revision setting have been encouraging, and this procedure may help achieve pain relief and incorporation of bone graft. However, additional study is needed with longer follow-up and assessment of long-term survivorship, allograft incorporation, and biomechanical properties of the allograft before widespread use of this technique can be recommended.

The Glenoid: Implantation Versus Hemiarthroplasty

Good and excellent results at early and midterm follow-up for shoulder arthroplasty have been reported in the literature. Despite an increase in the number of reports on shoulder replacement surgery over the last decade, the indications for resurfacing of the glenoid are not yet clearly defined, and various reports have described good results with routine use of either total shoulder arthroplasty or humeral head replacement alone.[35,57] Consequently, the value of using a glenoid component and the anatomic factors that affect outcome are still being debated. This ongoing controversy has confused and exasperated many orthopaedic surgeons, leaving uncertain the advisability of prosthetic replacement without resurfacing of the glenoid. Although clinical loosening of the glenoid does not commonly occur, radiographic evidence of radiolucent lines at the bone-cement interface are common, with an incidence ranging from 30% to 90%.[57] In one study with an unprecedented mean follow-up of 12 years (range, 5 to 17 years), 75 glenoid components (84%) had radiographic evidence of radiolucencies at the bone-cement interface, and 39 glenoid implants (44%) demonstrated definite radiographic loosening. Even more concerning was the statistically significant association between radiographic evidence of glenoid implant loosening and pain ($P = 0.0001$). Moreover, with increasing duration of follow-up, the number of patients reporting satisfactory pain relief declined from 92% to 82%.[44]

When compared with shoulder arthroplasty, it has been shown that hemiarthroplasty has the advantages of decreased complexity, operating time, blood loss, and cost, but does it provide favorable effectiveness and outcome?[35] A prospective randomized study involving shoulder arthroplasty with or without resurfacing of the glenoid in patients with osteoarthritis demonstrated slightly superior results in the total shoulder arthroplasty group. Specifically, total shoulder arthroplasty provided significantly better pain relief and internal rotation than hemiarthroplasty. The total shoulder arthroplasty group also demonstrated better results in the specific areas of patient satisfaction, function, and strength, although none of these differences were found to be significant. The authors noted, however, that evaluation using the University of California at Los Angeles and American Shoulder and Elbow Surgeons scoring systems revealed no significant differences in outcomes between the two groups.[35]

A recent multicenter clinical study of shoulders with primary osteoarthritis evaluated the influence of preoperative factors on outcome of shoulder arthroplasty.[58] Glenoid erosion, humeral head subluxation, and severe preoperative loss of passive motion of the shoulder were found to have significant effects on outcome, whereas a repairable full-thickness tear of the rotator cuff isolated to the

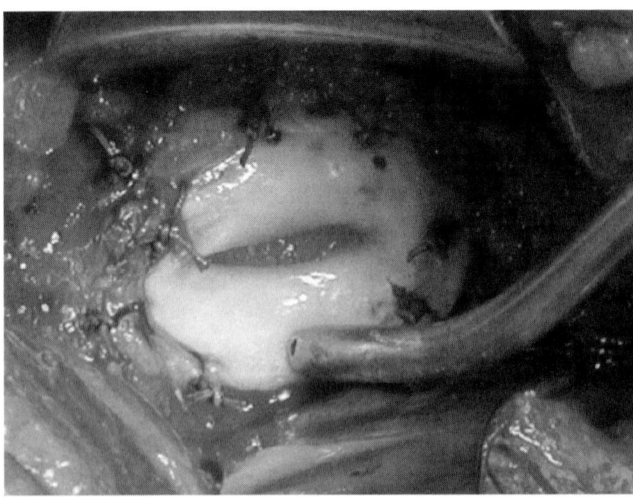

Figure 9 Photograph of a meniscal allograft secured to the glenoid with nonabsorbable sutures.

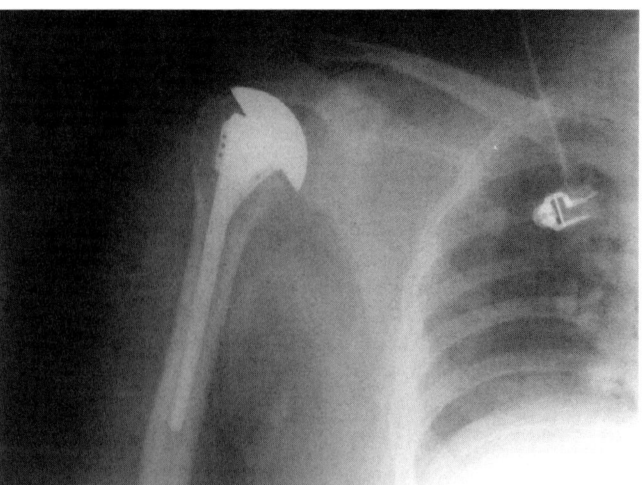

Figure 10 AP radiograph of a patient who underwent hemiarthroplasty and meniscal allograft glenoid resurfacing. Note the restored joint space.

Table 1
Indications for Prosthetic Humeral Shoulder Arthroplasty Without Glenoid Resurfacing

The humeral joint surface is degenerative but the cartilaginous surface of the glenoid is intact, and there is sufficient glenoid arc to stabilize the humeral head.
When there is insufficient bone to support a glenoid component (for example, after severe medial erosion of the glenoid in rheumatoid arthritis).
Rotator cuff tear arthropathy associated with fixed upward displacement of the humeral head relative to the glenoid.
Shoulders that are subject to heavy demands (such as certain motion disorders or an anticipated heavy loading from occupation, sport, or lower extremity paresis).
When used in conjunction with biologic resurfacing of the glenoid in young patients with glenohumeral arthritis.
Several reports from the literature have also described the results of proximal humeral prosthetic replacement for patients with osteonecrosis, osteoarthritis, rheumatoid arthritis, and posttraumatic degenerative arthritis.

supraspinatus tendon did not affect outcome. In 29 shoulders with moderate to severe eccentric posterior erosion, active external rotation and forward flexion were better after total shoulder arthroplasty than after hemiarthroplasty. Humeral head subluxation consistently resulted in a less favorable outcome regardless of whether a hemiarthroplasty or a total shoulder arthroplasty had been performed. On the basis of these data, the authors recommended the use of a glenoid component in shoulders with glenoid erosion and in the presence of a small repairable tear of the supraspinatus tendon when there is coexistent glenoid arthritis.

Hemiarthroplasty in conjunction with biologic resurfacing of the glenoid has been used as an alternative to total shoulder arthroplasty in selected younger patients. A variety of soft-tissue interpositional materials has been used, including anterior capsule, autogenous fascia lata, and Achilles tendon allograft to improve the results of hemiarthroplasty alone. More recently, soft-tissue interposition using a meniscal allograft has been used as a biologic means of resurfacing the glenoid in younger patients with glenohumeral arthritis (Figures 9 and 10). The reported advantages of meniscal allografts over other methods of biologic resurfacing include the evidence of synovial-based healing when used in the knee, improved structural characteristics, and a wedge shape that compensates for glenoid wear while contributing to the concavity-compression mechanism of shoulder stability. A review of current literature suggests that prosthetic humeral shoulder arthroplasty without resurfacing of the glenoid is indicated for the conditions listed in Table 1. Several reports from the literature in the past decade have also described the results of using proximal humeral prosthetic replacement to treat patients with osteonecrosis, osteoarthritis, rheumatoid arthritis, and posttraumatic degenerative arthritis.

For the treatment of osteonecrosis, hemiarthroplasty has provided consistently good pain relief in 90% to 100% of patients, and the range of motion approaches normal. When hemiarthroplasty is used to treat patients with rheumatoid arthritis, osteoarthritis, or posttraumatic glenohumeral arthrosis, satisfactory pain relief is less consistently achieved, but is still quite acceptable. Range of motion tends to be less, ranging from one third to three fourths that of normal.[18]

The literature comparing hemiarthroplasty and total shoulder arthroplasty favors the former to manage certain conditions of the shoulder, including inadequate glenoid bone (revision procedures or rheumatoid arthritis with moderate to severe medial glenoid erosion), irreparable rotator cuff tears associated with fixed upward displacement of the humeral head relative to the glenoid, glenohumeral arthrosis in younger patients when used in conjunction with biologic resurfacing of the glenoid, and osteonecrosis of the humeral head associated with an intact cartilaginous surface of the glenoid.

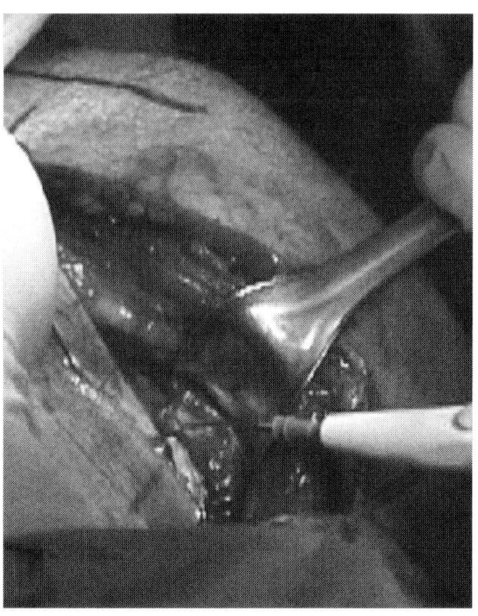
Figure 11 Photograph showing release of the upper pectoralis major during initial exposure. A Darrach retractor is placed under the tendon to protect deep structures, and then the upper 3 to 4 cm is incised.

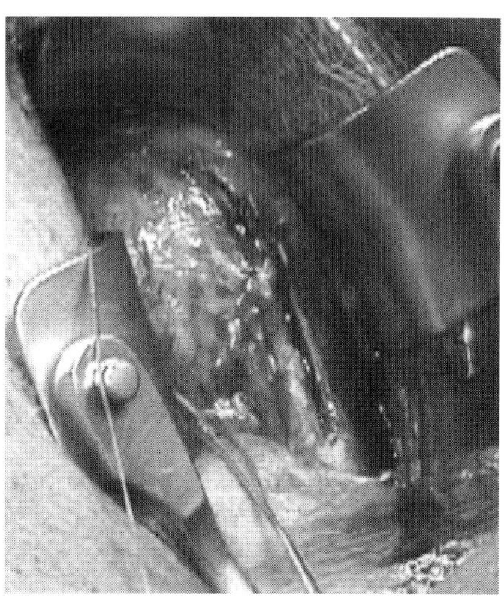
Figure 12 Photograph showing the bicipital groove that serves as a landmark to find and release the rotator interval. The transverse humeral ligament is incised and the release extended proximally into the rotator interval. At this point the biceps tendon is tenotomized at the origin.

Surgical Technique

Total shoulder arthroplasty is relatively uncommon, with the average orthopaedic surgeon performing less than five of these procedures per year. Therefore, the surgical technique is generally considered difficult in comparison with the more commonly performed knee and hip arthroplasties. Several important surgical technical considerations during humeral and glenoid exposure can greatly decrease the difficulty of the technique and thus improve the reproducibility of the procedure for less experienced surgeons.

For total shoulder arthroplasty, the shoulder is generally approached through a deltoid pectoral incision. The patient is placed in a modified beach chair position, in which the back is inclined to a 45° angle. The arm must be draped free so that a large degree of extension is possible to allow anterior dislocation of the humeral head. The incision should begin at the anterior aspect of the clavicle and extend distally directly over the coracoid process toward the insertion of the deltoid. The average incision is approximately 14 to 15 cm long, but with surgeon experience, it can start at the coracoid process and extend distally as little as 7 to 8 cm. The standard deltoid pectoral approach is then used, dissecting the deltoid laterally and the pectoralis major inferomedially.

It is advisable at this point to release approximately 3 or 4 cm of the superior portion of the pectoralis major (Figure 11). The superior, sternal head tendon should be released all the way into the substance of the upper fibers of the clavicular head. Subdeltoid dissection should be done until the fibers of the deltoid insertion are visualized distally.

As a matter of routine in those people with primary osteoarthritis and intact rotator cuffs, the medial origin of the coracoid acromial ligament is released from the coracoid to allow better access to the rotator interval. This release is then followed down inferiorly with blunt dissection, achieving a subcoracoid plane below the short head of the biceps and coracoid brachialis and superficial to the subscapularis. The humeral head is then rotated until the bicipital groove is central in the exposure.

The biceps tendon is released through the transverse humeral ligament into the rotator interval, exposing the origin (Figure 12). Tenotomy is performed from the origin and the biceps tendon is allowed to retract out of the shoulder joint. This allows significantly better exposure to the humeral head for later in the procedure.

Because the rotator interval has been opened, the upper portion of the subscapularis is easily appreciated. The inferior leash of the anterior humeral circumflex vessels is suture ligated, and the subscapularis is tagged with sutures. Tenotomy of the subscapularis is then performed approximately 1 cm medial to its lesser tuberosity insertion. This tenotomy is taken from the rotator interval and extends inferiorly, directly parallel to the biceps tendon group.

Release of the subscapularis should proceed in a distal and lateral direction,

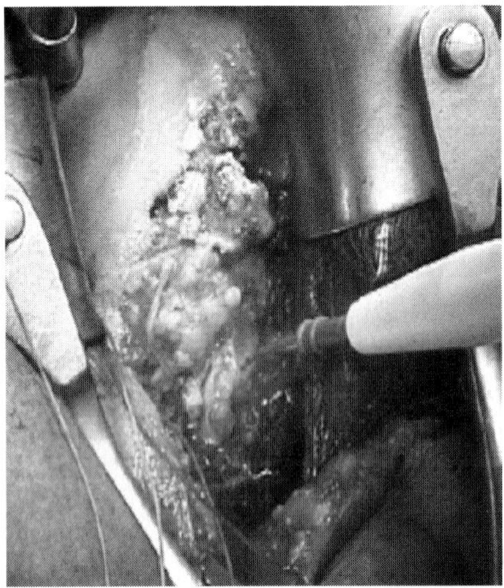

Figure 13 Photograph showing tenotomy of the subscapularis and release of the lateral capsule proceeding laterally in a direction parallel to the bicipital groove. It is extended distally past the upper fibers of the latissimus dorsi and then taken subperiosteally in a medial direction around the humeral neck.

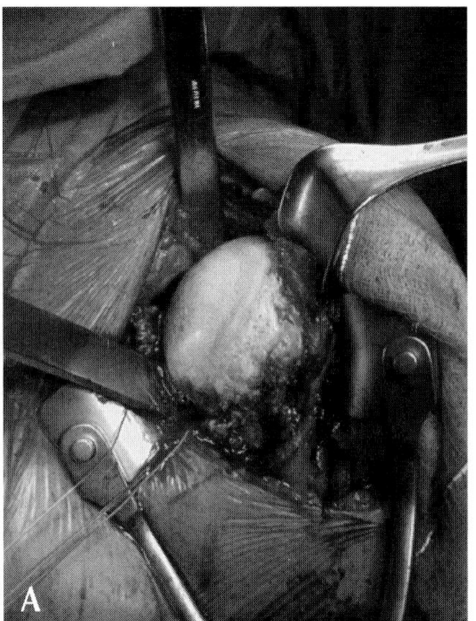

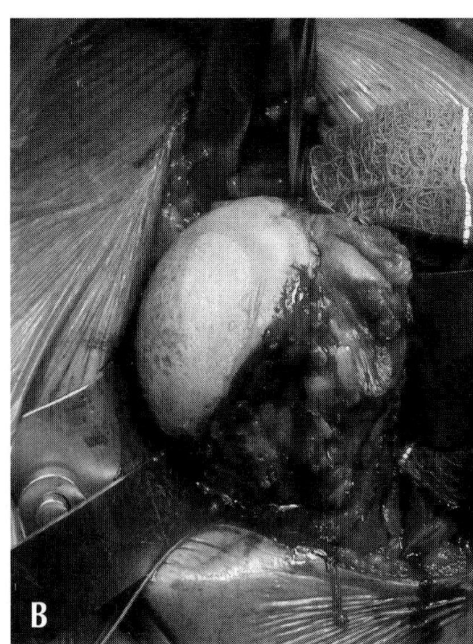

Figure 14 A, Photograph during initial exposure of humeral head showing retained osteophytes. **B,** Photograph after osteotome removal of the osteophytes. Note the more anatomic appearance of the humeral head.

parallel to the line of the biceps tendon and not the line of the anatomic neck. This release should be extended until the upper centimeter of the latissimus dorsi/teres major insertion to the humerus is released (Figure 13). The farther the inferior subscapularis release, the better the exposure for inferior capsular release later in the procedure.

The capsular release should be performed with the arm adducted and externally rotated. As the dissection proceeds inferiorly and extends posteriorly, the arm should be flexed and externally rotated further. Dissection should then be taken around the humeral neck from anterior toward posterior, extending well distally. With adduction, external rotation of the humeral head, and then forward flexion of the arm, a release of the inferior capsule can be achieved at times on the posterior side of the humeral head. If large anterior and inferior osteophytes are encountered, these should be removed before releasing any capsule posteriorly because this will improve the safety of the exposure. Once the inferior ligaments are released, the humeral head can be dislocated anteriorly, with extension of the arm and external rotation. A retractor is placed posterior to the humeral head and levered against the coracoid to help the humeral head anterior. A pointed tip retractor is then placed along the anatomic neck just in front of the rotator cuff to expose the superior portion of the humeral head. Any osteophytes are removed from the humeral head to achieve a more anatomic appearance (Figure 14). The surgeon should be well acquainted with the appearance of a normal humeral head to recognize appropriate osteophyte removal. Aggressive osteophyte removal improves exposure and subscapularis tension upon closure.

Following osteophyte removal, a humeral neck cut is performed, according to the instrumentation. Generally, modern instrumentation allows use of an intramedullary device to perform an osteotomy cut of the humerus exactly at the angle of the prosthesis. To restore the normal geometry of the humerus, it is very important that the osteotomy angle match the angle of the prosthesis. Following osteotomy of the humerus, the canal is generally prepared according to the instrumentation of any given prosthesis. It is important that the humeral head removed from the osteotomy be used as a helpful guide, but it should not be used as the absolute indicator of head size. Generally, head size is best determined by the thickness rather than the circumference of the removed head. Choice of a humeral head size should err toward the smaller size whenever two sizes are considered.

The humeral head is then generally retracted posteriorly using a posterior glenoid retractor, and subscapularis release is performed. The superior glenohumeral ligament and coracohumeral ligament can be released by simply removing any adhesions between the upper rolled edge of the subscapularis and the coracoid base. The middle glenohumeral ligament is generally visible as a thick band of tissue, traversing across the rolled edge of the subscapularis at the level of the glenoid. This band of tissue is sharply

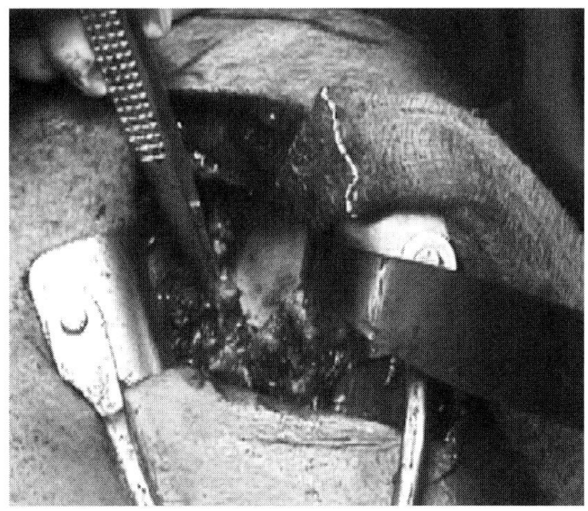

Figure 15 Photograph showing the anterior and lateral edge of the inferior capsule after release of the rotator interval and middle glenohumeral ligament. It can be lifted up with forceps and blunt dissection proceeds deep to free the axillary nerve. A moist sponge can be inserted into this space to improve exposure.

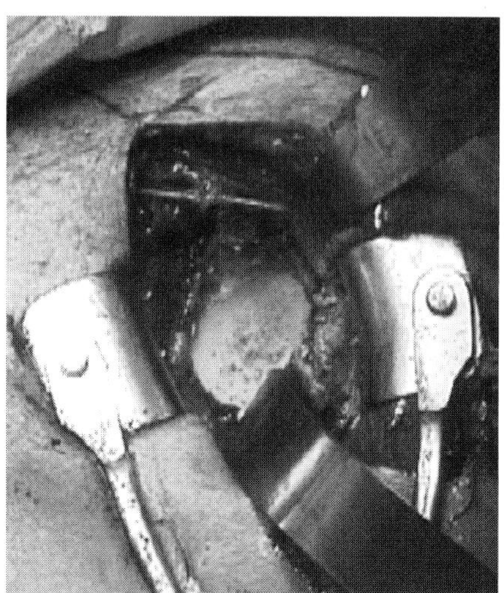

Figure 16 Photograph showing complete capsular release allowing a perpendicular exposure to the glenoid, which permits the use of straight drills and reamers.

incised. Attention is then focused on the inferior capsule, the most important portion of the release. The inferior capsule can usually be elevated laterally by lifting it with a pair of forceps and placing a moist sponge directly inferior (Figure 15). The sponge is pushed gently medially, pushing the axillary nerve inferior and medial. The axillary nerve can be palpated just inferior to the inferior capsule and its location verified to be out of harm's way. Once the inferior capsule is dissected away from the axillary nerve, it is incised directly to the glenoid rim and around the glenoid anteriorly to remove any remaining adhesions from the subscapularis to the glenoid. An adequate release would allow placement of the surgeon's finger along the anterior neck of the glenoid until the neck of the scapular body can be palpated. Once these releases are performed, a perpendicular exposure to the glenoid should be achievable (Figure 16). Glenoid preparation can be obtained using straight reamers. Placement of the central drill hole should be keyed off of the anterior rim of the glenoid because this is typically the best preserved portion of bone in a patient with primary osteoarthritis.

The glenoid is implanted first. Meticulous attention should be placed on cementation technique. Repeat pressurization of cement is generally very effective in placing cement deep within the cancellous bony matrix of the glenoid vault. It is also very helpful for controlling bleeding from the glenoid. Cement is commonly injected into either the keel or peg holes and repeatedly compressed with either the use of sponges or provided instrumentation. The glenoid is then inserted, achieving a 1.5-mm mantle behind the base plate in addition to the keel or peg holes cement mantle. Transosseous sutures are then placed into the humerus for subscapularis repair. The assembled humeral component is then cemented into place. Use of cement allows the greatest latitude to obtain an anatomic placement of the humeral head. Standard closure over drains is then performed.

Arthroplasty in Rotator Cuff-Deficient Shoulders

Rotator cuff-deficient shoulders with degenerative joint disease are a treatment challenge. Most patients will present primarily because of shoulder pain. Shoulder function can be varied even with significant chronic rotator cuff deficiency. The arthritic condition of the shoulder as a result of a chronic rotator cuff tear is called rotator cuff tear arthropathy. This is characterized clinically by pain, poor active motion, near-normal passive motion, crepitus, weakness, and occasionally significant fluid production seen under the deltoid.[59] Radiographically, this condition is characterized by elevation of the humeral head, a new acromiohumeral articulation that has been formed, loss of joint space at the glenohumeral joint, and adaptive changes on the acromion and the humeral head. In patients with advanced disease, there can be collapse of the humeral head.

No staging or classification systems have yet been developed to categorize the radiographic changes or clinical features such as active motion versus passive motion associated with rotator cuff tear arthropathy. Not every patient with an irreparable rotator cuff tear goes on to experience painful symptomatic arthropathy. The pattern of radiographically detectable degenerative changes can be varied. Typically, predominantly superior wear with the acromiohumeral articulation can be seen, and the humeral head has a new fulcrum under the coracoacromial arch. Centralized wear into the glenoid with medialization of the humeral head can also be seen. There is also a florid arthropathic destruction that can be encountered. It is unclear at this time whether these are different stages of the same degenerative process or different patterns of degeneration occurring in response to rotator cuff deficiency.

To determine the prognostic factors for treatment in the different patterns of degenerative change in patients with rotator cuff deficiency, an attempt was made recently to classify the changes to the acromion and glenoid.[60] Patients were treated with either hemiarthroplasty or a reverse prosthesis. Risk factors for poorer results were identified in patients with a superior sloping glenoid in both the hemiarthroplasty and reverse prosthesis groups. A thinned and atrophic acromion was also associated with poorer results in the hemiarthroplasty group. Although this has been the only attempt to categorize the degenerative changes associated with rotator cuff deficiency and correlate them with clinical results in rotator cuff tear arthropathy, more detailed analysis, a larger series of patients, and longer follow-up will be necessary to categorize them further. Because the population is getting older and staying active longer, rotator cuff deficiency with arthritis will likely be an increasing problem. The more detailed analysis and information available regarding this condition can only lead to better treatment.

Although new devices are becoming available in the United States, the best currently available treatment option for chronic rotator cuff deficiency with arthritis (rotator cuff tear arthropathy) seems to be hemiarthroplasty.[61-63] This treatment is typically used for the patient who has had no previous coracoacromial arch surgery and has pain that is unresponsive to conservative treatment. Conservative treatment should have included the use of nonsteroidal anti-inflammatory drugs and possibly a cortisone injection. Basic physical therapy emphasizing the internal rotators, external rotators, and the anterior deltoid should also have been implemented. If patients still have unremitting pain after conservative treatment, then hemiarthroplasty should be discussed.

Although hemiarthroplasty has been shown to predictably relieve pain, it is a procedure with limited goals. Functional ability, specifically active elevation, has been less predictable with hemiarthroplasty; thus, shoulder function after hemiarthroplasty for rotator cuff tear arthropathy is never normal. At best, patients and surgeons should expect approximately 90° of active elevation on average.[59,61-63] It is unclear why some patients do better than others with regard to active elevation and shoulder function. No prognostic factor has been identified that correlates with a better outcome. However, poorer results are associated with patients with previous rotator cuff repair attempts, previous coracoacromial arch surgery (acromioplasty), or the use of a total shoulder arthroplasty.[61-63]

As a result in part of the unpredictable functional improvement after hemiarthroplasty, other treatment options have been attempted to treat patients with rotator cuff deficiency. One such option is the bipolar hemiarthroplasty, which has been shown to achieve pain relief comparable to that of hemiarthroplasty. Functional improvement in terms of active elevation has been poorer, however.[64] Problems with overstuffing the joint and subscapularis attenuation have been noted to occur. This has also been noted to occur with monoblock hemiarthroplasty when an oversized head is used. In patients with rotator cuff tear arthropathy, therefore, bipolar hemiarthroplasty holds no advantage over standard hemiarthroplasty. Bipolar hemiarthroplasty may possibly be beneficial in the treatment of patients with extensive medialization of the glenoid, in which instance this procedure can provide lateral offset to the humeral shaft in relation to the eroded glenoid and thereby help the lever arm of the deltoid (provided overstuffing is avoided).

Currently, the most acceptable treatment for rotator cuff deficiency and arthritis of the shoulder is hemiarthroplasty; however, if the coracoacromial arch has been violated by previous surgery, the results of hemiarthroplasty become less predictable and actually become unsatisfactory with regard to pain relief and functional restoration. If patients have robust acromial bone stock and active elevation to at least 60° preoperatively, hemiarthroplasty can be a good treatment option. However, if patients have pseudoparalysis and poor active motion, hemiarthroplasty alone will not restore function. The reverse ball-and-socket arthroplasty, as described by Grammont and Baulot,[65] was developed in an attempt to improve functionality in patients with rotator cuff-deficient arthritis. Currently, one type of the reverse ball-and-socket arthroplasty prosthesis has been approved by the US Food and Drug Administration, but experience in the United States is limited.

This prosthesis incorporated a new design concept with regard to reverse shoulder arthroplasty by moving the center of rotation of the glenoid component medial and inferior.[65] This improved the deltoid lever arm in patients with rotator cuff-deficient shoulders and, more importantly, moved the center of rotation of the prosthetic glenoid implant component medially within the bone of the scapula. This theoretically places less force on the glenoid component-bone interface, resulting in less chance of implant loosening. Previous reverse designs were more constrained and had a much more lateral center of rotation.[66-68] Thus, the forces on the glenoid component and the interface between the glenoid component and scapula were magnified, resulting in loosening and failures. This medialization and inferior placement of the center of rotation of the glenoid component has produced midterm results in Europe showing durability on the glenoid side.[65,69]

Indications and Contraindications for Reverse Shoulder Arthroplasty

Patients with chronic rotator cuff deficiency and arthritis with poor active elevation and shoulder dysfunction are candidates for reverse shoulder arthroplasty. Although this procedure is done primarily to relieve pain, it can also restore function and active elevation over and above that which a traditional hemiarthroplasty can provide. Favard[70] has shown that a reverse shoulder arthroplasty for rotator cuff tear arthropathy averages 40° more forward elevation and a 20-point increase in average Constant score[71] compared with hemiarthroplasty.[72] Patients with rotator cuff deficiency for other reasons, such as multiply failed rotator cuff repairs, will usually not have good results with a hemiarthroplasty because of the violation of the coracoacromial arch. These patients will likely experience anterosuperior instability, which will cause the humeral head to subluxate superiorly between the acromion and the coracoid with attempted active elevation. This scenario is functionally disabling. Patients with rotator cuff tear arthropathy for whom hemiarthroplasty was not successful are better suited to undergo a reverse shoulder arthroplasty than another attempt at hemiarthroplasty. Patients with postfracture arthrosis with significant greater tuberosity loss or malunion will also likely have poor active elevation and function with traditional hemiarthroplasty and therefore may be better suited to undergo reverse shoulder arthroplasty.

Reverse shoulder arthroplasty is currently indicated for patients with rotator cuff tear arthropathy and pseudoparalysis. Included in this group are patients with multiply failed rotator cuff repairs with extremely poor function and anterosuperior instability, those with failed hemiarthroplasty and anterosuperior instability, and potentially those with significant loss of tuberosity bone or malunited tuberosity bone after fracture. To be a candidate for reverse shoulder arthroplasty, patients must have an intact deltoid, adequate glenoid bone stock to support the glenoid component, and no evidence of infection. Moreover, there should be no neurologic components to the symptoms (for example, peripheral neuropathy, stroke, or Parkinson's disease), and no excessive demand should be placed on the shoulder (for example, a wheelchair-bound patient). Because of the late effects of forces across the glenoid component, there has been concern that patients younger than 70 years may not be suitable candidates for the reverse shoulder arthroplasty.[69] Nonetheless, younger patients typically have other reconstructive options available.

The contraindications for reverse shoulder arthroplasty are either absolute or relative. Absolute contraindications are loss or inactivity of the anterior deltoid and significant glenoid bone stock deficiency that would not allow a glenoid component to be securely implanted. Glenoid bone stock deficiency could be the result of degenerative bone loss or significant bone loss caused by a loose glenoid component from a previous total shoulder arthroplasty. Rheumatoid arthritis is a relative contraindication. Reports on reverse prosthesis in patients with rheumatoid arthritis have shown good pain relief, but there is concern with glenoid loosening.[72] This is probably a bone stock issue because of the systemic nature of the rheumatoid arthritis and the medicines needed to treat it. Age, as mentioned previously, is also a relative contraindication, as is the ability of the patient to understand the nature of the surgery and the rehabilitation involved. Realistic expectations for outcomes and realistic assessment of shoulder arthroplasty experience should be maintained.

Anterosuperior instability of the shoulder is a clinical finding that has not been widely discussed. By definition, for patients to have anterosuperior instability, significant rotator cuff deficiency must be present. This is almost always a chronic condition, with adaptive changes involving the humeral head, acromion, and glenoid. The anterosuperior instability can occur with an intact coracoacromial arch, but most often there has been violation of the coracoacromial arch through previous surgery, degenerative wear or thinning, or an insufficiency fracture of the acromion. Anterosuperior instability can occur after multiply failed rotator cuff repairs with loss of rotator cuff and now violation of the coracoacromial arch. Anterosuperior instability can occur after implant surgery such as hemiarthroplasty to treat rotator cuff arthropathy or after arthroplasty to treat fractures. Thus, rotator cuff deficiency can be caused by chronic degeneration (as with rotator cuff tear arthropathy), failed rotator cuff repair with retear, or the loss of the tuberosities and the associated rotator cuff after humeral head replacement for fracture. This type of shoulder instability is functionally disabling because of the loss of a fulcrum for active shoulder elevation. It can be associated with pain and, as the name implies, the humeral head is drawn in the anterosuperior direction with any attempted active motion of the shoulder.

The causes of anterosuperior instability can be thought of as a combination of what is missing and what is left in the shoulder, which has significant implications on treatment options and functional results. What is missing can include most of the rotator cuff. Usually only the teres minor and subscapularis muscles are intact, and the subscapularis can also be deficient. The coracoacromial arch is usually violated; thus, the superior fulcrum that might have provided resistance to anterosuperior instability is absent. The tuberosities can be deficient, atrophic, or malunited after fractures. The native articular surface can be absent because of fracture and/or having undergone arthroplasty. The anterior deltoid is typically intact, but it may be weakened from previous surgery. This allows the middle and posterior deltoid to be potentially more powerful, which pulls the arm into extension with attempted elevation and helps produce the anterosuperior migration of the humeral head with attempted elevation.

The only real salvage procedure currently available to treat anterosuperior instability is reverse shoulder arthroplasty. Attempts at reconstructing the coracoacromial arch, hooded glenoid components, and muscle-tendon transfers have not been able to restore function as well as reverse shoulder arthroplasty. Patients with anterosuperior instability are extremely challenging to treat. For total shoulder arthroplasty, surgeons should be experienced in all types of shoulder surgery, particularly shoulder arthroplasty and revision shoulder arthroplasty.

Summary

The decisions confronting the surgeon performing contemporary shoulder arthroplasty are far more complex than those of a few decades ago. Early on, knowing if the patient had a rotator cuff tear and if the cartilage on the glenoid was worn were sufficient information to determine indications for a Neer arthroplasty. Subsequently, a modular implant became another option to consider. As glenoid problems become increasingly apparent, the exact role of glenoid resurfacing became less unclear. Currently, the surgeon must have a sophisticated understanding of the extent of any compromise to the patient's rotator cuff function, the integrity of the remaining glenoid bone, and a familiarity with an extensive and expanding array of prosthetic options, including reverse shoulder arthroplasty.

References

1. Ballmer FT, Sidles JA, Lippitt SB, Matsen FA III: Humeral prosthetic arthroplasty: Surgically relevant considerations. *J Shoulder Elbow Surg* 1993;2:296-304.
2. Boileau P, Walch G: The three-dimensional geometry of the proximal humerus, implications for surgical technique and prosthetic design. *J Bone Joint Surg Br* 1997;79:857-865.
3. Boileau P, Walch G, Liotard JP: Cineradiographic study of active elevation of the prosthetic shoulder. *J Orthop Surg* 1992;6:351-359.
4. Pearl ML, Volk AG: Coronal plane geometry of the proximal humerus relevant to prosthetic arthroplasty. *J Shoulder Elbow Surg* 1996;5:320-326.
5. Pearl ML, Volk AG: Retroversion of the proximal humerus in relationship to prosthetic replacement arthroplasty. *J Shoulder Elbow Surg* 1995;4:286-289.
6. Roberts SNJ, Foley APJ, Swallow HM, Wallace WA, Coughplan DP: The geometry of the humeral head and the design of prostheses. *J Bone Joint Surg Br* 1991;73:647-650.
7. Pearl ML, Kurutz S: Geometric analysis of commonly used prosthetic systems for proximal humeral replacement. *J Bone Joint Surg Am* 1999;81:660-671.
8. Pearl ML, Kurutz S, Robertson DD, Yamaguchi K: Geometric analysis of selected press fit prosthetic systems for proximal humeral replacement. *J Orthop Res* 2002;20:192-197.
9. Karduna AR, Williams GR, Williams JL, Iannotti JP: Kinematics of the glenohumeral joint: Influences of muscle forces, ligamentous constraints, and articular geometry. *J Orthop Res* 1996;14:986-993.
10. Williams GR Jr, Wong KL, Pepe MD, et al: The effect of articular malposition after total shoulder arthroplasty on glenohumeral translations, range of motion, and subacromial impingement. *J Shoulder Elbow Surg* 2001;10:399-409.
11. Harryman DT, Sidles JA, Harris SL, Lippitt SB: The effect of articular conformity and the size of the humeral head component on laxity and motion after glenohumeral arthroplasty: A study in cadavera. *J Bone Joint Surg Am* 1995;77:555-563.
12. Karduna AR, Williams GR, Williams JL, Iannotti JP: Joint stability after total shoulder arthroplasty in a cadaver model. *J Shoulder Elbow Surg* 1997;6:506-511.
13. Kronberg M, Broström LA, Soderlund V: Retroversion of the humeral head in the normal shoulder and its relationship to the normal range of motion. *Clin Orthop* 1990;253:113-117.
14. Pearl ML, Volk AG: Retroversion of the proximal humerus relevant to prosthetic replacement arthroplasty. *J Shoulder Elbow Surg* 1995;7:286-289.
15. Robertson D, Yan J, Bigliani L, Yamaguchi K, Flatow E: Three dimensional analysis of the proximal humerus: relevance to arthroplasty, in *Program and Abstracts of the American Shoulder and Elbow Surgeons, 15th Open Meeting*. Anaheim, CA, 1999.
16. Iannotti JP, Gabriel JP, Schneck SL, Evans BG, Misra S: The normal glenohumeral relationships. *J Bone Joint Surg Am* 1992;74:491-500.
17. Jobe CM, Iannotti JP: Limits imposed on glenohumeral motion by joint geometry. *J Shoulder Elbow Surg* 1995;7:281-285.
18. Ballmer FT, Sidles JA, Lippitt SB, Matsen FA III: Total shoulder arthroplasty: Some considerations related to glenoid surface contact. *J Shoulder Elbow Surg* 1994;3:299-306.
19. Neer CS II: Replacement arthroplasty for glenohumeral osteoarthritis. *J Bone Joint Surg Am* 1974;56:1-13.
20. Cofield RH: Total shoulder arthroplasty with the Neer prosthesis. *J Bone Joint Surg Am* 1984;66:899-906.
21. Hawkins RJ, Bell RH, Jallay B: Total shoulder arthroplasty. *Clin Orthop* 1989;242:188-194.
22. Neer CS II, Watson KC, Stanton FJ: Recent experience in total shoulder replacement. *J Bone Joint Surg* 1982;64:319-337.
23. Franklin JL, Barrett WP, Jackins SE, Matsen FA III: Glenoid loosening in total shoulder arthroplasty: Association with rotator cuff deficiency. *J Arthroplasty* 1988;3:39-46.
24. Churchill RS, Brems JJ, Kotschi H: Glenoid size, inclination, and version: An anatomic study. *J Shoulder Elbow Surg* 2001;10:327-332.
25. Friedman R, LaBerge M, Dooley RL, O'Hara AL: Finite element modeling of the glenoid component: Effect of design parameters on stress distribution. *J Shoulder Elbow Surg* 1992;1:261-270.
26. Warner JJ, Bowen MK, Deng XH, Hannafin JA, Arnoczky SP, Warren RF: Articular contact patterns of the normal glenohumeral joint. *J Shoulder Elbow Surg* 1998;7:381-388.
27. Soslowsky LF, Flatow EL, Bigliani LU, Mow VC: Articular geometry of the glenohumeral joint. *Clin Orthop* 1992;285:181-190.
28. Ibarra C, Dines DM, McLaughlin JA: Glenoid replacement in total shoulder arthroplasty. *Orthop Clin North Am* 1998;29:403-413.
29. Iannotti JP, Williams GR: Total shoulder arthroplasty: Factors influencing prosthetic design. *Orthop Clin North Am* 1998;29:377-391.
30. Harryman DT, Sidles JA, Clark JM, McQuade KJ, Matsen FA: Translation of the humeral head on the glenoid with passive glenohumeral motion. *J Bone Joint Surg Am* 1990;72:1334-1343.
31. Amstutz HC, Sew Hoy AL, Clarke I: UCLA anatomic total shoulder arthroplasty. *Clin Orthop* 1981;155:7-20.
32. Gristina AG, Romano RL, Kammire GC, Webb LX: Total shoulder replacement. *Orthop Clin North Am* 1987;18:445-453.
33. Neer CS II: Articular replacement for the humeral head. *J Bone Joint Surg Am* 1955;37:215-228.
34. Boyd AD Jr, Thomas WH, Scott RD, Sledge CB, Thornhill TS: Total shoulder arthroplasty versus hemiarthroplasty. *J Arthroplasty* 1990;5:329-336.
35. Gartsman GM, Roddey TS, Hammerman SM: Shoulder arthroplasty with or without resurfacing of the glenoid in patients who have

osteoarthritis. *J Bone Joint Surg Am* 2000;82: 26-34.

36. Hawkins RJ, Greis PE, Bonutti PM: Treatment of symptomatic glenoid loosening following unconstrained shoulder arthroplasty. *Orthopedics* 1999;22:229-234.

37. Conner PM, Bigliani LU: Prosthetic replacement for osteoarthritis: Hemiarthroplasty versus total shoulder replacement. *Semin Arthroplasty* 1997;8:268-277.

38. Collins D, Tencer A, Sidles J Matsen F III: Edge displacement and deformation of glenoid components in response to eccentric loading: The effect of preparation of the glenoid bone. *J Bone Joint Surg Am* 1992;74:501-507.

39. Norris BL, Lachiewicz PF: Modern cement technique and the survivorship of total shoulder arthroplasty. *Clin Orthop* 1996;328:76-85.

40. Orr TE, Carter DR, Schurman DJ: Stress analyses of glenoid component designs. *Clin Orthop* 1988;232:217-224.

41. Stone KD, Grabowski JJ, Cofield RH, Morrey BF, An KN: Stress analyses of glenoid components in total shoulder arthroplasty. *J Shoulder Elbow Surg* 1999;8:151-158.

42. Wallace AL, Phillips RL, MacDougal GA, Walsh WR, Sonnabend DH: Resurfacing of the glenoid in total shoulder arthroplasty: A comparison, at a mean of five years, of prostheses inserted with and without cement. *J Bone Joint Surg Am* 1999;81:510-518.

43. Anglin C, Wyss UP, Pichora D: Mechanical testing of shoulder prostheses and recommendations for glenoid design. *J Shoulder Elbow Surg* 2000;9:323-331.

44. Torchia ME, Cofield RH, Settergren CR: Total shoulder arthroplasty with the Neer prosthesis: Long-term results. *J Shoulder Elbow Surg* 1997;6:495-505.

45. Giori NJ, Beaupre GS, Carter DR: The influence of fixation peg design on the shear stability of prosthetic implants. *J Orthop Res* 1990;8:892-898.

46. Lazarus MD, Jensen KL, Southworth C, Matsen FA III: The radiographic evaluation of keeled and pegged glenoid component insertion. *J Bone Joint Surg Am* 2002;84:1174-1182.

47. Rodosky MW, Bigliani LU: Indications for glenoid resurfacing in shoulder arthroplasty. *J Shoulder Elbow Surg* 1996;5:231-248.

48. Sperling JW, Cofield RH, Rowland CM: Neer hemiarthroplasty and Neer total shoulder arthroplasty in patients fifty years old or less: Long-term results. *J Bone Joint Surg Am* 1998;80:464-473.

49. Neer CS II, Morrison DS: Glenoid bone-grafting in total shoulder arthroplasty. *J Bone Joint Surg Am* 1988;70:1154-1162.

50. Antuna SA, Sperling JW, Cofield RH, Rowland CM: Glenoid revision surgery after total shoulder arthroplasty. *J Shoulder Elbow Surg* 2001;10:217-224.

51. Cofield RH: Total shoulder arthoplasty: Complications and revision surgery. *Instr Course Lect* 1990;39:449-462.

52. Petersen SA, Hawkins RJ: Revision of failed total shoulder arthroplasty. *Orthop Clin North Am* 1998;29:519-533.

53. Steinmann SP, Cofield RH: Bone grafting for glenoid deficiency in total shoulder replacement. *J Shoulder Elbow Surg* 2000;9:361-367.

54. Hill JM, Norris TR: Long-term results of total shoulder arthroplasty following bone-grafting of the glenoid. *J Bone Joint Surg Am* 2001;83: 877-883.

55. Burkhead WZ Jr, Hutton KS: Biologic resurfacing of the glenoid with hemiarthroplasty of the shoulder. *J Shoulder Elbow Surg* 1995;4:263-270.

56. Wainwright D: Glenoidectomy: A method of treating the painful shoulder in severe rheumatoid arthritis. *Ann Rheum Dis* 1974;33:110.

57. Wirth MA, Rockwood CA Jr: Complications of shoulder arthroplasty. *Clin Orthop* 1994;307: 47-69.

58. Iannotti JP, Norris TR: Influence of preoperative factors on outcome of shoulder arthroplasty for glenohumeral osteoarthritis. *J Bone Joint Surg Am* 2003;85-A:251-258.

59. Neer CS II, Craig EV, Fukuda H: Cuff-tear arthropathy. *J Bone Joint Surg Am* 1983;65:1232-1244.

60. Oudet D, Favard L, Lautmann S, et al: La Prothese D'Epaule Aequalis dans les Omarthroses avec Rupture Massive et non Reparable de la Coiffe, in Walch G, Boileau P, Mole D (eds): *2000 Shoulder Prostheses: Two to Ten Year Follow-up*. Montpelier, France, Sauramps Medical, 2001, pp 241-246.

61. Field LD, Dines DM, Zabinski SJ, Warren RF: Hemiarthroplasty of the shoulder for rotator cuff arthropathy. *J Shoulder Elbow Surg* 1997;6:18-23.

62. Sanchez-Sotelo J, Cofield RH, Rowland CM: Shoulder hemiarthroplasty for glenohumeral arthritis associated with severe rotator cuff deficiency. *J Bone Joint Surg Am* 2001;83:1814-1822.

63. Williams GR Jr, Rockwood CA Jr: Hemiarthroplasty in rotator cuff-deficient shoulders. *J Shoulder Elbow Surg* 1996;5:362-367.

64. Worland RL, Jessup DE, Arredondo J, Warburton KJ: Bipolar shoulder arthroplasty for rotator cuff arthropathy. *J Shoulder Elbow Surg* 1997;6:512-515.

65. Grammont PM, Baulot E: Delta shoulder prosthesis for rotator cuff rupture. *Orthopedics* 1993;16:65-68.

66. Coughlin MJ, Morris JM, West WF: The semiconstrained total shoulder arthroplasty. *J Bone Joint Surg Am* 1979;61:574-581.

67. Laurence M: Replacement arthroplasty of the rotator cuff deficient shoulder. *J Bone Joint Surg Br* 1991;73:916-919.

68. Post M, Haskell SS, Jablon M: Total shoulder replacement with a constrained prosthesis. *J Bone Joint Surg Am* 1980;62:327-335.

69. Boulahia A, Edwards TB, Walch G, Baratta RV: Early results of a reverse design prosthesis in the treatment of arthritis of the shoulder in elderly patients with a large rotator cuff tear. *Orthopedics* 2002;25:129-133.

70. Favard L, Lautmann S, Sirveaux F, et al: Hemiarthroplasty versus reverse arthroplasty in the treatment of osteoarthritis with massive rotator cuff tear, in Walch G, Boileau P, Mole D (eds): *2000 Shoulder Prostheses: Two to Ten Year Follow-up*. Montpelier, France, Sauramps Medical, 2001, pp 261-268.

71. Constant CR, Murley AH: A clinical method of functional assessment of the shoulder. *Clin Orthop* 1987;214:160-164.

72. Rittmeister M, Kerschbaumer F: Grammont reverse total shoulder arthroplasty in patients with rheumatoid arthritis and nonreconstructible rotator cuff lesions. *J Shoulder Elbow Surg* 2001;10:17-22.

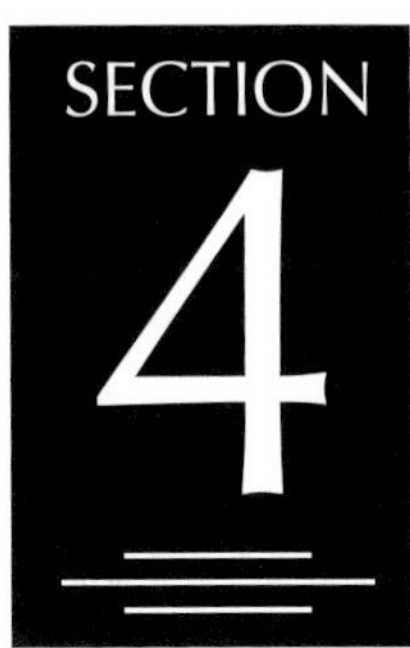

Shoulder Fractures

Shoulder Fractures

Fractures of the proximal humerus represent a difficult clinical challenge for the practicing orthopaedic surgeon. Imaging is difficult as radiographs are easily distorted by arm rotation or improper beam alignment, yet much less time is available than in reconstructive cases for extensive tests and consultations, and subspecialty referral may be difficult in a multiply injured emergency patient. Classification schemes have been shown to be unreliably applied by different surgeons, and even when they agree, tremendous controversy exists as to the best treatment modality. The authors in this section bring a tremendous depth of experience to this difficult topic and provide a clear, yet detailed review that will be helpful to both the general orthopaedist taking trauma call and the shoulder specialist treating referral patients.

In recent years, there has been tremendous interest in new and innovative methods of fixing proximal humerus fractures. In the last decades of the last century, many authors reported disappointment with the results of large anterograde nails and traditional plate-and-screw fixation of these injuries, fueling growth in the use of humeral head replacement. In their chapter on nonprosthetic management, Iannotti and associates masterfully survey the many changes that have led to a renaissance of internal fixation. The authors emphasize proper imaging and identification of fracture patterns, especially assessing bone quality and comminution and understanding deforming forces (eg, internal rotation of the head segment by the intact lesser tuberosity in a three-part fracture). They provide a clear discussion of the importance of recognizing the valgus impacted four-part fracture, which is more amenable to repair than the classic four-part fracture-dislocation. The former has an intact medial soft-tissue sleeve and a lower risk of osteonecrosis. Furthermore, it is an almost ideal indication for newer methods of minimally invasive repair, which the authors detail nicely. The use of percutaneous pins and cannulated screws has revolutionized the care of many, if not most, proximal humerus fractures, and stiffness is rare when open approaches are avoided. Even when open reduction is needed, the newer implants such as fixed-angle ("locking") plates have improved the reproducibility of internal fixation, even when bone quality is poor. Finally, even when osteonecrosis ensues, the clinical result may be acceptable if an anatomic reduction has been achieved, as Christian Gerber has demonstrated.

Michael Wirth beautifully reviews the late sequelae of proximal humerus fractures. He draws considerable attention to the problem of stiffness, which can be a devastating problem. It is easy to focus on the bone fragments, visible on radiographs, but neglect the capsule and rotator cuff, an error that can lead to severely impaired function. Dr. Wirth presents clear evidence that a physician-directed rehabilitation program is essential to recovery of shoulder motion after either nonsurgical care or surgical treatment.

Osteonecrosis occurs more often with complex fractures and after open surgery with soft-tissue stripping and may require shoulder arthroplasty. The problem of malunion is discussed in appropriate detail, emphasizing that displacement of the greater tuberosity, which can catch on the acromion if superior or abut on the glenoid edge if posterior, is less well tolerated than displacement or angulation of the surgical neck, for which shoulder motion can compensate to some degree. The poorest results generally ensue when malunion is compounded by articular loss through posttraumatic osteoarthritis or osteonecrosis, and Dr. Wirth notes that prosthetic arthroplasty in these cases is often plagued by extensive scarring, deltoid weakness, unreliable pain relief, and a higher rate of complications. He also discusses the challenges posed by nonunions, which can lead to bone resorption and head cavitation. There has been much controversy since the references cited here about the best treatment for those nonunions symptomatic enough to require surgery. Some authors have rejected humeral head replacement as prone to complications and failure, especially if tuberosity osteotomy is used, whereas we have reported success if a calcar bone graft is used to promote healing and the tuberosities are protected. Whenever the head is preserved, fixation and grafting are preferred.

The final chapters in the section survey humeral head replacement for proximal humerus fractures. Phipatanakul and Norris nicely review the indications for this procedure, especially severe fractures with loss of soft-tissue attachments to the head segment in older patients with poor bone quality. This discussion, taken together with the earlier chapter by Iannotti and associates, presents much helpful information on this difficult decision: fix or replace. Kwon and Zuckerman expertly distill the available data on the results of humeral head replacement for fracture, pointing out that pain relief has been far more reliable than motion and function. Younger patients and those treated without delay appear to fare better. The discussion about the prime prognostic role of anatomic tuberosity healing is excellent. Indeed, these lessons have led to many recent innovations designed to improve the accuracy and security of tuberosity healing, including the use of cerclage suturing methods, stronger sutures or even cables, bone grafting the tuberosity-shaft junction, implants specially designed for fractures with less proximal metal (leaving more room for bone grafting and tuberosity healing), reduced retroversion to decrease pull on the greater tuberosity when the arm is internally rotated in a sling, and slower rehabilitation to protect the repair.

The articles by Lervick and associates and by Plausinis and associates review the prevention, recognition, and treatment of complications of humeral head replacement for fracture. Infection, nerve injury, periprosthetic fracture, instability, tuberosity malunion and nonunion, stiffness and heterotopic ossification, glenoid erosion, loosening, and prosthetic malposition may present singly or in combination. There is increasing use of revision with a reverse arthroplasty in the setting of failed humeral head replacement with tuberosity pull-off. Indeed, some trials are underway in Europe comparing primary reverse arthroplasty with conventional humeral head replacement as the initial treatment for severe proximal humerus fractures.

These articles cover a challenging topic with great clarity and yet rich detail. Even though replacement arthroplasty will continue to have a role as a salvage procedure for difficult cases, the indications for internal fixation of proximal humerus fractures will likely continue to evolve, driven by improved devices and broader dissemination of the techniques for percutaneous repair. Orthopaedic surgeons who care for proximal humerus fractures will find much useful information in this excellent section.

Evan L. Flatow, MD
Lasker Professor and Interim Chair
Department of Orthopaedic Surgery
Mount Sinai School of Medicine
New York, New York

Nonprosthetic Management of Proximal Humeral Fractures

Joseph P. Iannotti, MD, PhD
Matthew L. Ramsey, MD
Gerald R. Williams, Jr, MD
Jon J.P. Warner, MD

Abstract

Many proximal humeral fractures can be treated without the need for hemiarthroplasty. Treatment choice is affected by fracture location and pattern, as well as by patient factors including age, activity level, quality of bone, and ability to comply with a regimen of therapy. Successful diagnosis and treatment of proximal humeral fractures is dependent on good-quality radiographs, but in some cases, intraoperative assessment of the fracture pattern is required for a complete and accurate diagnosis of the fracture pattern and severity. A discussion of nonsurgical and surgical treatment options and techniques needed to achieve anatomic reduction and stable fixation is important.

Indications and Diagnosis

Most proximal humeral fractures are not sufficiently displaced or angulated to require surgical management. It is estimated that 20% of all proximal humeral fractures should be treated surgically,[1] and humeral head replacement is the preferred method of treatment of many of those fractures. An indication for hemiarthroplasty is the classic four-part fracture or four-part fracture-dislocation, particularly when the articular segment of the humeral head is separated from the tuberosities and the humeral shaft, because of the expected high risk of osteonecrosis. Other indications for hemiarthroplasty are fragmentation of the articular surface and severe osteoporosis. On the other hand, reduction and internal fixation can be accomplished for displaced fractures associated with an intact humeral head with good quality bone. The indications for open or closed reduction and internal fixation are related to the fracture pattern, the quality of the bone, the status of the rotator cuff, and the age and activity level of the patient. The goal of reduction and fixation of a proximal humeral fracture is to obtain nearly anatomic reduction and stable fixation to allow an early range of motion.[2] Recently, there has been an emphasis on the use of less invasive open procedures for reduction and fixation, thereby minimizing periarticular scarring and decreasing the risk of vascular insult to the articular humeral head segment from the surgical exposure.[3-5]

Accurate diagnosis and effective management of proximal humeral fractures require good quality radiographs in at least two orthogonal planes. In general, basic radiographs include an AP view, an axillary view, and a scapular lateral (Y) view. Sometimes, in an emergency department setting, it is not easy to obtain all three of these views with sufficient quality to make a clear diagnosis and define the best treatment options. A CT scan can be of value when the plain radiographs do not clearly define the size of the fragments or the degree of displacement. Although MRI is rarely needed, it is indicated when the patient has symptoms suggestive of a preinjury shoulder disorder such as a rotator cuff tear. It can

One or more of the authors or the departments with which they are affiliated have received something of value from a commercial or other party related directly or indirectly to the subject of this chapter.

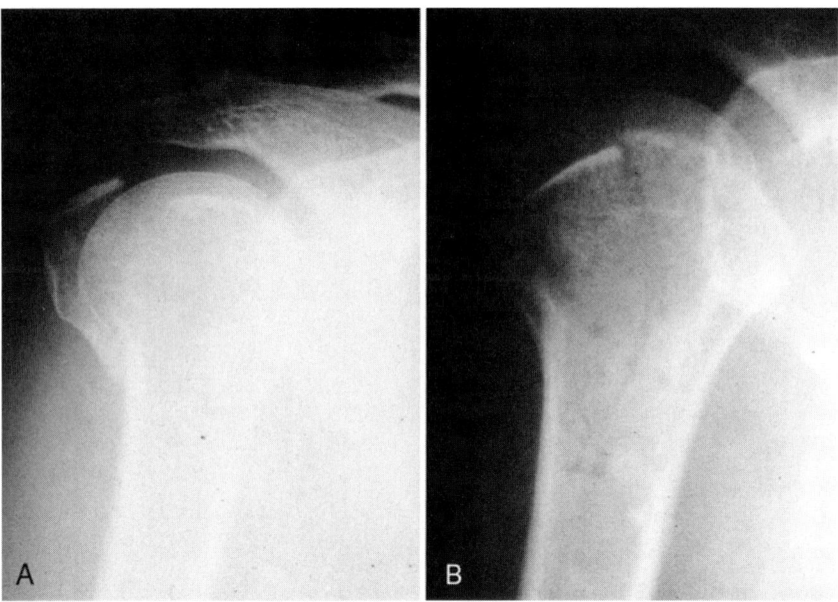

Figure 1 A small fragment of the greater tuberosity treated with a figure-of-8 suture technique through a deltoid-splitting incision. Sutures are passed through the tendon-bone insertion of the rotator cuff and then into the diaphyseal cortical bone. **A,** Preoperative radiograph. **B,** Postoperative radiograph.

also be useful in the evaluation of the rotator cuff when the patient has persistent pain after the fracture has healed.

Isolated Fracture of the Greater Tuberosity

Fractures of the greater tuberosity can be associated with an acute glenohumeral dislocation or a tear of the rotator cuff. When associated with a glenohumeral dislocation, the greater tuberosity fracture fragment is usually small and lies in a satisfactory position after reduction of the dislocation of the humeral head. In these cases, the size of the fragment, the amount of residual displacement, and the presence of a full-thickness rotator cuff tear determine the need for surgical management. In Neer's review of displaced proximal humeral fractures, 1 cm or more of displacement was considered an indication for surgical management.[1,6] This general guideline may not apply to all cases of greater tuberosity fracture. Nonsurgical treatment is usually recommended for such fractures that have less than 0.5 cm of superior displacement or less than 1 cm of posterior displacement. The difference between the amount of allowable superior displacement and the amount of allowable posterior displacement is because of the greater likelihood of symptoms associated with subacromial impingement when there is superior displacement. Patient age and activity level influence the decision to reduce and internally fix a displaced fracture of the greater tuberosity as nonsurgically treated fractures are likely to cause more pain in active individuals.

Results of Surgery

Flatow and asssociates[7] evaluated the results in 12 patients in whom an isolated acute fracture of the greater tuberosity had been treated with open reduction and internal fixation with use of a deltoid-splitting approach and suture fixation. The results were uniformly good or excellent. In that study, 0.5 cm of superior displacement was considered to be a sufficient indication for open reduction and internal fixation.

Surgical Technique

The superior surgical approach, such as splitting of the deltoid, is ideal for smaller fracture fragments and for fractures associated with a rotator cuff tear. This approach allows direct exposure and repair of both the rotator cuff and the greater tuberosity (Figure 1). The innervation of the deltoid by the axillary nerve limits the distal extent of the superior approach to approximately 5 cm from the lateral aspect of the acromion. A large fracture fragment with diaphyseal extension is difficult to mobilize, reduce, and fix through the superior approach without undue risk to the axillary nerve and should be managed surgically through a deltopectoral approach. The deltopectoral approach enables distal placement of sutures, a plate, or screws into the fragment with less risk of injury to the axillary nerve. When a large fragment of the greater tuberosity is displaced posteriorly and is behind the humeral head, a bone hook can be used to pull the fragment into the surgical field. Then, placement of a traction suture into the rotator cuff to control and manipulate the fragment allows the fragment to be anatomically reduced to the proximal part of the humerus.

A fragment of the greater tuberosity is excised only when it is less than 1 cm in size. If the fragment is larger, excision makes rotator cuff repair very difficult, if not impossible. Therefore, most displaced fragments of the greater tuberosity should be saved and treated with open reduction and internal fixation. The method of fixation depends on several factors, including the size of the fragment, the quality of the bone, the degree of comminution, and the presence of an associated rotator cuff tear. Suture fixation with use of the rotator cuff for proximal fixation is preferable, particularly for smaller and comminuted fragments or for osteoporotic bone. Most fractures of the greater tuberosity are secured with a figure-of-8 suture as well as an intraosseous suture with No. 5 or larger nonabsorbable suture material. Cancellous bone screws can be used for large noncomminuted fragments when the bone is of good quality. Bone screw fixation is often supplemented with a figure-of-8 suture (Figure 2).

Malunions

Persistent pain as a result of malunion of the greater tuberosity can occur with as little as 0.5 cm of superior displacement. The symptoms result from subacromial impingement. Such subacromial pain can be treated with subacromial decompression if the displacement is less than 1 cm. If the displacement is minimal and the fragment is 1 cm or smaller in size, excision of the osseous prominence that is causing impingement followed by rotator cuff repair can yield a satisfactory result. When the greater tuberosity is displaced more than 1 cm, an osteotomy of the fragment is the preferred treatment (Figure 3). The fragment is then mobilized by dissection and release of scar tissue and the underlying capsule associated with the torn and scarred rotator cuff. Mobilization of the retracted rotator cuff tissue is required to reduce the greater tuberosity fragment to an anatomic position. Mobilization of the rotator cuff requires release of the rotator interval and the underlying capsule at the site of the fracture.

Beredjiklian and associates[8] evaluated the results at an average of 44 months after surgical management of a proximal humeral malunion in 39 patients, 11 of whom had an isolated malunion of a fracture of the greater tuberosity. These 11 malunions were treated with a combination of osteotomy and fixation of the tuberosity or subacromial decompression and excision of a portion of the impinging fracture fragment. When the tuberosity was osteotomized, capsular release was required to obtain a full passive arc of motion and to achieve cuff repair. Nine patients had a satisfactory result. The results of the surgical management of malunions of the greater tuberosity have been reported to be less favorable than the results of reduction and fixation of acute fractures.[9] However, the results of surgical management of an isolated greater tuberosity malunion are generally more favorable than the results of surgical management of malunions that also involve the surgical neck or both tuberosities (three- and four-part malunions).

Surgical Neck Fractures

Surgical neck fractures are often undertreated and are associated with a relatively high risk of malunion or nonunion. Malunion can be fairly well tolerated if the relationship of the articular surface and the tuberosities is not distorted. Fracture classifications, although very good, tend to underestimate or overestimate the severity of the fractures because the quality of the bone or the health and understanding of the patient are not always considered.[1,10,11] With this in mind, one can define two distinct patient groups who should be treated with different approaches, even when the fracture is the same.[12]

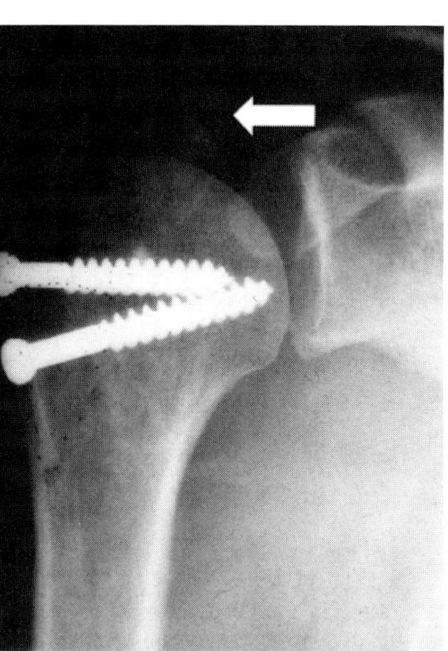

Figure 2 A fracture of the greater tuberosity associated with anterior dislocation of the humerus was treated with two screws with good fixation and an anatomic reduction. Three weeks after the surgery, the patient had a minor fall and sustained a fracture of the greater tuberosity proximal to the superior screw (*arrow*). Supplemental figure-of-8 fixation through the tendon-bone insertion reduces this complication with isolated screw fixation.

One group consists of young patients, more often male, who sustain high-energy trauma. This sometimes causes fragments to be impacted, but more often than not there is comminution. Typically, the bone quality is good with thick cortices and dense cancellous structure. The patient is usually able to comply with postoperative therapy. This group can be treated with a variety of surgical methods, including open reduction and internal fixation.

The second group consists of elderly patients, more often female. Minor trauma, such as a fall, causes impaction or comminution of thin cortices and porous cancellous bone. An unstable configuration of thin bone fragments is the rule. Elderly

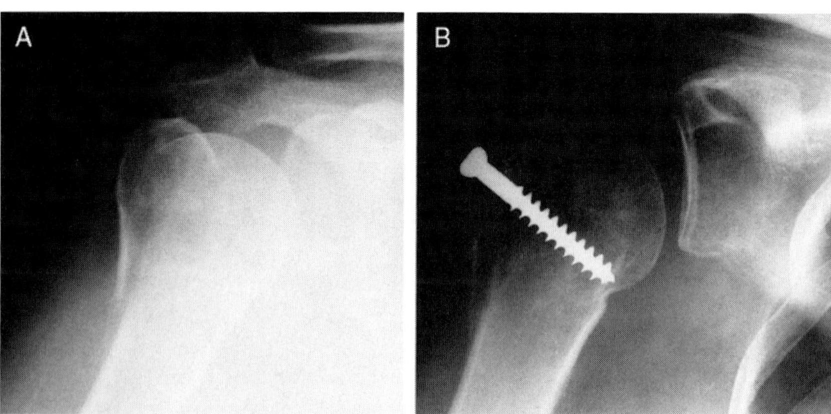

Figure 3 A, A radiograph of a malunion of the greater tuberosity. **B,** The malunion was treated with an osteotomy, reduction, and internal fixation.

patients sometimes have a poor understanding of the nature of the surgery or their role in postoperative rehabilitation, may have comorbid medical conditions that adversely affect the outcome, and often are frail and have a limited social support system to aid in postoperative recovery. Rigid internal fixation devices often fail when applied to thin porous bone, so fixation options may be more limited in these patients. In some cases, it is better to perform a hemiarthroplasty because of poor-quality bone.

Indications for stabilization of a surgical neck fracture include a displaced unstable fracture, multiple trauma, association with other upper extremity fractures, vascular injury, and a patient who will comply with a postoperative regimen.

Percutaneous internal fixation is an excellent option for a displaced two-part fracture that can be reduced with closed manipulation. While this technique can be difficult and tedious, it offers several advantages. There is almost no dissection of the soft tissues, which minimizes the risk of the articular segment becoming avascular.

Surgical Technique

The technique of closed reduction and percutaneous fixation of proximal humeral fractures was originally described by Bohler[13] for the treatment of fractures in children, but it has become a standard treatment method for displaced two-part fractures when the patient has good-quality bone and minimal comminution.

There are several pitfalls with this treatment. The first is improper patient selection. The ideal indication is a displaced two-part fracture of the surgical neck that can be reduced by closed manipulation with the patient under anesthesia. Marked comminution or the inability to reduce the fracture are contraindications to this technique. Another pitfall is related to patient positioning, draping, and fluoroscope placement in the operating room. The patient should be positioned on the operating table so that the arm is free to be manipulated and biplanar fluoroscopic image intensification is possible. While use of a fluoroscopic operating table is preferred by some, we prefer to place the patient supine onto a long bean bag that can be contoured around the scapula, allowing the patient to be moved sufficiently laterally for C-arm visualization. The C-arm is brought in from a cranial direction, and a closed reduction, confirmed in two planes, is performed before preparation and draping of the shoulder for surgery (Figure 4).

A third pitfall is related to the reduction maneuver. Usually, two-part fractures have an apex anterior angulation. In such cases, some longitudinal traction is applied while posteriorly directed pressure on the humerus is used to correct the anterior angulation. It is helpful to have a sterile arm-positioner to hold the arm in place of an assistant. Once the reduction is confirmed, the arm is prepared in a sterile fashion and fixation pins are placed under image-intensification control. Two and a half-millimeter terminally threaded pins (AO; Synthes, Paoli, PA) are preferred for the internal fixation. The terminal threads of these pins help to prevent migration. In some patients, cannulated 4.0-mm screws can be used to fix the fracture.

The pinning technique has been described in detail previously.[14] After the fracture has been reduced, a pin is held in front of the shoulder and an image in the AP plane confirms proper orientation. A small stab incision is then made, and a straight clamp is used to spread the soft tissue down to the lateral humeral cortex. Two pins are then inserted, from inferior and lateral up into the articular fragment, and biplanar confirmation of proper pin placement is performed. Next, a third pin is placed from a more anterior and distal orientation. In the case of a three-part fracture with an unstable greater tuberosity fragment, one or two additional pins can be placed through this fragment and down into the humeral shaft (Figure 5). The pins are

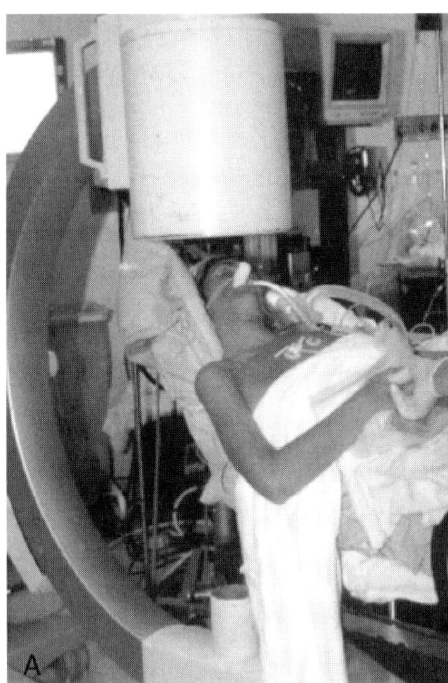

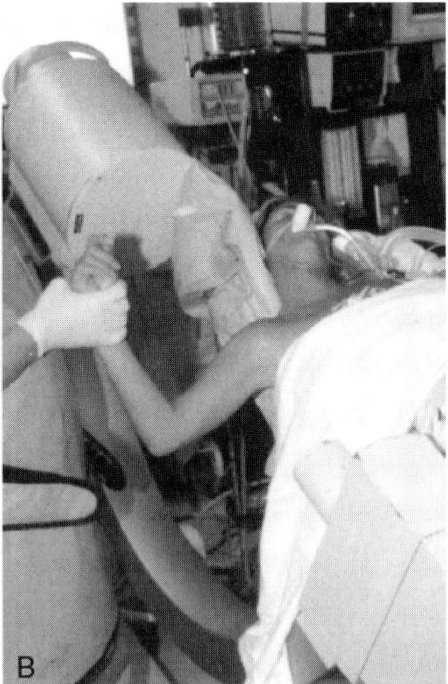

Figure 4 A, A patient positioned in the beach-chair position, with the body held in place with a large bean bag. The image intensifier is placed at the head of the table. **B,** The image intensifier can be positioned for both AP and axillary views of the proximal part of the humerus.

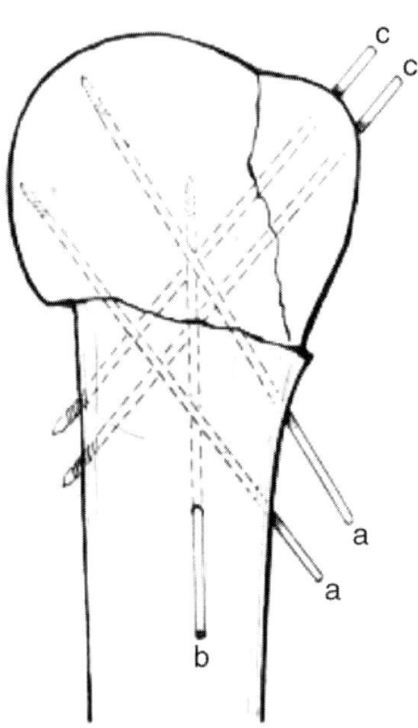

Figure 5 Two pins (a) are inserted from inferior and lateral up into the articular segment, and biplanar confirmation of proper placement is performed. A third pin (b) is placed from a more anterior and distal orientation. Two additional pins (c) can be used to stabilize a greater tuberosity fragment. (Reproduced with permission from Jaberg H, Warner JJ, Jakob RP: Percutaneous stabilization of unstable fractures of the humerus. *J Bone Joint Surg Am* 1992;74;508-515.)

trimmed so that they lie underneath the skin, and then all incisions are closed with sutures. The shoulder is placed in an immobilizer, which the patient wears for 4 to 6 weeks. Pendulum exercises are instituted immediately after treatment of two-part fractures. When a proximal pin was used to secure a greater tuberosity fragment, no motion is begun until 3 weeks after the surgery, at which time the proximal pins are removed and pendulum exercises are begun. The patient should be evaluated weekly in the physician's office for the first 2 postoperative weeks to ensure that the pins do not become prominent as the soft-tissue swelling around the pins subsides. Serial radiographs are made at each visit to monitor for movement of the pins. If the pins do become prominent, they should be trimmed back to a subcutaneous position. The pins are usually removed between 4 and 6 weeks after surgery, either in the physician's office or in an operating room. After the pins have been removed, active motion is commenced. In general, stiffness is not a problem as the joint was not violated by surgical dissection.

Intramedullary fixation with use of combinations of rods, wires, and sutures to treat two-part fractures of the surgical neck has also been described.[15] Although this method has been successful when it has been performed properly by some surgeons, there are concerns about torsional rigidity and the risk of displacement. Furthermore, impingement by a prominent rod can be a problem (Figure 6).

An elderly patient with a two-part fracture of the surgical neck may have osteoporotic bone, precluding rigid fixation. To address this, Banco and associates[16] described a method of fixation termed the "parachute technique." With this method, heavy sutures of 5-mm Dacron are placed through the rotator cuff tendons and then through drill holes in the humeral shaft distal to the fracture so that stability is achieved through impaction and compression of the fracture (Figure 7).

A displaced comminuted surgical neck fracture associated with good-quality bone can be treated successfully with a special blade-plate (Figure 8). Preoperative planning is essential, especially when there is extensive comminution, so that length can be restored. Long arm radiographs of both humeri allow the surgeon to determine the proper length and to restore the fractured humerus

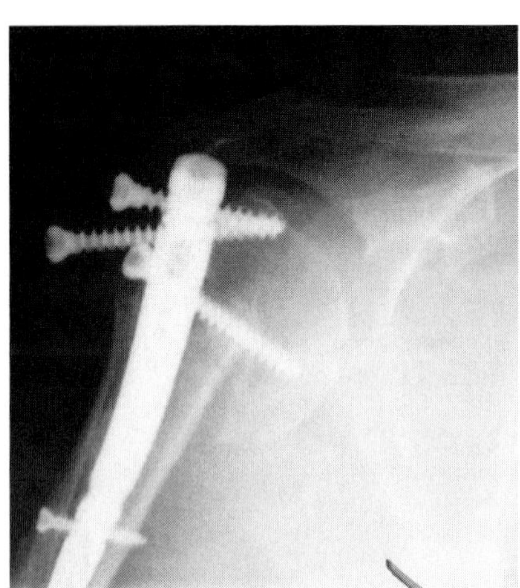

Figure 6 Nonunion of the surgical neck treated with a locking intramedullary rod. Failure of fixation and reduction lead to healing in varus malunion and prominent hardware in the subacromial space.

to match the humerus on the contralateral side. An AO distractor can be used to restore length, and then the blade-plate can be applied. Because no dissection is required in the region of the medial soft tissues adjacent to the bicipital groove, the risk of devascularizing the humeral head fragment is reduced.

Three-Part Fractures

The muscles that are attached to the fracture fragments create deforming forces. Awareness of the common patterns of three-part proximal humeral fractures and an understanding of the muscle forces that act on the fracture fragments allow one to adjust the treatment of each patient.

Deforming Forces

In three-part fractures, fracture lines occur through the surgical neck and the greater or lesser tuberosity. Involvement of the greater tuberosity is much more common than involvement of the lesser tuberosity. The greater tuberosity is displaced superiorly and posteriorly by the pull of the attached supraspinatus, infraspinatus, and teres minor. The degree of displacement depends largely on the location of the fracture line with respect to the rotator cuff insertion. The humeral head fragment is pulled into internal rotation by the attached subscapularis, and the shaft is displaced anteriorly and medially by the pull of the pectoralis major. These forces, combined with the proximal pull of the deltoid, produce retroversion of the humeral head.

With a three-part fracture with a lesser tuberosity fragment, the lesser tuberosity is displaced medially by the attached subscapularis. The humeral head and the greater tuberosity fragment are pulled into adduction and external rotation. The shaft is pulled anteriorly and medially by the pectoralis major and proximally by the deltoid.

An understanding of the deforming forces is critical because these forces must be neutralized to achieve a satisfactory reduction of the fracture and the fixation devices must be capable of withstanding the continuous muscle forces. The options for internal fixation include interfragmentary fixation with sutures or wire, percutaneous pinning, plate-and-screw fixation, and intramedullary fixation with and without suture supplementation.

Surgical Technique

Regardless of the method of fixation, adequate surgical exposure is critical. For most three-part fractures, an extended deltopectoral approach provides the exposure necessary to mobilize and fix the surgical neck and tuberosity components of the fracture. The fracture of the greater tuberosity is more easily managed through a superior deltoid-splitting approach, but fixation of the surgical neck portion of a three-part fracture through this approach is possible only with an intramedullary rod.

There are two goals in the surgical management of three-part proximal humeral fractures. The first is to obtain an anatomic reduction of the fracture fragments, and the second is to neutralize the deforming forces to prevent displacement of the fragments following fixation. Often these two goals can be achieved simultaneously within the fixation construct. However, several techniques achieve these goals independently.

Interfragmentary Fixation Interfragmentary fixation with suture or wires is an established method for fixing three-part fractures of the proximal part of the humerus.[17,18] Neutralization of the forces about the humerus requires achievement of both horizontal and vertical stability across the fracture. To obtain adequate suture fixation in osteopenic bone or comminuted tuberosity fragments, the sutures must be passed at the tendon-bone junction of the tuberosity. Accurate placement of the sutures into the humeral head in the anterior-to-posterior and superior-to-inferior directions is imperative. When the sutures that have been passed through the tuberosity are then passed into the humeral head fragment, they must be placed at the margin of the fracture bed because, when they are placed in the fracture site, the tuberosity fragment tends to be displaced as the sutures are tied. The same is true for the sutures directed in the superior-to-inferior direction. Superior displacement of the tuberosity fragment should be avoided because it can cause subacromial impingement.

The sutures form a figure-of-8 tension-band configuration. Heavy nonabsorbable suture is recommended. We currently use No. 2 fiberwire suture (Arthrex, Naples, FL). Drill holes are made in the shaft

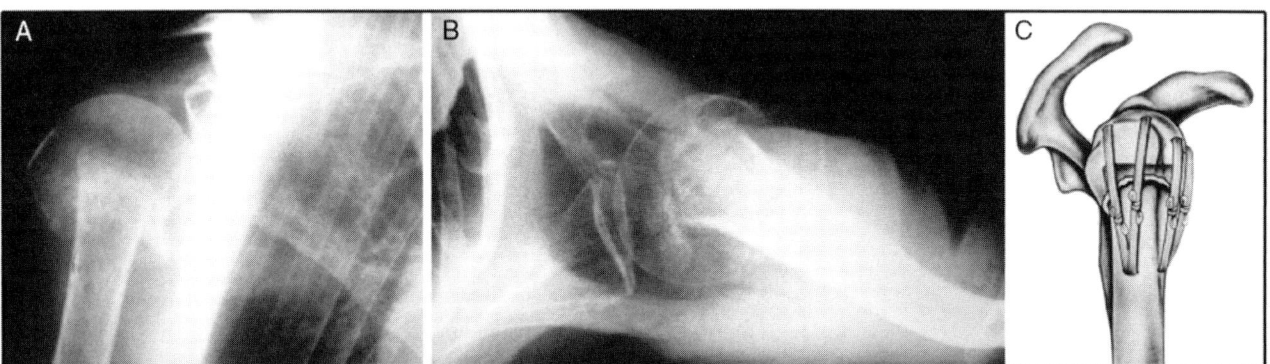

Figure 7 AP **(A)** and axillary **(B)** radiographs of a surgical neck fracture treated with the "parachute technique" of fixation described by Banco and associates.[16] **C,** Heavy sutures have been placed through the rotator cuff tendons and then through drill holes in the humeral shaft distal to the fracture.

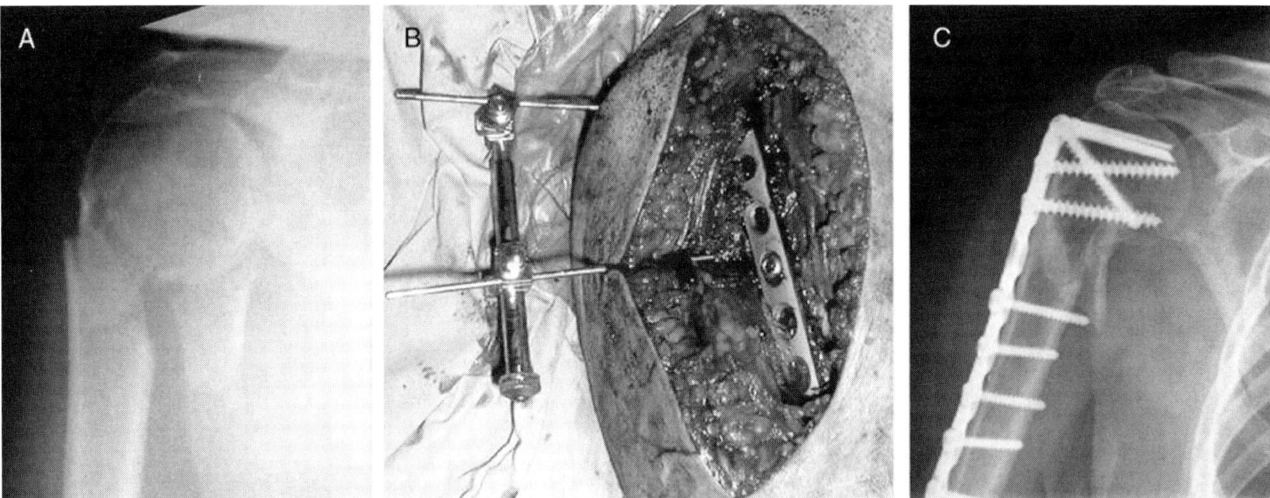

Figure 8 A, Preoperative AP radiograph of a comminuted surgical neck fracture with loss of humeral length. **B,** Intraoperative exposure with use of an AO distractor to restore length. A blade-plate is then applied. **C,** Postoperative AP radiograph showing restoration of humeral length, anatomic reduction, and excellent fixation of both major fragments.

fragment about 1 to 2 cm distal to the fracture site along the medial and lateral ridges of the bicipital groove. Horizontal sutures are then passed through the fractured tuberosity fragment at the bone-tendon junction and through the intact tuberosity of the humeral head fragment. Finally the sutures are crossed and passed through the drill holes in the shaft fragment, forming a figure-of-8. As these sutures are tied, the major deforming forces across the fracture are neutralized (Figure 9).

A potential complication associated with use of the figure-of-8 tension-band technique as the only means of fixation is overlap of the fracture fragments as the sutures are tied. To maintain the fracture reduction as the sutures are tied, interfragmentary sutures can be placed through the fracture site.[12] Drill holes are placed at the fracture margins, on corresponding sides of the fracture fragments, and a figure-of-8 suture is passed with the suture crossing at the fracture site. This prevents the fracture fragments from overlapping when the tension-band neutralization suture is tightened.

Hawkins and associates[17] reported satisfactory results in 12 of 14 patients treated with a wire tension-band construct. However, forward elevation was limited to approximately 120°, and osteonecrosis of the humeral head developed in two patients.

Percutaneous Pinning Percutaneous pinning of three-part proximal humeral fractures requires advanced

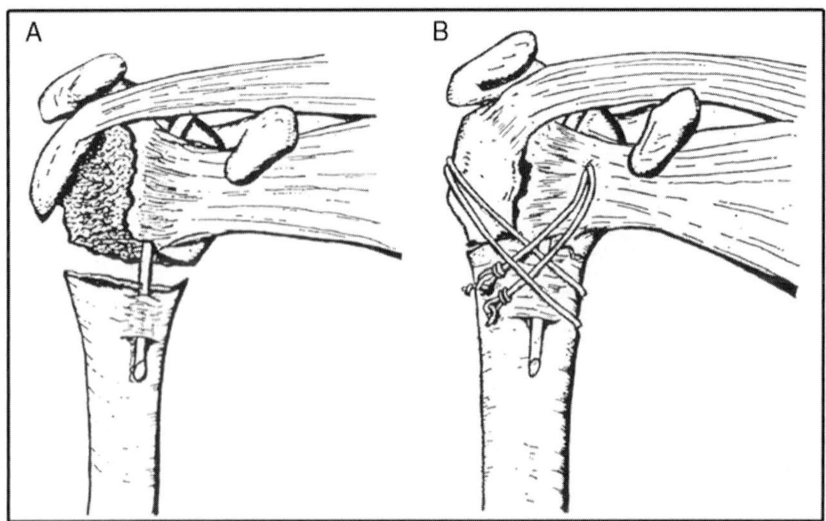

Figure 9 Displaced three-part proximal humeral fracture **(A)** treated with a figure-of-8 fixation suture **(B)** as described by Hawkins and associates.[17] (Reproduced with permission from Hawkins RJ, Bell RH, Gurr K: The three-part fracture of the proximal part of the humerus: Surgical treatment. *J Bone Joint Surg Am* 1986;68;1410-1414.)

skills; good bone stock; minimal comminution, particularly of the tuberosity fragment; and a patient who is able and willing to cooperate with treatment. A retrograde lateral pin, a retrograde anterior pin, or a retrograde anterolateral pin can be used. The retrograde anterolateral pin is most commonly used to achieve percutaneous fixation of the shaft to the humeral head. A fourth option, an antegrade superolateral pin, can supplement the retrograde pin if instability is a problem, but it will slow rehabilitation because it will impinge on the acromion.

Necessary equipment includes a C-arm and image intensifier, 2.5-mm terminally threaded pins, a pin cutter, a small cannulated-screw system, a small- to medium-sized periosteal elevator, and a reduction pick or hook. A knowledgeable assistant is always helpful, and a skillful radiology technician to operate the C-arm and image intensifier is mandatory.

The patient is placed in the beach-chair position with the back of the operating table elevated approximately 30°. The C-arm is positioned so that AP and axillary images can be made. Through a stab incision at the level of the surgical neck, the humeral head is elevated with a reduction tool, reestablishing the neck-shaft angle. The retrograde pins are placed to obtain fixation of the humeral head to the humeral shaft. The greater tuberosity fragment is reduced to the head-shaft composite with use of a reduction pick and is provisionally fixed with a guide-wire for the 4.0-mm cannulated screw set. When the tuberosity has been reduced satisfactorily, a screw of appropriate length is placed.

Percutaneous pinning of three-part fractures of the proximal part of the humerus is technically demanding. A transitional step before performing the fully percutaneous technique is performing open reduction and internal fixation of the greater tuberosity fragment through a superior deltoid-splitting approach followed by percutaneous pinning of the surgical neck component of the fracture. The deltoid split is performed between the anterior and middle thirds of the deltoid, with the anterior third of the deltoid released in continuity with its periosteal sleeve from the acromion. The tuberosity fragment is then fixed to the head fragment with an interfragmentary suture technique. The surgical neck component can be anatomically reduced through the superior deltoid split. Under fluoroscopic guidance, the surgical neck component can then be fixed percutaneously. Once the surgeon has become comfortable with this technique, he or she can transition to a fully percutaneous technique.

Resch and associates[5] reported good to very good functional results with percutaneous pinning of three-part proximal humeral fractures. At 24 months, no patient in their study showed radiographic evidence of necrosis of the humeral head. The expertise required to obtain such outstanding results of the treatment of these difficult fractures cannot be overstated.

Plate-and-Screw Fixation The results of plate-and-screw fixation of three-part proximal humeral fractures have been mixed. Although some authors have reported excellent results,[19,20] this approach has typically been associated with a high complication rate, particularly in elderly patients.[21-25] Earlier implants were poorly designed, and placement of those implants required extensive soft-tissue stripping, which placed the vascular supply to the humeral head at risk. Currently, there is a renewed interest in plate-and-screw fixation with the development of better implants, including the fixed-angle blade-plate and the locking anatomic proximal humeral plates.

The indication for plate-and screw fixation is a comminuted fracture, particularly one involving the tuberosity and the surgical neck and requiring rigid fixation. An extended deltopectoral incision is used to approach the fracture, and the tuberosity fragment is first reduced to the humeral head with interfragmentary sutures. If a blade-plate is used, a guide-wire is advanced into the humeral head under fluoroscopic guidance and a plate of appropriate length is selected. If an anatomic proximal humeral locking plate is chosen, it is placed along the greater tuberosity and diverging, locked screws are placed into the humeral head. Then, the head is anatomically reduced to the shaft, and bicortical shaft fixation is performed.

If bone quality is a concern, neutralization sutures can be placed at the bone-tendon junction and passed through one of the holes of the plate to counteract the pull of the rotator cuff on the head and tuberosity fragments.

Intramedullary Fixation There are two types of intramedullary fixation of three-part proximal humeral fractures: (1) intramedullary fixation as the sole means of fixation,[2] and (2) intramedullary fixation with Ender rods supplementing a tension band. The second type is the preferred method of intramedullary fixation because it provides longitudinal and rotational stability to the fracture.

These methods are technically demanding. Because the fracture line in the greater tuberosity fragment is at the articular margin, insertion of an intramedullary rod at the articular margin may displace the fragment. When there is a fracture of the lesser tuberosity, the entry point for the medullary canal is unaffected. Therefore, intramedullary fixation is probably better for three-part fractures with a fracture of the lesser tuberosity than it is for those with a fracture of the greater tuberosity.

Management of the Ender rods and sutures can be cumbersome, even in two-part fractures of the proximal part of the humerus. The application of this technique to three-part proximal humeral fractures requires, in addition, management of the tuberosity fragment.

The peril associated with Ender rod fixation of three-part fractures involving the greater tuberosity is the need for a bone bridge between the margin of the tuberosity fracture and the articular margin to place the rods into the medullary canal. It has been recommended that the Ender rods be modified by creation of an additional hole above the manufactured hole through which to place sutures and keep the rod distal to the level of the greater tuberosity[15] (Figure 10). The superior hole is used to form a tension-band construct that neutralizes the deforming forces across the surgical neck. Two additional sutures are placed through the lower hole, with one limb of each suture coming out of drill holes placed in the shaft fragment. These sutures counteract the tension band suture that is trying to pull the Ender rod out of the medullary canal.

Valgus Impacted Four-Part Fractures

The valgus impacted four-part fracture is characterized by impaction of the lateral aspect of the humeral articular surface through a fracture of the anatomic neck.[3-5,26,27] This lateral impaction results in a valgus deformity of the humeral head such that the articular surface faces superiorly, toward the acromion, rather than medially, toward the glenoid. As the articular surface is imploded into the proximal humeral metaphysis, the greater and lesser tuberosities typically displace from each other as well as from the humeral shaft through intertubercular and surgical neck fractures lines.

Although this displacement pattern may fit Neer's criteria for four-part fractures,[1] the fracture does not behave as such because of at least two important factors. First, true valgus impacted four-part fractures are characterized by little or no displacement (ie, translation) of the medial aspect of the humeral articular surface with respect to the medial aspect of the shaft. Second, the shaft, periosteum, displaced tuberosities, glenohumeral joint capsule, and rotator cuff form a single continuous sleeve of tissue.[3-5,26,27] The lack of displacement between the medial aspect of the humeral articular surface and the shaft preserves the inferomedial part of the periosteum and its associated vessels. Therefore, the prevalence of necrosis of the humeral head (5% to 10%) is much lower than that associated with standard four-part fractures.[3-5,26,27] Moreover, the continuous sleeve of tissue connecting the shaft, tuberosities, glenohumeral joint capsule, and rotator cuff imparts substantial stability and encourages anatomic or nearly anatomic reduction of the tuberosities when the head is reduced.[3-5,26,27]

Radiographic Features

Initial radiographs should include an AP view in the scapular plane, a transscapular lateral view (the Y view), and an axillary view.[1] At first glance, the severity of valgus impacted four-part fractures may be underestimated. Closer inspection reveals the humeral articular surface to be facing superiorly. The displacement of the greater and lesser tuberosities (especially the greater tuberosity) may seem severe,

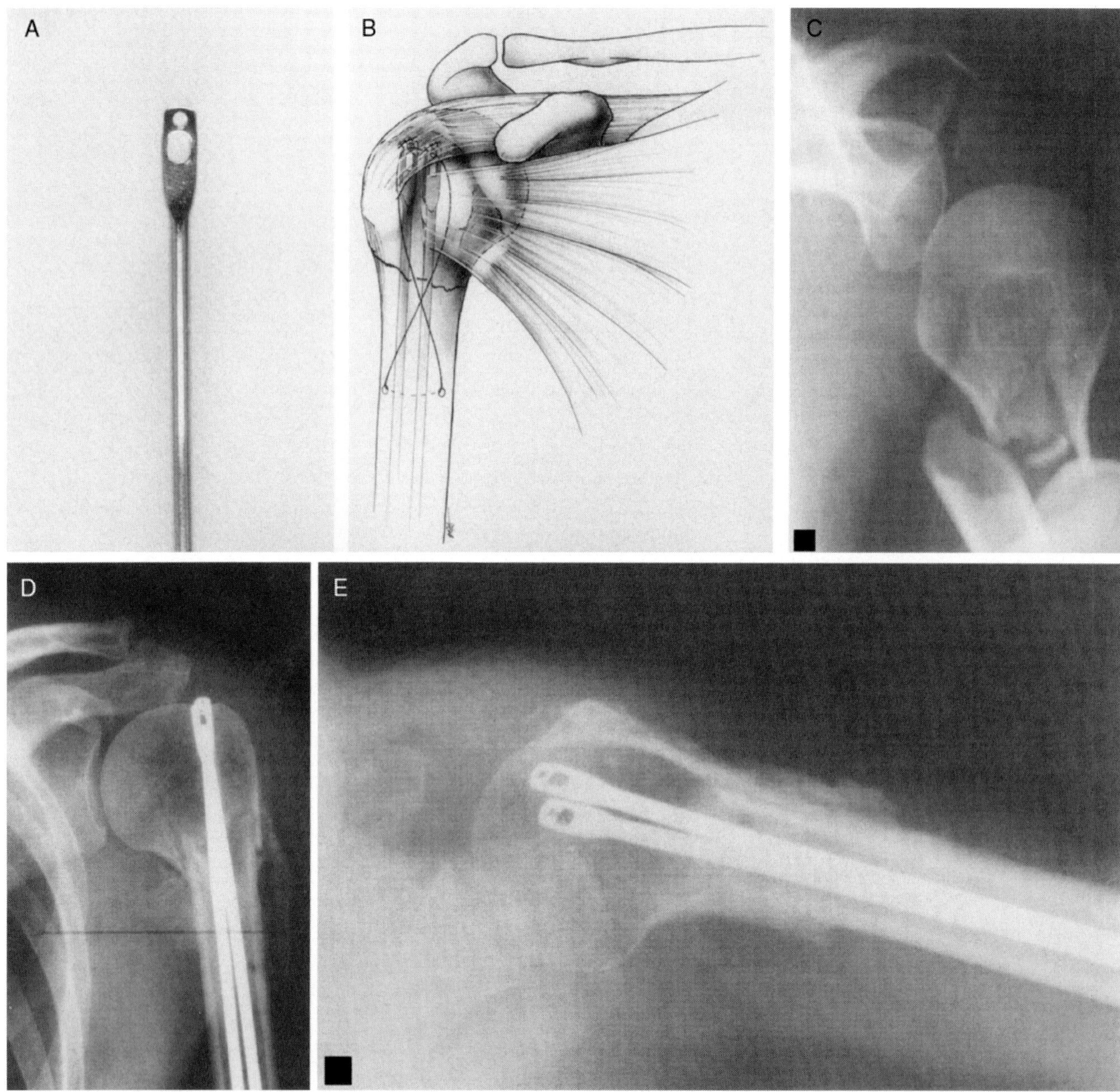

Figure 10 A and **B,** Modified Ender rod with figure-of-8 suture fixation. **C,** Preoperative AP radiograph of an unstable three-part fracture. **D** and **E,** Postoperative radiographs. (Reproduced with permission from Cuomo F, Flatow EL, Maday MG, Miller SR, McIlveen SJ, Bigliani LU: Open reduction and internal fixation of two- and three-part displaced surgical neck fractures of the proximal humerus. *J Shoulder Elbow Surg* 1992;1;287-295.)

but the relative tuberosity displacement is primarily the result of the valgus impaction of the humeral head (Figure 11). The intertubercular fracture line is typically posterior to the bicipital groove. This is an important consideration when surgical reduction is being contemplated.

Treatment Options

Potential treatment options include early mobilization, percutaneous reduction and internal fixation, open reduction and internal fixation, and hemiarthroplasty. The vast majority of valgus impacted four-part fractures are amenable to percutaneous reduction and internal fixation. Nonsurgical treatment often results in painful malunion and therefore is indicated only for elderly, sedentary patients with medical comorbidities that preclude surgical treatment. Percutaneous reduction and internal fixation is an excellent option for patients who

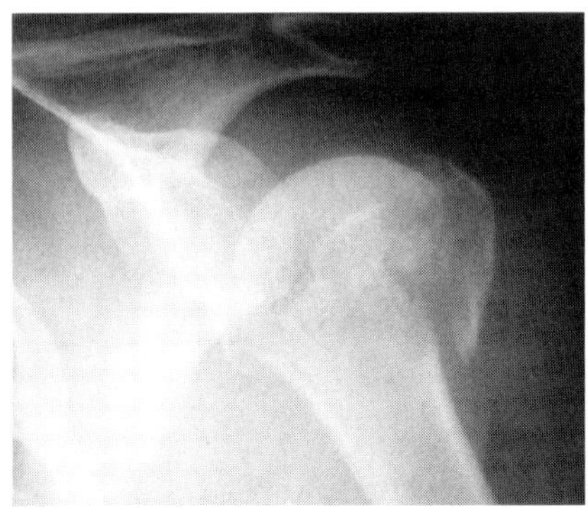

Figure 11 AP radiograph of a classic valgus impacted four-part fracture. The displacement of the tuberosities is secondary to the valgus impaction of the articular segment. There is unimportant displacement of the humeral shaft in relation to the humeral head consistent with an intact medial periosteal soft-tissue sleeve and an intact blood supply in this area.

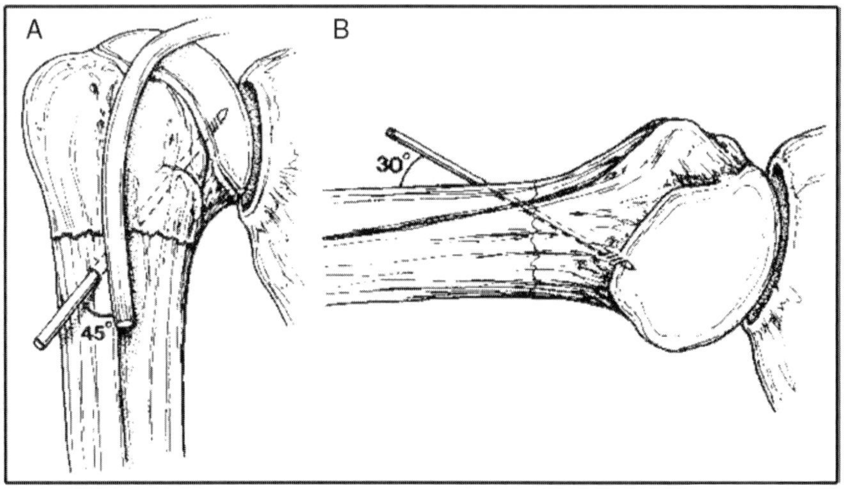

Figure 12 Percutaneous fixation of the head fragment with two pins. First, the pin is placed on the anterolateral surface of the humerus and advanced to within 1 cm of the subchondral surface of the head under fluoroscopic guidance. Accurate placement typically requires the pin to be angled 45° medially **(A)** and 30° posteriorly **(B)**. A second pin is then placed parallel and slightly superior or inferior to the first.

have an acute injury (7 to 10 days old), good bone quality, and minimal comminution and can be relied on to cooperate with treatment. Open reduction and internal fixation is primarily indicated for acute fractures that are not reducible by closed means, for severe osteopenic bone, for extensive comminution, or for fractures that are between 10 days and 4 months old. Hemiarthroplasty is reserved for fractures that are more than 4 months old or the rare acute fracture in an elderly, sedentary patient with severe osteopenia.

Percutaneous Reduction and Internal Fixation The patient is positioned so that radiographs can be made in two orthogonal planes. This should be verified before sterile preparation and draping. The optimal patient position is semirecumbent in a beach-chair configuration, with the back of the table elevated 30° to 45°. The affected extremity should be positioned off the edge of the table to allow adequate C-arm access. The anesthesia equipment is moved to the opposite side of the table to allow the C-arm to enter the surgical field from superior with the plane of the C-arm parallel to the table's edge (Figure 4). The arm and shoulder are then prepared and draped.

Successful percutaneous reduction and internal fixation may be accomplished by following a series of individual steps: percutaneous reduction of the articular segment, fixation of the head, reduction and fixation of the greater tuberosity, and reduction and fixation of the lesser tuberosity.[1] Reduction and fixation is not always required for both tuberosities. This decision is made after reduction and fixation of the head.

A small Cobb periosteal elevator is used to reduce the humeral head on the shaft through a small incision in the skin. With the arm held in 20° to 30° of abduction and neutral rotation, the level of the intertubercular fracture is identified with fluoroscopy. A 1.5- to 2.0-cm incision is made on the anterolateral surface of the arm over the fracture. The elevator is placed through this incision, through the deltoid, and into the fracture under fluoroscopic guidance. It is then placed under the lateral portion of the humeral head. This position is again verified radiographically. A superiorly directed force is applied to the undersurface of the head with use of the elevator. This maneuver should be done carefully to avoid overreduction or translation of the humeral head. In acute fractures, the head usually reduces very easily and stays in the reduced position after the elevator is removed.

Once the head fragment is reduced, it is fixed in that position with percutaneously placed 2.5-mm terminally threaded pins. Two retrograde anterolateral pins are usually sufficient. The first pin is placed on the skin, its relationship to the humerus is visualized radiographically, and the entry site is located. The pin enters the arm midway between the anterior and lateral surfaces. After the skin incision is made, a hemostat

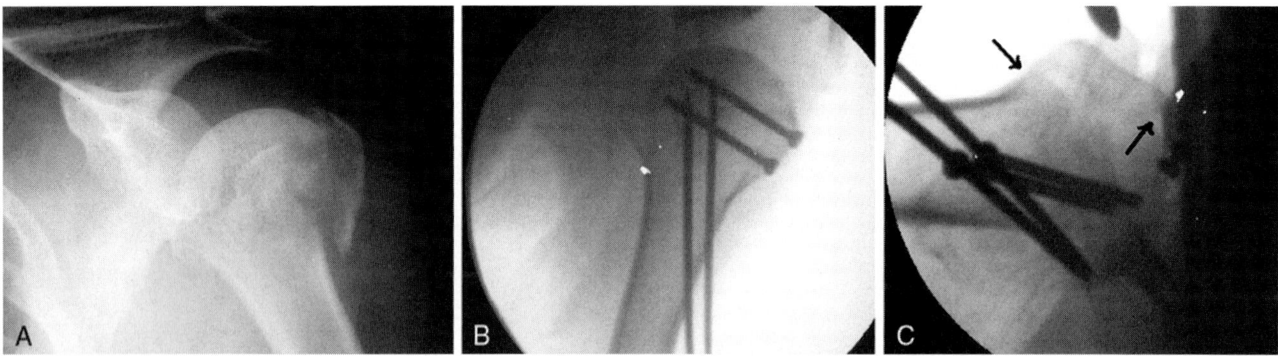

Figure 13 A, AP radiograph of a four-part humeral head fracture. **B,** AP fluoroscopic view of the fracture after reduction and fixation of the head and greater tuberosity fragments. **C,** Axillary fluoroscopic view of the fracture with mild residual displacement of the lesser tuberosity fragment.

is used to spread the soft tissues bluntly until the bone is identified. This lessens the risk of injury to the axillary nerve. The pin is placed on the anterolateral surface of the humerus and advanced to within 1 cm of the subchondral surface of the head under fluoroscopic guidance. Accurate pin placement typically requires angling of the pin 45° medially and 30° posteriorly (Figure 12). A second pin is placed parallel and slightly superior or inferior to the first one. At least 1 cm should separate the pins at their site of entry into the bone. Accurate placement of the pins and the quality of the reduction are evaluated by rotating the humerus in a 90° arc of motion while continuously visualizing the humerus under fluoroscopy.

The greater tuberosity is often found to be anatomically reduced after the head has been reduced. If the tuberosity is anatomically reduced and is stable with motion (as assessed fluoroscopically), it should not need additional fixation. If reduction and fixation of the greater tuberosity is required, a 5-mm incision is made at the midpart of the acromion, approximately 2 to 3 cm distal to the lateral acromial border. A reduction hook or a small elevator is placed through this incision, through the deltoid, and down to the tuberosity surface. The tuberosity is reduced by pulling it forward and slightly distally. A guidewire from a small cannulated-screw set is then placed percutaneously through the greater tuberosity approximately 1 cm inferior to its most superior edge. The guide-wire is then passed across the humerus and into the subchondral bone of the humeral head at an approximately 90° angle with the shaft. Accurate placement of the guide-wire is verified radiographically in two planes (by rotating the humerus). After measurement of the length of the screw, an appropriately sized cannulated screw is placed. Initial predrilling and tapping of the humerus usually is not necessary. A second, parallel screw is placed in a similar fashion approximately 1.5 cm distal to the first. Accurate screw placement is verified fluoroscopically.

The lesser tuberosity is visualized by rotating the C-arm, without moving the humerus. Residual displacement of the lesser tuberosity is better tolerated than is residual displacement of the greater tuberosity; therefore, it is important to visualize these relationships accurately[1,2] (Figure 13). A nonanatomic relationship between the lesser tuberosity and the articular surface may be misinterpreted as displacement of the tuberosity rather than residual displacement of the head. If the problem is residual displacement of the head, the relationship between the shaft and the lesser tuberosity will be normal, despite displacement between the head and the lesser tuberosity. Under these circumstances, it is probably better to accept a small (0.5- to 1.0-cm) amount of residual head displacement than to redo the previously placed fixation. If there is residual displacement of the lesser tuberosity, reduction is achieved with a reduction hook placed through the previously made anterolateral incision. Percutaneous screw fixation can be achieved through an anterior incision. Two parallel AP screws are placed with use of the same technique as used for the greater tuberosity.

The pins are cut under the skin, and the wounds are closed in a standard fashion. Pendulum exercises are instituted the next day. Passive flexion and external rotation with the patient supine are begun during the third postoperative week. The pins are removed at 3 to 4 weeks. More aggressive passive stretching and strengthening are instituted at 6 weeks after reduction.

Open Reduction and Internal Fixation Open reduction and internal fixation usually is not required for acute four-part fractures, except when an acceptable reduction could not be attained percutaneously. Under these circumstances, the patient and the C-arm are positioned as described above. The fracture is exposed through a standard deltopectoral incision. The head is then reduced by placing an elevator through the intertubercular fracture line under direct visualization. Percutaneously placed pins are then used as described above to fix the head and shaft fragments. Next, the tuberosities are sutured to themselves with interfragmentary nonabsorbable sutures.

Subacute fractures more than 10 days but less than 4 months old are routinely treated with open reduction and internal fixation. Patient and C-arm positioning is identical to that described above. The fracture is exposed through a standard deltopectoral approach. The intertubercular fracture line is identified and may need to be recreated with an osteotome. The greater and lesser tuberosities are levered open to make them more mobile and to allow access to the undersurface of the valgus impacted head fragment. A small osteotome is used to score the medial junction of the head fragment and the shaft. Care is taken to avoid complete perforation of the medial cortex. The head is then elevated with a small elevator. In the subacute situation, there is a tendency for the head to redisplace into valgus. Therefore, allograft cancellous chips are packed under the elevated head. Fixation of the head can be performed with several devices. A humeral blade-plate is an excellent option in this setting because of its rigidity (Figure 14).

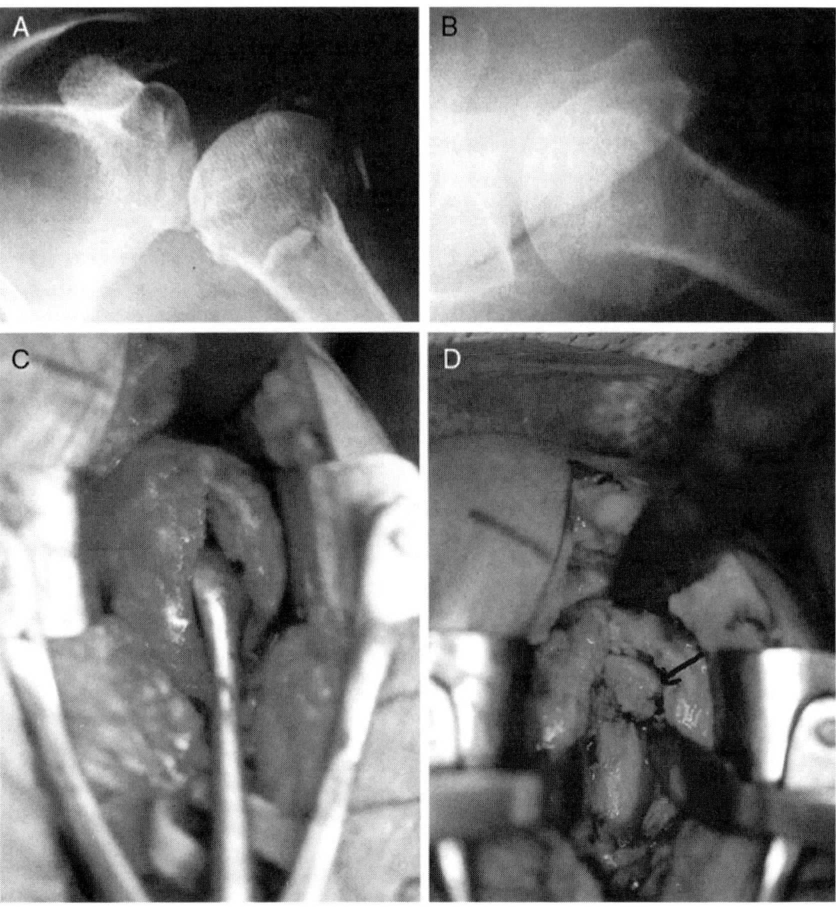

Figure 14 A and **B,** AP and axillary radiographs made 16 days after the patient sustained a subacute valgus impacted fracture. **C,** A Cobb elevator is used to reduce the humeral articular fragment. **D,** A corticocancellous bone graft was placed to maintain the reduction and fill the void. Then, an AO humeral blade-plate was inserted above the graft into the articular fragment, and the side-plate was fixed to the humeral shaft with screws.

Pendulum exercises are instituted on the first postoperative day. Passive flexion and external rotation exercises with the patient supine are added at 7 to 10 days. More aggressive stretching and strengthening exercises are started at 6 weeks after surgery.

References

1. Neer CS II: Displaced proximal humeral fractures: II. Treatment of three-part and four-part displacement. *J Bone Joint Surg Am* 1970;52:1090-1103.
2. Mouradian WH: Displaced proximal humeral fractures: Seven years' experience with a modified Zickel supracondylar device. *Clin Orthop* 1986;212:209-218.
3. Resch H, Beck E, Bayley I: Reconstruction of the valgus-impacted humeral head fracture. *J Shoulder Elbow Surg* 1995;4:73-80.
4. Resch H, Hubner C, Schwaiger R: Minimally invasive reduction and osteosynthesis of articular fractures of the humeral head. *Injury* 2001;32(suppl 1): SA25-SA32.
5. Resch H, Povacz P, Frohlich R, Wambacher M: Percutaneous fixation of three- and four-part fractures of the proximal humerus. *J Bone Joint Surg Br* 1997;79:295-300.
6. Neer CS II: Displaced proximal humeral fractures: I. Classification and evaluation. *J Bone Joint Surg Am* 1970;52:1077-1089.

7. Flatow EL, Cuomo F, Maday MG, Miller SR, McIlveen SJ, Bigliani LU: Open reduction and internal fixation of two-part displaced fractures of the greater tuberosity of the proximal part of the humerus. *J Bone Joint Surg Am* 1991;73:1213-1218.
8. Beredjiklian PK, Iannotti JP, Norris TR, Williams GR: Operative treatment of malunion of a fracture of the proximal aspect of the humerus. *J Bone Joint Surg Am* 1998;80:1484-1497.
9. Norris TR, Green A, McGuigan FX: Late prosthetic shoulder arthroplasty for displaced proximal humerus fractures. *J Shoulder Elbow Surg* 1995;4:271-280.
10. Siebenrock KA, Gerber C: The reproducibility of classification of fractures of the proximal end of the humerus. *J Bone Joint Surg Am* 1993;75:1751-1755.
11. Sidor ML, Zuckerman JD, Lyon T, Koval K, Cuomo F, Schoenberg N: The Neer classification system for proximal humeral fractures: An assessment of interobserver reliability and intraobserver reproducibility. *J Bone Joint Surg Am* 1993;75:1745-1750.
12. Gerber C, Warner J: Alternatives to hemiarthroplasty for complex proximal-humeral fractures, in Warner JJ, Iannotti JP, Gerber C (eds): *Complex* and *Revision Problems in Shoulder Surgery.* Philadelphia, PA, Lippincott-Raven, 1997, pp 215-243.
13. Bohler J: Les fractures recentes de l'epaule. *Acta Orthop Belg* 1964;30:235-242.
14. Jaberg H, Warner JJ, Jakob RP: Percutaneous stabilization of unstable fractures of the humerus. *J Bone Joint Surg Am* 1992;74:508-515.
15. Cuomo F, Flatow EL, Maday MG, Miller SR, McIlveen SJ, Bigliani LU: Open reduction and internal fixation of two- and three-part displaced surgical neck fractures of the proximal humerus. *J Shoulder Elbow Surg* 1992;1:287-295.
16. Banco SP, Andrisani D, Ramsey M, Frieman B, Fenlin JM Jr: The parachute technique: Valgus impaction osteotomy for two-part fractures of the surgical neck of the humerus. *J Bone Joint Surg Am* 2001;83(suppl 2):38-42.
17. Hawkins RJ, Bell RH, Gurr K: The three-part fracture of the proximal part of the humerus: Operative treatment. *J Bone Joint Surg Am* 1986;68:1410-1414.
18. Hawkins RJ, Kiefer GN: Internal fixation techniques for proximal humeral fractures. *Clin Orthop* 1987;223:77-85.
19. Esser RD: Open reduction and internal fixation of three- and four-part fractures of the proximal humerus. *Clin Orthop* 1994;299:244-251.
20. Esser RD: Treatment of three- and four-part fractures of the proximal humerus with a modified cloverleaf plate. *J Orthop Trauma* 1994;8:15-22.
21. Cofield RH: Comminuted fractures of the proximal humerus. *Clin Orthop* 1988;230:49-57.
22. Kristiansen B, Christiensen SW: Plate fixation of proximal humeral fractures. *Acta Orthop Scand* 1986;57:320-323.
23. Lee CK, Hansen HR: Post-traumatic avascular necrosis of the humeral head in displaced proximal humeral fractures. *J Trauma* 1981;21:788-791.
24. Paavolainen P, Bjorkenheim JM, Slatis P, Paukku P: Operative treatment of severe proximal humeral fractures. *Acta Orthop Scand* 1983;54:374-379.
25. Svend-Hansen H: Displaced proximal humeral fractures. A review of 49 patients. *Acta Orthop Scand* 1974;45:359-364.
26. Habermeyer P, Schweiberer L: Corrective interventions subsequent to humeral head fractures. *Orthopade* 1992;21:148-157.
27. Jakob RP, Miniaci A, Anson PS, Jaberg H, Osterwalder A, Ganz R: Four-part valgus impacted fractures of the proximal humerus. *J Bone Joint Surg Br* 1991;73:295-298.

Late Sequelae of Proximal Humerus Fractures

Michael A. Wirth, MD

Abstract

Proximal humerus fractures, both minimally displaced and complex, are subject to the development of complications. Late sequelae of such injuries include refractory shoulder stiffness, osteonecrosis, malunion, nonunion, and heterotopic bone formation. A prompt, accurate diagnosis and proper treatment protocol can decrease the occurrence and severity of such complications. When complications do occur, treatment options to improve outcome should be implemented.

Instr Course Lect 2003;52:13-16.

Fractures of the proximal humerus account for 4% to 5% of all fractures.[1,2] Approximately 60% to 80% of these injuries are minimally displaced (so-called one-part fractures) and can be satisfactorily treated with a sling and early range-of-motion exercises. Contrary to popular belief, the seemingly innocuous nature of these minimally displaced fractures does not preclude the development of complications. In general, late sequelae of fractures of the proximal humerus include refractory shoulder stiffness, osteonecrosis, malunion, nonunion, and heterotopic bone formation. The aftereffects of proximal humerus fractures, both minimally displaced and more complex multipart injuries, can be the result of the injury itself or the treatment. Consequently, it is imperative to make an accurate diagnosis so that the most appropriate treatment can be promptly instituted.

Refractory Shoulder Stiffness

One of the most common aftereffects of fractures of the proximal humerus is shoulder stiffness. Factors that contribute to this complication include the severity of the initial injury, prolonged immobilization, articular surface malunion, and patient noncompliance with rehabilitation. In a functional outcome study of 104 patients with minimally displaced proximal humerus fractures, the percentage of good and excellent results was significantly greater when supervised physical therapy was instituted less than 14 days after injury.[3] Shoulder stiffness also has a negative effect on displaced three- and four-part proximal humerus fractures. The results of late arthroplasty for these complex fractures are inferior to the results achieved with acute humeral head replacement, mainly because of the effects of fixed soft tissue.[4-6] In this situation, soft-tissue scarring and contractures markedly limit functional range of motion in this normally compliant joint. Numerous studies have emphasized the importance of an early physician-directed rehabilitation program to minimize refractory shoulder stiffness for both nonsurgically treated and surgically treated patients in the postoperative period.[3,7-10]

Osteonecrosis

In general, the incidence of osteonecrosis is proportional to the complexity of the proximal humerus fracture and the extent of the surgical dissection of soft tissue. Osteonecrosis is usually associated with three- and four-part fractures and fracture dislocations and infrequently occurs following two-part fractures (Fig. 1). Osteonecrosis occurs in 3% to 14% of patients after closed reduction of displaced three-part fractures and in 13% to 34% after closed reduction of four-part fractures.[11-17] One series reported a 34% incidence of osteonecrosis in a series of patients treated with open reduction and internal fixation (ORIF) with a T-plate.[18] The pathology may be first detected by MRI before it is seen with conventional radiography. Later, osteoporosis or osteosclerosis may be seen on plain radio-

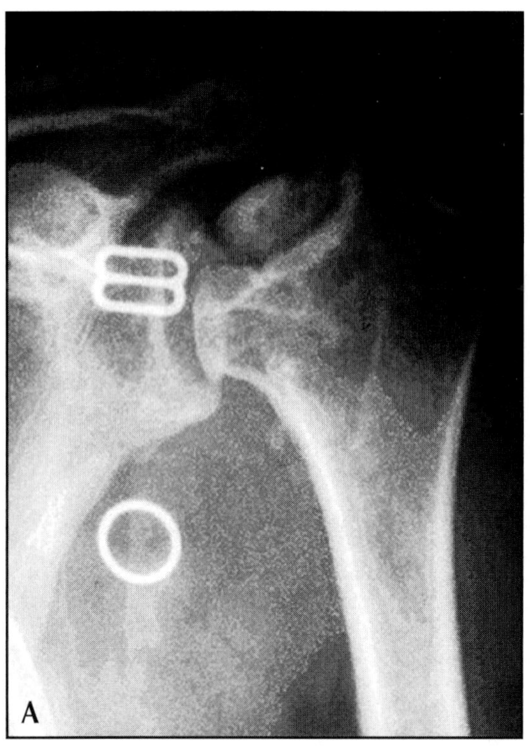

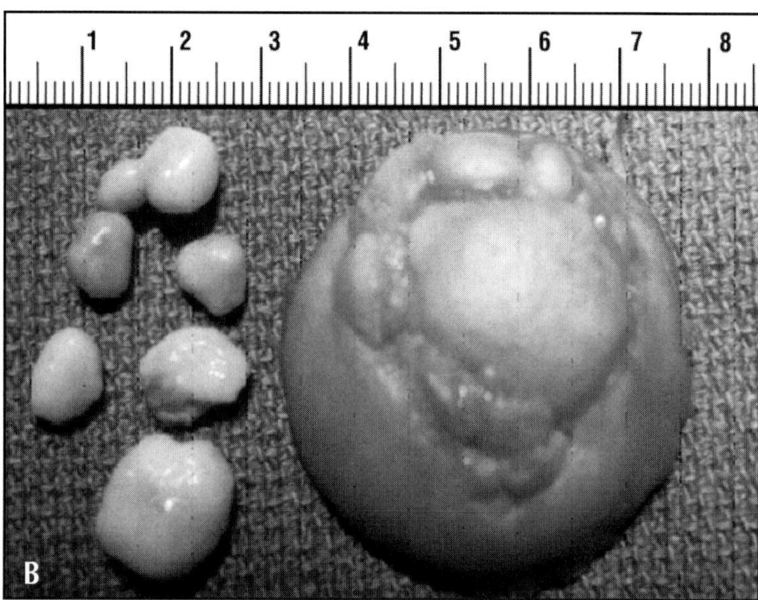

Fig. 1 A, AP radiograph of a patient who sustained an impaction fracture of the humeral head 2 years prior, as the result of a motorcycle accident. **B,** Appearance of the humeral head and multiple loose bodies at the time of humeral head replacement surgery.

graphs. In end-stage osteonecrosis, collapse of the subchondral bone occurs and the irregular humeral head eventually destroys the glenoid articular cartilage and results in secondary degenerative joint disease. Prosthetic arthroplasty is the primary surgical option when major pain and functional loss are present.

Malunion

Malunion results when closed reduction or ORIF fails to restore the normal anatomic relationships between the humeral head and shaft, tuberosities, and glenohumeral joint (Fig. 2). Malunion of the greater tuberosity is usually superior, posterior, or both. Superior displacement that encroaches on the subacromial space will result in pain, weakness, and a mechanical block to overhead elevation. When the displacement is predominantly posterior, external rotation is limited because of abutment with the posterior glenoid. When pain and functional limitations are present, osteotomy is indicated if displacement exceeds 5 mm. Fixed soft-tissue contractures make it difficult to adequately immobilize and fix the tuberosity to restore the dynamic quality of the rotator cuff muscle-tendon unit. Thorough preoperative counseling to discuss reasonable expectations is essential as functional results often are modest. Two-part surgical neck fractures infrequently result in pain or functional limitation that would necessitate surgical intervention. Occasionally, a varus malunion causes impingement between the acromion and the superiorly displaced greater tuberosity. In many patients, this type of malunion can be adequately treated by open or arthroscopic acromioplasty with or without an osteotomy of the greater tuberosity. Humeral head articular malunions associated with joint incongruity and subsequent degenerative changes are the result of malunited three- and four-part proximal humerus fractures. Prosthetic arthroplasty is generally required for this type of late sequelae. The prognosis is less favorable than for fractures treated acutely because of extensive scarring, deltoid weakness, inferior pain relief, and a higher rate of complications.

Nonunion

Nonunion of the proximal humerus usually occurs in elderly patients with osteoporosis.[19-22] The incidence of this late sequela is difficult to determine but may occur in up to 23% of surgical neck fractures in the elderly.[23] Factors associated with nonunion of the proximal humerus include soft-tissue interposition, hanging arm casts, inadequate ORIF, patient alcoholism, and comorbidities such as diabetes mellitus.[10,24-31] Many patients with nonunion of the proximal humerus have minimal pain and a functional range of motion that obviates the need for surgery.[10,22,32-40] Closed methods of treatment that require prolonged immobilization or extremes of positioning are inappropriate because they can result in functionally disabling arthrofibrosis. For patients with pain and functional disability, surgical treatment options are mainly based on the quality of bone, the stability of the

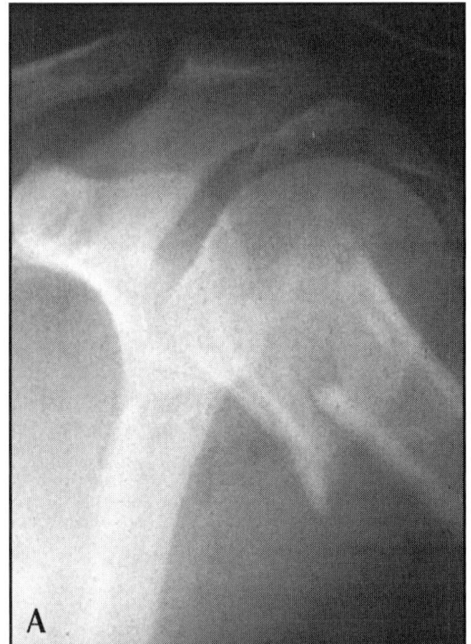

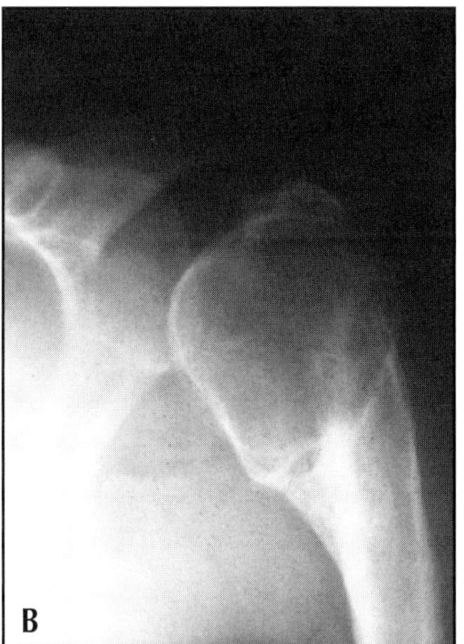

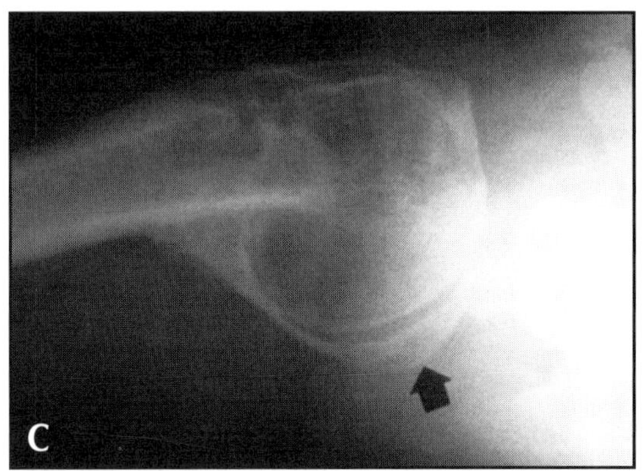

Fig. 2 A, AP radiograph showing a three-part fracture of the proximal humerus. **B,** AP radiograph showing malunion of the proximal humerus several months after injury. Note the varus position of the head/shaft fracture components and the superior displacement of the greater tuberosity. **C,** Axillary lateral radiograph showing posterior displacement of the greater tuberosity (*arrow*).

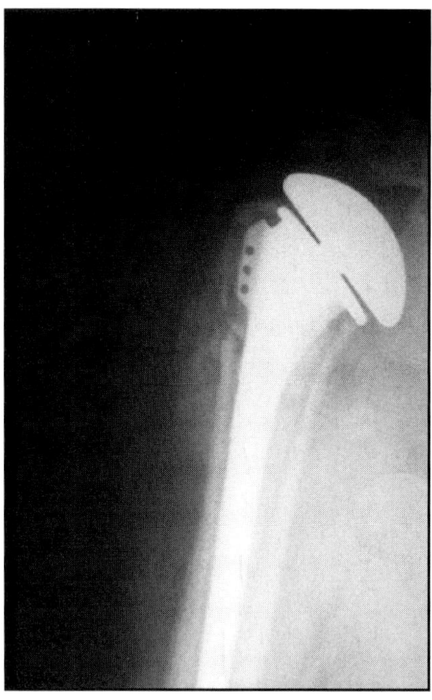

Fig. 3 Heterotopic bone is seen on this AP radiograph taken 12 months after hemiarthroplasty was done on a patient with a four-part proximal humerus fracture. The patient had good motion and excellent functional outcome.

surgical construct at the time of surgery, the integrity of the humeral head and glenoid articular surfaces, and the vascularity of the humeral head. ORIF with bone grafting is the preferred method of treatment when adequate bone quality and quantity allow secure fixation that permits early rehabilitation while avoiding the complications associated with prolonged immobilization. Unfortunately, many surgical neck nonunions are associated with resorption of the humeral head fragment and cavitation, which results in severe bone loss.

Heterotopic Bone Formation

The formation of ectopic bone about the proximal humerus after fracture is common and there is usually little clinical relevance to the patient's functional outcome.[41,42] In 1970, Neer[42] presented results from a series of 117 consecutive patients with three- and four-part fractures and fracture dislocations. Ectopic ossification occurred in 12% of patients, including three patients treated with closed reduction, five treated with ORIF, and six who had a hemiarthroplasty. Predisposing factors for the development of ectopic ossification include the extent of soft-tissue injury, the number of repeated manipulations, and the delay of reduction by more than 7 days. In the majority of patients, ectopic bone formation represents an incidental radiographic finding (Fig. 3). Only rarely does the bone formation bridge the glenohumeral space resulting in limited motion; surgical resection is then recommended to restore a functional range of motion.

Summary

Although complications such as refractory shoulder stiffness, osteonecrosis, malunion, nonunion, and heterotopic bone formation can occur following proximal humerus fractures, prompt treatment should be instituted to improve outcome. Nonsurgical treatment such as a physician-directed rehabilitation program, and surgical treatment such as prosthetic arthroplasty or ORIF with bone grafting usually yield favorable results.

References

1. Lind T, Kroner K, Jensen J: The epidemiology of fractures of the proximal humerus. *Arch Orthop Trauma Surg* 1989;108:285-287.

2. Stimson BB (ed): *A Manual of Fractures and Dislocations*, ed 2. Philadelphia, PA, Lea & Febiger, 1947, pp 241-260.
3. Koval KJ, Gallagher MA, Marsicano JG, Cuomo F, McShinawy A, Zuckerman JD: Functional outcome after minimally displaced fractures of the proximal part of the humerus. *J Bone Joint Surg Am* 1997;79:203-207.
4. Frich LH, Sojbjerg JO, Sneppen O: Shoulder arthroplasty in complex acute and chronic proximal humeral fractures. *Orthopedics* 1991;14: 949-954.
5. Neer CS II: Glenohumeral arthroplasty, in Neer CS II (ed): *Shoulder Reconstruction*. Philadelphia, PA, WB Saunders, 1990, pp 143-271.
6. Tanner MW, Cofield RH: Prosthetic arthroplasty for fractures and fracture-dislocations of the proximal humerus. *Clin Orthop* 1983;179: 116-128.
7. Bertoft ES, Lundh I, Ringqvist I: Physiotherapy after fracture of the proximal end of the humerus: Comparison between two methods. *Scand J Rehabil Med* 1984;16:11-16.
8. Brostrom F: Early mobilization of fractures of the upper end of the humerus. *Arch Surg* 1943;46:614-615.
9. Ekström T, Lagergren C, von Schreeb T: Procaine injections and early mobilisation for fractures of the neck of the humerus. *Acta Chir Scand* 1965;130:18-24.
10. Gristina AG: Management of displaced fractures of the proximal humerus. *Contemp Orthop* 1987;15:61-93.
11. Fourier P, Martini A: Post-traumatic avascular necrosis of the humeral head. *Int Orthop* 1977;1:187-190.
12. Geneste R, Durandeau A, Gauzere JM, Roy J: The treatment of fracture–dislocation of the humeral head by blind pinning. *Rev Chir Orthop Reparatrice Appar Mot* 1980;66:383-386.
13. Hägg O, Lundberg B: Aspects of prognostic factors in comminuted and dislocated proximal humeral fractures, in Bateman JE, Welsh RP (eds): *Surgery of the Shoulder*. Philadelphia, PA, BC Decker, 1984, pp 51-59.
14. Jakob RP, Kristiansen T, Mayo K, Ganz R, Müller ME: Classification and aspects of treatment of fractures of the proximal humerus, in Bateman JE, Welsh RP (eds): *Surgery of the Shoulder*. Philadelphia, PA, BC Decker, 1984, pp 330-343.
15. Knight RA, Mayne JA: Comminuted fractures and fracture-dislocations involving the articular surface of the humeral head. *J Bone Joint Surg Am* 1957;39:1343-1355.
16. Kristiansen B, Christensen SW: Plate fixation of proximal humeral fractures. *Acta Orthop Scand* 1986;57:320-323.
17. Lee CK, Hansen HR: Post-traumatic avascular necrosis of the humeral head in displaced proximal humeral fractures. *J Trauma* 1981;21: 788-791.
18. Sturzenegger M, Fornaro E, Jakob RP: Results of surgical treatment of multifragmented fractures of the humeral head. *Arch Orthop Trauma Surg* 1982;100:249-259.
19. Rose SH, Melton LJ III, Morrey BF, Ilstrup DM, Riggs BL: Epidemiologic features of humeral fractures. *Clin Orthop* 1982;168:24-30.
20. Neer CS II: Displaced proximal humeral fractures: Part I. Classification and evaluation. *J Bone Joint Surg Am* 1970;52:1077-1089.
21. Neer CS II: Four-segment classification of displaced proximal humeral fractures. *Instr Course Lect* 1975;24:160-168.
22. Sorensen KH: Pseudarthrosis of the surgical neck of the humerus: Two cases, one bilateral. *Acta Orthop Scand* 1964;34:132-138.
23. Neer CS II: Nonunion of the surgical neck of the humerus. *Orthop Trans* 1983;7:389.
24. Coventry MB, Laurnen EL: Ununited fractures of the middle and upper humerus: Special problems in treatment. *Clin Orthop* 1970;69:192-198.
25. Ray RD, Sankaran B, Fetrow KO: Delayed union and non-union of fractures. *J Bone Joint Surg Am* 1964;46:627-643.
26. Rooney PJ, Cockshott WP: Pseudarthrosis following proximal humeral fractures: A possible mechanism. *Skeletal Radiol* 1986;15:21-24.
27. Epps CH Jr, Cotler JM: Complications of treatment of fractures of the humeral shaft, in Epps CH Jr (ed): *Complications in Orthopaedic Surgery*, ed 2. Philadelphia, PA, JB Lippincott, 1986, pp 277-304.
28. Mayer PJ, Evarts CM: Nonunion, delayed union, malunion, and avascular necrosis, in Epps CH Jr (ed): *Complications in Orthopaedic Surgery*, ed 2. Philadelphia, PA, JB Lippincott, 1986, pp 207-230.
29. Muller ME, Thomas RJ: Treatment of nonunion in fractures of long bones. *Clin Orthop* 1979;138:141-153.
30. Neviaser JS: Complicated fractures and dislocations about the shoulder joint. *J Bone Joint Surg Am* 1962;44:984-998.
31. Paavolainen P, Bjorkenheim JM, Slatis P, Paukku P: Operative treatment of severe proximal humeral fractures. *Acta Orthop Scand* 1983;54:374-379.
32. Leach RE, Premer RF: Nonunion of the surgical neck of the humerus: Method of internal fixation. *Minn Med* 1965;48:318-322.
33. Neer CS II, Rockwood CA Jr: Fractures and dislocations of the shoulder: Part I. Fractures about the shoulder, in Rockwood CA Jr, Green DP (eds): *Fractures in Adults*, ed 2. Philadelphia, PA, JB Lippincott, 1984, pp 675-721.
34. DePalma AF, Cautilli RA: Fractures of the upper end of the humerus. *Clin Orthop* 1961;20:73-93.
35. Dingley A, Denham R: Fracture-dislocation of the humeral head: A method of reduction. *J Bone Joint Surg Am* 1973;55:1299-1300.
36. Drapanas T, McDonald J, Hale HW Jr: A rational approach to classification and treatment of fractures of the surgical neck of the humerus. *Am J Surg* 1960;99:617-624.
37. Keene JS, Huizengia RE, Engber W.D, et al: Proximal humeral fractures: A correlation of residual deformity with long-term function. *Orthopedics* 1983;6:173-178.
38. Perkins G: Rest and movement. *J Bone Joint Surg Br* 1953;35:521-539.
39. Young TB, Wallace WA: Conservative treatment of fractures and fracture-dislocations of the upper end of the humerus. *J Bone Joint Surg Br* 1985;67:373-377.
40. Laing PG: The arterial supply of the adult humerus. *J Bone Joint Surg Am* 1956;38:1105-1116.
41. Wirth MA, Rockwood CA Jr: Complications of shoulder arthroplasty. *Clin Orthop* 1994;307: 47-69.
42. Neer CS II: Displaced proximal humeral fractures: Part II. Treatment of three-part and four-part displacement. *J Bone Joint Surg Am* 1970;52:1090-1103.

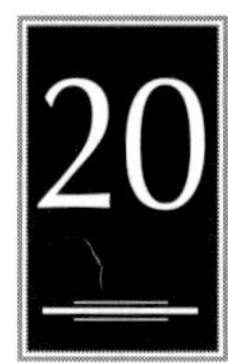

Indications for Prosthetic Replacement in Proximal Humeral Fractures

Wesley P. Phipatanakul, MD
Tom R. Norris, MD

Abstract

Prosthetic replacement is a good treatment option in osteoporotic patients with four-part fractures, fracture-dislocations, head-split fractures with more than 40% articular surface involvement, anatomic neck fractures, dislocations present for longer than 6 months, and selected three-part fractures. Early prosthetic replacement of proximal humeral fractures has a better outcome than late reconstructive prosthetic management. Prosthetic design features specific for fracture care have led to a reduction in complications. Techniques will continue to improve as prosthetic design features specific for fractures evolve.

Most fractures of the proximal humerus are relatively nondisplaced and can be treated nonsurgically. Displaced two-part fractures and many three-part fractures generally are not considered for prosthetic replacement because good results are achieved with osteosynthesis. Certain fracture patterns often preclude the ability to use internal fixation techniques to reconstruct the proximal humerus, particularly in elderly patients with osteoporosis. This problem is compounded in patients with comminution and poor bone quality. The literature supports prosthetic replacement as a definitive treatment option in patients with four-part fractures and fracture-dislocations, head-split fractures with greater than 40% articular surface involvement, anatomic neck fractures, dislocations present for 6 months or longer in which the cartilage has softened, and selected three-part fractures in patients with osteopenia that precludes secure internal fixation.[1-3]

The preferred concept is to perform the most reliable procedure in the initial management. The idea of treating all fractures initially with internal fixation with the thought of prosthetic management as the salvage procedure is not a recommended algorithm. Malunions are very difficult to treat. Reconstruction of malunions is one of the most challenging procedures and is associated with a higher rate of complications.[1,4] The literature clearly shows that early prosthetic replacement of proximal humeral fractures has a better outcome than late prosthetic management.[5-11] In addition, late prosthetic surgery for failed early treatment is more technically difficult. Factors to consider in surgical decision making include the risk of nonunion, malunion, or osteonecrosis, bone quality, time from injury, and the need for future surgery and revision.

Anatomic Neck Fracture

Anatomic neck fractures are quite rare. In fact, there are no series in the literature dealing exclusively with this fracture pattern; therefore, much of the management is based intuitively. The fracture location is medial to the rotator cuff insertion and thus the humeral head is devoid of soft-tissue attachment. It is logical to conclude a higher rate of osteonecrosis in this rare fracture pattern. In cadaver studies, it has been shown that displaced anatomic neck fractures completely disrupt the blood flow to the articular portion of the humeral head.[12] Hertel and associates[13] in a recent study identified factors that predict humeral head ischemia following proximal humeral fractures. Their classification scheme divided fractures into 12 types based on five basic fracture planes that can be identified by answering the following questions: Is there a fracture between the greater tuberosity and either the head and/or shaft? Is there a fracture between the lesser tuberosity and the head and/or shaft? Is there a fracture between the lesser and the greater

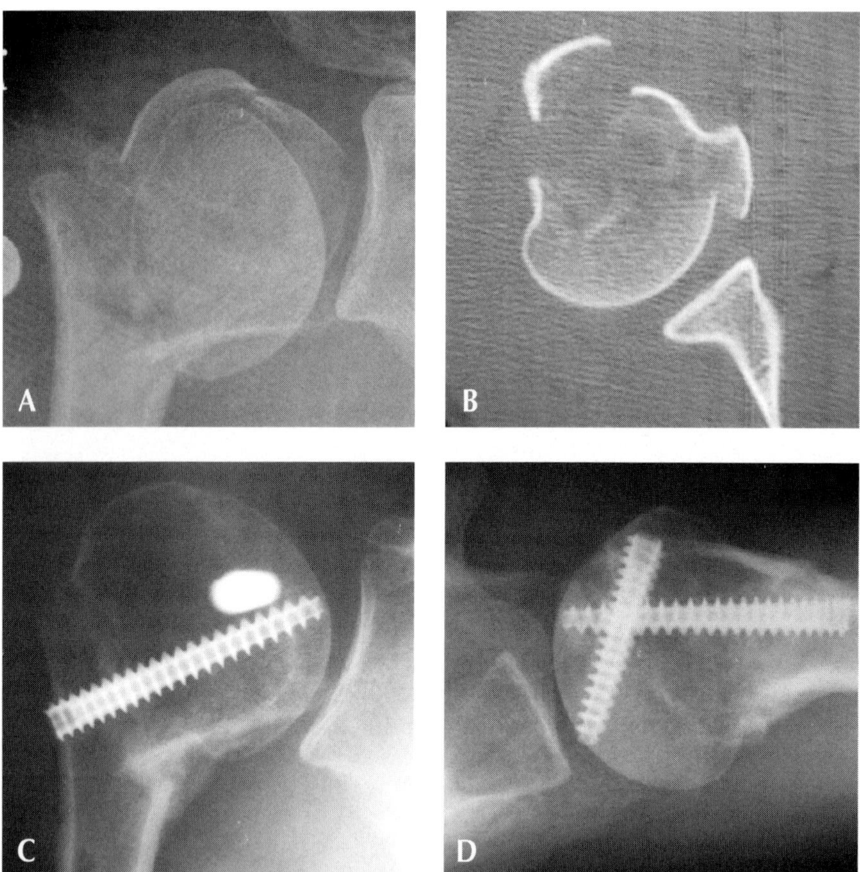

Figure 1 AP radiograph **(A)** and axial CT scan **(B)** demonstrating a four-part proximal humeral fracture with a head-splitting component in a 32-year-old woman. **C** and **D,** Follow-up radiographs demonstrating healed fracture without humeral head collapse. Osteosynthesis should be considered in young patients provided an anatomic reduction can be achieved.

tuberosity? They found that the most relevant predictors of ischemia were the length of the dorsomedial metaphyseal extension with the humeral head; the integrity of the medial hinge; and the basic fracture type determined with the binary description system. In particular, those types with fracture planes between the humeral head and other anatomic structures, that is, variations of the anatomic neck fracture, were at highest risk. By combining the above criteria (anatomic neck, short calcar, disrupted hinge), positive predictive values for ischemia of up to 97% could be obtained. Moderate and poor predictors of ischemia, in descending order, were fractures consisting of four fragments, angular displacement of the head, the amount of dislocation of the tuberosities, glenohumeral dislocation, head-split components, and fractures consisting of three fragments.[13] Acute prosthetic replacement is an appropriate treatment option in this fracture pattern where solid fixation may be difficult to achieve in addition to a high likelihood of head collapse. Attempts at internal fixation should be reserved for the younger population (Figures 1 and 2).

Three-Part Fractures

Good results with internal fixation of three-part fractures have been reported.[14] However, osteosynthesis of three-part fractures in elderly patients has revealed poorer results. A series of elderly patients were randomized to either conservative treatment or tension band osteosynthesis.[15] No differences in functional outcomes were observed between the two groups. Major complications occurred in the surgically treated group only. Prosthetic management of three-part fractures should be considered in the older patient with osteoporotic bone that prevents stable fixation. A prosthesis may provide immediate stability and decrease the need for secondary procedures because of hardware failure or fracture nonunion/malunion. Head collapse is not the major issue in three-part fractures. In fact, it is unusual to develop osteonecrosis in a three-part fracture because the intact lesser tuberosity preserves the arcuate artery by keeping the intertubercular groove intact. The fracture pattern is usually posterior to the groove and involves the greater tuberosity and the surgical neck. The arcuate artery is a branch off the anterior circumflex artery that supplies the majority of the blood supply to the humeral head and has been shown to have a constant insertion point in the groove.[16]

Four-Part Fractures and Fracture-Dislocation

Treatment of four-part fractures remains controversial. This fracture pattern is much more problematic than the three-part fracture. The articular portion is completely separated from its blood supply.[12] Neer[17,18] found a 75% incidence of osteonecrosis in four-part fractures. Internal fixation of these fracture types in the past has generally been poor.[17,19] Mild osteonecrosis does not necessarily preclude a good outcome. Gerber and associates[20] reviewed 25 patients with post-traumatic osteonecrosis analyzed at 7.5 years follow-up. The patients were divided into two groups: those with anatomic reduction versus those with malunions. Those with anatomic reduction fared significantly better; 62% had good function-

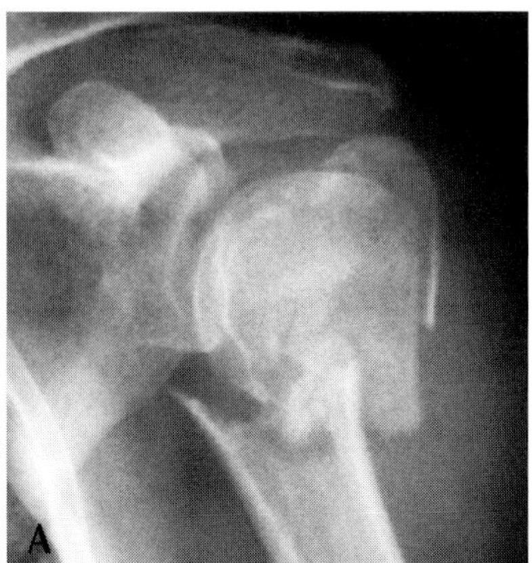

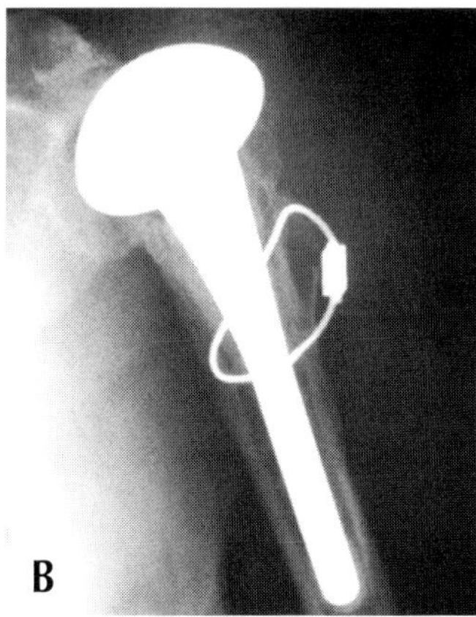

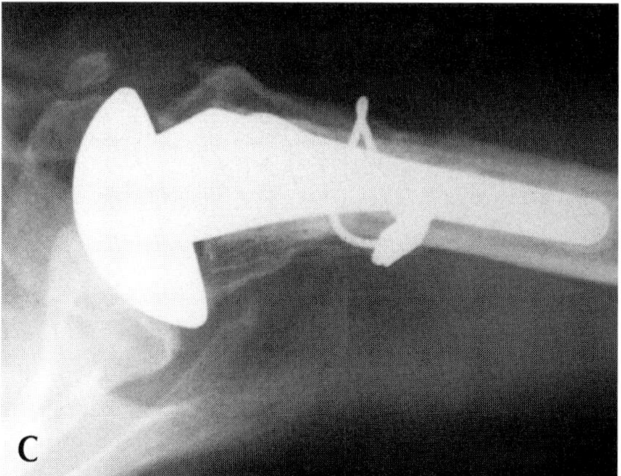

Figure 2 **A**, Radiograph showing a fracture pattern suggestive of a three-part fracture in a 73-year-old patient. **B** and **C**, Follow-up radiographs with the prosthetic component in place. Intraoperatively, a four-part fracture with head split was discovered. With this same fracture pattern in an older patient with poorer bone quality, a prosthetic replacement is a good treatment option.

al results versus 16% in the other group. When committing to osteosynthesis of a proximal humeral fracture, obtaining an anatomic or near-anatomic reduction, especially in three- and four-part fractures, is paramount. If the fracture pattern doesn't allow for achievement of this goal, then prosthetic replacement should be considered. Recently, one series documented 87% good results using the Constant score with open reduction and internal fixation.[21] However, the patients in that series were younger (average age 48 years), and nearly half of the patients were excluded either because they died or because they required conversion to arthroplasty as a result of failed osteosynthesis. Despite their enthusiasm with osteosynthesis, the authors recommended considering prosthetic replacement for the elderly. Others have found primary prosthetic replacement in four-part fractures to be superior to osteosynthesis.[22]

The results of percutaneous treatment have also been disappointing. One study reported a 75% poor result with this technique secondary to osteonecrosis, and thus concluded that percutaneous pinning is not a good option in four-part fractures.[23] With poor outcomes with surgical fixation of four-part fracture, multiple series documenting improved results with prosthetic management have emerged. Satisfactory results range mostly in the 60% to 90% range, with good pain relief in about 80% to 85%.[5,6,11,24-28] A joint dislocation further complicates the blood supply. The incidence of osteonecrosis is higher in this situation. A recent report found a 39% incidence of osteonecrosis in three-part fracture-dislocation, and 89% in four-part fracture-dislocation.[21] Another series found that internal fixation in four-part fracture-dislocation resulted in 100% failure and recommended prosthetic management.[29] Patients must be informed that prosthetic treatment is designed to be a pain-relieving operation. Multiple reports document excellent pain relief with functional gains less predictable.[6,25,30,31] Therefore, acute prosthetic management of four-part fractures in the elderly is recommended, particularly because the literature has shown reliable reproducible results in several series using this technique (Figure 3). This indication extends to both the three- and four-part fracture-dislocations in the elderly. Prosthetic replacement in the younger patient causes concern about the longevity of the implant. Recent studies have shown good survivorship of the prosthesis in a fracture situation, over 90% at 10 years.[32] Osteosynthesis should be reserved for the younger patient. However, when considering osteosynthesis as the initial treatment, it should be remembered that functional outcomes of acute prosthetic replacement are better than those of replacement for either delayed or failed internal fixation.[10] One report found prosthetic replacement within 4 weeks of injury to produce superior results,[5] whereas others have found intervention within 2 weeks to be better.[8,11] Thus, although it is prudent to proceed with treatment sooner rather than later, a 2- to 4-week time period allows enough time for surgical planning and patient optimization.

Impression Fracture and Chronic Dislocation

Impression fractures are often associated with dislocation. More than 40% to 50% involvement of the articular surface can be considered a contraindication to osteosynthesis. In one series it was determined that a head-split fracture with more than 40% articular involvement was an appropriate indication for prosthetic management.[2] Another report recommended arthroplasty if the head involvement was more than 45% or dislocation was present for longer than 6 months.[3]

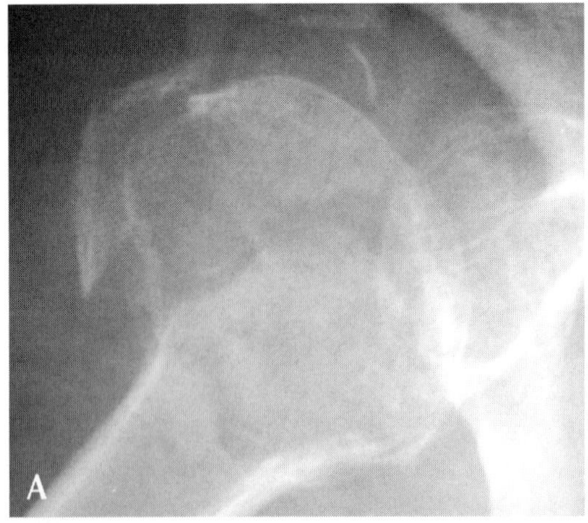

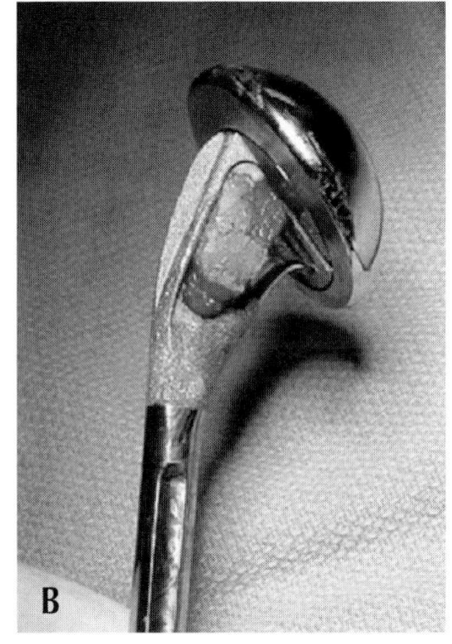

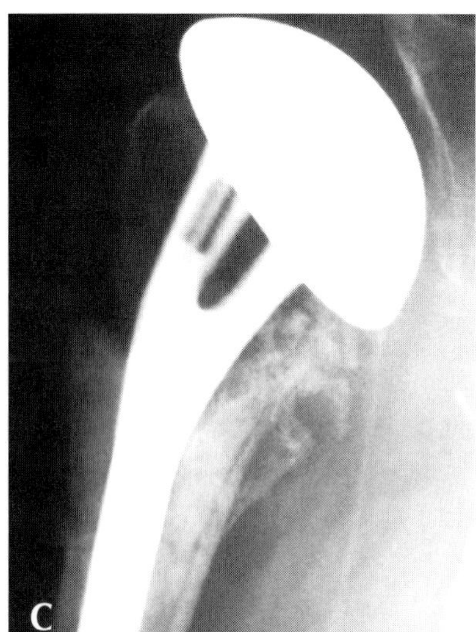

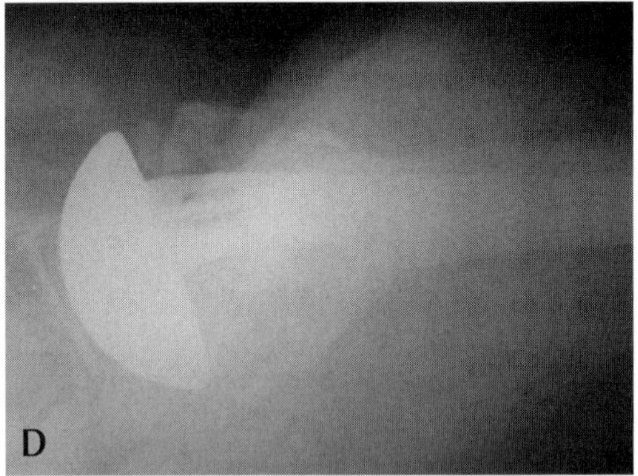

Figure 3 A, An AP radiograph demonstrates a proximal humeral fracture in an elderly patient. **B,** Photograph of a fracture-prosthesis with a bone graft from the patient's removed articular segment in place. **C** and **D,** Follow-up radiographs demonstrate consolidation of the tuberosities with the prosthesis in place.

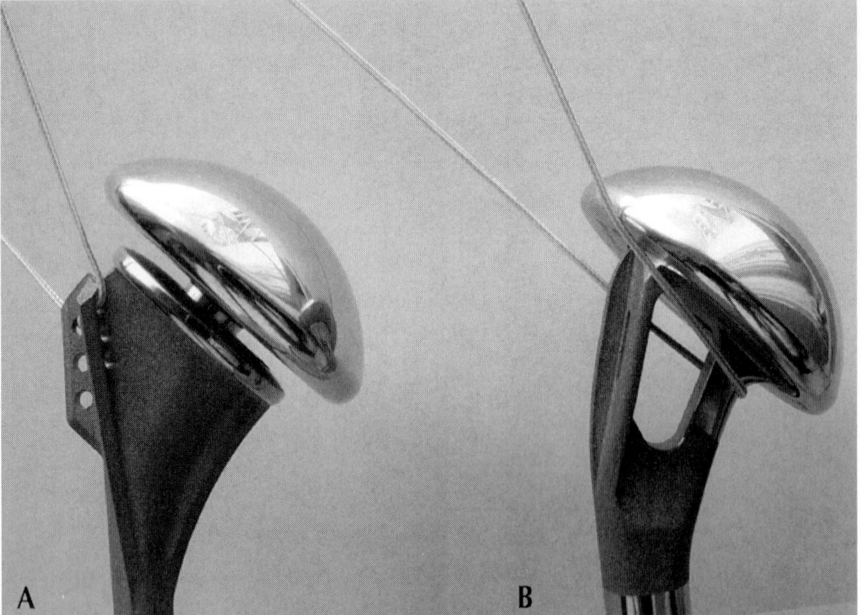

Figure 4 A, This fracture-prosthesis has a smooth medial collar, which facilitates placement of circumferential cerclage sutures without a stress riser. Biomechanical data have found that this configuration is more stable compared with placing sutures through a hole in a prosthetic fin **(B)**.

Valgus Impacted Four-Part Fracture

This fracture pattern behaves differently than the true four-part fracture and must be distinguished because this can change the treatment options. The humeral head is impacted without lateral displacement, and thus the periosteum medially leading up to the humeral head is intact and preserves the blood supply for the most part. This is a unique four-part fracture not necessarily requiring prosthetic replacement. Good results are reported with open reduction, bone grafting, and limited internal fixation. However, functional outcome is correlated with obtaining an anatomic reduction.[33]

Summary

Prosthetic replacement of acute proximal humeral fractures is a good treatment option. Osteosynthesis is a poor choice if the fracture environment precludes stability and an anatomic reduction. It is important to initially perform the procedure that will provide the most predictable outcome, because secondary surgery is more technically demanding with outcomes clearly inferior to primary treatment. The literature supports that prosthetic management is a good indication in the older population with complex fracture patterns. When surgical treatment is indicated, early management has produced superior results, with pain relief more predictable than functional gains. The treatment of the younger population is not as clear. Factors associated with lower functional scores included increasing patient age, alcohol and tobacco use, neurologic deficit, and a poorly positioned prosthesis.[32] Although these factors do not preclude prosthetic use, this information can help better inform patients on outcome expectations. Changes in the technical aspect of prosthetic surgery will continue to affect the indications for its use. A recent report demonstrated that the most significant factor associated with poor result of humeral head replacement for acute fracture was tuberosity migration.[34] This has led to modifications of the prosthetic design specific for fracture care (Figure 4). These changes include less metal at the proximal part of the prosthesis and a smooth medial calcar to allow placement of a circumferential medial cerclage. These changes facilitate tuberosity osteosynthesis. Biomechanical data have shown that a circumferential medial cerclage adds significant stability to the tuberosity construct, while incorporating sutures into a prosthetic fin did not.[35] These prosthetic design changes have led to a reduction in tuberosity migration by a factor of two.[36] Techniques will continue to improve as prosthetic design features specific for fractures evolve and prevention of tuberosity dehiscence diminishes.

References

1. Antuna SA, Sperling JW, Sanchez-Sotelo J, Cofield RH: Shoulder arthroplasty for proximal humeral malunions: Long-term results. *J Shoulder Elbow Surg* 2002;11:122-129.
2. Compito CA, Self EB, Bigliani LU: Arthroplasty and acute shoulder trauma: Reasons for success and failure. *Clin Orthop* 1994;307:27-36.
3. Hawkins RJ, Neer CS II, Pianta RM, Mendoza FX: Locked posterior dislocation of the shoulder. *J Bone Joint Surg Am* 1987;69:9-18.
4. Beredjiklian PK, Iannotti JP, Norris TR, Williams GR: Operative treatment of malunion of a fracture of the proximal aspect of the humerus. *J Bone Joint Surg Am* 1998;80:1484-1487.
5. Bosch U, Skutek M, Fremerey RW, Tscherne H: Outcome after primary and secondary hemiarthroplasty in elderly patients with fractures of the proximal humerus. *J Shoulder Elbow Surg* 1998;7:479-484.
6. Dimakopoulos P, Potamitis N, Lambiris E: Hemiarthroplasty in the treatment of comminuted intraarticular fractures of the proximal humerus. *Clin Orthop* 1997;341:7-11.
7. Becker R, Pap G, Machner A, Neumann WH: Strength and motion after hemiarthroplasty in displaced four-fragment fracture of the proximal humerus: 27 patients followed for 1-6 years. *Acta Orthop Scand* 2002;73:44-49.
8. Demirhan M, Kilicoglu O, Altnel L, Eralp L, Akalin Y: Prognostic factors in prosthetic replacement for acute proximal humerus fractures. *J Orthop Trauma* 2003;17:181-189.
9. Frich LH, Sojbjerg JO, Sneppen O: Shoulder arthroplasty in complex acute and chronic proximal humeral fractures. *Orthopedics* 1991;14:949-954.
10. Norris TR, Green A, McGuigan FX: Late prosthetic shoulder arthroplasty for displaced proximal humerus fractures. *J Shoulder Elbow Surg* 1995;4:271-280.
11. Moeckel BH, Dines DM, Warren RF, Altchek DW: Modular hemiarthroplasty for fractures of the proximal part of the humerus. *J Bone Joint Surg Am* 1992;74:884-889.
12. Brooks CH, Revell WJ, Heatley FW: Vascularity of the humeral head after proximal humeral fractures: An anatomical cadaver study. *J Bone Joint Surg Br* 1993;75:132-136.
13. Hertel R, Hempfing A, Stiehler M, Leunig M: Predictors of humeral head ischemia after intracapsular fracture of the proximal humerus. *J Shoulder Elbow Surg* 2004;4:427-433.
14. Hawkins RJ, Bell RH, Gurr K: The three-part fracture of the proximal part of the humerus: Operative treatment. *J Bone Joint Surg Am* 1986;68:1410-1414.
15. Zyto K, Ahrengart L, Sperber A, Tornkvist H: Treatment of displaced proximal humeral fractures in elderly patients. *J Bone Joint Surg Br* 1997;79:412-417.
16. Gerber C, Schneeberger AG, Vinh TS: The arterial vascularization of the humeral head: An anatomical study. *J Bone Joint Surg Am* 1990;72:1486-1494.
17. Neer CS II: Displaced proximal humeral fractures: II. Treatment of three-part and four-part displacement. *J Bone Joint Surg Am* 1970;52:1090-1103.
18. Neer CS II: Displaced proximal humeral fractures: I. Classification and evaluation. *J Bone Joint Surg Am* 1970;52:1077-1089.
19. Kristiansen B, Christensen SW: Proximal humeral fractures: Late results in relation to classification and treatment. *Acta Orthop Scand* 1987;58:124-127.
20. Gerber C, Hersche O, Berberat C: The clinical relevance of posttraumatic avascular necrosis of the humeral head. *J Shoulder Elbow Surg* 1998;7:586-590.
21. Wijgman AJ, Roolker W, Patt TW, Raaymakers EL, Marti RK: Open reduction and internal fixation of three and four-part fractures of the proximal part of the humerus. *J Bone Joint Surg Am* 2002;84:1919-1925.
22. Schai P, Imhoff A, Preiss S: Comminuted humeral head fractures: A multicenter analysis. *J Shoulder Elbow Surg* 1995;4:319-330.
23. Soete PJ, Clayson PE, Costenoble VH: Transitory percutaneous pinning in fractures of the proximal humerus. *J Shoulder Elbow Surg* 1999;8:569-573.
24. Tanner MW, Cofield RH: Prosthetic arthroplasty for fractures and fracture-dislocations of the proximal humerus. *Clin Orthop* 1983;179:116-128.
25. Goldman RT, Koval KJ, Cuomo F, Gallagher MA, Zuckerman JD: Functional outcome after humeral head replacement for acute three- and four-part proximal humeral fractures. *J Shoulder Elbow Surg* 1995;4:81-86.
26. Boileau P, Trojani C, Walch G, Krishnan SG, Romeo A, Sinerton R: Shoulder arthroplasty for the treatment of the sequelae of fractures of the proximal humerus. *J Shoulder Elbow Surg* 2001;10:299-308.
27. Boss AP, Hintermann B: Primary endoprosthesis in comminuted humeral head fractures in patients over 60 years of age. *Int Orthop* 1999;23:172-174.
28. Zyto K, Wallace WA, Frostick SP, Preston BJ: Outcome after hemiarthroplasty for three- and four-part fractures of the proximal humerus. *J Shoulder Elbow Surg* 1998;7:85-89.
29. Darder A, Darder A Jr, Sanchis V, Gastaldi E, Gomar F: Four-part displaced proximal humeral fractures: Operative treatment using Kirschner wires and a tension band. *J Orthop Trauma* 1993;7:497-505.
30. Kay SP, Amstutz HC: Shoulder hemiarthroplasty at UCLA. *Clin Orthop* 1988;228:42-48.
31. Wretenberg P, Ekelund A: Acute hemiarthroplasty after proximal humerus fracture in old patients: A retrospective evaluation of 18 patients followed for 2-7 years. *Acta Orthop Scand* 1997;68:121-123.
32. Robinson CM, Page RS, Hill RM, Sanders DL, Court-Brown CM, Wakefield AE: Primary hemiarthroplasty for treatment of proximal

humeral fractures. *J Bone Joint Surg Am* 2003;85:1215-1223.

33. Resch H, Beck E, Bayley I: Reconstruction of the valgus-impacted humeral head fracture. *J Shoulder Elbow Surg* 1995;4:73-80.

34. Boileau P, Kirshnan SG, Tinsi L, Walch G, Coste JS, Mole D: Tuberosity malposition and migration: Reasons for poor outcomes after hemiarthroplasty for displaced fractures of the proximal humerus. *J Shoulder Elbow Surg* 2002;11:401-412.

35. Frankle MA, Ondrovic LE, Markee BA, Harris ML, Lee WE III: Stability of tuberosity reattachment in proximal humeral hemiarthroplasty. *J Shoulder Elbow Surg* 2002;11:413-420.

36. Boileau P: Prosthetic shoulder replacement for fracture: Results of the multicentre study, in Walch G, Boileau P, Mol D (eds): *2000 Shoulder Prostheses: Two to Ten Year Follow Up*. Paris, France, Sauramps Medical, 2001, pp 561-569.

Outcome After Treatment of Proximal Humeral Fractures With Humeral Head Replacement

Young W. Kwon, MD, PhD
Joseph D. Zuckerman, MD

Abstract

After its initial description by Neer and associates, humeral head replacement has been widely used to treat complex fractures of the proximal humerus. Many studies have confirmed that the treatment of proximal humeral fractures with humeral head replacement is associated with reliable pain relief as well as good patient satisfaction. A limited number of studies have also suggested that the prostheses have reasonable longevity, with the rate of prosthesis survival at 83% to 94% at 10 years. The functional outcome after the procedure, however, has not been as predictable. Using various outcomes scoring instruments, multiple studies have reported a wide range of results. Some authors have reported mostly disappointing outcomes, whereas others have reported generally satisfactory results. The most critical factor influencing the long-term outcome appears to be the position of the greater tuberosity. Other factors that are also associated with a good outcome include younger age, minimal delay between the traumatic event and the surgical procedure, and the absence of any neurologic deficit. For young patients with a complex proximal humeral fracture, humeral head replacement still remains a viable treatment option. However, whenever possible, most authors favor open reduction and internal fixation because of the issues affecting the longevity of the prosthesis. By understanding and minimizing the risk factors leading to a poor result, a reasonable functional outcome, reliable pain relief, and a high rate of patient satisfaction can be expected after treatment of proximal humeral fractures with humeral head replacement.

In the 1950s, Neer described the use of a metallic humeral head replacement for the treatment of complex proximal humeral fractures.[1-2] Subsequently, Neer and associates[3-5] expanded on their experience and provided the general guidelines for treating proximal humeral fractures with a prosthesis. Other investigators have also reported their experiences with humeral head replacement to treat patients with comminuted and/or displaced proximal humeral fractures. Functional outcomes reported in these articles have been inconsistent, with some authors reporting satisfactory results and others reporting mostly disappointing results.

When attempting to analyze the data presented in these studies, it is often difficult to identify the specific indications for humeral head replacement that were used. Thus, it is unclear whether similar types of fracture patterns were treated in a similar manner by the individual surgeons. In general, the indications (guidelines) used by most surgeons when electing to proceed with humeral head replacement are to treat patients with (1) severely comminuted fractures not amenable to stable internal fixation; (2) displaced three- or four-part fractures with dislocation of the humeral head; (3) humeral head splitting fractures (Figure 1); and (4) a poor outcome after initial treatment without a prosthesis.

Another difficult task associated with comparison of the results from various reports is the variability in the outcome assessment. Multiple patient-based as well as surgeon-based outcomes instruments have been used to assess the functional result after humeral head replacement. These outcome scoring systems include the American Shoulder and Elbow Surgeons Score, the Constant Score, the University of California at Los Angeles (UCLA) Shoulder Rating Score, the Hospital for Special Surgery (HSS) Shoulder Scoring System, and the Neer Scoring system.[3,6-8] All of these outcome instruments attempt to evaluate and integrate all or some combination of the following factors: pain, range of motion, strength, functional use, and patient satisfaction. Unfortunately, different scoring systems place variable emphasis on each of these factors, which precludes a direct and simple conversion of one system to another.

Despite these limitations, an attempt will be made to review and integrate the data presented in the relevant studies. The review will focus primarily on the

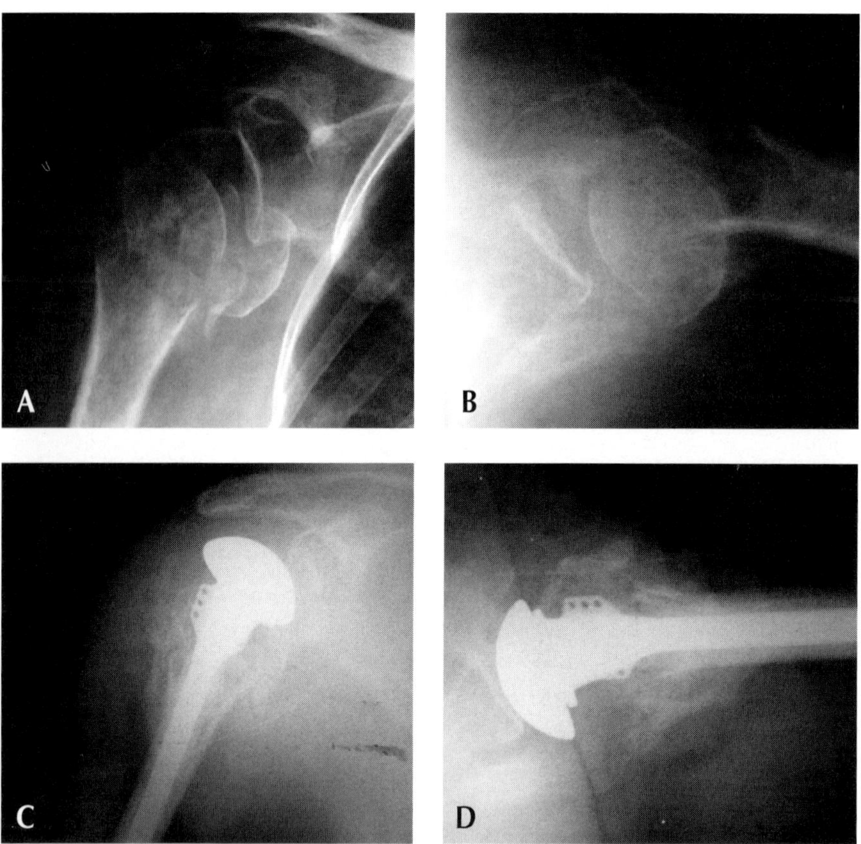

Figure 1 Preoperative AP **(A)** and axillary **(B)** radiographs of a 70-year-old woman with a proximal humeral fracture treated with humeral head replacement reveal comminuted head splitting fracture of the proximal humerus. Postoperative AP **(C)** and axillary **(D)** radiographs of the same patient reveal an abundance of new bone formation with anatomic placement of the tuberosities.

recent literature (over the past 10 years) when the indications, techniques, and instrumentation for humeral head replacement have become more standardized. The data will be analyzed to formulate a general outcome that can be expected after using humeral head replacement to treat patients with proximal humeral fractures. Specific emphasis will also be placed on the identification of preoperative and postoperative factors that closely correlate with the overall outcome.

Results After Humeral Head Replacement

Among the different studies reporting on the results of treating proximal humeral fractures with humeral head replacement, perhaps the most reproducible aspect of the outcome is the level of pain after the procedure. In a retrospective 42-month follow-up study of 18 elderly patients, Wretenberg and Ekelund[9] reported that approximately 61% of the patients were completely pain free. Of the remaining patients, none reported pain scores higher than 28 out of 100 on a visual analog scale for pain. Similarly, Compito and associates[10] reviewed their series of 70 patients at an average follow-up of 33 months. They found that 73% of the patients were completely pain free and that 95% of the patients had either minimal or no pain at the time of their latest evaluation. Other studies have also reproduced these low levels of pain in patients who were treated with humeral head replacement for their proximal humeral fractures. Among the various reports, good to excellent pain relief was found in 73% to 97% of the treated patients.[11-14]

Partly because of the reliably low levels of pain, the rate of patient satisfaction after the procedure is also quite high. In one series of 27 patients, a 70% rate of patient satisfaction was reported, whereas in another series of 32 patients, a satisfaction rate of 75% was reported.[13,15] These rates were actually modest in comparison with other reports. In five other studies assessing 9 to 38 patients, the rates of patient satisfaction were significantly higher at 80% to 92%.[11,16-19] To estimate the overall rate of patient satisfaction, the raw data from these seven studies were combined. The analysis, based on the number of patients and their rate of satisfaction, revealed that more than 80% of the patients who underwent primary humeral head replacement expressed satisfaction with their treatment.

Despite the consistently low levels of pain and the high rate of patient satisfaction, reported functional outcomes after humeral head replacement have been more variable. Lack of a universally accepted shoulder outcome assessment instrument has limited the ability to easily compare and/or combine the raw data from one study with others. Therefore, interpretation of the published results must be performed with some caution. Nevertheless, some studies have reported disappointing results, whereas others have reported generally good outcomes. In most of the patients with a poor result, their dissatisfaction appeared to be largely related to the limitations in shoulder motion and to the decreased ability in performing activities of daily living.

Few of the published studies used the UCLA score to assess outcome in patients who underwent primary humeral head replacement. This instrument incorporates pain, function, range of motion, strength of forward flexion, and patient satisfaction on a 35-point scale.[6] Hawkins and Switlyk[11] reported in their series of 20 patients that 6 patients (30%) had a poor outcome based on the UCLA scoring system. At 40 months after the procedure, average active elevation was limited to 72°, whereas active external rotation was limited to 16°. Overall UCLA score for the entire group was 24, which was considered to be a fair outcome.[11] In the series of 25 patients reported by Bosch and associates,[20] 11 patients underwent immediate humeral head replacement for proximal humeral fractures. The UCLA score for these patients ranged from 17 to 34 with an average of 27, which was also considered to be a fair outcome. Average forward flexion in these patients was slightly better at 94°. However, there was great variability among the patients in their ranges of motion. Some patients reported active flexion to only 30°, whereas others were able to flex their shoulders to 140°.

Another more commonly used outcome assessment instrument is the Constant score, which measures four clinical modalities (pain, range of motion, power, and activities of daily living) on a 100-point scale.[7] Some authors have slightly modified this instrument to reflect age/sex of patient, and strength of the unaffected extremity. With this instrument, six recent studies have reported functional outcome in patients whose proximal humeral fractures were treated with primary humeral head replacement. Scores from these series, each containing 11 to 138 patients, varied widely from 38 to 68.[13-15,20-22] In a report of 18 patients treated with primary humeral head replacement, Movin and associates[21] cited one of the worst reported outcomes to date. At an average follow-up of 37 months, the average Constant score for these patients was only 38. The authors also noted a marked reduction in the patients' ability to perform activities of daily living. The authors suggested, however, that compliance with the postoperative therapy regimen may not have been adequate in the elderly population in the study and that the poor rehabilitation may have contributed to the disappointing overall results. In contrast to this study, Demirhan and associates[13] followed 32 patients for an average period of 35 months and observed an average Constant score of 68 and average active elevation of 113°. Despite these reasonable values, wide variability in their results was noted. Thus, the Constant score and the active elevation among the patients ranged from 19 to 98 and from 30° to 180°, respectively. In one of the largest observational studies reported to date, Robinson and associates[14] documented the results of 138 consecutive patients treated with primary humeral head replacement for proximal humeral fractures. The average 12-month Constant score in this series was 64. The authors observed consistently low levels of pain in their patients. However, similar to other reports, variable levels of function, strength, and motion were noted.

To estimate the overall functional outcome in patients treated with humeral head replacement for proximal humerus fractures, Constant scores from six recent studies were combined.[13-15,20-22] Based on the number of patients and the Constant score from each of these studies, the calculated Constant score was 59.6. It appears that the overall functional outcome after this procedure, as assessed by the Constant score, is fair. In addition, there also appears to be a wide variability in outcomes, with some patients reporting excellent results and others reporting disappointing results.

Factors Influencing Outcome

Preoperative factors that appear to influence long-term outcome include patient age, delay in the time to treatment, and the presence of a neurologic deficit. Correlation between patient age and the eventual outcome has been noted in multiple studies. They suggest that younger patients typically have a more satisfactory functional outcome after humeral head replacement than their older counterparts.[12,14,16,23] Using the HSS scoring system, which assesses the levels of pain, function, power, and range of motion, Moeckel and associates[16] evaluated functional outcome in 22 patients who underwent primary humeral head replacement. The HSS score for patients younger than 70 years was 91 on a 100-point scale. In contrast, the average score for patients older than 70 years dropped significantly, to 74, after similar treatment. The authors suggested that the superior condition of the rotator cuff tissues as well as the ability to participate in appropriate rehabilitation may have contributed to the improved outcome in the younger patients. Similarly, Goldman and associates[12] noted that the patients younger than 70 years exhibited significantly improved active forward flexion, internal rotation, and external rotation when compared with their older counterparts. In addition, the younger patients also reported noticeably improved function at the time of their final evaluation.

Another preoperative factor that appears to influence the eventual outcome is a delay in the surgical treatment. As noted by several authors, a shorter interval between the traumatic event and the procedure was clearly associated with an improved outcome.[13,16,18,22] Less well defined, however, is the specific interval of delay that leads to the deteriorating outcome. Becker and associates[22] demonstrated an inverse relationship between the interval to treatment and the resulting outcome. Using the Neer scoring system, the most pronounced difference in the outcome was found between groups who were treated before or after a 7-day delay. Patients who underwent surgery within the first 7 days had an average Neer score of 97, and patients who

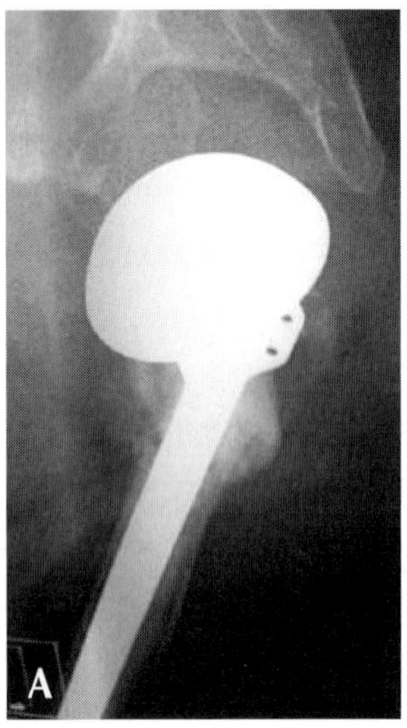

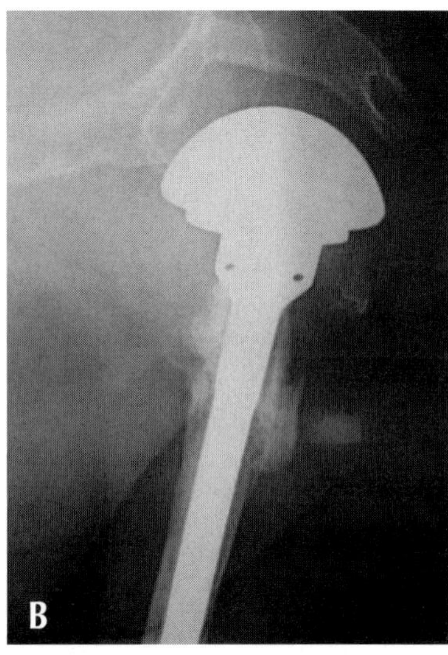

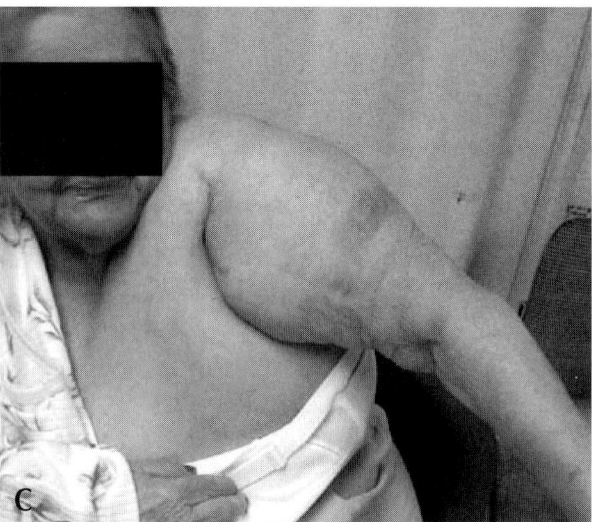

Figure 2 Radiographs (**A** and **B**) of a 72-year old woman obtained 18 months after undergoing humeral head replacement to treat a proximal humeral fracture reveal tuberosity malposition and resorption. As a result, the patient had a poor functional outcome, with limited active range of motion (**C**) and difficulties with activities of daily living. (*Photographs courtesy of N. Tejwani, MD.*)

underwent the surgical procedure 2 to 4 weeks after the trauma had an average Neer score of 88.[22] Others authors have analyzed the outcome in groups of patients who underwent the procedure before or after a 2-week delay and found that those in the earlier treatment group also showed significantly improved outcomes.[13,16] When this interval is increased to 30 days, however, the difference in the long-term outcome appears to be less distinct. Several authors have reported minimal to no significant difference in the eventual outcome between groups of patients who were treated before or after a 30-day delay.[18-19,22]

After this initial treatment period, patients who require a delayed or a secondary humeral head replacement for the treatment of proximal humeral fractures typically are those who are dissatisfied with their original treatment or have developed a sequelae from their injury. These patients are likely to experience worse outcomes than those who underwent the procedure as the primary treatment during the acute period. Results from several different studies have supported this concept. In general, patients who underwent delayed or secondary shoulder arthroplasty for a previously failed treatment of proximal humeral fractures exhibited inferior results when compared with those patients who underwent primary humeral head replacement.[20-21,24-28]

The postoperative factor that is most significantly associated with long-term outcome is the position of the greater tuberosity. Tuberosity malposition, as demonstrated in a cadaver model, can lead to a significant limitation in range of motion as well as a significant increase in the force required to induce motion.[29] Hence, patients with a malpositioned tuberosity are likely to experience significant limitations in motion as well as strength (Figure 2). These limitations can lead to a noticeable compromise of function. This hypothesis has been confirmed in multiple clinical studies.[13-14,23] Boileau and associates[23] followed 66 patients for an average period of 27 months after humeral head replacement for their proximal humeral fractures and found that 50% of the patients exhibited tuberosity malposition. The malposition occurred as a result of incorrect intraoperative placement of the tuberosity or after postoperative migration of the fragment. The authors defined greater tuberosity malposition based on the following radiographic criteria: (1) at least 5 mm above the top of the prosthetic head, (2) at least 10 mm below the top of the prosthetic head, or (3) posterior to the neck of the prosthesis. Using this definition, they noted that tuberosity malposition in any direction was associated with a significantly inferior functional outcome.[23]

In addition to its position, secure fixation of the tuberosity can also affect the eventual outcome. Boileau and associates[23] noted that 23% of the patients in their series experienced tuberosity detachment and migration during the initial postoperative period.[23] The migration occurred whether or not the initial placement of the tuberosity was anatomically accurate. The authors also observed that the complication occurred more frequently in women older than 75 years and suggested a possible link to osteopenia.[23] Biomechanically, use of a cerclage suture or wire to bind the tuberosities onto the humeral prosthesis appears to improve the stability of the construct.[30]

This fixation technique, therefore, may minimize the risk of subsequent tuberosity migration.

Another postoperative factor that influences the long-term outcome is the ability to participate in early supervised rehabilitation. This ability, however, may be dependent on other preoperative and postoperative factors. As discussed earlier, age and tuberosity fixation can influence the postoperative rehabilitation regimen. In addition, concomitant neurologic deficit is also likely to affect the patient's ability to participate in rehabilitation.[14] Nevertheless, many different reports have emphasized the need for aggressive and early postoperative rehabilitation to ensure a successful outcome, especially as it relates to the range and strength of shoulder motion.[10-11,13,17,23]

Humeral Head Replacement for the Young Patient

Treatment of complex proximal humeral fractures in the young patient can be difficult. Several studies have demonstrated that patients younger than 70 years who have undergone humeral head replacement generally have a more favorable outcome than their elderly counterparts.[12,14,16,24] Superior condition of the rotator cuff tissues, reduced perioperative morbidity, improved bone quality, and the ability to participate in early rehabilitation are all factors likely to contribute to improved outcome in young patients. Despite these favorable prognostic factors, age as well as increased activity level can also contribute to excessive and possibly premature wear on the prosthesis. Thus, the potential for young patients to outlive or out use their prostheses must be considered when deciding to proceed with a humeral head replacement.

There is little information in the literature regarding this specific topic. Sperling and associates[31] reported on their experience with 74 patients who underwent humeral head replacement before age 50 years, with an average follow-up of 12.3 years. The procedure was performed on patients whose average age was 39 years. The indications for the procedure included both fracture and nonfracture pathology. Using the Neer criteria, the authors considered the result to be satisfactory only if the patient had minimal pain, active external rotation greater than 20°, active abduction greater than 90°, and was satisfied with the result. Within these parameters, it was noted that 35 of the 74 patients (47%) had either an unsatisfactory or an unsuccessful result. However, it was also noted that the prosthesis had a reasonable rate of survival. At 10 and 15 years after the surgery, the rates of prosthesis survival were found to be 83% and 73%, respectively. In comparison to the patients with rheumatoid arthritis who presumably had a lower physical demand from their shoulders, the rate of prosthesis survival in patients with a previous trauma was noticeably lower.

A recent study by Robinson and associates[14] also presented data regarding long-term outcome after humeral head replacement. A 13-year observational cohort study of 163 consecutive patients who were treated with humeral head replacement for proximal humerus fractures was performed. Average age of these patients was 68 years with a range of 30 to 90 years. Thus, application of these data to a younger population of patients must be performed with some caution. Nevertheless, these authors noted excellent survival rates of the implanted prosthesis. At 5 and 10 years after the procedure, the prosthesis survival rates were 95.3% and 93.9%, respectively.[14]

Despite this reasonable longevity, other treatment options are typically considered for the young patient before proceeding with humeral head replacement. When anatomic reduction and sufficient fixation is possible, many authors have reported good to excellent results after opern reduction and internal fixation (ORIF).[4,32-33] A direct comparison between ORIF and primary humeral head replacement for the treatment of proximal humerus fractures is difficult because the indications for each procedure differ. Typically, humeral head replacement is reserved for displaced three- to four-part fractures and fracture-dislocations in which the likelihood of subsequent sequelae such as malunion, nonunion, and osteonecrosis is unacceptably high.

In a recent article, Wijgman and associates[33] reported on their experience treating three- and four-part proximal humeral fractures with ORIF. Sixty patients were assessed after an average period of 120 months; 87% good to excellent results and 85% patient satisfaction were reported. Seventy-seven percent of the patients with radiographic evidence of osteonecrosis still reported a satisfactory outcome. Therefore, the development of osteonecrosis did not preclude the possibility of obtaining a good long-term result. These results compare favorably with those from patients who underwent primary humeral head replacement for the treatment of three- and four-part fractures. It should be noted, however, that patients with a fracture pattern not amenable to stable internal fixation underwent a primary hemiarthroplasty and were excluded from this series.

After undergoing primary ORIF, patients with a poor outcome may then undergo humeral head replacement as a secondary procedure. Again, these patients are more likely to experience a worse outcome when compared with patients who underwent primary humeral head replacement during the acute period. A limited number of studies have confirmed this suspicion. Thirteen of the 23 patients reported by Norris and associates[25] were originally treated with ORIF for their proximal humeral fractures. At an average of 19.7 months after the fracture, these patients then underwent hemiarthroplasty or total shoulder arthroplasty as a salvage procedure for failed ORIF. Good pain relief was noted after shoulder arthroplasty, as 78% of these patients reported minimal to no pain. However, only 44% of the patients were able to perform shoulder level activity. In a series of 27 patients reported by Bosch and associates,[20] 5 had undergone a previous ORIF. After humeral head replacement, these patients also reported a fair functional outcome with an average UCLA score of 23.4 and an average Constant score of 45.6. In contrast, patients who underwent humeral head replacement as the primary treatment in the same series exhibited average UCLA and Constant scores of 25.1 and 65.6, respectively.[20] Finally, in patients with nonunions after attempted ORIF, treatment with shoulder arthroplasty only yielded 50% satisfactory results per the Neer criteria.[28] These studies suggest that patients who undergo secondary shoulder arthroplasty for failed proximal humerus ORIF are likely to experience a worse outcome than those who undergo primary humeral head replacement.

Despite the data presented, the issue of whether ORIF is preferable to humeral head replacement remains unanswered. Many authors favor and recommend primary ORIF whenever possible and reserve humeral head replacement only for those fracture patterns in which anatomic reduction and stable fixation are not possible. This recommendation appears to have increased support among orthopaedic surgeons when treating younger patients who may either outlive or outuse their prostheses. Unfortunately, few scientific data address this specific issue to guide the surgeon and the patient.

Summary

The decision to proceed with humeral head replacement for the treatment of proximal humeral fractures must be made on an individual basis. Several factors including patient age, expectations, and anticipated result should be considered and discussed with the patient to increase the likelihood of a satisfactory outcome. Although most patients will experience good pain relief and high satisfaction, the functional outcome can vary greatly. In order to increase the likelihood of a satisfactory outcome, risk factors associated with a poor result should be minimized.

References

1. Neer CS: Articular replacement for the humeral head. *J Bone Joint Surg Am* 1955;37:215-228.
2. Neer CS: Indications for replacement of the proximal humeral articulation. *Am J Surg* 1955;89:901-907.
3. Neer CS: Displaced proximal humerus fractures: Part I. Classification and evaluation. *J Bone Joint Surg Am* 1970;52:1077-1089.
4. Neer CS: Displaced proximal humerus fractures: Part II. Treatment of three part and four part displacement. *J Bone Joint Surg Am* 1970;52:1090-1103.
5. Neer CS, McIlveen SJ: Recent results and techniques of prosthetic replacement for four-part proximal humeral fractures. *Orthop Trans* 1986;10:475.
6. Ellman H, Hanker G, Bayer M: Repair of the rotator cuff: End result study of factors influencing reconstruction. *J Bone Joint Surg Am* 1986;68:1136-1144.
7. Constant CR, Murley AH: A clinical method of functional assessment of the shoulder. *Clin Orthop* 1987;214:160-164.
8. McCoy SR, Warren RF, Bade HA, Ranawat CS, Inglis AE: Total shoulder arthroplasty in rheumatoid arthritis. *J Arthroplasty* 1989;4:105-113.
9. Wretenberg P, Ekelund A: Acute hemiarthroplasty after proximal humerus fracture in old patients. *Acta Orthop Scand* 1997;68:121-123.
10. Compito CA, Self EB, Bigliani LU: Arthroplasty and acute shoulder trauma. *Clin Orthop* 1994;307:27-36.
11. Hawkins RJ, Switlyk P: Acute prosthetic replacement for severe fractures of the proximal humerus. *Clin Orthop* 1993;289:156-160.
12. Goldman RT, Koval KJ, Cuomo F, Gallagher MA, Zuckerman JD: Functional outcome after humeral head replacement for acute three and four part proximal humerus fractures. *J Shoulder Elbow Surg* 1995;4:81-86.
13. Demirhan M, Kilicoglu O, Altinel L, Eralp L, Akalin Y: Prognostic factors in prosthetic replacement for acute proximal humerus fractures. *J Orthop Trauma* 2003;17:181-188.
14. Robinson CM, Page RS, Hill RMF, Sanders DL, Court-Brown CM, Wakefield AE: Primary hemiarthroplasty for treatment of proximal humerus fractures. *J Bone Joint Surg Am* 2003;85:1215-1223.
15. Zyto K, Wallace WA, Frostick SP, Preston BJ: Outcome after hemiarthroplasty for three and four part fractures of the proximal humerus. *J Shoulder Elbow Surg* 1998;7:85-89.
16. Moeckel BH, Dines DM, Warren RF, Altchek DW: Modular hemiarthroplasty for fractures of the proximal part of the humerus. *J Bone Joint Surg Am* 1992;74:884-889.
17. Dimakopoulos P, Potamitis N, Lambiris E: Hemiarthroplasty in the treatment of comminuted intraarticular fractures of the proximal humerus. *Clin Orthop* 1997;341:7-11.
18. Skutek M, Fremerey RW, Bosch U: Level of physical activity in elderly patients after hemiarthroplasty for three and four part fractures of the proximal humerus. *Arch Orthop Trauma Surg* 1998;117:252-255.
19. Prakash U, McGurty DW, Dent JA: Hemiarthroplasty for severe fractures of the proximal humerus. *J Shoulder Elbow Surg* 2002;11:428-430.
20. Bosch U, Skutek M, Fremerey RW, Tscherne H: Outcome after primary and secondary hemiarthroplasty in elderly patients with fractures of the proximal humerus. *J Shoulder Elbow Surg* 1998;7:479-484.
21. Movin T, Sjoden GOJ, Ahrengart L: Poor function after shoulder replacement in fracture patients. *Acta Orthop Scand* 1998;69:392-396.
22. Becker R, Pap G, Machner A, Neumann WH: Strength and motion after hemiarthroplasty in displaced four fragment fracture of the proximal humerus. *Acta Orthop Scand* 2002;73:44-49.
23. Boileau P, Krishnan SG, Tinsi L, Walch G, Coste JS, Mole D: Tuberosity malposition and migration: Reasons for poor outcomes after hemiarthroplasty for displaced fractures of the proximal humerus. *J Shoulder Elbow Surg* 2002;11:401-412.
24. Dines DM, Warren RF, Altchek DW, Moeckel BH: Post traumatic changes of the proximal humerus: Malunions, nonunions, and osteonecrosis. Treatment with modular hemiarthroplasty or total shoulder arthroplasty. *J Shoulder Elbow Surg* 1993;2:11-21.
25. Norris TR, Green A, McGuigan FX: Late prosthetic shoulder arthroplasty for displaced proximal humerus fractures. *J Shoulder Elbow Surg* 1995;4:271-280.
26. Boileau P, Trojani C, Walch G, Krishnan SG, Romeo A, Sinnerton R: Shoulder arthroplasty for the treatment of the sequelae of fractures of the proximal humerus. *J Shoulder Elbow Surg* 2001;10:299-308.
27. Antuna SA, Sperling JW, Sanchez-Sotelo J, Cofield RH: Shoulder arthroplasty for proximal humeral malunions: Long-term results. *J Shoulder Elbow Surg* 2002;11:122-129.
28. Antuna SA, Sperling JW, Sanchez-Sotelo J, Cofield RH: Shoulder arthroplasty for proximal humeral nonunions. *J Shoulder Elbow Surg* 2002;11:114-121.
29. Frankle MA, Greenwald DP, Markee BA, Ondrovic LE, Lee WE: Biomechanical effects of malposition of tuberosity fragments on the humeral prosthetic reconstruction for four part

proximal humerus fractures. *J Shoulder Elbow Surg* 2001;10:321-326.

30. Frankle MA, Ondrovic LE, Markee BA, Harris ML, Lee WE: Stability of tuberosity reattachment in proximal humeral hemiarthroplasty. *J Shoulder Elbow Surg* 2002;11:413-420.

31. Sperling JW, Cofield RH, Rowland CM: Neer hemiarthroplasty and Neer total shoulder arthroplasty in patients fifty years old or less. *J Bone Joint Surg Am* 1998;80:464-473.

32. Cofield RH: Comminuted fractures of the proximal humerus. *Clin Orthop* 1988;230: 49-57.

33. Wijgman AJ, Roolker W, Patt TW, Raaymakers ELFB, Marti RK: Open reduction and internal fixation of three and four part fractures of the proximal part of the humerus. *J Bone Joint Surg Am* 2002;84:1919-1925.

Complications After Hemiarthroplasty for Fractures of the Proximal Humerus

Gregory N. Lervick, MD
Raymond M. Carroll, MD
William N. Levine, MD

Abstract

Humeral head replacement is frequently used in the treatment of selected fractures of the proximal humerus. This technique is usually successful in terms of pain relief and patient satisfaction. However, complications may occur and can adversely affect outcome. Careful preoperative planning, meticulous surgical technique, and appropriate postoperative rehabilitation are the best methods to promote a successful result. Potential complications and methods to avoid them at initial surgery should be reviewed.

Over the past 50 years, prosthetic humeral head replacement (HHR) has become a valued technique in the surgical management of complex fractures of the proximal humerus.[1-24] The fractures for which hemiarthroplasty is the indicated treatment include Neer four-part fractures, head-splitting fractures, and some three-part fractures in elderly patients when the bone quality is poor.[1,12,14,15,25-27] Although some authors have advocated open reduction and internal fixation (ORIF) of three- and four-part fractures, particularly in young patients,[28,29] HHR is a more viable option for most older or lower demand patients.

Although HHR has produced satisfactory results in a high percentage of patients, complications may occur. These complications can lead to prolonged disability and are costly for both the patient and the health care system. Subsequent surgical or prolonged nonsurgical treatment may be required. In this chapter, the most common complications associated with hemiarthroplasty for treating complex fractures of the proximal humerus will be outlined, with special emphasis on appropriate techniques at the time of initial surgery because their use is the most prudent means of avoiding complications. Specific treatment options for failed hemiarthroplasty in this clinical setting will also be discussed.

Evaluation

History

As with any condition about the shoulder, obtaining a complete patient history is crucial to making an accurate diagnosis. In elderly patients who have had previous surgery, a complete history may be difficult to obtain because these patients may be unable to recall specific events of their postoperative course. However, valuable information can be obtained from referring physicians, family members, and physical or occupational therapists.

The most important aspect of the history is the identification of the patient's specific complaint. Pain, stiffness, weakness, and instability are all potential complaints that often coexist. In particular, it should be determined whether the patient failed to progress following the initial procedure or deteriorated over time after having early function. Adverse events such as subsequent trauma or medical illness should be noted.

Careful attention should be paid to the previous surgical procedure, postoperative rehabilitation, subsequent trauma, and possible signs of infection. Previous surgical notes should be reviewed to determine the initial fracture type, surgical approach, type and size of the implant, method of implant fixation (cement versus cementless), and method of tuberosity fixation. These issues are critical when considering surgical revision. Also, postoperative physician's notes and physical therapist's notes should be reviewed.

Examination

The physical examination is the next critical step in the evaluation of the symptomatic patient following unsuccessful hemiarthroplasty. The location of the previous surgical incision should be documented, along with atrophy of the shoulder girdle musculature. Particular attention is paid to the status of the deltoid, which may have been injured in previous surgery. Deltoid dehiscence or severe dysfunction can be catastrophic and remains an unsolved clinical problem. A complete neurologic evaluation should be performed.

Next, range of motion of the shoulder is assessed and documented. Active forward elevation and external and internal rotation at the side and in abduction are determined. Functional range of motion, such as the ability to place the hand to the mouth, behind the head, to the back pocket, to the contralateral axilla, and to the middle of the back, should be observed. Subsequently, passive range of motion, typically in the supine position, is evaluated. Particular note is made of discrepancies between active and passive range of motion because such discrepancies may relate to numerous factors, including pain, tuberosity nonunion or malunion, neurologic dysfunction, and instability.

Laboratory Studies

Laboratory studies must supplement the workup of the patient with a persistent painful hemiarthroplasty. Infection should be ruled out in any patient with chronic or acute pain following previous arthroplasty. A complete blood cell count with differential and measurement of erythrocyte sedimentation rate (ESR) and C-reactive protein (CRP) are recommended. In patients with an abnormally elevated white blood cell count, ESR, and/or CRP, aspiration of the glenohumeral joint is recommended to rule out sepsis. A joint aspiration may also be considered in the setting of normal laboratory studies if the clinical suspicion remains high.

Imaging

A standard shoulder trauma series consisting of three AP views in the scapular plane (neutral, external, and internal rotation), a scapular Y view (lateral view in the scapular plane), and an axillary lateral view should be obtained. Implant size and position, tuberosity healing, evidence of implant loosening, bony or prosthetic fracture, and condition of the glenoid are all noted. In some situations adjuvant tests can be obtained. CT scans may be helpful in determining implant position, tuberosity healing or malposition, and glenoid erosion. Bone scans also provide useful information when the clinical and laboratory evaluations remain uncertain. MRI may be helpful in assessing the tuberosities and rotator cuff, although special sequencing is required to minimize the interference of the metal implant.

Other Tests

When neurologic injury is suspected, an electromyogram (EMG) and nerve conduction velocity studies should be obtained. These studies can help pinpoint the affected area because the clinical examination may be confusing in the setting of previous surgery and persistent symptoms.

Functional Outcome

Important measures of functional outcome include pain, range of motion, ability to perform activities of daily living (ADL), complications, and the need for further nonsurgical or surgical treatment. A variety of outcome measurements are described in the literature and emphasize certain aspects of outcome more than others; as a result, the success and complication rates tend to be variable.[2-10,13-15,18-20,22-24,30]

The results of many series with respect to pain relief are generally quite good. Although different methods have been used to assess pain, most series demonstrate successful outcomes at short- to medium-term follow-up in the range of 71% to 93%.[2,4-10,15,21,22,24] However, outcome with regard to motion and performance of ADL is considerably less predictable. Neer[31] described a rating system that emphasized strength, range of motion, and functional performance in addition to pain relief. His initial description of 91% satisfactory results in 43 patients led to the widespread acceptance of humeral head replacement for three- and four-part proximal humeral fractures. Although some studies have demonstrated less successful outcomes,[7,23,30] most recent series have reproduced the early success with hemiarthroplasty, especially with regard to patient satisfaction.[2-6,8,9,12,22,24] However, satisfaction does not always correlate with functional ability. In one series of 26 hemiarthroplasties performed for acute proximal humeral fractures, 73% of patients had difficulty with at least 3 of the 15 functional tasks on the American Shoulder and Elbow Surgeons rating system. In particular, lifting and using the hand above shoulder level were problematic. Despite these deficiencies, however, the patients remained pain free and satisfied with outcome.[8]

Several studies have investigated the results of acute versus delayed treatment of proximal humeral fractures. Tanner and Cofield[22] found that hemiarthroplasty for proximal humeral malunions or nonunions is not as successful as acute treatment. A more recent study included 23 chronic proximal humeral fractures treated with HHR or total shoulder replacement at an average of 15 months from injury. The authors demonstrated a higher rate of complications and revision surgery and less predictable function than that typically seen with acute hemiarthroplasty. Results of many series including both acute and chronic fractures have indicated that there is poorer function and a higher risk of complications with delayed treatment.[2,3,6,7,20]

Complications

Tuberosity Failure

Numerous studies cite failure of tuberosity healing as a major factor in poor outcome following hemiarthroplasty. Complications related to tuberosity fixation and healing include frank nonunion, malunion, tuberosity resorption, and rotator cuff insufficiency. The lack of a clearly accepted radiographic or clinical definition of tuberosity failure has resulted in the variable rates of failure (0% to 50%) reported in the literature.[2,5-7,9,10,13-15,19,22,24]

Tuberosity nonunion is usually related to inadequate reduction and fixation at the time of initial surgery (Fig. 1). In one large series there was a 25% rate of tuberosity nonunion at short-term follow-up in patients treated for acute proximal humeral fractures. All patients had poor function; one patient required revision and had minimal improvement.[22] The authors also described an association between excessive tuberosity resection and tension overload of the rotator cuff tendons, possibly leading to insufficiency of the rotator cuff or nonunion/malunion of the tuberosities. Although tuberosity failure is more frequently reported in the treatment of acute fractures, it has also been reported with delayed treatment, particularly when one or both of the tuberosities require osteotomy.[2,19,22]

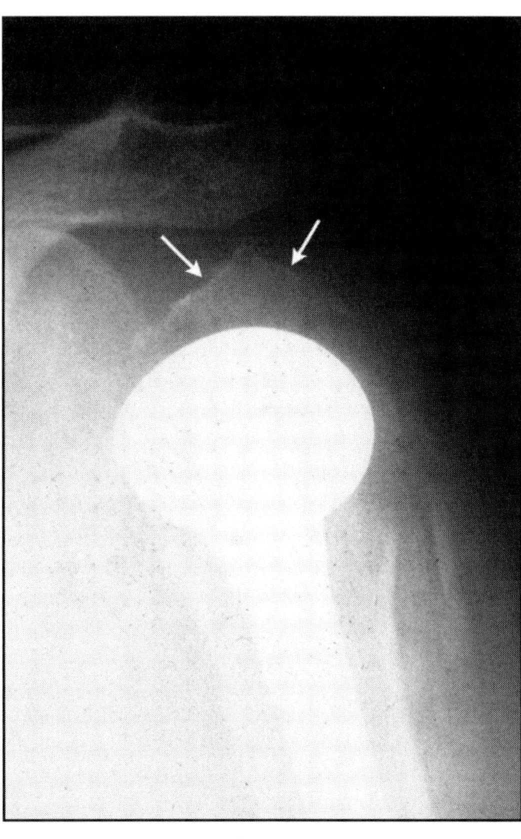

Fig. 1 Neutral rotation AP radiograph of a 68-year-old man who presented 3 months after undergoing hemiarthroplasty for a four-part left proximal humerus fracture. Despite initial postoperative pain relief, the patient failed to progress with continued physical therapy and had severely limited active elevation and external rotation. Nonunion of the greater tuberosity with displacement superior to the humeral head component in the acromiohumeral interval is demonstrated (*arrows*). The patient required revision open reduction and internal suture fixation of the displaced tuberosity.

Despite having initial good relief of discomfort, these patients typically fail to progress in the ensuing months of rehabilitation. They have pain, stiffness, and limited ability to actively move the arm. These symptoms are due either to the nonfunctional rotator cuff or to displacement of the nonunited or malunited tuberosities creating a mechanical block to motion beneath the acromion or against the glenoid rim.

Attention to detail at the time of the initial surgery minimizes the risk of tuberosity failure. The first step is accurate identification of the tuberosities, which may be difficult depending on fracture configuration and extent of comminution. The long head of the biceps is a useful anatomic landmark that can help with orientation because the lesser tuberosity is medial and the greater tuberosity lateral to the tendon. Once identified, the tuberosities are then secured with heavy nonabsorbable sutures through the associated rotator cuff tendons at the bone-tendon junction. The rotator cuff tendons will usually provide adequate holding power and provide for tuberosity mobilization even when the tuberosities are badly comminuted. Intra-articular or extra-articular releases are performed to allow complete mobilization of the tuberosity fragments and provide for tension-free reduction.

The method of tuberosity fixation has improved over time. Initially, most authors described wire fixation, but problems with breakage and migration have led most surgeons to use heavy nonabsorbable suture materials to repair the tuberosities.[4,8-10,21,22,31] The tuberosities should be reduced and fixed to the humeral shaft through drill holes in a reduced position using a combination of No. 2 and No. 5 nonabsorbable sutures. This procedure guarantees adequate tuberosity-to-shaft apposition to allow bony healing. The fin holes on the prosthesis are never used as the sole source of tuberosity fixation. Also, the resected humeral head is used as a source of autogenous bone graft. This bone graft is placed in the intramedullary canal between the tuberosities and the shaft and is both osteoinductive and osteoconductive. After the cement is placed in the canal, care should be taken to remove excess cement from the tuberosity-proximal shaft interface because it may interfere with bony healing. The final position of the tuberosities relative to the implant-

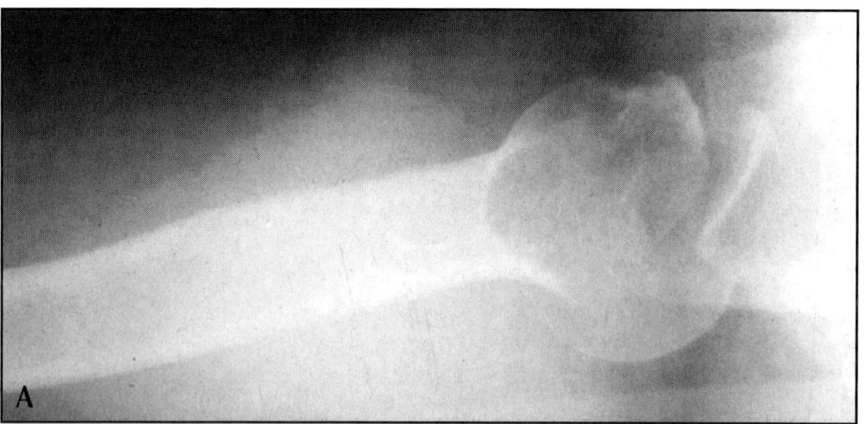

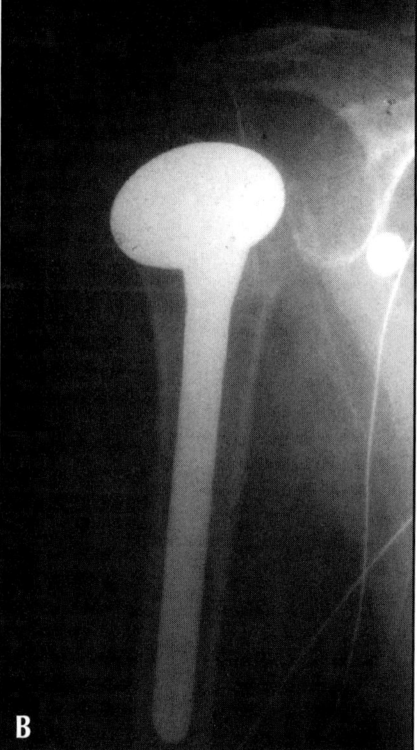

Fig. 2 A, Preoperative axillary radiograph of a 59-year-old woman with a comminuted posterior fracture dislocation of the right proximal humerus. The patient underwent HHR. **B,** Neutral rotation postoperative AP radiograph demonstrates excessive retroversion of the humeral component, leading to symptomatic posterior instability. The patient underwent revision HHR with soft-tissue balancing to restore stability.

ed humeral head should be carefully noted. The tuberosities should be reduced below the level of the prosthetic humeral head. Intraoperative fluoroscopy can be used in situations in which the reduction is uncertain.

Prosthesis Malposition

Very few published case series indicate component malposition alone as a major reason for clinical failure. However, in two series of failed hemiarthroplasties, malposition has been reported as a factor in poor outcome, suggesting its occurrence may be more frequent than originally believed.[5,14,32] In a series of 29 acute and 9 chronic proximal humeral fractures, one patient was reported to have component malposition, but the report did not describe the patient's clinical result or any need for revision.[6] In another series, one symptomatic posterior subluxation and glenoid erosion that required revision to total shoulder arthroplasty was reported. At the time of revision, excessive retroversion of the humeral component was noted.[13] It is likely that improper positioning of the humeral component is an underlying cause of several more frequently reported complications, including tuberosity failure, tuberosity malunion, subacromial impingement, rotator cuff insufficiency, and glenohumeral instability.

The potential malpositions seen clinically are excess anteversion or retroversion, inappropriate prosthetic height, and inappropriate prosthetic humeral head size. The treating surgeon should be aware of these potential complications and how to avoid them. The best method for avoiding poor component position and/or sizing is precise technique at the time of initial surgery. Preoperative radiographs of the contralateral uninjured shoulder are also obtained for preoperative planning. Inappropriate version of the component may lead to instability of the shoulder and should be avoided. This complication is more likely to occur in fractures with associated glenohumeral dislocation, in particular chronic posterior glenohumeral fracture-dislocations (Fig. 2). In this situation, soft tissues are either contracted or redundant and accommodate the deformity. If the position of the soft tissues is not recognized, placing the humeral component in the standard 30° to 40° of retroversion may lead to posterior instability. Therefore, the prosthesis should be placed in less than typical retroversion, for instance, 10° to 20°. The temptation to place the humeral component in neutral rotation, however, should be resisted because this placement can lead to anterior instability. The use of surgical instrumentation that allows assessment of version can be a tremendous help in fracture surgery during which normal anatomic orientation is often lost. Finally, the posterior soft tissues should be thoroughly assessed because capsular plication or cuff tensioning procedures may be required to correct any residual instability.

Improper height of the prosthesis is another avoidable technical error. Positioning the humeral head too high or proud relative to the tuberosities places abnormal tension on the tendons of the rotator cuff and can lead to mechanical impingement beneath the coracoacromial arch. This impingement may contribute to later subacromial impingement and rotator cuff insufficiency, and it may increase the risk of tuberosity failure.[1] An acromioplasty should not be performed in this situation because disruption of the coracoacromial arch may result in anterosuperior instability of the prosthesis (Fig. 3). However, abnormally low positioning of the head functionally shortens the humerus, alters the tension in the rotator cuff and deltoid myofascial sleeve, and weakens the mechanical advantage (lever arm) of the shoulder.[33] This placement usually results in limitation of active motion, weakness, and impingement of the now prominent tuberosities.

The final error related to component position is the size of the prosthetic humeral head. An excessively large humeral head component overstuffs the joint and often will lead to limited motion and persistent pain. On the other hand, undersizing the humeral head decreases humeral offset and, therefore, weakens the functional lever arm of the shoulder.[33] Undersizing the head also can be a contributing factor in postoperative glenohumeral instability. Proper head sizing has been greatly facilitated by the intraoperative use of modular prosthetic design, which enables the surgeon to try various head heights and diameters, including some with offset or eccentric head shapes. The push-pull method of testing humeral head stability is recommended. Using this intraoperative manual assessment, the humeral head should translate approximately 50% of the glenoid articular diameter in both the AP and superoinferior directions. The hand should also be adducted to the contralateral axilla without excessive tension.

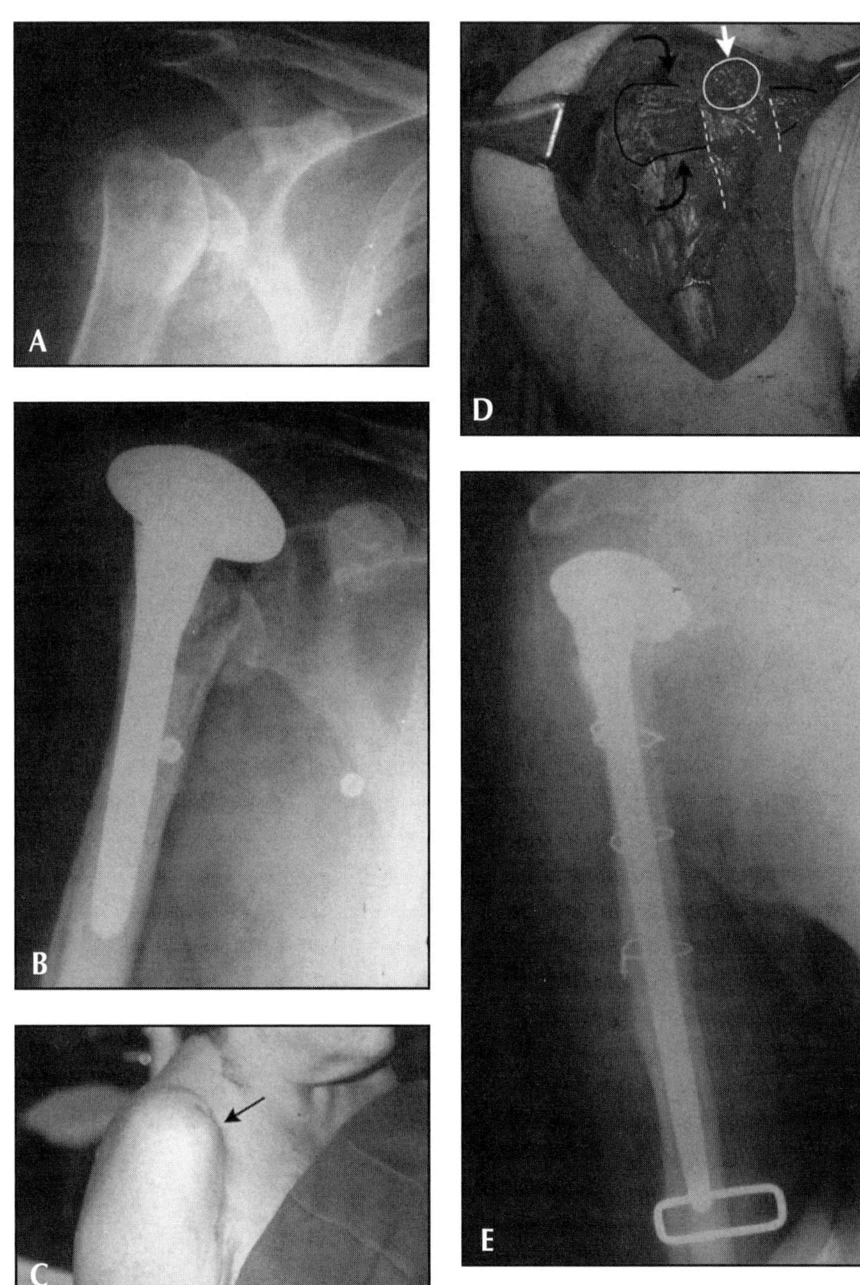

Fig. 3 A, AP radiograph of a 62-year-old woman demonstrates a comminuted four-part fracture of the right proximal humerus. A hemiarthroplasty was performed that was complicated by proximal migration **(B)** of the humeral component. Subacromial impingement related to the prominent component was the diagnosis. She later underwent arthroscopic subacromial decompression with release of the coracoacromial ligament, resulting in further proximal migration of the component and severe anterosuperior instability. The subcutaneous position of the implant **(C)** is demonstrated by the black arrow. The patient ultimately required revision of the humeral component and subcoracoid pectoralis major transfer (**D** and **E**) (white outline/arrow = coracoid process; white dashed outline = strap muscles; black outline/arrows = pectoralis major). She had significant pain relief and reasonable improvement in function using limited goals criteria.

Poor Rehabilitation

The relationship between satisfactory functional outcomes and a structured rehabilitation program has been emphasized previously.[15,34] Many authors have reported unsatisfactory results, which they ascribe to poor compliance with postoperative rehabilitation.[5,9,10,22,30] In 1983, Tanner and Cofield[22] suggested that patients whose physical therapy was delayed more than 2 weeks postoperatively achieved less than ideal motion. Compito and associates[5] noted that 6 of 11 (55%) unsatisfactory results in their primary series were directly related to noncompliance with rehabilitation and activity restrictions.

The relationship of increasing age, associated medical problems, and poor compliance with rehabilitation is also well documented.[6,9,10,30] Several authors have noted that despite limited function, these patients are pain free and pleased with their result.[9,10] Excellent functional outcome, in terms of strength and range of motion, may not be a realistic goal in this population regardless of treatment modality; however, a painless stiff shoulder is likely better than a painful stiff shoulder. We use the three-phase protocol of shoulder rehabilitation initially outlined by Hughes and Neer.[34] Phase I begins on postoperative day 1 and consists of pendulum exercises, and passive forward elevation and external rotation in the supine position. The allowed range of motion is gradually increased during the first 6 weeks, and pulley exercises are avoided until radiographic evidence of tuberosity healing is demonstrated. Phase II starts approximately 6 to 8 weeks following surgery and includes pulley exercises, active exercises in the supine and erect positions, and deltoid isometrics. Phase III begins 12 weeks after surgery and includes light resistance exercises and stretching. The protocol is individualized depending on associated injuries, confidence in tuberosity fixation, and patient compliance.

Instability

Variable rates of postoperative instability have been reported in most series of hemiarthroplasties performed for proximal humeral fractures. Definition of the clinical problem is critical in reviewing the true incidence of symptomatic instability. Reports of the occurrence of posterior or anterior dislocation are rare. Tanner and Cofield[22] reported 2 patients from a group of 27 with delayed treatment of a proximal humeral fracture who had early postoperative dislocations. Both were treated nonsurgically with closed reduction and no ultimate compromise of the clinical result. Despite obvious concerns for malpositioning of the humeral component, recurrent unidirectional (anterior or posterior) instability appears to be a very rare problem. In one series, an 18% rate of recurrent instability was reported in a subset of chronic proximal humeral fractures.[7] Recurrent unidirectional instability has been reported more frequently following hemiarthroplasty performed on a delayed basis.[2,7]

The most frequent instability pattern seen is one of anterosuperior migration or subluxation of the humeral head. This pattern of proximal migration has been reported by numerous authors and has been shown to adversely affect outcome.[3,13,22] This finding was first emphasized by Tanner and Cofield,[22] who found some degree of anterosuperior instability in 49% of their patients. In our experience, proximal migration may be associated with rotator cuff insufficiency, failure of tuberosity fixation, improper component position or size, and/or neurologic injury. The effect of anterosuperior migration on functional outcome is likely to depend on the magnitude of displacement. Small amounts of proximal head displacement are frequently seen and typically do not require surgical revision. However, marked superior displacement of the humeral component, occasionally to a subcutaneous location, severely limits function and is extremely difficult to treat.

The best method of treatment is avoidance of this devastating complication. Strict attention to version of the humeral component is critical, as outlined previously. Also, particular emphasis is placed on safe positions of immobilization after surgery. When an early dislocation does occur, closed reduction and immobilization of the arm in a position that will avoid the direction of instability is recommended.

Neurologic Injury

Nerve injury is a relatively common complication of comminuted proximal humeral fractures. Stableforth[21] reported a 6.1% incidence of brachial plexus injury in a series of 81 patients with four-part fractures. Reported cases of nerve injury occurring as the result of hemiarthroplasty for proximal humeral fractures are fortunately relatively uncommon.[3,10,24]

An EMG-nerve conduction velocity study should be obtained if the examination suggests a neurologic injury. The sensitivity of the physical examination for identifying nerve injury in this setting is often poor. In one series of failed arthroplasties for proximal humeral fracture, 30% had EMG-documented nerve injury.[7] It is not known whether these injuries were a result of the initial injury or the procedure.

Aseptic Loosening

Symptomatic, aseptic loosening is an uncommon complication in hemiarthroplasty for proximal humeral fractures. Compito and associates[5] reported 11 patients with symptomatic, aseptic loosening in cementless arthroplasties in their series of failed arthroplasties. The average time from the primary surgery to symptomatic loosening was not reported. Muldoon and Cofield[14] reported one patient with a cementless prosthesis who had symptomatic loosening at 11 years. The modest numbers of aseptic loosenings reported in the literature may well be related to the relative short-term follow-up periods of the published series. Symptomatic aseptic loosening was not described in cemented prostheses in any of the reviewed papers.

Many authors have reported radiolucent lines adjacent to both cemented and cementless humeral prostheses.[3,8-11,13,14,22] In cemented prostheses, the radiolucency is at the bone-cement interface. Although some authors describe progressive radiolucency, there is currently no proven relationship between radiolucency and symptomatic loosening. Again, longer-term follow-up may establish a relationship between radiolucent lines and ultimate symptomatic loosening.

Infection

Infection remains a particular concern at the time of initial surgery, as well as in the subacute and late postoperative phases. As with other major joint arthroplasties, infection most likely results from bacterial contaminants at the time of original surgery. Very few studies in which infection occurred after humeral head replacement have focused on the etiologic organism(s). A recent review described six patients from a series of patients with 28 acute and 55 delayed treatment proximal humeral fractures who developed infections. Two of the patients with acute infections (early postoperative phase) were successfully treated with intravenous antibiotics. The remaining four patients presented with subacute deep infections and were treated with resection arthroplasties. Of the six, four grew *Staphylococcus aureus*, one grew *S epidermidis*, and one was culture negative.[14]

Theoretically, patients undergoing humeral head arthroplasty for proximal humeral fracture are at risk for postoperative infection for two reasons. First, the patients are often elderly and debilitated, have a poor nutritional state, and have multiple medical problems. They sometimes have other bacterial sources such as the upper respiratory tract and urinary tract. Second, joint replacement in the setting of acute fracture hematoma and associated soft-tissue injury presents an environment that may be favorable for bacterial growth. In the series reported to date there is a 0% to 18% rate of infection following hemiarthroplasty for proximal humeral fracture.[3,4,6-11,13-16,20,22-24,30] It should be realized, however, that these series typically involve small numbers of patients, and deep infections and acute superficial wound complications are often grouped together when reporting results. The rate of chronic deep infection is likely quite small, but when it does occur, prosthetic resection or staged revision are frequently required.

Attention to sterility and atraumatic technique at the time of initial surgery are crucial components of the surgical plan. Care should be taken to avoid prolonged retraction of the soft tissues, including the skin. Excessive stripping of fracture fragments destroys vascularity, increases the risk of infection, and should be avoided unless necessary for anatomic reduction of the tuberosities to the shaft. Prophylactic antibiotics (first-generation cephalosporin or alternative) are administered prior to surgery and are continued in the perioperative period for 48 hours. We also routinely close the wound over a medium-sized suction-drainage device, which is typically discontinued 24 to 48 hours postoperatively.

Glenoid Erosion

Glenoid erosion is infrequently cited as a cause of failure.[5,9,13] Compito and associates[5] reported approximately eight failures related to glenoid erosion in their series of failed prostheses. No clear method of quantifying glenoid erosion is offered in any of the published reports. It is also unclear whether glenoid erosion occurs without the influence of component malposition or instability.

More commonly, radiographic changes related to glenoid arthritis are reported.[10,14,22] In one review article, six patients with glenoid arthritis were reported at an average follow-up of 56 months.[14] One of the six was reported to have severe glenoid arthritis at 7-year follow-up but remained asymptomatic. Only one patient required revision at 11 years. These data suggest that glenoid arthritis may be part of the natural history of hemiarthroplasty for proximal humeral fractures.

Heterotopic Ossification

Ectopic bone formation following fracture of the proximal humerus is a frequent radiographic finding. Six patients of 43 treated with hemiarthroplasty were found to have developed heterotopic ossification at follow-up in Neer's initial series. An association with fracture-dislocation, repeated attempts at reduction, and delayed fracture treatment were noted.[15] Numerous studies since have discussed the frequent occurrence of heterotopic ossification in proximal humeral fractures treated with hemiarthroplasty.[3,6,8,22,24] The diagnosis can usually be made with standard radiographs. There have been classification schemes devised for heterotopic ossification in the region of the proximal humerus.[13,22] Neither system was found to have any correlation with postoperative function. Although it often is noted radiographically, a review of the existing literature suggests heterotopic ossification rarely adversely affects outcome.[2,7-11,13-16,20,22-24,29-36] In the studies specifically addressing the issue, no patients required reoperation.

Tuberosity Prominence and Subacromial Impingement

Prominence of the tuberosities following fracture treatment with HHR has been described. The problem is multifactorial and relates to many of the complications previously discussed, namely failure of tuberosity fixation and/or reduction, inappropriate component height, and heterotopic ossification. Published reports of few series specifically mention impingement syndrome as a complication following HHR. Also, reports of the series on failed hemiarthroplasties have confirmed a relatively infrequent incidence of impingement syndrome.[5,14,32] The effect of superior tuberosity displacement on outcome remains somewhat unclear. A series of patients with 20 acutely treated fractures included one patient diagnosed with subacromial impingement; however, that patient also had nonunion of the greater tuberosity and required revision ORIF and rotator cuff repair.[13] In another study, little correlation was found between tuberosity prominence and outcome; three patients were noted to have at least 1.5 cm of greater tuberosity displacement on postoperative radiographs but all of them had acceptable functional results.[24] However, a recent review of arthroscopy after glenohumeral arthroplasty included four patients initially treated for four-part fractures of the proximal humerus or fracture dislocations. Three of the four required arthroscopic subacromial decompression; all had improvement in their postoperative motion and functional scores, suggesting that impingement syndrome may be a correctable condition following hemiarthroplasty.[37]

Analysis of Failures: New York Orthopaedic Hospital Experience

A series of failed hemiarthroplasties for acute proximal humeral fractures has previously been reported.[5] This series of patients represents a large group of patients with unsatisfactory results typically seen in a tertiary care referral center. A total of 27 patients (29 shoulders) were reviewed; average patient age was 63 years (range, 37 to 79 years). Most of these patients (79%) were referred from outside institutions. Approximately 75% of the patients in this series had their initial surgery within 15 days of the injury. Overall, 18 patients required revision surgery due to one or more complications.

Analysis of the mode of clinical failure demonstrated the multifactorial nature of the problem. Eighty-three percent of the affected shoulders had more than one complication as the underlying cause of failure. Tuberosity malunion or nonunion was by far the most common complication (15 shoulders, 52%). Other frequent causes of poor results included improper rehabilitation (41%), neurologic injury (31%), component malposition (31%), and glenoid erosion (24%).

Treatment

Nonsurgical

As with any condition, nonsurgical options should be considered in the initial treatment of the symptomatic patient. Every patient should have a complete workup with appropriate diagnostic studies (including imaging and laboratory evaluation) prior to embarking on a course of nonsurgical treatment. Judicious use of anti-inflammatory medication, physical therapy, and corticosteroid injections may occasionally be helpful in the management of these difficult fractures. However, both the patient and treating physician should be realistic in their expectations of the proposed treatment method.

Surgical

Patients with identifiable problems diagnosed using imaging or laboratory evaluation will frequently require surgical intervention. Numerous potential surgical treatment options are available to the surgeon depending on the clinical situation. It must be noted, however, that surgical treatment has a guarded prognosis. To our knowledge, no series exists that is dedicated to the surgical treatment of failed hemiarthroplasty for proximal humerus fracture.

The treatment of nonunion or malunion of the tuberosities requires mobilization and revision ORIF of the tuberosities and must be augmented with autogenous or allograft bone graft. If malposition of the component has contributed to the failure of tuberosity healing, limited motion, instability, or glenoid erosion, the humeral component should be revised. Occasionally, tuberosity malunion resulting in impingement alone can be treated successfully with arthroscopic or open acromioplasty and subacromial decompression, with or without tuberoplasty. Arthroscopic treatment with or without manipulation under anesthesia might be considered in the setting of excessive stiffness not explained by improper component size or position, but only if adequate clinical and radiographic healing can be documented.

The treatment of symptomatic instability is complex and depends on many factors including bone quality, component malposition, neurologic injury, and direction or pattern of instability. Component malposition should be corrected with revision. Soft-tissue procedures such as capsular plication, tendon repair, or tendon transfer can be considered when inappropriate component position is ruled out.

In particular, we have found the treatment of severe anterosuperior instability to be challenging. When small to moderate amounts of proximal component migration are seen, we recommend avoiding acromioplasty or decompression of the coracoacromial arch. Release of the coracoacromial ligament in this setting is potentially disastrous because it removes the last remaining soft-tissue constraint to superior migration of the humeral head. In situations where anterosuperior instability of the humeral component is severe and the coracoacromial arch is compromised, use of an Achilles allograft to reconstruct the coracoacromial arch has been described.[38] We have not found static reconstructions of the coracoacromial arch to be successful.[39] Dynamic attempts to treat anterosuperior instability include transfer of the pectoralis major tendon and have been performed as an alternative to the static reconstructions.[36,40] These are salvage situations, and it is reasonable to consider these procedures. However, the procedures should be considered as a pain-relieving measure only because any significant functional benefit, in terms of restoration of motion and strength, has yet to be demonstrated.

The treatment of infection can be problematic. Surgical treatment options include irrigation and débridement with retention of components, one-stage reimplantation, two-stage reimplantation, and resection arthroplasty. To our knowledge, no series of any of these techniques have been published. Consideration should also be given to suppressive antibiotic therapy in patients who are poor surgical candidates for medical reasons.

The indications for surgical treatment of neurologic dysfunction are unclear. Nerve exploration and grafting has infrequently been described, and its role and effectiveness are uncertain. Tendon or muscle transfers may be helpful in certain situations. However, as a general rule, nonsurgical management is recommended.

Symptomatic glenoid erosion, as mentioned previously, has not been a significant problem in the short term. A recent series of HHRs treated with conversion to total shoulder replacement included 10 patients out of 22 who initially had proximal humeral fractures as their presenting diagnosis. In that study, improvements in range of motion and pain scores were demonstrated, although functional improvement was more limited. No analysis of the posttraumatic subset of patients was performed.[35]

Summary

HHR for the treatment of complex proximal humeral fractures has gained acceptance over the past 50 years. Despite good results in the acute setting with regard to pain relief and patient satisfaction, complications can and do occur and may adversely affect the surgical outcome. The most reliable means of avoiding these complications is an accurate preoperative diagnosis and strict attention to surgical technique. Failure of the operation is often multifactorial and may require surgical revision, the results of which are far less predictable than those of primary hemiarthroplasty. Any patient with persistent pain or unacceptable limitation of function requires a thorough diagnostic evaluation to determine the etiology of the problem. The surgeon should educate the patient about the limited goals of treatment in this situation so that realistic expectations can be achieved with either nonsurgical or surgical treatment.

References

1. Bigliani LU, McCluskey GM III: Prosthetic replacement in acute fractures of the proximal humerus. *Semin Arthroplasty* 1990;1:129-137.
2. Boileau P, Trojani C, Walch G, Krishnan SG, Romeo A, Sinnerton R: Shoulder arthroplasty for the treatment of the sequelae of fractures of the proximal humerus. *J Shoulder Elbow Surg* 2001;10:299-308.
3. Bosch U, Skutek M, Fremerey RW, Tscherne H: Outcome after primary and secondary hemiarthroplasty in elderly patients with fractures of the proximal humerus. *J Shoulder Elbow Surg* 1998;7:479-484.
4. Boss AP, Hintermann B: Primary endoprosthesis in comminuted humeral head fractures in patients over 60 years of age. *Int Orthop* 1999;23:172-174.
5. Compito CA, Self EB, Bigliani LU: Arthroplasty and acute shoulder trauma: Reasons for success and failure. *Clin Orthop* 1994;307:27-36.
6. Dimakopoulos P, Potamitis N, Lambiris E: Hemiarthroplasty in the treatment of comminuted intraarticular fractures of the proximal humerus. *Clin Orthop* 1997;341:7-11.
7. Frich LH, Sojbjerg JO, Sneppen O: Shoulder arthroplasty in complex acute and chronic proximal humeral fractures. *Orthopedics* 1991;14: 949-954.
8. Goldman RT, Koval KJ, Cuomo F, Gallagher MA, Zuckerman JD: Functional outcome after humeral head replacement for acute three- and four-part proximal humeral fractures. *J Shoulder Elbow Surg* 1995;4:81-86.
9. Green A, Barnard L, Limbird RS: Humeral head replacement for acute, four-part proximal humerus fractures. *J Shoulder Elbow Surg* 1993;2:249-254.
10. Hawkins RJ, Switlyk P: Acute prosthetic replacement for severe fractures of the proximal humerus. *Clin Orthop* 1993;289:156-160.
11. Kay SP, Amstutz HC: Shoulder hemiarthroplasty at UCLA. *Clin Orthop* 1988;228:42-48.
12. Levine WN, Connor PM, Yamaguchi K, et al: Humeral head replacement for proximal humeral fractures. *Orthopedics* 1998;21:68-75.
13. Moeckel BH, Dines DM, Warren RF, Altchek DW: Modular hemiarthroplasty for fractures of the proximal part of the humerus. *J Bone Joint Surg Am* 1992;74:884-889.
14. Muldoon MP, Cofield RH: Complications of humeral head replacement for proximal humeral fractures. *Instr Course Lect* 1997;46:15-24.
15. Neer CS II: Displaced proximal humeral fractures: Part II. Treatment of three-part and four-part displacement. *J Bone Joint Surg Am* 1970;52:1090-1103.
16. Neer CS II, Watson KC, Stanton FJ: Recent experience in total shoulder replacement. *J Bone Joint Surg Am* 1982;64:319-337.
17. Neer CSI: Articular replacement for the humeral head. *J Bone Joint Surg Am* 1955;37:215-228.
18. Neer CSI: Recent results and techniques of prosthetic replacement for 4-part proximal humeral fractures. *Orthop Trans* 1986;10:475.
19. Norris TR, Green A, McGuigan FX: Late prosthetic shoulder arthroplasty for displaced proximal humerus fractures. *J Shoulder Elbow Surg* 1995;4:271-280.
20. Schai P, Imhoff A, Preiss S: Comminuted humeral head fractures: A multicenter analysis. *J Shoulder Elbow Surg* 1995;4:319-330.
21. Stableforth PG: Four-part fractures of the neck of the humerus. *J Bone Joint Surg Br* 1984;66:104-108.
22. Tanner MW, Cofield RH: Prosthetic arthroplasty for fractures and fracture-dislocations of the proximal humerus. *Clin Orthop* 1983;179: 116-128.
23. Willems WJ, Lim TE: Neer arthroplasty for humeral fracture. *Acta Orthop Scand* 1985;56:394-395.
24. Zyto K, Wallace WA, Frostick SP, Preston BJ: Outcome after hemiarthroplasty for three- and four-part fractures of the proximal humerus. *J Shoulder Elbow Surg* 1998;7:85-89.
25. Cofield RH: Comminuted fractures of the proximal humerus. *Clin Orthop* 1988;230:49-57.
26. Connor PM, D'Alessandro DF: Role of hemiarthroplasty for proximal humeral fractures. *J South Orthop Assoc* 1995;4:9-23.
27. Dines DM, Warren RF: Modular shoulder hemiarthroplasty for acute fractures: Surgical considerations. *Clin Orthop* 1994;307:18-26.
28. Darder A, Darder A Jr, Sanchis V, Gastaldi E, Gomar F: Four-part displaced proximal humeral fractures: Operative treatment using Kirschner wires and a tension band. *J Orthop Trauma* 1993;7:497-505.
29. Esser RD: Open reduction and internal fixation of three- and four-part fractures of the proximal humerus. *Clin Orthop* 1994;299:244-251.
30. Kraulis J, Hunter G: The results of prosthetic replacement in fracture-dislocations of the upper end of the humerus. *Injury* 1976;8: 129-131.

31. Neer CS II: Displaced proximal humeral fractures: Part I. Classification and evaluation. *J Bone Joint Surg Am* 1970;52:1077-1089.

32. Bigliani LU, Flatow EL, McCluskey GW, Fischer RA: Failed prosthetic replacement in dsiplaced proximal humerus fractures. *Orthop Trans* 1991;15:747-748.

33. Rietveld AB, Daanen HA, Rozing PM, Obermann WR: The lever arm in glenohumeral abduction after hemiarthroplasty. *J Bone Joint Surg Br* 1988;70:561-565.

34. Hughes M, Neer CS II: Glenohumeral joint replacement and postoperative rehabilitation. *Phys Ther* 1975;55:850-858.

35. Sperling JW, Cofield RH: Revision total shoulder arthroplasty for the treatment of glenoid arthrosis. *J Bone Joint Surg Am* 1998;80:860-867.

36. Klepps SJ, Galatz L, Yamaguchi K: Subcoracoid pectoralis major transfer: A salvage procedure for irreparable subscapularis deficiency. *Tech Shoulder Elbow Surg* 2001;2:85-91.

37. Hersch JC, Dines DM: Arthroscopy for failed shoulder arthroplasty. *Arthroscopy* 2000;16: 606-612.

38. Dines DM, Warren RF, Font-Rodriguez D: Revision shoulder arthroplasty. *Tech Shoulder Elbow Surg* 2001;2:26-37.

39. Flatow EL, Connor PM, Levine WN, Arroyo JS, Pollock RG, Bigliani LU: Coracoacromial arch reconstruction for anterosuperior instability. *Proceedings of the 13th Open Meeting of the American Shoulder and Elbow Surgeons*. San Francisco, CA, 1997.

40. Wirth MA, Rockwood CA Jr: Complications of total shoulder-replacement arthroplasty. *J Bone Joint Surg Am* 1996;78:603-616.

Complications of Humeral Head Replacement for Proximal Humeral Fractures

Derek Plausinis, MASc, MD
Young W. Kwon, MD, PhD
Joseph D. Zuckerman, MD

Abstract

Humeral head replacement has been widely used for the treatment of complex proximal humeral fractures. The procedure is associated with a high rate of patient satisfaction as well as reliable relief of pain. The functional outcomes, however, have been variable. Reported complications include infection, neurologic injury, intraoperative fracture, instability, tuberosity malunion and nonunion, rotator cuff tear, heterotopic ossification, glenoid erosion, and stiffness. When technical factors such as tuberosity malunion or component malpositioning are considered as postoperative complications, the incidence of complications is relatively high. This high rate of complications, in turn, may be related to the wide range of reported functional outcomes.

Instr Course Lect 2005;54:371-380.

Results after humeral head replacement for the treatment of acute proximal humeral fractures have been mixed. The variability in the reported outcomes reflects the technical factors related to the reconstruction, the timing of the surgery, the nature of the patient population, and the different methods of assessing the results. Hemiarthroplasty for the treatment of proximal humeral fractures provides good to excellent pain relief in 73% to 97% of patients.[1-5] Patients are generally satisfied with the procedure, as reflected by the 70% to 92% satisfaction rates in most series.[1,4,6-10] Functional outcomes, however, have been variable. One of the more commonly used outcome instruments is the Constant score, which measures four clinical parameters, including pain, range of motion, power, and activities of daily living, on a 100-point scale. Using this system, some authors have reported average scores as low as 38 points whereas others have reported average scores as high as 68 points.[3-5,10-12] Within each series, however, there has been a broad range of results, with excellent outcomes in some patients and poor results in others.[4,5,9,11,13,14]

Perioperative complications are the most important factors affecting outcome. The reported prevalence of complications after humeral head replacement for treatment of acute proximal humeral fractures has varied substantially from one series to another. This variability is a result, in part, of the differences in the definition of what constitutes a complication. For example, one series may include superficial infection as a complication whereas in another series it may be considered only as a minor inconvenience. The duration of clinical follow-up has also varied, further confounding the reported rates of complications. In general, longer follow-up is associated with an increased prevalence of complications.

Complications after humeral head replacement for the treatment of proximal humeral fractures include infection, neurologic injury, intraoperative fracture, instability, tuberosity malunion and nonunion, rotator cuff tear, component malpositioning, heterotopic ossification, glenoid erosion, and stiffness.[1-27] These reported complications are summarized in Table 1; no attempt was made to combine the raw data from the retrospective series because many complications, such as superficial infection or stiffness, are likely to be underappreciated and underreported.

Infections and Wound Problems

Prevention of infection after a humeral head replacement requires meticulous surgical technique, particularly because of the potential contamination from the axilla. Perioperative antibiotics should be

Table 1
Complications Following Humeral Head Replacement for Acute Proximal Humeral Fractures

Complication	Range of Reported Prevalence in Literature*
Infection	
Superficial	0 to 6%
Deep	Usually < 2%; 1 of 16 in one series
Preoperative nerve palsy	
Axillary	0 to 13%
Radial	< 1%
Median	< 1%
Musculocutaneous	Uncommon, 1 of 44†
Brachial plexus	0 to 6%
Postoperative nerve palsy	
Transient	
Axillary	0 to 5%
Radial	Uncommon, 1 of 29†
Permanent	Uncommon‡
Intraoperative fracture	Uncommon, 1 of 11†
Postoperative periprosthetic fracture	0 to 2%
Instability	
Excessive AP translation	0 to 7%
Dislocation	0 to 5%
Tuberosity problems	
Intraoperative malpositioning	0 to 27%
Detachment and migration	0 to 23%
Resorption	0 to 7.0%
Nonunion	0 to 17%
Malunion	0 to 39%
Rotator cuff tear or proximal migration	0 to 23%
Humeral component problems	
Retroversion > 40°	0 to 39.1%
Anteversion > 0°	0%
Prosthetic height (humeral length)	
Prosthesis >10 mm too long	0 to 26%
Prosthesis >10 mm too low	0 to 36%
Radiolucent lines	0 to 32%
Revision for aseptic loosening of cemented stem	0 to 1%
Heterotopic ossification	
Brooker grade 1 or 2	0 to 17%
Brooker grade 3 or 4	0 to 7%
Glenoid degenerative changes	
Radiographic changes	0 to 35%
Requiring revision	0 to 4%
Stiffness requiring release	Uncommon, 1 of 64†
Reflex sympathetic dystrophy	0 to 4%

*The broad range of results reflects the different patient populations, methods of reporting, and numbers of patients in the series; in addition, most authors did not report the presence or absence of many of the listed complications
† This complication was reported in only one series
‡ See text for details

used routinely. Careful handling of the soft tissues is essential, particularly for elderly patients, whose tissues are more sensitive to traumatic insults.

Recognized risk factors for infection include previous shoulder surgery, increased surgical time, and patient comorbidities. Compromised immune function such as that caused by immunosuppressive therapy, rheumatoid arthritis, diabetes mellitus, and malignant lesions may also predispose patients to a postoperative infection. Other risk factors include infection at another site, chronic renal failure being treated with dialysis, radiation therapy, poor nutrition, and obesity.[28-31]

Infections include acute postoperative infections occurring within 30 days after the surgery, subacute infections occurring within 6 months after the surgery, and late infections occurring 6 months or more after the surgery. Both acute and subacute infections usually originate from the initial surgery. Late infections represent hematogenous seeding of the surgical site. Subacute and late infections often present as early prosthetic loosening and usually are not associated with wound drainage or breakdown (Figure 1).

Most authors have not commented specifically on superficial infections, but in one study the prevalence was 5.5%.[5] Most of these infections can be treated successfully with antibiotics alone. Deep infection during the acute postoperative period is relatively uncommon, with no more than one acute deep infection reported in several studies that included from 16 to 72 patients.[2,12,15,19] In the largest series published to date, only two deep infections were found in 138 patients.[5] One of those patients was treated successfully with surgical débridement alone, whereas the other patient required revision of the prosthesis.

Management of infections following shoulder arthroplasty has been largely extrapolated from the hip and knee arthroplasty literature.[28,29,32-36] As such, the treatment is determined, in part, by the time of presentation. An acute deep postoperative infection should be treated with urgent irrigation and débridement. Every effort should be made to maintain the security of the tuberosity fixation. After surgical débridement, the patient is treated with intravenous antibiotics. The choice of antibiotic should be determined from the results of the intraoperative culture. Early consultation with an infectious disease specialist is encouraged. If the initial débridement is not successful, the implant and the cement mantle should be removed and an antibiotic-impregnated cement spacer should be inserted.[33,36] During the procedure, the tuberosities should be secured to the shaft in anticipation of implantation of a new prosthesis at a later date.

Delayed infections should be treated with surgical débridement, removal of the implant, and insertion of an antibiotic-impregnated cement spacer (Figure 2). Treatment of late hematogenous infections is variable. For example, a patient in whom an "acute" shoulder infection develops following a urinary tract or periodontal infection can be treated with surgical débridement alone if the radiographs and the intraoperative examination suggest that the bone-cement interface is not involved. If the initial débridement is not successful, however, a more extensive débridement and removal of the prosthesis are necessary.

Treatment of an infection at the site of a prosthesis is more likely to be successful when the involved organism has a high sensitivity to standard intravenous antibiotics. Pseudomonal infections are particularly difficult to treat because of the organisms' slow rate of replication and resistance to many antibiotics.[37] Although the subject is somewhat controversial, other gram-negative organisms have also been considered to be difficult to eradicate.[37]

In addition to infections, other soft-tissue complications may also occur, at a very low rate. To the authors' our knowledge, only one superficial wound dehiscence has been reported in the literature; it was successfully managed with local wound care.[3] In addition, only a few symptomatic hematomas have been reported.[5,18,19] Typically, awareness and prompt recognition provide the basis for successful management of these complications.

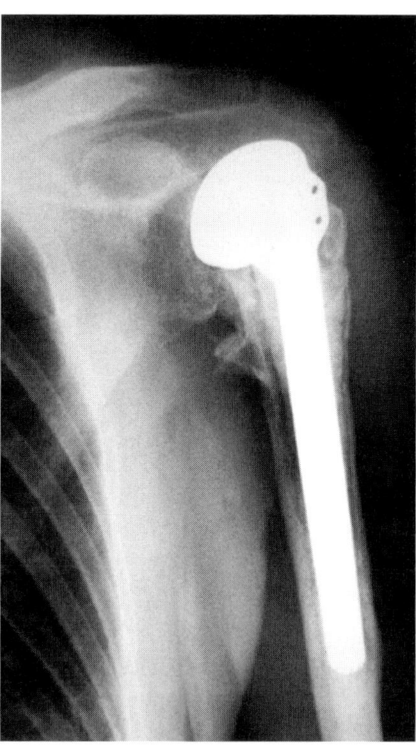

Figure 1 AP radiograph of the shoulder showing a loose humeral prosthesis 6 months following a hemiarthroplasty. Blood work and glenohumeral arthrocentesis confirmed septic loosening.

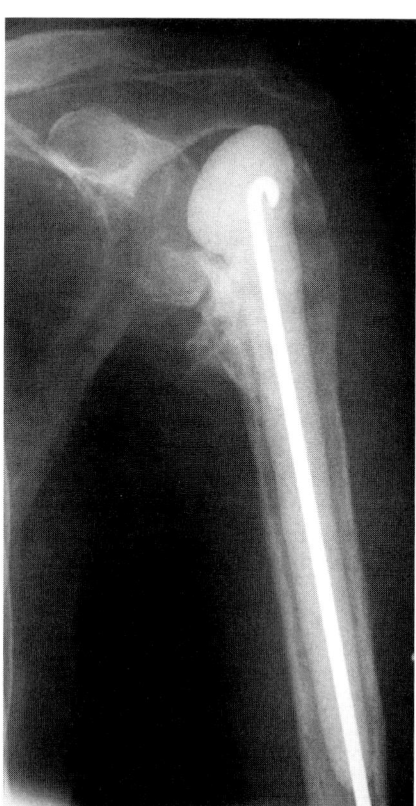

Figure 2 Septic loosening treated with removal of the prosthesis and insertion of an antibiotic-impregnated cement spacer.

Nerve Injury

Neurologic injury from proximal humeral fractures is an underappreciated complication. The prevalence of neurologic injury reported in the literature has been based on the initial clinical assessment. When electrodiagnostic studies have been done, however, nerve injury has been identified in up to 67% of patients with a proximal humeral fracture.[38,39] Preoperative clinical recognition of a neurologic injury has been reported in up to 15% of patients requiring hemiarthroplasty.[5] Nerve injuries that occur during the surgical procedure are much less common. When they do occur, most are transient and rarely result in a permanent deficit. The distinction between a nerve injury that occurs after the initial trauma from one that occurs during the surgery is important for patient management as well as for medicolegal reasons.

The axillary nerve is the most commonly injured nerve, with the rate of injury being as high as 12.5% in one series.[5,26,27] The second most common nerve injury involves the brachial plexus. These injuries have been reported in up to 6.1% of cases.[5,6,19] Isolated radial or median nerve palsies have been reported, but their prevalence is less than 1%.[5] In an earlier study, Neer and McIlveen[20] reported higher rates of median and radial nerve injuries as well as one musculocutaneous and two ulnar nerve injuries. However, those injuries were believed to have occurred during the initial attempts at reduction before the hemiarthroplasty.[20] To the authors' knowledge, no other reports of isolated musculocutaneous or suprascapular nerve injuries exist in the literature. The lack of such reported injuries seems to be the result of the difficulty in recognizing the deficit in an acutely injured patient. When electrodiagnostic studies have been performed in patients with a proximal humeral fracture, the prevalence of abnormalities in the musculocutaneous and suprascapular nerves have been reported to be 29% and 48%, respectively.[39]

Surgical management of proximal humeral fractures is associated with a low risk of nerve injury. Transient axillary nerve palsy related to the surgical procedure occurs in less than 5% of cases.[1,4,5,14,26] The injury typically occurs at the inferior aspect of the glenohumeral joint as the nerve passes in an anterior-to-posterior direction. This area must be explored carefully with clear visualization. Often, the injury is caused by a misplaced retractor or overly aggressive retraction. Continuous awareness of the location of the nerve, usually through palpation or direct visualization, is crucial to avoiding injury. The musculocutaneous nerve may also be injured by inappropriate retraction, particularly if the retraction is applied more distally on the undersurface of the conjoined tendon. Most injuries of the suprascapular nerve occur during surgery for a chronic fracture that requires extensive mobilization of the tuberosities and/or rotator cuff. Direct injury to the suprascapular nerve can occur when dissection and mobilization are performed more than 1 cm medial to the superior and posterior glenoid margin. Isolated radial nerve injury during humeral head replacement is rare and has been reported only once.[14]

Although most injuries are neurapraxias, permanent nerve injuries may occur after the initial trauma or after the surgery. If there are concerns that a direct nerve injury (such as a laceration) has occurred, electrodiagnostic studies should be performed. If the study indicates a disruption of the nerve, early exploration and repair should be considered. Unfortunately, there are insufficient data regarding the prevalence of permanent nerve injury. In the largest reported series to date, 21 of 138 patients (15%) had preoperative neurologic symptoms, with 9 (6.5%) having persistent symptoms after 6 weeks.[5]

Intraoperative Fractures

The prevalence of intraoperative fractures has been reported to be 1% to 3% during total shoulder arthroplasty[40] and even lower during hemiarthroplasty for proximal humeral fractures. To the authors' knowledge, only one report of an intraoperative fracture during the treatment of an acute proximal humeral fracture exists.[16] However, when the surgery has been performed to treat the late complications of these fractures, the prevalence of intraoperative fracture has been as high as 5.5%.[24] Because some intraoperative fractures may be unrecognized and stabilized by the cement mantle, it is possible that they are underreported in the acute setting.

Treatment of an intraoperative fracture depends on the location and the extent of propagation. Fractures in the proximal portion of the shaft that do not extend beyond the distal tip of the humeral stem can usually be treated with cerclage wire fixation. If the fracture extends distal to the standard humeral component, a long-stem component should be used. The prosthesis should extend at least two cortical diameters distal to the fracture, and a cerclage wire should be used for supplementary fixation. If a long-stem component is not available, a plate or a biologic strut graft across the fracture site can be applied. During the insertion of the prosthesis, care must be taken to prevent extravasation of the cement through the fracture site, as the heat from the curing process may damage the nearby neurovascular structures.[41]

In most instances, intraoperative fractures can be prevented by using meticulous surgical technique. Forced manipulation of the shaft should be avoided. Proper positioning of the patient on the operating table to allow full extension of the humerus provides adequate exposure for the insertion of the humeral component. In addition, drill holes in the humeral shaft for the fixation of the tuberosities should be placed distally to minimize the possibility of fracture propagation. In severely osteopenic bone, a cement restrictor may not be appropriate because excessive pressurization within the canal may occur.

Instability

The definition of instability of the glenohumeral joint after humeral head replacement has been inconsistent in the literature. Thus, the reported rates of this complication have been variable. Some authors have defined superior subluxation as instability, whereas others have considered it to be a complication related to the rotator cuff. Inferior instability is also not well defined because inferior subluxation is a common postoperative finding thought to be related to deltoid atony. Inferior subluxation usually resolves spontaneously. Persistent inferior subluxation may represent a nerve injury or malpositioning of the prosthesis and usually does not cause the sensation of instability.

Anterior and posterior instability usually presents with the typical symptoms of subluxation or dislocation. Even in the absence of a documented dislocation, excessive translation in the anterior-posterior direction has been found in up to 7.1% of patients.[6,10,24] Dislocation after humeral head replacement is less common. Hawkins and Switlyk[1] reported one dislocation in their series of 20 patients, and Robinson and associates[5] reported three dislocations (2.2%) in their series of 138 patients.

Factors that increase the risk of joint instability include failure to restore the physiologic version and height of the humeral head component, compromise of the rotator cuff, and problems related to the tuberosities. Often, instability develops as a result of resorption or migration of a tuberosity. Detachment of the lesser tuberosity compromises the anterior shoulder restraint and may lead to anterior instability, especially with external rotation. Detachment of the greater tuberosity can result in superior migration of the humeral head as well as anterior instability. Although posterior instability can occur, it is less common.

Treatment of glenohumeral joint instability after humeral head replacement is based on the severity of the symptoms. For patients with no gross structural defects or component malposition, rehabilitation and activity modification may be sufficient. If the symptoms persist or if there are structural abnormalities, surgical intervention must be considered. The goal of these procedures is to restore the normal anatomy and the constraints of shoulder stability. In rare instances, the procedure may require the use of allografts or autografts to augment the surrounding structures.[42]

Complications Related to the Tuberosities and the Rotator Cuff

Reconstruction of the tuberosities has been increasingly recognized as a crucial element influencing the clinical outcome.[10,12,26] Many complications are associated with improper function of the tuberosities and the rotator cuff. They include postoperative migration, nonunion, malunion, and resorption of the tuberosities.

Migration and Nonunion

Postoperative migration of the tuberosities is a common complication that substantially increases the likelihood of a poor functional outcome[26] (Figure 3). The prevalence of tuberosity migration has been reported to be between 2% and 23%.[4-6,9,10,18,24,26] The method of tuberosity attachment and the ability to obtain secure fixation are the key elements influencing tuberosity stability and subsequent union. Overall bone quality has also been suggested to influence the likelihood of tuberosity migration.[26] The clinical importance of postoperative migration appears to be determined by the degree of migration. Minimal migration and displacement frequently result in weakness and a decreased range of motion whereas, with more displacement, instability and pain may also be present. In this clinical setting, surgical management should be considered, with the goals of mobilizing the tuberosities and obtaining a secure reattachment. Given the high rate of tuberosity migration, it is not surprising that the prevalence of tuberosity nonunion has been as high as 17%.[6,10,24,26] Although the clinical relevance may vary among individuals, this complication is usually associated with an inferior outcome. For patients with substantial symptoms, surgical intervention to reattach the tuberosities should be considered. In some patients, this may be difficult because the factors that resulted in the original nonunion may still be present.

During the surgery, all attempts should be made to provide maximal stability to the tuberosity fixation. The concept of defining fixation in the longitudinal and transverse directions has been described previously.[43] After contact between the tuberosities and the shaft has been confirmed, sufficient longitudinal fixation should be placed to allow early rehabilitation. For transverse fixation, the tuberosities should be in contact with each other and should be stabilized with cerclage fixation that encompasses both of the tuberosities and the humeral component. Multiple sutures should be used to maximize the stability. It is recommended that, when possible, cancellous bone graft from the removed humeral head be used to enhance the healing potential.

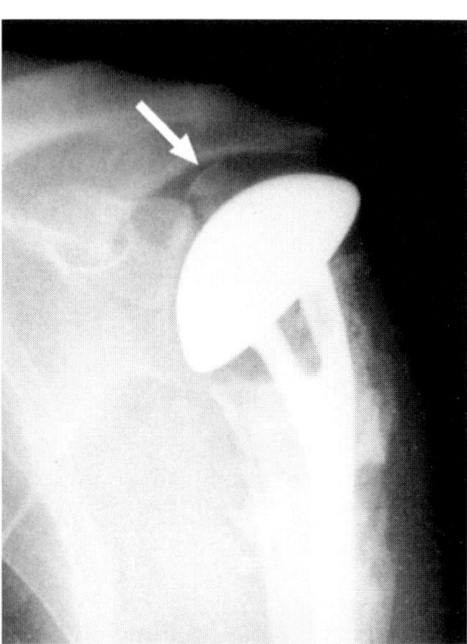

Figure 3 An AP radiograph of the shoulder made 6 weeks postoperatively showing failure of tuberosity fixation with migration of the greater tuberosity (*arrow*).

Malunion

Malunion of the tuberosities may occur as a result of improper intraoperative positioning or after tuberosity migration. Proper positioning of the tuberosities has been critically evaluated only recently.[4,12,26] In one recent series, the prevalence of tuberosity malunion was reported to be as high as 39%.[26] When the initial postoperative radiographs were critically appraised, initial malpositioning of the tuberosity was found in 27% of those patients.[26] In the coronal plane, the greater tuberosity was positioned either too inferiorly (> 10 mm inferior to the top of the humeral head) or too superiorly (< 5 mm inferior to the top of the humeral head) in 18% of the patients. In the sagittal plane, horizontal malpositioning was found in 23% of the patients. Mighell and associates,[12] who used slightly different criteria to define malreduction in their series, found that the tuberosities were malpositioned in 21% of their 72 patients.

When malunited, the lesser tuberosity often heals medial to its original position. This medialization can cause limitations in internal rotation strength. However, malunion of the lesser tuberosity does not usually cause substantial clinical symptoms. In contrast, malunion of the greater tuberosity is associated with a substantially inferior outcome.[10,12,26] If the greater tuberosity is too superior, it will impinge against the acromion as well as limit forward elevation and abduction. If the tuberosity is too posterior, there may be substantial loss of external rotation. Treatment of tuberosity malunion should be guided by the clinical symptoms and the extent of functional impairment. A revision operation typically consists of osteotomy, mobilization, and reattachment in the anatomic position.[44] The scar tissue generated from the previous injury and surgery makes surgical exposure and identification of the tuberosity fragment difficult. In addition, the osteotomized fragment must be adequately mobilized to obtain a tension-free reconstruction, although this may not be possible in patients with severe rotator cuff muscle contractures. Finally, the presence of the humeral head prosthesis can interfere with the placement of transosseous fixation. If a modular humeral component is present, it may be possible to exchange the humeral head for a smaller one to reduce tension on the tuberosities.

For certain patients in whom the greater tuberosity is too superior, isolated subacromial decompression can be considered.[45,46] However, this procedure does not correct the underlying deformity and should be considered only when the superior displacement is limited. In addition, subacromial decompression may lead to rupture of the coracoacromial ligament. Without a competent coracoacromial arch, anterosuperior instability may ensue and cause additional clinical symptoms.

Tuberosity Resorption and Rotator Cuff Tears

Compromise of the rotator cuff may be identified at the time of the initial operation or it may be inferred at follow-up from radiographs showing resorption of the greater tuberosity and superior migration of the humeral head.[1,3,4,6-8,12,14,24,26] Typically, the patient exhibits a lack of recovery or a gradual loss of active motion. It is often difficult to determine whether the compromise of the rotator cuff is a result of progressive tissue degeneration or is secondary to the loss of tuberosity fixation. Uncommonly, a patient who had regained good active motion and function may sustain an injury that results in a rotator cuff tear. Even in the absence of trauma, an acute rotator cuff injury must be considered if a patient has a sudden loss of active motion.

The diagnosis of acute rotator cuff tears is based on clinical examination with confirmation by radiographic studies. Both MRI[47] and ultrasound[48] have been used for diagnosis. However, interpretation of these studies often requires considerable expertise and experience. Another useful radiographic study is arthrography, as it can clearly demonstrate a full-thickness rotator cuff tear. If an acute full-thickness tear is confirmed, surgical repair should be considered. However, it is important to emphasize that this should be considered only for a patient with an acute tear. Patients with a chronic tear with or without tuberosity resorption are usually not candidates for surgery. To the authors' knowledge, there is no information regarding this specific issue in the literature. Thus, management of this complication should be individualized and based on established principles.

Surgical management provides only limited benefits for patients with a gradual loss of rotator cuff function and possible tuberosity resorption. Nonsurgical treatment, including pain management, a limited-goal therapy program, and supportive care, is the preferred approach. There may be a role for the reverse design shoulder prosthesis for patients with this difficult complication.[49] However, the clinical efficacy of this revision surgery has not yet been documented.

Component-Related Complications

Malpositioning

Insertion of the humeral component in anatomically appropriate amounts of version and height is critical to the outcome. In most instances, anatomic landmarks can be used to place the humeral component in 20° to 40° of retroversion. The humeral head should interact concentrically with the glenoid surface such that the superior tip of the metallic head is roughly equivalent to the top of the glenoid. Ideally, the top of the humeral head should also be 4 to 6 mm superior to the top of the greater tuberosity. Component positioning had not been critically reviewed in the literature until recently, when Boileau and associates,[26] using postoperative CT, found that 9 of the 23 patients (39%) in their series had the humeral component placed in more than 40° of retroversion. Comparison with radiographs of the uninjured limbs as controls for humeral length revealed that 26% of the humeral stems had been placed more than 10 mm too superiorly and 36% of the stems had been placed more than 10 mm too inferiorly.[26]

Identifying the proper version and height of the humeral component may be difficult in some instances because of the limited exposure and the lack of anatomic landmarks. In addition, component version and height may also be inadvertently altered when the prosthesis is finally inserted into the cement mantle. Although techniques that do not use cement have been described, it is the authors' belief that cement is mandatory to maintain proper positioning and provide rotational stability. If substantial component malpositioning is identified, either intraoperatively or postoperatively, and is thought to result in instability, the component should be revised.

Loosening

The prevalence of radiolucent lines around the humeral prosthesis is variable, with reported rates of between 0 and 32%.[1-3,5,6,8-12,14,15,24,26] Despite the presence of radiolucent lines, symptomatic aseptic loosening requiring revision is an uncommon problem, occurring in fewer than 2% of patients.[12] Prostheses inserted without the aid of a cement mantle are associated with a higher rate of aseptic loosening.[1] Loosening of the humeral component is usually associated with progressive radiolucency at the bone-cement interface (Figure 4). The diagnosis of loosening is established by using criteria similar to those for femoral component loosening after total hip arthroplasty.[50] Definitive loosening is thought to have occurred if the prosthesis has changed position, the cement mantle has fragmented or fractured, there is a progressive radiolucent line at the cement-prosthesis interface (debonding), or the prosthesis is broken or bent. If the component is loose, the patient must be evaluated for the presence of an underlying deep infection. This evaluation may include joint aspiration as well as laboratory tests such as a white blood cell count and determination of the erythrocyte sedimentation rate and C-reactive protein level. Other sources of shoulder pain and discomfort must also be considered. If component loosening is the primary source of symptoms, revision surgery should be considered. If possible, the entire cement mantle should be removed, and the new prosthesis should be inserted with careful attention to cementing techniques. Use of a long-stem component can be considered if there are substantial endosteal bone defects. Although insertion of a cementless implant may be considered, lack of metaphyseal bone support often precludes this option.

Heterotopic Ossification

Heterotopic ossification following a humeral replacement is relatively common, occurring in 25% to 56% of cases.[11,12] Mighell and associates[12] reported that mild heterotopic ossification (grade I or II)[51] was found in 17% of their patients and more extensive heterotopic ossification (grade III or IV)[51] was found in only 7%. Other authors have also observed heterotopic ossification in their patients, but their reported rates have been variable.[1,3,4,6,7,10,15,26]

Several patient-related factors predispose to the formation of heterotopic bone. Ankylosing spondylosis, diffuse idiopathic skeletal hyperostosis, and a history of heterotopic bone formation have all been associated with an increased risk.[52] Other independent risk factors include high-energy injuries and a delay in the treatment beyond 10 to 14 days.[20,21,28] It has also been found that heterotopic ossification can develop when a revision procedure is performed following an early failure of internal fixation, especially when the second procedure is performed 2 to 4 weeks after the initial procedure.

Fortunately, most patients with heterotopic ossification in the shoulder exhibit minimal symptoms.[53] If, however, the heterotopic bone is excessive, it can adversely affect the range of motion. Surgical excision should be considered when a patient demonstrates functional limitations. Excision should be attempted only after the ossification process has matured and the radiographic margins are clearly defined. For most patients, this requires a period of at least 6 months after the initial surgery.[52] In addition to the standard radiographs, CT is usually necessary for accurate localization of the ossification. Bone within or bridging the subacromial space is typically easy to locate and excise. If the bone has formed within the rotator cuff, the excision must be combined with a repair of any full-thickness defects in the rotator cuff tendons. Excessive bone that is overlying the glenohumeral joint may be in close proximity to the axillary nerve and other branches of the brachial plexus. Therefore, bone excision in this area requires meticulous dissection.

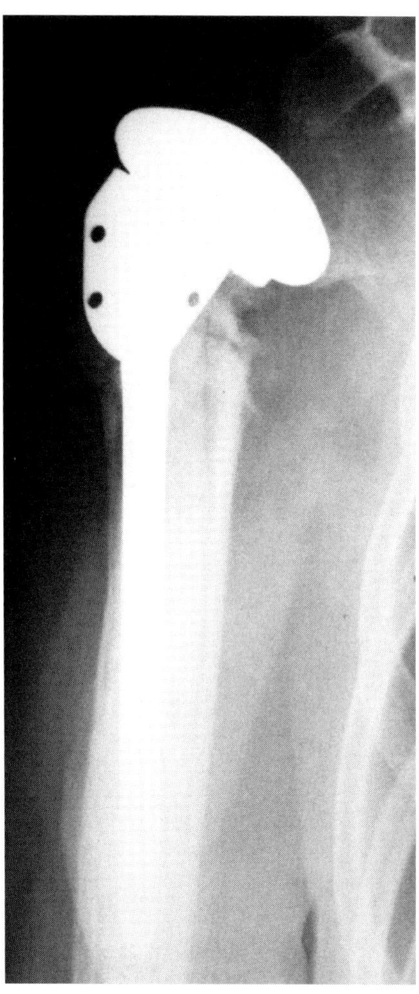

Figure 4 Aseptic loosening of the humeral stem. Note the radiolucent line completely surrounding the cement mantle.

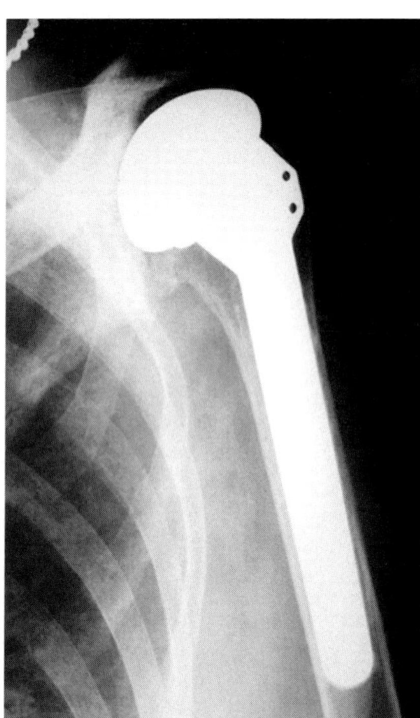

Figure 5 Medial migration of the prosthetic humeral head as the result of glenoid erosion.

The initial humeral head replacement as well as the excision of heterotopic ossification requires meticulous technique to minimize soft-tissue trauma. In addition, these procedures should be performed at the appropriate time, and the "at risk" period should be avoided. For patients considered to be at high risk for heterotopic bone formation, prophylaxis with indomethacin or radiation therapy should be considered.

Glenoid Complications

As the radiographic appearance of degenerative changes in the glenoid is subject to interpretation, the reported prevalence of such changes has been variable. In general, glenoid wear requiring revision surgery is fairly uncommon. Mighell and associates[12] reported that in their series of 72 patients, only 3 had glenoid degeneration requiring revision surgery. This low rate of glenoid wear may be caused in part by the relatively low activity level of the typical patient who sustains a proximal humeral fracture. Factors that contribute to the development of glenoid degeneration include preexisting loss of cartilage before the surgery, unrecognized injury or additional injury at the time of the surgery, and the activity level of the patient.[12] The duration of follow-up may also influence the prevalence of this complication, as glenoid degeneration is more likely to develop over time.

The treatment of loss of glenoid articular cartilage is generally determined by the severity of the symptoms. When there is evidence of glenoid degeneration (Figure 5), it must first be confirmed that the symptoms are from the glenoid and not from other sources. An intra-articular injection of lidocaine can help to confirm this diagnosis. If the symptoms are mild or moderate, anti-inflammatory medications and activity modification may be sufficient. If there is substantial pain and disability, however, revision surgery with insertion of a glenoid component should be considered. Preoperative radiographs must be scrutinized to ensure that adequate bone stock is present to support a glenoid component.

Stiffness

Stiffness is difficult to define because many of the other complications discussed above result in decreased range of motion. Patients with good passive motion but poor active motion may have musculotendinous, neurologic, or tuberosity-related complications as discussed previously. For the purpose of this chapter, stiffness is defined as loss of both active and passive motion that compromises function. The prevalence of clinically relevant stiffness is relatively low: only one case requiring surgical release has been reported in the literature.[2]

The initial treatment of stiffness is aggressive rehabilitation. If disability persists, soft-tissue release can be considered. The release can be performed after an open exploration or through an arthroscopic approach. Arthroscopic release minimizes soft-tissue dissection, but it can be technically demanding. Initial steps involve intra-articular circumferential capsular release. The subacromial space is then addressed with complete bursectomy and release of scar tissue. Gliding of the rotator cuff tendon within the subacromial space must be restored. In most instances, a release of the coracoacromial ligament as well as a limited acromioplasty are recommended. Upon completion of the procedure, a gentle manual manipulation of the shoulder is performed to gain additional motion. The degree of motion obtained in the operating room is the long-term postoperative goal. A structured and supervised rehabilitation program is essential to maintain any improvements. Typically, the patient is admitted to the hospital for 2 to 3 days to initiate this therapy program. Postoperative analgesia can be augmented with an interscalene block on the first and second postoperative days to allow aggressive rehabilitation with minimal pain.

Summary

Humeral head replacement is an acceptable, and often preferred, method of treatment of complex proximal humeral fractures. Although the procedure is associated with reliable relief of pain as well as a high rate of patient satisfaction, the functional outcomes can vary. This variability is related in part to postoperative complications, many of which are related to technical errors during the surgery. Detailed surgical planning and meticulous surgical technique minimize the risk of these complications, which in turn improves the outcome for the patient.

References

1. Hawkins RJ, Switlyk P: Acute prosthetic replacement for severe fractures of the proximal humerus. *Clin Orthop* 1993;289:156-160.

2. Compito CA, Self EB, Bigliani LU: Arthroplasty and acute shoulder trauma:

Reasons for success and failure. *Clin Orthop* 1994;307:27-36.

3. Goldman RT, Koval KJ, Cuomo F, Gallagher MA, Zuckerman JD: Functional outcome after humeral head replacement for acute three- and four-part proximal humeral fractures. *J Shoulder Elbow Surg* 1995;4:81-86.

4. Demirhan M, Kilicoglu O, Altinal L, Eralp L, Akalin Y: Prognostic factors in prosthetic replacement for acute proximal humerus fractures. *J Orthop Trauma* 2003;17:181-189.

5. Robinson CM, Page RS, Hill RM, Sanders DL, Court-Brown CM, Wakefield AE: Primary hemiarthroplasty for treatment of proximal humeral fractures. *J Bone Joint Surg Am* 2003;85:1215-1223.

6. Moeckel BH, Dines DM, Warren RF, Altchek DW: Modular hemiarthroplasty for fractures of the proximal part of the humerus. *J Bone Joint Surg Am* 1992;74:884-889.

7. Dimakopoulos P, Potamitis N, Lambiris E: Hemiarthroplasty in the treatment of comminuted intraarticular fractures of the proximal humerus. *Clin Orthop* 1997;341:7-11.

8. Skutek M, Fremerey RW, Bosch U: Level of physical activity in elderly patients after hemiarthroplasty for three- and four-part fractures of the proximal humerus. *Arch Orthop Trauma Surg* 1998;117:252-255.

9. Zyto K, Wallace WA, Frostick SP, Preston BJ: Outcome after hemiarthroplasty for three-and four-part fractures of the proximal humerus. *J Shoulder Elbow Surg* 1998;7:85-89.

10. Prakash U, McGurty DW, Dent JA: Hemiarthroplasty for severe fractures of the proximal humerus. *J Shoulder Elbow Surg* 2002;11:428-430.

11. Becker R, Pap G, Machner A, Neumann WH: Strength and motion after hemiarthroplasty in displaced four-fragment fracture of the proximal humerus: 27 patients followed for 1-6 years. *Acta Orthop Scand* 2002;73:44-49.

12. Mighell MA, Kolm GP, Collinge CA, Frankle MA: Outcomes of hemiarthroplasty for fractures of the proximal humerus. *J Shoulder Elbow Surg* 2003;12:569-577.

13. Bosch U, Skutek M, Fremerey RW, Tscherne H: Outcome after primary and secondary hemiarthroplasty in elderly patients with fractures of the proximal humerus. *J Shoulder Elbow Surg* 1998;7:479-484.

14. Movin T, Sjoden GO, Ahrengart L: Poor function after shoulder replacement in fracture patients: A retrospective evaluation of 29 patients followed for 2-12 years. *Acta Orthop Scand* 1998;69:392-396.

15. Neer CS II: Displaced proximal humeral fractures: II. Treatment of three-part and four-part displacement. *J Bone Joint Surg Am* 1970;52:1090-1103.

16. Kraulis J, Hunter G: The results of prosthetic replacement in fracture-dislocations of the upper end of the humerus. *Injury* 1976;8:129-131.

17. Des Marchais JE, Benazet JP: Evaluation of Neer's hemi-arthroplasty in the treatment of humeral fractures. *Can J Surg* 1983;26:469-471.

18. Tanner MW, Cofield RH: Prosthetic arthroplasty for fractures and fracture-dislocations of the proximal humerus. *Clin Orthop* 1983;179:116-128.

19. Stableforth PGL: Four-part fractures of the neck of the humerus. *J Bone Joint Surg Br* 1984;66:104-108.

20. Neer CS II, McIlveen SJ: Recent results and technique of prosthetic replacement for 4-part proximal humeral fractures. *Orthop Trans* 1986;10:475.

21. Neer CS II, McIlveen SJ: Humeral head replacement with reconstruction of the tuberosities and the cuff in 4-fragment displaced fractures: Current results and techniques. *Rev Chir Orthop Reparatrice Appar Mot* 1988;74(suppl 2):31-40.

22. Neumann K, Muhr G, Breitfuss H: Primary humerus head replacement in dislocated proximal humeral fracture: Indications, technique, results. *Orthopade* 1992;21:140-147.

23. Pietu G, Deluzarches P, Gouin F, Letenneur J: Complex injuries of the proximal humerus treated with humeral head prosthesis: Apropos of 21 cases reviewed after a median 4-year follow-up. *Acta Orthop Belg* 1992;58:159-169.

24. Muldoon MP, Cofield RH: Complications of humeral head replacement for proximal humeral fractures. *Instr Course Lect* 1997;46: 15-24.

25. Wretenberg P, Ekelund A: Acute hemiarthroplasty after proximal humerus fracture in old patients: A retrospective evaluation of 18 patients followed for 2-7 years. *Acta Orthop Scand* 1997;68:121-123.

26. Boileau P, Krishnan SG, Tinsi L, Walch G, Coste JS, Mole D: Tuberosity malposition and migration: Reasons for poor outcome after hemiarthroplasty for displaced fractures of the proximal humerus. *J Shoulder Elbow Surg* 2002;11:401-412.

27. Christoforakis JJ, Kontakis GM, Katonis PG, et al: Relevance of the restoration of humeral length and retroversion in hemiarthroplasty for humeral head fractures. *Acta Orthop Belg* 2003;69:226-232.

28. Brown TD, Bigliani LU: Complications with humeral head replacement. *Orthop Clin North Am* 2000;31:77-90.

29. Brems JJ: Complications of shoulder arthroplasty: Infections, instability, and loosening. *Instr Course Lect* 2002;51:29-39.

30. Tsukayama DT, Goldberg VM, Kyle R: Diagnosis and management of infection after total knee arthroplasty. *J Bone Joint Surg Am* 2003;85(suppl 1):S75-S80.

31. Zimmerli W, Ochsner PE: Management of infection associated with prosthetic joints. *Infection* 2003;31:99-108.

32. Robbins GM, Masri BA, Garbuz DS, Duncan CP: Primary total hip arthroplasty after infection. *J Bone Joint Surg Am* 2001;83:602-614.

33. Seitz WH Jr, Damacen H: Staged exchange arthroplasty for shoulder sepsis. *J Arthroplasty* 2002;17(suppl 1):36-40.

34. Langlais F: Can we improve the results of revision arthroplasty for infected total hip replacement? *J Bone Joint Surg Br* 2003;85:637-640.

35. Mitchell PA, Masri BA, Garbuz DS, Greidanus NV, Duncan CP: Cementless revision for infection following total hip arthroplasty. *Instr Course Lect* 2003;52:323-330.

36. Jerosch J, Schneppenheim M: Management of infected shoulder replacement. *Arch Orthop Trauma Surg* 2003;123:209-214.

37. Salvati EA, Gonzalez Della Valle A, Masri BA, Duncan CP: The infected total hip arthroplasty. *Instr Course Lect* 2003;52:223-245.

38. de Laat EA, Visser CP, Coene LN, Pahlplatz PV, Tavy DL: Nerve lesions in primary shoulder dislocations and humeral neck fractures: A prospective clinical and EMG study. *J Bone Joint Surg Br* 1994;76:381-383.

39. Visser CP, Coene LN, Brand R, Tavy DL: Nerve lesions in proximal humeral fractures. *J Shoulder Elbow Surg* 2001;10:421-427.

40. Williams GR, Iannotti JP: Management of periprosthetic fractures: The shoulder. *J Arthroplasty* 2002;17(suppl 1):14-16.

41. Lynch NM, Cofield RH, Silbert PL, Hermann RC: Neurologic complications after total shoulder arthroplasty. *J Shoulder Elbow Surg* 1996;5:53-61.

42. Iannotti JP, Antoniou J, Williams GR, Ramsey ML: Iliotibial band reconstruction for treatment of glenohumeral instability associated with irreparable capsular deficiency. *J Shoulder Elbow Surg* 2002;11:618-623.

43. Zuckerman JD, Cuomo F, Koval KJ: Proximal humeral replacement for complex fractures: Indications and surgical technique. *Instr Course Lect* 1997;46:7-14.

44. Boileau P, Trojani C, Walch G, Krishnan SG, Romeo A, Sinnerton R: Shoulder arthroplasty for the treatment of the sequelae of fractures of the proximal humerus. *J Shoulder Elbow Surg* 2001;10:299-308.

45. Bigliani LU, D'Alessandro DF, Duralde XA, McIlveen SJ: Anterior acromioplasty for subacromial impingement in patients younger than 40 years of age. *Clin Orthop* 1989;246:111-116.

46. Porcellini G, Campi F, Paladini P: Articular impingement in malunited fracture of the humeral head. *Arthroscopy* 2002;18:E39.

47. Sperling JW, Potter HG, Craig EV, Flatow E, Warren RF: Magnetic resonance imaging of painful shoulder arthroplasty. *J Shoulder Elbow Surg* 2002;11:315-321.

48. Sofka CM, Adler RS: Original report: Sonographic evaluation of shoulder arthroplasty. *AJR Am J Roentgenol* 2003;180:1117-1120.

49. Boulahia A, Edwards TB, Walch G, Baratta RV: Early results of a reverse design prosthesis in the treatment of arthritis of the shoulder in elderly patients with a large rotator cuff tear. *Orthopedics* 2002;25:129-133.

50. Barrack RL, Mulroy RD Jr, Harris WH: Improved cementing techniques and femoral component loosening in young patients with hip arthroplasty: A 12-year radiographic review. *J Bone Joint Surg Br* 1992;74:385-389.

51. Brooker AF, Bowerman JW, Robinson RA, Riley LH Jr: Ectopic ossification following total hip replacement: Incidence and a method of classification. *J Bone Joint Surg Am* 1973;55:1629-1632.

52. Iorio R, Healy WL: Heterotopic ossification after hip and knee arthroplasty: Risk factors, prevention, and treatment. *J Am Acad Orthop Surg* 2002;10:409-416.

53. Sperling JW, Cofield RH, Rowland CM: Heterotopic ossification after total shoulder arthroplasty. *J Arthroplasty* 2000;15:179-182.

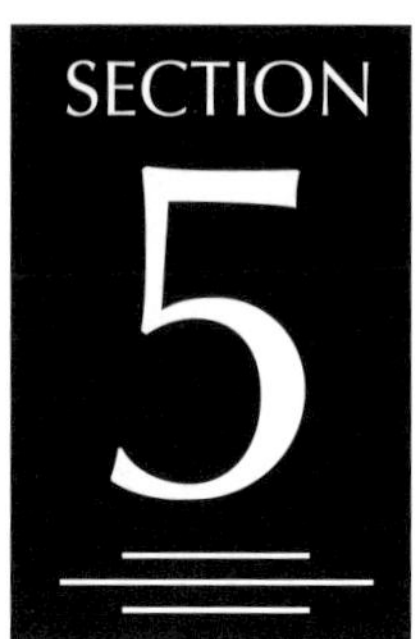

Miscellaneous Conditions About the Shoulder

Miscellaneous Conditions About the Shoulder

The five articles in this section provide an overview of some common and uncommon conditions of the shoulder. The articles provide excellent information that both the general orthopaedic surgeon and the shoulder specialist will find interesting and clinically useful. The principles stressed in each review should be applied into practice.

In their article on the management of the diabetic stiff shoulder, Scarlat and Harryman provide an insightful review of the current understanding of diabetes mellitus and how it affects the shoulder and the treatment options currently available. The authors describe the two major types of stiffness: frozen shoulder (adhesive capsulitis) and posttraumatic stiffness. The region of the rotator interval is a key site of the fibrogenesis.

The authors also briefly review the differences between type 1 and type 2 diabetes and stress the importance of working with a primary care physician or a diabetes specialist to ensure that the patient's blood glucose is well controlled. When nonsurgical management fails, manipulation or surgical release of the capsule is recommended. In contrast to other reports, these authors advise manipulation as an option for those individuals whose symptoms have been present for 6 months or less; however, they clearly do not recommend manipulation for patients with long-standing, refractory, posttraumatic, or postoperative stiffness. Most experts agree that patients with long-standing stiffness or those with severely restricted motion are best treated surgically, with either open or preferably arthroscopic capsular release. Both open and arthroscopic releases are described.

In the second article in this section, Bennett and Allan present a detailed overview of the many surgical options available for treating the sequelae of obstetrical brachial plexus palsy. Obstetrical birth palsy occurs in up to 1 in 250 births as a result of traction and usually resolves without operative intervention. Surgery is typically reserved for the most severe cases.

Joint preservation is stressed, and joint mobilization is important once the diagnosis is made. MRI or CT can be helpful to assess joint congruity in patients with restricted motion.

The authors clearly outline the prerequisites for successful tendon transfer, particularly emphasizing the importance of a supple joint that is concentric and reduced. The choice of transfer must not interfere with existing function, and the donor muscle must have at least grade 4 of 5 strength, as one full grade loss in strength is to be expected postoperatively. The authors also include an excellent review of the biomechanical considerations of tendon transfers and how to optimize the biomechanics when performing tendon transfers in the shoulder.

The indications for and techniques of latissimus dorsi transfer, and combined latissimus dorsi / teres major transfers are described. This article is especially relevant because many of these techniques, which were initially developed for use in children, are now being used in adult reconstructive surgery to salvage irreparable rotator cuff tears, and this article provides an excellent foundation for understanding the principles of functional muscle transfers.

In the second part of this article, the authors describe tendon transfers about the elbow. The merits and limitations of the proximal transfer of the flexor pronator group (Steindler), the anterior transfer of the triceps (Carroll Hill), the bipolar pectoralis major transfer, and the bipolar latissimus transfer are described. Microvascular techniques, such as the free gracilis, and techniques to restore triceps function also are discussed. Obstetrical brachial plexus palsy is a common problem with significant historic relevance. Many of the basic principles of tendon transfer were pioneered in the treatment of this condition. Obstetrical brachial plexus palsy obviously remains a complex and challenging clinical problem largely because of the myriad presentations and limited studies that compare different surgical techniques. The authors highlight the importance of outcomes studies to further define the best options for the specific nerve and muscle deficits.

In the third article in this section, Medvecky and Zuckerman review disorders of the sternoclavicular (SC) joint. Although infrequently injured, this joint can be quite difficult to treat because of its unique anatomy and its proximity to the mediastinum and great vessels. The authors provide an excellent review of the anatomy and biomechanics of this joint. Epidemiology, mechanisms of injury, and typical clinical presentation of patients with SC disorders are also described. Imaging typically includes chest radiographs, which allow side-to-side comparison, and special SC views such as the Hobbs view. Three-dimensional imaging studies (MRI and CT) are also helpful in assessing the direction and degree of injury.

SC joint disorders can be divided into traumatic, atraumatic, degenerative, inflammatory, and other miscellaneous types. Traumatic injuries include sprains, anterior dislocations, posterior dislocations, medial clavicular physeal injuries, chronic dislocations, and intra-articular disk injuries. A key point highlighted in the article is that the medial clavicular physis remains open until age 23 to 25. Because of the poor ligamentous supports, closed treatment of anterior dislocations often is ineffective. Posterior dislocations are often associated with significant compression of the trachea, esophagus, or great vessels, and a thoracic surgery consultation should be obtained before any attempts at reduction. The authors advise against closed reduction for dislocations older than 7 days because of potential retro-sternal adhesions. Atraumatic SC injuries include spontaneous anterior subluxation or posterior dislocation. Nonsurgical management is recommended for this category of injury unless thoracic compromise is suspected.

The SC joint can have degenerative osteoarthritis, which is usually treated nonsurgically. Excision of the medial clavicle can be performed in refractory cases. Inflammatory conditions include monoarticular noninfectious subacute arthritis, septic arthritis, and rheumatoid arthritis Treatment for this category is both medical and surgical.

The final disorder described is SC hyperostosis, which is characterized by hyperossification of the sternum, clavicle, ribs, and soft tissues. Patients often present with swelling, redness, and pain. This disorder is much more common in women. The etiology is unknown, although treatment with antibiotics has resulted in faster improvement in some series, which suggests an infectious cause.

The final two articles describe how to recognize and manage complications of shoulder surgery. Guttmann and associates provide a timely review of the complications of treatment of complete acromioclavicular joint (AC) dislocations. Because of the high failure rates with the Weaver Dunn techniques, new anatomic techniques to repair the injured coracoclavicular and AC ligaments have been suggested. The authors describe problems associated with nonsurgical treatment, specifically skin problems, osteolysis, and posttraumatic arthritis.

Neurologic symptoms also may develop in some patients as a result of a medialized scapula and thoracic outlet compromise. In these situations, many patients opt for surgical repair or reconstruction. The article also describes the complications of the Weaver Dunn procedure, which relies on the coracoacromial ligament to reconstruct the coracoclavicular ligaments. Care must be taken when harvesting and preparing the coracoacromial ligament to avoid technical problems such as inadequate length and inappropriate tensioning. Regardless of the technique, the most common postoperative complication is loss of reduction, a problem that can be very difficult to treat. In certain instances, nonsurgical management may be the best option.

Another complication of AC joint surgery is failure of the hardware, particularly when coracoclavicular screws are used. Infection, implant migration, and other less common complications also have been reported. The authors do not discuss horizontal AC joint instability, but this condition, in which the clavicle moves posteriorly to abut on the spine of the scapula, can cause localized pain in this region. Preservation of the AC ligaments is thought to prevent this problem; however, when it occurs, ligament reconstruction may be the best treatment option.

The final article by Gill and associates is an exhaustive case-based review of the myriad complications of shoulder surgery. In the last decade, we have learned a lot about the causes of these complications, and fortunately many can now be completely avoided by careful patient selection and appropriate surgical technique. The article starts with a discussion of the complications of instability surgery. The most common are recurrent instability, stiffness, arthrosis, and hardware-related problems. The authors discuss neurovascular problems and rupture of the subscapularis. Fortunately, some of these problems have been obviated and others minimized by new techniques, particularly arthroscopic surgery.

The article then describes complications of rotator cuff surgery such as failure of healing or recurrent tear, infection, and stiffness. Again, as arthroscopic techniques improve, some of these complications have become less common. For example, stiffness and infection rates seem to be much lower with arthroscopic techniques, and deltoid detachment is virtually eliminated with arthroscopic rotator cuff repair. The problem of recurrent tears or failure of tendon healing remains a significant problem that requires further study.

Shoulder arthroplasty and its inherent complications are then described, including the problems associated with glenoid loosening. Clearly, we have made strides in this area, and with better cement techniques, better prosthetic designs, and better instrumentation, such as concentric reamers, glenoid components will have better longevity and durability. Instability after shoulder arthroplasty most commonly occurs anteriorly and has multiple causes. Improvements have been made with better and stronger techniques for subscapularis repair, such as the new lesser tuberosity osteotomy techniques that reduce the risk of rupture, and with better implant designs that allow more anatomic placement of the components, place less stress on the subscapularis repair, and run less risk of overstuffing the joint.

Similarly, other complications of shoulder arthroplasty, such as rotator cuff tears, which frequently occur from poor humeral placement or inappropriate implant design, can be prevented entirely with improved restoration of the anatomy. When rotator cuff tears do occur in the setting of a total shoulder arthroplasty, they can now be treated more effectively with either primary repair or new alternative implants such as the reverse shoulder arthroplasty. The authors also describe complications of fracture surgery such as neurovascular injury, osteonecrosis, and tuberosity failure. Again, new surgical techniques, implants, and strategies are being developed to address each of these problems. The complications of arthrodesis and frozen shoulder are also discussed.

The authors conclude with a section on the complications of shoulder arthroscopy, particularly complications unique to this minimally invasive surgery. Fluid is a necessary component for arthroscopy, and its management is critical to avoid the problems associated with excessive extravasation of fluid, such as soft-tissue swelling and compartment syndrome. Minimizing fluid pressure and using cautery for hemostasis allow the arthroscopist to see clearly and work expeditiously and safely. Nerve injuries are historically among the most common complications of arthroscopic surgery and can be related to positioning, the type of anesthesia, or technique.

Complications, unfortunately, are inevitable in shoulder surgery. However, with careful attention to detail and better understanding of their causes, many can be avoided altogether. When complications do occur, the best course of action is early reognition, a frank, honest discussions with the patient, and appropriate treatment.

Peter J. Millett, MD, MSc
Shoulder Service
Steadman Hawkins Clinic
Vail, Colorado

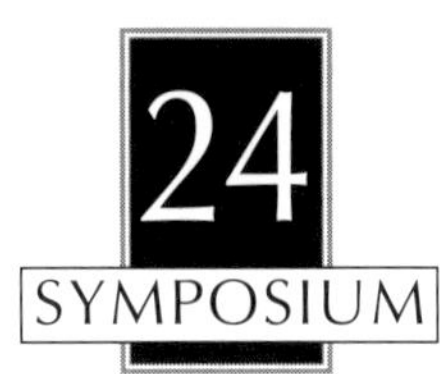

Management of the Diabetic Stiff Shoulder

Marius M. Scarlat, MD
Douglas T. Harryman II, MD

Introduction

Although there are numerous musculoskeletal side effects associated with diabetes mellitus, stiffness of major joints is one of the most common and yet possibly one of the most easily avoided.[1–21] All patients with any degree of diabetes mellitus should perform regular daily stretching exercises to maintain flexibility of their joints. In no case should anyone attempt to limit joint motion because of minor discomfort or for injuries that are not associated with displacement of bone fragments. No matter what pathomechanism initiated painful stiffness, it is critical that the painful joint be moved early on through a full range of motion.[2,8–10,18]

The primary purpose of this chapter is to discuss the current understanding of how diabetes mellitus affects the shoulder and the treatment available for those affected by this condition. Shoulder stiffness, with or without diabetes mellitus, remains a disabling condition.[8–10,22–26] It causes significant unrelenting pain that acutely or chronically inhibits full functional use of the affected extremity and limits all daily activities. Patients complain of difficulty sleeping at night and of restricted extremity use for reaching, pushing, pulling, lifting, carrying, driving, and maintaining routine daily activities (often including daily hygiene). Because this painful condition typically is long lasting and also responds poorly to ordinary over-the-counter medications, afflicted patients usually seek potent analgesia from clinicians to diminish irritability, but physicians must resist routinely administering narcotics.

Classification of the Diabetic Stiff Shoulder

Shoulder stiffness presents in 2 major categories. We define these 2 categories, in line with others,[2,8–10,18,26,27] as (1) the frozen shoulder and (2) the posttraumatic stiff shoulder. The condition referred to as frozen shoulder is often also called adhesive capsulitis. These 2 names, and others, denote a condition of painful global restriction of both active and passive motion caused by capsular fibrosis and contracture of the surrounding musculotendinous units. On the other hand, the posttraumatic stiff shoulder, defined as a condition of shoulder stiffness due to a specific injury from trauma or surgical intervention, typically presents with limited active and passive motion as a result of capsular and/or humeroscapular motion interface fibrosis. There may be overlap between these 2 types of stiffness, because neither condition is exclusive of the other. Rarely do both of these conditions exist in the same patient, whether or not the patient also has diabetes mellitus.

Diabetic Frozen Shoulder Pathophysiology

Limited Joint Motion Syndrome

Epidemiology As we mentioned earlier, patients with diabetes mellitus are at much greater risk for developing limited motion in all joints.[1–3,6,13,15,18,21] Limited joint motion syndrome has been described as a condition that presents with joint stiffness in the hands and other major articulations. Generally, this condition is more frequent in those who have been insulin-dependent for many years.[1,2,5,14–16,18] Its cause has been attributed to high-circulating blood-glucose levels, which are thought to accelerate aging of certain body proteins. This aging process triggers a series of chemical reactions in proteins that then accumulate irreversible cross-links between adjacent molecules, such as long collagen chains.[2,6,13,28–31] This pathway, which is considered nonenzymatic glycosylation, appears irreversible, and with time leads to arthrofibrosis.

The term cheirarthropathy is used to describe waxy thickening and induration of the skin associated with contractures of the fingers. Sherry and associates[21] found that joint stiffening was more common in patients who demonstrated skin changes. Fisher and associates[6] noted a higher incidence of not only idiopathic frozen shoulder but also bilateral shoulder involvement in 13 of 29 patients with cheirarthropathy. In this study, 10 patients had bilateral frozen shoulder. The authors also observed an increased frequency of microvascular complications, including neuropathy and advanced retinopathy, in diabetic patients with cheirarthropathy compared with controls.

Shoulder stiffness has also been

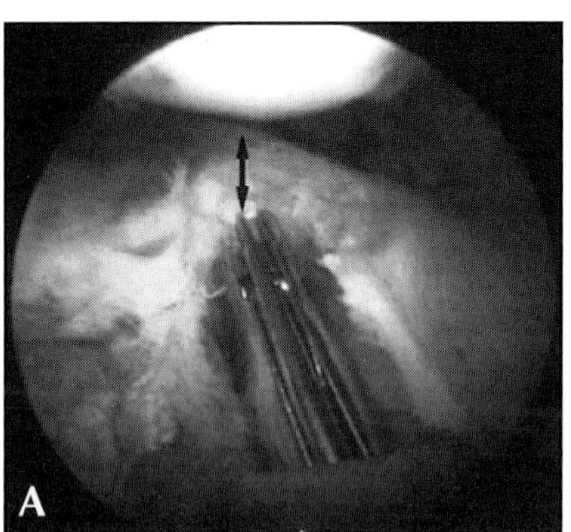

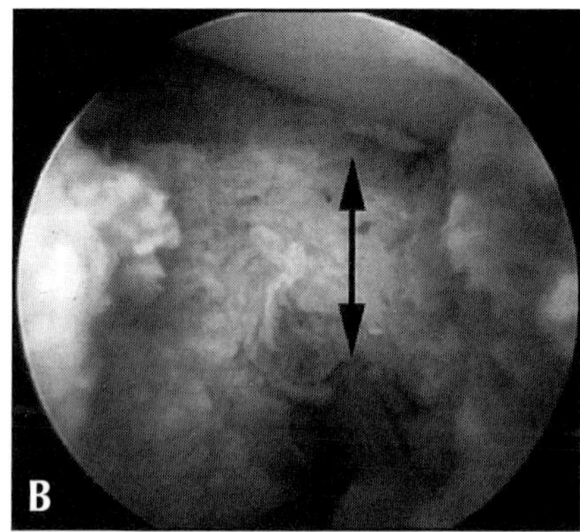

Fig. 1 A, Note the relative thickness of the inferior capsular sling in an idiopathic frozen shoulder (3 mm) compared to the thickness of the capsule in B. **B,** Note the thick (10 mm) inferior capsular sling, which is much thicker in this diabetic frozen shoulder with long-standing severe capsular fibrosis.

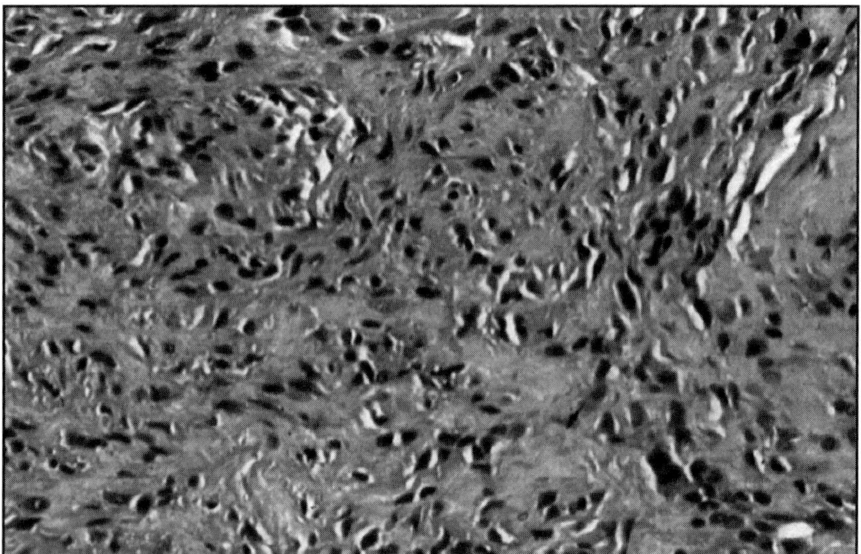

Fig. 2 Histopathology showing dense irregular collagen and fibrocytes in the articular capsule of a diabetic frozen shoulder. This pathologic photomicrograph is identical to the pathology found in Dupuytren's palmar fascia contractures of the hand.

reported to antedate the symptoms of diabetes and other comorbidities.[2,3,13–15,18,32] It is generally accepted that long-term use of supplemental insulin and fluctuating levels of glucose increase the risk of developing shoulder stiffness.[13] Furthermore, patients who have had a long duration of supplemental insulin dependency also have greater potential for resistance to all treatment modalities[2,13,14,18,20] Up to 36% of patients with insulin-dependent diabetes are likely to develop shoulder stiffness, compared to 3% of the general population.[33]

Pathophysiology Investigators have proposed that the glenohumeral joint capsule may develop a contracture in response to cytokine, lymphocyte, or monocyte products. The site of predilection seems to be the rotator interval capsule.[14,33–35] Certain chemotactic factors, such as platelet-derived growth factor, are potent mitogenic polypeptides that stimulate mesenchymal cells. Although there is a component of inflammation in the adjacent glenohumeral synovium even in patients who have insulin-dependent diabetes, the fibrogenic response within the underlying glenohumeral capsule is excessive in the insulin-dependent diabetic shoulder when compared with the similar condition in the nondiabetic idiopathic frozen shoulder (Fig. 1). The capsule responds by forming thick, dense collagen fibers that histopathologically look similar, if not identical, to Dupuytren's contracture of palmar fascia in the hand (Fig. 2). When this fibrous tissue response to cytokines and the nonenzymatic glycosylization of capsular glycosaminoglycans such as hyaluronic acid are coupled, the end result is transformation of compliant glenohumeral joint capsule into a thick inflexible tissue.

Description of Type 1 and Type 2 Diabetes Mellitus

Orthopaedic surgeons who plan to treat patients with diabetes must also know the basic differences between type 1 and type 2 diabetes mellitus. Diabetes mellitus is defined as a group of metabolic diseases characterized by hyperglycemia. Diabetes may result from a defect in insulin secretion and/or tissue response to the action of insulin. The vast majority of diabetes fall into 2 broad etiopathogenic categories.

Type 1 diabetes presents in individuals who demonstrate a deficiency of insulin secretion that may result from an autoimmune process affecting the pancreatic islets of Langerhans. The more common diabetic condition is type 2, which is often characterized by a combination of tissue resistance to insulin action and an inadequate compensatory insulin secretory response.[36]

According to the National Health Interview Survey, the number of people with diagnosed diabetes increased 5-fold between 1958 and 1993. A similar report in 1989 indicated that 43% of people with

Table 1
Comparison between asymptomatic shoulder ranges of motion in diabetics versus nondiabetics*

Asymptomatic Side Motion Measurement	Age (years)	FE degrees	ERS degrees	ERA degrees	IRA degrees	IRB spinal segment	XBA cm span
Nondiabetic (n = 129)	47 ± 11	169 ± 7	68 ± 14	93 ± 9	78 ± 15	15 ± 2	14 ± 5
Diabetic (n = 45)	47 ± 9	163 ± 12	57 ± 18	86 ± 11	71 ± 13	13 ± 3	16 ± 5
Difference	none	6	11	7	7	2	2

* FE = forward elevation; ERS = external rotation at the side; ERA = external rotation in coronal plane abduction; IRA = internal rotation in coronal plane abduction; IRB = internal rotation up the back; XBA = cross-body adduction

diagnosed diabetes were treated with insulin. Of these, 7% could be differentiated as type 1, and the remaining majority as type 2. In addition to these diagnosed cases, as many as 7 million undiagnosed cases of type 2 diabetes were present in the United States in 1989. In addition, 11% of adults when tested by an oral glucose challenge have impaired glucose intolerance as reported in the 1976–1980 Second National Health and Nutrition Examination Survey.

In summary, the prevalence of both type 1 and type 2 diabetes mellitus is frequent in the United States and appears to be increasing across all racial and ethnic categories. The prevalence significantly increases with age, from 1.3% between the ages of 18 and 44 years to as high as 10.4% over the age of 65 years.[37]

Presentation: Sufficient Diagnostic Criteria

As in all conditions, it is essential to complete a thorough history and physical examination prior to supportive laboratory and radiographic tests or advocating therapeutic intervention. The physician must consider a complete differential diagnosis to exclude the possibility of extrinsic pathology or other conditions that may present with symptoms similar to the diabetic frozen shoulder. For example, a patient with long-standing, insulin-dependent diabetes may have limited motion associated with degenerative conditions such as rotator cuff tears, arthritis, or even cervical disk disease. Clinical clues should be available to differentiate between these etiologies.

History The history of a diabetic frozen shoulder is typically idiopathic, with an insidious onset or minimal evidence of trauma that leads to painful shoulder motion.

Examination The examination demonstrates global restrictions in all planes and rotations, with the most significant restriction in glenohumeral rotation as compared with the opposite side or normal shoulder motion. It should be noted that in adult diabetic patients who are age matched to controls, all shoulder motions are significantly reduced by an average of 6° to 11° (Table 1). This points out the importance of measuring a patient's opposite side and noting whether symptoms are present unilaterally or bilaterally. These patient data include over 170 refractory stiff shoulders followed prospectively for surgical treatment since May 1991.

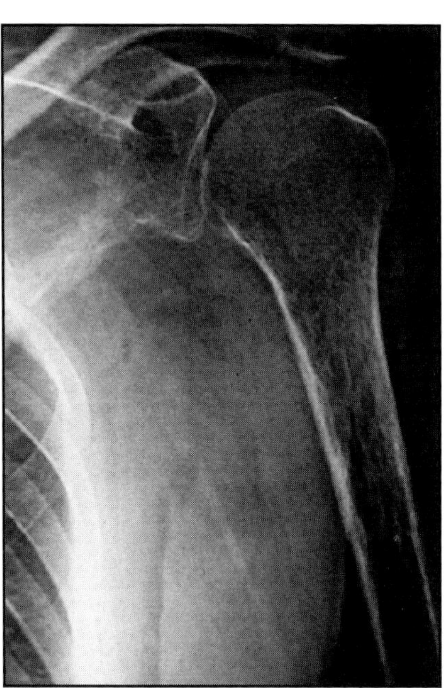

Fig. 3 An example of severe osteopenia in a patient who developed a diabetic frozen shoulder. A period of immobilization was prescribed presumably to reduce pain.

Radiography Routine radiographic and/or diagnostic laboratory tests should be obtained prior to instituting interventional therapeutic measures. Two routine orthogonal views showing the glenohumeral joint, one perpendicular to the plane of the scapula and also an axillary lateral, are typically absent of pathology with the exception of occasional disuse osteopenia (Fig. 3). Bone scintigraphy may be positive due to localized hypervascularity, but this type of scan is not useful for gauging the severity of disease or the response to therapy.[8] Its major usefulness is to rule out the presence of a tumor. Arthrography has been recommended in the past by some clinical investigators to simply make the diagnosis of a limited joint capacity secondary to the condition of adhesive capsulitis, but it is not necessary.

Laboratory Occasionally, the orthopaedic surgeon might identify a patient with undiagnosed type 2 diabetes melli-

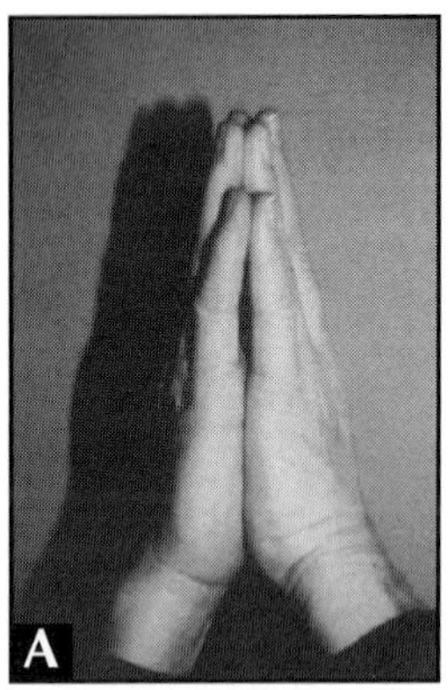

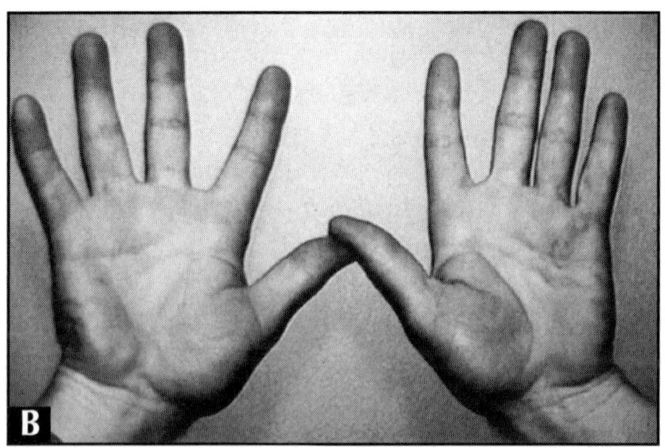

Fig. 4 A, Example of mild clinodactyly in the fourth and fifth fingers which when coupled with a Dupuytren's contracture leads to a positive prayer sign. **B,** Evidence of Dupuytren's contracture with cheirarthropathy, a waxy thickening of the fingers. The Dupuytren's palmar fascia contracture is nonprogressive and typically found in association with the fourth finger of the hand.

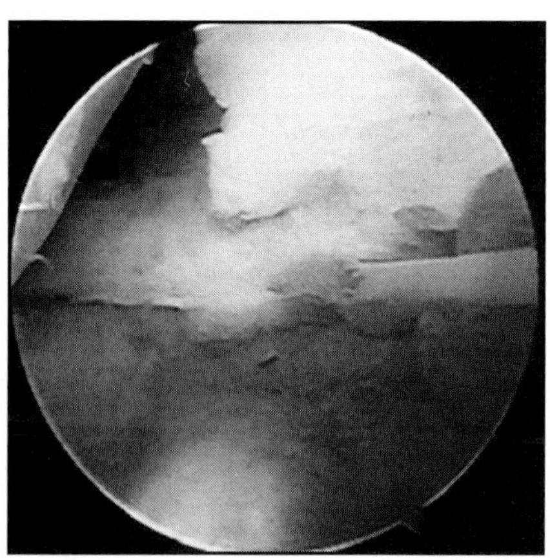

Fig. 5 Arthroscopic view of the posterosuperior capsule with evidence of inflamed synovium covering the posterior capsule and a rare adhesion in the posterior recess. The synovium produces cytokines, which cause a proliferative fibroblastic response.

tus. If a patient has clinical manifestations of clinodactylia with a positive prayer sign (Fig. 4) or has evidence of cheirarthropathy or Dupuytren's palmar fascial contracture, the clinician may want to request an oral glucose tolerance test. Lequesne and associates[38] found 17 of 60 new patients with glucose intolerance and idiopathic frozen shoulder. Generally it is best to ask a family practitioner or diabetologist to evaluate and manage blood glucose levels for those with suspected diabetic frozen shoulder. It is important that the diabetes be well controlled while proceeding with management of shoulder stiffness.

Treatment

Nonsurgical Treatment

Prevention It is incumbent on the clinician to inform or remind patients with diabetes or other immunologic collagen-vascular disorders prone to joint stiffness, that prevention, simply by stretching, is the key. Any shoulder condition presenting in a diabetic patient should reflexively cause the treating provider to encourage mobilization instead of extremity immobilization. Immobilization simply augments stiffness. Of course, mobilization should only be administered after a thorough history, physical examination, and acceptable radiographs. For example, we would only encourage early mobilization after an acute proximal humeral fracture when healing is evident. The mainstay of effective nonoperative treatment begins with gentle active-assisted and passive stretching range of motion exercises.

Harryman and associates[34] have demonstrated that a simple home-stretching program is an effective treatment for shoulder stiffness. This home program includes 4 stretches; forward elevation, external rotation at the side, internal rotation up the back, and cross-body adduction. We call this the Jackin's Stretching Exercise Program. Given the propensity for shoulder stiffness in one fifth to one third of patients with diabetes, these and other maintenance stretching exercises should be performed daily.

In addition to the stretching exercise program, some benefit may be achieved by using analgesics, such as nonsteroidal anti-inflammatory medications, or intra-articular steroid injections. Shoulder pain preventing the performance of the stretching exercise program is best relieved by an intra-articular steroid injection. Steroids effectively reduce pain and inflammation on a temporary basis.[2,8,10,13,14,18,26,27,34] The interior of the glenohumeral joint in these patients is lined by inflamed synovium (Fig. 5). Synovitis may be typical in any frozen shoulder but our data do not demonstrate a statistically significant reduction in the severity of synovitis with longer duration of symptoms.

In addition to understanding the basic condition of diabetes mellitus, a treating physician must consider the wide range of cardiac, renal, neural, ophthalmologic, peripheral-vascular, and musculoskeletal comorbidities. It is important to work together with your patient's primary care physician when administering medications that modulate the serum glucose and/or interfere with nonsurgical and/or surgical intervention. Treatment may challenge any or all systems essential for your patient's survival.

Surgical Treatment

Manipulative Intervention Under Anesthesia Shoulder stiffness, like diabetes, comes in varying degrees of severity. We have found that manipulation is most successful for patients whose stiff shoulder symptoms have been present for less than 6 months.[8,9,34] Manipulation is less beneficial for patients who present with posttraumatic or postsurgical stiffness. Janda and Hawkins[10] have recommended against manipulation under anesthesia for patients with insulin-dependent diabetes because of frequent recurrent contracture and persistent stiffness. In contrast, we have found that patients with a milder degree of stiffness and those with a shorter duration of symptoms readily respond to a gentle manipulation under anesthesia and an intra-articular injection of steroid.

Patients who present with long-term insulin-dependent refractory diabetic frozen shoulder or diabetic postsurgical stiffness do not respond well to either nonsurgical stretching or manipulation under anesthesia. In our prospective study, 37 symptomatic diabetic stiff shoulder patients failed to respond to nonsurgical treatment and underwent a total of 44 primary procedures (7 bilateral). Manipulation under anesthesia was initially attempted in all cases. A successful increase in motion was achieved in 25%. All shoulders, including those with an improved range of motion under anesthesia, were also treated with surgical arthroscopic capsular release. The method of manipulation under anesthesia in the diabetic frozen shoulder is not different from that previously reported.[8,9] The manipulation must not be forceful, because if too much torque is applied, complications, such as humeral or greater tuberosity fracture or a rotator cuff tear, may occur. The clinician should recognize that even with a successful manipulation, some residual contracture of the musculotendinous units must often be accepted, which will only respond to frequent and persistent stretching that requires effort on the part of the patient. We always perform our manipulation after administration of an interscalene long-acting anesthetic block plus sedation. Whenever full range is achieved using manipulation alone, arthroscopic capsular release is unnecessary.

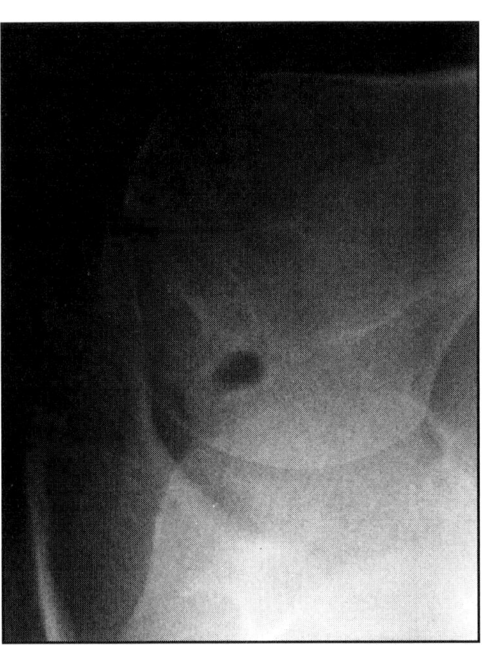

Fig. 6 Anteroposterior radiograph showing a circular defect in the humeral head secondary to improper forceful introduction of the arthroscopic trocar which entered the humeral head instead of the joint.

We also instill inside the joint 40 mg of methylprednisolone mixed with marcaine and epinephrine. After manipulation, continuous passive motion is started immediately.

Surgical Arthroscopic or Combined Open Release When a painful stiff shoulder has been refractory to nonsurgical stretching measures, we recommend early surgical intervention to include gentle manipulation and immediate arthroscopic or combined arthroscopic and open release. Surgical options and risks are discussed with the patient prior to treatment. Because manipulation is often unsuccessful or only partially successful, we encourage these stiff shoulder patients to undergo surgical release. We recommend an interscalene block as the primary anesthetic or as an adjunct to sedation or general anesthesia. The block provides the advantage of comfortable postoperative motion on a continuous passive motion device.

Arthroscopic Capsular Release Technique[39] We begin by performing a bilateral range of motion examination under anesthesia. We then attempt a gentle manipulation. Next, the patient is placed in a beach chair position and a posterior superior portal is created after marking the surgical anatomy. The glenohumeral joint is entered by inserting a tapered-tip trocar through the soft spot at the posterior-superior aspect of the joint. Heavy-handed force must be avoided, because a hard push in the wrong location could cause the trocar to enter the humeral head, especially when the bone may be less resistant than the articular capsule (Fig. 6). Occasionally, we use a sharp trocar to pierce the thickened posterior capsule and immediately switch back to the blunt tapered tip before advancing into the joint.

When manipulation is partially successful, irrigation with epinephrine solution helps to wash blood from the joint. Once visualization is possible, the biceps tendon is identified. The scope is advanced toward the rotator interval. In very stiff shoulders there is no room below the biceps tendon, but the scope can be advanced above the biceps tendon toward the rotator interval capsule. A Wissinger rod can be used to create an anterosuperior portal from inside out. Alternatively, this portal is created out-

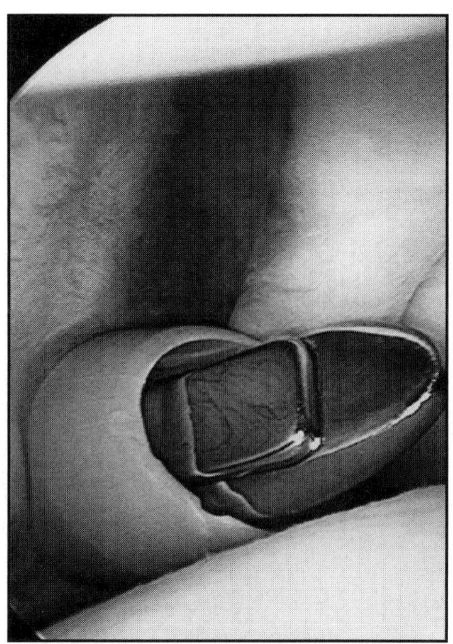

Fig. 7 Arthroscopic capsular release forceps (Smith-Nephew-Acufex-Dyonics) are used to resect a wide bite of articular capsule leaving the rotator cuff musculature entirely intact. The design of these forceps includes a long tapered nose that can help develop an extracapsular plane to avoid injury to muscle, nerve, or vessels.

side-in by making a portal 1.5 cm anterior to the acromioclavicular joint and passing a sharp trocar through the rotator interval capsule under direct visualization. A 30° arthroscope is inserted through the anterosuperior portal to visualize the posterosuperior capsule adjacent to the glenoid labrum.

Initial observation in the anterosuperior and posterior aspects of the joint typically reveals synovial inflammation and synovitis on the labrum and biceps tendon (Fig. 5). In 93% of our cases, synovitis was found inside the joint in these locations. It is important that the surgeon resist the temptation to debride synovitis.

Now, retract the posterior cannula to release the contracted posterosuperior capsule using capsular release forceps. These forceps are specially designed to free the capsule from the subjacent rotator cuff musculature and to widely resect the thick capsule. The labrum should be left entirely intact. We prefer capsular release forceps to electrocautery, because the forceps can mechanically separate a plane and cleanly excise a wide section of tissue to prevent recurrent contractures. Unipolar or bipolar cautery is effective at cutting the capsule, but bubbles may obscure visibility and the depth of cautery penetration is not as easy to control. Electrocautery also caramelizes tissue and may injure rotator cuff fibers, however, injury to neurovascular structures rarely occurs with the use of these devices. After the posterosuperior quadrant has been released, the posterior capsule is released in an inferior direction as far as visibility will allow.

The arthroscope is then exchanged in position and the anterosuperior rotator interval capsule is completely excised. Again we warn against the temptation to use a motorized shaver for debridement except for sucking out pieces of capsule, because use of this device can cause additional bleeding. Little to no bleeding will occur when the capsule is mechanically resected using the capsular release forceps (Fig. 7). Next, the anterior capsule is resected further inferiorly, continuing with the middle glenohumeral ligament and extending toward the anterior-inferior glenohumeral ligament. Alternatively, a 70° arthroscope can be used to assist in visualizing the release in an inferior direction.

The arthroscope is then retracted posteriorly to visualize the intact and contracted posteroinferior capsule. A pin-portal converter is used to create a second posterior-inferior portal for placement of a second posterior cannula. Once portal access is established, the capsular release forceps are inserted and the cannula is retracted. Because the axillary nerve is adjacent to the capsule in the posteroinferior quadrant, we close the capsular release forceps and separate the rotator cuff musculature and neurovascular structures from the external surface of the contracted capsule before resection of capsular tissue. The cannula must be inserted and retracted alternatively with the capsular release forceps. The suction shaver is used effectively to extract tissue fragments. The cutting orifice of the motorized shaver must always be directed toward the labrum to avoid nerve or vascular injury.

The inferior capsular release should be performed no more than 1 cm from the inferior labrum to avoid risk to the neurovascular structures. The inferior release of the capsule continues using the maximum length of the angulated capsular release forceps. As the release continues from posterior to anterior, the inferior border of the subscapularis will be encountered. The release continues into the anteroinferior quadrant. In this location the inferior glenohumeral ligament is quite thick.

Next, the arthroscope is positioned to visualize the upper rolled border of the subscapularis tendon, and a second anteroinferior portal is placed from outside to inside just above the subscapularis tendon. Once the portal is inserted, the anterosuperior portal is used for arthroscopic visualization and the capsular release forceps are positioned through the anteroinferior portal to resect the inferior glenohumeral ligament from the deep surface of the subscapularis muscle. The thick capsuloligamentous structure must be released completely, until a direct connection is made between the anterior and posterior release. The humeral head will not drop inferiorly and will not fully rotate until the inferior glenohumeral ligament is completely divided.

Once the release has been connected circumferentially about the joint, it is important to finish with a synovectomy and wide resection of the capsular margins and the synovectomy to prevent early scar formation and restricted capsular volume. In our experience, repeat arthroscopic capsular releases for diabetic stiff shoulders have been required for patients in whom we performed (1) an isolated posterior capsular release, (2) incomplete capsular release, or (3) did not adequately release the humeroscapular motion interface. We have repeated 8 releases to thoroughly resect all capsular contractures and improve postoperative motion.

Once the intra-articular capsular release is complete, we visualize the subacromial space. Usually, significant adhesion contractures of the humeroscapular motion interface are seen only in patients with prior surgical intervention (Fig. 8). These adhesions connect the deep surface of the deltoid to the rotator cuff and, because they prevent rotating or gliding motions, limit the shoulder range.

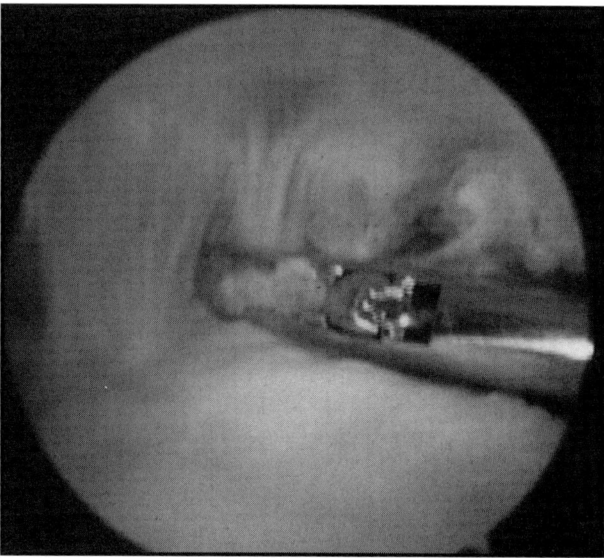

Fig. 8 Arthroscopic view of the subacromial space where significant adhesions are present in this patient who had prior open rotator cuff repair. These adhesions prevent relative motion between rotator cuff and overlying coracoacromial arch or deltoid. The entire humeroscapular motion interface must glide to allow patients recovery of fully rotational motion.

Combined Release Technique Shoulders with a prior open surgical procedure are best treated after arthroscopic capsular release with an axillary deltopectoral approach to perform a complete lysis of adhesions between the bursal surface around the proximal humerus and surfaces of the entire rotator cuff, coracoacromial arch, coracoid base, and conjoint tendon. This arthroscopic and open procedure is termed a combined release. Combined release leaves the entire musculotendinous units of the rotator cuff completely intact and ready for stretching. Prior to closure of the deltopectoral interval, hyaluronic acid derivatives are placed throughout the humeroscapular motion interface. After surgery, there are no restrictions for both active assisted and passive motions of the shoulder.

Postoperative Management At the end of the surgical procedure, we routinely instill 40 mg of methylprednisolone inside the joint. It is important to warn diabetics that their circulating blood glucose levels may fluctuate for up to 5 days. The patients should check their blood sugar more frequently than usual. After surgery, the patient's operated extremity is connected to a continuous passive motion device. Later that day, while the regional interscalene block is effective, we range the extremity to demonstrate the achieved extremes while the patient observes. This maneuver reinforces their confidence to maximally push the extremity.

Our patients are discharged the day after surgery once the therapist reinforces the Jackin's Stretching Exercise Program. We recommend reexamination within 3 weeks. The stretching exercises must be performed in all 4 quadrants, 5 times a day, with 5 repetitions of each stretching maneuver. In our study, 15 of 52 diabetic releases required remanipulation and reinjection 3 to 4 weeks after surgical release. Remanipulation generally recovers the motion achieved at the time of release if it is performed within 4 weeks after the procedure.

Results

Demographics

In our study of 37 diabetic patients with refractory frozen shoulder, a total of 52 surgical procedures were performed. Average age was 47 ± 9 years (range 34 to 67 years). Over one third (14 of 37, 38%) had bilateral shoulder stiffness, and 7 underwent bilateral surgical treatment. Eight shoulders of the initial 44 primary releases eventually underwent revision arthroscopic capsular release, for a total of 52 procedures. At the time of this review, follow-up of the diabetic patients averaged 3.5 ± 2 years (range 1.2 to 8.4 years).

Duration of Symptoms

Our 37 diabetic patients were extracted from a prospective study that began in 1991 to assess arthroscopic management of the stiff shoulder. The symptomatic duration prior to arthroscopic surgical capsular release averaged 26 ± 25 months (range 4 to 131 months).

Patients with a long duration (> 18 months) of painful stiffness prior to surgical release were found to have a significantly lower impression of their own general health (SF-36 evaluation) both before surgery and at follow-up (p = 0.007 for both cases). In contrast, duration of symptoms did not relate to severity of stiffness as measured at presentation or after release for all 6 ranges of motion. There were, however, specific motion differences for forward elevation on the asymptomatic side in patients who initially presented with bilateral shoulder stiffness when compared to nondiabetics who had an opposite asymptomatic shoulder (146 ± 22° versus 165 ± 9°, p = 0.0003).

Type 1 Versus Type 2

In our patient population, 20 primary cases were diagnosed with type 1 and 24 with type 2 diabetes. The average duration of all diabetic conditions was 20.4 ± 10 years (range, 1 to 36 years). The average age of patients with type 1 diabetes was 44 ± 7.4 years and their diabetes had been diagnosed for 24 ± 9 years. For type 2, it was 49 ± 9.5 years of age and duration of diabetic condition was 17 ± 10 years. These differences in age and duration of symptoms were significant between the 2 groups ($p = 0.046$ and $p = 0.03$, respectively). In summary, patients with type 1 diabetes were younger but had diabetes mellitus longer than those with type 2. The duration of symptoms prior to arthroscopic capsular release, however, was not significantly different between type 1 and type 2 (type 1–24.4 months and type 2–27.1 months).

We differentiated characteristics of shoulder function and health status at presentation and after arthroscopic capsular release for those with type 1 and type 2 diabetes. We found that at presentation, type 1 patients indicated better shoulder function and health status than did those patients with type 2 diabetes mellitus. For example, patients with type 1 diabetes answered on presentation affirmatively to 5.4 ± 2.8 questions on the Simple Shoulder Test (SST) as compared to 3.3 ± 2.7 with type 2 diabetes ($p = 0.02$). Similar results were found on the initial presentation as assessed by the SF-36. Those with type 1 diabetes were found to have much higher scores for physical function ($p = 0.02$), emotional role ($p = 0.02$), mental health ($p = 0.02$), and comfort ($p = 0.002$). After surgical release, however, there were absolutely no differences on the SST or SF-36 Health Status scores between those with type 1 or type 2 diabetes.

Associated Musculoskeletal Manifestations

Our study patients often exhibited musculoskeletal manifestations of long-term diabetes mellitus such as we have described earlier (Dupuytren's contracture, Prayer sign, clinodactyly, cheirarthropathy, and limited joint motion syndrome). We attempted to differentiate patients with these manifestations and the severity of shoulder stiffness. We identified that 43% of our primary cases (19 of 44) had an associated Dupuytren's contracture and 45% had a positive Prayer sign (20 of 44). There was no correlation between the severity of measured shoulder stiffness, the isolated or multiple presentation of findings of limited joint motion syndrome, and the SST or SF-36 scores ($p = 0.75$). A highly significant correlation, however, was found when relating the presentation of nontraumatic onset of diabetic stiffness and bilateral shoulder stiffness (Fisher's exact, $p = 0.009$). Accordingly, no patient with bilateral shoulder stiffness had a history of traumatic injury onset.

Traumatic Injury or Surgery

Seventy-five percent of our primary cases presented with refractory diabetic frozen shoulder and no significant trauma. The patients, however, often indicated that some minor degree of trauma or surgical intervention initiated the onset of symptoms. Twelve shoulders (27%), had undergone an arthroscopic or open surgical procedure to that shoulder prior to our capsular release intervention. This group of 12, who had had a prior surgical procedure, was significantly older (age 51 versus 45, $p = 0.041$) and had been using insulin for a much shorter duration (15 versus 26 years, $p = 0.023$) when compared with those patients who had not had prior surgery. We also found that this prior surgery group had been symptomatic for more than twice the time (42 versus 20 months, $p = 0.009$) than those who had not had prior surgery before capsular release. It also follows that these patients had undergone physical therapy for an extended period of up to an average of nearly 2 years, which was greater than those who had not had prior surgery (23 versus 9 months, $p = 0.009$). Seven patients (16%) had either a partial- or full-thickness rotator cuff tear or a prior cuff repair in advance of their arthroscopic capsular release. Although these had prior surgery, no differences were found on SST or SF-36 before release or at follow-up compared with those without surgery. In contrast, those who attributed the origin of their symptoms to an injury were found to have significantly lower preoperative scores of physical function ($p = 0.04$) and comfort ($p = 0.001$) when compared with those who had no history of an injury.

Work

The majority of our patients (32) were of working age. Only 5 were retired, medically or otherwise. Of those able to work, 43% had a job and 45% were required to perform physically demanding manual work (12% moderate physical demand). At the time of presentation, 22 of 32 were not working because of painful stiffness symptoms related to their diabetic frozen shoulder. After arthroscopic capsular release and at long-term follow-up, a total of 29 patients were not retired, and, of these, 23 had returned to work. The average age of those patients who returned to work was significantly younger (43 versus 51 years, $p = 0.008$) than those who were considered retired. Of interest, we found that patients who were significantly limited in their ability to reach up their back were also less likely to return to work (preflexibility ratio 0.31 versus 0.57, $p =$ 0014).

Surgical Findings

Surgical findings, including the severity of synovitis and other associated findings such as a rotator cuff or labral tears, had no relationship to the degree of limited range, stiffness, duration of symptoms, length of treatment, or the degree of functional limitation on SST prior to the arthroscopic capsular release. There was, however, a direct relationship between those patients who exhibited diffuse synovitis (grade 3) and significantly diminished range of external rotation at the side and in abduction compared with those patients who only had 2 areas of synovitis (grade 2) on follow-up motion examination after capsular release ($p = 0.0003$).

The arthroscopic finding of significant humeroscapular motion interface adhesions was associated with a shorter duration (12 years) of insulin usage compared with those who did not have adhesions outside of the joint (24 years). These humeroscapular motion interface adhesions were present in shoulders with a history of trauma, especially from prior surgery.

In more than one third of our primary cases (16 of 44), we observed other pathology, such as a partial-thickness rotator cuff or biceps tendon tear, labral tear, or prior acromioplasty. In this group, the duration of insulin usage was shorter, 15 ± 10 years as compared to 28 ± 8 years for those that did not have any associated pathology ($p = 0.009$). A significant number of patients from this associated pathology group also required additional surgery other than a capsular release.

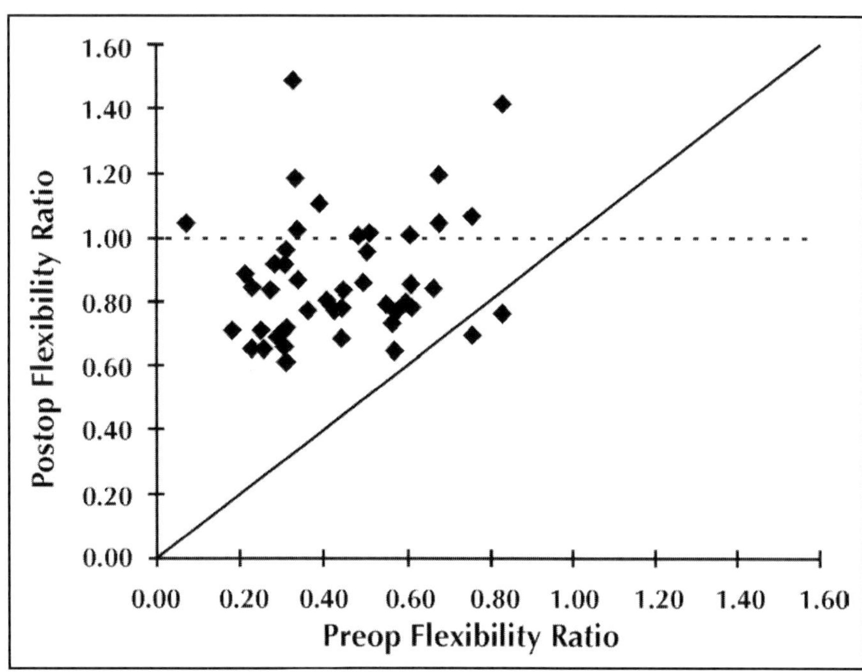

Fig. 9 Graphic representation of preoperative and postoperative ratios for range of motion in each patient.[8,34] Note the flexibility ratio of 1.0 (dotted line), which means symmetric motion between the operative and opposite side. All 6 motion measurements were used for calculating the flexibility ratio. After surgery, the operative shoulder often exhibited greater flexibility than the nonoperative shoulder (as evidenced by standard deviations of greater than 1.0). Points along the oblique line indicate no change between preoperative and postoperative flexibility ratio for each shoulder.

Outcome Measurement

Range of Motion Paired comparisons were completed for all 6 range of motions measured at presentation and at specific intervals of follow-up after arthroscopic capsular release. The 6 motions—forward elevation, external rotation at the side and in abduction, internal rotation in abduction, up the back, and cross-body adduction—were all remarkably improved ($p < 0.0001$, Fig. 9). Although these objective measurements for range of motion demonstrated such a highly significant level of improvement, the patient's perspective in terms of health status as measured by the SF-36 questionnaire was unremarkable.

Simple Shoulder Test Shoulder function, as measured by the SST, also demonstrated a highly significant improvement at long-term follow up after arthroscopic capsular release (Fig. 10). The average preoperative SST score of total affirmatives (4.2 ± 2.9) doubled at follow-up to 7.9 ± 3.4 ($p < 0.0001$). On review of each specific question answered on the SST, we found that 10 out of 12 questions were significantly improved by the Wilcoxon sign-rank test. Only questions 8 and 9, which related to carrying 20 pounds at the side and tossing a softball underhand 20 yards with the affected extremity, failed to show a significant level of improvement. Questions 1 and 2, which relate to comfort at rest or sleep, revealed a highly significant improvement ($p = 0.01$ and $0 = 0.003$, respectively). Questions 3, 4, 5, and 11, which related to motion, were also significantly improved at follow-up (tuck your shirt, $p = 0.007$; place hand behind head, $p = 0.008$; reach to shelf at shoulder level, $p = 0.008$; wash back of opposite shoulder, $p = 0.007$).

SST questions related to strength demonstrated significant improvement (Question 6—lift 1 pound to shoulder level, $p = 0.04$; 7—lift 8 pounds to shoulder level, $p = 0.007$), with the exception of question 8, which related to carrying 20 pounds at the side ($p = 0.09$). As mentioned previously with regard to employment, a significant majority of patients were able to return to work at their regular job ($p = 0.04$).

SF-36 Health Status Questionnaire Eight scores are generated by the SF-36 health status questionnaire, but the only significant improvement was demonstrated by the comfort score ($p = 0.0002$,

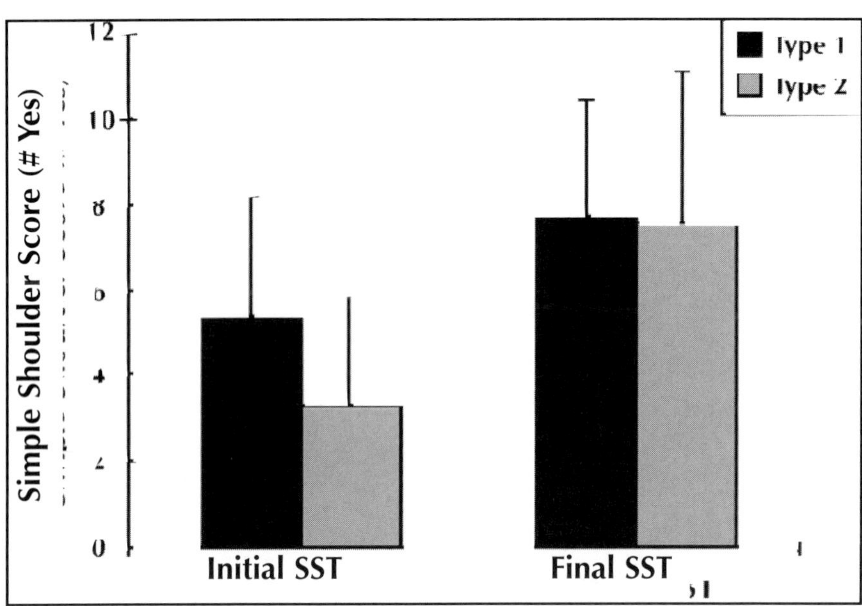

Fig. 10 Note the initial significant difference at presentation between type 1 and type 2 diabetes in total number of affirmative answers on the Simple Shoulder Test (SST). Postoperatively, there was no difference in the long-term functional outcome.

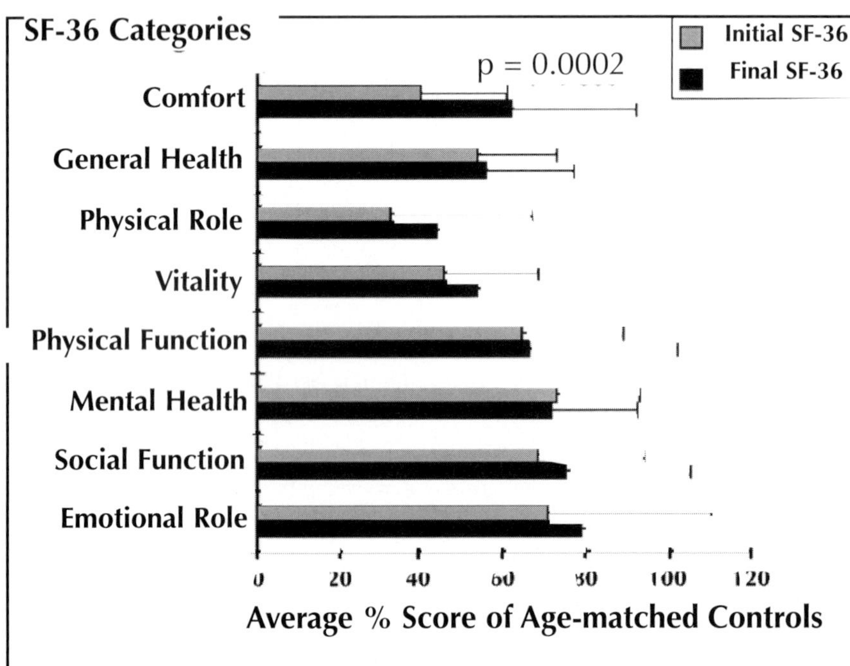

Fig. 11 Graph that displays the initial and final outcome for all 8 scores on the SF-36 health status instrument. Note that only the comfort score was improved after arthroscopic capsular release. Seven of 8 functions were essentially unchanged.

Fig. 11). Surprisingly, no other scores were improved at the $p = 0.05$ level.

Subsequent Problems

Eight patients underwent repeat arthroscopic capsular releases. All 8 patients also had bilateral shoulder stiffness. Four patients who required repeat release also had severe humeroscapular motion interface adhesions secondary to a prior open surgical procedure. One patient with insulin-dependent diabetes and scleroderma underwent 1 open and 3 arthroscopic procedures on the same shoulder over a 10-year period. Her latest procedure was a combined release of the joint capsule and humeroscapular motion interface to improve range of motion.

There was 1 surgical complication among the 52 procedures. This complication included inadvertent insertion of the arthroscopic trocar into the humeral head (Fig. 6), which later collapsed and required a hemiarthroplasty replacement. There were no other complications, other than patients who developed recurrent painful stiffness and functional limitation at long-term follow-up. Five patients continued to exhibit significant stiffness and a final SST score lower than or the same as the initial preoperative SST score.

Patients who required additional surgery, such as either repeat manipulation or arthroscopic capsular release, after the initial procedure, were found to have a significantly lower postoperative SST score (5.3 ± 3.3 versus 8.7 ± 2.9, $p = 0.01$). These patients also demonstrated a lower physical function and vitality score on the SF-36 health status questionnaire ($p = 0.02$ and $p = 0.005$, respectively).

Discussion

In summary, the efficacy of arthroscopic capsular release is documented both in terms of range of motion and function, as assessed by the SST. The follow-up and outcome are documented in greater detail than in prior studies regarding the diabetic stiff shoulder. The efficacy of complete arthroscopic and/or combined release is recorded and, so far, the results have not diminished with time. To our knowledge, this is the first prospective study concerning surgical management for diabetic shoulder stiffness.

We further summarize the following conclusions from this study: (1) Patients with diabetes mellitus are more susceptible to developing shoulder stiffness to the extent of bilateral involvement, especially those with type 1 diabetes mellitus. We recommend a daily prophylactic range of motion stretching program to prevent stiff shoulders. (2) Manipulation is only partially effective for insulin-dependent patients and is more effective for those who have a shorter duration of symptoms. (3) Patients who have a long duration of symptoms have a lower perspective of their own health status both before treatment and at long-term follow-up after arthroscopic capsular release. Therefore, early release of the refractory diabetic stiff shoulder is recommended. (4) Patients with type 1 diabetes mellitus, according to SST and SF-36 scores, maintain a better functional level than do patients with type 2 diabetes mellitus. There were no differences, however, after arthroscopic capsular release at long-term follow-up. (5) The diabetic stiff shoulder can recover excellent function and range of motion after treatment with manipulation and arthroscopic capsular release, but these results do not necessarily change the overall health status other than comfort scores. (6) Patients with diabetes mellitus and an incomplete arthroscopic release or post-surgical stiffness may require repeat surgical release but do not necessarily end up with a poorer result at long-term follow-up. (7) We recommend early treatment with manipulation and complete arthroscopic release to prevent chronic painful symptoms, prolonged disability, long-term expensive therapy, and loss of work or sequelae of permanent muscle contractures about the shoulder.

References

1. Arkkila PE, Kantola IM, Viikari JS: Dupuytren's disease: Association with chronic diabetic complications. *J Rheumatol* 1997;24: 153–159.
2. Arkkila PE, Kantola IM, Viikari JS, Ronnemaa T: Shoulder capsulitis in type I and II diabetic patients: Association with diabetic complications and related diseases. *Ann Rheum Dis* 1996;55:907–914.
3. Bridgman JF: Periarthritis of the shoulder and diabetes mellitus. *Ann Rheum Dis* 1972;31: 69–71.
4. Buchanan WW, Kean WF, Rooney PJ: Some metabolic aspects of arthritis. *S Afr Med J* 1982; 61:467–471.
5. Chammas M, Bousquet P, Renard E, Poirier JL, Jaffiol C, Allieu Y: Dupuytren's disease, carpal tunnel syndrome, trigger finger, and diabetes mellitus. *J Hand Surg* 1995;20A:109–114.
6. Fisher L, Kurtz A, Shipley M: Association between cheiroarthropathy and frozen shoulder in patients with insulin-dependent diabetes mellitus. *Br J Rheumatol* 1986;25:141–146.
7. Florack TM, Miller RJ, Pellegrini VD, Burton RI, Dunn MG: The prevalence of carpal tunnel syndrome in patients with basal joint arthritis of the thumb. *J Hand Surg* 1992;17A:624–630.
8. Harryman DT II, Lazarus M, Rozencwaig R: The stiff shoulder, in Rockwood CA Jr, Matsen FA III, Wirth MA, Harryman DT II (eds): *The Shoulder*, ed 2. Philadelphia, PA, WB Saunders, 1998, vol 2, pp 1064–1112.
9. Harryman DT II: Shoulders: Frozen and stiff, in Heckman JD (ed): *Instructional Course Lectures 42*. Rosemont, IL, American Academy of Orthopaedic Surgeons, 1993, pp 247–257.
10. Janda DH, Hawkins RJ: Shoulder manipulation in patients with adhesive capsulitis and diabetes mellitus: A clinical note. *J Shoulder Elbow Surg* 1993;2:36–38.
11. Koh WH, Seah A, Chai P: Clinical presentation and disease associations of gout: A hospital-based study of 100 patients in Singapore. *Ann Acad Med Singapore* 1998;27:7–10.
12. Lundberg BJ: The frozen shoulder: Clinical and radiographical observations. The effect of manipulation under general anesthesia: Structure and glycosaminoglycan content of the joint capsule. Local bone metabolism. *Acta Orthop Scand* 1969; 119(suppl):1–59.
13. Moren-Hybbinette I, Moritz U, Schersten B: The clinical picture of the painful diabetic shoulder: Natural history, social consequences and analysis of concomitant hand syndrome. *Acta Med Scand* 1987;221:73–82.
14. Ogilvie-Harris DJ, Myerthall S: The diabetic frozen shoulder: Arthroscopic release. *Arthroscopy* 1997;13:1–8.
15. Pal B, Anderson J, Dick WC, Griffiths ID: Limitation of joint mobility and shoulder capsulitis in insulin- and non-insulin-dependent diabetes mellitus. *Br J Rheumatol* 1986;25: 147–151.
16. Pal B, Griffiths ID, Anderson J, Dick WC: Association of limited joint mobility with Dupuytren's contracture in diabetes mellitus. *J Rheumatol* 1987;14:582–585.
17. Reeves B: The natural history of the frozen shoulder syndrome. *Scand J Rheumatol* 1975;4: 193–196.
18. Rosenbloom AL, Silverstein JH: Connective tissue and joint disease in diabetes mellitus. *Endocrinol Metab Clin North Am* 1996;25: 473–483.
19. Rosenbloom AL, Silverstein JH, Lezotte DC, Riley WJ, Maclaren NK: Limited joint mobility in diabetes mellitus of childhood: Natural history and relationship to growth impairment. *J Pediatr* 1982;101:874–878.
20. Sattar MA, Luqman WA: Periarthritis: Another duration-related complication of diabetes mellitus. *Diabetes Care* 1985;8:507–510.
21. Sherry DD, Rothstein RR, Petty RE: Joint contractures preceding insulin-dependent diabetes mellitus. *Arthritis Rheum* 1982;25:1362–1364.
22. Baslund B, Thomsen BS, Jensen EM: Humero-scapular periarthrosis. *Ugeskr Laeger* 1991;153:170–173.
23. Bulgen DY, Binder AI, Hazleman BL, Dutton J, Roberts S: Frozen shoulder: Prospective clinical study with an evaluation of three treatment regimens. *Ann Rheum Dis* 1984;43:353–360.
24. Helbig B, Wagner P, Dohler R: Mobilization of frozen shoulder under general anaesthesia. *Acta Orthop Belg* 1983;49:267–274.
25. Matsen FA III , Lippitt SB, Sidles JA, Harryman DT II (eds): *Practical Evaluation and Management of the Shoulder*. Philadelphia, PA, WB Saunders, 1994.
26. Ogilvie-Harris DJ, Biggs DJ, Fitsialos DP, MacKay M: The resistant frozen shoulder: Manipulation versus arthroscopic release. *Clin Orthop* 1995;319:238–248.
27. Pollock RG, Duralde XA, Flatow EL, Bigliani LU: The use of arthroscopy in the treatment of resistant frozen shoulder. *Clin Orthop* 1994;304: 30–36.
28. Baird KS, Alwan WH, Crossan JF, Wojciak B: T-cell mediated response in Dupuytren's disease. *Lancet* 1993;341:1622-1623.
29. Bucala R, Makita Z, Koschinsky T, Cerami A, Vlassara H: Lipid advanced glycosylation: Pathway for lipid oxidation in vivo. *Proc Natl Acad Sci USA* 1993;90:6434–6438.
30. Hogan M, Cerami A, Bucala R: Advanced glycosylation endproducts block the antiproliferative effect of nitric oxide: Role in the vascular and renal complications of diabetes mellitus. *J Clin Invest* 1992;90:1110–1115.
31. Makita Z, Radoff S, Rayfield EJ, et al: Advanced glycosylation end products in patients with diabetic nephropathy. *N Engl J Med* 1991;325:836–842.
32. Siebold JR: Digital sclerosis in children with insulin-dependent diabetes mellitus. *Arthritis Rheum* 1982;25:1357–1361.

33. Bunker TD, Anthony PP: The pathology of frozen shoulder: A Dupuytren-like disease. *J Bone Joint Surg* 1995;77B:677–683.

34. Harryman DT II, Matsen FA III, Sidles JA: Arthroscopic management of refractory shoulder stiffness. *Arthroscopy* 1997;13:133–147.

35. Ozaki J, Nakagawa Y, Sakurai G, Tamai S: Recalcitrant chronic adhesive capsulitis of the shoulder: Role of contracture of the coracohumeral ligament and rotator interval in pathogenesis and treatment. *J Bone Joint Surg* 1989;71A:1511–1515.

36. Conference TADAC: Classification of diabetes mellitus. *Diabetes Care* 1998;1(suppl 1):4–8.

37. Harris M: *Descriptive Epidemiology in Diabetes in America.* NIH, Boston, MA, 1995, vol 2, p 1468.

38. Lequesne M, Dang N, Bensasson M, Mery C: Increased association of diabetes mellitus with capsulitis of the shoulder and shoulder-hand syndrome. *Scand J Rheumatol* 1997;6:53–56.

39. Harryman DT II: Arthroscopic management of shoulder stiffness. *Oper Tech Sports Med* 1997;5:264–274.

Tendon Transfers About the Shoulder and Elbow in Obstetrical Brachial Plexus Palsy

James B. Bennett, MD
Christopher H. Allan, MD

Table 1
Options for tendon release, tendon or muscle transfer, and osseous procedures by site

Lesion	Procedure
Shoulder	
Adduction and internal rotation contracture	Release or recession of subscapularis muscle
Isolated abduction contracture	Release or recession of deltoid muscle
Abduction and external rotation contracture	Transfer of infraspinatus tendon to teres minor tendon; release or recession of infraspinatus and supraspinatus tendons with or without release of deltoid muscle
Dysfunction of supraspinatus or infraspinatus muscle	Transfer of latissimus dorsi tendon to greater tuberosity
Dysfunction of anterior and middle parts of deltoid muscle (partial reinnervation of paralyzed deltoid muscle)	Anterior transfer of posterior part of deltoid muscle
Dysfunction of deltoid muscle	Transfer of trapezius muscle with bone to lateral aspect of humerus; bipolar transfer of latissimus dorsi muscle
Dysfunction of subscapularis muscle	Transfer of serratus anterior muscle; transfer of pectoralis major tendon
Combined deficits	Variable (multiple tendon and muscle transfers as described by Ober[23] and by Harmon;[15] see text)
Internal or external rotation deformity with incongruent glenohumeral joint	Humeral derotation osteotomy
Severe dysfunction of shoulder with pain or instability	Glenohumeral arthrodesis
Elbow	
Dysfunction of biceps muscle	Unipolar or bipolar transposition of pectoralis major muscle; bipolar transposition of latissimus dorsi muscle; free microvascular transfer of gracilis rectus muscle; modified Steindler flexorplasty; anterior transfer of triceps tendon
Dysfunction of triceps muscle	Transfer of latissimus dorsi muscle

Obstetrical or birth palsy of the brachial plexus occurs in as many as 1 in 250 births.[1,2] Predisposing factors include high birth weight, prolonged labor, breech presentation, and shoulder dystocia. The actual lesion is produced by traction on the neural elements; for example, stretching of the brachial plexus with forced lateral flexion of the head and neck. Most of these injuries resolve without operative intervention. For patients who are more severely affected, however, a variety of procedures are available (Table 1). The treatment algorithm to maximize each child's long-term functional recovery is continuously evolving (Table 2).

Table 2
Timing of surgical procedures in patients who have obstetrical brachial plexus palsy

Age (mos.)	Procedure
3–9	Exploration and repair of brachial plexus
12–24	Release of contractures
24–60*	Tendon and muscle transfers
> 60 (and incongruent joint)	Osseous procedures

**As long as the glenohumeral joint is congruent, tendon and muscle transfers may be performed at a later date, but they should be considered at these earlier times to maximize functional recovery*

In the earliest phase of treatment, exploration, neurolysis, and operative repair or reconstruction of the injured brachial plexus may be undertaken. The decision to intervene with an operation depends on the time that has elapsed since the injury, the recovery of function to that point, and the surgeon's personal philosophy regarding the likelihood of additional gains with nonoperative treatment. Most surgeons perform such procedures, when appropriate, in infants between three and nine months of age.[3,4] Joint mobilization and range of motion exercises performed by the parents and guided by a physical or occupational therapist can help to maintain a congruent glenohumeral joint and to minimize contractures.

Patients with incomplete recovery who are seen more than 6 months after birth frequently have muscle contractures due to unopposed muscle forces and are no longer candidates for direct repair of the plexus. These children can often benefit from releases of the contractures to maintain a congruent joint and to maximize the range of motion. Releases are usually performed between the ages of 12 and 24 months, but they may be useful in older patients if the glenohumeral joint is congruent.

Waters and associates made the point that glenohumeral deformity occurs along a spectrum of severity, with less severe changes being potentially reversible with soft-tissue joint relocation procedures, a situation that is analogous to the joint remodeling seen in children managed for congenital dysplasia of the hip.[5] The decision as to whether to perform tendon transfers or osseous procedures is therefore difficult when the deformity is not clearly at one end of the spectrum or the other, and it is based on assessment of the congruence of the glenohumeral joint. Plain radiographs may be inadequate for the evaluation of joint congruence in order to select treatment, since the glenoid is incompletely ossified at the age when these decisions must be made. Pearl and Edgerton[6] recently reported their experience with the intraoperative use of axillary glenohumeral arthrography to assist with selection of the appropriate operative procedure. Waters and associates described the preoperative use of computed tomography or magnetic resonance imaging to better depict the glenohumeral deformity.[5]

Tendon transfers are generally performed between the ages of 2 and 5 years, although some authorities advocate attempts at soft-tissue joint realignment in children as old as 9 or 10 years if the glenohumeral joint is congruent.[6] Waters and Peljovich[7] recently compared the results of tendon transfers with those of humeral derotation osteotomies; the patients who were managed with soft-tissue procedures had an average age of 4.9 ± 2.5 years at the time of the operation, whereas those managed with osteotomies had an average age of 8.4 ± 3.7 years.

In addition to an assessment of joint congruence, muscle grading is necessary before tendon transfer, to ensure that the transferred muscle will provide adequate power. Adequate power requires a grade of at least 4 of 5, which corresponds to active movement against gravity and some resistance but not normal power. Accurate muscle grading is not possible until optimum strength has been achieved, usually with the assistance of therapy, and the child is old enough to comply with testing.

Osseous procedures are usually performed in patients who are first seen when they are older than 5 years of age since, as we noted, joint incongruity tends to increase with the patient's age. Appropriate procedures for severely incongruent joints include humeral rotational osteotomy for persistent internal rotation contracture and glenohumeral arthrodesis in the setting of severe pain, instability, or arthritic changes. When posterior dislocation of the humeral head has occurred, posterior capsular plication may be necessary to prevent recurrent posterior instability.[8]

While each of these components of operative treatment has its role, the present discussion will be limited to release of contractures and tendon transfers and will specifically consider procedures that aim to restore function of the shoulder and elbow.

Biomechanics of Shoulder Stability

The longitudinal, proximal pull of the deltoid muscle (as well as the long head of the triceps, the pectoralis minor, and the coracobrachialis muscles) on the humerus is counteracted by the depressor force of the rotator cuff muscles. The line of action of this force is medial and slightly downward. The rotator cuff plays its greatest role as a stabilizer between 30° and 75° of humeral elevation, with its role diminishing thereafter until, at 120° of elevation, it no longer contributes to stability of the glenohumeral joint. In the absence of an intact rotator cuff, the inferior portion of the pectoralis major muscle, along with the latissimus dorsi muscle, may resist superior translation of the humeral head in the glenoid fossa.

The subscapularis muscle also functions to resist anterior glenohumeral instability. The long head of the biceps muscle assists in this. The subscapularis muscle may also prevent posterior translation through its anterior pull. Posterior stability is also provided by the infraspinatus muscle and the posterior aspect of the capsule of the glenohumeral joint.

Inferior stability is provided by the posterior part of the deltoid muscle, the supraspinatus muscle, and the superior portion of the glenohumeral joint capsule. The pull of the serratus anterior muscle on the scapula tilts the glenoid from a more vertical to a more horizontal position with humeral elevation; this provides an osseous shelf resisting inferior translation as well.[9]

Muscle Contracture

The most commonly encountered birth palsy involves the fifth and sixth cervical nerve roots (713 of 1,486 patients [48%] in Gilbert's series had such involvement[10]) or the fifth, sixth, and seventh roots (431 of 1,486 patients [29%] in Gilbert's series), with diminished or absent abduction and external rotation leading to an adduction and internal rotation contracture. The chief difference between these 2 patterns of involvement is the complete elbow extension due to intact triceps function in the first pattern. Other patterns involve more caudad nerve roots (the eighth cervical and first thoracic nerve roots) or whole plexus injury. The more caudad nerve root injuries tend to affect function of the hand and wrist and are not discussed here.

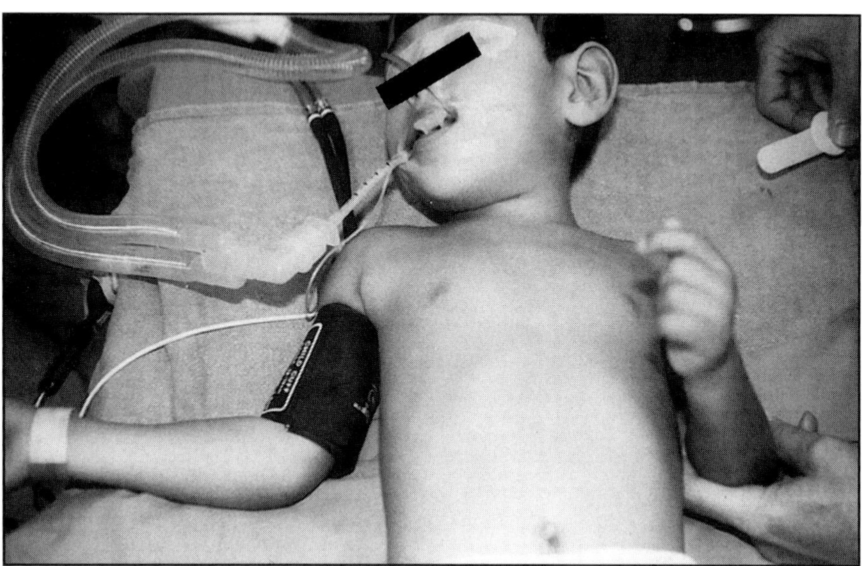

Fig. 1 Release of the subscapularis muscle as described by Carlioz and Brahimi.[12] Photograph demonstrating a preoperative adduction contracture of the left shoulder with an internal rotation contracture of approximately 20°.

Release of the Subscapularis Muscle

Release or recession of the subscapularis muscle, probably first described by Sever in 1918,[11] has withstood the test of time and is still performed in various modified forms in patients who have an internal rotation contracture of the shoulder (Fig. 1). The pectoralis major muscle does not usually result in contracture and therefore does not require release.

Most often the entire origin of the subscapularis muscle is released from the anterior aspect of the scapula, as described by Carlioz and Brahimi;[12] this allows the humerus to be externally rotated and splinted in this position. An advantage to this method compared with earlier techniques that involved the release of the insertion of the subscapularis tendon is the avoidance of anterior instability of the shoulder. The deformity recurs if the period of immobilization is inadequate. Our protocol dictates that the splint be worn full-time for 3 months and then at night for an additional 3 months; the splint is applied with the humerus in external rotation and the shoulder in 30° to 45° of abduction. The strength of the external rotator muscles may recover or transfers may be required to provide active external rotation.

Technique The patient is placed in lateral decubitus with use of a beanbag or another type of support. The affected shoulder and torso are prepared to the midline anteriorly and posteriorly. A longitudinal incision is made along the lateral border of the scapula, and dissection is carried out down to the latissimus dorsi muscle, the fibers of which cover the lateral aspect of the scapula. This muscle is retracted inferiorly, and the inferior angle of the scapula is identified and stabilized with towel clips. The subscapularis muscle is readily identified and is elevated in its entirety from the anterior surface of the scapula with use of electrocautery or a periosteal elevator (Fig. 2). Dissection is performed in a subperiosteal fashion, progressing from the inferior angle upward. The scapula is manipulated as needed with use of the towel clips. An external rotatory force on the humerus is applied gently throughout the release to confirm adequate release of the muscle and elimination of the contracture (Fig. 3). Care must be taken to avoid injury of the subscapular artery and nerve running anteromedial to the glenoid neck and anterior to the subscapularis muscle as well as injury of the suprascapular artery and nerve running from anterior to posterior over the scapular notch. After complete release of the subscapularis muscle, the wound is closed over a suction drain. A splint, made preoperatively, is applied to maintain the arm in abduction and external rotation (Fig. 4). The patient wears the splint full-time for 3 months, removing it only to bathe and for gentle range-of-motion exercises, which are begun at 6 weeks. The patient then wears the splint only at night for an additional 3 months. At 6 months postoperatively, treatment with the splint is discontinued.

Transfer of the Infraspinatus Tendon to the Teres Minor Tendon

In the less common situation involving a combined external rotation and abduction contracture, it may be necessary to release the supraspinatus and infraspinatus tendons, as described by Zancolli and Zancolli.[4] Release of the insertion of the

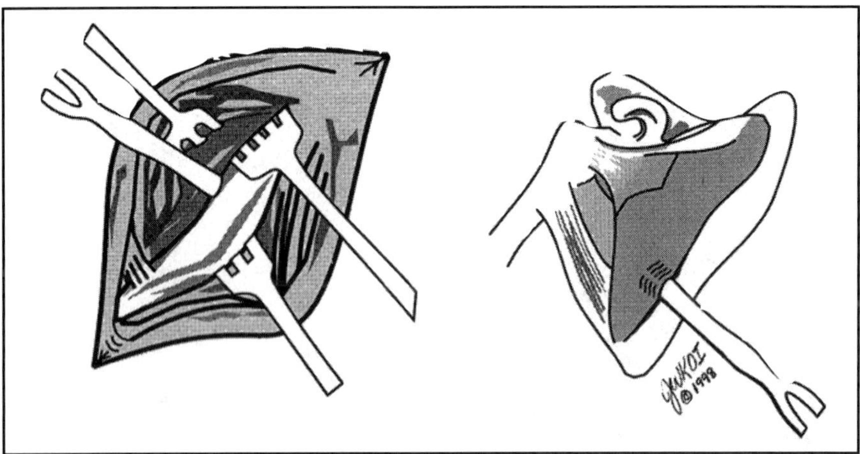

Fig. 2 Drawings illustrating the release of the subscapularis muscle described by Carlioz and Brahimi.[12] The drawing on the left shows the approach to the left subscapularis muscle. The fibers of the latissimus dorsi muscle are split and retracted to the upper left and the lower right by 2 separate retractors. The upper right retractor stabilizes the lateral border of the scapula. Below the upper left retractor is a periosteal elevator elevating the subscapularis muscle off the anterior surface of the scapula. The drawing on the right shows the right subscapularis muscle being elevated off the anterior surface of the scapula by an osteotome.

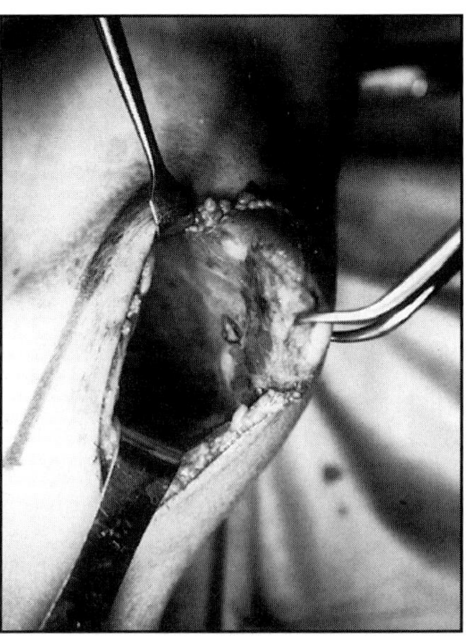

Fig. 3 Intraoperative photograph showing recession of the subscapularis (held in the towel clip) off of the anterior surface of the scapula.

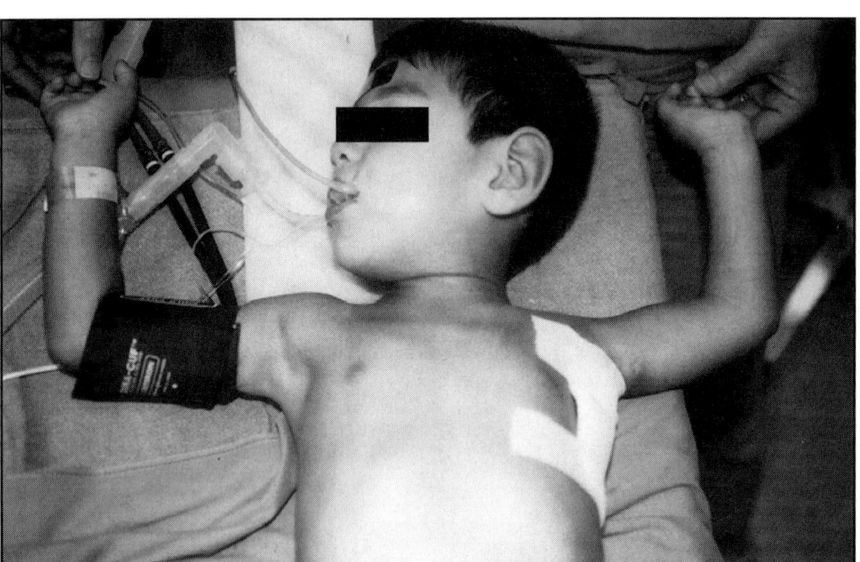

Fig. 4 Postoperative photograph made after release of the subscapularis muscle, demonstrating external rotation of approximately 45°. (This is the same patient as is shown in Fig. 1.)

deltoid muscle on the humerus may also be necessary. An anterior dislocation of the humeral head is often associated with this contracture. The glenohumeral joint is reduced after division of the tendons of the external rotators, step-cut lengthening of the infraspinatus tendon, and transfer of that tendon to the teres minor tendon. Anterior capsular plication may be necessary to tighten the lax anterior glenohumeral ligaments. It should be noted that some authors[4] think that this lesion occurs only as a complication of excessive splinting in the so-called Statue of Liberty position (marked abduction and external rotation), first described by Fairbank,[13] rather than secondary to birth injury.

Technique A posterior approach to the shoulder is used, with a longitudinal skin incision made from superior to inferior overlying the glenohumeral joint. The posterior part of the deltoid muscle is identified and elevated, revealing the underlying contracted infraspinatus and teres minor muscles. The tendon of the infraspinatus is divided several centimeters medial to its insertion on the greater tuberosity of the humeral head. The tendon of the teres minor is divided at its insertion and then sutured to the infraspinatus tendon attachment, thereby lengthening the course of the teres minor by several centimeters. The infraspinatus muscle is now closed to the reattached teres minor. The combined effect is to lengthen the external rotator complex. The arm is splinted in adduction and internal rotation; the patient wears the splint full-time for 3 months and only at night for an additional 3 months. Physical therapy for active and passive motion is performed with the splint off beginning at 6 weeks. As an alternative to the procedure just described, some authors have advocated recession or muscle slide of the supraspinatus, infraspinatus, and teres minor muscles, as described by Debeyre and associates.[14]

Tendon Transfers About the Shoulder

Principles

The principles of tendon transfer are similar regardless of location.

The involved joint must have a functional range of motion. Achievement of such motion most often requires the involvement of therapists working with the child's parents to maintain a supple joint before the operation. The program can include dynamic splinting and stretching to improve passive motion. In addition, as we already discussed, joint contractures must be released and the joint must be congruent and reduced. Skin must be supple without constricting scars.

In an already injured extremity, the surgeon must ensure that the choice of the donor muscle-tendon unit or units will not interfere with existing function.

Adequate strength (a grade of at least 4 of 5) of the donor muscle must be confirmed. Preoperative and postoperative strengthening programs are routinely employed. Most transfers result in the loss of approximately 1 muscle grade, and this must be planned for. It is best to avoid transferring a tendon when the muscle of that tendon was previously paralyzed and has now recovered.

The excursion of the donor muscle-tendon unit must be adequate. In some patients, amplitude can be increased by the addition of a segment of fascia lata or by regional fascial extension. For example, intercostal fascia can be used to lengthen a latissimus dorsi muscle transfer, or rectus sheath can be used with a pectoralis major muscle transfer.

Each tendon should perform only one function. The transfer should employ a straight line of pull.

When possible, synergy should be employed such that the simultaneous contractions of different muscles combine to achieve a desired function. To this end, manual or electrodiagnostic testing to check for in-phase firing of planned donors with nearby, uninvolved motors should be performed preoperatively, to ensure that transferred motors and intact motors do not act as antagonists and prevent active motion. Reinnervation patterns of the brachial plexus may also result in cocontraction of antagonistic muscle groups.

Biomechanics

Shoulder elevation is most efficiently performed in the plane of the scapula. The glenohumeral joint has its greatest stability and mobility (150°) in this position. Tendon transfers to restore shoulder elevation should therefore be done in the plane of the scapula when possible. Shoulder elevation involves both the supraspinatus and the deltoid muscle. Both muscles are active throughout the full range of elevation, although the supraspinatus muscle is most efficient in the first 45° of this motion. The results of studies of the deltoid muscle are divided as to whether its efficiency is maximum at 90° of elevation or at full elevation.[9]

The deltoid muscle behaves as if it were several smaller muscles pulling in slightly different directions and contracting separately in a sequential fashion. The middle part of the deltoid contracts first and, as it is most nearly in line with the plane of the scapula, has the greatest effect on elevation. The anterior fibers cause more flexion and the posterior fibers cause more extension than the middle portion. Some authors have concluded that transfer of the anterior or posterior portion of the deltoid muscle to a more lateral position is therefore justified in order to increase elevation.[9]

The most important scapular motor is the inferior portion of the serratus anterior muscle. This muscle positions the glenoid slightly beneath the humeral head during elevation through its pull laterally and inferiorly on the scapula and thereby stabilizes the glenohumeral joint. This function must be present if transfers are to be performed to restore elevation.

Because the humeral head has a greater diameter, tendons transferred to the humeral head (or to the rotator cuff) in order to bring about rotation are more efficient (have a greater lever arm) than transfers to the shaft of the humerus.[9]

Tendon transfers about the shoulder are most commonly performed for lesions of the fifth and sixth cervical nerve roots involving the suprascapular and axillary nerves and for deficits of the nerve to the subscapularis secondary to shoulder instability. Involved muscles include the supraspinatus and infraspinatus, all or part of the deltoid, and the subscapularis.

Suprascapular Nerve and Supraspinatus and Infraspinatus Muscles (Fifth and Sixth Cervical Nerve Roots)

Weak or absent function of the supraspinatus and infraspinatus muscles leads to decreased external rotation of the humerus and the characteristic internal rotation contracture of obstetric brachial plexus palsy (Fig. 5). This problem is commonly addressed either with transfer of the latissimus dorsi tendon to the posterior aspect of the rotator cuff or the greater tuberosity, as described by Hoffer and associates[15] (Fig. 6), or with a shift of its insertion from anterior to posterior, converting it to an external rotator, as described originally by L'Episcopo[16] and as modified by Covey and associates.[17]

Transfer of the Latissimus Dorsi Tendon to the Posterior Aspect of the Rotator Cuff The procedure described by Hoffer and associates[15] has the advantage of increasing glenohumeral abduction as well as external rotation if function of the deltoid muscle is present. The transfer increases the stabilizing function of the

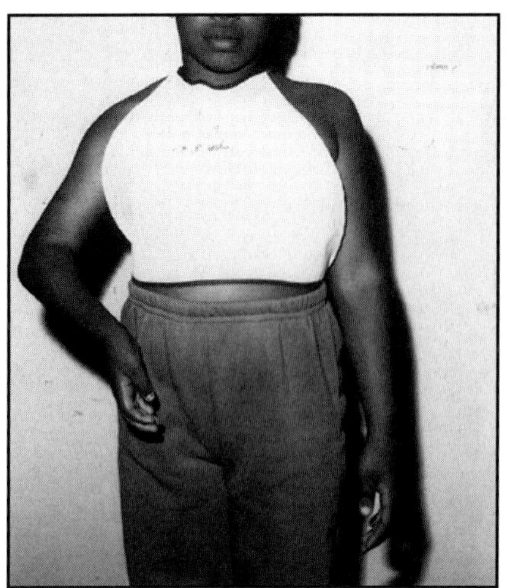

Fig. 5 Preoperative photograph showing loss of external rotation and abduction of the shoulder.

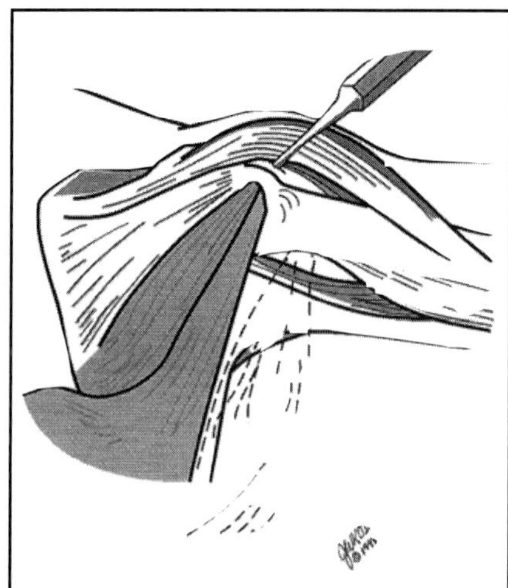

Fig. 6 Drawing illustrating the modification, described by Hoffer and associates,[15] of the transfer of the latissimus dorsi tendon to the greater tuberosity or the rotator cuff. A retractor elevates the deltoid muscle. The shaded muscles are the transposed latissimus dorsi (below) and the teres major (above). These muscles are taken from their previous position (dotted lines) to a new site of attachment into the rotator cuff over the greater tuberosity, so that the muscles are converted from internal to external rotators and provide abduction.

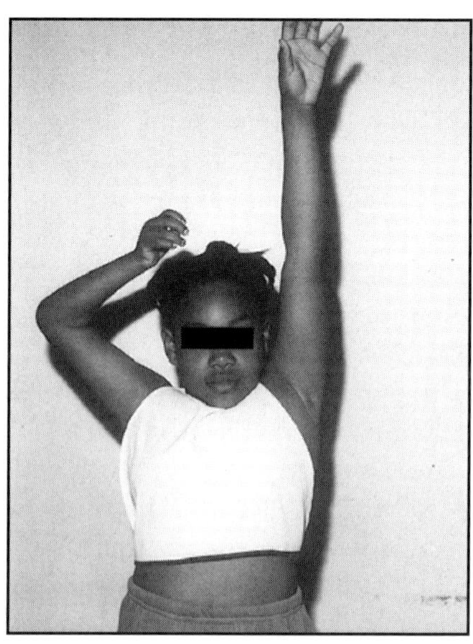

Fig. 7 Postoperative photograph showing external rotation and abduction of the shoulder with weak function of the triceps muscle.

rotator cuff, providing a secure glenohumeral fulcrum around which the deltoid can direct its pull on the lateral aspect of the humerus. Triceps function must be present to allow extension of the elbow when the shoulder is abducted and externally rotated.

Technique The patient is placed in lateral decubitus, and the affected extremity is prepared and draped free. An anterior axillary incision is made, and the pectoralis major tendon insertion is identified and, if necessary, released. If the pectoralis major muscle is not contracted (and the senior author [J.B.B.] believes that it rarely is), then a single posterior incision is used. The subscapularis muscle may be released, as described earlier, if indicated. The tendons of the latissimus dorsi and teres major are identified through a separate, posterior incision. These tendons are released as well, with protection of the radial nerve and the contents of the quadrilateral space throughout. The interval between the posteroinferior margin of the deltoid muscle and the rotator cuff is then developed, and the arm is maximally abducted and externally rotated. The released tendons of the latissimus dorsi and the teres major are next transferred posterior to the long head of the triceps muscle and sutured as superiorly as possible to the rotator cuff. Two longitudinal incisions are made in the cuff, and the tendons are pulled through these incisions and sutured to themselves, thereby converting the latissimus dorsi and teres major muscles into external rotators of the shoulder. Postoperatively, a shoulder spica splint is applied with the shoulder in 60° to 90° of abduction and external rotation. This splint is worn full-time for 3 months and only at night for an additional 3 months (Fig. 7).

Posterolateral Transfer of the Latissimus Dorsi and Teres Major Tendons to the Humeral Shaft With the modification[17] of the L'Episcopo procedure,[16] the latissimus dorsi is transected at its musculotendinous junction and sutured to the teres major tendon, which has been taken directly off bone. The remaining latissimus tendon, still attached to the humeral shaft, is rerouted posterolaterally, while the combined latissimus muscle and teres major tendon are taken posteromedially. These are sutured together posterolateral to the shaft of the humerus, converting both muscles into external rotators.

Technique The patient is placed in lateral decubitus. The arm is draped free, and an axillary incision 5 to 6 cm in length is made transversely from the anterior to the posterior axillary fold. The latissimus dorsi and teres major tendons are identified. The latissimus dorsi is dissected free from the teres major and transected at its musculotendinous junction, and its tendon, still attached to bone, is tagged. A 3-cm lateral incision is made over the proximal part of the lateral aspect of the deltoid muscle. The latissimus muscle belly is sutured to the teres major muscle, which is then released from its humeral insertion. With use of tag sutures, the combined latissimus and teres major muscle group is tunneled posterior to the humerus. The tagged latissimus tendon is taken anterior to the humerus and out through the lateral deltoid incision. The tagged latissimus and teres major muscles are tied to the tagged latissimus tendon, and its course anterior to the humerus and then posterolateral converts the muscles to external rotators. Care is taken throughout to avoid the axillary nerve, particularly in patients who have intact deltoid function. A spica splint is applied with the shoulder in 30° to 45° of abduction and external rotation and is used for 3 months, after which time gentle range of motion and strengthening exercises are begun. The patient wears the splint only at night for another 3 months.

Axillary Nerve and Deltoid Muscle (Fifth and Sixth Cervical Nerve Roots)

There are several procedures that can be used to replace some portion of the function of the deltoid muscle.

Anterior Transfer of the Posterior Third of the Deltoid In patients in whom the anterior and middle thirds of the deltoid are nonfunctional but the posterior third is intact, an anterior transfer of the posterior third can be performed. As first described by Harmon[18] for the treatment of deficits secondary to poliomyelitis, the posterior third of the deltoid muscle is freed from its scapular origin and sutured anteriorly along the lateral aspect of the clavicle, in the region of the nonfunctional anterior and middle deltoid muscle fibers.

Technique A superoposterior incision is made, beginning at the middle third of the clavicle and extending posteriorly to the middle of the scapular spine. Full-thickness flaps are raised superiorly and inferiorly, revealing the posterior third of the deltoid muscle. The muscle is detached subperiosteally from its origin and freed for about half its length from underlying tissue. Care must be exercised to protect underlying branches of the axillary nerve. The outer third of the clavicle is exposed subperiosteally as well, and the free former origin of the posterior third of the deltoid muscle is sutured to this new location. Wounds are closed, and the arm is splinted in 60° to 90° of abduction and forward elevation. The splint is worn full-time for 3 months, after which time gentle active and passive range of motion exercises are begun and the splint is worn for another 3 months at night only.

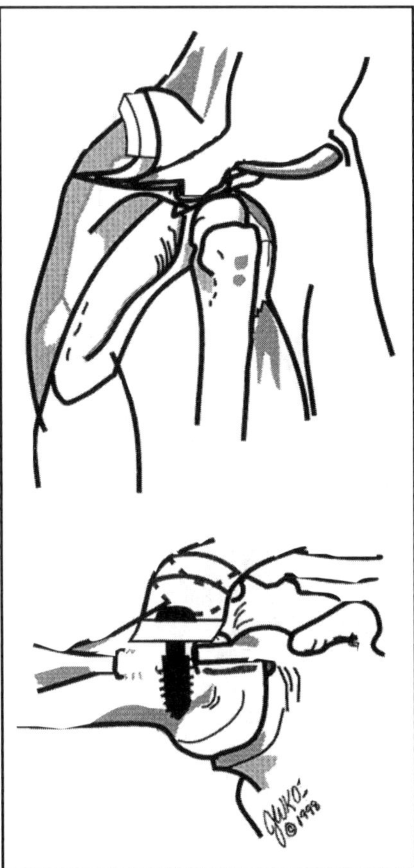

Fig. 8 Drawings illustrating the procedure. The upper drawing shows a lateral view of the right shoulder, with the acromial bone block and attached trapezius muscle elevated. The lower drawing shows the acromial bone block with attached trapezius muscle secured with screw fixation to the roughened lateral aspect of the proximal part of the humerus distal to the greater tuberosity. (Modification of Mayer's[19] transfer of the trapezius muscle attached to an acromial bone block.)

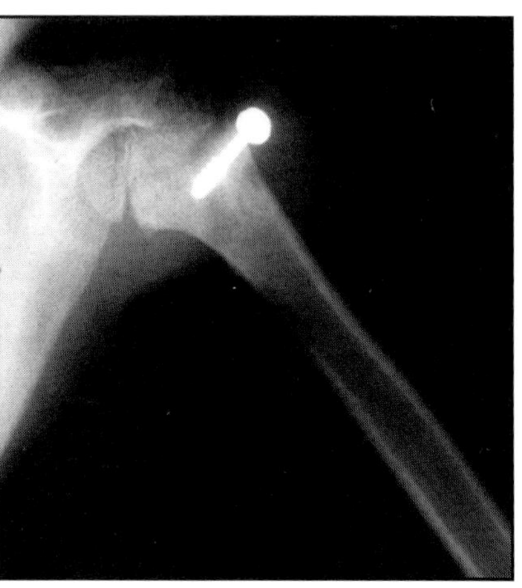

Fig. 9 Radiograph made after performance of the transfer to restore shoulder abduction. (Modification of Mayer's[19] transfer of the trapezius muscle attached to an acromial bone block.)

Transfer of the Trapezius Muscle to the Lateral Aspect of the Humeral Shaft Alternatively, a modification of Mayer's[19] transfer of the trapezius muscle can be performed (Fig. 8). Mayer's original procedure involved dissection of the trapezius muscle free of its insertion along the acromion, scapular spine, and lateral aspect of the clavicle; attachment of a segment of fascia lata rolled into a tube; and suture into a bone tunnel in the region of the deltoid tuberosity on the lateral aspect of the humerus. A modification in which a portion of the acromion is removed to allow for a more straight-line pull is now more commonly used. The lateral aspect of the acromion and its attached trapezius is removed, and its undersurface is roughened with a rasp. Fixation with a screw and washer secures the acromion and trapezius transfer to the proximal part of the humeral shaft (Fig. 9).

Technique A saber-cut incision is made from the inferior border of the anterior axillary fold over the anterior aspect of the shoulder to a point a few centimeters lateral to the medial border of the scapula and just distal to the scapular spine. The trapezius muscle is exposed by careful flap dissection along its entire insertion—that is, anterior, lateral, and posterior. Extensive mobilization of the proximal and middle parts of the trapezius muscle provides an increase of 5 or 6 centimeters in length.[20] The fibrotic deltoid muscle is split longitudinally to allow proximal exposure of the humeral head and shaft. The lateral aspect of the trapezius muscle with its underlying acromion is separated from surrounding tissue. Osseous cuts are made through the lateral aspect of the scapular spine posteriorly. Bone with its attached trapezius muscle is rasped on its undersurface and pulled distally to the lateral aspect of the abducted humerus. The selected site of insertion, distal to the tuberosity, is also rasped, and the bone-and-muscle transfer is secured with a screw over a washer. The arm is then abducted to 60° to 90° and splinted. The splint is worn full-time for 3 months, until bone-healing occurs, and then only at night for another 3 months, during which time physical therapy is given for improvement of the range of motion and for strengthening.

Bipolar Transfer of the Latissimus Dorsi Muscle for Dysfunction of the Deltoid Finally, bipolar transfer of the latissimus dorsi muscle (both ends of the muscle are rotated) on its neurovascular pedicle, as described by Itoh and associates,[21] can be used to treat dysfunction of the deltoid. The procedure involves transection of both the origin and the insertion of the latissimus dorsi muscle. The flat tendon that was originally the humeral insertion is sutured to the insertion of the deltoid muscle, and the broad muscular end is sutured to the periosteum of the acromion and the distal part of the clavicle or to the insertion of the trapezius muscle, thereby substituting for the nonfunctional deltoid muscle.

Technique The patient is placed in lateral decubitus, with the involved side up, and three incisions are made. First, a longitudinal axillary incision is made over the lateral border of the latissimus dorsi muscle, extending up to the distal half of the deltopectoral groove; second, an anterolateral incision is made over the insertion of the deltoid muscle on the humerus; and, third, a curvilinear incision is made along the lateral third of the clavicle and the anterior and lateral aspects of the acromion. The anterior border of the latissimus dorsi muscle is bluntly elevated from the chest wall, with care taken to identify and protect the neurovascular bundle. This is followed proximally, with ligation of communicating branches. Subcutaneous tissue is cleared from the latissimus dorsi muscle for approximately 20 centimeters distal from its humeral insertion. Marking sutures are placed 10 centimeters apart in the body of the muscle as a guide to its resting tension. The muscle is then taken off the inferior angle of the scapula and separated from the teres major muscle. Care must be taken to preserve the thoracodorsal vascular pedicle beneath these muscles. The humeral insertion is divided. The lumbodorsal fascia is then cut near the origin of the latissimus dorsi muscle and at least 20 cm from its humeral insertion. The entire latissimus dorsi muscle can then be raised, with its neurovascular bundle still attached, and rotated so that the undersurface with its attached neurovascular bundle is superficial. A superficial tunnel connecting the incision over the deltoid muscle insertion with that over the anterolateral aspect of the acromion and clavicle is then created. The latissimus dorsi muscle is again rotated in order to allow the flat tendon of insertion to be passed distally down the subcutaneous tunnel in the arm and sutured to the deltoid muscle insertion. The broad muscle end taken from the lumbodorsal fascia is rotated up to the acromioclavicular incision. The arm is flexed to 70° to 80° and abducted to 60°, and the proximal end of the transferred latissimus dorsi muscle is sutured to the periosteum of the anterolateral aspect of the acromion and clavicle or to the trapezius muscle insertion. The position of the neurovascular bundle must be checked frequently to be sure that no excessive torsion or traction is applied; at the completion of the transfer, the bundle should rest anterolaterally on the proximal border of the pectoralis major muscle. Again, a splint is worn for 3 months with the arm abducted to 60° to 90°, after which the splint is worn only at night and range of motion exercises are begun. The splint is worn at night for 3 months.

Subscapularis Nerve and Muscle (Fifth and Sixth Cervical Nerve Roots)

The subscapularis nerve and muscle are usually functioning in brachial plexus palsy affecting the fifth and sixth cervical nerve roots, but occasionally the muscle's function is decreased, resulting in anterior glenohumeral instability. The subscapularis muscle's function as an internal rotator can be replaced by transfer either of the pectoralis major tendon or of the serratus anterior tendon to the lesser tuberosity of the humerus. It should be noted that the transferred pectoralis major tendon must be passed posterior to the conjoined tendon to duplicate the function of the subscapularis muscle; otherwise, anterior instability may result.

Transfer of the Serratus Anterior Tendon to the Lesser Tuberosity

Technique The patient is placed in lateral decubitus with the involved side up. Through a saber-cut incision over the shoulder, the trapezius muscle is reflected up and back, exposing the superomedial angle of the scapula. The levator scapulae muscle is taken off its insertion here, and the underlying serratus anterior muscle is identified. The insertion of the proximal 2 digitations of the serratus anterior muscle merges with the medial limit of the subscapularis muscle on the anterior aspect of the scapula. These are separated with sharp dissection. The 2 muscular slips are now rolled into a tube and held with suture; the tube is left long for rerouting. The arm is then elevated to 60° to 90°, and an incision is made along the posterior wall of the axilla. The neurovascular bundle is retracted upward and laterally, and blunt dissection is used to open a path proximal to the superior border of the serratus anterior muscle to the first rib. The tube consisting of the proximal two digitations is passed anteriorly with use of the attached suture and is sewn into the tendinous tissue over the lesser tuberosity of the humerus.[20] The arm is splinted with the shoulder maintained in an internally rotated position and the forearm against the trunk, and the splint is worn full-time for 3 months. It is then worn only at night for another 3 months, and range of motion exercises are begun during this period.

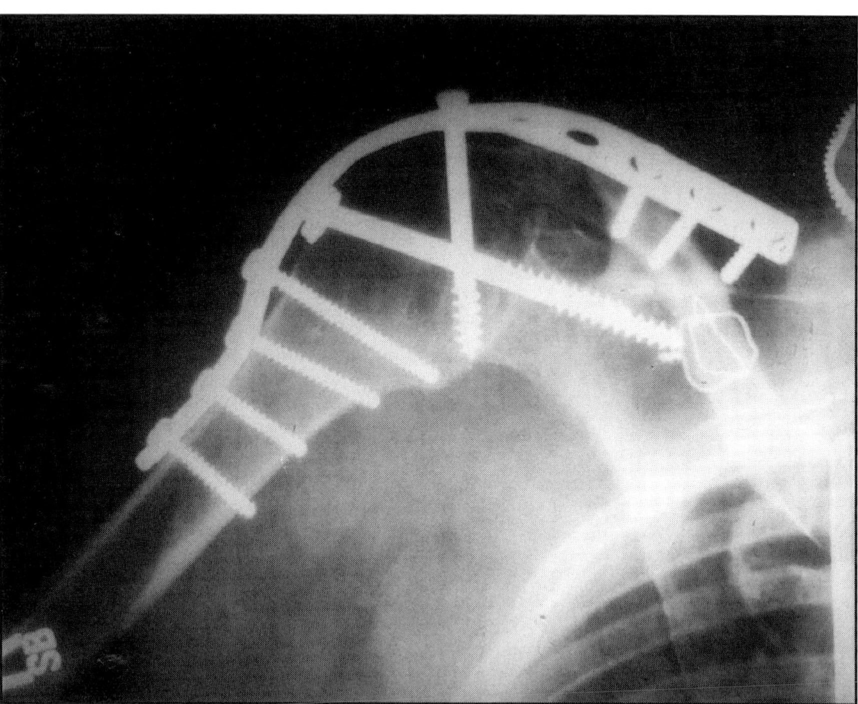

Fig. 10 Radiograph made after a shoulder arthrodesis performed with a 4.5-mm AO dynamic compression plate.

Multiple Nerve Deficits

Occasionally, multiple transfers are required for multiple nerve deficits. These procedures most commonly involve some combination of the biceps-triceps-latissimus dorsi tendon transfers described by Harmon[22] (first used in the treatment of functional losses secondary to poliomyelitis) and based on Ober's earlier work.[23] Transfers performed in combination include transfer of the posterior third of the deltoid muscle to the lateral aspect of the clavicle, as described, together with transfer of the tendinous origins of the long head of the triceps muscle and the short head of the biceps muscle to the lateral aspect of the acromion, to aid in abduction, and transfer of the latissimus dorsi and teres major tendons or of the tendinous insertion of the clavicular head of the pectoralis major muscle posteriorly, to provide external rotation of the humerus. Multiple options are available, and one common combination will be described.

Multiple Transfers of the Biceps, Triceps, and Latissimus Dorsi Tendons

Technique Through a saber-cut incision, the posterior third of the deltoid muscle is taken off the scapular spine. The tendon of the long head of the triceps muscle is released from the scapula, and the latissimus dorsi tendon is taken off its insertion on the humerus. The tendon of the short head of the biceps muscle is removed from the coracoid process. The arm is held in 90° of abduction and 30° of external rotation. The tendon of the short head of the biceps muscle is passed through the anterior third of the deltoid muscle and sutured to the anterior aspect of the acromion with the elbow flexed to 90°. The tendon of the long head of the triceps muscle is then sutured to the posterolateral aspect of the acromion with the elbow flexed to 30°. The released tendon of the latissimus dorsi muscle is sutured under tension to the insertion of the infraspinatus muscle. The released posterior third of the deltoid muscle is then sutured over these structures to the anterolateral aspect of the acromion and the lateral aspect of the clavicle. The arm is splinted in 60° to 90° of abduction, 30° of external rotation, and 90° of elbow flexion.

Arthrodesis

When a patient has severe combined lesions and the surgeon cannot reasonably expect to achieve glenohumeral stability with any of the described soft-tissue procedures, it may be necessary to perform a glenohumeral arthrodesis to treat pain, instability, or arthritis (Fig. 10). Arthrodesis of the shoulder requires scapular stability and functional scapular muscles. Instability or incongruity of the shoulder should not be addressed if the arm or hand is nonfunctional. However, shoulder arthrodesis can enhance the power of weak elbow flexion or extension transfers by isolating the forces of the transfer to the elbow.

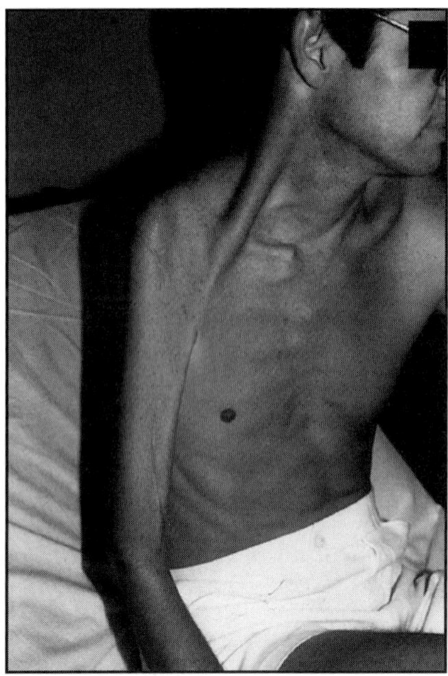

Fig. 11 Photograph showing extension after transfer of the sternocleidomastoid muscle to the biceps tendon lengthened with a fascia lata graft.

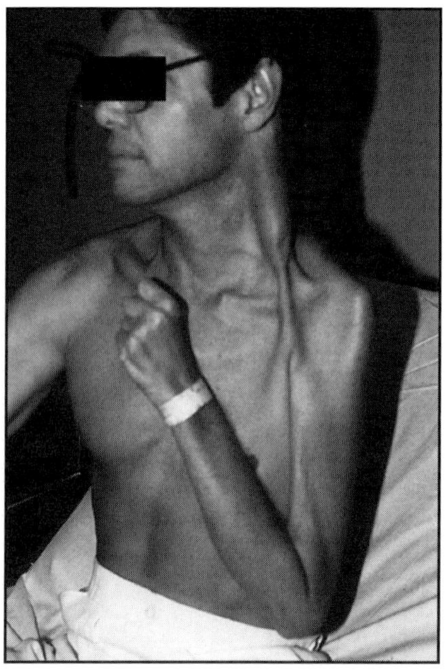

Fig. 12 Photograph showing flexion after transfer of the sternocleidomastoid muscle to the biceps tendon lengthened with a fascia lata graft.

Tendon Transfers About the Elbow

Elbow flexion is frequently absent or diminished in obstetrical brachial plexus palsy involving the musculocutaneous nerve (the fifth and sixth cervical nerve roots) and therefore impairing the function of the biceps and brachialis muscles. Numerous procedures to restore this function have been described, with one of the earliest being the proximal reattachment of the origin of the flexor-pronator muscle group as outlined by Steindler.[24] Despite later modifications to reduce some of the unwanted sequelae (for example, pronation deformity) of this transfer, other transfers are now often preferred to the Steindler flexorplasty, although it has the benefit of being simple to perform. Another procedure that was used more widely in the past is anterior transfer of the triceps tendon insertion, which provides better strength of elbow flexion than the Steindler transfer does but leaves the patient unable to actively extend the elbow on the side of the operation in order to use crutches or to assist in transfer from bed to chair. An early but cosmetically unacceptable procedure was transfer of the sternocleidomastoid muscle (Figs. 11 and 12), which involves detaching this muscle from its insertion and linking it to the insertion of the biceps muscle by means of a long strip of fascia lata. This transfer is now generally avoided.

Proximal Transfer of the Origin of the Flexor-Pronator Muscle Group

Technique A curvilinear incision is made at the posteromedial aspect of the elbow, passing behind the medial epicondyle and angling laterally (radially) both proximal and distal to this level. The medial antebrachial cutaneous nerve is identified and protected. The ulnar nerve is transposed anteriorly. The median nerve is identified between the 2 heads of the pronator teres muscle and mobilized from surrounding tissue, with protection of the branches to the pronator teres muscle. An osteotome is used to remove a piece of the medial epicondyle that is less than 1 cm in thickness with its attached origin of the flexor-pronator muscle group. This mass is reflected distally, and the muscles are mobilized from inferior attachments, with their innervation protected as the dissection progresses. The elbow is then flexed to 130°, and the flexor mass and the epicondyle are pulled proximally and radially several centimeters to the anterior humeral cortex. The site is chosen such that the elbow can be flexed to 60° with the wrist and fingers fully flexed. An attachment site then is prepared, with a roughened spot made on the humerus. The epicondylar segment is placed in this spot, and the transfer is secured with a screw inserted over a washer. The epicondyle can be predrilled for ease of fixation. The anterolateral fixation prevents the pronation deformity that was seen after early versions of the transfer, which involved a more medial attachment. The arm is then splinted with the elbow flexed to 90° and the forearm in full supination, and this position is maintained for 4 to 6 weeks. Gentle range of motion exercises are then begun to regain all but the terminal 30° of elbow extension for 8 weeks; then, full extension is slowly regained with continued therapy.

Anterior Transfer of the Triceps Tendon

As described by Carroll and Hill,[25,26] this procedure was designed for patients in whom paralysis or injury had left the flexor-pronator mass unusable for transfer.

Technique The patient is placed in lateral decubitus with the arm draped free. A posterior incision is made, curving slightly around the tip of the olecranon. The ulnar nerve is identified medially. The lateral intermuscular septum is exposed. The triceps tendon insertion is taken off the ulna with a longitudinal extension of periosteum. The muscle is carefully elevated off the posterior part of the humerus for 10 to 15 cm, with protection of both the radial nerve as it courses anteriorly through the lateral intermuscular septum and the previously identified ulnar nerve medially. The triceps insertion with attached periosteum is then rolled into a tube. Next, an anterior incision is made to identify the biceps tendon insertion. The interval between the brachioradialis and pronator teres muscles is developed, with protection of the anterior neurovascular bundle, and the bicipital tuberosity is identified. A tunnel lateral to the radius is created from back to front, and the tube consisting of the triceps and attached periosteum is pulled anteriorly, superficial to the radial nerve. The elbow is flexed to 90°, and the forearm is supinated fully. The triceps is pulled to maximum tension, and the tube of tendon and attached periosteum is sutured to the biceps tendon near its insertion. The arm is splinted in this position for 4 to 6 weeks, after which time active range of motion exercises are begun.

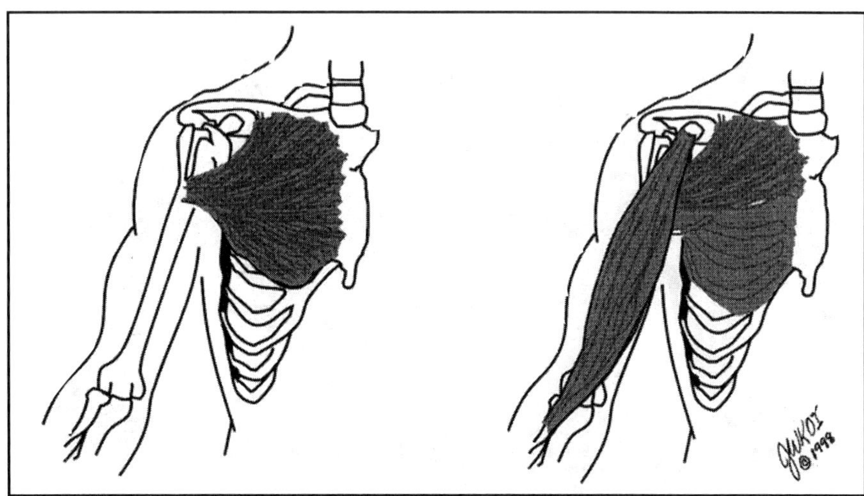

Fig. 13 Drawings illustrating the bipolar pectoralis major flexorplasty as described by Schottstaedt and associates.[28] The drawing on the left shows the sternal and clavicular origins of the pectoralis major muscle. The drawing on the right illustrates how only the sternal origin is taken down, rolled into a tube, and tunneled under the skin to be attached to the insertion of the biceps tendon. The insertion of the pectoralis major muscle is taken off the humerus and is either attached to the coracoid process (sutured to the conjoined tendon) or, for greater shoulder stability, sutured through drill holes in the anterior aspect of the acromion.

Bipolar Transposition of the Pectoralis Major Muscle

Clark,[27] in 1946, described a transfer of the inferior aspect of the sternal origin of the pectoralis major muscle to the biceps tendon with good restoration of elbow flexion in one patient. Schottstaedt and associates[28] modified this procedure, releasing both the origin and the insertion of the inferior two thirds of the muscle. The senior author (JBB) prefers this complete transposition. The procedure requires a grade of at least 4 of 5 for the strength of the sternal head of the pectoralis major muscle.

Technique The patient is placed supine, and the affected extremity and ipsilateral side of the chest are prepared and draped. An oblique incision is made from the axilla downward and medially, and the chondrosternal two thirds of the pectoralis major muscle is identified and elevated from the ribs and sternum. Care is taken, as the dissection progresses cephalad, to identify and preserve the neurovascular bundle entering the underside of the muscle from beneath the clavicle. Electrocautery facilitates elevation of the muscle from the underlying ribs and intercostal muscles. As dissection of the pectoralis major muscle progresses, the intercostal perforating arteries are encountered near the sternum. These must be cauterized or ligated; otherwise, they may retract and cause bleeding within the thoracic cavity. The humeral insertion of the chondrosternal portion of the muscle is released through the same incision. The insertion of the superior third of the pectoralis major muscle (originating from the clavicle) is left intact. A second incision is made over the biceps tendon insertion in the volar aspect of the proximal part of the forearm, and a subcutaneous tunnel is bluntly created, joining the 2 incisions along the anterolateral aspect of the arm. The origin of the pectoralis major muscle released from the ribs and sternum is rolled into a tube and passed down this tunnel into the second incision. With the elbow flexed to 90°, the tube consisting of the muscle origin is secured to the distal part of the biceps tendon or the bicipital tuberosity on the radius. One method is to use nonabsorbable suture passed in a crisscross weave through the muscle-end tube, pulled through drill holes in the radial neck with use of straight free needles, and tied through a small dorsal incision. The free humeral insertion of the pectoralis major muscle is drawn upward and sutured to the conjoined tendon at the coracoid process (Fig. 13). The neurovascular bundle must be kept free from any torsion or traction. Postoperatively, the arm is splinted with the elbow flexed to 90°; the splint is worn full-time for 3 months and then only at night for another 3 months. A program of active flexion is begun at 6 weeks.

Bipolar Transfer of the Latissimus Dorsi Muscle

A second option is to transfer the latissimus dorsi muscle, as described by

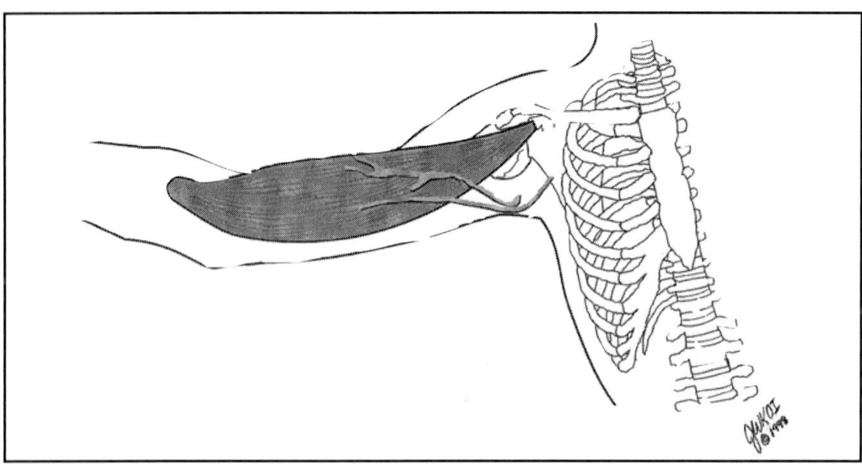

Fig. 14 Drawing illustrating how the spinous origin of the latissimus dorsi muscle is rolled into a tube and tunneled subcutaneously to the biceps tendon insertion. The humeral insertion of the latissimus dorsi tendon is taken down and reattached, as is done with a transfer of the pectoralis major muscle, either to the conjoined tendon origin on the coracoid process or to the anterior aspect of the acromion. Bipolar latissimus dorsi flexorplasty as described by Hovnanian.[17]

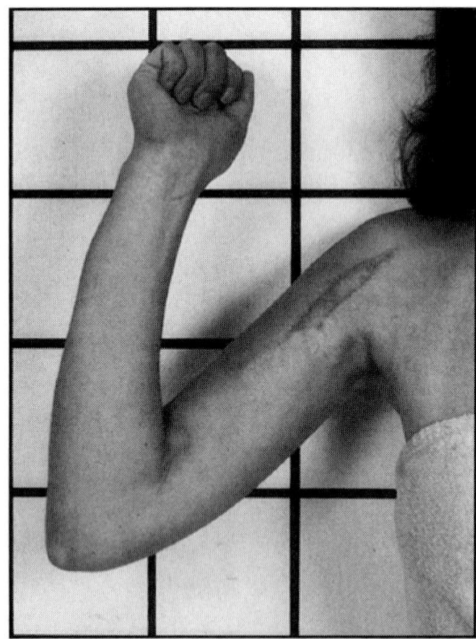

Fig. 15 Photograph showing elbow flexion after bipolar latissimus dorsi flexorplasty as described by Hovnanian.[29]

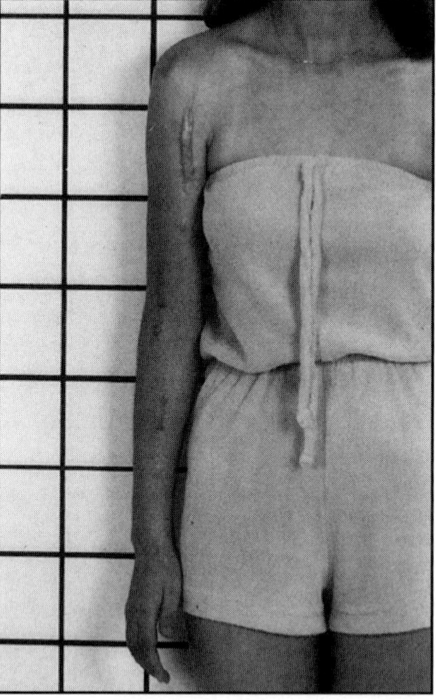

Fig. 16 Photograph showing elbow extension after bipolar latissimus dorsi flexorplasty described by Hovnanian.[29]

Hovnanian.[29] This procedure also requires a grade of 4 of 5 for the strength of the donor muscle. Like the transfer of the bipolar pectoralis major muscle, the procedure is technically demanding but results in moderate elbow flexion superior to that seen with other techniques.

Technique The patient is placed in lateral decubitus, and the affected arm and hemithorax are prepared and draped. A long incision is made beginning over the origin of the latissimus dorsi muscle, following its anterolateral margin, and crossing the axillary fold to proceed down the medial border of the arm to the antecubital fossa. The origin of the latissimus dorsi muscle with its fascial investment is released. The proximal margin is cut across its muscle fibers posteriorly. The neurovascular bundle enters in the proximal third and is carefully preserved. Gradual dissection with electrocautery frees the muscle from surrounding tissue, with communicating vessels cauterized or ligated as required. The thoracodorsal nerve is readily identified entering the undersurface of the muscle and coursing from the apex of the axilla. Once the entire muscle has been freed, the only remaining attachments are its humeral insertion and the neurovascular bundle. The muscle origin is taken to the distal aspect of the arm and sutured to the biceps tendon and the radial tuberosity. The insertion is released and sutured to the conjoined tendon origin on the coracoid process or the anterior aspect of the acromion (Fig. 14). The wounds are closed, and the arm is splinted with the elbow flexed to 90°. The splint is worn full-time for the first 3 months, except when range of motion exercises are performed, and it is worn only at night for another 3 months. Active flexion and extension are begun at 6 weeks (Figs. 15 and 16), but passive extension is avoided for 3 months.

Free Microneurovascular Transfer of the Gracilis Muscle

A free microneurovascular muscle transfer may be performed[30,31] in a limited number of patients. The most commonly selected donor muscle is the gracilis.[32] This procedure is indicated when no functional muscles are available for transfer in a child who has a good passive range of elbow motion and no or very weak active elbow flexion.

Technique A medial thigh incision is made, extending longitudinally from a point 2 cm distal to the pubic tubercle to a point 10 cm proximal to the adductor tubercle of the femur. Dissection is carried down to the longitudinal fibers of the gracilis muscle. Several vascular pedicles enter the muscle, but the dominant pedicle, comprising branches from the medial femoral circumflex artery and vein, along with the motor branch to the gracilis from the anterior division of the obturator nerve, can be found on the undersurface of the muscle, approximately one-quarter of the distance from the pubis to the adductor tubercle. The tendon of insertion is sectioned from the femur. Lesser vascular pedicles are ligated as the muscle is elevated from distal to proximal. The dominant neurovascular pedicle is then ligated and transected as close to the exit of the nerve and vessels from their main trunks as can be safely performed. The proximal part of the tendon is divided, and the muscle is taken from the donor site to the affected arm. An anterior axillary incision is made, and dissection is carried out to the level of the insertion of the pectoralis major tendon on the humerus. The tendon of origin of the free gracilis muscle is passed deep to the pectoralis major tendon and fixed to the coracoid process with interosseous wiring or is attached to the conjoined tendon with nonabsorbable suture. Additional attachments to surrounding fascia, the clavicle, or the second rib are performed as necessary with suture fixation. A second incision is made over the anterior aspect of the proximal part of the forearm, and the biceps tendon insertion is identified. The distal end of the free gracilis muscle transfer is tunneled subcutaneously down the anterior aspect of the arm and woven into the biceps tendon insertion with the elbow flexed to 110°. An anterior incision is next made on the chest in line with the fourth rib, and the intercostal nerves beneath the third, fourth, and fifth ribs are identified. The nerves are sectioned anteriorly and taken posterior to the midaxial line, where the intercostal nerves of the fourth and fifth thoracic nerve roots are sutured into the motor nerve to the gracilis, and the intercostal nerve of the third thoracic nerve root is implanted directly into the muscle in neurotization fashion. Arterial anastomosis is made with use of the lateral thoracic, thoracodorsal, or thoracoacromial artery. Venous outflow is through the thoracoacromial or cephalic vein. Postoperative vascular assessment is critical to the successful application of this transfer as ischemia or decreased outflow may require reexploration of the microvascular anastomoses. Postoperative rehabilitation requires a reinnervation time of 6 months to 1 year for maximum functional return.

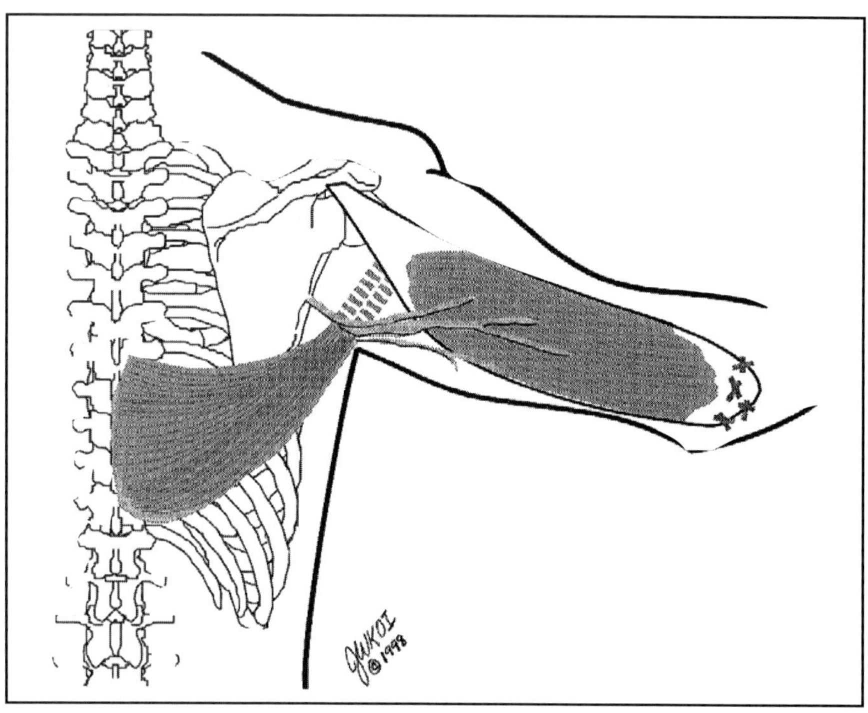

Fig. 17 Drawing illustrating bipolar latissimus dorsi tricepsplasty as described by Hovnanian.[29] The spinous origin of the muscle is tunneled subcutaneously down the posterior aspect of the arm and reattached into either the triceps tendon or the olecranon. The tendinous insertion is taken off the humerus and reattached to the posterior aspect of the acromion.

Bipolar Latissimus Dorsi Tricepsplasty

Function of the triceps muscle may be restored in selected patients with transfer of the latissimus dorsi muscle (Fig. 17) as described by Hovnanian[29] and previously in this chapter. Gravity provides adequate extension for patients who have unilateral brachial plexus palsy. Involvement of the lower extremity or bilateral involvement of the upper extremity may require forceful extension for walking with crutches or for weight transfer.

Deformity of the Elbow

As first summarized by Aitken,[33] a series of changes in the proximal parts of the radius and ulna is frequently seen in patients who have obstetrical brachial plexus palsy. These changes tend to occur in patients who have some, although incomplete, recovery. The commonly observed sequence begins with increased curvature of the ulna and slight backward displacement of the proximal part of the radius. The radial epiphysis becomes obliquely oriented with respect to the shaft. Left untreated, complete posterior dislocation of the radius occurs, a conical deformity of the radial head develops, and the head articulates with an abnormally flattened capitellum. Aitken suggested that the changes in the ulna are due to the uneven pull of the triceps muscle against the nonfunctional biceps and brachialis muscles, complicated by splinting of the elbow in flexion for too long a period of time. The radial dislocation may be related to splinting in supination against the pull of the pronator teres and a contracted interosseous membrane. In his series, Aitken reduced elbow flexion to 45° at the first sign of such changes, and he weaned patients from splinting if and when biceps and brachialis function returned.

Other authors[1,34] have described the common occurrence of flexion contractures at the elbow in brachial plexus palsy. This can occur with overactivity of the biceps and brachialis. Medial and lateral instability can occur as well, necessitating augmentation or reefing of soft tissues. Incompetence of the annular ligament may necessitate reconstruction with a triceps tendon slip or fascia lata graft.[35]

Overview

Obstetrical brachial plexus palsy remains a challenging clinical problem, with few data regarding the outcomes of the wide variety of surgical procedures that have been described. Until recently, there have been no controlled clinical studies (of which we are aware) comparing different techniques, and surgeons have had to rely on reports summarizing results of individual procedures as compared with the natural history of the deformity. Rigorous and reproducible standardized outcomes measures are lacking, in part because of the wide variability in the severity of involvement of affected individuals, and this lack has made comparison difficult as well. The recent heightened interest in outcomes assessment appears to be leading to more work in this area, which will be crucial to the optimization of the care of patients who have this complicated disorder.

References

1. Tachdjian MO (ed): *Pediatric Orthopaedics,* ed 2. Philadelphia, PA, WB Saunders, 1990, vol 3, pp 2009–2082.
2. Waters PM: Obstetric brachial plexus injuries: Evaluation and management. *J Am Acad Orthop Surg* 1997;5:205–214.
3. Clarke HM, Curtis CG: An approach to obstetrical brachial plexus injuries. *Hand Clin* 1995;11:563–581.
4. Zancolli EA, Zancolli ER Jr: Palliative surgical procedures in sequelae of obstetric palsy. *Hand Clin* 1988;4:643–669.
5. Waters PM, Smith GR, Jaramillo D: Glenohumeral deformity secondary to brachial plexus birth palsy. *J Bone Joint Surg* 1998;80A:668–677.
6. Pearl ML, Edgerton BW: Glenoid deformity secondary to brachial plexus birth palsy. *J Bone Joint Surg* 1998;80A:659–667.
7. Waters PM, Peljovich AE: Shoulder reconstruction in patients with chronic brachial plexus birth palsy: A case control study. *Clin Orthop* 1999;364:144–152.
8. Troum S, Floyd WE III, Waters PM: Posterior dislocation of the humeral head in infancy associated with obstetrical paralysis: A case report. *J Bone Joint Surg* 1993;75A:1370–1375.
9. Comtet JJ, Herzberg G, Naasan IA: Biomechanical basis of transfers for shoulder paralysis. *Hand Clin* 1989;5:1–14.
10. Gilbert A: Long-term evaluation of brachial plexus surgery in obstetrical palsy. *Hand Clin* 1995;11:583–595.
11. Sever JW: The results of a new operation for obstetrical paralysis. *Am J Orthop Surg* 1918;16:248–257.
12. Carlioz H, Brahimi L: Place of internal disinsertion of the subscapularis muscle in the treatment of obstetric paralysis of the upper limb in children. *Ann Chir Infant* 1971;12:159–167.
13. Fairbank HAT: Birth palsy: Subluxation of the shoulder-joint in infants and young children. *Lancet* 1913;1:1217–1223.
14. Debeyre J, Patte D, Elmelik E: Repair of ruptures of the rotator cuff of the shoulder: With a note on advancement of the supraspinatus muscle. *J Bone Joint Surg* 1965;47B:36–42.
15. Hoffer MM, Wickenden R, Roper B: Brachial plexus birth palsies: Results of tendon transfers to the rotator cuff. *J Bone Joint Surg* 1978;60A:691–695.
16. L'Episcopo JB: Tendon transplantation in obstetrical paralysis. *Am J Surg* 1934;25: 122–125.
17. Covey DC, Riordan DC, Milstead ME, Albright JA: Modification of the L'Episcopo procedure for brachial plexus birth palsies. *J Bone Joint Surg* 1992;74B:897–901.
18. Harmon PH: Anterior transplantation of the posterior deltoid for shoulder palsy and dislocation in poliomyelitis. *Surg Gynecol Obstet* 1947;32:117–120.
19. Mayer L: Transplantation of the trapezius for paralysis of the abductors of the arm. *J Bone Joint Surg* 1927;9:412–420.
20. Saha AK: Surgery of the paralysed and flail shoulder. *Acta Orthop Scand* 1967;97(suppl): 5–90.
21. Itoh Y, Sasaki T, Ishiguro T, Uchinishi K, Yabe Y, Fukuda H: Transfer of latissimus dorsi to replace a paralysed anterior deltoid: A new technique using an inverted pedicled graft. *J Bone Joint Surg* 1987;69B:647–651.
22. Harmon PH: Surgical reconstruction of the paralytic shoulder by multiple muscle transplantations. *J Bone Joint Surg* 1950;32A:583–595.
23. Ober FR: An operation to relieve paralysis of the deltoid muscle. *JAMA* 1932;99:2182.
24. Steindler A: Tendon transplantation in the upper extremity. *Am J Surg* 1939;44:260–271.
25. Carroll RE: Restoration of flexor power to the flail elbow by transplantation of the triceps tendon. *Surg Gynecol Obstet* 1952;95:685–688.
26. Carroll RE, Hill NA: Triceps transfer to restore elbow flexion: A study of fifteen patients with paralytic lesions and arthrogryposis. *J Bone Joint Surg* 1970;52A:239–244.
27. Clark JMP: Reconstruction of biceps brachii by pectoral muscle transplantation. *Br J Surg* 1946;34:180–181.
28. Schottstaedt ER, Larsen LJ, Bost FC: Complete muscle transposition. *J Bone Joint Surg* 1955;37A:897–919.
29. Hovnanian AP: Latissimus dorsi transplantation for loss of flexion or extension at the elbow: A preliminary report on technic. *Ann Surg* 1956;143:493–499.
30. Chuang DC, Epstein MD, Yeh MC, Wei FC: Functional restoration of elbow flexion in brachial plexus injuries: Results in 167 patients (excluding obstetric brachial plexus injury). *J Hand Surg* 1993;18A:285–291.
31. Chuang DCC: Functioning free muscle transplantation, in Peimer CA (ed): *Surgery of the Hand and Upper Extremity.* New York, NY, McGraw-Hill, 1996, vol 2, pp 1901–1910.
32. Krakauer JD, Wood M: Adult injuries and salvage, in Peimer CA (ed): *Surgery of the Hand and Upper Extremity.* New York, NY, McGraw-Hill, 1996, pp 1411–1442.
33. Aitken J: Deformity of the elbow joint as a sequel to Erb's obstetrical paralysis. *J Bone Joint Surg* 1952;34B:352–365.
34. Leffert RD (ed): *Brachial Plexus Injuries.* New York, NY, Churchill Livingstone, 1985, pp 189–235.
35. Oner FC, Diepstraten AF: Treatment of chronic post-traumatic dislocation of the radial head in children. *J Bone Joint Surg* 1993;75B: 577–581.

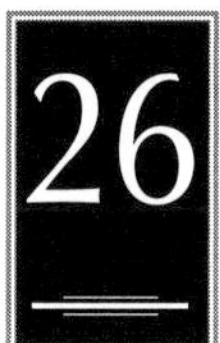

Sternoclavicular Joint Injuries and Disorders

Michael J. Medvecky, MD
Joseph D. Zuckerman, MD

Introduction

The sternoclavicular joint (SCJ) is injured infrequently because of its medial location. However, indirect forces transmitted medially from the shoulder can result in sprains, fractures, or dislocations. Difficulty with diagnosis may be a result of limitations of standard radiography as well as the relative rarity of the injury. Conditions common to all synovial joints, including osteoarthritis, rheumatoid arthritis, or sepsis, may also affect this joint. The proximity of vital neurovascular and visceral structures makes thorough evaluation and accurate diagnosis imperative. The purpose of this chapter is to review the diverse injuries and disorders that can affect the SCJ and discuss the rationale for diagnostic and treatment options.

Anatomy

Osseous Structure

The SCJ is the only true articulation between the axial skeleton and the appendicular skeleton (Fig. 1). This diarthrodial joint has the least amount of bony stability of any major joint in the body.[1,2] The medial end of the clavicle is concave front to back and convex vertically and is relatively incongruous with the clavicular notch of the sternum. Less than half of the medial clavicle articulates with the upper portion of the sternum.[3,4] The anatomic configuration of the bony structure provides minimal inherent stability.

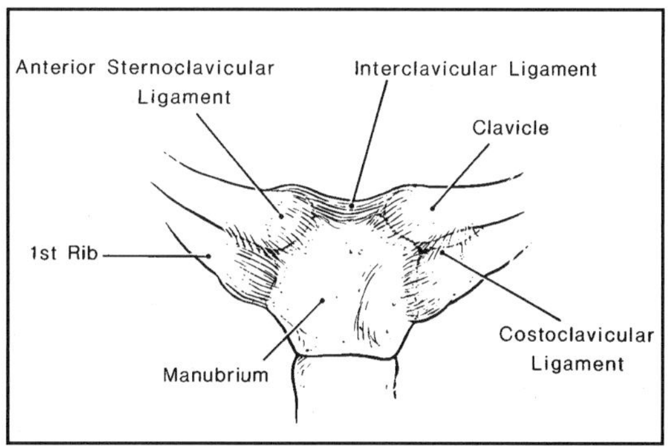

Fig. 1 Gross osseous anatomy of the sternoclavicular joint and ligamentous supports.

Intra-articular Disk

The intra-articular disk is a fibrocartilaginous structure that arises from the synchondral junction of the first rib. It passes between the medial end of the clavicle and the lateral aspect of the manubrium and inserts onto the superior and posterior aspects of the medial clavicle.[5] Anteriorly and posteriorly, the disk blends into the fibers of the capsular ligament. It divides the SCJ into 2 synovial spaces, and acts as a checkrein against medial displacement of the clavicular head.[5]

Ligamentous Supports

The costoclavicular ligament or rhomboid ligament attaches the supermedial aspect of the first rib and its adjacent synchondral junction with the sternum to the inferior surface of the medial end of the clavicle. It consists of an anterior and a posterior fasciculus, which are directed laterally and medially, respectively, and provides stability during rotation and elevation of the medial clavicle.[6,7]

The interclavicular ligament connects the superior aspect of the clavicles to the superior aspect of the manubrium and the capsular ligaments.

The capsular ligament represents the thickenings of the anterosuperior and posterior joint capsule. The clavicular attachment is primarily into the epiphysis of the medial clavicle with some secondary blending of the fibers into the metaphysis.[2,5,6] In a cadavaric ligament-sectioning study, Bearn[6] demonstrated that the capsular ligament is the most important structure in preventing upward displacement of the medial clavicle. Sectioning of the interclavicular, costoclavicular, and intra-articular disk ligaments had no effect on clavicular position. However, division of the capsular ligament alone resulted in downward depression of the clavicle under its own weight.

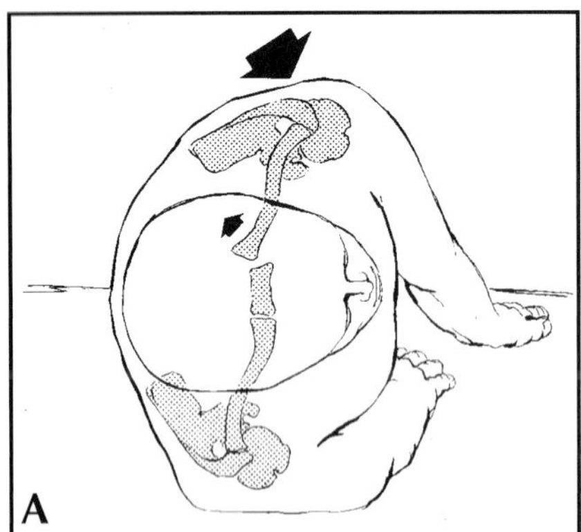

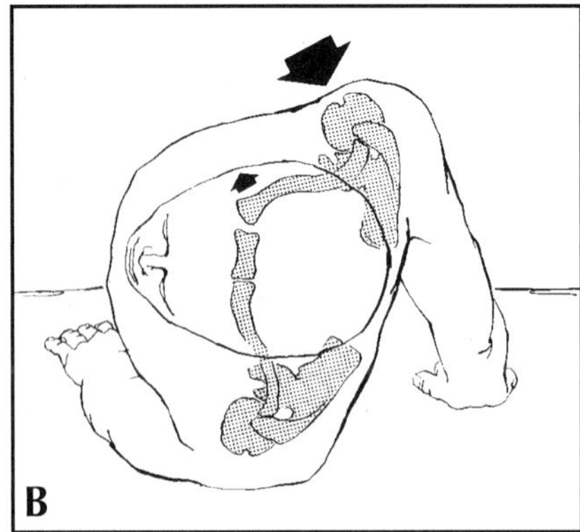

Fig. 2 Mechanisms that produce anterior and posterior sternoclavicular joint dislocations. **A,** An anteromedially directed force applied to the posterolateral aspect of the shoulder results in reciprocal posterior displacement of the medial clavicle. **B,** A posteromedially directed force applied to the anterolateral aspect of the shoulder results in reciprocal anterior displacement of the medial clavicle. (Reproduced with permission from Rockwood CA Jr, Wirth MA: Injuries to the sternoclavicular joint, in Rockwood CA Jr, Green DP, Bucholz RW, Heckman JD (eds): *Rockwood and Green's Fractures in Adults*, ed 4. Philadelphia, PA, Lippincott-Raven, 1996, vol 2, pp 1415–1471.)

Ossification Pattern

The clavicle is the first long bone of the body to ossify (fifth intrauterine week), but the epiphysis at the medial end of the clavicle is both the last in the body to appear and the last to close. The medial clavicular epiphysis ossifies between the 18th and 20th years and fuses with the shaft of the clavicle between the 23rd and 25th years.[2,5,8,9] This is important when evaluating medial clavicle injuries in patients younger than 25 years of age.

Biomechanics of the Sternoclavicular Joint

The shoulder consists of 4 distinct articulations—glenhumeral, acromioclavicular, scapulothoracic, and sternoclavicular—that allow the arm to be positioned in space and provide a range of motion that exceeds that of any other joint.[3] Because most scapulothoracic motion occurs through the SCJ, rigid fixation or fusion would greatly limit shoulder motion.[2,4,5,9]

The SCJ is divided into 2 functional units. Anterior and posterior translation (clavicular protraction and retraction) occurs between the sternum and the meniscus. Superior and inferior translation (clavicular elevation and depression) takes place between the clavicle and the meniscus.[3] The clavicle can also rotate about its long axis. Inman and associates[10] noted 4° of clavicular elevation for every 10° of arm elevation through the first 90° of motion. Beyond 90° of forward elevation, there was negligible sternoclavicular motion. The clavicle is capable of approximately 40° of rotation along its longitudinal axis. Reciprocal motion occurs at the SCJ and acromioclavicular joints during clavicular protraction or retraction and elevation or depression, but not with rotation. The role each ligament plays in providing stability to the SCJ depends on the sternal and clavicular position as well as the arm position and the applied load. However, little quantitative information exists. Bearn's study demonstrated the dominant role of the capsular ligament in maintaining shoulder "poise," but only with an applied vertical load.[6] The role that each ligament and the osseous architecture contribute to the stability of the SCJ has yet to be determined using variously applied loads and differential glenhumeral positioning.

Sternoclavicular Joint Injuries

Incidence

Dislocations of the SCJ are exceedingly rare injuries. In 1958, Cave[11] reported on over 1,600 dislocations occurring around the shoulder. Only 3% of these injuries were SCJ dislocations. Anterior SCJ dislocations occur much more frequently than do posterior dislocations. Rockwood and Wirth[2] reported 50 posterior dislocations out of 185 traumatic SCJ injuries, whereas Nettles and Linscheid[12] reported 3 posterior dislocations in a series of 60 SCJ dislocations. In total, only 102 posterior SCJ dislocations have been reported in the English-language literature over the past 65 years.[13]

Mechanism of Injury

SCJ dislocations may result from either a direct or an indirect mechanism. The direct mechanism consists of a blow applied to the anteromedial aspect of the clavicle resulting in a posterior dislocation of the SCJ; however, a direct mechanism is not associated with an anterior dislocation. The indirect mechanism occurs when an anteriorly directed force is applied to the posterolateral aspect of the shoulder resulting in reciprocal posterior displacement of the medial clavicle (Fig. 2, *A*), leading to a posterior dislocation. A posteriorly directed force applied to the anterolateral aspect of the shoulder will result in reciprocal anterior displacement of the medial clavicle (Fig. 2, *B*), producing anterior dislocation. During anterior dislocation, the first rib may contribute to the instability by acting as a fulcrum, levering the sternal end of the clavicle.

Clinical Presentation

Patients with injury to the SCJ may present with complaints of pain localized to this area. The arm usually is held across the chest, occasionally with the support of the contralateral arm, and any glenohumeral or scapulothoracic movement may exacerbate the pain. If a dislocation has occurred, the shoulder may appear

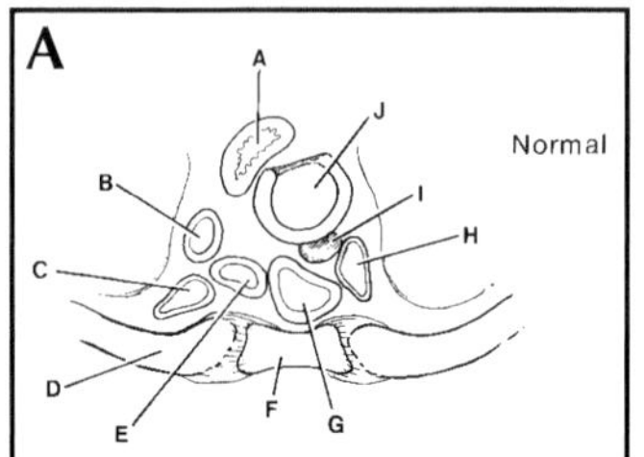

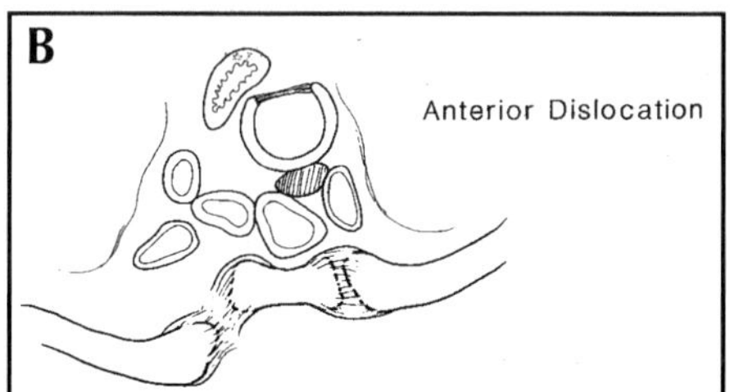

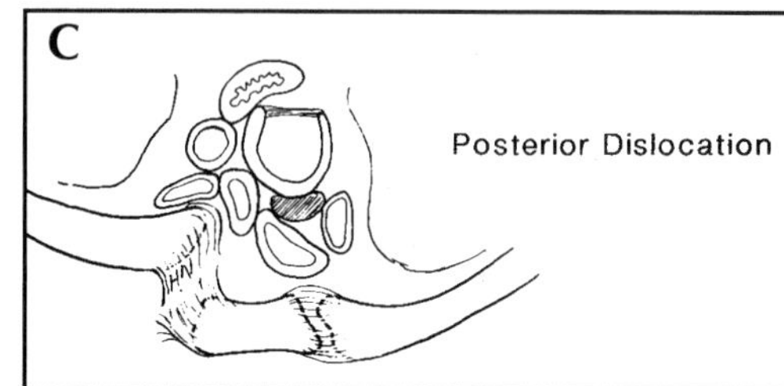

Fig. 3 Cross-sectional anatomy through the sternoclavicular joint. **A,** A: esophagus, B: left subclavian artery, C: left subclavian vein, D: clavicle, E: left common carotid artery, F: manubrium, G: right innominate artery, H: right subclavian vein, I: lymph node, J: trachea. **B,** Anterior sternoclavicular dislocation. **C,** Posterior sternoclavicular dislocation demonstrating compression of mediastinal structures. (Reproduced with permission from Zuckerman JD, Buchalter JS: Shoulder injuries, in Zuckerman JD (ed): *Comprehensive Care of Orthopaedic Injuries in the Elderly.* München, Germany, Urban & Schwarzenberg, 1990, p 292.)

shortened, and the head may be tilted to the ipsilateral side and rotated to the contralateral side secondary to sternocleidomastoid muscle spasm. With an anterior dislocation, the medial clavicle may be visible, prominent, and easily palpable anterior to the manubrium (Fig. 3, *B*). With posterior dislocation, there may be a sulcus of the SCJ region, and the lateral border of the manubrium may be easily palpable inferior to the sternal notch (Fig. 4). However, the degree of deformity associated with posterior dislocations can be quite subtle. Swelling over the SCJ may mask a posterior dislocation. The pain associated with posterior dislocations is usually more severe than with anterior dislocations. In addition, there may be symptoms of dyspnea, dysphagia, or a sensation of tightness in the throat. Signs of venous congestion may be present in the neck or upper extremities, or there may be asymmetric pulses compared with the contralateral limb. These symptoms result from compression of the vascular and visceral structures within the mediastinum (Fig. 3, *C*).

Radiologic Examination

Routine chest radiographs may demonstrate asymmetry of the SCJ compared with the contralateral side (Fig. 5, *B* and *C*). Rockwood[9] described the 40° cephalic-tilt or "serendipity view" that is a true caudocephalic view of both SCJs and the medial clavicles (Fig. 5, *A*). The affected clavicle will appear superior when an anterior dislocation is present and inferior when a posterior dislocation is present (Fig 5, *D*).

The Hobbs view is obtained by having the patient lean forward over the x-ray table with the arms straddling the cassette.[2,5,14] The X-ray beam passes through the neck. Patients in severe pain may be intolerant of this positioning. The image resembles a lordotic chest view, and in a posterior SCJ dislocation, the medial end of the clavicle is projected inferiorly.

The Heinig view is obtained in the supine position with the X-ray beam directed tangential to the joint and parallel to the opposite clavicle.[2,5] This view projects a lateral image of the manubrium with the clavicle articulating from its superior position. Anterior and posterior dislocations can be identified by their relationship to the manubrium.

Computed Tomography/Magnetic Resonance Imaging

Computed tomography (CT), by nature of its axial images and resolution quality, facilitates the characterization of injuries to the SCJ.[15,16] It clearly delineates the direction and degree of instability and at the same time can identify associated medial clavicle fractures or physeal injuries (Fig. 5, *E*). Magnetic resonance imaging (MRI) has the added benefit of delineating soft-tissue findings, that is, compression of mediastinal structures, that may accompany posterior dislocations (Fig. 5, *F*).

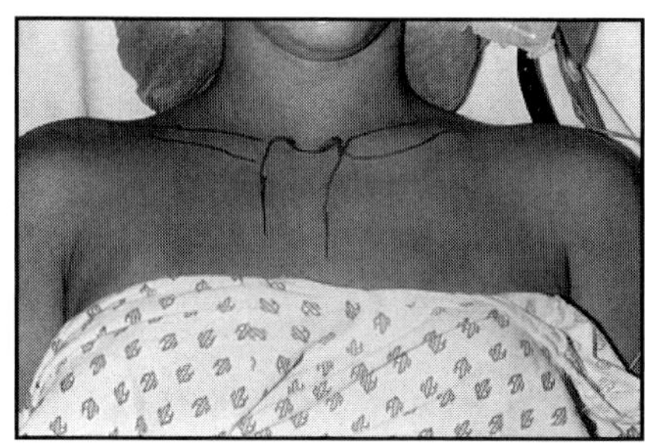

Fig. 4 Clinical photograph of a 30-year-old woman shown 1 week after being injured in a motor vehicle accident. The patient complains of pain localized to the right sternoclavicular joint. (Reproduced with permission from Rockwood CA Jr, Wirth MA: Injuries to the sternoclavicular joint, in Rockwood CA Jr, Green DP, Bucholz RW, Heckman JD (eds): *Rockwood and Green's Fractures in Adults,* ed 4. Philadelphia, PA, Lippincott-Raven, 1996, vol 2, pp 1415–1471.)

Sternoclavicular Sprain

Acute sprains of the SCJ may be classified as type I (mild), type II (moderate), or type III (severe, ie, dislocation) depending on the degree of injury to the supporting ligaments and joint capsule. In a type I injury, the ligaments are intact although some stretching of the fibers may occur. The clavicle appears in

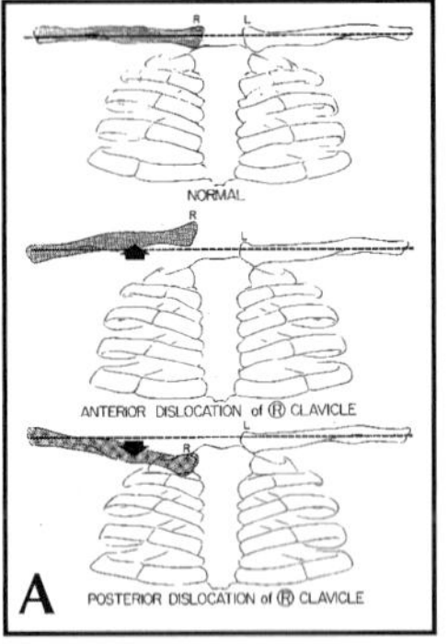

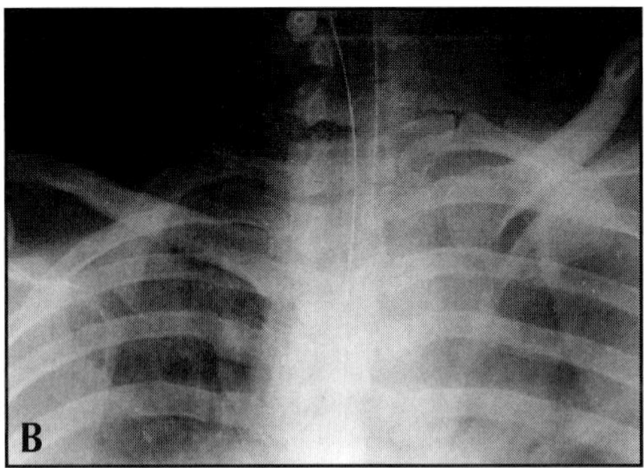
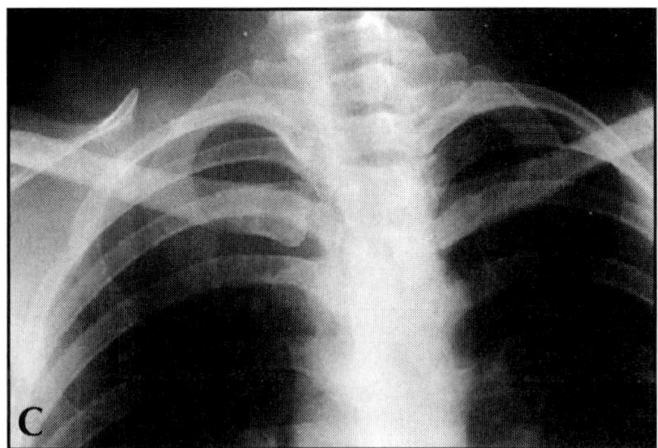
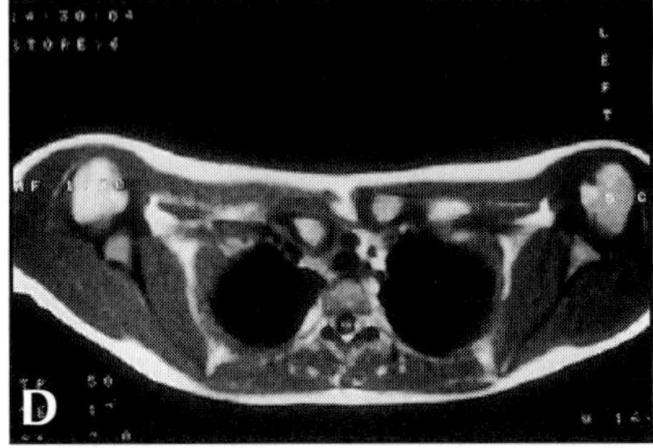
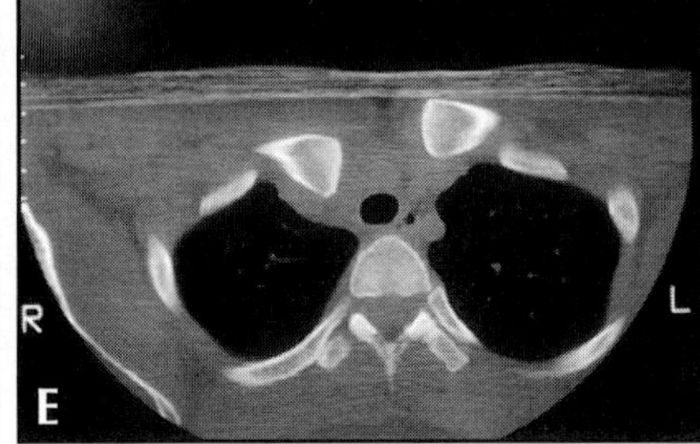
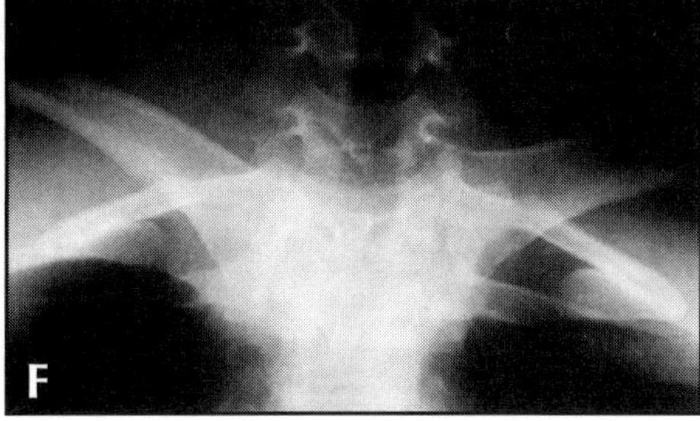

Fig. 5 A, Schematic of the "serendipity view" demonstrating position of the clavicle with anterior and posterior sternoclavicular joint (SCJ) dislocation. (Reproduced with permission from Rockwood CA Jr, Wirth MA: Injuries to the sternoclavicular joint, in Rockwood CA Jr, Green DP, Bucholz RW, Heckman JD (eds): *Rockwood and Green's Fractures in Adults*, ed 4. Philadelphia, PA, Lippincot-Raven, 1996, vol 2, pp 1415–1471.) **B,** Anteroposterior (AP) view of the chest demonstrating widening of the left SCJ and superior displacement of medial clavicle = anterior SCJ dislocation. **C,** AP view of the chest demonstrating left posterior SCJ dislocation. **D,** Serendipity view demonstrating right posterior SCJ dislocation. Note inferior displacement of medial clavicle relative to the manubrium. **E,** Computed tomography scan demonstrating posterior SC joint dislocation. Medial clavicular physes closed. **F,** Magnetic resonance image of medial clavicles just cephalad to sternal notch. Posterior SCJ dislocation is clearly delineated. Right subclavian vein, trachea, and esophagus do not appear to be compressed.

anatomic position with respect to its medial articulation. Only symptomatic treatment is necessary, which usually consists of local modalities (ice followed by heat) and analgesics for the first few days. A sling provides support for the upper extremity for 7 to 10 days, after which time a gradual return to full activities is encouraged.

In type II sprains, there is incomplete disruption of the ligamentous support and some degree of subluxation occurs that can be anterior or posterior. Symptomatic treatment is preferred, with local modalities and short-term immobilization. For anterior injuries, a simple sling is sufficient. For posterior injuries, some authors have recommended a figure-of-8 clavicle strap. The duration of immobilization should be 3 to 6 weeks, depending on the symptoms. However, activities should be limited for 8 to 10 weeks to prevent further injury.

A type III sprain or dislocation is the result of complete disruption of the supporting ligamentous structures. Anterior and posterior dislocation will be discussed separately.

Acute Anterior Dislocation

The vast majority of SCJ dislocations occur anteriorly, and most occur in young men as the result of motor vehicle accidents or athletic injuries.[2,5,9,12,17] Associated neurovascular injuries are rare, but a careful evaluation is mandatory.[18–21] With these injuries, the treatment options are closed reduction or, in unusual circumstances, open reduction and stabilization. Closed reductions often are unsuccessful with immediate redisplacement of the medial clavicle. This problem has led some authors to recommend the use of a sling as the definitive treatment.

Closed reduction may be done in the emergency department with use of narcotics and/or muscle relaxants or may require the use of general anesthesia in the operating room. The patient is placed supine with a bolster placed between the scapulae, and the affected arm placed off the edge of the bed. Traction is applied to the arm, which is positioned in approximately 90° of abduction and slight extension. Gentle pressure applied over the medial clavicle may assist in the reduction. However, once the pressure is released or the arm is brought back to the side, redisplacement usually occurs. If the medial clavicle remains unstable and redislocates, we prefer to use a sling as definitive treatment to support the arm until symptoms subside. However, if the medial clavicle remains reduced with the shoulder retracted, the use of a figure-of-8 dressing, a clavicle strap harness, or a plaster figure-of-8 cast may be successful in maintaining the reduction. Radiographs are obtained to assess the reduction. Immobilization should be maintained for a period of 6 weeks' follow-up.

In 1990, de Jong and Sukul[22] reported 5-year follow-up data on 10 patients with traumatic anterior SCJ dislocation. The next most common associated injury was craniofacial trauma. Nonsurgical treatment consisted of analgesics and immobilization with a sling or clavicle strap. Results of this treatment were good in 7 patients, fair in 2, and poor in 1 patient, and only the associated injuries had a negative effect on the functional outcome of the patient.

Open reduction of anterior dislocation is rarely indicated. It has been attempted using different approaches ranging from soft-tissue reconstruction to use of hardware for transfixion.[23–26] Most techniques have been associated with an unacceptably high incidence of redisplacement. In some situations, catastrophic and life-threatening complications have occurred with the use of pins for fixation.[27,28] In 1990, Lyons and Rockwood[28] reported on the complications of migration of pins used in shoulder surgery. Their literature review identified 49 complications in 47 patients. Twenty-one of the 47 patients had pins inserted for the treatment of SCJ dislocation. All of the SCJ dislocations were anterior, and pinning for the treatment of this injury resulted in the most serious consequences.

Migrated pins included smooth and threaded Kirschner wires (K-wires), K-wires bent at the skin surface, and Hagie pins. Seventeen pins migrated to major vascular structures, including the heart, ascending aorta, and subclavian and pulmonary arteries. Eight patients died, including 6 sudden deaths. All deaths occurred in patients who had fixation of the SCJ, and all patients died within 3 months after the surgery. Another 6 patients who had SCJ fixation survived cardiac tamponade only after a surgical intervention. The risk of pin migration and the disastrous complications that can ensue absolutely contraindicate the use of pins to secure the SCJ in surgical stabilizations.

Acute Posterior Dislocations

Of the 102 cases of posterior dislocations reported in the English-language literature over the past 65 years, 30% resulted in complications related to compression of the trachea, esophagus, brachial plexus, or great vessels, with 3 reported fatalities.[13] Because of the morbidity and mortality associated with posterior dislocations, a thorough examination should be performed and documented. Signs of dysphagia, dyspnea, venous congestion, carotid bruit, and arterial compromise are all indications of compression of vital structures.[18–21, 29–34] Complete radiographic studies should be used, including CT, MRI, and angiography if indicated. There should be coordination with thoracic or trauma surgery consultants before any reduction maneuvers. **(CD-35.1)**

Closed reduction (after physeal closure) is recommended for posterior dislocations in all patients older than 23 to 25 years of age who present within 7 days of the injury. Closed reductions should be avoided after 7 days because of the adhesions that can develop with retrosternal structures. The abduction-traction technique described for anterior dislocations also should be used for posterior dislocations. Application of traction to the ipsilateral upper extremity in a position of abduction and extension will usually elevate the medial clavicle, freeing it from its position behind the sternum. If this maneuver is not successful, the adduction method can be used. In this method, traction is applied to the adducted and slightly extended extremity. The downward traction on the arm may be more effective in elevating the medial clavicle. Either method can be assisted by manually manipulating the clavicle forward as the maneuver is performed. If these methods are not successful, Rockwood[9] has described a technique of reduction under general anesthesia in which the clavicle is grasped with a towel clip percutaneously. As the reduction maneuver is performed, traction on the towel clip facilitates reduction. Most closed reductions are stable. However, the reduction should be confirmed radiographically. **(CD-35.2)**

Buckerfield and Castle[17] described a technique of closed reduction in which caudal traction was applied to the adducted arm while both shoulders were forced posteriorly by direct pressure. They brought about a closed reduction in 6 patients who failed closed reduction with the abduction-traction technique. This maneuver attempts to use the first rib as a fulcrum, levering the clavicle superiorly. Following successful closed reduction, a figure-of-8 dressing or figure-of-8 clavicle strap should be applied to maintain the shoulders in retraction for approximately 6 weeks to allow for soft-tissue healing. Radiographs should be repeated 1 and 2 weeks later to confirm the reduction.

If closed reduction is unsuccessful, the reduction is not stable, or the dislocation occurred more than 7 days previously, open reduction and stabilization is indicated. This procedure should be performed in association with a thoracic surgeon because of the proximity of the mediastinal structures. The patient should be in the supine position with a bolster between the scapulae. The ipsilateral upper extremity should be prepped to allow manipulation intraoperatively. An oblique incision is made over the SCJ. Subcutaneous flaps are developed, and the anterior capsule is exposed. The capsule is divided in line with the medial clavicle with preservation of superior and inferior flaps. The medial clavicle is iden-

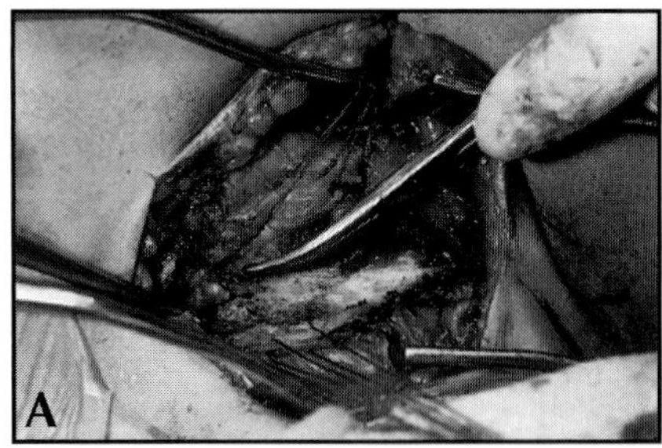
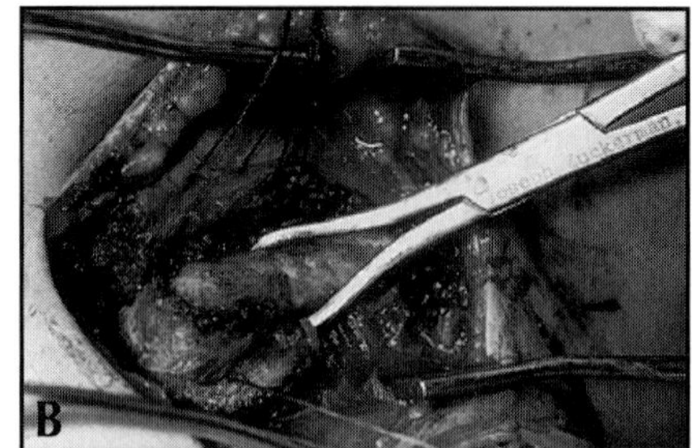
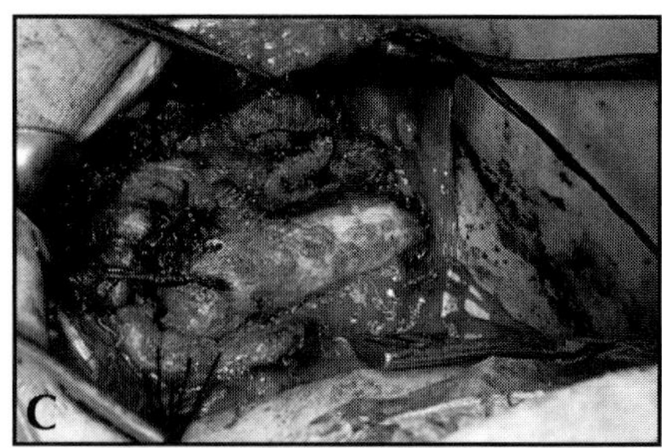

Fig. 6 Surgical photographs of open reduction of chronic posterior dislocation. **A,** The clamp is pointing to the retrosternal position of the clavicular head. **B,** A towel clip is being used to reduce the medial clavicle from its retrosternal position. **C,** Reconstruction completed; sutures (#5 Ethibond) through drill holes used to reconstruct the sternoclavicular and costoclavicular ligaments.

tified, exposed, and followed medially as it passes behind the sternum (Fig. 6, *A*). The superior and inferior cortices should be exposed so that a towel clip or bone clamp can be placed. In addition, the posterior cortex should be freed of any soft-tissue adhesions. The thoracic surgeon will be helpful during this dissection. With the towel clip or clamp in place, a reduction maneuver is performed with traction on the upper extremity and manipulation of the medial clavicle up and over the superior aspect of the sternum (Fig. 6, *B*). In acute dislocations, the reduction usually is stable and soft-tissue reconstruction is not necessary, as in chronic dislocations. This closure should include secure repair of the anterior capsule. Postoperative immobilization can use a sling or figure-of-8 strap. Radiographs should be obtained 1 week later to confirm reduction.

Medial Clavicular Physeal Injury

Knowledge of the ossification and fusion pattern of the medial clavicular epiphysis is important, because many so-called SCJ dislocations may actually be fractures involving the medial clavicular physis. Accurate diagnosis and classification go beyond academic interests and have important treatment implications.

Patients younger than age 25 years who present with injury localized to the SCJ should be suspected of having an injury to the medial clavicular epiphysis. The clinical presentation is similar to that seen in adults, with signs and symptoms varying with the direction of displacement. Physeal separation may not be evident on plain radiographs if the medial clavicular physis has not yet ossified. The axial images provided by CT scan allow for documentation of the malposition of the medial clavicle and can identify an ossified epiphysis articulating with the manubrium.[16]

Earlier reports of SCJ injuries, which included injuries to children and adolescents, did not classify these as transphyseal injuries, and they were treated similarly to adult injuries.[17,30,35–37] Open reduction occasionally was performed if retrosternal dislocation persisted after attempted closed reduction. Brooks and Henning[35] performed open reduction and internal fixation using smooth K-wires. Buckerfield and Castle[17] performed closed reduction on 7 patients, 2 of whom demonstrated signs of thoracic outlet compression. Selesnick and associates[30] asserted that the treatment is the same for an adult retrosternal dislocation and a medial clavicular physeal posterior fracture-dislocation.

More recent recommendations are to observe anterior physeal injuries. Closed reduction should be attempted for posterior physeal injuries that are seen within 10 days of the injury. Only if signs of thoracic outlet obstruction are present should open reduction be performed, without placement of hardware.[37,38] After this 10-day period, expectant management is recommended, provided there is no evidence of neurovascular or visceral compromise. Many[2,5,8,38–41] believe that remodeling along an intact periosteal sleeve will eliminate most of the bony deformity or displacement.

Chronic Dislocation of the Sternoclavicular Joint

Chronic anterior SCJ dislocation[2,5,42,43] usually results in little functional limitation and most patients remain asymptomatic. A nonsurgical approach is the treatment of choice because this dislocation has a benign natural history. If degenerative changes develop at the SCJ, 6 to 12 months of nonsurgical treatment have been exhausted, and injection of local anesthetic relieves the symptoms, a medial clavicle resection with reconstruction of the costoclavicular ligament may provide effective pain relief.

Chronic posterior dislocation requires the same thorough evaluation needed for acute SCJ dislocations. The chronicity of the injury and the degree of displacement may produce an obvious sulcus at the lateral border of the manubrium. Standard radiographs and a CT scan should be obtained to evaluate the retrosternal space for compression of the neurovascular and visceral structures. Angiography or barium gastrointestinal studies may also be needed. As described previously, posterior SCJ dislocations have up to 30% incidence of complications involving the trachea, esophagus, brachial plexus, or great vessels, and a meticulous workup is necessary. Consultation with a thoracic surgeon is required. Because of the risk of chronic compression and/or adhesions of the mediastinal structures, open reduction and stabilization is necessary in the setting of a chronic dislocation. The technique is similar to the one previously described for open reduction of acute dislocations. However, the reduction generally is not stable, and reconstruction of the costoclavicular and sternoclavicular ligaments is necessary. We prefer to use #5 nonabsorbable suture passed through drill holes in the sternum, medial clavicle, and first rib (Fig. 6, C).

Atraumatic Spontaneous Anterior Subluxation

In 1989, Rockwood and Odor[43] reviewed the natural history of spontaneous atraumatic anterior subluxation. The average age at presentation was 18 years, with males and females equally represented and 80% demonstrating generalized ligamentous laxity. All patients sought care because the medial end of the clavicle suddenly became prominent during a simple overhead elevation of the arm. None of the patients could voluntarily sublux the SCJ with the arm in adduction, and subluxation occurred only with flexion or combined flexion, abduction, and external rotation. Subluxation produced little discomfort, if any, and most patients presented with concerns over appearance or anxiety as to the nature of the problem. Twenty-nine of 37 patients were treated nonsurgically, and at the most recent follow-up, none reported any limitation in activity or alteration in their lifestyle as the result of the subluxation of the joint. Ninety percent of the patients treated nonsurgically reported intermittent episodes of subluxation. Seventy-nine percent of patients reported absolutely no associated discomfort, and 21% had only minimal discomfort.

In contrast, all patients treated surgically reported an unsatisfactory result. Complications in the reconstructive group included residual pain and recurring instability, clavicular fracture and nonunion, need for a repeat resection arthroplasty, painful scar, and thoracic outlet syndrome, which was treated with resection of the entire residual clavicle.

Nonsurgical treatment for spontaneous atraumatic anterior subluxation consists of education and reassurance of the patient and the family.[43,44] Supportive measures may include local modalities and analgesics followed by gradual and progressive strengthening exercises for the shoulder, with advancement back to unrestricted activity as tolerated. Surgical treatment is rarely if ever indicated because of the high incidence of unsatisfactory results and complications.

Atraumatic Posterior Dislocation

Atraumatic posterior dislocation of the SCJ is an extremely rare event, with only 4 cases reported in the literature. In 1993, Martin and associates[45] described the first radiographically documented atraumatic posterior dislocation in a 50-year-old woman, who experienced severe right shoulder pain on awakening from sleep and reported new-onset dysphagia. She underwent unsuccessful closed reduction under general anesthesia; afterward, she developed new-onset dyspnea and worsening dysphagia with cross-chest adduction of her arm. A repeat CT scan demonstrated continued posterior dislocation of the SCJ. After 2 weeks, the patient had complete resolution of her dyspnea and dysphasia, and noted mild resolution of her pain. A repeat CT scan at this time demonstrated continued posterior displacement of the medial clavicle. Nonsurgical treatment was recommended. At follow-up 1 year later, the patient was completely asymptomatic. Because of close proximity to the neurovascular structures with a posterior sternoclavicular dislocation, a high index of suspicion for neurovascular, tracheo-esophageal, or pulmonary complications should be maintained. Although this condition is rare, it should be classified and treated in a similar manner as traumatic posterior sternoclavicular dislocations.

Intra-articular Disk Injury

Following injury to the upper extremity, a patient may complain of a painful popping or clicking sensation at the SCJ that is otherwise stable to examination. Consideration should be given to possible injury of the intra-articular disk or an intra-articular medial clavicle fracture. Analogous to a meniscal tear of the knee or triangular fibrocartilage complex tear of the wrist, this injury can be disabling.[2,8,46] MRI and MR arthrography have been recommended to delineate irregularities of the intra-articular disk.[47] Duggan[46] reported a case of a patient with persistent popping at the SCJ. Excision of the loose intra-articular disk and capsular repair resulted in resolution of the patient's symptoms. Care must be taken not to overlook degenerative changes of the inferomedial or articular aspect of the clavicle.

Degenerative Disorders

Osteoarthritis

Osteoarthritis of the SCJ is uncommon, but the incidence does rise with advancing age.[42] Kier and associates[48] evaluated 55 cadaveric SCJs for the presence of characteristic radiographic signs of osteoarthritis including joint space narrowing, osteophyte and/or cystic formation, and sclerosis. These findings were uncommon in patients younger than age 40 years, but were present in 53% of those older than age 60 years. Changes were typically bilateral and were most severe along the inferomedial portion of the articular margin of the clavicle.

Patients will typically complain of pain about the SCJ. They may also be

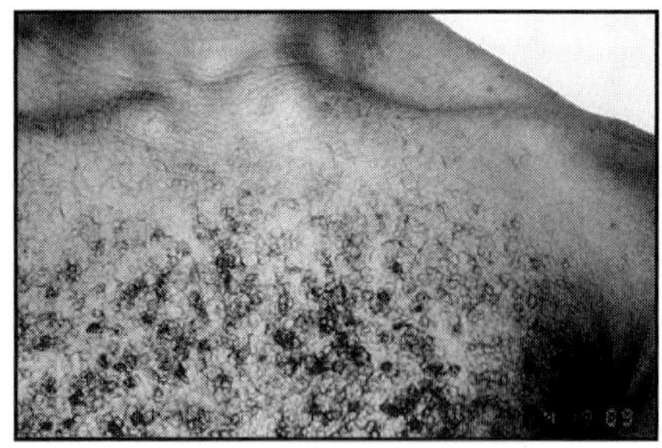

Fig. 7 Clinical photograph of the upper chest of a 48-year-old man with degenerative arthritis of the left sternoclavicular joint. The patient complains of long-standing pain, swelling, and prominence.

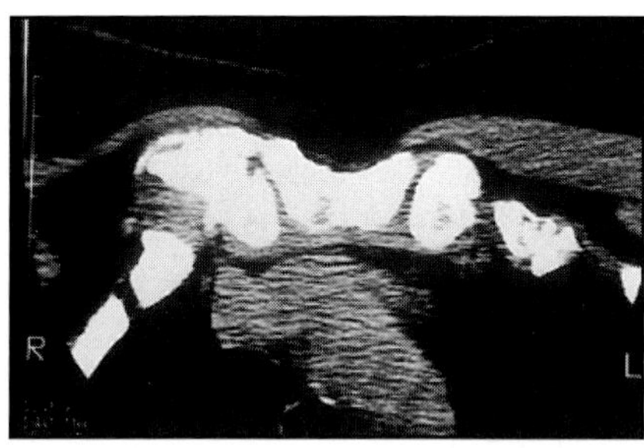

Fig. 8 Computed tomography scan demonstrating changes consistent with degenerative sternoclavicular joint arthritis, including joint space narrowing and osteophyte formation.

aware of a painful clicking. Findings include swelling and tenderness on palpation over the joint (Fig. 7). There may be a prominence evident secondary to either osteophyte formation or subluxation (Fig. 8). Range of motion of the ipsilateral shoulder may cause pain, particularly with adduction type movements and elevation above the horizontal.

Symptoms will generally respond to nonsurgical measures consisting of rest, nonsteroidal anti-inflammatory drugs (NSAIDs), or local injection of corticosteroids. Patients with persistent severe symptoms that have not responded to 6 months or more of nonsurgical treatment may be considered candidates for medial clavicle resection. Patients can expect significant symptomatic relief with this procedure. However, it is essential to maintain the integrity of the costoclavicular ligament for joint stability.

Monoarticular Noninfective Subacute Arthritis

Bremner[49] described a monoarticular noninfective arthritis affecting the SCJ of women with an average age of 56 years. There was neither a history of injury nor evidence of other joint involvement. Patients developed tenderness and swelling over the joint. Swelling may be present with slight erythema, which initially raised concerns about an infectious etiology. The white blood cell count and the erythrocyte sedimentation rate were normal. Radiographs showed evidence of erosion of the articular surfaces. The natural history, as reported, consisted of persistent swelling for a few months followed by gradual resolution over a period of several months up to a year. The symptoms generally disappeared despite continued swelling. The condition carries an excellent prognosis, and no patient had involvement of the other joint in the manifestations of generalized rheumatoid disease.

Infection: Septic Arthritis

Patients who present with swelling and tenderness localized to the SCJ should always have infection included in the differential diagnosis. Unlike septic arthritis of other joints, bacterial infection of the SCJ is usually insidious in onset.[50] However, similar to septic arthritis of other joints, erythema, warmth, and edema are usually present. There is no pain on active and passive shoulder motion. Wohlgethan and associates[51] noted a band of induration parallel to and below the clavicle, corresponding to the path of the superficial lymphatic drainage. The white blood cell count usually is not elevated but the erythrocyte sedimentation rate and a C-reactive protein may be markedly elevated. Aspiration will confirm the diagnosis. Numerous organisms have been isolated from SCJ sepsis, with *Staphylococcus aureus* most common in patients without a history of drug abuse. *Pseudomonas aeruginosa* is most frequently isolated from intravenous drug abusers.[50] In most cases, surgical management is indicated, consisting of joint debridement with medial clavicle resection and a course of intravenous antibiotics based on the organisms involved.

Wohlgethan and associates[51] found a 20% incidence of abscess formation in these patients. This complication did not correlate either with a history of drug abuse or a specific underlying organism. Because of the risk of retrosternal spread and abscess formation, they recommend an initial and follow-up CT scan in all cases.

Rheumatoid Arthritis

The SCJ is a synovial joint and, as such, can be involved in the rheumatoid process. Occasionally, involvement of the SCJ can be the presenting finding, but more commonly it is one component of a polyarticular process. In a radiographic review of patients with rheumatoid arthritis, 33 of 105 patients had either subchondral or marginal erosions of the SCJ documented by tomography.[52] Treatment primarily is optimal medical management of the rheumatoid process. In selected patients with symptoms refractory to medical management, medial clavicle resection can result in significant improvement of symptoms.

Sternocostoclavicular Hyperostosis

Sternocostoclavicular hyperostosis (SCCH) is a disorder characterized by hyperossification of the sternum, clavicles, upper ribs, and surrounding soft tissues.[34,53–55] It is encountered predominantly in the fifth and sixth decades of life, and is more common in women. There is a high incidence of pustulosis of the palms and soles that suggests a common etiologic factor.[34,53,55] Pain and tenderness in the upper anterior part of the chest are the most common complaints. One study found that the severity of the pustulosis was directly proportional to the intensity of the chest pain.[53] Laboratory findings may include leukocytosis, an elevated erythrocyte sedimentation rate, an elevated antistreptolysin-O titer, a positive test for C-reactive protein, and negative tests for antinuclear antibodies, rheumatoid factor, and histocompatibility antigen B-27. Bone and tissue cultures are almost invariably negative,[34] although Edlund and associates[55] reported positive cultures of *Proprionibacterium acnes* in 7 of 15 patients with this disorder. The histopathology is consistent with chronic inflammation. The natural history of the disorder is uncertain, and the treatment is symptomatic with NSAIDs providing effective pain relief. The association of SCCH with pustulosis and the observation that antibiotics as well as surgical removal of focal infections suppressed skin eruptions have led to the use of antibiotics in the treatment of SCCH. Chigira and associates[53] observed that antibiotics were more effective than NSAIDs in relieving pain in 8 of 11 patients. Pustulosis and chest pain diminished after antibiotic therapy in most patients.[53] However, the etiology of the disorder and the optimal treatment have yet to be determined.

References

1. Cope R, Riddervold HO, Shore JL, Sistrom CL: Dislocations of the sternoclavicular joint: Anatomic basis, etiologies, and radiologic diagnosis. *J Orthop Trauma* 1991;5:379–384.
2. Rockwood CA Jr, Wirth MA: Injuries to the sternoclavicular joint, in Rockwood CA Jr, Green DP, Bucholz RW, Heckman JD (eds): *Rockwood and Green's Fractures in Adults*, ed 4. Philadelphia, PA, Lippincot-Raven, 1996, vol 2, pp 1415–1471.
3. Zuckerman JD, Matsen FA III: Biomechanics of the shoulder, in Nordin M, Frankel VH (eds): *Basic Biomechanics of the Musculoskeletal System*, ed 2. Philadelphia, PA, Lea & Febiger, 1989, pp 225–247.
4. Flatow EL: The biomechanics of the acromioclavicular, sternoclavicular, and scapulothoracic joints, in Heckman JD (ed): *Instructional Course Lectures 42*. Rosemont, IL, American Academy of Orthopaedic Surgeons, 1993, pp 237–245.
5. Rockwood CA Jr, Wirth MA: Disorders of the sternoclavicular joint, in Rockwood CA Jr, Matsen FA III (eds): *The Shoulder*. Philadelphia, PA, WB Saunders, 1990, pp 477–525.
6. Bearn JG: Direct observations on the function of the capsule of the sternoclavicular joint in clavicular support. *J Anat* 1967;101:159–170.
7. Cave AJE: The nature and morphology of the costoclavicular ligament. *J Anat* 1961;95: 170–179.
8. Wirth MA, Rockwood CA Jr: Acute and chronic traumatic injuries of the sternoclavicular joint. *J Am Acad Orthop Surg* 1996;4:268–278.
9. Rockwood CA Jr: Dislocations of the sternoclavicular joint, in Evans EB (ed): American Academy of Orthopaedic Surgeons *Instructional Course Lectures XXIV.* St Louis, MO, CV Mosby, 1975, pp 144–159.
10. Inman VT, Saunders JB, Dec M, Abbott LC: Observations on the function of the shoulder joint. *J Bone Joint Surg* 1944;26A:1–30.
11. Cave EF (ed): *Fractures and Other Injuries*: Chicago, IL, Year Book Publishers, 1958.
12. Nettles JL, Linscheid RL: Sternoclavicular dislocations. *J Trauma* 1968;8:158–164.
13. Ono K, Inagawa H, Kiyoto K, Terada T, Suzuki S, Maekawa K: Posterior dislocation of the sternoclavicular joint with obstruction of the innominate vein: Case report. *J Trauma* 1998;44:381–383.
14. Hobbs DW: Sternoclavicular joint: A new axial radiographic view. *Radiology* 1968;90:801.
15. Levinsohn EM, Bunnell WP, Yuan HA: Computed tomography in the diagnosis of dislocations of the sternoclavicular joint. *Clin Orthop* 1979;140:12–16.
16. Cope R, Riddervold HO: Posterior dislocation of the sternoclavicular joint: Report of two cases, with emphasis on radiologic management and early diagnosis. *Skeletal Radiol* 1988;17:247–250.
17. Buckerfield CT, Castle ME: Acute traumatic retrosternal dislocation of the clavicle. *J Bone Joint Surg* 1984;66A:379–385.
18. Borrero E: Traumatic posterior displacement of the left clavicular head causing chronic entrinsic compression of the subclavian artery. *Phys Sports Med* 1987;15:87–89.
19. Gale DW, Dunn ID, McPherson S, Oni OO: Retrosternal dislocation of the clavicle: The "stealth" dislocation. *Injury* 1992;23:563–564.
20. Jougon JB, Lepront DJ, Dromer CE: Posterior dislocation of the sternoclavicular joint leading to mediastinal compression. *Ann Thorac Surg* 1996;61:711–713.
21. Wasylenko MJ, Busse EF: Posterior dislocation of the clavicle causing fatal tracheoesophageal fistula. *Can J Surg* 1981;24:626–627.
22. de Jong KP, Sukul DM: Anterior sternoclavicular dislocation: A long-term follow-up study. *J Orthop Trauma* 1990;4:420–423.
23. Booth CM, Roper BA: Chronic dislocation of the sternoclavicular joint: An operative repair. *Clin Orthop* 1979;140:17–20.
24. Burrows HJ: Tenodesis of subclavius in the treatment of recurrent dislocation of the sterno-clavicular joint. *J Bone Joint Surg* 1951;33B:240–243.
25. Eskola A, Vainionpää S, Vastamäki M, Slätis P, Rokkanen P: Operation for old sternoclavicular dislocation: Results in 12 cases. *J Bone Joint Surg* 1989;71B;63–65.
26. Lunseth PA, Chapman KW, Frankel VH: Surgical treatment of chronic dislocation of the sterno-clavicular joint. *J Bone Joint Surg* 1975;57B:193–196.
27. Daus GP, Drez D Jr, Newton BB Jr, Kober R: Migration of a Kirschner wire from the sternum to the right ventricle: A case report. *Am J Sports Med* 1993;21:321–322.
28. Lyons FA, Rockwood CA Jr: Migration of pins used in operations on the shoulder. *J Bone Joint Surg* 1990;72A:1262–1267.
29. Howard FM, Shafer SJ: Injuries to the clavicle with neurovascular complications: A study of fourteen cases. *J Bone Joint Surg* 1965;47A:1335–1346.
30. Selesnick FH, Jablon M, Frank C, Post M: Retrosternal dislocation of the clavicle: Report of four cases. *J Bone Joint Surg* 1984;66A: 287–291.
31. Worman LW, Leagus C: Intrathoracic injury following retrosternal dislocation of the clavicle. *J Trauma* 1967;7:416–423.
32. Paterson DC: Retrosternal dislocation of the clavicle. *J Bone Joint Surg* 1961;43B:90–94.
33. Gangahar DM, Flogaites T: Retrosternal dislocation of the clavicle producing thoracic outlet syndrome. *J Trauma* 1978;18:369–372.
34. Saghafi M, Henderson MJ, Buchanan WW: Sternocostoclavicular hyperostosis. *Semin Arthritis Rheum* 1993;22:215–223.
35. Brooks AL, Henning GD: Abstract: Injury to the proximal clavicular epiphysis. *J Bone Joint Surg* 1972;54A:1347–1348.
36. Tyer HDD, Sturrock WDS, Callow FMcC: Retrosternal dislocation of the clavicle. *J Bone Joint Surg* 1963;45B:132–137.
37. Lewonowski K, Bassett GS: Complete posterior sternoclavicular epiphyseal separation: A case report and review of the literature. *Clin Orthop* 1992;281:84–88.
38. Lemire L, Rosman M: Sternoclavicular epiphyseal separation with adjacent clavicular fracture. *J Pediatr Orthop* 1984;4:118–120.
39. Zaslav KR, Ray S, Neer CS II: Conservative management of a displaced medial clavicular physeal injury in an adolescent athlete: A case report and literature review. *Am J Sports Med* 1989;17:833–836.
40. Asher MA: Dislocations of the upper extremity in children. *Orthop Clin North Am* 1976;7: 583–591.
41. Eidman DK, Siff SJ, Tullos HS: Acromioclavicular lesions in children. *Am J Sports Med* 1981;9:150–154.

42. Wirth MA, Rockwood CA Jr: Chronic conditions of the acromioclavicular and sternoclavicular joints, in Chapman MW, Madison M (eds): *Operative Orthopaedics*, ed 2. Philadelphia, PA, JB Lippincott, 1993, pp 1673–1693.

43. Rockwood CA Jr, Odor JM: Spontaneous atraumatic anterior subluxation of the sternoclavicular joint. *J Bone Joint Surg* 1989;71A: 1280–1288.

44. Sadr B, Swann M: Spontaneous dislocation of the sterno-clavicular joint. *Acta Orthop Scand* 1979;50:269–274.

45. Martin SD, Altcheck D, Erlanger S: Atraumatic posterior dislocation of the sternoclavicular joint: A case report and literature review. *Clin Orthop* 1993;292:159–164.

46. Duggan N: Recurrent dislocation of the sternoclavicular cartilage. *J Bone Joint Surg* 1931;13: 365.

47. Brossman J, Stabler A, Preidler KW, Trudell D, Resnick D: Sternoclavicular joint: MR imaging-anatomic correlation. *Radiology* 1996;198: 192–198.

48. Kier R, Wain SL, Apple J, Martinez S: Osteoarthritis of the sternoclavicular joint: Radiographic features and pathologic correlation. *Invest Radiol* 1986;21:227–233.

49. Bremner RA: Monarticular, non-infective subacute arthritis of the sterno-clavicular joint. *J Bone Joint Surg* 1959;41B:749–753.

50. Yood RA, Goldenberg DL: Sternoclaviculur joint arthritis. *Arthritis Rheum* 1980;23:232–239.

51. Wohlgethan JR, Newberg AH, Reed JI: The risk of abscess from sternoclavicular septic arthritis. *J Rheumatol* 1988;15:1302–1306.

52. Kalliomaki JL, Viitanen SM, Virtama P: Radiographic findings of sternoclavicular joints in rheumatoid arthritis. *Acta Rheumatol Scand* 1968;14:233–240.

53. Chigira M, Maehara S, Nagase M, Ogimi T, Udagawa E: Sternocostoclavicular hyperostosis: A report of nineteen cases, with special reference to etiology and treatment. *J Bone Joint Surg* 1986;68A:103–112.

54. Hallas J, Olesen KP: Sterno-costo-clavicular hyperostosis: A case report with a review of the literature. *Acta Radiol* 1988;29:577–579.

55. Edlund E, Johnson U, Lidgren L, et al: Palmoplantar pustulosis and sternoclavicular arthro-osteitis. *Ann Rheum Dis* 1988;47: 809–815.

Reference to Video

Wirth MA, Rockwood CA Jr: Surgical Management of Posterior Sternoclavicular Dislocations. San Antonio, TX, The University of Texas Health Science Center, 1994.

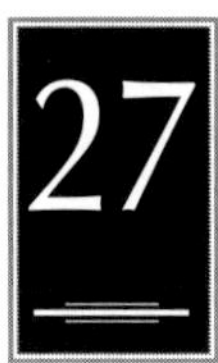

Complications of Treatment of Complete Acromioclavicular Joint Dislocations

Dan Guttmann, MD
Nader E. Paksima, DO
Joseph D. Zuckerman, MD

Introduction

The treatment of complete acromioclavicular (AC) joint dislocations ranges from a period of sling immobilization to complex joint stabilization techniques. The complexity of this subject can be reflected in a quote by Urist,[1] who stated that the treatment of AC joint injuries "ranges from the neatest and smallest, to the largest and most grotesque in the whole field of traumatic and orthopaedic surgery." Consequently, the reported complications of the wide spectrum of treatments for AC joint dislocations range from minor skin irritation to instability and degenerative arthritis of the AC joint to potentially devastating compromise of the thoracic cavity and mediastinum.

This chapter will not be a review of all the different treatment options available but rather a discussion of the complications that can occur in association with nonsurgical and surgical treatment of complete AC joint dislocations.

Anatomy

The AC joint is a diarthrodial joint involving the medial facet of the acromion and the distal clavicle. Its articular surfaces are covered with hyaline cartilage with an interposed fibrocartilaginous disk (meniscus). A thin capsule surrounds the joint and is stabilized by anterior and posterior as well as superior and inferior ligaments. The AC ligaments, the coracoclavicular (CC) ligaments, and the muscular envelope stabilize the AC joint. The AC ligaments provide primary horizontal stability (anteroposterior) for both small and large displacements.[2,3] The AC ligament capsular attachment on the clavicle is approximately 1.5 cm from the joint. Therefore, an AC resection of 2 cm or more would potentially compromise anteroposterior stability.[4] The CC ligaments include the conoid and trapezoid ligaments. The conoid ligament provides vertical stability (superoinferior) at large displacements, and the trapezoid ligament functions to stabilize compressive forces. The AC joint can have an angle of inclination that is variable in both the sagittal and coronal planes.[5]

Classification

AC joint injuries have been classified into 6 different types. The type of injury and the activity level of the patient are the most important factors to consider when assessing treatment options.

Type I injuries involve a sprain of the AC ligament with intact AC and CC ligaments and a stable joint. In type II injuries, the AC ligaments are disrupted, and the CC ligaments remain intact. Type III injuries involve disruption of both the AC and CC ligaments, which results in a complete dislocation of the AC joint and an unstable joint. Type IV injuries involve a posterior displacement of the clavicle; often the distal clavicle becomes interposed within the fibers of the trapezius muscle. Type V injuries are characterized by marked superior displacement of the distal clavicle. Type VI injuries also involve tearing of both the AC and CC ligaments, but the displacement is inferior with the clavicle in a subacromial or subcoracoid position.

Nonsurgical treatment is commonly the approach for types I and II AC joint injuries. Treatment of type III AC injuries is somewhat more controversial, especially for injuries in athletes and heavy laborers. The discussion that follows refers mainly to complications that are associated with complete AC joint dislocations, specifically types III, IV, and V. Type VI is a very rare injury, and the limited incidence precludes a meaningful discussion of its complications.

Complications of Nonsurgical Treatment

Nonsurgical management has generally used 2 approaches: a simple arm sling and a harness type device. In the sling approach, the deformity generally is accepted, and the sling is worn until the discomfort subsides sufficiently to allow increased use and participation in a reha-

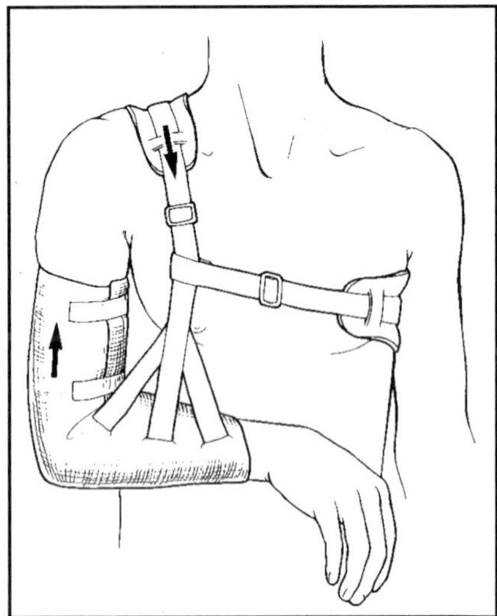

Fig. 1 The Kenny Howard sling is a harness-type device designed to support the arm and apply downward pressure on the lateral clavicle. (Reproduced with permission from Rockwood CA, Williams GR, Young DC: Injuries to the clavicular joint, in Rockwood CA, Green DP, Bucholz RW (eds): *Rockwood and Green's Fractures in Adults*, ed 3. Philadelphia, PA, JB Lippincott, 1991, p 1207.)

bilitation program. The harness approach uses a device designed to immobilize the lateral clavicle in a reduced position as soft-tissue healing occurs and must be worn for 3 to 6 weeks. Currently, the simple sling is used more commonly. Complications of nonsurgical treatment include skin and wound problems, osteolysis of the clavicle, posttraumatic arthritis and loss of function, and neurovascular injury.

Skin and Wound Problems

The mechanism of injury most commonly is a fall onto the point of the shoulder. This fall often results in an abrasion of the skin overlying the shoulder. Subsequent treatment using a harness-type device (Kenny Howard sling) can be problematic because of the pressure of the harness over the area of skin injury (Fig. 1). For harness devices to work, as the arm is supported, downward pressure must be placed on the lateral clavicle. Pressure on this area of skin injury can lead to breakdown (Fig. 2). Twenty percent of patients have required abandonment of this treatment method for this reason.[6] The true incidence of noncompliance with sling harness devices is unknown, but many patients are unable to tolerate 3 weeks or more of continuous sling and strap therapy.

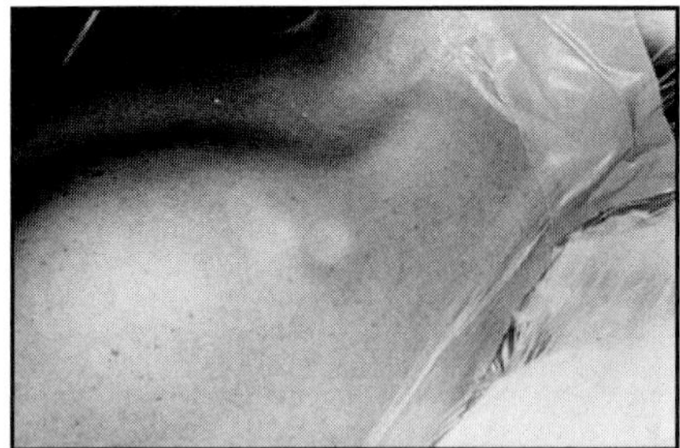

Fig. 2 Skin abrasions may occur from the injury that caused the acromioclavicular dislocation.

Osteolysis of the Clavicle

Another complication of AC joint injuries is osteolysis of the distal end of the clavicle, which can occur after an acute injury and has been referred to as posttraumatic osteolysis[7,8] (Fig. 3). Others have reported cases of osteolysis in athletes who did not have an acute injury.[9]

A technetium bone scan and a Zanca view (15° cephalic tilt with 50% decrease in penetrance) radiograph can aid in the diagnosis. Radiographic findings include osteopenia, tapering, osteolysis, or osteophyte formation at the distal clavicle. The symptom is pain, especially with flexion and abduction of the arm. The condition usually is self-limiting in most cases, and symptoms frequently subside within 1 year. Rest and activity modifications are the initial conservative treatment methods. The distal clavicle has been reported to reconstitute itself. Pain that does not respond to conservative measures is treated with excision of the distal clavicle.

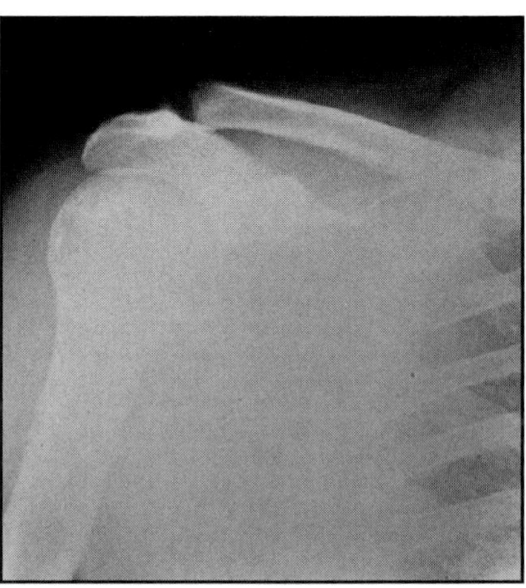

Fig. 3 Another complication of acromioclavicular joint injuries is osteolysis of the distal end of the clavicle.

Posttraumatic Arthritis and Loss of Function

Injuries to the AC joint may eventually lead to degenerative changes and residual instability, ranging from subluxation to complete dislocation. Patients may complain of activity-related pain and weakness as well as a significant and noticeable deformity. In addition, tissues may be interposed in the AC joint. Prolonged immobilization may also provoke joint stiffness. The literature is controversial concerning the long-term outcome of AC joint injuries treated nonsurgically.

Several studies have questioned whether types I and II injuries treated nonsurgically have significant sequelae. Patients with these injuries may develop degenerative changes and related pain and disability over time.[7,8,10] Bergfeld and associates[11] found a significant incidence of late symptoms and radiographic evidence of arthritis following types I and II injuries. Cox[10] reported on persistent symptoms following type II injuries in 1981 and found that symptomatic degenerative changes occur with mild degrees of AC injury. Cook and Heiner[12] reported degenerative changes as high as 24% in their review.

Nonsurgical management of posttraumatic arthritis typically involves activity modification, oral nonsteroidal anti-inflammatory drugs, and judicious use of intra-articular steroid injections. Surgical treatment may be indicated when symptoms persist. Lateral clavicle resection should be combined with CC stabilization when any residual instability exists. This is certainly true for types III, IV, and V injuries and should be considered for type II injuries. In these situations, lateral clavicle resection alone will not provide satisfactory outcomes and should be reserved for residuals of type I injuries[13] (Fig. 4).

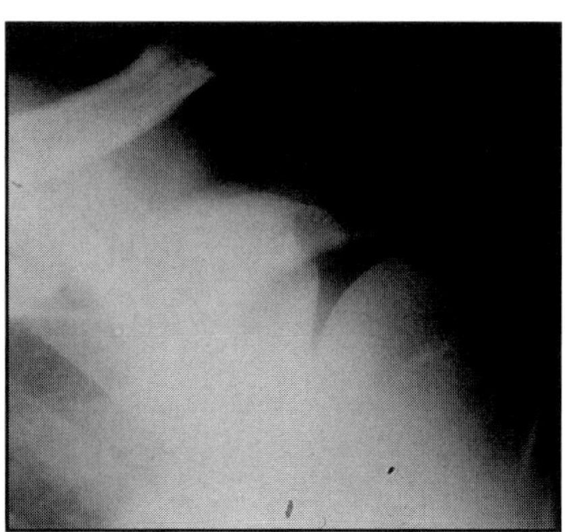

Fig. 4 Excessive lateral clavicle resection may lead to further clinical instability, pain, and cosmetic deformity.

Neurovascular Injury

Some patients with chronic AC joint instability develop arm weakness and paresthesias that may present like a vague brachial plexopathy.[4] In these patients, the instability of the shoulder girdle can produce a traction effect on the brachial plexus, resulting in neurologic symptoms. Meislin and associates[14] reported on a patient who had a brachial plexus neurapraxia that developed 8 years after a type III AC separation. In some situations, vascular symptoms may be present, suggesting thoracic outlet symptoms. Stabilization of the AC joint can be successful in resolving these symptoms.

Complications of Surgical Treatment

The complications of surgical treatment of AC joint injuries are potentially much greater and more serious than those of nonsurgical therapy and can be divided into preoperative, intraoperative, and postoperative complications. Preoperative complications include skin and wound breakdown and associated injuries. Intraoperative complications include inadequate ligament length, compromise of the coracoid attachment, excessive lateral clavicle resection, and neurovascular injury. Postoperative complications include loss of reduction, fracture, failure of hardware and/or suture, implant migration, infection, delayed neurovascular injury, hypertrophic scar formation and hypersensitivity, muscle detachment, ossification, osteolysis of the clavicle, and postoperative AC arthritis.

Preoperative Complications

Preoperative problems usually involve skin abrasions and/or tenting of the skin and associated injuries. Abrasions overlying areas where surgical incisions are planned should be completely healed before exposure. Skin tenting is most commonly encountered in type V injuries. Early surgery may be necessary in the case of significant tenting of the skin to limit pressure necrosis. In all cases, great care should be taken to handle the skin and soft tissues very cautiously and to avoid excessive undermining. In addition, incisions made over compromised areas of skin increase the risk of postoperative infection and skin breakdown.

It is also important to rule out any other associated injuries with complete AC dislocations. Barber[15] reported a patient with a type IV AC injury who also sustained a contralateral pneumothorax and ipsilateral pulmonary contusion. Bernard and associates[16] reported on the rare AC dislocation associated with a coracoid process fracture. To detect the fracture, the orthopaedist should obtain an axillary lateral radiograph or tomogram. Coracoid process fractures should be suspected with all AC dislocations occurring in the first 3 decades of life.[16] AC dislocations may also be associated with fractures involving the midclavicle, the distal clavicle into the AC joint, and the acromion process.[17] The presence of such a fracture may complicate either nonsurgical or surgical results.

Intraoperative Complications

Intraoperative problems often depend on the type of repair used. The most common surgical procedure described in the literature for complete AC joint dislocation is some form of modified Weaver-Dunn procedure.[18] The key element in this procedure involves detachment of the acromial origin of the coracoacromial ligament and transfer to the lateral clavicle for stabilization. The lateral clavicle is resected after mobilization of the coracoacromial ligament to ensure adequate length of the ligament transfer. More length can often be gained by partially releasing the coracoid attachment.

The Weaver-Dunn procedure may be complicated by inadequate ligament length, compromise of its coracoid attachment, and excessive lateral clavicle resection after the ligament is mobilized. In cases where an excessive amount of clavicle is resected, or the ligament length or attachment is compromised, use of CC stabilization using a heavy nonabsorbable suture is preferred.

Other potential intraoperative sources of complications include neurovascular injuries to the subclavian and axillary arteries and veins as well as the musculocutaneous nerve or other branches of the brachial plexus. Injuries to these structures may occur while passing suture material or instruments around the undersurface of the coracoid. Specially designed, curved suture-passing instruments have helped to make this potentially difficult maneuver easier (Fig. 5). It is

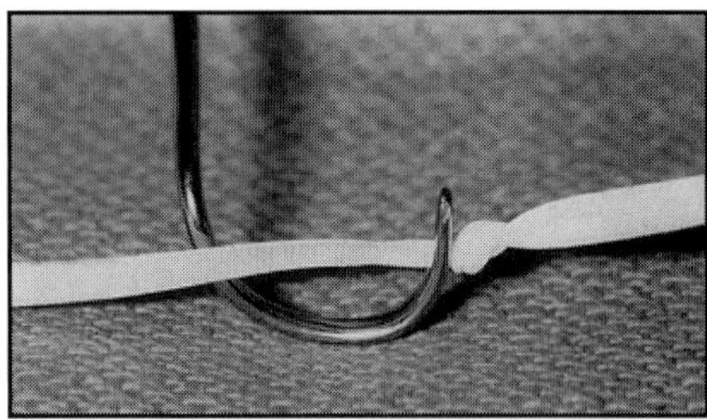

Fig. 5 Specially designed, curved instruments are used to aid in passing sutures or tape around the coracoid, as well as to help to avoid injuring neurovascular structures.

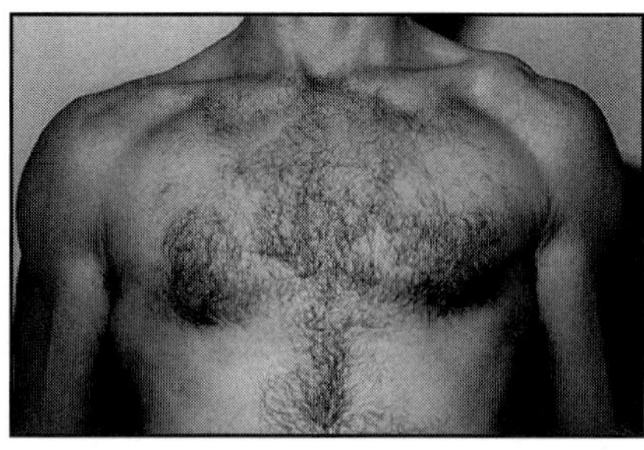

Fig. 6 Loss of reduction is evident 8 months following acromioclavicular repair in this patient with previous anterior shoulder repair for recurrent instability. Patient had only mild symptoms and did not require further treatment.

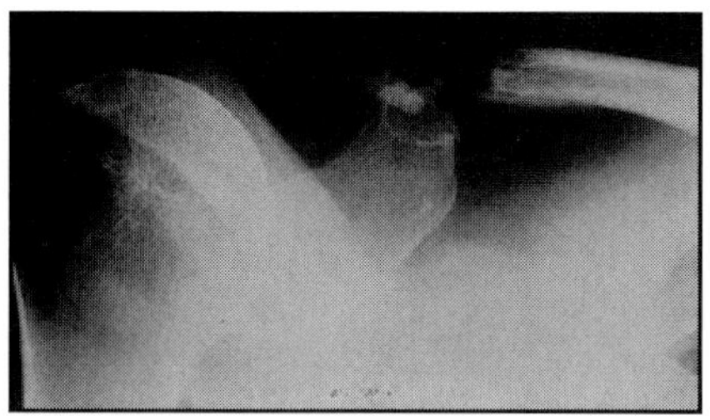

Fig. 7 Following reconstruction, erosion of suture or tape through the clavicle may occur, producing a fracture.

vital for the surgeon to stay as close to the bone as possible as the instrument or tape is passed and not to plunge when drilling or placing screws into the coracoid.

Postoperative Complications

Loss of Reduction and Fracture The incidence of loss of reduction (Fig. 6) has been reported to be as high as 44%, despite an initial anatomic reduction. Stam and Dawson[19] reported on a series of 20 surgical reconstructions using Dacron tape in which 9 had residual dislocation on stress views and 14 had erosion of the clavicle by the tape. Six of the 14 required surgical release of the Dacron tape to prevent the erosion from producing a fracture. One fracture did occur from this mechanism[19] (Fig. 7).

CC repair using wire or nonabsorbable sutures through drill holes or around the clavicle may also lead to gradual erosion and possible fracture.[20–22] If the AC injury has healed, the fractured clavicle can be treated as a type II lateral clavicle fracture. Fracture of the coracoid has also been reported following the use of merselene tape to reconstruct the CC ligaments. However, this is less likely to result in displacement.

Loss of reduction is known to occur after all types of successful reconstructions. This loss can occur acutely from loss of fixation or fracture or gradually as the repair fatigues and stretching occurs. The decision to reoperate must be made on an individual basis with each patient evaluated carefully. In many patients, progressive loss of reduction is not associated with significant symptoms, and reoperation would not be indicated. However, acute loss of reduction, particularly when associated with fracture or hardware failure, may require reoperation. This also should be assessed carefully, especially with respect to whether a successful outcome can be achieved.

Failure of Hardware The use of hardware has been associated with breakage, migration, and fixation failure. In a classic study, Larsen and associates[23] compared nonsurgical and surgical treatment of acute AC dislocations. Forty-one patients were operated on and 43 patients were treated conservatively. After 13 months there was no difference in the clinical results. Half of the patients who were operated on, however, had problems with the metallic device, such as breakage or migration of the pins, or both, and 6 patients had a superficial infection.[23]

Screws may be used to supplement the ligament transfer and to maintain the reduction of the lateral clavicle. In 1949, Bosworth[24] described a technique of percutaneous insertion of a screw through the clavicle into the coracoid to compress the CC space. Tsou[25] reported on a series of 53 AC joint dislocations treated with a percutaneous technique. Thirty-two percent had technical complications that included 2 cases of screws missing the coracoid, 4 cases of late screw pullout, 6 cases of subluxation after screw removal, and 2 cases of persistent serous drainage. MacDonald and associates[26] reported pullout as the patient was improperly awakened from anesthesia. Recent modifications of this technique use cannulated screws that are placed using an open reduction technique. Fluoroscopic guidance may be helpful. Both cortices of the coracoid must be engaged.

If loss of reduction or screw pullout is noted in the immediate postoperative period, reoperation to correct the problem usually is indicated. When the loss of reduction occurs over a period of weeks to months, then underlying infection must be ruled out and reinsertion of the screw may not give optimal results.

Other reported complications of use of the CC screw include fracture of the coracoid and lateral clavicle and overpenetration of the screw causing neurovascular complications. Strict adherence to proper techniques and fluoroscopic guidance can prevent these complications. Screw breakage can be a late complication from fatigue failure and can be avoided with screw removal at the proper time.

The use of suture anchors placed into the base of the coracoid obviates the need to pass sutures and instruments underneath the coracoid. However, suture anchors carry their own risk of complications, which include overpenetration as well as pullout and migration. Once again, adherence to proper insertion technique and careful evaluation of the fixation of each anchor can decrease the incidence of these problems.

Infection Many authors have reported using absorbable or nonabsorbable tape or suture to reconstruct the CC ligaments. Neault and associates[27] reported 3 cases of deep infection following the use of Dacron tape. All patients responded to removal of the foreign material, debridement, and antibiotic therapy. None of the patients required an additional stabilization procedure, and all were reported to have full and painless range of motion. These authors believed that the use of a nonabsorbable suture might act as a nidus for infection, which may occur acutely or even years later.[27]

Fullerton[28] presented a case of the failure of a Dacron graft 14 months after reconstruction. There were no signs of infection, and failure had occurred in the substance of the graft near the knot. The patient was treated with a modified Weaver-Dunn procedure.[28]

Skjeldal and associates[29] performed a coracoid transfer, which has been used to treat complete dislocations of the AC joint, in 17 patients. Eleven patients subsequently needed reoperation to remove the internal fixation screw; 2 had deep infections. In 3 patients the coracoid tip fragmented during the operation. As a result they have not recommended using this procedure for treatment for acute AC joint injuries.[29]

Implant Migration Transfixion pins have also been used in the treatment of AC dislocations and have been associated with potentially devastating complications. There have been numerous reports of migration of transfixion pins into areas of vital organs including the lung, liver, neck, spinal canal, subclavian artery, and the aorta.[30-33] Smooth Kirschner wires, threaded pins, Steinmann pins, and Hagie pins have all been reported to migrate. Several authors have recommended bending the lateral end of the wires and/or using a tension band technique to prevent migration. These maneuvers will not absolutely prevent migration. The pins also have a tendency to break medial to the bend, leaving the medial piece free to migrate. Overall, use of transfixation hardware should be avoided to prevent these potentially significant complications (Fig. 8).

Delayed Neurovascular Complications Neurovascular complications, although rare, may also occur postoperatively. When they occur, they can be quite serious. Injuries to the musculocutaneous nerve have been reported as a complication of transfer of the tip of the coracoid to the anterior clavicle. Caspi and associates[34] reported on 3 such cases in their series of 54 patients. The transfer acts as a dynamic stabilizer, exerting a downward force on a clavicle. All patients had spontaneous recovery within 5 months.[34] Sethi and Scott[35] have reported on the migration of a Hagie pin that lacerated the subclavian artery. Grauthoff and Klammer[36] reported on the migration of pins into the subclavian artery and the aorta.

Hypertrophic Scar Formation and Hypersensitivity Painful incisions, hypertrophic scar formation, and soft-tissue sensitivity have all been reported following these procedures. Areas of skin and subcutaneous tissue adherent to the clavicle are often hypersensitive and can pose cosmetic problems. Women often report discomfort from bra straps on the area or from the use of shoulder bags. These skin problems can be difficult to manage. Most improve over time with simple measures like massage for desensitization. Revision surgery is unlikely to result in significant improvement and, therefore, should probably be avoided.

Muscle Detachment After a reconstruction it is critical to adequately repair the deltoid and trapezius attachments. Deltoid and trapezius detachment can be a devastating problem. Although this complication has not been reported in the literature as occurring after AC reconstruction, it is certainly a potential complication.

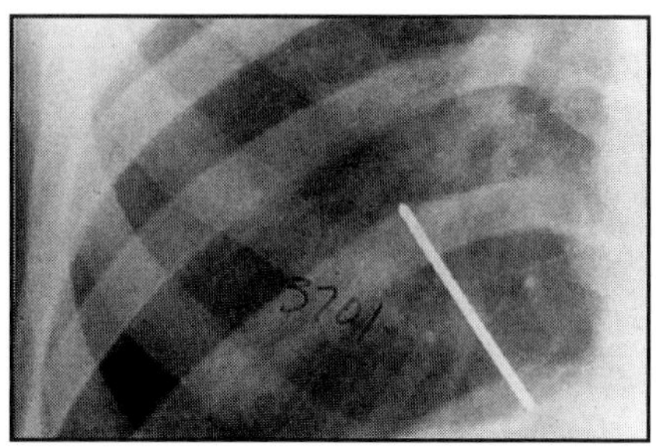

Fig. 8 Migration of a transfixion pin into the lung is fortunately infrequent but can have devastating consequences. (American Academy of Orthopaedic Surgeons Shoulder Educators Course. Newport, RI, May 1985.)

Coracoclavicular Ossification Ossification in the region of the CC ligaments has been reported after AC injuries treated surgically or nonsurgically and may appear as early as the third week.[37,38] Arner and associates[39] reported that ossification of the AC or CC ligament is the rule rather than the exception. The incidence of ossification of the CC interval has been reported to range from 50% to 85%. Ossification has also occurred in association with reconstruction of the CC ligament with synthetic material. Goldberg and associates[40] reported on a case of transient brachial plexus injury caused by calcification around a Dacron graft. In most series, however, there has been no correlation between the presence of ossification in the CC interval and symptoms or compromise of shoulder function[38,41] (Fig. 9).

Osteolysis of the Lateral Clavicle Osteolysis of the lateral clavicle has also been reported following surgical repair. This most often is associated with procedures that require transfixion of the AC joint. Eskola and associates[42,43] found that when screws are used to transfix the AC joint there is a much higher incidence of

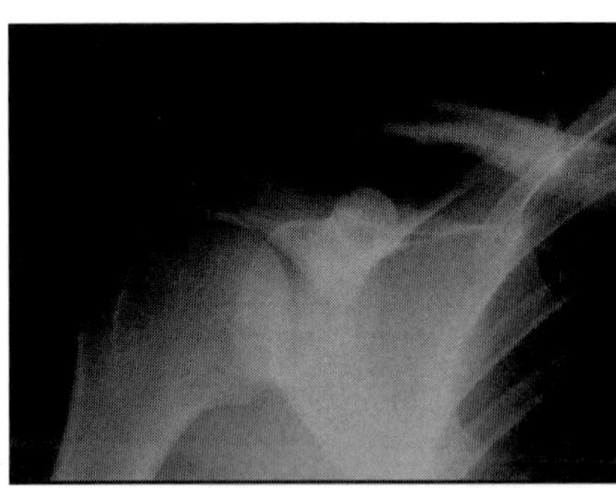

Fig. 9 Ossification may occur in the region of the coracoclavicular ligaments following acromioclavicular injuries treated nonsurgically or surgically.

osteolysis. This complication emphasizes the importance of using surgical techniques that do not require intra-articular transfixation of the AC joint.

Postoperative Acromioclavicular Arthritis Arthritis may also develop in the AC joint following surgical reconstruction. Henkel and associates[44] have reported on the use of a new temporary fixation device in 19 patients with acute AC dislocations. They used a clavicle hook-plate combined with suture of the ligaments. Radiologic signs of AC arthritis were found in 21% of the patients, but only 1 patient had a painful AC joint. Two superficial wound infections (10.5%) were treated successfully with antibiotics without removal of the implant. Neither breakage nor loosening of the clavicle hook-plate was observed.[44]

Broos and associates[45] reported on the long-term results of 87 patients with complete AC dislocations treated surgically with a Bosworth screw or a Wolter plate. Sixteen percent had implant failures; redislocation was seen in 25% of the patients, calcifications in 39%, and arthritis in 41%. Their end results were good or excellent in only 60% of the patients and fair or bad in 40%.[45]

Conclusion

Treatment of AC injuries can be extremely challenging. Most patients do well with nonsurgical treatment and regain acceptable shoulder function. Complications of nonsurgical management are relatively uncommon. Complications following surgical management are more common but the overall incidence remains low. In general, careful choice of the procedure to be performed and strict adherence to proper technique will decrease the risk of intraoperative and postoperative complications. The treatment of postoperative complications, particularly those that result in loss of reduction, should be evaluated carefully, particularly with respect to the need for reoperation.

References

1. Urist MR: The treatment of dislocations of the acromioclavicular joint: A survey of the past decade. *Am J Surg* 1959;98:423–431.
2. Urist MR: Complete dislocations of the acromioclavicular joint: The nature of the traumatic lesion and effective methods of treatment with an analysis of forty-one cases. *J Bone Joint Surg* 1946;28A:813–837.
3. Salter EG Jr, Nasca RJ, Shelley BS: Anatomical observations on the acromioclavicular joint and supporting ligaments. *Am J Sports Med* 1987;15:199–206.
4. Nuber GW, Bowen MK: Acromio clavicular joint injuries and distal clavicle fractures. *J Am Acad Orthop Surg* 1997;5:11–18.
5. Richards RR: Acromioclavicular joint injuries, in Heckman JD (ed): *Instructional Course Lectures 42*. Rosemont, IL, American Academy of Orthopaedic Surgeons, 1993, pp 259–269.
6. Allman FL Jr: Fractures and ligamentous injuries of the clavicle and its articulation. *J Bone Joint Surg* 1967;49A:774–784.
7. Madsen B: Osteolysis of the acromial end of the clavicle following trauma. *Br J Radiol* 1963;36:822–828.
8. Murphy OB, Bellamy R, Wheeler W, Brower TD: Post-traumatic osteolysis of the distal clavicle. *Clin Orthop* 1975;109:108–114.
9. Cahill BR: Atraumatic osteolysis of the distal clavicle: A review. *Sports Med* 1992;13:214–222.
10. Cox JS: The fate of the acromioclavicular joint in athletic injuries. *Am J Sports Med* 1981;9:50–53.
11. Bergfeld JA, Andrish JT, Clancy WG: Evaluation of the acromioclavicular joint following first-and second-degree sprains. *Am J Sports Med* 1978;6:153–159.
12. Cook DA, Heiner JP: Acromioclavicular joint injuries. *Orthop Rev* 1990;19:510–516.
13. Flatow EL, Duralde XA, Nicholson GP, Pollock RG, Bigliani LU: Arthroscopic resection of the distal clavicle with a superior approach. *J Shoulder Elbow Surg* 1995;4:41–50.
14. Meislin RJ, Zuckerman JD, Nainzadeh N: Type III acromioclavicular joint separation associated with late brachial-plexus neurapraxia. *J Orthop Trauma* 1992;6:370–372.
15. Barber FA: Complete posterior acromioclavicular dislocation: A case report. *Orthopedics* 1987;10:493–496.
16. Bernard TN Jr, Brunet ME, Haddad RJ Jr: Fractured coracoid process in acromioclavicular dislocations: Report of four cases and review of the literature. *Clin Orthop* 1983;175:227–232.
17. Wurtz LD, Lyons FA, Rockwood CA Jr: Fracture of the middle third of the clavicle and dislocation of the acromioclavicular joint: A report of four cases. *J Bone Joint Surg* 1992;74A:133–137.
18. Weaver JK, Dunn HK: Treatment of acromioclavicular injuries, especially complete acromioclavicular separation. *J Bone Joint Surg* 1972;54A:1187–1194.
19. Stam L, Dawson I: Complete acromioclavicular dislocations: Treatment with a Dacron ligament. *Injury* 1991;22:173–176.
20. Kappakas GS, McMaster JH: Repair of acromioclavicular separation using a Dacron prosthesis graft. *Clin Orthop* 1978;131:247–251.
21. Nelson CL: Abstract: Repair of acromioclavicular separations with knitted Dacron graft. *Clin Orthop* 1979;143:289.
22. Park JP, Arnold JA, Coker TP, Harris WD, Becker DA: Treatment of acromioclavicular separations: A retrospective study. *Am J Sports Med* 1980;8:251–256.
23. Larsen E, Bjerg-Nielsen A, Christensen P: Conservative or surgical treatment of acromioclavicular dislocation: A prospective, controlled, randomized study. *J Bone Joint Surg* 1986;68A:552–555.
24. Bosworth BM: Complete acromioclavicular dislocation. *N Engl J Med* 1949;241:221–225.
25. Tsou PM: Percutaneous cannulated screw coracoclavicular fixation for acute acromioclavicular dislocations. *Clin Orthop* 1989;243:112–121.
26. MacDonald PB, Alexander MJ, Frejuk J, Johnson GE: Comprehensive functional analysis of shoulders following complete acromioclavicular separation. *Am J Sports Med* 1988;16:475–480.

27. Neault MA, Nuber GW, Marymont JV: Infections after surgical repair of acromioclavicular separations with nonabsorbable tape or suture. *J Shoulder Elbow Surg* 1996;5:477–478.

28. Fullerton LR Jr: Recurrent third degree acromioclavicular joint separation after failure of a Dacron ligament prosthesis: A case report. *Am J Sports Med* 1990;18:106–107.

29. Skjeldal S, Lundblad R, Dullerud R. Coracoid process transfer for acromioclavicular dislocation. *Acta Orthop Scand* 1988;59:180–182.

30. Eaton R, Serletti J: Computerized axial tomography: A method of localizing Steinmann pin migration. A case report. *Orthopedics* 1981;4: 1357–1360.

31. Mazet R Jr: Migration of a Kirschner wire from the shoulder region into the lung: Report of two cases. *J Bone Joint Surg* 1943;25A: 477–483

32. Norrell H Jr, Llewellyn RC: Migration of a threaded Steinmann pin from an acromioclavicular joint into the spinal canal: A case report. *J Bone Joint Surg* 1965;47A:1024–1026.

33. Lindsey RW, Gutowski WT: The migration of a broken pin following fixation of the acromioclavicular joint: A case report and review of the literature. *Orthopedics* 1986;9:413–416.

34. Caspi I, Ezra E, Nerubay J, Horoszovski H: Musculocutaneous nerve injury after coracoid process transfer for clavicle instability: Report of three cases. *Acta Orthop Scand* 1987;58: 294–295.

35. Sethi GK, Scott SM: Subclavian artery laceration due to migration of a Hagie pin. *Surgery* 1976;80:644–646.

36. Grauthoff H, Klammer HL: Complications due to migration of a Kirschner wire from the clavicle. *RFO Fortschr Geb Rontgenstr Nuklearmed* 1978;128:591–594.

37. Millbourn E: On injuries to the acromio-clavicular joint: Treatment and results. *Acta Orthop Scand* 1950;19:349–382.

38. Weitzman G: Treatment of acute acromioclavicular joint dislocation by a modified Bosworth method: Report on twenty-four cases. *J Bone Joint Surg* 1967;49A:1167–1178.

39. Arner Ö, Sandahl U, Ohrling H: Dislocation of the acromio-clavicular joint: Review of the literature and a report on 56 cases. *Acta Chir Scand* 1957;113:140–152.

40. Goldberg JA, Viglione W, Cumming WJ, Waddell FS, Ruz PA: Review of coracoclavicular ligament reconstruction using Dacron graft material. *Aust N Z J Surg* 1987;57:441–445.

41. Alldredge RH: Abstract: Surgical treatment of acromioclavicular dislocation. *Clin Orthop* 1969;63:262–263.

42. Eskola A, Vainionpaa S, Korkala O, Rokkanen P: Acute complete acromioclavicular dislocation. A prospective randomized trial of fixation with smooth or threaded Kirschner wires or cortical screw. *Ann Chir Gynaecol* 1987;76: 323–326.

43. Eskola A, Vainionpaa S, Korkala S, Santavirta S, Gronblad M, Rokkanen P: Four-year outcome of operative treatment of acute acromioclavicular dislocation. *J Orthop Trauma* 1991;5:9–13.

44. Henkel T, Oetiker R, Hackenbruch W: Treatment of fresh Tossy III acromioclavicular joint dislocation by ligament suture and temporary fixation with the clavicular hooked plate. *Swiss Surg* 1997;3:160–166.

45. Broos P, Stoffelen D, Van de Sijpe K, Fourneau I: Surgical management of complete Tossy III acromioclavicular joint dislocation with the Bosworth screw or the Wolter plate: A critical evaluation. *Unfallchirurgie* 1997;23:153–160.

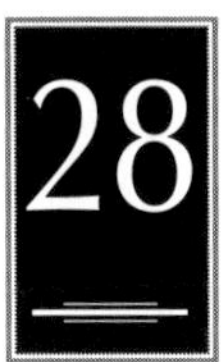

Complications of Shoulder Surgery

Thomas J. Gill, MD
Russell F. Warren, MD
Charles A. Rockwood, Jr, MD
Edward V. Craig, MD
Robert H. Cofield, MD
Richard J. Hawkins, MD

Introduction

This chapter will discuss some of the common and more serious complications associated with surgery around the shoulder. It is arranged in a case presentation format that is similar to that used in the symposium. Topics for discussion include complications related to instability surgery, rotator cuff surgery, arthroplasty, and fracture surgery, with special sections on arthrodesis (versus resection arthroplasty) and arthroscopy. Miscellaneous topics such as frozen shoulder and hardware complications are also presented.

Complications of Open Surgery for Instability

In treating shoulder instability, the 3 aims of reconstructive surgery are to restore stability, maintain pain-free mobility, and avoid complications. In the past, surgeons have concentrated on stability, selecting the simplest procedures by which to achieve that objective with a low recurrence rate.[1] More recent studies have demonstrated that patients are more concerned with full mobility and function, even to the exclusion of absolute stability.[2] Complications after surgical stabilization may imply that the direction of the instability was not recognized, that an anterior repair may be too tight, and that pain after stabilization may be caused by impingement.[1]

Loss of Motion Without Arthrosis

A 24-year-old man had a repair for anterior instability of his shoulder. Six months postoperatively, he still has some pain and there is only 0° of external rotation despite rigorous rehabilitation. Radiographs are normal, but the patient is unhappy with the functional outcome.

Loss of external rotation is a complication that is seen with stabilizations for anterior instability. A loss of rotation at 0° abduction with good rotation at 90° implies that the limitation in external rotation rests with the subscapularis, which moves above the center of joint rotation at 90° of abduction. Loss of external rotation at both 0° and 90° of abduction indicates that the capsule is tight as well. The choice of approach depends on the previous procedure. If the patient still cannot perform external rotation past 0° after 6 months of rehabilitation from a Bankart-type repair with capsular or rotator interval tightening, an arthroscopic capsular release and subacromial debridement should be performed. A wait longer than 6 months increases the risk of glenohumeral arthrosis from increased glenohumeral contact pressure, sometimes with posterior subluxation of the head. Arthroscopic release of the anterior capsule, including the subscapularis, until the desired amount of external rotation is achieved was the preferred approach. Releasing the inferior capsule arthroscopically does endanger the axillary nerve, although by staying sufficiently lateral in the pouch, injury to this nerve is rare.

An open Z-lengthening of the subscapularis should be considered if rotation is still restricted following the arthroscopic release, or if the surgeon prefers an open release. In general, 20° of rotation is gained for every 1 cm of lengthening. At least 30° of external rotation and 50° of elevation can typically be gained using this approach. If not, the subdeltoid and subcoracoid spaces should also be released. Leaving the patient with an internal rotation contracture will increase the joint compressive forces with attempted rotation while causing posterior translation of the humeral head over time. Such a combination often leads to degenerative wear in the posterior aspect of the joint and/or posterior instability in rare instances. The goals of performing a capsular release as early as 6 months postoperatively are relief of pain, improved function, and prevention of osteoarthrosis. Arthroscopic releases are preferred, but those less familiar with applications of the arthroscope prefer an open approach.

Loss of Motion With Glenohumeral Arthrosis

A 48-year-old man had a repair for anterior instability 10 years ago. He now has a significant internal rotation deformity of his arm. Although the patient's other motions are acceptable, pain persists and radiographs show osteoarthritis.

Glenohumeral arthrosis following surgery for instability is the result of excessively tight reconstructions. Samilson and Prieto[3] correlated limitation of external rotation with severity of arthrosis after surgical stabilization. Another cause of arthrosis following instability surgery has been malplacement or loosening of hardware.[3–7] Bone transplants at the anterior glenoid rim have also been associated with arthrosis,[8,9] as have osteotomies that enter the joint.

Osteoarthrosis of the glenohumeral joint is particularly common after a Putti-Platt capsulorrhaphy or Bristow procedure.[8,10] It has also been described after the Magnuson-Stack and duToit procedures.[9] In fact, arthrosis may result from any procedure that makes the shoulder too tight and limits motion. Following a Putti-Platt procedure, disabling pain is typically seen 10 to 13 years postoperatively in association with substantial limitation of motion.[9–12] The limitation of motion is frequently disabling, and is often as much as a 30° to 40° internal rotation contracture. Treatment of this complication depends on the degree of functional limitation, the amount of pain, and the extent of the arthrosis. Mild symptoms and mild arthrosis are treated with an alteration in activities, physiotherapy, and anti-inflammatory medications. If the symptoms and arthrosis are moderate, an arthroscopic anterior release or open Z-plasty lengthening of the subscapularis and capsule can be performed, as previously described.[10,11] Arthroscopic releases can be very successful under these circumstances, helping to diminish pain, increase function, and slow the progression of the arthrosis.

Marked joint degeneration (as seen on an axillary radiograph) or failure of soft-tissue release are indications for prosthetic replacement. A soft-tissue procedure to increase rotation must be performed at the same time as the arthroplasty. Options include an anterior Z-plasty lengthening, a 360° release, and/or an anterior interval release. The use of a smaller prosthetic humeral head and more medial reattachment of the subscapularis and capsule can also improve motion. Anteroposterior radiographs alone frequently underestimate the extent of joint space narrowing.

Hemiarthroplasty is performed if the glenoid is concentric, moderately degenerative, and the humeral head is centered on the axillary radiographic view. If the glenoid is flattened with posterior erosion, a hemiarthroplasty or, more commonly, a total shoulder arthroplasty might be performed with a posterior capsular plication and less retroversion than normal. The osteoarthrosis that results from the limitation of external rotation is likely the result of increased joint contact pressures and shear forces with continued attempts at rotation.

Late degenerative arthrosis has been documented following Bankart reconstruction.[2,4] In 1 study,[4] 14 of 33 shoulders had minimal changes, 3 had moderate changes, and 1 had severe changes at 15-year follow-up. There was a relationship between degenerative radiographic changes, length of follow-up, and restriction of external rotation with the arm abducted 90°.

Of the various options for open surgical anterior stabilization, Bankart reconstruction appears to have the lowest incidence of osteoarthrosis. In a long-term outcome study, Gill and associates[2] described a single case of osteoarthrosis in a group of 60 shoulders at 12 years follow-up. As with other techniques, the arthrosis was associated with a substantial postoperative loss of external rotation. Regardless of the instability procedure performed, preservation of motion is not only critical to the functional outcome and satisfaction of the patient, but it appears to be important in the prevention of arthrosis.

Complications of Hardware and Osteoarthrosis

A 46-year-old woman who underwent a Bristow procedure for recurrent anterior instability 3 years ago now complains of pain and limited motion. Although the patient has not experienced any instability since surgery, she has never been pain-free.

Complications of failed Bristow procedures include recurrent painful anterior instability, articular degeneration, nonunion of the coracoid transfer, loosening of the screw fixation, neurovascular injury, and posterior instability, with an overall complication incidence ranging from 14% to 48%.[7,8,13–15] Articular damage may be the result of direct contact of the humeral head with the transferred coracoid and screw. The screw may be found intra-articularly or impinging on the humeral head with motion. The risk of complications is lowered with proper technique for placement of the coracoid transplant.[15] As a result, the Bristow procedure is not recommended for the primary treatment of symptomatic anterior instability.[8]

The placement of hardware near the glenohumeral joint should be performed with caution. Screws and staples can produce complications that require reoperation and are capable of causing a permanent loss of joint function. Zuckerman and Matsen[7] identified 4 implant-related complications: (1) incorrect placement; (2) migration after placement; (3) loosening; and (4) breakage of the device. Patients with implant-related complications present with anterior shoulder pain, stiffness, crepitus, or radiating paresthesias. The average time from the original operation to the onset of symptoms averaged 16 months in 1 study. Staples are not recommended for rotator cuff repair because of their tendency to migrate. There is often a considerable delay in the diagnosis of implant-related complications. Adequate surgical exposure and careful placement of the implant are essential when these devices are used around the shoulder.

If at all possible, hardware should not be used around the glenohumeral joint. If complications do occur in this instance, the implant should be removed and the joint debrided. If significant osteoarthrosis has resulted from the use of hardware, an arthroplasty may be performed.

Neurovascular Injury

A 23-year-old woman complains of limited motion following a Putti-Platt procedure. Physical examination reveals full passive elevation, abduction, and rotation, but marked weakness in forward elevation and abduction.

Brachial plexus injuries have been sustained during Putti-Platt and Bristow procedures.[13] Suture material has been retrieved from around or within the musculocutaneous, ulnar axillary, and median nerves. Lacerations to the axillary artery have also been reported. These complications are caused by inadequate knowledge of regional anatomy, blind clamping of vascular lacerations, and the use of axillary incisions with limited exposure. During a Putti-Platt repair, abduction should be minimized and sutures placed under direct vision to avoid neurovascular injury.

A Bristow procedure presents a slightly different situation. The musculocutaneous nerve is at risk with the coracoid transfer, and it has been suggested that the musculocutaneous nerve be identified and mobilized.

Once an injury is discovered following a stabilization procedure, the indication for immediate exploration is the surgeon's decision based on knowledge of the events of the procedure. Most neurologic injuries following such surgery spontaneously resolve. A musculocutaneous injury following a Bristow procedure may be an indication for immediate surgical exploration. The neurologic structures involved should be explored at 3 to 6 months if there is no recovery by clinical and electromyographic examination, because there is a high likelihood of structural neurologic injury.[13] In general, good recovery of motor function with variable sensory return can generally be expected following nerve surgery.

Subscapularis Ruptures

A 19-year-old man who is a college football player underwent open Bankart repair for recurrent anterior instability 6 months ago. He complains of instability and pain during tackling drills with the affected arm.

Recurrent instability following a stabilization procedure may be related to several factors. First, a new traumatic event can precipitate a "new" instability, even after an effective previous repair. Second, rupture of the subscapularis can lead to recurrent anterior instability and weakness in internal rotation. Third, the previous procedure can fail. Fourth, there may have been a failure to identify an associated posterior or multidirectional component to the previous instability for which an anterior stabilization was performed.

It is important to identify the cause of the recurrent instability before surgical treatment is attempted. If an arthroscopic Bankart repair has failed with minimal new trauma, consideration should be given to performing a revision open Bankart procedure. If an open Bankart procedure fails after a new traumatic event, a second revision open Bankart procedure could be performed. Arthroscopic examination prior to the open procedure can confirm that a new Bankart lesion is the cause of the instability. The results following revision Bankart procedures are very good, with over 85% good and excellent results to be expected. If the recurrent instability is a result of previously missed posterior or multidirectional pathology, these other directions should be addressed at the time of the revision stabilization.

In the case presented, the subscapularis had torn. This diagnosis can be suggested on physical examination by the presence of increased external rotation compared to the opposite shoulder, weak internal rotation, and a positive lift-off test. Magnetic resonance imaging (MRI) can confirm the diagnosis. Rupture of the subscapularis can occur when the tendon has been released from the lesser tuberosity for surgical exposure in Bankart reconstruction; this is particularly true when the subscapularis and capsule are released together as a single flap. Tendon rupture can lead to recurrent instability, weakness, and pain. In order to prevent this complication, a meticulous repair of the subscapularis should be performed during the closure. The tenotomy should be made at least 10 to 15 mm from the insertion at the lesser tuberosity to allow an adequate soft-tissue stump for later repair. Strong nonabsorbable sutures should be used for repair, and external rotation should be limited to neutral for the first 2 weeks postoperatively in order to minimize stress on the healing anterior tissues.

Early repair of a torn subscapularis tendon is important. If the diagnosis of a torn subscapularis is made late, or if there is a delay of several months before the patient is taken to surgery, the subscapularis may be retracted far medially. This may be the reason that only 2 out of 3 subscapularis repairs appear to do well. If the tendon is not repairable or is of poor quality, a pectoralis transfer can be performed. It is important to ensure that the pectoralis is transferred under tension by placing the tendon lateral to the bicipital groove if stability and internal rotation are to be restored.

Failed Surgery for Multidirectional Instability

A 27-year-old woman who has had 4 previous stabilizations performed for multidirectional instability complains of severe pain with scapular winging. Electromyograms are negative, and translational testing in all 3 directions reveals instability, with a reproduction of the patient's symptoms.

Failed surgery for multidirectional instability poses a difficult therapeutic dilemma. It is important to spend time getting to know these patients and understanding their emotional and physical condition. Assuming there are no psychiatric issues, the previous surgeries and surgical reports should be reviewed to determine what approaches (anterior versus posterior) and what soft tissues were used.

Typically, the results of surgery for multidirectional instability are poor, with less than a 50% success rate. An examination under anesthesia and arthroscopic examination may be helpful to determine the extent of shoulder instability, and whether there are any structural problems, such as a Bankart lesion, that can be addressed. Further attempts at stabilization must be made cautiously. If the patient's clinical complaints become life-altering, glenohumeral arthrodesis may be considered. Some surgeons have noted that patients may still complain of instability even after a successful fusion, although this was not our experience.

Complications of Rotator Cuff Surgery

Complications can be minimized during rotator cuff surgery by following several basic principles. One of the most important aspects of rotator cuff surgery is preservation of the deltoid origin. Deltoid detachment can be minimized by avoiding extensive coronal detachments. The axillary nerve is protected by limiting the deltoid split to 5 cm or less.[16] A simple longitudinal split with medial and lateral subperiosteal elevation allows a strong side-to-side closure with braided, nonabsorbable suture, and avoids the need for reattachment through drill holes. If the deltoid muscle does pull off during the postoperative period, it should be reattached immediately in order to salvage the function of the muscle. Once the avulsed muscle has retracted, repair is almost impossible.

The acromion should not be shortened in order to maintain the proper fulcrum for deltoid function. Only the required amount of the anterior/inferior acromion should be resected to relieve impingement, with particular attention paid to any bone spurs present. Not only will deltoid dysfunction be minimized, but acromial fracture will be prevented as well. A strong, tension-free repair of the cuff tissue, including intimal tears, is important. To achieve this, fixation to bone is almost always required. Finally, the question remains as to how "heroic" we should be in trying to repair massive rotator cuff tears, with most of us agreeing that there is more reticence to attempts at a massive repair than in the past.

Failed Cuff Repair

A 67-year-old man complains of decreased motion and weakness 6 months after having undergone a rotator cuff repair. The patient denies any new trauma or acute onset of pain.

One of the most common complications of rotator cuff surgery is rerupture of the cuff, especially following a large or massive repair. Rerupture can occur even after the most technically well-performed reconstructions. Even so, several technical points should be considered. Although arthroscopic rotator cuff repairs are slowly becoming more popular, we decided to use an open approach with heavy, nonabsorbable sutures (#2 or #3 Ethibond sutures using a Mason-Allen or similar technique) that are then brought through drill holes into a bony trough. Suture anchors, although growing in popularity, had not as yet been used by any of us. Hypertrophied bursal tissue should not be mistaken for rotator cuff tissue when performing the repair. If the repair is believed to have excessive tension, an abduction pillow may be used for 4 to 6 weeks, allowing passive motion above the pillow. Early passive motion can be achieved in this manner and postoperative stiffness can be minimized, even for massive tears.

The results following revision cuff repairs are variable and depend on the size of the tear, quality of the tissue, and chronicity of the rupture. Other factors influencing the outcome following cuff repair include a high-riding humeral head and greater than 50% fatty infiltration of the cuff muscles. MRI can show whether the cuff muscles have been replaced by fat or are significantly retracted. If so, rehabilitation alone may be the best option. If the tear cannot be repaired at the time of revision, clinical improvement can sometimes be obtained by performing a simple debridement and removal of bone spurs followed by an appropriate postoperative rehabilitation program.

Rotator cuff repairs or revisions should not be performed under excessive tension. A methodical mobilization of tissue can be performed by releasing the coracohumeral ligament and subdeltoid adhesions. If further release is needed, the superior capsule can be sharply released and elevated from the superior glenoid neck above the origin of the long head of the biceps in order to free the supraspinatus. In general, the supraspinatus should not be advanced more than 2 cm to prevent injury to the suprascapular nerve. A Bankart lesion can be made to mobilize the subscapularis or release the capsule off the glenoid neck outside the labrum.

The results following revision rotator cuff repair depend on the initial procedure and how it was done. If a patient had done well for 2 years following repair and rerupture occurs, a revision rotator cuff repair can be expected to have a good outcome. If the patient had never had good results after the first procedure, a favorable outcome can be expected less often. If the original procedure was not done adequately (eg, failing to secure the cuff to a bony trough using a strong suturing technique), revision cuff repair may be helpful.

Rotator Cuff Infection

A 60-year-old man who underwent reconstruction of a 5-cm tear 3 weeks ago has had increasing pain, fever, chills, and a draining incision.

One of the most serious complications following repair of large and massive cuff tears is postoperative infection. There must be a high index of suspicion for infection in the patient who returns with pain and limited mobility following this procedure. Early identification and treatment is the best chance for a reasonable functional outcome. Aspiration may be helpful, as are routine laboratory tests. An MRI may be helpful to identify any sequestered areas outside of the joint. If there is any doubt, surgical exploration and debridement should be performed as soon as possible, especially in the setting of a draining wound.

Once a thorough lavage and debridement are completed, every attempt should be made to repair the torn cuff as soon as possible, even at the primary debridement. Repairs done more than several days later are less likely to be possible because of the presence of muscle retraction, scarring, and adhesions. Multiple debridements over several days may be required, depending on the chronicity of the infection and the organism involved. Primary closure of the wound should be done and it should not be left to granulate.

Intravenous antibiotics are generally used for 4 to 6 weeks with an indwelling catheter, followed by oral antibiotics for 2 weeks. The functional outcome is quite variable, but a fair outcome with minimal pain can generally be expected if the infection is treated early. If continued pain and functional disability result, arthrodesis is a consideration.

Perhaps even more important than repairing the rotator cuff is maintaining a functional deltoid. Patients with an irreparable cuff after debridement for an infection can still have a functional shoulder if the deltoid can be salvaged.

Loss of Motion

A 60-year-old woman has a stiff shoulder 8 months after rotator cuff repair.

A captured shoulder is a potential complication of rotator cuff surgery[17] and is characterized by subdeltoid adhesions and capsular scarring. The normal rolling motion of the humeral head on the glenoid is restricted, while the contribution of the supraspinatus in shoulder abduction is magnified, compressing the humeral head against the glenoid and possibly resulting in chondral wear. A lengthy period of rehabilitation is indicated, given the potential to rupture the cuff with a manipulation. An arthroscopic release may be safer than a manipulation, especially during the first 6 months following repair. Arthroscopy should also be used for recalcitrant cases. Treatment involves arthroscopic release of the subdeltoid adhesions, capsular releases, and appropriate soft-tissue debridement.

Arthroplasty

Total shoulder arthroplasty is associated with numerous complications. In order of frequency, these include prosthetic loosening, glenohumeral instability, rotator cuff tears, periprosthetic fracture, infection, implant failure or dissociation, deltoid dysfunction, and neurovascular injury.[18] Coupled with the fact that the average age of patients who have a total shoulder arthroplasty is the lowest among those for all major joint replacements, a thorough understanding of the biomechanical and technical considerations that pertain to shoulder replacement surgery is important.

The rate of complications inherent to historically applied constrained total shoulder arthroplasty ranges from 8% to 100%.[19,20] Complications have been the result of biomechanical considerations, including mechanical loosening, instability, and implant fracture, deformation, or dissociation.[18] These problems are the result of fundamental design flaws, and a lack of understanding of forces around the shoulder. These forces approximate body weight during unrestricted active elevation of the shoulder. Because of this fact, Wirth and Rockwood[18] question the use of constrained systems even as a salvage procedure. Currently, do not use constrained systems.

Complications such as loosening, instability, infection, and periprosthetic fracture are less common after unconstrained total shoulder arthroplasty. According to Neer and associates,[21] 4 factors must be addressed to minimize complications: (1) osseous deficiency of the humeral head or glenoid; (2) defective rotator cuff; (3) deficient/dysfunctional deltoid muscle; and (4) chronic instability.

Glenoid Loosening

A 71-year-old man who underwent a total shoulder arthroplasty 5 years ago now complains of increasing pain and decreased motion.

Radiographic loosening of the glenoid or humeral component is common and represents nearly one third of all complications associated with total shoulder arthroplasty.[18] Most cases of clinically significant loosening involve the glenoid. The diagnosis can be difficult, with a differential diagnosis that includes cuff tears, subscapularis ruptures, instability, infection, and even fracture. To complicate the matter, radiolucent lines are frequently seen after surgery as a result of suboptimal cementing technique. Torchia and Cofield[22] reported an 84% rate of glenoid radiolucencies at 12 years, with 44% definite radiologic loosening. Clinical loosening is less common,[21,23–25] with most series reporting a glenoid revision rate of less than 2%. Even so, the high incidence of radiographic glenoid loosening has led some authors to recommend primary hemiarthroplasty for glenohumeral osteoarthrosis.[26]

A variety of methods can be used to diagnose a loose glenoid component. Physical examination is very helpful, with patients reporting increased pain on motion testing, a restricted arc of motion, and the occasional presence of a "clunk" with motion. Sequential radiographs and/or arthrograms may document a change in position of the component, while fluoroscopically positioned spot views of the glenoid can show the bone-cement interface quite accurately. More recently, arthroscopy is becoming the procedure of choice to assess the stability of the glenoid.

Once it has been determined that the glenoid is loose, it should be removed. Bony defects in the glenoid may be grafted. The decision whether to reimplant a glenoid must be made on an individual basis. In general, the glenoid can be left out with a conversion to a hemiarthroplasty. The grafting procedure will permit the rare insertion of the glenoid in the future if symptoms dictate.

Several technical modifications can improve fixation and durability of the glenoid component.[18] The subchondral plate should be preserved using concentric spherical reaming for optimum osseous support,[27] new glenoid designs and biomaterials[28] are available, and mismatching of the diameters of the glenoid and humeral head[29,30] may be advantageous. The use of cemented, pegged polyethylene glenoid components is preferred. Epinephrine-soaked thrombin sponges are placed prior to cementing to keep the bony surface as dry as possible for interdigitation of the cement.

Humeral loosening is rarely a problem. Cofield[24] reported that lucent lines around a humeral prosthesis do not indicate future clinical problems. Radiolucent lines have been more frequently reported around uncemented humeral components. However, clinical loosening is rare.[24,31] A press-fit of the humeral component in the medullary canal is preferred. Occasionally, bone graft from the humeral head can be used to help fill a capacious canal. Cement is reserved for cases in which a stable press-fit cannot be obtained, or in fracture management (for example, 4-part fractures).

Arthroplasty Instability

A 56-year-old woman who underwent a total shoulder arthroplasty 7 months ago now complains of instability and pain.

Glenohumeral instability is the second most common complication following total shoulder arthroplasty, ranging from 0%[32] to 29%.[22] Anterior instability is usually the result of humeral component malrotation, anterior deltoid dysfunction,[26] or rupture of the repaired subscapularis.[33] Clinically obvious anterior subluxation or dislocation does not occur without an incompetent subscapularis or coracoacromial arch.[18,26] Disruption of the subscapularis repair can result from poor surgical technique, poor tissue quality, inappropriate physical therapy, or the use of oversized components. When performing the subscapularis tenotomy, an adequate stump of tendon left laterally is helpful for reattachment. The repair is later performed using interrupted, heavy, nonabsorbable sutures. Medializing the subscapularis and capsule to the osteotomy cut requires meticulous tendon to bone suturing, and can be quite difficult. In order to protect the subscapularis repair, external rotation may be restricted for the first 3 weeks.

Superior instability is associated with rotator cuff dysfunction, failed cuff repair, rotator cuff rupture, an incompetent coracoacromial arch, and an excessive acromioplasty. It is not directly related to the development of discomfort or impending component failure.[34] However, the potential for glenoid loosening is certainly increased because of edge loading at the superior glenoid rim.[23] Anterosuperior instability is a nearly unsolvable problem. Attempts to reconstruct the coracoacromial ligament or obtain coverage of the humeral component have limited success.

Posterior instability is typically associated with a glenoid component that is retroverted more than 20°, or a humeral component that is retroverted more than 45°.[18,25] A tight anterior closure or posterior glenoid erosion can also lead to posterior instability, as can arthroplasty for locked posterior dislocations. Chronic osteoarthrosis frequently causes erosion of the posterior aspect of the glenoid. If unrecognized at surgery, the component can be inserted with excessive retroversion. Minor bony deficiencies can be compensated for by careful reaming of the anterior rim, or by alteration of the humeral version so that the combined glenohumeral retroversion equals 30°. For example, in the presence of a chronic, locked posterior dislocation, neutral version may be needed to prevent posterior instability. Severe deficiencies may require posterior bone grafting.[35] Computed tomography is helpful to assess the extent of bony deficiency. Posterior capsulorrhaphy is helpful to prevent posterior instability in this setting.

Inferior instability is typically found after arthroplasty for proximal humeral fractures, revision arthroplasty procedures, or previous osteosynthesis.[18,21,36] Inferior subluxation impedes the ability to elevate the arm because of shortening of the humerus and subsequent weakening of the deltoid. The resting tension of the deltoid and rotator cuff must be preserved during shoulder arthroplasty. In general, the head of the humeral component should be higher than the greater tuberosity after insertion. In cases of severe comminution, indirect reduction of the fracture fragments with longitudinal traction can temporarily restore humeral length to allow proper positioning of the humeral component to be assessed and marked prior to insertion.

If inferior instability does occur, several treatments can be attempted. Inferior subluxation caused by muscle atony presents the most difficult challenge, and is generally addressed through rehabilitation. A Kenny Howard sling can be used in cases of prolonged inferior instability in order to maintain reduction. The neurologic status of the deltoid and brachial plexus should be assessed. An inferior capsular shift and superior reconstruction may be attempted if nonsurgical measures are unsuccessful.

Recurrent Cuff Tear

One year after undergoing a total shoulder arthroplasty, a 64-year-old man complains of pain, decreased motion, and weakness in his shoulder.

Postoperative tearing of the rotator cuff occurs in 1% to 13% of cases.[18,26] The natural history is similar to that seen in the general population, and pain is not a universal feature.[26] The diagnosis can be difficult. MRI may not be helpful, and arthrograms and arthroscopy are usually not. Surgical exploration following a high index of suspicion is the best method of diagnosis. Surgical cuff repair following arthroplasty poses a significant challenge. Emphasis should be placed on rehabilitation of the deltoid, the remaining cuff, and scapular stabilizers.

Periprosthetic Fracture

A 75-year-old man who underwent a total shouder arthroplasty 6 years ago falls while walking down the stairs and sustains a fracture at the tip of the humeral prosthesis.

Periprosthetic fracture has been reported in 3% of shoulder arthroplasties,[18,26,37] and accounts for 20% of all complications.[38] Intraoperative fractures are the result of excessive and/or maldirected reaming, forceful humeral component insertion, or manipulation of the humerus during surgery to enhance exposure.[39] It is important during patient positioning to ensure that the arm is free to extend over the side of the table in order to facilitate humeral preparation. A bone hook is used to dislocate the humeral head to minimize the torque and forces necessary to deliver the humeral head. Power reamers are avoided, particularly in osteopenic bone. The humeral component is placed from a superolateral position to allow direct insertion into the humeral canal. Adequate surgical exposure and retractor placement also avoids the need for excessive humeral manipulation for visualization during glenoid preparation. If an intraoperative fracture does occur, immediate open reduction and internal fixation is recommended. Cerclage wiring with possible exchange of the humeral component to a long-stem prosthesis may be performed. Bone grafting is optimal.

Postoperative fractures also occur following total shoulder arthroplasty. Advocates of immediate open reduction and internal fixation[39,40] point out that the advanced age of many patients, marked osteopenia, and poor soft-tissue quality make nonsurgical treatment less attractive. In addition, a faster return to function has been reported with immediate fixation. Others believe that nonsurgical treatment with bracing can be successful.[18,37] If satisfactory alignment and/or healing cannot be obtained in a brace, open reduction and internal fixation with grafting as needed should be performed. **(CD-43.1)**

Infection

A 58-year-old man who underwent total shoulder arthroplasty 3 weeks ago now has increasing pain, fever, and chills. Infection following total shoulder arthroplasty is a rare but serious complication. The presence of comorbidities such as diabetes mellitus, rheumatoid arthritis, collagen vascular disorders and previous surgeries will increase the chance of infection.[18] The use of immunosuppressive drugs such as corticosteroids has also been associated with an increased risk of sepsis.

Laboratory tests such as a complete blood count, an erythrocyte sedimentation rate, and a C-reactive protein may help to confirm the diagnosis, but cannot definitively rule out infection. Radioisotope scanning and joint aspiration may also be helpful. In reality, sepsis becomes a clinical diagnosis based on a detailed history and physical examination. Once a diagnosis is made, options for treatment include antibiotic suppression, irrigation and debridement, removal of the implant with reimplantation, resection arthroplasty, and possible arthrodesis.

The type of treatment depends on the length of time from the index arthroplasty, the virulence of the offending organism, the stability of the implants, and the comorbidities of the patient. An aggressive approach to suspected infections is recommended. Early surgical exploration is performed, and appropriate cultures are taken. Frozen tissue sections can give additional information. In the absence of obvious purulence with a stable prosthesis, an extensive debridement with copious antibiotic irrigation is performed, and the implant retained.

If the implant is loose or a gram-negative organism is isolated, the implant is removed and antibiotic beads are placed. One-stage reimplantation is seldom indicated. Parenteral antibiotics are generally administered for 4 weeks, followed by 3 weeks of oral therapy. Staged reimplantation can be done at about 3 months. Consideration can be given to converting a total shoulder arthroplasty to a hemiarthroplasty at that time. If the organism was virulent, gram-negative, and debridements have failed, resectional arthroplasty may be the treatment of choice. Following resectional arthroplasty, pain relief can be expected in two thirds of patients, and active elevation of 70° can be achieved. Arthrodesis is also an option in this setting, but the huge amount of bone loss and graft that would be needed make it a less attractive alternative.

Neurologic Injury

A 41-year-old woman with rheumatoid arthritis has no biceps function with an absent biceps reflex on the first day after a total shoulder arthroplasty.

Nerve injury following total shoulder arthroplasty is rare, with an incidence ranging from less than 1%[25] to 4%.[41] The upper and middle trunks of the brachial plexus are most commonly affected. The long deltopectoral approach leaving the deltoid attached to the clavicle has been found to be associated with nerve injury, as have shorter surgical times and the use of methotrexate.[41] Most complications involving peripheral nerves in total shoulder arthroplasty are neurapraxias caused by compression or traction. Laceration of an axillary nerve has been reported.[42]

All patients should have a careful neurologic examination following total shoulder arthroplasty. When a deficit is noted, there is little indication for immediate exploration unless an intraoperative incident that could be related to the deficit is suspected. Otherwise, passive motion should be maintained during the recovery period. Temporary static splinting may be helpful. If a hematoma is suspected, an MRI scan may be helpful. If there is no improvement after 6 weeks, electromyography is performed to help determine whether the injury is to an isolated peripheral nerve (the musculocutaneous in this case) or to the brachial plexus. In addition, an electromyogram can assess the extent and degree of injury, that is, whether the injury is complete or incomplete. Surgical exploration should be performed in the rare event that there is no spontaneous improvement by clinical or electromyographic examination after 3 to 6 months. Neurologic injury after total shoulder arthroplasty has little effect on the long-term result.[41]

Miscellaneous Complications of Arthroplasty

A variety of complications related to the prosthesis have been reported in total shoulder arthroplasty (SD Martin, MD, CB Sledge, MD, WH Thomas, MD, TS Thornhill, MD, 1995, unpublished data). These include dissociation of modular humeral components,[43] dissociation of the polyethylene liner from its metal-backed glenoid component,[44,45] fracture of the glenoid keel or metal-backing,[44] and fracture of the glenoid fixation screws.[46]

Neer and Kirby[47] reported on the complications associated with revision shoulder arthroplasty. The most common causes of failure were preoperative conditions such as neuromuscular problems, infection, or systemic arthritis; surgical complications such as detachment of the deltoid muscle, nonunion of the greater tuberosity, or loosening/breakage of the components; and postoperative problems such as glenohumeral instability and insufficient rehabilitation. Loss of external rotation was also common. The results of revision arthroplasty were inferior to the results of primary arthroplasty.

There are many factors that contribute to a favorable outcome following total shoulder arthroplasty. Perhaps the most important element is maintenance of good deltoid function, which is essential to the success of total shoulder arthroplasty.[18]

Complications of Fracture Management

A variety of complications have been reported to follow closed or open treatment of proximal humeral fractures.[48,49] These include infection, neurovascular injury, malunion, nonunion, hardware failure, joint stiffness, heterotopic ossification, and cuff deficiency. Osteonecrosis is a specific complication of displaced proximal humerus fractures.[48] Infection occurs infrequently after open reduction and internal fixation of proximal humerus fractures because of an excellent vascular supply with good soft-tissue coverage.

The rate of nonunion is dependent on the fracture pattern, but is significantly increased with excessive soft-tissue stripping at surgery. Joint stiffness following surgery can be minimized by avoiding prolonged immobilization and prominent hardware. Heterotopic ossification is minimized by avoiding repetitive forceful attempts at closed reduction, operating within 7 days of injury, and the use of adequate irrigation during surgery to debride bone fragments.

Neurovascular Injury

A 31-year-old man collides with a tree while skiing and sustains a 3-part proximal humerus fracture. Evaluation in the emergency department reveals that the patient is neurologically intact. Open reduction and internal fixation are performed, but biceps function is absent in the recovery room.

Neurovascular injury following open reduction of proximal humeral fractures has been reported, with an incidence of axillary artery compromise up to 5% and a 6% incidence of brachial plexus injuries.[50,51] Vascular injuries are generally the result of the initial trauma and typically occur at the junction of the anterior humeral circumflex and axillary arteries. However, the axillary artery can be injured during open reduction through manipulation of the fracture fragments as well. The axillary nerve is vulnerable at the inferior aspect of the capsule, where it can be closely adherent with the altered fracture anatomy, or with excessive deltoid-splitting for exposure.[52] If the location of the nerve is unclear, it should be explored and protected. Overzealous retraction of the conjoined muscle to gain exposure can injure the musculocutaneous nerve as well.

In this case, it is not completely clear whether the musculocutaneous injury was caused in the operating room or at the time of the initial trauma, although intraoperative retraction is the most likely source. An electromyogram may be obtained at 6 weeks to document the extent and degree of injury. If there is no evidence of functional or electromyographic return, the nerve may be explored at 3 to 6 months.

Osteonecrosis

A 46-year-old woman who has a 3-part proximal humerus fracture undergoes open reduction and internal fixation using plates and screws. The fracture pattern was difficult to assess and reduce, and wide exposure was necessary to perform the internal fixation. One year later, the patient has shoulder pain and increased humeral head density on radiographs.

Osteonecrosis is one of the most severe complications following some 2-part fractures, displaced 3-part fractures, and 4-part fractures. The incidence ranges from 3% to 25% in 3-part fractures, and is as high as 90% in 4-part fractures.[48,53] The incidence of osteonecrosis is higher in patients who undergo open reduction and internal fixation than those treated closed.

In order to minimize this complication, a technique of open reduction and internal fixation that involves minimal soft-tissue stripping is recommended. After the superficial dissection, exposure of the entire proximal humerus is not performed. Instead, visualization and anatomic landmarks can be obtained through the fracture lines themselves. Indirect reduction through longitudinal traction while using a Freer elevator for gentle fragment manipulation is often all that is necessary to perform an adequate reduction. A tension-band wire technique[54] can be used for fracture fixation of 3-part and some 4-part fractures that minimizes soft-tissue stripping and provides adequate support for early postoperative motion.

If osteonecrosis does develop, a correlation with patient symptoms must be assessed, because not all osteonecrosis causes pain. Hemiarthroplasty can be performed in the setting of painful osteonecrosis, following open reduction and internal fixation of a proximal humerus fracture. A glenoid component may be necessary in long-standing cases if secondary destruction of the glenoid has occurred.

Cuff-Tuberosity Failure

A vigorous 69-year-old man falls and sustains a 4-part fracture of the proximal humerus. A hemiarthroplasty is performed. Postoperatively, the patient continues to complain of limited motion and pain despite months of appropriate rehabilitation. Range of motion testing reveals pain with active elevation to 80°. Radiographs show inferior subluxation of the humeral head with the tuberosities above the level of the prosthetic head.

Immediate prosthetic replacement for 4-part fractures has met with varied success and a host of complications. Neer[48] reported consistently good and excellent results, whereas the results of other authors have been less favorable.[55] Failures are generally the result of an inability to reconstruct the rotator cuff, failure to obtain bony union (not soft-tissue attachment) of the tuberosities to the shaft, failure to reproduce the anatomic humeral offset and length that provides the necessary lever arm for the rotator cuff and deltoid muscles, and failure to recreate the appropriate glenohumeral retroversion to help insure joint stability. Axillary nerve palsy has been reported, as has instability of the implant.[56]

A good functional result following prosthetic replacement is directly related to the surgeon's ability to obtain union of the rotator cuff and its attached tuberosities to the humeral shaft. Techniques that can enhance this outcome include: (1) the use of cement, placing the humeral prosthesis in the appropriate resting length with 30° to 40° of retroversion; (2) secure fixation of the tuberosities to the humeral shaft (not the prosthesis); and (3) bone graft underneath the tuberosities, as needed.[56] If there is difficulty assessing the version of the prosthesis, a simple test can determine its accuracy. The hand and forearm should be placed in neutral rotation with the elbow adducted at the side. In this position, the humeral head should point to the glenoid. If the bicipital groove can be found, the lateral flange should be placed 7 mm posterior to it. Failure to achieve union of the tuberosities to the shaft results in a cuff-deficient shoulder. Early reconstruction allows the best chance at salvaging shoulder function. Late reconstruction is extremely challenging.

In the case presented, the humeral component has been placed in an inferior position. Humeral length has not been reestablished, and impingement is resulting from the tuberosities that have been repaired in a position superior to the humeral head. If the patient is able to live with the pain and limited motion, further rehabilitation is all that should be done. If not, consideration might be given to a revision arthroplasty using a cemented humeral prosthesis to regain humeral length.

Application of Arthrodesis for Complications of Shoulder Surgery

Glenohumeral arthrodesis is indicated for the multiply operated rotator cuff patient with pain who remains disabled, and the multiply operated instability patient who remains unstable with recalcitrant, chronic pain that has not responded to more traditional measures. Failed and/or infected total shoulder arthroplasties can also be considered for arthrodesis, although resection arthroplasty may be the preferred option in these cases because of the technical challenge and generally poor outcomes that follow attempts at arthrodesis. Arthrodesis is a late salvage procedure in the patient with an extremely painful shoulder and without any other surgical options. Under such circumstances, patients will usually opt to live with the pain, and this may be the best option. A trial of immobilization for 1 to 2 weeks that greatly diminishes pain might suggest the outcome from glenohumeral fusion. Resection arthroplasty as an alternative to arthrodesis may be a better option following arthroplasty failure.

Malrotation of the Arthrodesis

A 27-year-old woman has an arthrodesis of her dominant shoulder for intractable multidirectional instability despite repeated attempts at surgical stabilization. The surgeon tells the patient that the arthrodesis was "successful" at 6 months because of radiographic evidence of union at the glenohumeral joint. However, the patient is functionally disabled, and is unable to feed herself, use a computer, or perform rectal hygiene.

The most common complication following glenohumeral arthrodesis is malrotation of the shoulder.[57] Nonunion, wound infection, iliac crest wound hematomas, and fracture below the implant also occur. Malposition is defined as fusion in more than 15° of flexion or abduction, or rotation of less than 40° or more than 60°. If the shoulder is in excessive abduction or flexion, it cannot hang comfortably when the arm is at the side. The scapula becomes medially or posteriorly rotated, resulting in periscapular muscle strain and chronic pain. Rotation must allow the patient to reach his or her mouth and opposite axilla, the front of his or her shirt, belt buckle, and buttocks. Reconstructive osteotomy as described by Groh and associates[57] is the procedure of choice to eliminate pain and improve function.

Frozen Shoulder

A 38-year-old woman in whom impingement is the diagnosis has an arthroscopic subacromial decompression. Four months later, there is global loss of motion in all planes with a firm endpoint on passive testing. The patient complains of pain, insomnia, and an inability to perform activities of daily living.

Frozen shoulder can be a postoperative complication rather than a primary, idiopathic condition. In this setting, a specific diagnosis as to the cause of the motion loss must be made. Typically, motion is restricted more in one plane than others. For example, loss of external rotation following instability surgery is generally caused by tight anterior soft tissues. In this setting, manipulation is not likely to be helpful. Arthroscopic release or an open release with subscapularis lengthening would be appropriate. In contrast, loss of elevation following an acromioplasty is more often the result of subacromial and/or subdeltoid adhesions, and should be treated with an appropriate release or manipulation.

The diagnosis of frozen shoulder must be differentiated from true adhesive capsulitis. True adhesive capsulitis is a primary pathology of the joint capsule that typically results in a global loss of motion in all planes. The treatment of this condition involves rehabilitation with terminal stretch exercises. Manipulation under anesthesia is a useful adjunct in expediting the return to motion, especially if no improvements in motion are seen after 3 weeks of therapy. If a full range of motion is not restored at the time of closed manipulation, arthroscopic release is indicated.[58] A global release can be performed, beginning at the rotator interval and continuing anteriorly and inferiorly through the anterior capsule and subscapularis. The axillary pouch and posterior capsule are released as well, with care taken inferiorly to avoid the axillary nerve. Results following this treatment have been excellent.

Complications of manipulation include humeral fracture, dislocation, rotator cuff tearing, or rarely, neurovascular injury. Excessive force should be avoided during manipulation. If motion does not return using a judicious amount of force, arthroscopic release is generally a safer option.

Arthroscopy

In general, arthroscopy of the shoulder is a safe procedure. Of 21 experienced arthroscopists polled, only 9 complications were revealed out of over 1,100 cases.[59] Staple capsulorrhaphy had the highest complication rate (3.3%). Major complications, such as neurologic and vascular injuries, were extremely rare. Less common general complications included severe iatrogenic cartilage damage during instrument insertion, instrument breakage, and reflex sympathetic dystrophy.[60]

Septic arthritis following shoulder arthroscopy is rare. Reported rates range from 0.04% to 3.4%.[61,62] The use of perioperative antibiotics has been reported to be beneficial, with up to a 4-fold reduction in infection rates.[61,63] Strict adherence to antiseptic techniques and the reduction of surgical time are also important.

Patient Positioning

A 21-year-old man has an arthroscopic Bankart procedure performed for anterior instability. A general anesthetic is used. The patient is noted to have a musculocutaneous nerve palsy in the recovery room.

Patient positioning, particularly of the head in the beach chair position, must be checked before and during any arthroscopic procedure. All bony prominences must be well padded. An axillary roll can help prevent compression of the brachial plexus against the thorax by the humeral head.[64] Excessive extension, rotation, and lateral flexion of the neck toward either side should be avoided to minimize tension on the plexus. Allowing the arm to hang off the table increases strain on the plexus by placing the arm in an abducted, externally rotated and extended position, as can happen with the use of an oversized shoulder roll. Adduction of the arm keeps the axillary and musculocutaneous nerves more medial with respect to the shoulder, thus allowing a safer area of instrumentation lateral to the coracoid. Traction with forward flexion of 20° minimizes plexus strain. Extreme arm extension and abduction should be avoided.

Proper patient positioning is essential to lessen the potential for pressure and traction neurapraxias.[60] Brachial plexus injury caused by malpositioning of the patient during surgery is a rare but documented complication.[64] In the lateral decubitus position, brachial plexus strain is most common. Although this is generally considered a rare complication, an incidence as high as 30% has been reported, with resolution of symptoms occurring in 6 to 12 weeks.[65,66] Pitman and associates[66] demonstrated that the incidence of subclinical neurapraxias is high, most likely related to arm positioning, joint distension, and traction. The musculocutaneous nerve was most vulnerable as it enters the conjoined muscles, particularly with the combination of traction and abduction. While in the lateral decubitus position, the patient's dependent arm should be placed anterior to the thorax and a roll placed in the axilla to avoid plexus compression. Balanced longitudinal skin traction not to exceed 10 to 15 lb should be anchored on the operating table instead of a fixed point on the floor.[64] The arm should be flexed 10° to 20° with no more than 70° of abduction. Some authors[60,67] have advocated the beach chair position to reduce the incidence of traction neurapraxias.

Once a neurologic injury is documented, it is almost always a neurapraxia. Full recovery is generally seen with expectant treatment.

Fluid Extravasation

A surgeon is performing an arthroscopic subacromial decompression when the surgical field becomes filled with blood. The surgeon increases the pressure of the arthroscopic pump in order to obtain hemostasis. Once the field clears, the pressure is left elevated. The procedure has been going on for over 90 minutes when the assistant notices that the patient's shoulder is greatly swollen. The surgery is rapidly completed and the arthroscope removed.

Extravasation of fluid can complicate shoulder arthroscopy.[60] All landmarks and portals should be marked prior to inserting the arthroscope to facilitate proper orientation if edema does occur. The pressure sensor should be attached to the arthroscope, and the pump pressure closely monitored. If extravasation does occur, it seldom poses a risk to the patient. Ogilvie-Harris and Boynton[68] demonstrated that the pressure in the deltoid muscle drops to baseline levels minutes after finishing a procedure with no clinical or electromyographic evidence of muscle damage. This is in direct contrast to arthroscopy of the knee, where extravasation of fluid can cause a compartment syndrome. Therefore, if extravasation does occur, turn off the fluid for 10 minutes. If the swelling persists, expedite the completion of the procedure.

Intraoperative bleeding can be minimized during shoulder arthroscopy by maintaining irrigation fluids at the recommended height or pressure, using a solution containing 10 ml of epinephrine (1:300,000 to 1:3,000,000) diluted in a 3-l bag, infiltrating portals with a marcaine and epinephrine solution, and the use of hypotensive anesthesia.[60] Hypotensive anesthesia is especially helpful during subacromial decompressions to prevent bleeding from the bursal capillaries as well as the exposed cancellous bed of the acromion. The use of electrocautery devices prior to and during shaving in the subacromial space is also recommended to prevent excessive soft-tissue bleeding. If a bleeding vessel is identified, it should be cauterized.

Complications Related to Subacromial Space Procedures

A 32-year-old man who is a football player has an arthroscopic subacromial decompression for impingement. He returns to contact drills at 6 weeks postoperatively, and notices sharp pain in his shoulder and a return of his impingement symptoms after practice. Radiographs demonstrate a displaced acromial fracture.

Arthroscopic subacromial space procedures are generally safe, with favorable short-term results and a complication rate less than 1%.[59,60,69–71] Complications include intraoperative bleeding, instrument breakage, transient neurapraxias, and acromial fracture. Proper patient selection is essential.

Acromial burring should be performed cautiously to avoid fracture resulting from aggressive resection. If there is any doubt regarding the adequacy of resection, the lateral portal can be extended by 1 to 2 cm to allow digital palpation of the subacromial space. Any remaining bony prominences, particularly at the anterolateral corner of the acromion, can be identified and resected without removing more bone from adequately decompressed areas. This is especially helpful early in the learning curve with this procedure. The incidence of failure resulting from inadequate decompression can be minimized by using this technique without introducing any added morbidity. The presence of partial- or full-thickness rotator cuff tears can also be assessed using digital palpation. If a displaced fracture involving a significant portion of the acromion occurs as in this case, open reduction internal fixation using a tension-band technique should be performed.

Other complications of subacromial decompression include hematoma and traction neuropathy,[69] infection, acromial fracture,[72] reflex sympathetic dystrophy,[72,73] and instrument breakage. Heterotopic bone was reported postoperatively in 10 cases in 1 series,[74] with recurrent impingement occurring in 8. Patients at risk, such as those with hypertrophic pulmonary arthropathy, obesity, or diabetes, should be considered for heterotopic ossification prophylaxis. An increased rate of complications can be expected in patients with additional preoperative pathologic conditions, such as neck pain or restricted motion, and in a workers' compensation population.[73]

Complications Related to Arthroscopic Instability Surgery

A 25-year-old woman undergoes an arthroscopic Bankart procedure performed for recurrent anterior instability. Six months postoperatively, she returns to competitive kayaking, but sustains a dislocation in the high-post position (abduction, external rotation).

For an arthroscopic stabilization procedure to be accepted, it must parallel the results obtained with open stabilization of the same problem. Aside from high failure rates with arthroscopic stabilizations, the possibility of nerve injury may be greater.[75,76] In fact, the highest complication rate (3.2%) in shoulder arthroscopy has been reported with staple capsulorrhaphy,[59] and recurrence is more likely than with open repairs. Migration of hardware and articular damage is not uncommon.[7] As a result, we do not perform this procedure for the treatment of instability of the glenohumeral joint.

The approach to arthroscopic stabilization procedures has changed significantly over the past 2 years since the introduction of laser and heat probe techniques. In the past, a contributing factor to the high rate of unsuccessful arthroscopic Bankart procedures was a failure to address the capsular redundancy that typically accompanies traumatic Bankart lesions. Although this redundancy is able to be successfully addressed during open Bankart repairs,[2] simply suturing the anterior capsule/labrum back to the glenoid rim arthroscopically does not achieve the same goal. In order to address this problem, an anterior thermal capsulorrhaphy can be added to the vast majority of arthroscopic Bankart procedures. Postoperative stability is generally excellent, and has paralleled the results of open reconstructions at short-term follow-up. Restriction of motion has been minimal with this technique, averaging about 5° less external rotation on the operated shoulder. Complications with this technique have been minimal.

For glenohumeral instability without a Bankart lesion, a thermal capsulorrhaphy rather than an open inferior capsular shift can be considered. As with the arthroscopic Bankart procedures, early results have been very encouraging. Mild to moderate instabilities are immobilized for 1 week following the procedure, reserving 2- to 3-week immobilizations for severe unidirectional and most multidirectional instabilities. Altough anecdotal reports of axillary nerve injuries have been reported following thermal shrinkage of the axillary pouch, this complication has not been seen by us.

Even so, nerve injury can occur during arthroscopic procedures.[66,77,78] The suprascapular nerve is vulnerable with transglenoid techniques as it descends in the posterior aspect of the glenoid neck. The axillary nerve is at risk with thermal shrinkage of the inferior aspect of the axillary pouch, or with inferior instrument placement. A recent anatomic study has demonstrated a margin of safety of 1 cm with surgery to the inferior capsule (CL Eakin, MD, RJ Hawkins, MD, 1997, unpublished data). The axillary nerve is also vulnerable from a low posterior portal placement. The cannula should not be placed lower than 2 cm from the posterolateral border of the acromion to avoid damage to the nerve.[79] Finally, the musculocutaneous nerve can be damaged by placing an anterior portal too low or too medial. In general, the anterior portal must not be placed inferior or medial to the coracoid process.

Correct portal placement is essential to avoid nerve injury. The posterior portal is located approximately 2 cm distal and 1 cm medial to the posterolateral corner of the acromion. Distal placement can injure the axillary nerve. The cannula is inserted in the direction of the coracoid. More medial insertion can injure the suprascapular neurovascular bundle. The anterior portal is placed just distal to the acromioclavicular joint. It must remain lateral and proximal to the coracoid process. It can be established under direct visualization using a spinal needle, or via a Wissinger rod passed through the posterior cannula positioned in the superior interval. Passage of the rod below the subscapularis can injure the brachial plexus and axillary sheath. The musculocutaneous nerve is at risk of injury because of an excessively medial anterior portal placement. The lateral portal is placed 2 cm from the lateral border of the acromion. Inferior placement can damage the axillary nerve.

Nerve injuries during shoulder arthroscopy can also occur during joint distension, fluid extravasation, positioning, manipulation, excessive traction,[66] and portal placement.[80] Traction can be applied either parallel or perpendicular to the long axis of the arm. Perpendicular traction minimizes abduction and therefore neurapraxias.[81] In general, no more than 10 to 15 lb of traction is necessary and it should be attached to the operating table rather than applied by a fixed object. An assistant can also be used. The brachial plexus is at risk because it is attached at 2 points along its course (the prevertebral fascia at the transverse processes and the axillary fascia in the arm). As longitudinal traction increases the distance between these 2 fixed points, injury can occur. The freely moving humeral head and clavicle can also cause injury with malpositioning.

In general, proper patient selection and attention to technical detail will decrease the incidence of complications in shoulder arthroscopy. Careful patient and extremity positioning lessens the potential for pressure and traction neurapraxias. Electrosurgical instruments and adequate distension pressure helps to minimize intraoperative bleeding and improves visualization.

Conclusion

In general, the results following shoulder surgery are somewhat more variable than those obtained in other aspects of orthopaedic surgery. A significant reason for this is the failure to establish an accurate diagnosis prior to surgery. Seldom should the surgeon be in a position where the joint is being 'explored' in order to determine the source of pain. Diagnoses such as instability, impingement, acromioclavicular arthritis, and biceps tendinitis can rarely be made in this fashion. Instead, a careful history and physical examination coupled with appropriate imaging and laboratory tests will generally reveal the source of pathology. The difficulty in diagnosis around the shoulder is compounded by the fact that many problems, such as rotator cuff disease and instability, exist along a spectrum of severity, and are not mutually exclusive of other pathology. By having a clear understanding of the pathophysiology that affects the shoulder and making carefully selected surgical decisions, the incidence of complications surrounding surgery to the shoulder can be significantly diminished.

Once the decision to perform surgery has been made, knowledge of potential intraoperative and postoperative complications can significantly lower their incidence. For example, the use of hand reamers instead of power reamers and minimizing rotational torque during humeral preparation in total shoulder arthroplasty can minimize the potential for fracturing the humerus. The clinician should have a high index of suspicion when evaluating for potential postoperative complications such as infection. Early recognition and aggressive treatment will allow the optimal functional outcome. Lastly, the surgeon must know what can and cannot help. Surgery for a failed Bankart procedure can yield excellent results, but attempting to operate on superior instability following total shoulder arthroplasty is more likely to be futile.

References

1. Hawkins RH, Hawkins RJ: Failed anterior reconstruction for shoulder instability. *J Bone Joint Surg* 1985;67B:709–714.
2. Gill TJ, Micheli LJ, Gebhard F, Binder C: Bankart repair for anterior instability of the shoulder: Long-term outcome. *J Bone Joint Surg* 1997;79A:850–857.
3. Samilson RL, Prieto V: Dislocation arthropathy of the shoulder. *J Bone Joint Surg* 1983;65A:456–460.
4. Rosenberg BN, Richmond JC, Levine WN: Long-term followup of Bankart reconstruction: Incidence of late degenerative glenohumeral arthrosis. *Am J Sports Med* 1995;23:538–544.
5. O'Driscoll SW, Evans DC: Long-term results of staple capsulorrhaphy for anterior instability of the shoulder. *J Bone Joint Surg* 1993;75A:249–258.
6. Sisk TD, Boyd HB: Management of recurrent anterior dislocation of the shoulder: Du Toit-type or staple capsulorrhaphy. *Clin Orthop* 1974;103:150–156.
7. Zuckerman JD, Matsen FA III: Complications about the glenohumeral joint related to the use of screws and staples. *J Bone Joint Surg* 1984:66A:175–180.
8. Young DC, Rockwood CA Jr: Complications of a failed Bristow procedure and their management. *J Bone Joint Surg* 1991;73A:969–981.
9. Lusardi DA, Wirth MA, Wurtz D, Rockwood CA Jr: Loss of external rotation following anterior capsulorrhaphy of the shoulder. *J Bone Joint Surg* 1993;75A:1185–1192.
10. Hawkins RJ, Angelo RL: Glenohumeral osteoarthrosis: A late complication of the Putti-Platt repair. *J Bone Joint Surg* 1990;72A:1193–1197.
11. MacDonald PB, Hawkins RJ, Fowler PJ, Miniaci A: Release of the subscapularis for internal rotation contracture and pain after anterior repair for recurrent anterior dislocation of the shoulder. *J Bone Joint Surg* 1992;74A:734–737.
12. Leach RE, Corbett M, Schepsis A, Stockel J: Results of a modified Putti-Platt operation for recurrent shoulder dislocations and subluxations. *Clin Orthop* 1982;164:20–25.
13. Richards RR, Hudson AR, Bertoia JT, Urbaniak JR, Waddell JP: Injury to the brachial plexus during Putti-Platt and Bristow procedures: A report of eight cases. *Am J Sports Med* 1987;15:374–380.
14. Hill JA, Lombardo SJ, Kerlan RK, et al: The modified Bristow-Helfet procedure for recurrent anterior shoulder subluxations and dislocations. *Am J Sports Med* 1981;9:283–287.
15. Hovelius L, Korner L, Lundberg B, et al: The coracoid transfer for recurrent dislocation of the shoulder: Technical aspects of the Bristow-Latarjet procedure. *J Bone Joint Surg* 1983;65A:926–934.
16. Post M: Complications of rotator cuff surgery. *Clin Orthop* 1990;254:97–104.
17. Mormino MA, Gross RM, McCarthy JA: Captured shoulder: A complication of rotator cuff surgery. *Arthroscopy* 1996;12:457–461.
18. Wirth MA, Rockwood CA Jr: Complications of total shoulder-replacement

arthroplasty. *J Bone Joint Surg* 1996;78A: 603–616.

19. Laurence M: Replacement arthroplasty of the rotator cuff deficient shoulder. *J Bone Joint Surg* 1991;73B:916–919.
20. Post M: Constrained arthroplasty of the shoulder. *Orthop Clin North Am* 1987;18: 455–462.
21. Neer CS II, Watson KC, Stanton FJ: Recent experience in total shoulder replacement. *J Bone Joint Surg* 1982;64A:319–337.
22. Torchia ME, Cofield RH: Long-term results of Neer total shoulder arthroplasty. *Orthop Trans* 1994;18:977.
23. Barrett WP, Franklin JL, Jackins SE, Wyss CR, Matsen FA III: Total shoulder arthroplasty. *J Bone Joint Surg* 1987;69A:865–872.
24. Cofield RH: Total shoulder arthroplasty with the Neer prosthesis. *J Bone Joint Surg* 1984;66A:899–906.
25. Hawkins RJ, Bell RH, Jallay B: Total shoulder arthroplasty. *Clin Orthop* 1989; 242:188–194.
26. Wirth MA, Rockwood CA Jr: Complications of shoulder arthroplasty. *Clin Orthop* 1994:307:47–69.
27. Collins D, Tencer A, Sidles J, Matsen F III: Edge displacement and deformation of glenoid components in response to eccentric loading: The effect of preparation of the glenoid bone. *J Bone Joint Surg* 1992;74A:501–507.
28. Wirth MA, Basamania C, Rockwood CA Jr: Fixation of glenoid component: Keel versus pegs. *Op Tech Orthop* 1994;4: 218–225.
29. Harryman DT, Sidles JA, Harris SL, Lippitt SB, Matsen FA III: The effect of articular conformity and the size of the humeral head component on laxity and motion after glenohumeral arthroplasty: A study in cadavera. *J Bone Joint Surg* 1995; 77A:555–563.
30. Severt R, Thomas BJ, Tsenter MJ, Amstutz HC, Kabo JM: The influence of conformity and constraint on translational forces and frictional torque in total shoulder arthroplasty. *Clin Orthop* 1993;292: 151–158.
31. Brenner BC, Ferlic DC, Clayton ML, Dennis DA: Survivorship of unconstrained total shoulder arthroplasty. *J Bone Joint Surg* 1989;71A:1289–1296.
32. McCoy SR, Warren RF, Bade HA III, Ranawat CS, Inglis AE: Total shoulder arthroplasty in rheumatoid arthritis. *J Arthroplasty* 1989;4:105–113.
33. Moeckel BH, Altchek DW, Warren RF, Wickiewicz TL, Dines DM: Instability of the shoulder after arthroplasty. *J Bone Joint Surg* 1993;75A:492–497.
34. Boyd AD Jr, Thomas WH, Scott RD, Sledge CB, Thornhill TS: Total shoulder arthroplasty versus hemiarthroplasty: Indications for glenoid resurfacing. *J Arthroplasty* 1990;5:329–336.
35. Neer CS II, Morrison DS: Glenoid bone-grafting in total shoulder arthroplasty. *J Bone Joint Surg* 1988;70A:1154–1162.
36. Frich LH, Sojbjerg JO, Sneppen O: Shoulder arthroplasty in complex acute and chronic proximal humeral fractures. *Orthopedics* 1991;14:949–954.
37. Groh GI, Heckman MM, Curtis RJ, Rockwood CA Jr: Treatment of fractures adjacent to humeral prosthesis. *Orthop Trans* 1994;18:1072.
38. Wirth MA: Part I: Periprosthetic fractures of the upper extremity, in Rockwood CA Jr, Green DP, Bucholz RW, Heckman JD (eds): *Rockwood and Green's Fractures in Adults*, ed 4. Philadelphia, PA, Lippincott-Raven, 1996, pp 540–576.
39. Bonutti PM, Hawkins RJ: Fracture of the humeral shaft associated with total shoulder replacement arthroplasty of the shoulder: A case report. *J Bone Joint Surg* 1992 ;74A:617–618.
40. Boyd AD Jr, Thornhill TS, Barnes CL: Fractures adjacent to humeral prostheses. *J Bone Joint Surg* 1992;74A:1498–1504.
41. Lynch NM, Cofield RH, Silbert PL, Hermann RC: Neurologic complications after total shoulder arthroplasty. *J Shoulder Elbow Surg* 1996;5:53–61.
42. Cofield RH: Unconstrained total shoulder prostheses. *Clin Orthop* 1983;173: 97–108.
43. Cooper RA, Brems JJ: Recurrent disassembly of a modular humeral prosthesis: A case report. *J Arthroplasty* 1991;6: 375–377.
44. Cofield RH, Daly PJ: Total shoulder arthroplasty with a tissue-ingrowth glenoid component. *J Shoulder Elbow Surg* 1992;1:77–85.
45. Driessnack RP, Ferlic DC, Wiedel JD: Dissociation of the glenoid component in the Macnab/English total shoulder arthroplasty. *J Arthroplasty* 1990;5:15–18.
46. McElwain JP, English E: The early results of porous-coated total shoulder arthroplasty. *Clin Orthop* 1987;218:217–224.
47. Neer CS II, Kirby RM: Revision of humeral head and total shoulder arthroplasties. *Clin Orthop* 1982;170:189–195.
48. Neer CS II: Displaced proximal humeral fractures: Part II. Treatment of three-part and four-part displacement. *J Bone Joint Surg* 1970;52A:1090–1103.
49. Schlegel TF, Hawkins RJ: Displaced proximal humerus fractures: Evaluation and treatment. *J Am Acad Orthop Surg* 1994;2: 54–66.
50. Stableforth PG: Four-part fractures of the neck of the humerus. *J Bone Joint Surg* 1984;66B:104–108.
51. Zuckerman JD, Flugstad DL, Teitz CC, King HA: Axillary artery injury as a complication of proximal humeral fractures: Two case reports and a review of the literature. *Clin Orthop* 1984;189:234–237.
52. Flatow EL, Cuomo F, Maday MG, Miller SR, McIlveen SJ, Bigliani LU: Open reduction and internal fixation of two-part displaced fractures of the greater tuberosity of the proximal part of the humerus. *J Bone Joint Surg* 1991;73A: 1213–1218.
53. Hägg O, Lundberg BJ: Aspects of prognostic factors in comminuted and dislocated proximal humeral fractures, in Bateman JE, Walsh RP (eds): *Surgery of the Shoulder.* Philadelphia, PA, BC Decker, 1984, pp 51–59.
54. Hawkins RJ, Bell RH, Gurr K: The three-part fracture of the proximal part of the humerus: Operative treatment. *J Bone Joint Surg* 1986;68A:1410–1414.
55. Tanner MW, Cofield RH: Prosthetic arthroplasty for fractures and fracture-dislocations of the proximal humerus. *Clin Orthop* 1983;179:116–128.
56. Hawkins RJ, Switlyk P: Acute prosthetic replacement for severe fractures of the proximal humerus. *Clin Orthop* 1993;289: 156–160.
57. Groh GI, Williams GR, Jarman RN, Rockwood CA Jr: Treatment of complications of shoulder arthrodesis. *J Bone Joint Surg* 1997;79A:881–887.
58. Warner JJP: Frozen shoulder: Diagnosis and management. *J Am Acad Orthop Surg* 1997;5:130–140.

59. Small NC: Complications in arthroscopic surgery performed by experienced arthroscopists. *Arthroscopy* 1988;4:215–221.

60. Bigliani LU, Flatow EL, Deliz ED: Complications of shoulder arthroscopy. *Orthop Rev* 1991;20:743–751.

61. D'Angelo GL, Ogilvie-Harris DJ: Septic arthritis following arthroscopy, with cost/benefit analysis of antibiotic prophylaxis. *Arthroscopy* 1988;4:10–14.

62. Johnson LL, Shneider DA, Austin MD, Goodman FG, Bullock JM, DeBruin JA: Two percent glutaraldehyde: A disinfectant in arthroscopy and arthroscopic surgery. *J Bone Joint Surg* 1982;64A:237–239.

63. Neu HC: Cephalosporin antibiotics as applied in surgery of bones and joints. *Clin Orthop* 1984;190:50–64.

64. Cooper DE, Jenkins RS, Bready L, Rockwood CA Jr: The prevention of injuries of the brachial plexus secondary to malposition of the patient during surgery. *Clin Orthop* 1988;228:33–41.

65. Klein AH, France JC, Mutschler TA, Fu FH: Measurement of brachial plexus strain in arthroscopy of the shoulder. *Arthroscopy* 1987;3:45–52.

66. Pitman MI, Nainzadeh N, Ergas E, Springer S: The use of somatosensory evoked potentials for detection of neuropraxia during shoulder arthroscopy. *Arthroscopy* 1988:4:250–255.

67. Skyhar MJ, Altchek DW, Warren RF, Wickiewicz TL, O'Brien SJ: Shoulder arthroscopy with the patient in the beach-chair position. *Arthroscopy* 1988;4:256–259.

68. Ogilvie-Harris DJ, Boynton E: Arthroscopic acromioplasty: Extravasation of fluid into the deltoid muscle. *Arthroscopy* 1990;6:52–54.

69. Ellman H: Arthroscopic subacromial decompression: Analysis of one- to three-year results. *Arthroscopy* 1987;3:173–181.

70. Altchek DW, Warren RF, Wickiewicz TL, Skyhar MJ, Ortiz G, Schwartz E: Arthroscopic acromioplasty: Technique and results. *J Bone Joint Surg* 1990;72A: 1198–1207.

71. Gartsman GM: Arthroscopic acromioplasty for lesions of the rotator cuff. *J Bone Joint Surg* 1990;72A:169–180.

72. Esch JC: Arthroscopic subacromial decompression and postoperative management. *Orthop Clin North Am* 1993;24: 161–171.

73. Hawkins RJ, Chris T, Bokor D, Kiefer G: Failed anterior acromioplasty: A review of 51 cases. *Clin Orthop* 1989;243:106–111.

74. Berg EE, Ciullo JV, Oglesby JW: Failure of arthroscopic decompression by subacromial heterotopic ossification causing recurrent impingement. *Arthroscopy* 1994;10:158–161.

75. Matthews LS, Vetter WL, Oweida SJ, Spearman J, Helfet DL: Arthroscopic staple capsulorrhaphy for recurrent anterior shoulder instability. *Arthroscopy* 1988;4: 106–111.

76. Morgan CD, Bodenstab AB: Arthroscopic Bankart suture repair: Technique and early results. *Arthroscopy* 1987;3:111–122.

77. Committee on Complications of the Arthroscopy Association of North America: Complications in arthroscopy: The knee and other joints. *Arthroscopy* 1986;2:253–258.

78. Andrews JR, Carson WG: Shoulder joint arthroscopy. *Orthopedics* 1983;6:1157–1162.

79. Bryan WJ, Schauder K, Tullos HS: The axillary nerve and its relationship to common sports medicine shoulder procedures. *Am J Sports Med* 1986;14:113–116.

80. Matthews LS, Zarins B, Michael RH, Helfet DL: Anterior portal selection for shoulder arthroscopy. *Arthroscopy* 1985;1:33–39.

81. Stanish WD, Peterson DC: Shoulder arthroscopy and nerve injury: Pitfalls and prevention. *Arthroscopy* 1995;11:458–466.

Reference to Video

Wirth MA, Rockwood CA: Revision Shoulder Arthroplasty. San Antonio, TX, University of Texas Health Science Center, 1997.

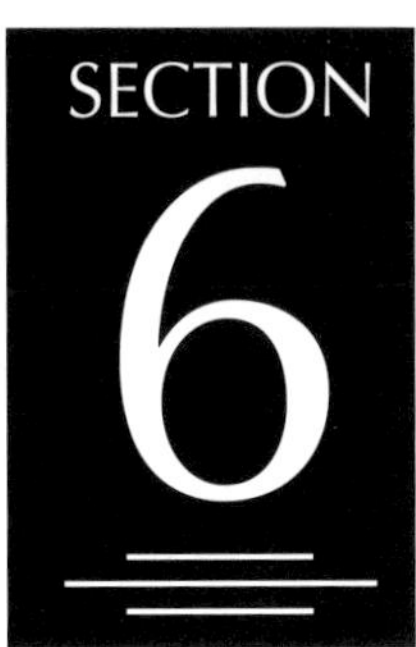

Elbow Arthroscopy and Sports Medicine

Elbow Arthroscopy and Sports Medicine

Elbow injuries, particularly in the athletic population, are the subject of increasing clinical and scientific interest, as reflected by the expanding body of literature in this area. Fueling this interest is increased awareness of these injuries, new diagnostic tools, new techniques for treatment, and better and reproducible surgical results. Importantly, elbow injuries in athletes may be performance hindering and/or career threatening. This section consists of six articles, which together, lay an excellent foundation for the evaluation and management of common elbow problems in the athletic population. In the first article, Lyons and asso-ciates review the basics of elbow arthroscopy. The next three articles address the elbow in the overhead throwing athlete, specifically (1) the medial collateral ligament (MCL); (2) posterior impingement; and (3) osteochondritis dissecans (OCD). Dr. Michael Ciccotti provides an excellent overview of epicondylitis, and Dr. Bernard Morrey shares his thoughts, vast experience, and work on distal biceps tendon injuries.

An estimated 10% of orthopaedic surgeons are believed to perform elbow arthroscopy, and only 2% of all arthroscopies are performed on the elbow. In their review of the fundamentals of elbow arthroscopy, Lyons and associates, who together represent wealth of knowledge and experience in elbow arthroscopy, review the indications, the options for patient positioning, and the common complications of elbow arthroscopy. They point out that many surgeons avoid elbow arthroscopy because of its potential risks, particularly for nerve injury. A fine discussion of elbow anatomy as it relates to portal positioning is included, as is a review of the authors' surgical technique.

In the second article, Williams and associates review MCL injuries in the throwing athlete. The repetitive loads of throwing put the MCL at risk for chronic attenuation or acute rupture, either of which can be disabling to the throwing athlete. The authors trace the history of this problem as it appears in the literature, beginning with Jobe's groundbreaking work on reconstruction of the MCL to newer generation reconstruction techniques. The anatomy and biomechanics of the elbow is reviewed with respect to the valgus stress seen with throwing sports. Evaluation of the elbow in the throwing athlete is then described, followed by a review of nonsurgical management, the indications for surgery, surgical technique, and finally the results of MCL reconstruction.

Posterior elbow impingement may result in a variety of individual factors, including repetitive hyperextension, degenerative osteophytes, and/or abutment of the proximal-medial olecranon within the medial olecranon fossa as a result of MCL laxity in throwers, or a combination of the above. Moskal and associates provide a clear review of this problem, differentiating the causes and describing the important factors in evaluation of the patient. Nonsurgical management as it relates to the underlying cause is described, followed by a discussion of the authors' arthroscopic approach to the elbow with posterior elbow impingement and valgus extension overload. Their experience wisely dictates arthroscopic assessment for valgus stability, before and after osteophyte excision, with the intention to reduce the need for reoperation, as first described by Timmerman and Andrews. They describe their rehabilitation protocol, and then report their published results as well as their large series results.

In the last of the articles addressing problems in the overhead throwing athlete, Yadao and associates provide a fine and comprehensive discussion of the difficult topic of OCD of the elbow. They help differentiate OCD from other lesions about the elbow that are often confused with OCD, concisely review the proposed etiologies, and discuss the evaluation and classification of this problem. Results of the different treatment strategies are then reviewed, with emphasis on the importance of staging and recommendation options based on the integrity of the overlying articular cartilage. The reader is appropriately cautioned about being overly optimistic about the prognosis for return to sports.

Michael Ciccotti's article on epicondylitis of the elbow is outstanding. This very common malady, affecting athletes and nonathletes alike, continues to remain something of an enigma, although it was first described more than 120 years ago. Dr. Ciccotti does a nice job identifying what is currently known about the condition as well as the controversies associated with medial (golfer's elbow) and lateral (tennis elbow) epicondylitis. He provides an overview about the proposed etiology and the evolution of the proposed pathophysiology. After a discussion about patient evaluation and the differential diagnosis, he nicely details the nonsurgical management of these problems. Although most of the published data are focused on the more common lateral epicondylosis, he describes the management of these problems similarly, beginning with the initial phase in which pain and inflammation are addressed and then progressing to the rehabilitation phase of stretching and strengthening. An evaluation of mechanics and equipment follows. Next he reviews the surgical technique of both types of epicondylitis, along with the postoperative course. He appropriately points out that even though most patients report a satisfactory outcome, a large proportion experience deficits in strength following lateral elbow surgery.

The last article in this section on distal biceps tendon injuries is by Bernard Morrey, who has done more to advance our knowledge about the elbow than most anyone; certainly this is true about our understanding and awareness of distal biceps tendon injury. The article begins with a comprehensive review of this uncommon injury, beginning with its incidence, the mechanism of injury and etiology, and patient evaluation. He reviews both single-incision and two-incision techniques; his modification (the Mayo modification) of the Boyd Anderson technique remains the gold standard. Potential complications and their management also are described. He concludes with his approach to delayed reconstruction of the distal biceps and management of partial ruptures of the distal biceps.

Marc R. Safran, MD
Director, Sports Medicine
Associate Professor,
Department of Orthopaedic Surgery
University of California,
San Francisco

Basics of Elbow Arthroscopy

Thomas R. Lyons, MD
Larry D. Field, MD
Felix H. Savoie III, MD

Introduction

Advances in arthroscopic technique and equipment over the last several years have made elbow arthroscopy an effective and safe alternative for the diagnosis and treatment of a variety of elbow disorders. The surgeon must have a precise knowledge of neurovascular anatomy to avoid injury to nerves and vessels around the elbow as well as extensive surgical experience to successfully perform elbow arthroscopy.

Current accepted indications for elbow arthroscopy include removal of loose bodies, treatment of synovitis and osteochondritis dissecans, capsular release, debridement of osteophytes, radial head excision, and assessment and treatment of instability.[1-4] With further refinements in surgical equipment and technique along with increasing clinical experience, new indications for elbow arthroscopy are likely to emerge. This chapter will outline options for patient positioning, discuss the pertinent anatomy and placement of arthroscopic portals, review surgical technique, and discuss the complications associated with elbow arthroscopy.

Anesthesia

Arthroscopy of the elbow is most commonly performed under general anesthesia. In addition to providing complete muscle relaxation, general anesthesia facilitates prone or lateral decubitus positioning, which may not be well tolerated in the awake patient. Scalene, axillary, or Bier blocks are options in patients in whom general anesthesia is contraindicated. Regional blocks may also be used in combination with general anesthesia for postoperative pain control.[5,6]

Patient Position

The position of the patient for elbow arthroscopy should allow adequate visualization of both anterior and posterior aspects of the joint, intraoperative manipulation of the elbow, and conversion to an open procedure when necessary. The supine, prone, and lateral decubitus positions each have distinct advantages and disadvantages. The position used ultimately depends on the surgeon's preference and experience.

Supine Position

In the supine position originally described by Andrews and Carson,[7] the patient lies supine with the shoulder over the edge of the operating table. The shoulder is abducted to 90° and the elbow is suspended by an overhead traction device attached to the hand or forearm. Alternatively, the arm is allowed to rest on arm boards and an assistant maintains the position of the elbow.

There are several advantages to the supine position for elbow arthroscopy.[5,7] Access to the patient's airway and administration of anesthesia is facilitated and intubation is not always required. Excellent visualization of the anterior aspect of the joint is achieved and conceptualization of intra-articular anatomy is facilitated in this position. In addition, the supine position allows ready conversion to an open procedure when required. Disadvantages of the supine position include poor access to the posterior aspect of the joint and difficulty in manipulation of the elbow if an overhead traction device is used. In addition, use of the supine position with the arm suspended may leave the elbow unstable and require the help of an assistant.[8]

Prone Position

The prone position, originally described by Poehling and associates,[9] addresses the shortcomings of the supine position. The patient is placed prone on the operating table over chest bolsters. The shoulder is abducted to 90° and the arm is supported by an arm positioner or arm board placed parallel to the operating table, allowing the elbow to rest in 90° of flexion. Advantages of the prone position include improved access to the posterior aspect of the joint and ease of elbow manipulation from full extension to near full flexion. In

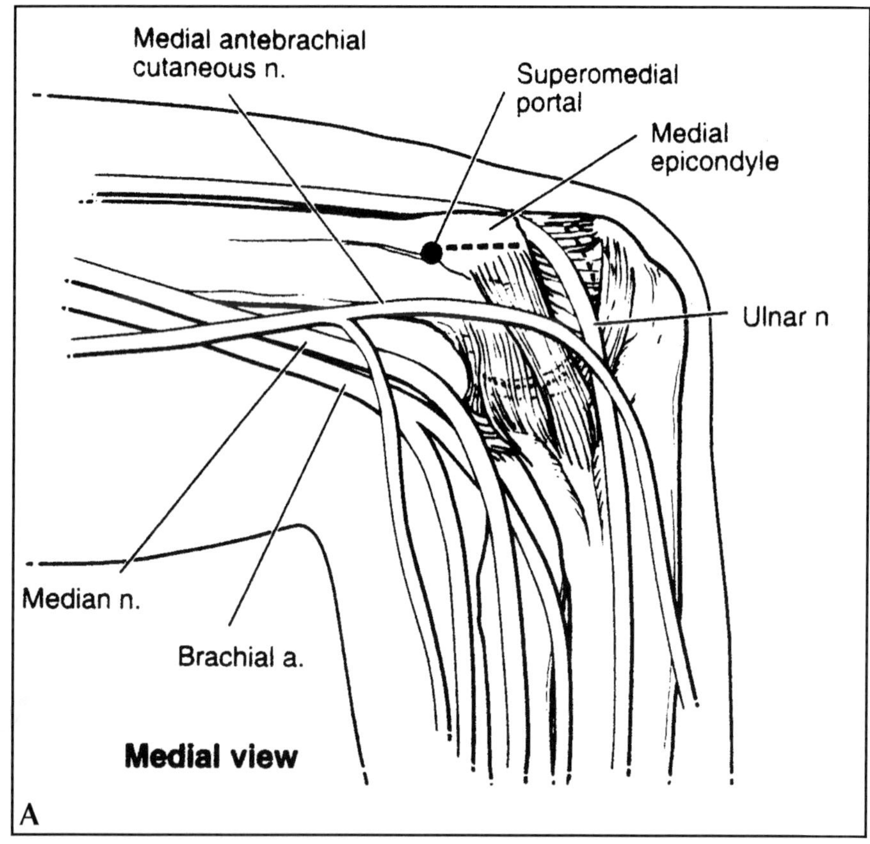

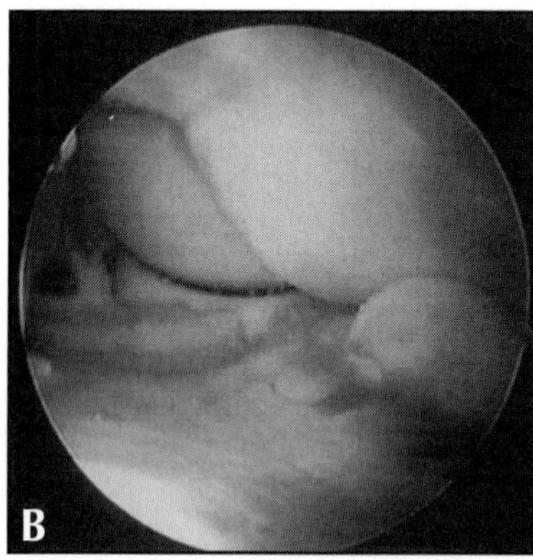

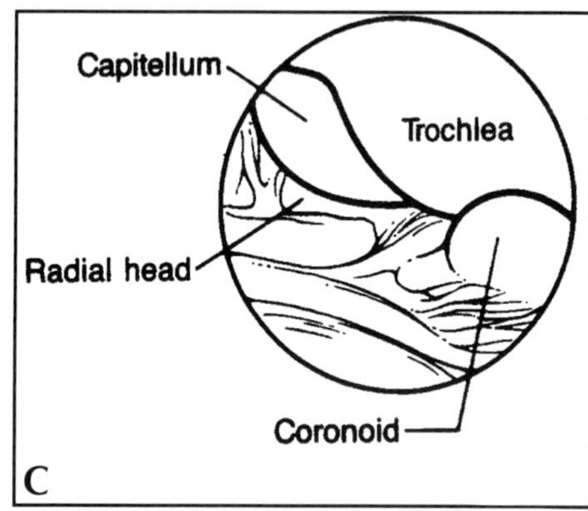

Fig. 1 A, Proximal medial portal. (Reproduced with permission from Plancher KD, Peterson RK, Brezenoff L: Diagnostic arthroscopy of the elbow: Set-up, portals, and technique. *Oper Tech Sports Med* 1998;6:2–10.) **B,** Arthroscopic view from proximal medial portal. **C,** Illustration of arthroscopic view from proximal medial portal. (Reproduced with permission from Savoie FH III, Field LD (eds): *Arthroscopy of the Elbow.* New York, NY, Churchill Livingstone, 1996.)

this position, gravity allows the neurovascular structures to displace anteriorly, providing additional safety when creating portals and operating in the anterior compartment. In addition, no traction device is needed and the elbow is maintained in a stable position. Like the supine position, the prone position allows an open procedure to be performed if necessary.[8,9] **(CD-23.1)**

Disadvantages of the prone position include difficulties in patient positioning and administration of anesthesia. Placement of the patient in the prone position necessitates padding of all prominences and careful handling of the head, neck, and face. If regional anesthesia is chosen, the prone position may not be well tolerated. If the regional block fails and general anesthesia becomes necessary, repositioning of the patient will be required. Although open approaches to the medial and lateral aspects of the joint are easily performed, an anterior approach may require patient repositioning.[5,6]

Lateral Decubitus Position

The lateral decubitus position described by O'Driscoll and Morrey[2] offer the advantages of both the prone and supine positions while avoiding some of their disadvantages. The patient is placed in the lateral decubitus position with the affected side up, the shoulder forward flexed 90° and internally rotated, and the elbow flexed 90° over a padded bolster.

Advantages of this position include those cited for the prone position but with easier patient positioning and better access to the airway for the anesthesiologist. Disadvantages of this position include the need for the bolster device and the occasional need to reposition the patient if an open procedure is required.[2,3]

Portal Placement

A thorough knowledge of neurovascular anatomy of the elbow is required to safely perform elbow arthroscopy. Surface landmarks, including the radial head, olecranon, lateral epicondyle, medial epicondyle, ulnar nerve, median nerve, and brachial artery, are marked on the skin. Prior to placement of the first portal, the joint is distended with 20 to 30 cc of sterile saline introduced through an 18-gauge spinal needle placed in the soft spot bounded by the lateral epicondyle, olecranon, and radial head. A distended joint facilitates initial portal placement as well as displaces the neurovascular structures away from the joint, providing an additional margin of safety.[10] **(CD-23.2)**

Anterior portals are created with the elbow in 90° of flexion while posterior portals require less flexion. A number 11 blade is used to incise the skin only, to avoid injury to superficial cutaneous nerves. A hemostat is then used to bluntly dissect to the joint capsule. To protect the articular surfaces, a blunt trocar is used to enter the joint. The egress of fluid from the cannula confirms intra-articular placement. Once a cannula is introduced into the joint, it is left in place throughout the operation to avoid the risks of multiple passes through the soft tissues and to decrease the likelihood of fluid extravasation. Several medial and lateral portals have been recommended for use as the initial portal in elbow arthroscopy.[7,9,11,12] The initial portal chosen, however, ultimately depends on the experience and preference of the surgeon.

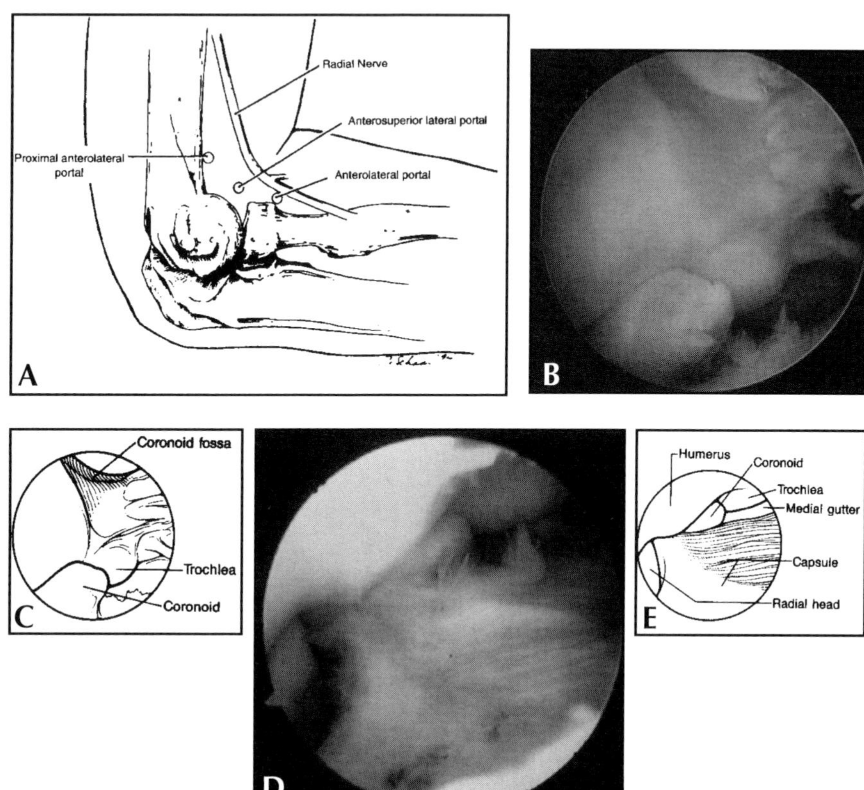

Fig. 2 A, Proximal lateral portal, preferred anterolateral portal, and standard anterolateral portal. **B,** Arthroscopic view from proximal lateral portal. **C,** Illustration of arthroscopic view from proximal lateral portal. **D,** Arthroscopic view from preferred anterolateral portal. **E,** Illustration of arthroscopic view from preferred anterolateral portal. (Reproduced with permission from Savoie FH III, Field LD (eds): *Arthroscopy of the Elbow.* New York, NY, Churchill Livingstone, 1996.)

Proximal Medial

The proximal medial portal, first described by Poehling and associates,[9] is located 2 cm proximal to the medial epicondyle and just anterior to the medial intermuscular septum (Fig. 1, *A*). Care must be taken to identify the medial intermuscular septum and remain anterior to it during surgery to avoid injury to the ulnar nerve. The blunt trocar is placed anterior to the septum and directed toward the radial head while maintaining contact with the anterior surface of the humerus to avoid injury to the median nerve and brachial artery. The trocar pierces the tendinous origin of the flexor-pronator group and medial capsule to enter the joint. A history of transposition of the ulnar nerve or subluxation of the ulnar nerve from its groove are contraindications to use of this portal.[6,8,12,13]

The proximal medial portal provides visualization of the entire anterior aspect of the joint including the anterior capsule, trochlea, capitellum, coronoid process, radial head, and medial and lateral gutters (Fig. 1, *B* and *C*). This portal is frequently used as the initial portal with the patient in the prone or lateral decubitus position.[8,9,12] Lindenfeld recommends use of a proximal medial portal initially because it offers safer access to the joint, allows better visualization, and results in less fluid extravasation than an anterolateral portal.[12] The posterior branch of the medial antebrachial cutaneous nerve, located on average 2.3 mm from the trocar, is at highest risk for injury.[13] The median nerve, located on average from 12.4 to 22.3 mm from the trocar with the elbow in flexion, is relatively safe.[12,13] The ulnar nerve, resting on average from 12 to 23.7 mm from the portal, is not at risk as long as the trocar remains anterior to the medial intermuscular septum.[12,13]

Proximal Lateral

The proximal lateral portal described by Stothers and associates,[13] Field and associates,[11] and Savoie and Field[14] is located 2 cm proximal and 1 cm anterior to the lateral epicondyle (Fig. 2, *A*). The blunt trocar is advanced toward the center of the joint while maintaining contact with the anterior humerus. The trocar pierces the brachioradialis and brachialis muscles before entering the joint through the lateral capsule.

This portal may be used as the initial portal and provides complete visualization of the anterior aspect of the joint,

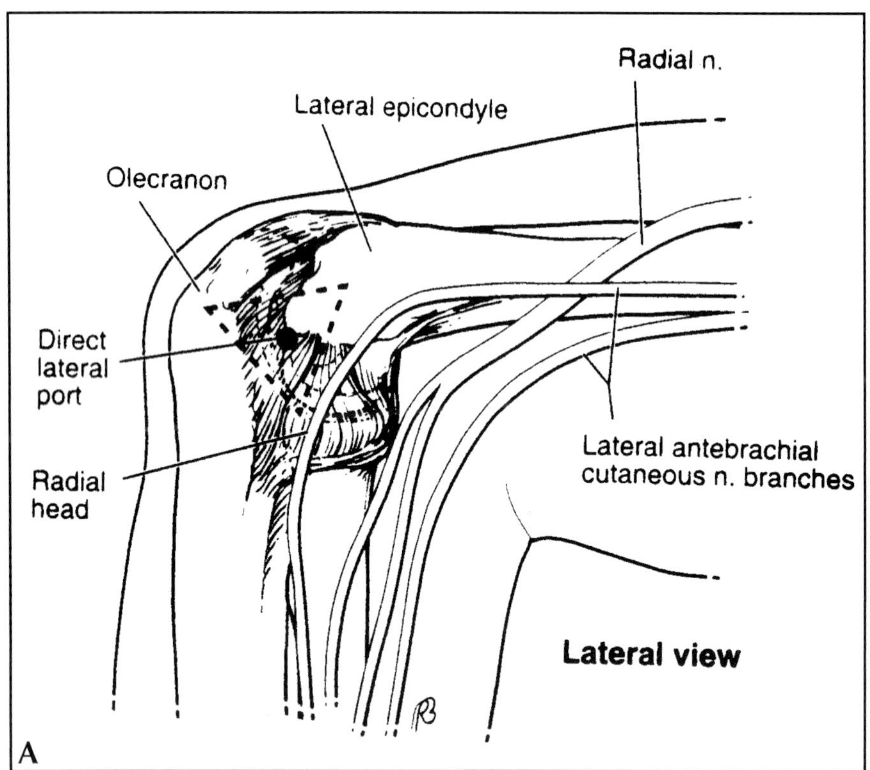

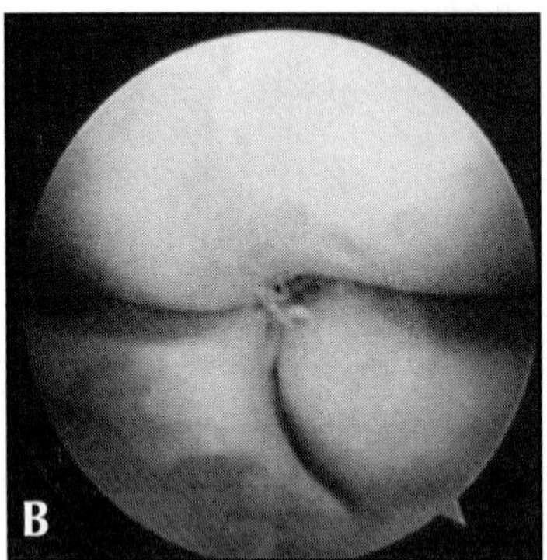

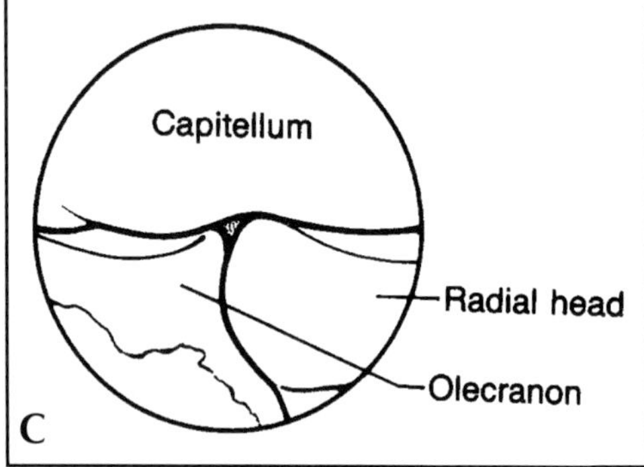

Fig. 3 A, Midlateral or direct lateral portal. (Reproduced with permission from Plancher KD, Peterson RK, Brezenoff L: Diagnostic arthroscopy of the elbow: Set-up, portals, and technique. *Oper Tech Sports Med* 1998;6:2–10.) **B,** Arthroscopic view from midlateral portal. **C,** Illustration of arthroscopic view from midlateral portal. (Reproduced with permission from Savoie FH III, Field LD (eds): *Arthroscopy of the Elbow.* New York, NY, Churchill Livingstone, 1996.)

including the anterior and lateral parts of the radial head and capitellum and lateral gutter[11,13,14] (Fig. 2, *B* and *C*). The posterior branch of the lateral antebrachial cutaneous nerve lies on average 6.1 mm from the trocar.[13] The radial nerve lies on average from 9.9 to 14.2 mm from the proximal lateral portal with the elbow in flexion, compared to 4.9 to 9.1 mm from the standard anterolateral portal.[11,13]

Anterolateral

The standard anterolateral portal described by Andrews and Carson[7] is located 3 cm distal and 1 cm anterior to the lateral epicondyle (Fig. 2, *A*). Anatomic studies have shown this portal to be located within 2 mm of the posterior antebrachial cutaneous nerve.[15] With the elbow in 90° of flexion and distended with fluid, the anterolateral portal is located on average from 4.9 to 9.1 mm from the radial nerve.[11,13] Anterolateral portal placement 3 cm from the lateral epicondyle results in placement that is excessively distal in most patients and places the radial nerve at increased risk. For this reason, some authors recommend a more proximal entry point for the anterolateral portal located at the sulcus between the radial head and capitellum[6] or directly anterior to the lateral epicondyle[11] (Fig. 2, *A*).

For anterolateral portal placement, the blunt trocar is aimed toward the center of the joint, passing through the extensor carpi radialis brevis muscle and lateral capsule into the joint. If a medial portal is used initially, the anterolateral portal may be created using an inside-out technique. With the arthroscope in the anteromedial or proximal medial portal, it is advanced to the capsule lateral to the radial head, and replaced with a blunt rod that tents the overlying skin. The skin is incised over the rod and a cannula is placed over the rod into the joint. In order to avoid radial nerve injury, care must be taken to enter the capsule lateral to the radial head rather than anterior to it.[6,12,13]

The medial aspect of the anterior joint, including the coronoid process, trochlea, coronoid fossa, and medial part of the radial head, is easily visualized (Fig. 2, *D* and *E*). For a better view of the radiocapitellar joint, the previously described proximal lateral portal is recommended.[11] In addition to allowing visualization of the anterior compartment, the anterolateral portal is a useful work portal with the arthroscope in the proximal medial portal.

Midlateral

The midlateral, soft spot, or direct lateral portal is located at the center of the triangle formed by the olecranon, lateral epicondyle, and radial head (Fig. 3, *A*). This portal is often used for distention of the joint prior to initial portal placement. The blunt trocar is pushed into the soft spot, through the anconeus muscle and capsule into the joint. Use of the midlateral portal poses minimal risk to neurovascular structures. Through this portal, the inferior aspect of the radial head and capitellum as well as the radioulnar articulation are well visualized (Fig. 3, *B* and *C*). The midlateral portal may be used for initial joint inspection, but leakage of fluid into the soft tissues often occurs. It may be advisable to delay use of this portal until the end of the operation.[4,6,13]

Anteromedial

The anteromedial portal as described by Andrews and Carson[7] lies 2 cm distal and 2 cm anterior to the medial epicondyle (Fig. 4, *A*). This portal may be established using an inside-out technique with the arthroscope in a lateral portal, or as recommended by Lindenfeld.[12] After incision through the skin only with the elbow flexed to 90° and distended with fluid, the blunt trocar is aimed at the center of the joint and pierces the flexor-pronator tendinous origin and the brachialis muscle before penetrating the joint capsule anterior to the medial collateral ligament.

The anteromedial portal permits visualization of the entire anterior compartment, particularly the lateral structures (Fig. 4, *B* and *C*). Cadaveric studies have shown that this portal lies on average 1 mm from the medial antebrachial cutaneous nerve.[13] The distance from the anteromedial portal to the median nerve is on average from 7 to 14 mm.[13,15] Lindenfeld recommends placement of a medial portal 1 cm proximal and 1 cm anterior to the medial epicondyle and reports an average distance from the portal to the median nerve of 22 mm.[12] Placement of the medial portal more proximally allows the trocar to be directed distally (parallel to the median nerve) rather than laterally (perpendicular and toward the median nerve).[12]

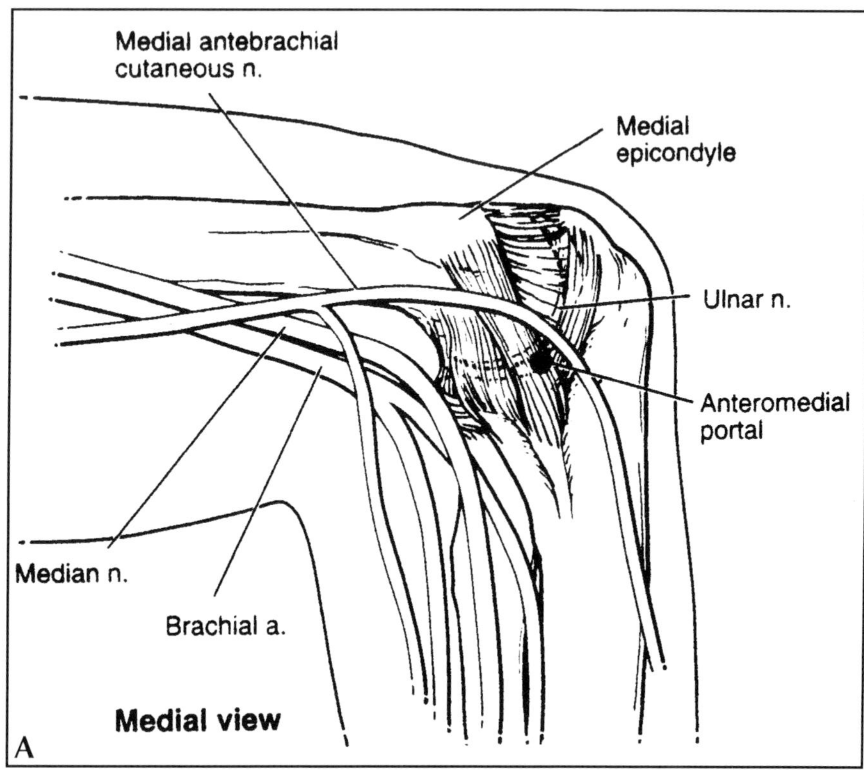

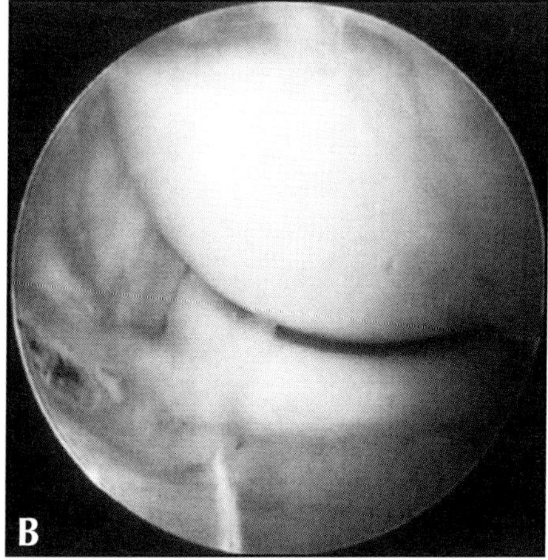

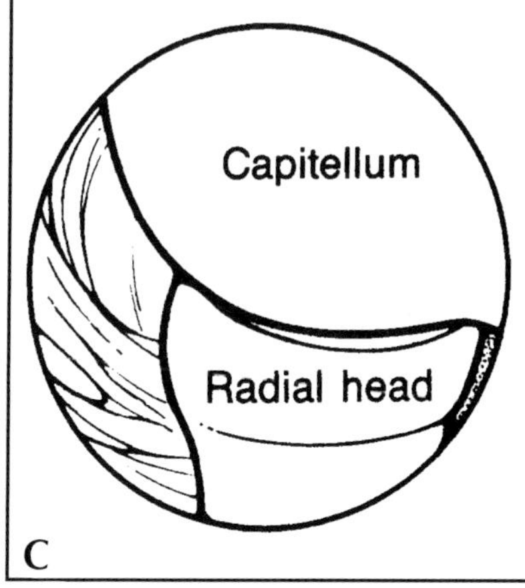

Fig. 4 A, Anteromedial portal. (Reproduced with permission from Plancher KD, Peterson RK, Brezenoff L: Diagnostic arthroscopy of the elbow: Set-up, portals, and technique. *Oper Tech Sports Med* 1998;6:2–10.) **B,** Arthroscopic view from anteromedial portal. **C,** Illustration of arthroscopic view from anteromedial portal. (Reproduced with permission from Savoie FH III, Field LD (eds): *Arthroscopy of the Elbow.* New York, NY, Churchill Livingstone, 1996.)

Posterolateral

The posterolateral portal is located 3 cm proximal to the olecranon tip and just lateral to the lateral edge of the triceps tendon (Fig. 5, *A*). With the elbow held in 45° of flexion to relax the triceps tendon and posterior capsule, a blunt trocar is directed toward the center of the olecranon fossa passing lateral to the triceps tendon to pierce the posterolateral capsule and enter

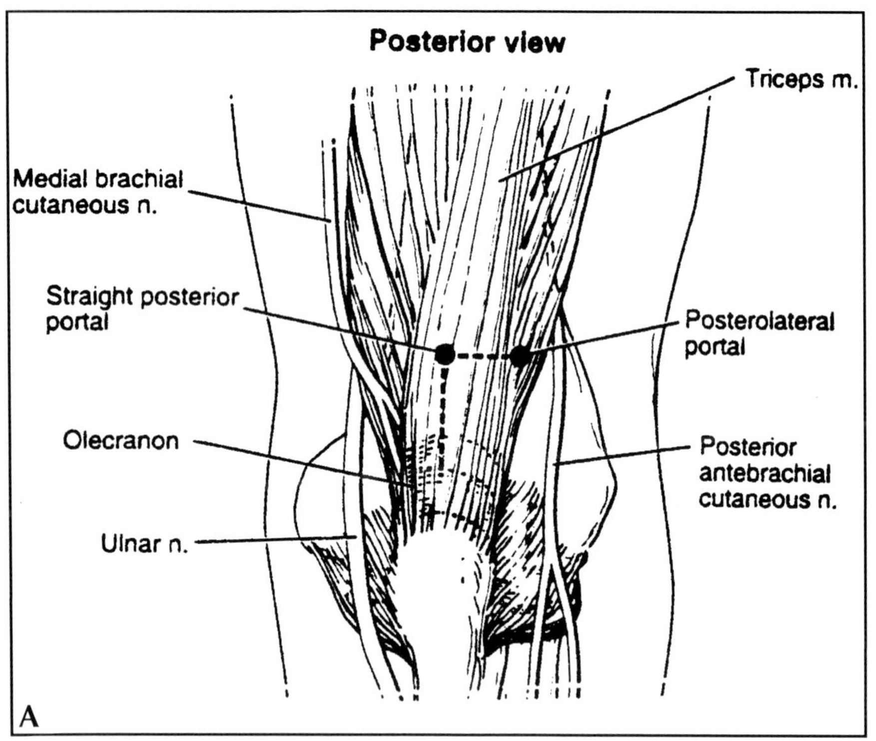

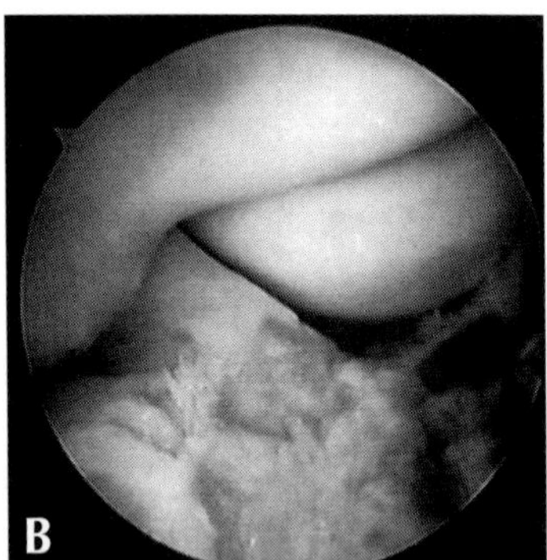

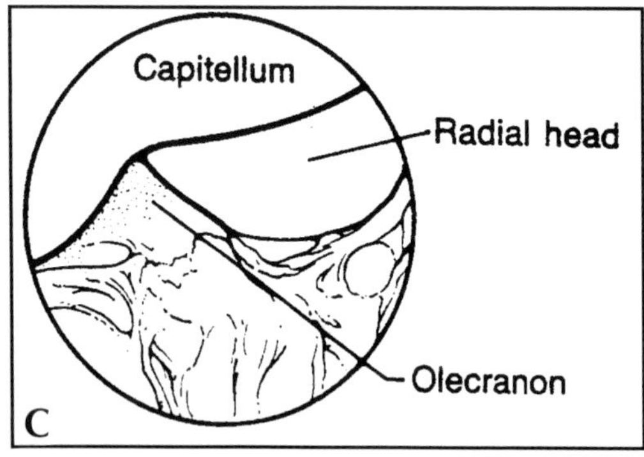

Fig. 5 A, Posterolateral and straight posterior portals. (Reproduced with permission from Plancher KD, Peterson RK, Brezenoff L: Diagnostic arthroscopy of the elbow: Set-up, portals, and technique. *Oper Tech Sports Med* 1998;6:2–10.) **B,** Arthroscopic view from posterolateral portal. **C,** Illustration of arthroscopic view from posterolateral portal. (Reproduced with permission from Savoie FH III, Field LD (eds): *Arthroscopy of the Elbow.* New York, NY, Churchill Livingstone, 1996.)

the joint.[13] This portal affords excellent access to the posterior aspect of the joint including the tip of the olecranon, olecranon fossa, and medial and lateral gutters (Fig. 5, *B* and *C*). Care must be taken when evaluating the medial gutter from this portal because the ulnar nerve lies just superficial to the medial capsule.[6,16]

Straight Posterior

The straight posterior or transtriceps portal located 3 cm proximal to the tip of the olecranon in the midline is used for instrumentation in the posterior aspect of the elbow[8,17] (Fig. 5, *A*). Again with the elbow in slight flexion, the blunt trocar is advanced anteriorly toward the olecranon fossa through the triceps tendon and posterior capsule into the joint. This portal, like the posterolateral portal, allows visualization of the entire posterior compartment. Limited access to the anterior compartment can be achieved using a transhumeral portal. After establishment of the straight posterior and posterolateral portals, fenestration of the distal humerus is carried out using a drill or burr through the straight posterior portal.[6]

Surgical Technique

A thorough preoperative evaluation is performed, including careful assessment of neurovascular function, range of motion, and stability. It is important to note the presence of a prior transposition of the ulnar nerve or other surgery on the elbow as the use of certain medial portals may be contraindicated in some situations.

Prior to induction of general anesthesia, many of our patients receive a scalene or axillary block to aid in postoperative pain control. The arm is supported in a commercially available arm holder (Instrument Makar) designed for this purpose (Fig. 6). The patient is placed prone on the operating table over chest bolsters with the shoulder abducted 90° and all bony prominences well padded (Fig. 7). The video monitor and other equipment are placed on a mobile cart on the contralateral side and a Mayo stand with the required instruments is placed next to the surgeon. A standard 4-mm, 30° arthroscope is routinely employed. Use of a 2.7-mm arthroscope may be necessary in small patients or in joints with limited motion. We use gravity inflow and have not found an arthroscopic pump necessary for adequate joint distention. A tourniquet is placed on the proximal arm and the extremity is prepared and draped in the usual fashion. A Coban bandage is wrapped around the hand and forearm to limit fluid extravasation. The extremity is exsanguinated and the tourniquet inflated. Surface landmarks are drawn on the skin at the radial head, medial and lateral epicondyles, olecranon, medial intermuscular septum, median nerve, and ulnar nerve as well as the planned arthroscopic portals. A spinal needle is placed into the soft spot bounded by the olecranon, radial head, and lateral epicondyle and 20 to 30 cc of sterile saline is injected. Distention of the joint is confirmed by elevation of the capsule and triceps tendon from the posterior elbow and return of fluid from the needle when the stylus is removed.

We use the proximal medial portal, described previously, as the initial portal. A spinal needle is directed along the anterior aspect of the humerus to enter the joint capsule; the return of fluid confirms needle placement into the joint. The needle is removed, the skin is carefully incised, and a blunt trocar is advanced along the same trajectory as the spinal needle. Intra-articular placement is again confirmed by the return of fluid from the cannula. The arthroscope is inserted and a systematic examination of the anterior compartment is performed. The capitellum and radial head are inspected; the forearm is rotated to evaluate the medial and lateral surfaces of the radial head. Next, the anterior and lateral aspects of the capsule are viewed. By withdrawing the arthroscope the trochlea, coronoid fossa, and coronoid process are examined.

The anterolateral portal is used for instrumentation and visualization of the medial aspect of the joint. The portal is established directly by placing a spinal needle into the joint just anterior to the radiocapitellar articulation. Care is taken to enter the capsule lateral to the joint rather than anterior to it in order to minimize the risk of radial nerve injury. The skin is incised and a blunt trocar advanced into the joint under direct vision. Alternatively, this portal can often be established using an inside-out technique. The arthroscope is moved to the anterolateral portal, and the medial capsule, trochlea, coronoid fossa, and coronoid process are evaluated.

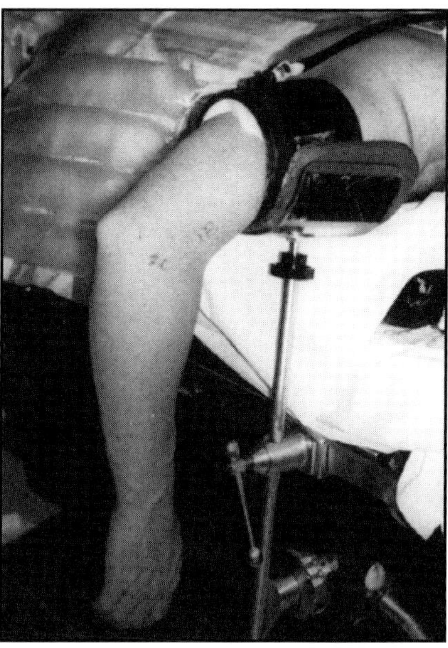

Fig. 6 Arm holder for use with patient in prone position (Instrument Makar).

Examination of the posterior compartment is initiated using the posterolateral portal. The medial and lateral gutters, olecranon tip, olecranon fossa, and posterior aspect of the radiocapitellar joint can be examined. If instrumentation is desired, a straight posterior portal is made. At the end of the procedure, the tourniquet is deflated and the joint irrigated. Depending on the procedure performed, drains may be placed through the cannulas. Local anesthetic is injected into the joint and cannulas are removed. The portals are left open, or adhesive strips are placed and a sterile soft dressing applied. **(CD-23.3)**

Complications

The most commonly reported complications of elbow arthroscopy are injuries to neural structures.[7,15,17–21] Although rare and often transient, nerve injuries can be devastating. Nerve complications can result from direct injury by arthroscopic trocars and instruments, compression caused by arthroscopic sheaths, overaggressive joint distention or fluid extravasation, or use of local anesthetic agents.[7,15,18]

The radial nerve is at risk during placement of the anterolateral portal. Injuries to the radial nerve, the superficial branch of the radial nerve, and the posterior interosseous nerve have been reported.[15,18,20,21] The median nerve is susceptible during placement of the anteromedial portal, and injuries to the median and anterior interosseous nerves have been documented.[7,15,19] Damage to the ulnar nerve after the use of multiple medial portals has been reported.[21] Injury to superficial cutaneous nerves resulting in neuroma formation has also been described.[15]

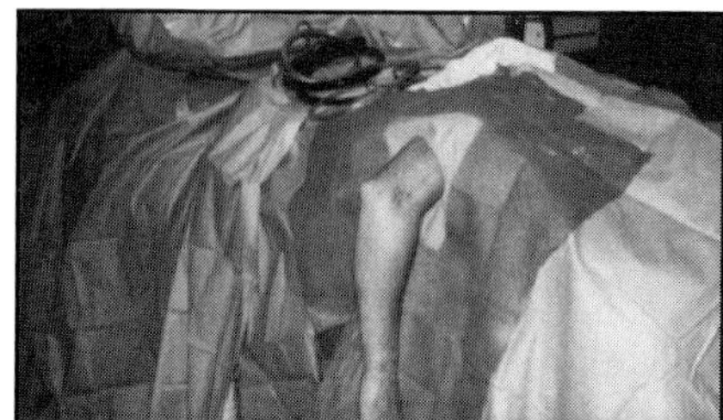

Fig. 7 Prone position.

Additional complications are similar to those of other arthroscopic procedures and include infection, instrument breakage, iatrogenic injury to articular cartilage, synovial fistula formation, and problems associated with use of a tourniquet. Other complications, such as arthrofibrosis and heterotopic bone formation, are unusual.[1,2,6,21]

The close proximity of portals to nerves and vessels places these structures at significant risk during elbow arthroscopy. We use the prone position, which allows the anterior neurovascular structures to fall away from portal sites. In addition, anterior portals are always created with the elbow in 90° of flexion and with the joint fully distended. A thorough knowledge of regional anatomy, use of meticulous surgical technique, and strict attention to detail will minimize the risk of neurologic complications.

Summary

With more innovation in arthroscopic equipment and surgical technique, elbow arthroscopy will continue to evolve and new indications will emerge. Strict adherence to the principles outlined above will allow the use of arthroscopy to treat a variety of elbow disorders in a safe and effective manner.

References

1. Marzo JM: Elbow arthroscopy: Indications and technique, in Peimer CA (ed): *Surgery of the Hand and Upper Extremity*. New York, NY, McGraw-Hill, 1996, pp 583–597.
2. O'Driscoll SW, Morrey BF: Arthroscopy of the elbow: Diagnostic and therapeutic benefits and hazards. *J Bone Joint Surg* 1992;74A:84–94.
3. O'Driscoll SW, Morrey BF: Arthroscopy of the elbow, in Morrey BF (ed): *The Elbow and Its Disorders*, ed 2. Philadelphia, PA, WB Saunders, 1993, pp 120–130.
4. Poehling GG, Ekman EF, Ruch DS: Elbow arthroscopy: Introduction and overview, in McGinty JB, Caspari RB, Jackson RW, Poehling GG (eds): *Operative Arthroscopy,* ed 2. Philadelphia, PA, Lippincott-Raven, 1996, pp 821–828.
5. Carson WG Jr, Meyers JF: Diagnostic arthroscopy of the elbow: Supine position surgical technique, arthroscopic and portal anatomy, in McGinty JB, Caspari RB, Jackson RW, Poehling GG (eds): *Operative Arthroscopy*, ed 2. Philadelphia, PA, Lippincott-Raven, 1996, pp 851–868.
6. Plancher KD, Peterson RK, Brezenoff L: Diagnostic arthroscopy of the elbow: Set-up, portals, and technique. *Oper Tech Sports Med* 1998;6:2–10.
7. Andrews JR, Carson WG: Arthroscopy of the elbow. *Arthroscopy* 1985;1:97–107.
8. Baker CL Jr: Normal arthroscopic anatomy of the elbow: Surgical technique with the patient prone, in McGinty JB, Caspari RB, Jackson RW, Poehling GG (eds): *Operative Arthroscopy*, ed 2. Philadelphia, PA, Lippincott-Raven, 1996, pp 869–876.
9. Poehling GG, Whipple TL, Sisco L, Goldman B: Elbow arthroscopy: A new technique. *Arthroscopy* 1989;5:222–224.
10. Miller CD, Jobe CM, Wright MH: Neuroanatomy in elbow arthroscopy. *J Shoulder Elbow Surg* 1995;4:168–174.
11. Field LD, Altchek DW, Warren RF, O'Brien SJ, Skyhar MJ, Wickiewicz TL: Arthroscopic anatomy of the lateral elbow: A comparison of three portals. *Arthroscopy* 1994;10: 602–607.
12. Lindenfeld TN: Medial approach in elbow arthroscopy. *Am J Sports Med* 1990;18: 413–417.
13. Stothers K, Day B, Regan WR: Arthroscopy of the elbow: Anatomy, portal sites, and a description of the proximal lateral portal. *Arthroscopy* 1995;11:449–457.
14. Savoie FH III, Field LD (eds): Anatomy, in *Arthroscopy of the Elbow.* New York, NY, Churchill Livingstone, 1996, pp 3–24.
15. Lynch GJ, Meyers JF, Whipple TL, Caspari RB: Neurovascular anatomy and elbow arthroscopy: Inherent risks. *Arthroscopy* 1986;2:190–197.
16. Andrews JR, Baumgarten TE: Arthroscopic anatomy of the elbow. *Orthop Clin North Am* 1995;26:671–677.
17. Poehling GG, Ekman EF: Arthroscopy of the elbow, in Jackson DW (ed): *Instructional Course Lectures 44.* Rosemont, IL, American Academy of Orthopaedic Surgeons, 1995, pp 217–228.
18. Papilion JD, Neff RS, Shall LM: Compression neuropathy of the radial nerve as a complication of elbow arthroscopy: A case report and review of the literature. *Arthroscopy* 1988;4:284–286.
19. Ruch DS, Poehling GG: Anterior interosseus nerve injury following elbow arthroscopy. *Arthroscopy* 1997;13:756–758.
20. Thomas MA, Fast A, Shapiro D: Radial nerve damage as a complication of elbow arthroscopy. *Clin Orthop* 1987;215:130–131.
21. Treacy SH, Field LD, Savoie FH III: Complications of elbow arthroscopy, in press.

Reference to Video

Savoie FH III: Basics of Elbow Arthroscopy. Jackson, MS, Mississippi Sports Medicine and Orthopaedic Center, 1998.

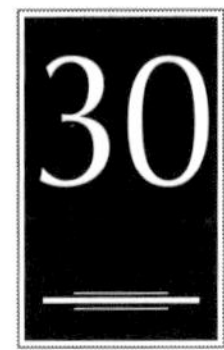

Medial Collateral Ligament Tears in the Throwing Athlete

Riley J. Williams III, MD
Erica Rowe Urquhart, MD, PhD
David W. Altchek, MD

Abstract

Medial collateral ligament (MCL) injuries of the elbow in throwing athletes are part of a spectrum of valgus extension overload injuries. Clinicians should consider reconstruction of the injured MCL in those patients who are unable to return to sports activities or work after an interval of rest and rehabilitation. Surgical treatment of this disorder has continued to evolve from the original technique developed by Jobe and associates. The authors' surgical technique involves reconstruction of the MCL using a single ulnar tunnel and single humeral tunnel that is performed through a muscle-splitting approach that usually obviates the need for ulnar nerve transposition. Knowledge of the biology and biomechanics of MCL function is important in the diagnosis and treatment of MCL injuries of the elbow in the throwing athlete.

Reconstruction of the medial collateral ligament (MCL) of the elbow has become widely accepted as a treatment option for medial elbow instability in the throwing athlete. It has been demonstrated that pitching a baseball results in angular velocity in excess of 3,000° per second at the elbow; this high velocity subsequently imparts a high load to the elbow.[1] These repetitive loads are typically resisted by the supporting structures of the medial elbow and can result in acute tearing or chronic attenuation of the MCL.[2] The resultant laxity of the MCL ultimately leads to elbow dysfunction and an inability to throw effectively. Understanding of this problem has progressed significantly over the past 20 years, and effective treatment strategies have been developed to facilitate a return to sports activity.

Historical Perspective

Prior to the groundbreaking work by Jobe and associates,[3] MCL tears were often unrecognized and left untreated. Patients who did not respond to nonsurgical treatment were forced to compete ineffectively, change position, or retire from sport.

In its earliest form, MCL reconstruction was performed using a harvested autograft tendon passed through multiple bony tunnels in both the distal humerus and proximal ulna.[3] Jobe described performing this procedure in association with a formal submuscular ulnar nerve transposition and complete elevation of the flexor mass from the medial humeral epicondyle. This method was effective in returning most elite level throwers (63%) to sports participation. However, the rate of complications was high (31%), and complications were typically related to postoperative dysfunction of the ulnar nerve.

As interest grew in this reconstructive procedure, studies began to focus on developing methods that might obviate the need for flexor mass elevation and ulnar nerve transposition. Smith and associates[4] reported on the "safe zone" of the medial elbow, whereby surgeons might expose the medial ulnohumeral articulation without interfering with local nerve function (Figure 1). This muscle-splitting approach (through the flexor carpi ulnaris) allowed for the development of second-generation MCL reconstruction methods that did not require ulnar nerve transposition and flexor mass detachment. The muscle split allowed for the successful modification of the original

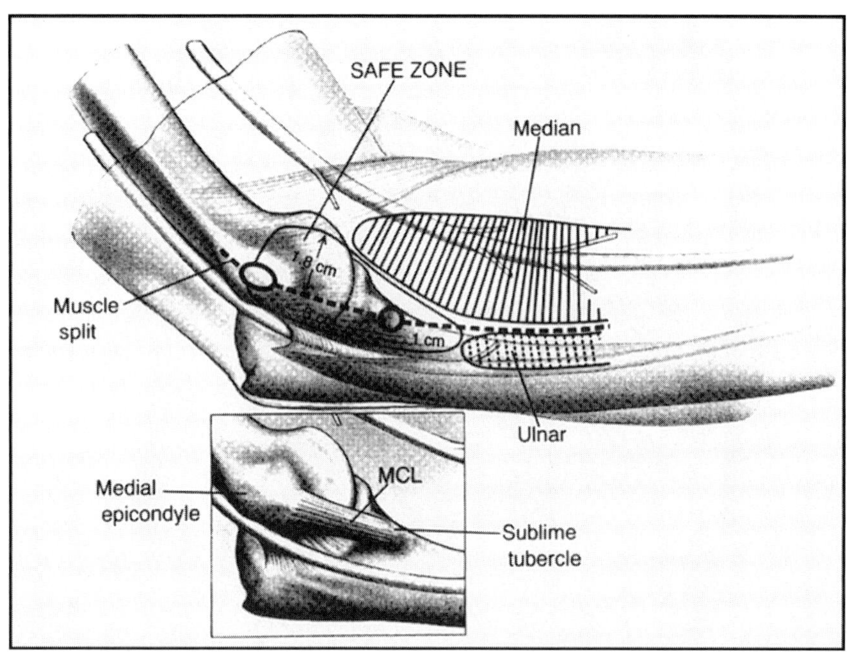

Figure 1 The medial elbow "safe-zone" for MCL reconstruction. (Reproduced with permission from Smith GR, Altchek DW, Pagnani MJ, Keeley JR: A muscle-splitting approach to the ulnar collateral ligament of the elbow: Neuroanatomy and operative technique. *Am J Sports Med* 1996; 24:575-580.)

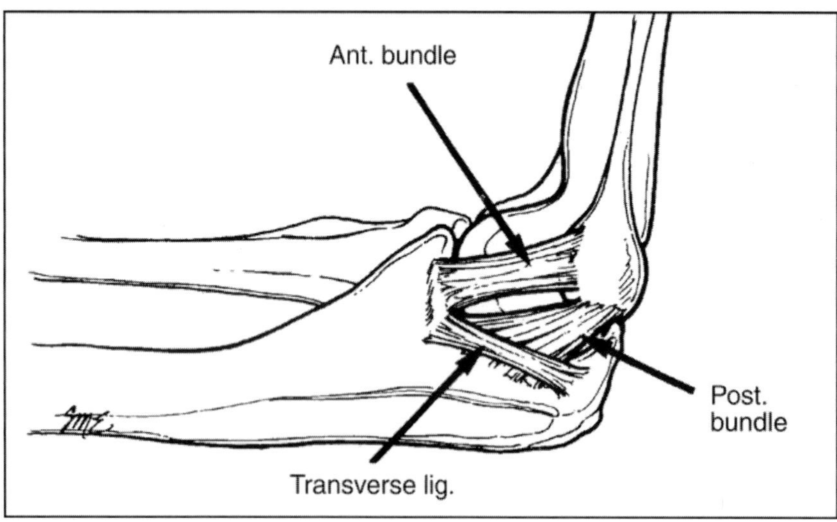

Figure 2 Medial (ulnar) complex of the elbow. (Reproduced with permission from Jobe FW, Elattrache NS: Diagnosis and treatment of ulnar collateral ligament injuries in athletes, in Morrey BF (ed): *The Elbow and Its Disorders*. Philadelphia, PA, WB Saunders, 1993, pp 566-572.)

Jobe technique as described by Thompson and associates.[5]

In the mid 1990s, attempts were made to further modify the technique of MCL reconstruction by using suture anchors to stabilize the transplanted MCL graft at the medial elbow; this method was soon abandoned following an early review that showed a failure rate of approximately 30% (DW Altchek, MD, personal communication, 2003). Despite its shortcomings, this reconstruction method demonstrated that both the ability to tension the graft and the placement of the graft within a bony tunnel were essential to its success. In 1996, the docking technique of MCL reconstruction was developed.[6] This technique is performed through a muscle-splitting approach, typically without ulnar nerve transposition, through bone tunnels, using a free graft. The three humeral bony tunnels that are required in the Jobe method make this procedure technically difficult and may predispose the medial epicondyle to fracture. Moreover, the figure-of-8 graft configuration does not allow for graft tensioning or rigid fixation. The docking technique uses a single humeral tunnel, and the triangular graft configuration facilitates the placement of a well-tensioned graft that is rigidly fixed.

Anatomy

The MCL is composed primarily of the anterior and posterior bundles (Figure 2). A transverse component of the MCL complex is occasionally present but is not considered a significant restraint to valgus stress. The anterior bundle of the MCL plays an important role in resisting valgus loads to the medial elbow. The anterior bundle originates from the lateral two thirds of the anteroinferior aspect of the medial epicondyle and inserts on the sublime tubercle of the ulna.[7] The posterior bundle originates from the posterior medial humeral epicondyle and inserts proximally and posteriorly to the sublime tubercle.[8] The anterior bundle is the strongest, stiffest portion of the MCL, with an average load to failure of 260 N. The anterior bundle is taut in elbow extension; the posterior bundle is taut in elbow flexion. The anterior band of the MCL is the primary restraint against valgus stress at 30°, 60°, and 90° of flexion. Valgus rotation increases with greater angles of elbow flexion, with the greatest instability at 90° of elbow flexion.[9] The importance of the anterior bundle is clear as the highest loads imparted to the elbow typically occur with the elbow at 90° of flexion during late cocking and early acceleration. Therefore, the anterior bundle should remain the focus of reconstruction for surgeons attempting to restore medial elbow stability following MCL injury.

Biomechanics

Elbow stability is maintained by both the bony articulations and collateral ligaments. At less than 20° of elbow extension and greater than 120° of flexion, the ulnohumeral articulation anatomy provides the greatest contribution to elbow stability against varus and valgus stress. However, between 20° and 120° of elbow flexion, the lateral collateral ligament and MCL serve as the primary stabilizers of the elbow joint against varus and valgus stress, respectively. The static function of the MCL is to serve as the primary restraint to valgus stress at this functional range of motion. Biomechanical analysis of the pitching motion has demonstrated arm rotational speeds in excess of 7,000° per second; elbow extension velocities of 2,300° per second have also been noted in high-level throwing athletes. The forces generated during the pitching motion are greatest at the medial elbow during the late cocking and early acceleration phases. At 90° of flexion, the MCL contributes 78% of the resistance to elbow distraction.[10] Thus, it is clear that MCL competency is critical to an effective throwing motion.

Table 1
Physical Examination of the Thrower's Elbow

Test/Maneuver	Clinical Relevance
Elbow range of motion	Extension loss common Loose bodies may cause crepitus
Resisted forearm pronation	Pain suggests flexor mass involvement
Ulnar nerve palpation at the cubital tunnel	Tenderness or Tinel's sign increases suspicion for involvement
Valgus stress to the elbow	Pain or laxity suggestive of MCL injury
Combined terminal elbow extension and forearm pronation	Pain indicative of posterior impingement

Indications

The primary indication for elbow MCL reconstruction in the throwing athlete is elbow pain associated with MCL incompetence that precludes participation in sports at preinjury levels. It is important to note that patients with MCL tears seldom report symptoms of instability. Typically, throwers report pain during the late cocking and acceleration phases of pitching. Pitchers are affected most often, but other baseball position players may also suffer injury. Acute MCL tears usually occur in association with a vigorous throwing effort (for example, an outfielder attempting to throw out a runner, or a javelin throw); following such an episode, the athlete usually cannot throw at all. However, most MCL tears occur over time, with patients reporting episodic elbow pain associated with the gradual deterioration of throwing ability. Ulnar nerve symptoms or posterior elbow pain may be reported as the condition becomes more chronic. A patient's history is of utmost importance in the evaluation of these athletes because the physical examination may be confusing. The history should attempt to determine pain location, symptom duration, the throwing phase during which pain is greatest, ulnar nerve involvement, and the effect (if any) of elbow injury on throwing velocity.

Examination

The entire neck and upper extremity should be evaluated; often, shoulder problems may contribute to the development of elbow problems in throwers over time. The elbow/forearm examination should be thorough and begin with inspection. Specific points to be included in the physical examination are listed in Table 1.

The valgus stress test for MCL injury remains a valuable part of the overall examination. However, it is sometimes difficult to effectively stabilize the humerus at angles greater than 30° of flexion. The manual valgus stress test is performed with the patient supine or sitting. Humeral rotation is controlled with one hand used as a lateral post. The opposite hand maximally pronates the forearm and places a valgus force on the elbow (Figure 3). If the valgus stress test reproduces the athlete's medial-sided elbow pain, or if laxity (usually minimal) is demonstrated by the examiner, the test is considered positive. The dynamic valgus stress test is also useful in evaluating suspected MCL injuries. In this maneuver, the examiner applies a valgus stress to the affected elbow and moves the forearm through a full arc of motion; the elicitation of pain during this test may increase suspicion of an MCL injury. It has been demonstrated that

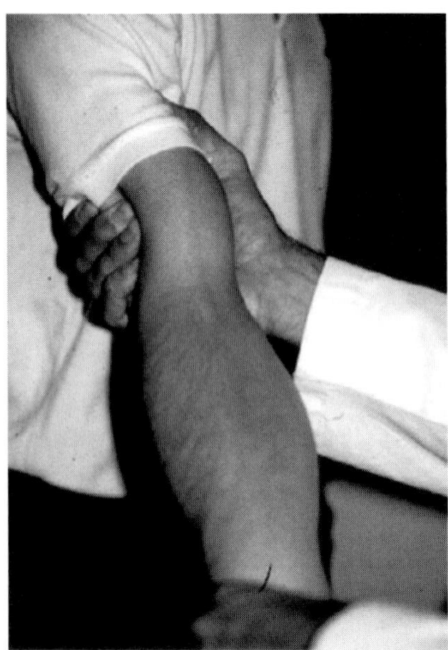

Figure 3 The valgus stress test.

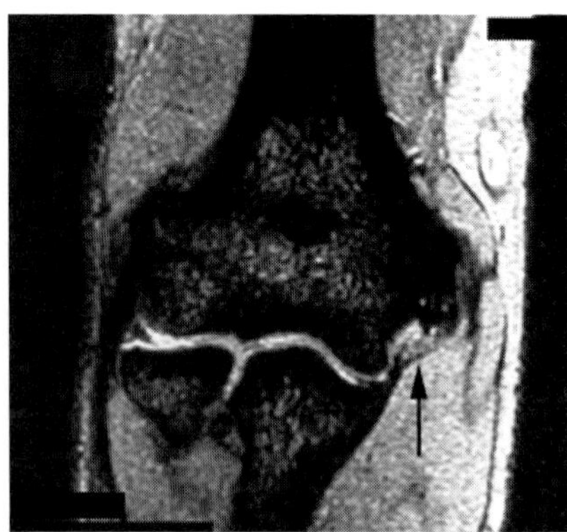

Figure 4 An MRI scan showing an MCL tear (*arrow*).

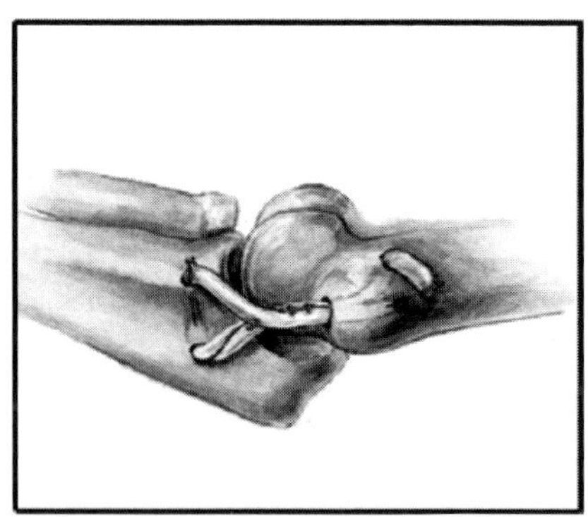

Figure 5 MCL reconstruction as developed by Jobe and associates.

chronic MCL laxity can result in the development of posterior olecranon osteophytes and intra-articular loose bodies.[11] Thus, assessment of the posterior elbow is critical for the successful treatment of the MCL-injured athlete.

Elbow radiographs are obtained during the initial assessment and include AP, lateral, and axial (oblique elbow view at 110° of elbow flexion) views. The axial view is most helpful in demonstrating the presence of posterior compartment loose bodies or osteophytes. Radiographic findings typically observed in patients with chronic MCL laxity include MCL calcification, medial ulnohumeral joint osteophytes, medial olecranon osteophytes, and loose bodies of the posterior compartment.

Other authors have advocated the use of stress radiographs in the diagnosis of MCL injuries. However, one series reported less than a 50% correlation between positive radiographic findings and the presence of MCL insufficiency.[12] CT arthrography scanning can also be used in the diagnosis of MCL injuries. Timmerman and associates[13] performed a prospective study on 25 baseball players with elbow pain in which CT arthrograms were 86% sensitive in confirming MCL injury.

Because MRI not only facilitates an assessment of the MCL but also permits the viewing of the articular surfaces and local anatomy, it is considered the primary modality for diagnosing MCL injury. A 1.5 Tesla MRI scan is used in combination with an elbow coil for optimal imaging. The elbow is imaged with the arm at the patient's side; the forearm is in supination and the elbow in full extension. Three-mm coronal views of the elbow result in a detailed image of the MCL (Figure 4). This MRI technique obviates the need for the use of contrast agents. MRI performed in this manner provides excellent contrast between subchondral bone, cartilage, and joint fluid.[14]

Recently, attention has been directed toward the use of ultrasound as a diagnostic tool in athletes with suspected MCL injuries. Sasaki and associates[15] used ultrasonography to evaluate the medial elbow compartment. Thirty baseball pitchers underwent elbow ultrasound evaluation with the elbow in 90° of flexion; the arm was subsequently subjected to a valgus gravitational stress. This study demonstrated that the medial joint space was significantly wider on the dominant throwing elbow than the contralateral elbow (2.7 mm and 1.6 mm, respectively). An angular deformity of the ulnar collateral ligament was noted in the dominant arm in a majority of these athletes. Moreover, increased medial joint space was associated with increased pain. The authors suggest that ultrasound may provide useful information on the condition of the ulnar collateral ligament and medial widening in the throwing athlete because this methodology allows the application of dynamic loads during elbow evaluation.[15]

MCL Reconstruction

All described methods of MCL reconstruction use a free autograft tendon that is placed in ulnar and humeral bone tunnels. As mentioned previously, the Jobe procedure uses three drill holes in the medial humeral epicondyle, two drill holes in the ulna, and a figure-of-8 tendon construct that is sutured to itself (Figure 5). In the docking technique, a free tendon autograft is placed in a triangular fashion with the graft passing through a single ulnar tunnel and the two free ends then being placed into a single medial epicondylar tunnel. Tension on the graft construct is maintained by tying sutures over a posterior humeral bone bridge; the resulting construct is rigid and firmly fixed. The authors' preferred method is described later in this chapter.

In the acutely injured elbow, control of pain and inflammation is prioritized. Early rehabilitation should focus on stretching and strengthening the rotator cuff, scapular stabilizers, and the flexor-pronator muscles of the forearm. Once elbow strength and flexibility have been restored, functional exercise, plyometrics, and a progressive throwing program are used to prepare the athlete for a return to sports activity.[11]

In general, MCL reconstruction is reserved for high-level athletes who are unable to throw effectively because of an incompetent MCL. Nonsurgical management of these athletes usually is not effective. Although it is possible for throwers to modify their pitching mechanics and successfully compensate for an unstable elbow, this outcome is not the norm. In a study of 31 throwing athletes with MCL tears, Rettig and associates[16] showed that only 42% of the athletes were able to return to a similar level of sports following a minimum 3-month rehabilitation trial. Moreover, the natural history of the thrower who continues to pitch with an MCL incompetent elbow is poor; posteromedial olecranon osteophytes, posterior impingement, and generalized osteoarthritic degeneration often occur over time.[17] In position players, nonsurgical management of MCL tears might be more effective. However, it is the ability of each athlete to compete effectively that ultimately determines the need for MCL reconstruction. Important issues in developing a preoperative plan are described in Table 2.

Table 2
Relevant Issues in Planning MCL Reconstruction

Issue	Points to Consider
Indications	Gross native MCL laxity not a prerequisite for MCL reconstruction; partial ligament injuries may cause disability and pain during throwing and not respond to conservative measures
Graft source	Ipsilateral palmaris tendon is typically used (variably present); may need to consider alternate graft source (eg, gracilis, plantaris, flexor carpi radialis strip)
Graft fixation and tension	Maximal graft tension and fixation is intuitively necessary for successful reconstruction—consider comfort level with method of reconstruction prior to proceeding
Ulnar nerve involvement	Must determine if the ulnar nerve is involved in the athlete's disability; nerve transposition is performed in these circumstances
Intra-articular pathology	The presence of loose bodies and/or posterior olecranon osteophytes can result in surgical failure if not addressed at the time of MCL reconstruction; these issues should be addressed during the elbow arthroscopy

Authors' Preferred Technique

Regional anesthesia is preferred. The surgical technique begins with elbow arthroscopy using an arm holder. The anterior compartment articular surfaces and synovium are evaluated, and an arthroscopic valgus stress test is performed at 70° of elbow flexion with the arm pronated. The anterior portion of the anterior band of the MCL may be visualized arthroscopically.[18] Valgus instability, implying MCL injury, may be confirmed upon distraction of the medial ulnohumeral joint (Figure 6); however, this finding is not present in all MCL-injured patients (such as those with partial tears). However, all intra-articular abnormalities (loose bodies, chondral defects, posterior osteophytes) are addressed before proceeding with ligament reconstruction. **(DVD-53.1)**

A tourniquet should be used. The ipsilateral palmaris longus tendon, or other graft source, is then harvested. If the palmaris longus muscle tendon is harvested, a transmuscular approach to the medial elbow is used to expose the native MCL. The antebrachial cutaneous branch of the median nerve often crosses the surgical field of the dissection of the flexor pronator mass and should be preserved. The anterior bundle of the MCL is incised longitudinally, the joint exposed, and valgus stress applied. MCL laxity is confirmed by observing separation of the joint surfaces by 3 mm or more. The ulna is exposed using a subperiosteal approach to protect the ulnar nerve. The ulnar tunnel holes are created anterior and posterior to the sublime tubercle using a No. 3 or No. 4 burr, depending on patient size. A small curved curet is used to connect the tunnels without violating the bony bridge. The anterior aspect of the medial epicondyle is exposed. A longitudinal tunnel is created up the epicondyle to a length of 15 mm with a No. 4 burr. Two small tunnels separated by 5 mm are created with a dental drill with a small bit (Figure 7). The native MCL is repaired, with the elbow in a reduced position. The graft is then passed from anterior to posterior through the ulnar tunnel, and one end of the graft is passed into the hu-

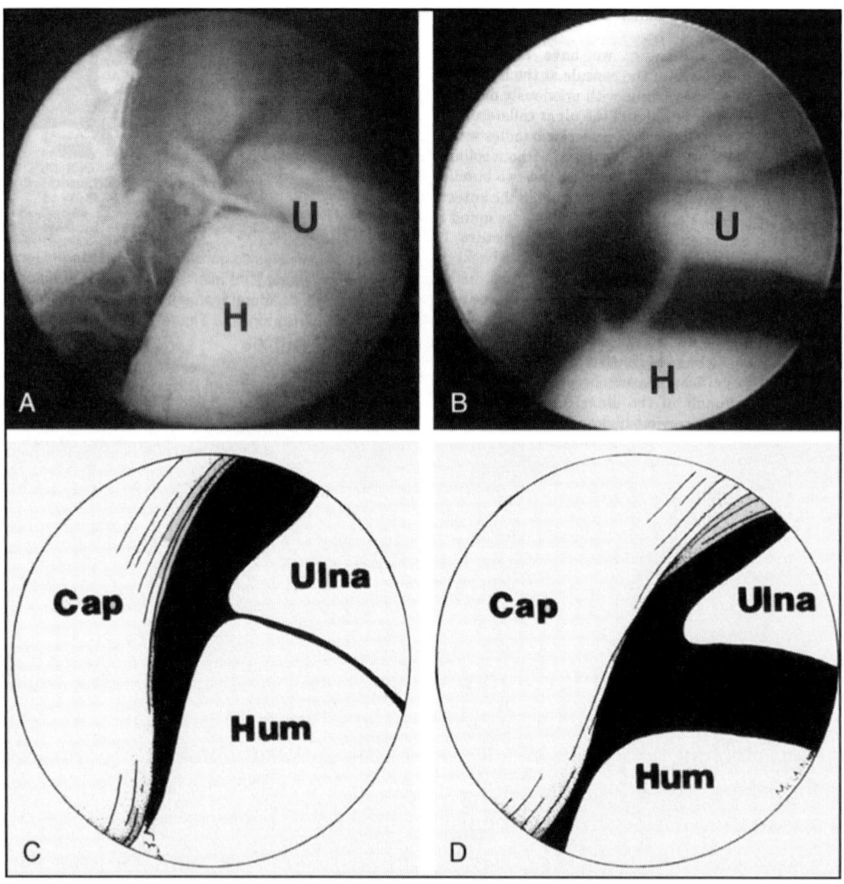

Figure 6 Arthroscopic views of the medial joint with the elbow at 70° of flexion after sectioning of the anterior bundle of the ulnar collateral ligament without valgus stress applied (**A**) and with valgus stress applied showing increased joint space between the coronoid process of the ulna and the humerus (**B**). H = humerus; U = ulna. Schematics showing increased distractions of the ulnohumeral joint after sectioning of the anterior bundle of the ulnar collateral ligament without valgus stress applied (**C**), and with valgus stress applied (**D**). Cap = capitellum; Hum = humerus.

meral tunnel. The elbow is further reduced with a varus stress and the forearm in supination. The elbow is then flexed and extended with tension on the graft to eliminate creep. The free end of the graft is placed adjacent to the humeral tunnel, sutures placed at the appropriate length necessary to facilitate graft tension once both graft ends lie within the humeral tunnel, and subsequently cut. The elbow is then again flexed and extended and the two sets of graft sutures are tied over the bony bridge, posteriorly on the humeral epicondyle (Figure 8). Following wound closure, the elbow is splinted in approximately 60° to 70° of flexion and relative forearm supination. Following wound dressing, the elbow is immobilized at approximately 70° to 90° of flexion, using a plaster splint.

The use of a hinged elbow brace is recommended 1 week after surgery because the biologic healing of the graft into the bone tunnels must precede vigorous throwing.[19] Motion is allowed between 45° and 90° of flexion. Gradual advancement to full range of motion takes place over the following 5 weeks. Physical therapy is initiated after the sixth week. At 12 weeks, bench pressing, weights, and more vigorous activities are allowed. At 4 months, an interval throwing program is initiated. By the ninth postoperative month, competitive pitching may begin.[11]

Results

Current methods of MCL reconstruction are supported by basic studies. One biomechanical study that used cadaveric elbows to assess valgus elbow stability demonstrated that an MCL-reconstructed elbow can withstand loads similar to that of the native MCL.[2] Each sample was secured to a testing frame, and 5 Nm valgus loads were applied at 30°, 60°, 90°, and 120° of flexion. MCL reconstruction restored medial elbow stability. Compared with the native ligament, mean medial elbow displacement in the MCL-reconstructed specimens was 99% (30°), 102% (60°), 97% (90°), and 89% (120°). This cadaveric study supports the idea that anterior bundle reconstruction restored the stability of the MCL through the full flexion arc.[2] Clinical outcomes studies on MCL reconstruction in high-level athletes confirm the successful restoration of medial elbow stability via the described methods of MCL reconstruction.

In the first study that described the clinical results of MCL reconstruction, Jobe and associates[3] reported on 16 high-level throwing athletes. During the surgical approach, the flexor mass was elevated and the ulnar nerve transposed in all patients. Ten patients (63%) returned to their previous level of sports; five patients retired from professional athletics. The authors also reported a high incidence of complications related to the ulnar nerve. Two patients had postoperative ulnar neuropathy; three patients reported some transient postoperative hypoesthesia. Although all of these nerve problems resolved, the authors cautioned clinicians on the use of this method because of the observed complication rate.[3]

These authors continued to analyze their results and published another study in 1992 that described the clinical results of 56 patients who underwent MCL reconstruction.[20] At a mean follow-up of approximately 6 years, 68% of the throwing athletes were able to return to sport at a level similar to their preinjury state. The authors noted a poorer rate of success in those patients who had undergone previous elbow surgery. Fifteen patients experienced ulnar neuropathy; nine of these patients required additional surgery.[20]

Thompson and associates[5] described the clinical results of the Jobe method used in conjunction with a muscle-splitting approach in 83 athletes. No ulnar nerve transposition was performed in these patients. Only 5% of patients experienced postoperative ulnar nerve symptoms; all resolved without the need for further surgery. Moreover, of the 33 patients who met a minimum follow-up criterion of 2 years, 93% had excellent clinical results and were able to return to throwing. Thus, the muscle-splitting approach, combined with eliminating the ulnar nerve transposition, significantly decreased the incidence of postoperative nerve dysfunction following the Jobe method of MCL reconstruction.

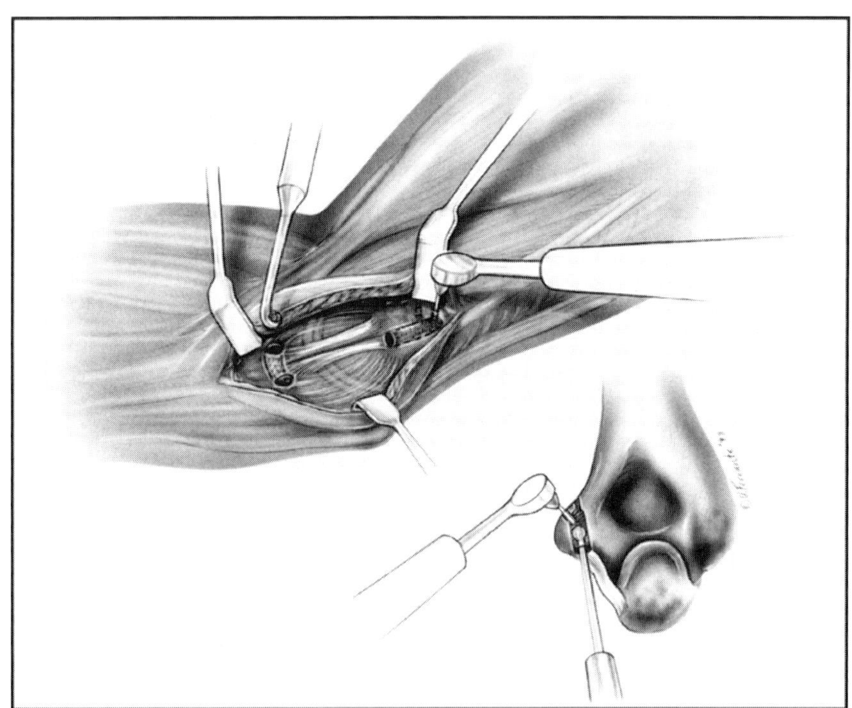

Figure 7 MCL reconstruction using the docking technique. The ulnar and humeral tunnels are used. (Reproduced with permission from Altchek D, Hyman J, Williams R, et al: Management of MCL injuries in throwers. *Tech Shoulder Elbow Surg* 2000;1: 73-81.)

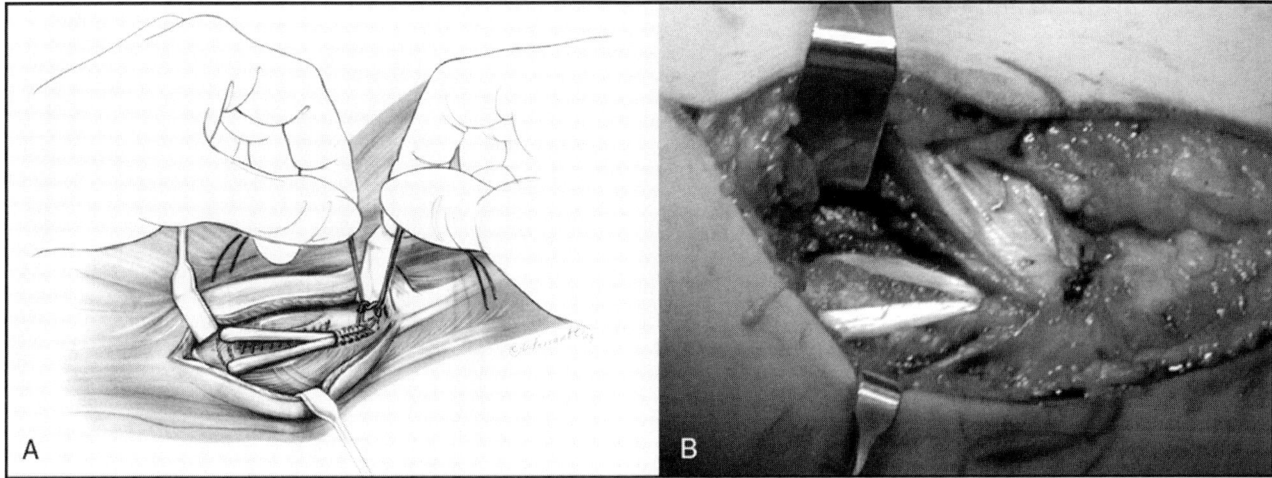

Figure 8 Final docking technique MCL construct. Drawing **(A)** and intraoperative photograph **(B)**. (Figure B is reproduced with permission from Altchek D, Hyman J, Williams R, et al: Management of MCL injuries in throwers. *Tech Shoulder Elbow Surg* 2000; 1:73-81.)

In another study, Azar and associates[21] described the successful application of the original Jobe method of MCL reconstruction in a group of high-level throwers over a 6-year period. After a mean follow-up period of 35 months, a success rate of 79% was reported in returning these athletes to competition. Ten patients had preoperative ulnar nerve findings; nine patients had complete resolution of symptoms after ulnar nerve transposition and MCL reconstruction. Overall, the mean interval to return to throwing competitively was 9.8 months.[21]

In another study, 36 elite-level throwers who underwent MCL reconstruction using the docking method were analyzed.[6] The surgical approach described previously was used for all patients. At a mean follow-up of 3.3 years, 92% of the athletes were able to return to sports activity at a level that met or exceeded their preinjury state for at least 1 year. No ulnar nerve dysfunction was observed in this group of patients. However, one patient experienced a postoperative medial antebrachial nerve neuroma that required excision, and another patient suffered fracture of the ulnar tunnel that necessitated revision MCL reconstruction. To date, the authors have performed more than 300 such procedures and continue to observe a high level of clinical success using this clinical approach.[6]

Summary

MCL tears are particularly disabling to the throwing athlete. MCL reconstruction may be indicated for symptomatic patients in whom conservative management has failed. Current methods of MCL reconstruction reliably enable treated athletes to return to sports activity following participation in an extensive physical therapy and throwing program. Our preferred surgical technique involves the use of elbow arthroscopy and reconstruction of the MCL through a muscle-splitting approach, without requiring ulnar nerve transposition. Clinical studies describing the results of both the Jobe and docking methods clearly demonstrate that affected individuals can reasonably expect a high return of elbow function 9 to 12 months after surgery.

References

1. Feltner M, Dapena J: Dynamics of the shoulder and elbow joints of the throwing arm during a baseball pitch. *J Sports Biomech* 1989;5:420-450.
2. Mullen DJ, Goradia VK, Parks BG, Matthews LS: A biomechanical study of stability of the elbow to valgus stress before and after reconstruction of the medial collateral ligament. *J Shoulder Elbow Surg* 2002;11:259-264.
3. Jobe FW, Stark H, Lombardo SJ: Reconstruction of the ulnar collateral ligament in athletes. *J Bone Joint Surg Am* 1986;68:1158-1163.
4. Smith GR, Altchek DW, Pagnani MJ, Keeley JR: A muscle-splitting approach to the ulnar collateral ligament of the elbow: Neuroanatomy and operative technique. *Am J Sports Med* 1996;24:575-580.
5. Thompson WH, Jobe FA, Yocum LA, Pink MM: Ulnar collateral ligament reconstruction in athletes: Muscle-splitting approach without transposition of the ulnar nerve. *J Shoulder Elbow Surg* 2001;10:152-157.
6. Rohrbough JT, Altchek DW, Hyman J, Williams RJ III, Botts JD: Medial collateral ligament reconstruction of the elbow using the docking technique. *Am J Sports Med* 2002;30:541-548.
7. O'Driscoll SW, Jaloszynski R, Morrey BF, An KN: Origin of the medial ulnar collateral ligament. *J Hand Surg Am* 1992;17:164-168.
8. Timmerman LA, Andrews JR: Histology and arthroscopic anatomy of the ulnar collateral ligament of the elbow. *Am J Sports Med* 1994;22:667-673.
9. Callaway GH, Field LD, Deng XH, et al: Biomechanical evaluation of the medial collateral ligament of the elbow. *J Bone Joint Surg Am* 1997;79:1223-1231.
10. Morrey BF, An KN: Articular and ligamentous contributions to the stability of the elbow joint. *Am J Sports Med* 1983;11:315-319.
11. Hyman J, Breazeale NM, Altchek DW: Valgus instability of the elbow in athletes. *Clin Sports Med* 2001;20:25-45.
12. Ellenbecker TS, Mattalino AJ, Elam EA, Caplinger RA: Medial elbow joint laxity in professional baseball pitchers: A bilateral comparison using stress radiography. *Am J Sports Med* 1998;26:420-424.
13. Timmerman LA, Schwartz ML, Andrews JR: Preoperative evaluation of the ulnar collateral ligament by magnetic resonance imaging and computed tomography arthrography: Evaluation in 25 baseball players with surgical confirmation. *Am J Sports Med* 1994;22:26-32.
14. Sofka CM, Potter HG: Imaging of elbow injuries in the child and adult athlete. *Radiol Clin North Am* 2002;40:251-265.
15. Sasaki J, Takahara M, Ogino T, Kashiwa H, Ishigaki D, Kanauchi Y: Ultrasonographic assessment of the ulnar collateral ligament and medial elbow laxity in college baseball players. *J Bone Joint Surg Am* 2002;84:525-531.
16. Rettig AC, Sherrill C, Snead DS, Mendler JC, Mieling P: Nonoperative treatment of ulnar collateral ligament injuries in throwing athletes. *Am J Sports Med* 2001;29:15-17.
17. Jobe FW, Elattrache NS: Diagnosis and treatment of ulnar collateral ligament injuries in athletes, in Morrey BF (ed): *The Elbow and Its Disorders*. Philadelphia, PA, WB Saunders, 1993, pp 566-572.
18. Field LD, Callaway GH, O'Brien SJ, Altchek DW: Arthroscopic assessment of the medial collateral ligament complex of the elbow. *Am J Sports Med* 1995;23:396-400.
19. Dillman CJ, Fleisig GS, Andrews JR: Biomechanics of pitching with emphasis on shoulder kinematics. *J Orthop Sports Phys Ther* 1993;18:402-408.
20. Conway JE, Jobe FW, Glousman RE, Pink M: Medial instability of the elbow in throwing athletes: Treatment by repair or reconstruction of the ulnar collateral ligament. *J Bone Joint Surg Am* 1992;74:67-83.
21. Azar FM, Andrews JR, Wilk KE, Groh D: Operative treatment of ulnar collateral ligament injuries of the elbow in athletes. *Am J Sports Med* 2000;28:16-23.

31

Arthroscopic Treatment of Posterior Elbow Impingement

Michael J. Moskal, MD
Felix H. Savoie III, MD
Larry D. Field, MD

Introduction

Posterior elbow impingement refers to a mechanical abutment of bony and soft tissues in the posterior compartment of the elbow that produces pain, stiffness, and/or locking. The clinical presentation is characterized by pain at the limits of elbow extension, with varying degrees of extension loss. In general, there are 3 broad categories of posterior elbow impingement. Posterior elbow impingement can be seen (1) as part of a primary osteoarthritic process; (2) abutment posteriorly with an intact ulnar collateral ligament, seen in athletes with hyperextension forces, and (3) bony abutment of the olecranon and the humerus, seen in overhand athletes with ulnar collateral ligamentous insufficiency. Although these categories are useful for diagnostic and treatment considerations, there is considerable overlap of the pathoanatomy encountered.

Posterior Elbow Impingement

Posterior elbow impingement in athletes occurs in 2 forms. Repetitive hyperextension of the elbow may produce posterior impingement. The pathologic entities are centrally located on the tip of the olecranon, and they usually will have reactive thickening of the bone bridge between the coronoid and olecranon fossae (Fig. 1). These lesions are seen in football linemen, gymnasts, rodeo participants, competitive weight lifters, and fast pitch softball pitchers. Radiographs in these patients are similar to those seen in patients who have primary osteoarthritis. There is usually no instability of the ligaments of the elbow, but these patients may have a mild capsular contracture anteriororly.

Instability may produce secondary posterior impingement between the outer edge of the olecranon and the inner edge of the olecranon fossae. Valgus instability produces changes on the medial side of the olecranon and the lateral aspect of the medial wall of the olecranon fossa. Varus and posterolateral instability produces lesions on the lateral aspect of the olecranon and the medial aspect of the lateral wall of the olecranon fossa (Fig. 2). Radiographs reveal eccentric changes in these areas, with no demonstrable thickening of the bone bridge between the olecranon and coronoid fossae of the distal humerus.

A significant number of competitive overhand throwers have more subtle forms of ulnar collateral ligament insufficiency. In a retrospective review of elbow surgery in professional baseball players, Andrews and Timmerman[1] noted that posterior extension injury was the most common diagnosis. However, ulnar collateral ligament injuries were underestimated and, of patients who required a second surgery, 25% required an ulnar collateral ligament reconstruction. They surmised that ulnar collateral ligament pathology would have been recognized more often with the arthroscopic valgus stress test[2] and recognition of undersurface tears.[3] Attenuation of the

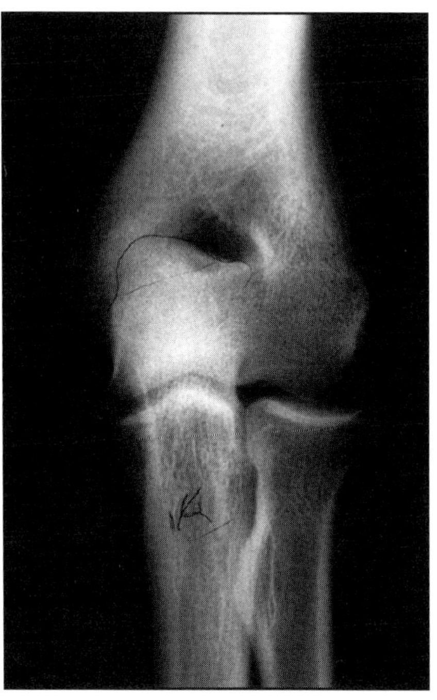

Fig. 1 Radiograph demonstrates the central spurring of the tip of the olecranon in a patient with posterior impingement.

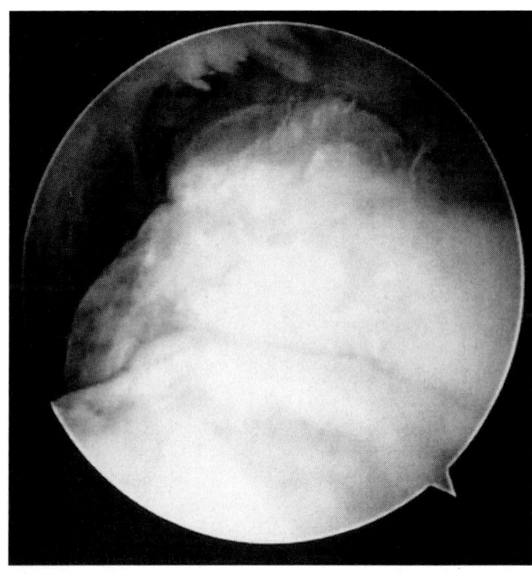

Fig. 2 Instability may produce eccentric spurring of the medial (valgus instability) or lateral (varus or posterolateral instability) olecranon.

medial stabilizing structures of the elbow allow increased valgus subluxation of the elbow during overhand throwing. Chronically, traction osteophytes along the medial aspect of the semilunar notch[4] and midsubstance calcifications of the ulnar collateral ligament[5] may develop. Increased compressive forces across the radiocapitellar joint from valgus instability can lead to chondromalacia and capitellar osteochondral lesions, in addition to posterior compartment lesions and loose bodies. In a throwing athlete, the presence of posterior impingement should focus the surgeon on instability. The arthroscopic stress test before and after spur resection should decrease the need for reoperation.

Posterior elbow impingement is also commonly encountered in degenerative and post-traumatic arthritis. Primary osteoarthritis may proceed with a predominately posterior involvement.[6] Patients are almost exclusively male and commonly present in the fourth to sixth decade of life. Mechanical abutment pain and diminished range of motion are caused by olecranon and coranoid osteophytes, decreased volume of the olecranon fossa, and loose bodies, which may or may not be imbedded in scar tissue. Crepitance and loss of elbow extension are common. Pain loss is typically more common at the extremes of extension than at flexion. Midrange pain is more common with advanced stages.

Arthroscopic treatment for posterior impingement has evolved from open techniques. Arthroscopic assessment and treatment allows the surgeon to evaluate and treat intra-articular pathology and offers significant advantages over open procedures, including limited soft-tissue dissection and increased visualization of both the anterior and posterior compartments. In our experience, as well as in that of others,[1] arthroscopic techniques in posterior compartment surgery have proven superior to open surgery. The essentials of treatment are removal of loose bodies, olecranon tip and coronoid process osteophyte excision, deepening[7] or fenestration[8] of the distal humerus, and excision of soft-tissue lesions, such as posterolateral plicae,[9] synovitis, and/or fat pad hypertrophy. Patient selection, technical expertise, and familiarity with both open and arthroscopic elbow surgery are all essential to success.

In addition, arthroscopic treatment for posterior impingement in throwers should also carefully assess posteromedial olecranon osteophytes with corresponding distal humeral lesions and overall humeral hypertrophy,[4] radiocapitellar degeneration,[10] posterolateral plicas,[9] and, most importantly, ulnar collateral ligament insufficiency.[11] The arthroscopic valgus stress test[2,12] before and after debridement is helpful to assess the integrity of the ulnar collateral ligament (Fig. 3).

Patient Evaluation

Information about the patient's age; occupational, athletic, and vocational activities; symptom onset; and its relation to these activities should be obtained. Patients with primary osteoarthritis are typically older, whereas patients with posterior impingement due to ulnar collateral insufficiency tend to be younger. Overhand athletes typically complain of increasing fatigue, numbness, and medial elbow pain during throwing. Overhand athletes may also complain of activity related pain in the posterolateral aspect of the radiocapitellar articulation.[13] Articular effusions are seen best posterolaterally in this radiocapitellar area. Range of motion may or may not be normal. Flexion contractures are common but are not uniformly present in patients with posterior elbow impingement.

Provocative testing is useful in the evaluation of posterior elbow impingement unrelated to primary osteoarthritis. In terminal extension, a valgus stress may be painful as the olecranon abuts against the humerus medially. Valgus stress testing can be performed with the patient sitting or

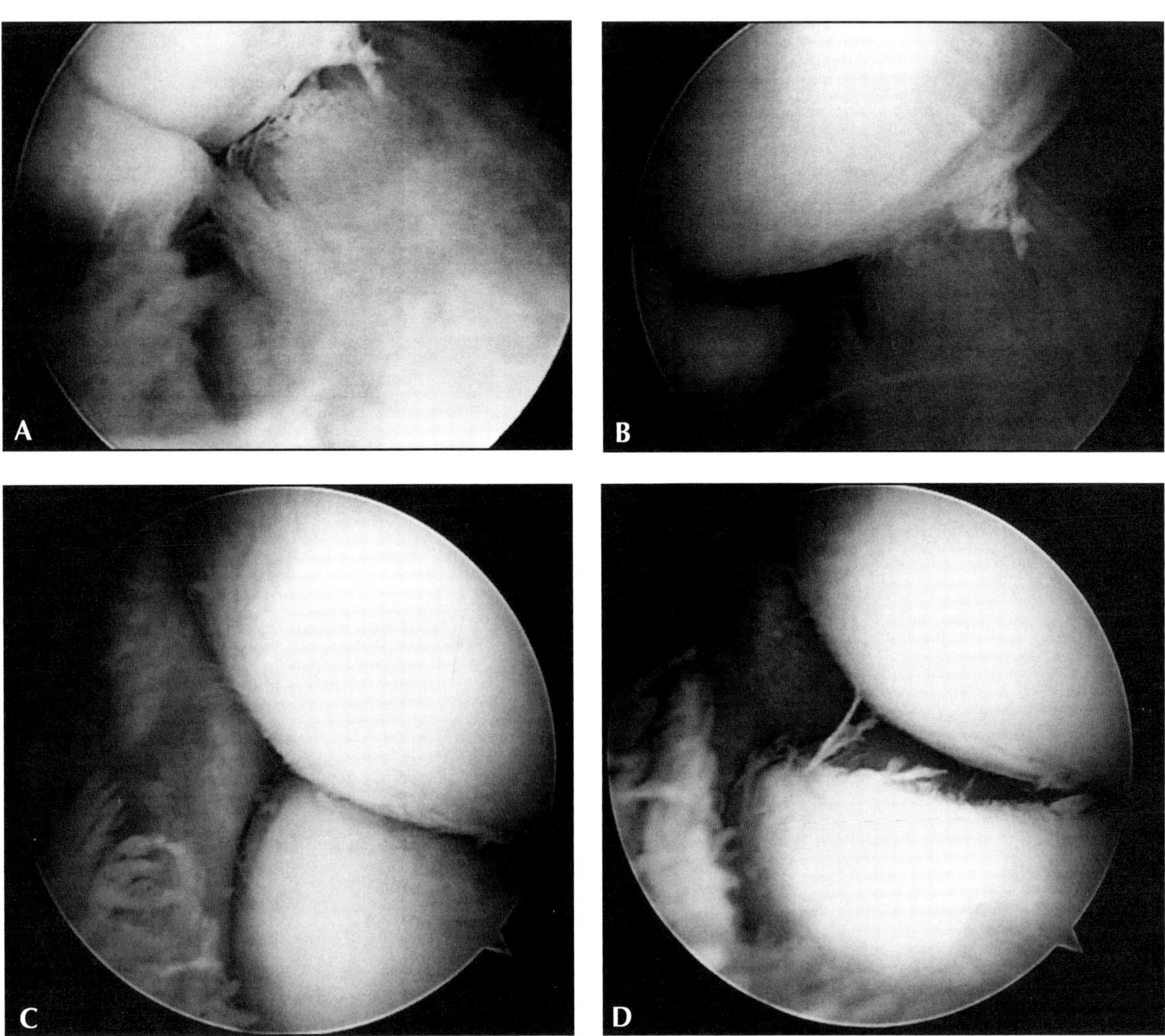

Fig. 3 Arthroscopy instability test may confirm the clinical diagnosis of valgus **(A, B)** or varus **(C, D)** instability.

lying prone. The examiner uses one hand to apply a valgus load while the other stabilizes the arm against the examining table and palpates the medial epicondyle, ulnar collateral ligament, ulnar groove, flexor-pronator origin, and the medial ulnohumeral joint. Valgus instability testing can be fairly subtle; complete anterior bundle sectioning may only increase valgus rotation by 3°.[14] Stability should be tested throughout the entire arc of motion, assessing for crepitance of the medial ulnohumeral and radiocapitellar joints as the olecranon seats into the olecranon fossa. Not all patients with posterior elbow pain have posterior impingement; for example, posterior pain can be caused by triceps tendinitis or olecranon stress fractures.[15]

Routinely, we obtain anteroposterior (AP) and lateral radiographs of the elbow; oblique and stress views are occasionally added to further assess the elbow. Loose bodies, medial epicondylar avulsion fractures, traction osteophytes of the medial semilunar notch, bony hypertrophy between the olecranon and coranoid fossae, coranoid and olecranon osteophytes are all common. Normal radiographs do not preclude symptomatic pathoanatomy, such as loose bodies and chrondral lesions. In fact, radiographs routinely underestimate the presence or numbers of loose bodies.[16,17] Computed tomography (CT) scans and magnetic resonance imaging (MRI) are occasionally helpful to further refine clinical diagnoses however, they are rarely indicated for osteoarthritic or degenerative conditions.[18]

Nonsurgical Management

The goal of treatment is the restoration of comfort and function. Patient education and nonsurgical treatment for posterior elbow impingement varies according to the primary etiology of the posterior elbow impingement and the functional requirements of the patient. The rehabilitation process for patients who have osteoarthritis as the primary etiology of posterior impingement is a gentle stretching and strengthening program. The gentle stretching program is designed to make modest gains. Patients and therapists are advised that aggressive stretching exacerbates symptoms and usually does not achieve any significant gains in motion or comfort. In general, to increase comfort after an acute injury, we recommend relative rest, cryotherapy, and, in some instances, a short term of nonsteroidal anti-inflammatory medications (NSAIDs).

After an acute injury, rest for a short period of time, to allow bleeding and swelling to subside, is beneficial. Gentle range of motion and stretching exercises, within mild pain limits are begun early. Cryotherapy diminishes pain[19] and may reduce bleeding and swelling[20] after an acute injury. The duration of ice application is limited by its potential harmful effects, such as thermal injury to subcutaneous nerves or rebound hyperemia after the cooling elements are removed.[21] NSAIDs seem to help diminish pain, but may not have a protective effect after injury.[22] We use NSAIDs for a limited time, carefully weighing their benefits against possible drug interactions and systemic side effects.

For overhand athletes, our nonsurgical and secondary postoperative rehabilitative program has evolved from the work of Wilson and associates[23] and Glousman and associates.[24] After an initial period of rest, with flexor and extensor muscle stretching, the athlete begins strengthening with low weight, high repetition isotonic exercises to build increase endurance. Isometric and isokinetic programs with gripping exercises are instituted to further increase conditioning and strengthening, advancing into plyometrics. Plyometric exercises induce a rapid transition from initial eccentric muscle contraction to concentric muscle contraction. In theory, muscle reeducation is enhanced as stretch reflexes cause the muscles to fire without conscious thought. Timing, proprioception, and muscle strength are improved. As rehabilitation continues, the rotator cuff and periscapular musculature are strengthened. As strength improves, the athlete returns to throwing using an interval throwing program.[25]

If nonsurgical therapy fails to restore comfort and function, surgical intervention is offered. The following arthroscopic surgical technique is a general approach to patients with limited motion and mechanical impingement associated with soft-tissue and bony lesions.

Surgical Technique

In all patients with a primary diagnosis of posterior elbow impingement, anterior compartment arthroscopy is performed as part of a complete arthroscopic exam. The patient is placed prone and the elbow is positioned as described by Poehling and associates.[26] Landmarks, including the medial and lateral epicondyles, olecranon tip, radiocapitellar joint and ulnar nerve, are outlined with a surgical marker. Preoperatively, we palpate the ulnar nerve to assess its stability within the cubital tunnel. We distend the elbow by injecting the joint with lactated ringers through the direct lateral (soft spot)[27] or posterocentral portal. If stiffness is significant, the average volume capacity and capsular compliance may be reduced, diminishing displacement of neurovascular structures.[28] During initial anterior portal placement, the elbow is flexed at 90° to maximize the displacement of neurovascular structures from the joint capsule. A proximal anteromedial portal is used for diagnostic evaluation of the anterior compartment (Fig. 3). Testing for varus and valgus instability is part of the initial assessment. The intra-articular pathology determines the placement of the lateral portal and the need for a transradiocapitellar inflow via the posterior soft spot.

To develop a proximal anterolateral portal an outside-in technique is the preferred method. This portal, which is placed just superior to the capitellum, is used for synovectomy, radiocapitellar joint debridement, coronoid osteophyte excision, and deepening the coronoid fossa. Viewing from the lateral portal, the proximal anteromedial portal is used as a surgical portal to excise trochlea spurs to complete the debridement. If indicated, radial head excision and/or anterior capsular release may be performed.

After anterior compartment arthroscopic surgery, the posterior compartment is evaluated using posterolateral and posterocentral portals. Inflow can be from a previous anterior portal, a posterior portal, or the viewing cannula. While viewing through the posterolateral portal, a full radius shaver is inserted through the posterocentral portal. The intervening adhesions and redundant posterior superior capsular scarring are debrided with the shaver from the posterior superior portion of the elbow and between the posterior humerus and triceps muscle. While an assistant flexes the elbow, the tip of the olecranon can be removed with mediolateral sweeps of a burr (Fig. 4). Care should be taken to avoid injury to the triceps insertion.

The medial and lateral gutters are evaluated next. The arthroscope is placed in the posterocentral portal and the shaver in the posterolateral portal. Excision of the adhesions in the lateral gutter is initiated proximally and continues distally. Occasionally, a straight lateral portal is needed to adequately debride the posterior radiocapitellar and radioulnar joints as well as a posterolateral plica, if present. The medial gutter is approached with the arthroscope in the posterolateral portal and operating from the posterocentral portal. A fully hooded shaver is used to protect the ulnar nerve during debridement. Extreme caution should be exercised, as the ulnar nerve is in close proximity normally.[29] Also, it can be displaced by scarring.

The olecranon fossa, which is frequently narrowed by bony hypertrophy, loose bodies, and scar tissue, is debrided using a combination of a shaver and burr. An ulnohumeral arthroplasty (fenestration) is initiated. A full-thickness pilot hole is made into the center of the olecranon fossa to the coranoid fossa with a 5-mm drill through the posterocentral portal, and viewing is done through the posterolateral portal. The initial pilot hole is enlarged with a burr through the posterocentral portal taking care to maintain the integrity of the medial and lateral humeral columns (Fig. 5). Adequate clearance of the coranoid and olecranon should be ensured.

In athletes who throw, increased bony clearance after posterior debridement can theoretically increase ulnohumeral opening, leading to valgus stress. According to Field and Altcheck,[12] medial ulnohumeral opening of 1 to 2 cm suggests complete anterior bundle insufficiency, whereas opening greater then 4-mm suggests complete medial collateral ligament insufficiency. In overhand athletes, we perform an arthroscopic valgus stress test after bony posterior debridement. We also specifically assess the trochlear notch in overhand athletes with posterolateral symptoms.[13]

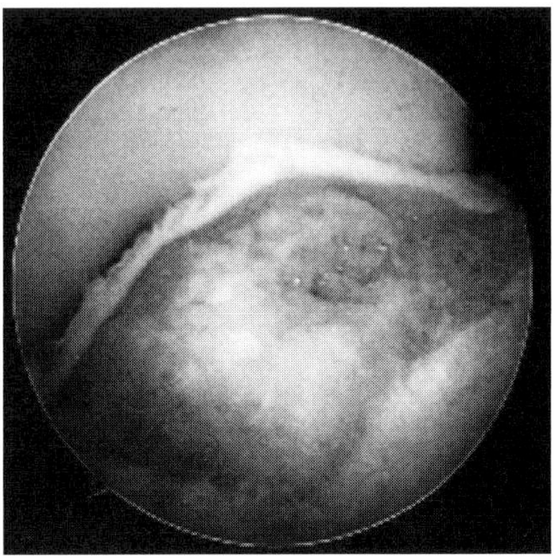

Fig. 4 Arthroscopic view of the olecranon after spur excision.

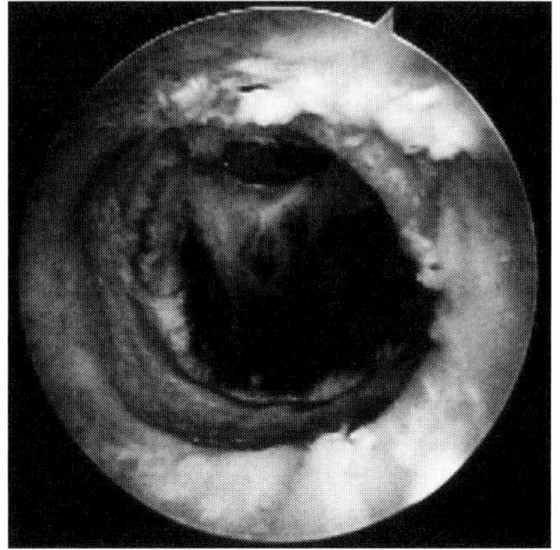

Fig. 5 Arthroscopic view of the olecranon fossa after fenestration for posterior impingement.

Postoperative Rehabilitation

Drains may be placed in the proximal anteromedial and the posterocentral or posterolateral portals. The straight lateral portal should be routinely sutured closed, because of the lack of soft-tissue layers between the skin and joint capsule. The other portals are left open. After application of sterile dressings, the elbow is splinted in extension and supination. Early motion is instituted, with or without continuous passive motion (CPM). Patients are monitored in the hospital for 1 to 3 days, depending on the extent of surgery and the severity of disease.

Specific therapy depends on the etiology of posterior impingement, functional requirements of the patient and secondary procedures performed. Static splinting or CPM is used at night usually for at least 3 weeks after surgery if motion gain is a significant postoperative goal. Organized therapy sessions may or may not be needed, and, again, these depend on the patient's progress and particular problem. Overhead throwers are started on a return-to-throw program that is similar to the secondary therapy described in the nonsurgical treatment section.

Results

Ogilvie-Harris and associates[30] reviewed 21 patients at an average of 35 months after arthroscopic surgery for posterior impingement due to degenerative arthritis. Anterior debridement and loose body removal was performed first, followed by posterior surgery, which consisted of removal of posterior loose bodies, removal of olecranon osteophytes, and debridement of the olecranon fossa to the point of fenestration. Significant reduction in pain, with increases in motion, strength and function, were noted. Results from arthroscopic surgery for osteoarthritis are generally good.[7,8] However, loose body removal alone does not typically improve patient's results; osteophyte excision is as important as loose body removal.[16,31]

In high-demand overhand athletes with posterior elbow impingement, reoperation rates may be high.[1] This high reoperation rate may be caused by the frequent high loads placed across the elbow, inadequate initial debridement, osteophyte reformation, unrecognized ulnar collateral insufficiency, and/or unrelated ligamentous attenuation postoperatively.

The senior author has reviewed his results of 53 arthroscopic debridements for arthrofibrosis of the elbow in 53 patients. On average, extension increased 41° (preoperative flexion contractures were reduced from 46° to 5° postoperatively) and flexion increased from 96° to 138°. Pronation increased on average 7° (75° to 82°) and supination increased 39° (47° to 86°). However, 1 patient ultimately underwent a successful elbow arthroplasty and 2 patients required a repeat arthroscopic debridement and release to maintain motion.

Conclusion

In properly selected patients, an arthroscopic approach to posterior impingement allows the surgeon to address both anterior and posterior intra-articular pathology. Arthroscopic evaluation and treatment of elbow pathology is particularly valuable because it increases visualization and diminishes soft-tissue trauma. Arthroscopic treatment of arthritic elbows is technically demanding. General techniques, as well as the sequence of procedures, should be dictated by pathology encountered during surgery and should not follow a rigid preoperative plan. Conversion to an open procedure does not represent failure.

References

1. Andrews JR, Timmerman LA: Outcome of elbow surgery in professional baseball players. *Am J Sports Med* 1995;23:407–413.
2. Timmerman LA, Andrews JR: Histology and arthroscopic anatomy of the ulnar collateral ligament of the elbow. *Am J Sports Med* 1994;22: 667–673.
3. Timmerman LA, Andrews JR: Undersurface tears of the ulnar collateral ligament in baseball players: A newly recognized lesion. *Am J Sports Med* 1994;22:33–36.
4. King J, Brelsford HJ, Tullos HS: Analysis of the pitching arm of the professional baseball pitcher. *Clin Orthop* 1969;67:116–123.
5. Jobe FW, Stark H, Lombardo SJ: Reconstruction of the ulnar collateral ligament in athletes. *J Bone Joint Surg* 1986;68A:1158–1163.
6. Morrey BF: Primary degenerative arthritis of the elbow: Treatment by ulnohumeral arthroplasty. *J Bone Joint Surg* 1992;74A:410–413.
7. Ward WG, Anderson TE: Elbow arthroscopy in a mostly athletic population. *J Hand Surg* 1993;18A:220–224.
8. Redden JF, Stanley D: Arthroscopic fenestration of the olecranon fossa in the treatment of osteoarthritis of the elbow. *Arthroscopy* 1993;9: 14–16.
9. Clarke RP: Symptomatic, lateral synovial fringe (plica) of the elbow joint. *Arthroscopy* 1988;4: 112–116.
10. DeHaven KE, Evarts CM: Throwing injuries of the elbow in athletes. *Orthop Clin North Am* 1973;4:801–808.
11. Morrey BF, Tanaka S, An KN: Valgus stability of the elbow: A definition of primary and secondary constraints. *Clin Orthop* 1991;265: 187–195.
12. Field LD, Altchek DW: Evaluation of the arthroscopic valgus instability test of the elbow. *Am J Sports Med* 1996;24:177–181.
13. Robla J, Hechtman KS, Uribe JW, Phillipon MS: Chondromalacia of the trochlear notch in athletes who throw. *J Shoulder Elbow Surg* 1996;5:69–72.
14. Callaway GH, Field LD, Deng XH, et al: Biomechanical evaluation of the medial collateral ligament of the elbow. *J Bone Joint Surg* 1997;79A:1223–1231.
15. Nuber GW, Diment MT: Olecranon stress fractures in throwers: A report of two cases and a review of the literature. *Clin Orthop* 1992; 278:58–61.
16. Ogilvie-Harris DJ, Schemitsch E: Arthroscopy of the elbow for removal of loose bodies. *Arthroscopy* 1993;9:5–8.
17. Ward WG, Belhobek GH, Anderson TE: Arthroscopic elbow findings: Correlation with preoperative radiographic studies. *Arthroscopy* 1992;8:498–502.
18. Ward WG, Anderson TE: Elbow arthroscopy in a mostly athletic population. *J Hand Surg* 1993;18:220–224.
19. Speer KP, Warren RF, Horowitz L: The efficacy of cryotherapy in the postoperative shoulder. *J Shoulder Elbow Surg* 1996;5:62–68.
20. Ho SS, Coel MN, Kagawa R, Richardson AB: The effects of ice on blood flow and bone metabolism in knees. *Am J Sports Med* 1994; 22:537–540.
21. Matsen FA III, Questad K, Matsen AL: The effect of local cooling on postfracture swelling: A controlled study. *Clin Orthop* 1975;109: 201–206.
22. Mishra DK, Friden J, Schmitz MC, Lieber RL: Anti-inflammatory medication after muscle injury: A treatment resulting in short-term improvement but subsequent loss of muscle function. *J Bone Joint Surg* 1995;77A:1510–1519.
23. Wilson FD, Andrews JR, Blackburn TA, McCluskey G: Valgus extension overload in the pitching elbow. *Am J Sports Med* 1983;11:83–88.
24. Glousman RE, Barron J, Jobe FW, Perry J, Pink M: An electromyographic analysis of the elbow in normal and injured pitchers with medial collateral ligament insufficiency. *Am J Sports Med* 1992;20:311–317.
25. Wilk KE, Arrigo C, Andrews JR: Rehabilitation of the elbow in the throwing athlete. *J Orthop Sports Phys Ther* 1993;17:305–317.
26. Poehling GG, Whipple TL, Sisco L, Goldman B: Elbow arthroscopy: A new technique. *Arthroscopy* 1989;5:222–224.
27. Morrey BF: Arthroscopy of the elbow, in Anderson LD (ed): American Academy of Orthopaedic Surgeons *Instructional Course Lectures XXXV*. St. Louis, MO, CV Mosby, 1986, pp 102–107.
28. Gallay SH, Richards RR, O'Driscoll SW: Intraarticular capacity and compliance of stiff and normal elbows. *Arthroscopy* 1993;9:9–13.
29. Marshall PD, Fairclough JA, Johnson SR, Evans EJ: Avoiding nerve damage during elbow arthroscopy. *J Bone Joint Surg* 1993;75B:29–131.
30. Ogilvie-Harris DJ, Gordon R, MacKay M: Arthroscopic treatment for posterior impingement in degenerative arthritis of the elbow. *Arthroscopy* 1995;11:437–443.
31. O'Driscoll SW: Elbow arthroscopy for loose bodies. *Orthopedics* 1992;15:855–859.

Osteochondritis Dissecans of the Elbow

Melissa A. Yadao, MD
Larry D. Field, MD
Felix H. Savoie III, MD

Abstract

Osteochondritis dissecans of the elbow is a localized condition of the articular surface that is commonly seen in the young athlete. This disorder refers primarily to lesions of the capitellum and can be difficult to treat. Although trauma and ischemia play significant roles, the exact etiology remains unknown. The natural history is poorly understood and long-term sequelae include degenerative arthritis. The integrity of the articular surface and the stability of the lesion can be carefully evaluated with MRI and arthroscopy. Management is based mainly upon these two factors, yet no good universal outcomes exist among the varied treatment options. Stable lesions identified early appear to have the best prognosis with conservative management. Indications for surgery include persistent or worsening symptoms despite prolonged conservative care, loose bodies, or evidence of instability. Whether to excise and débride or to fix an unstable fragment is a highly controversial topic. The clinician should recognize osteochondritis dissecans of the elbow as a potentially disabling condition where the prognosis for return to sport is guarded.

Osteochondritis dissecans of the elbow is a disorder commonly seen in the young athlete and can be a difficult condition to treat. It is a localized condition involving the articular surface, resulting in the separation of a segment of articular cartilage and subchondral bone. In addition to the elbow, this lesion is primarily found in the knee and ankle joints.[1] The etiology remains unclear, the clinical presentation can be vague, and the natural history is poorly understood. Moreover, management of these lesions often fails to achieve desired results.

The term osteochondritis dissecans was first used to describe the presence of loose bodies in knees in the absence of trauma. It was theorized that an inflammatory reaction of both bone and cartilage, followed by spontaneous necrosis, led to the separation of the articular surface and the formation of loose bodies. However, inflammatory cells were notably absent on later histopathologic studies and now most would agree that both trauma and ischemia play significant roles.[1-4]

The most common site of osteochondritis dissecans of the elbow is the capitellum. Lesions have been reported in the trochlea and radial head, as well as the olecranon and olecranon fossa.[5] Unfortunately, this condition has often been confused in the literature with other disorders affecting the immature elbow such as osteonecrosis, osteochondrosis, Panner's disease, little leaguer's elbow, osteochondral fracture or fragment, and hereditary epiphyseal dysplasia.[4-7]

Osteochondritis dissecans should be distinguished from Panner's disease, which is another disorder of the capitellum in the young patient. Panner's disease, also known as osteochondrosis of the capitellum, is focal osteonecrosis of the entire capitellum seen primarily in boys ages 7 to 12 years, peak age 9 years. Similar to Legg-Calvé-Perthes disease of the hip, this is a self-limited disease that is not associated with trauma.[8] Nonsurgical management is the mainstay of treatment with minimal morbidity.[9]

Osteochondritis dissecans, on the other hand, occurs in an older age group, generally athletes ages 11 to 21 years who report a history of overuse.[1,4] The osteonecrotic lesion involves only a segment of capitellum, located primarily at a central or anterolateral position.[2,10] Although MRI and arthroscopy have greatly improved the clinician's ability to evaluate osteochondritis dissecans, appropriate treatment of this disorder remains controversial. Often treated with benign neglect, this condition is a potentially sport-ending injury for an athlete, with long-term sequelae of degenerative arthritis.[10,11]

Etiology

The exact etiology of osteochondritis dissecans is unknown. Sporadic reports of osteochondritis dissecans in generations of families suggest genetic predisposition yet no convincing evidence exists.[12] Cases of bilateral involvement or in multiple locations have been reported as well.[4,13] In fact, this condition was once thought to be associated with multiple epiphyseal dysplasia, a rare inheritable disorder.[12] Beyond superficial similarities, these two disorders are very different.

Trauma

The prevalence of osteochondritis dissecans among male throwing athletes and female gymnasts lends credence to the roles of microtrauma and overuse. In these sports the elbow is subjected to compressive and/or shearing forces across the radiocapitellar joint.[1,4,10,12-17] Its prevalence among baseball pitchers has been closely examined. In pitchers, the valgus stresses during the early and late cocking phase of throwing significantly load the radiocapitellar joint in compression.[14,16,18,19] The exact mechanism in gymnasts is uncertain but it is believed that injuries occur with the arm extended.[4,13,20]

Biomechanically, the radiocapitellar joint acts as a secondary stabilizer of the elbow. Studies have shown that up to 60% of axial compression forces across the elbow are transmitted to the radiocapitellar joint.[21] Schenck and associates[22] have demonstrated mechanical differences between radial head and capitellar articular cartilage. The greater stiffness of the central radial head compared with the lateral capitellum could explain why the capitellum is a common site of osteochondritis dissecans and may contribute to the formation of this disorder.

Microtrauma and overuse can ultimately cause fatigue fracture of the subchondral bone of the capitellum. During the repair process, the healing subchondral bone is especially vulnerable.[23] Under continued shearing or compressive loads, the subchondral bone can no longer support the overlying articular surface, leading to breakdown and fragmentation of the involved segment of articular cartilage and subchondral bone. Failure of osseous repair results in bony resorption and separation, with the creation of loose bodies.[1,4,7,23]

Ischemia

A tenuous vascular supply to the distal humerus and capitellum support the belief that ischemia is a causative factor. Haraldsson[24] has shown that only one or two isolated vessels feed the capitellar epiphysis, entering posterior and traversing the compressible epiphyseal cartilage of the capitellum. No metaphyseal collateral flow exists. As in the hip and talus, injury such as repetitive compressive loading can set the stage for osteonecrosis.

Indeed, osteonecrosis of the subchondral bone is seen in the histopathology of osteochondritis dissecans. The earliest bony changes seen are hyperemia and edema while initially the articular surface remains intact and viable. At the interface between the necrotic subarticular segment and healthy bone, vascular granulation tissue absorbs the necrotic bone. Such reparative changes can be seen on plain radiographs as rarefaction at the periphery of the lesion.[7,23]

Following this stage, one of two events can occur. If the articular cartilage remains intact and the necrotic bone in situ, the necrotic bone will be absorbed and replaced by viable osseous tissue. As a result, the normal architecture of the capitellum is preserved. However, if the articular cartilage is disrupted, the necrotic segment can separate and form loose bodies. It is believed that the healing process, not the initial injury, is the pivotal stage of this disorder.[23]

Clinical Presentation

Osteochondritis dissecans is primarily a disorder of the young athlete and rarely occurs in adults. The typical patient is between the ages of 11 and 21 years (mean, 12 to 14 years).[1,4,9] Males are affected more often but this disorder is prevalent among female gymnasts. The dominant arm is almost always involved and bilateral involvement has been reported in 5% to 20% of patients.[12] A history of overuse is often described with common sport activities such as baseball, gymnastics, weightlifting, racquet sports, and cheerleading.[7]

Pain, the most common complaint, is usually insidious and progressive in nature and is associated with activities and relieved by rest. A patient may wait months before seeking medical attention. Pain is often localized over the lateral aspect of the elbow, but it may also be poorly defined.[12] Pain at night or at rest is usually indicative of other pathologic processes.[4]

Tenderness can be palpated laterally over the radiocapitellar joint. Range of motion is limited, particularly extension. It is not uncommon to see flexion contractures of 5° to 23°.[4,15,26-28] Loss of flexion is less likely while supination and pronation are rarely altered. Clicking, catching, grinding, or locking suggest fragment instability or loose bodies. Crepitus and swelling may be present as well.[1,4,7,12] Provocative tests such as the active radiocapitellar compression test may help confirm the diagnosis.[25] As the patient actively pronates and supinates the forearm with the elbow in full extension, dynamic muscle forces compress the radiocapitellar joint and reproduce the symptoms.

It is important to perform a thorough upper extremity examination to rule out other pathology. Osteochondritis dissecans is similar to other disorders affecting the immature elbow. Moreover, the throwing athlete can develop a variety of elbow injuries, which are loosely grouped together as the little leaguer's elbow. The excessive valgus forces during the cocking phase of throwing, which compress the lateral side, place tension on the medial aspect of the elbow. Injuries of the medial epicondyle and radial head, as well as injuries of the medial and lateral collateral ligaments are well documented.[4,18,19]

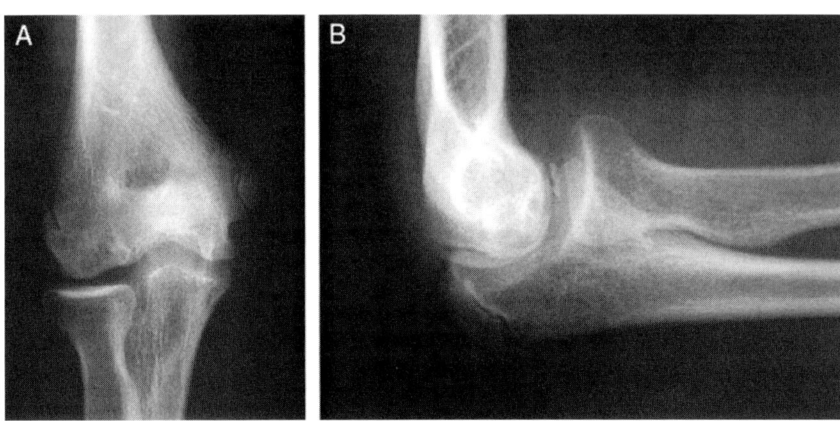

Figure 1 A, AP and **B,** lateral radiographs demonstrating radiolucency and rarefaction typical of osteochondritis dissecans of the elbow.

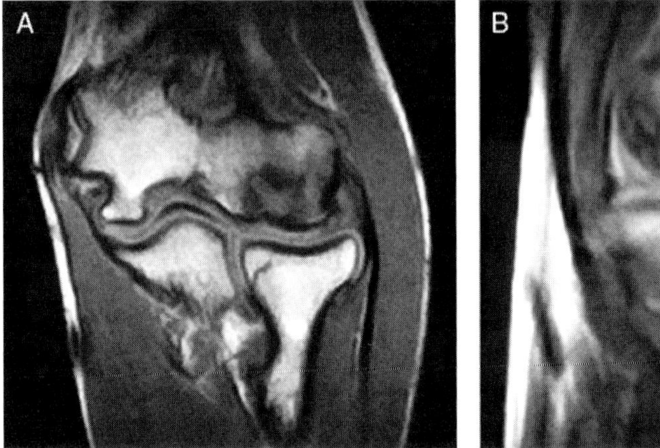

Figure 2 A, Coronal and **B,** sagittal MRI of the same lesion shown in Figure 1. Increased signal of the T2 image indicates disruption of the articular surface.

Diagnostic Evaluation

Radiology

Radiographs are the initial diagnostic test of choice. Standard AP and lateral views of the elbow will usually show the classic findings of radiolucency and rarefaction of the capitellum with flattening or irregularity of the articular surface. A rim of sclerotic bone often surrounds the radiolucent crater, which is typically located in the central or anterolateral aspect of the capitellum (Figure 1). Loose bodies may be present if the necrotic segment becomes detached. Supplemental views such as a 45° flexion AP or obliques may be helpful.[4,6,23]

Additional studies may be needed to further evaluate osteochondritis dissecans. CT is useful in determining the extent of the osseous lesion as well as presence and location of loose bodies. CT arthrography more accurately defines the integrity of the articular surface.[29] Ultrasound can reveal flattening and irregularity of the capitellum in early stages. However, this study is technician- and radiologist-dependent and its overall use limited.[23]

MRI has become the standard modality for additional evaluation.[4,23] Not only can MRI assess the articular surface, but it can also define both size and extent of the lesion (Figure 2). Early, stable lesions show changes on T1-weighted images, but T2-weighted images remain normal. On the other hand, advanced lesions show changes on both T1- and T2-weighted images.[4,30] Loose in situ lesions have a cyst under the lesion. Magnetic resonance arthrography can improve the diagnosis with leakage of dye beneath the disrupted cartilage.[23,30]

Recently, intravenous gadopentatedimeglumine has been advocated to evaluate the viability of the osteochondral fragment.[30,31] A diffuse lesion is highly suggestive of loosening and instability. Currently, determining if the fragment is viable has limited potential as long as controversy exists whether to fix or excise the fragment.

Progress and healing can be assessed via plain radiographs. If the fragment remains stable, the central sclerotic fragment gradually becomes less distinct and the surrounding area of radiolucency slowly ossifies. New bone formation can be seen as a relatively radiolucent bone fragment appearing over a flattened, sclerotic area of bone of the capitellum.[23] This healing process, however, may take several years.[12] A nonhealing lesion in a patient who remains symptomatic despite conservative treatment should prompt continued evaluation.[4,10]

An unstable fragment that detaches can transform into loose bodies and lead to degenerative changes. Medial osteophytes are sometimes present as well as irregularity of the capitellum and radial head. Compensatory changes, including radial head enlargement and premature closure of the proximal radial physis, can occur.[7,11]

Arthroscopy

Arthroscopy is gaining popularity as a diagnostic tool to evaluate the integrity of the articular surface. The lesion can be seen and palpated to determine if the articular surface is disrupted or the segment unstable. Associated pathology such as degenerative changes, radial head involvement, and instability can be evaluated as well.[5,27,28]

Classification

Several investigators have attempted to classify osteochondritic lesions of the capitellum. Minami and associates[32] first categorized lesions into three grades according to the anterior-posterior view of the elbow. Grade I lesions demonstrated a translucent cystic shadow in the lateral or middle capitellum. Grade II lesions showed a clear zone or split line between the lesion and the adjacent subchondral bone. The presence of loose bodies defined grade III lesions.

Bradley and Petrie[4] have modified Minami and associates' classification. Grade I lesions are separated into two groups based on radiographic and MRI findings. In type IA lesions, radiographs are normal and MRI demonstrates low signal on T1-weighted images and normal T2-weighted images. These findings are consistent with early osteochondritis dissecans lesions. Type IB lesions demonstrate classic radiographic findings of capitellar rarefaction, flattening, or sclerosis. MRI findings show increased signal on both T1- and T2-weighted images. Type IA lesions are believed to respond very well with conservative treatment whereas type IB lesions have less predictable outcomes. Another group, grade IV lesions, show evidence of radial head changes. Currently MRI cannot reliably identify these "bipolar" lesions and treatment options are controversial.[4]

Baumgarten and associates[27] devised an arthroscopic classification based on Ferkel and Chang's classification for osteochondritis dissecans of the talus. A grade I lesion has smooth but soft, ballottable articular cartilage. Fibrillations and fissuring of the articular cartilage are found in a grade 2 lesion. A grade 3 lesion shows exposed bone with a fixed osteochondral fragment. The fragment is loose but nondisplaced in a grade 4 lesion. However, in a grade 5 lesion, this unstable fragment is displaced with loose bodies present.[27]

To date, studies have not shown strong correlations between clinical presentation, classification, treatment, and outcome.[4,10,11,33]

Treatment

Treatment of osteochondritis dissecans is controversial, with options varying from nonsurgical measures to fragment excision to fixation of the fragment. Management decisions are based primarily on the integrity of the articular cartilage and status of the involved segment, whether it is stable, unstable but attached, or detached and loose.

Stable lesions with intact cartilage and in situ subchondral fragments are managed conservatively.[4,12,23] Sports and other aggravating activities are stopped for approximately 3 to 6 weeks until symptoms subside. The elbow can be protected in a hinged elbow brace without restriction. The brace can be locked for a short period should pain warrant temporary immobilization. Therapy begins after symptoms have abated and gradually incorporates stretching, strengthening, and plyometric training exercises. The athlete can usually return to unrestricted sports activity 3 to 6 months after treatment is begun.[7] Radiographs are not used to determine return to play because healing and other changes may take years to show up on radiographs.[12] Patients with intact lesions identified early and treated conservatively have the best prognosis. However, the clinician should inform the family of possible long-term sequelae.[10-13,20,23,26]

Surgical indications include persistent or worsening symptoms despite prolonged conservative care, loose bodies, or evidence of instability including violation of intact cartilage or detachment.[3-5,12] The only universally accepted regimen is the removal of loose bodies.[3-5,10-14,17,23,25-28,34] Otherwise, debate continues over two types of surgical management. One method is to excise the unstable fragment with or without subchondral drilling or abrasion chondroplasty.[3-5,7,10-15,20,23,27-28,33,34] The other method is attempted fixation of the segment with or without bone graft.[35-40]

Most clinicians surgically manage osteochondritic lesions with excision and some type of débridement. Following removal of any unstable fragments or loose bodies, the subchondral bone can be drilled or picked via microfracture technique to promote vascularization and healing.[4,12,17,26,34] Although much of the literature has focused on open procedures, arthroscopy has gained increasing popularity and the technique is well described.[5,27,28,33] Establishing the lateral portal is crucial for optimal visualization of and access to the lesion. Both the anterior and posterior compartments are carefully inspected for loose bodies and osteophytes. Various devices such as shavers, burrs, punches, and graspers are used to remove unstable or loose fragments (Figure 3).

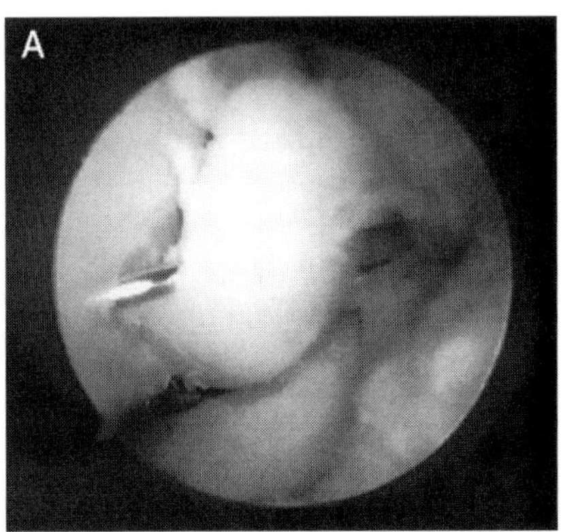

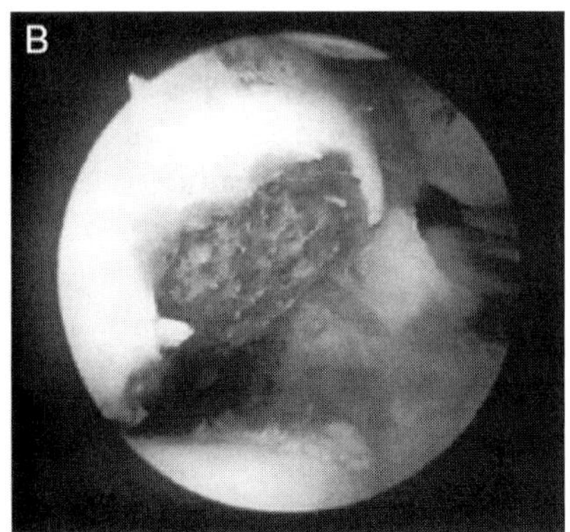

Figure 3 Arthroscopic management of a detached osteochondritic lesion of the capitellum viewed from the anteromedial portal. **A,** The loose fragment is temporarily stabilized with a spinal needle before being excised with a grasper from the anterolateral portal. **B,** The subchondral base after excision of the fragment and débridement with a shaver.

Fixation of the fragment remains controversial. Several techniques have been described, including Herbert screw fixation,[36] dynamic stapling,[37] Kirschner wires,[20] cancellous screws,[4] and bioabsorbable implants. Prior to reattachment, the débrided bone can be grafted to encourage healing. Other procedures include wedge osteotomies to unload the injured capitellar segment.[38,40] There is some concern about risking further injury to the articular surface or growth plate with fixation implants.[4] Although several studies have shown favorable results following reattachment of the fragment, none have clearly demonstrated marked improvement over excision and débridement alone.

Recent case reports describe techniques of cartilage repair and grafting used for other joints. Osteochondral grafting using rib has recently been reported.[39] Nakagawa and associates[40] studied a 13-year-old boy who played baseball who underwent a two-stage procedure for significant arthritis and limited motion from osteochondritis dissecans. The initial procedure comprised a wedge osteotomy and osteochondral grafting. The grafts appeared healed at the time of open débridement arthroplasty 10 months later. At 35 months follow-up, he had no elbow pain and no restrictions of daily living. Other future treatment techniques include periosteal grafting, perichondral grafting, and articular cartilage allograft transplant.[4,7,39,40]

Results

Clinical outcome studies reflect the general opinion that loose bodies should be excised. Long-term results suggest persistent limitation of activities.[10,11,17,26] However, the majority of the studies published are based on older diagnostic modalities, with surgical management using primarily open techniques. Outcomes following arthroscopy are promising but longer follow-up is needed.

Nonsurgical Management

Conservative treatment has shown favorable results when the lesion is detected early. Of three youth baseball players found to have osteochondritis dissecans via screening with MRI and ultrasound, the two players who temporarily stopped sports activity showed both clinical and radiographic resolution of the lesion. Both athletes returned to sports activity without problems, while the third player, who continued to pitch against medical advice, developed characteristic osteochondritis dissecans.[23]

Other studies with mixed results after nonsurgical treatment reflect the difficulty in identifying those lesions that may respond poorly to treatment. Takahara and associates[41] have reported on 24 patients (out of 91) treated conservatively for 6 months with average follow-up of 5.2 years. Patients were grouped according to initial radiographs: 17 had early lesions and 7 had advanced lesions. More than half of the patients continued to have pain with daily activities (53% with early lesions and 57% with advanced lesions). Although radiographic findings of little healing or improvement correlated with subjective poor results, the authors concluded that instability was hard to predict by radiographs alone.

In reviewing 66 elbows with an average follow-up of 13.6 years, Mitsunaga and associates[17] found that, of those patients treated nonsurgically, less than half of attached, stable lesions became detached and unstable. These patients did poorly with conservative measures and the authors recommended excision of loose lesions and drilling or curetting of subchondral bone.

Fragment Excision and Débridement

Currently in the literature the longest follow-up is an average 23 years (range, 11 to 35 years) on 31 patients.[11] In Bauer and associates' study, treatment consisted of fragment excision, loose body removal, and débridement with no attempt at reattachment. Forty percent of the patients continued to have pain on exertion and limited motion. Radiographic findings of degenerative joint disease, seen in 60% of patients, strongly correlated with persistent restricted motion. Additional procedures were not advocated.

Similarly, Woodward and Bianco[26] recommended the excision of loose bodies without drilling or reattachment in their outcome study on 42 male patients. With a mean follow-up of 12 years (range, 2 to 34 years), the overall prognosis was good. However, full motion could not be restored, with limitation of extension a common sequelae.

Arthroscopic excision with some form of débridement has shown favorable short-term results. Baumgarten and associates[27] reviewed 16 patients with average follow-up of 4 years (range, 2 to 6.2 years). Treatment varied according to the type of lesion: symptomatic stable lesions were drilled or débrided, unstable lesions underwent excision and abrasion chondroplasty, and loose bodies were excised. No attempts were made to reattach fragments. Range of motion improved, no patients developed degenerative arthritis, and 11 patients were able to return to sports activities. The authors advocated obtaining uniform bleeding at the lesion site.

Ruch and associates[28] reviewed results in 12 patients who underwent arthroscopic management for a mean follow-up period of 3.2 years. Partially or completely detached fragments were excised without any drilling or fixation. Eleven patients were satisfied but only three returned to competitive sports. Those patients whose radiographs showed a lateral capsule fragment had a significantly worse subjective outcome. Byrd and Jones[33] also noted poor prognosis with extension of the lesion to the lateral capitellum. Although Ruch and associates thought the lateral fragment was caused by avulsion injury, Byrd and Jones attributed this to the valgus loading forces.

Fixation

Most studies published in the literature about fixation of osteochondritic lesions have focused on baseball players. Kuwahata and Inoue[35] reported on six patients who underwent in situ stabilization of nondisplaced lesions with a minimum 12-month follow-up period. Having responded poorly to conservative management, all six patients underwent débridement, cancellous bone grafting, and fixation of the fragment with Herbert screws. All patients returned to sports activities by 1 year. Radiographic studies showed reossification of capitellar cyst and normal joint contouring.

Recently Takeda and associates[38] have described an open technique of bone grafting and pull-out wire fixation with favorable results in 11 male baseball players with an average follow-up of 57 months (range, 31 to 75 months). These patients failed 6 months of conservative treatment or had unstable lesions based on MRI or at the time of surgery. The fragment was reattached with a soft wire tied over a button on the nonarticular side to minimize injury to the articular surface. Nine patients had an excellent result, with all patients returning to their previous level of throwing ability at 7 to 14 months. Radiographs showed healing and minimal arthritis on all patients.

Prognostic Factors

Very few factors have been suggested as predictors of good or poor outcome. Although Pappas[9] suggested that younger patients had a better outcome, both Takahara and associates[10] and Ruch and associates[28] found no correlation with age. Several reports show advanced lesions with findings of degenerative arthritis tended to fare worse.[11,14,26] However, 32% of early lesions in another study did poorly.[41] In Takahara and associates' review of 53 patients with an average follow-up of 12.6 years, surgical findings of large chondral defects had poor subjective outcome: all large lesions, one third of moderate lesions, and no small lesions continued to be symptomatic.[10]

Return to Sports Activity

Although pain is usually diminished and range of motion improved, the ability to return to a competitive level of sports is difficult to predict. In Takahara's study, none of the patients treated conservatively and only half of the patients treated surgically were able to return to sports activity at the preinjury level.[10] Only one of seven elite gymnasts in the study by Jackson and associates[20] could return to competition. While only 4 of 10 baseball players in Baumgarten's study returned to organized baseball,[27] McManama and associates[15] reported 12 of 14 players competed at their previous level. All of the patients in Takeda and associates'[38] study returned to baseball, although one pitcher had to switch positions after 2 years.

Summary

The clinician should be suspicious osteochondritis dissecans in the young athlete with elbow pain. Early detection is one of the best weapons against unfavorable outcomes. Although MRI and arthroscopy have improved the ability to evaluate and manage this disorder, the question remains as to what to do with the acute in situ or partially detached fragment. At present most investigators advocate excising loose bodies or unstable lesions and drilling or abrading the underlying subchondral bone. Technical advances including osteochondral grafting and cartilage replacement may improve the outcome of this potentially disabling disorder, where currently half the patients continue to have pain and the prognosis for returning to competition is guarded.

References

1. Schenck RC Jr, Goodnight JM: Osteochondritis dissecans. *J Bone Joint Surg Am* 1996;78:439-456.
2. König F: Ueber freie Körper in den Gelenken. *Deutsche Zeitschr Chir* 1887;27:90-109.
3. Nagura S: The so-called osteochondritis dissecans of König. *Clin Orthop* 1960;18:100-122.
4. Bradley JP, Petrie RS: Osteochondritis dissecans of the humeral capitellum: Diagnosis and treatment. *Clin Sports Med* 2001;20:565-590.
5. Chess D: Osteochondritis, in Savoie FH III, Field LD (eds): *Arthroscopy of the Elbow*. New York, NY, Churchill Livingstone, 1996, pp 77-86.
6. Poehling GG: Osteochondritis dissecans of the elbow, in Norris TR (ed): *Orthopaedic Knowledge Update: Shoulder and Elbow.* Rosemont, IL, American Academy of Orthopaedic Surgeons, 1997, pp 363-367.
7. Peterson RK, Savoie FH III, Field LD: Osteochondritis dissecans of the elbow. *Instr Course Lect* 1999;48:393-398.
8. Panner HJ: A peculiar affection of the capitulum humeri, resembling Calve-Perthes' disease of the hip. *Acta Radiol* 1929;10:234-242.
9. Pappas AM: Osteochondrosis dissecans. *Clin Orthop* 1981;158:59-69.
10. Takahara M, Ogino T, Sasaki I, Kato H, Minami A, Kaneda K: Long term outcome of osteochondritis dissecans of the humeral capitellum. *Clin Orthop* 1999;363:108-115.
11. Bauer M, Jonsson K, Josefsson PO, Linden B: Osteochondritis dissecans of the elbow: A long-term follow-up study. *Clin Orthop* 1992;284:156-160.
12. Shaughnessy WJ: Osteochondritis dissecans, in Morrey BF (ed): *The Elbow and Its Disorders*, ed 3. Philadelphia, PA, WB Saunders, 2000, pp 255-260.
13. Singer KM, Roy SP: Osteochondrosis of the humeral capitellum. *Am J Sports Med* 1984;12:351-360.
14. Tivnon MC, Anzel SH, Waugh TR: Surgical management of osteochondritis dissecans of the capitellum. *Am J Sports Med* 1976;4:121-128.
15. McManama GB Jr, Micheli LJ, Berry MV, Sohn RS: The surgical treatment of osteochondritis of the capitellum. *Am J Sports Med* 1985;13:11-21.
16. Brown R, Blazina ME, Kerlan RK, Carter VS, Jobe FW, Carlson GJ: Osteochondritis of the capitellum. *J Sports Med* 1974;2:27-46.
17. Mitsunaga MM, Adishian DA, Bianco AJ Jr: Osteochondritis dissecans of the capitellum. *J Trauma* 1982;22:53-55.
18. Tullos HS, King JW: Lesions of the pitching arm in adolescents. *JAMA* 1972;220:264-271.
19. Adams JE: Injury to the throwing arm: A study of traumatic changes in the elbow joints of boy baseball players. *Calif Med* 1965;102:127-132.
20. Jackson DW, Silvino N, Reiman P: Osteochondritis in the female gymnast's elbow. *Arthroscopy* 1989;5:129-136.
21. An KN, Morrey BF: Biomechanics of the Elbow, in Morrey BF (ed): *The Elbow and Its Disorders*, ed 3. Philadelphia, PA, WB Saunders, 2000, pp 43-60.
22. Schenck RC Jr, Athanasiou KA, Constantinides G, Gomez E: A biomechanical analysis of articular cartilage of the human elbow and a potential relationship to osteochondritis dissecans. *Clin Orthop* 1994;299:305-312.
23. Takahara M, Shundo M, Kondo M, Suzuki K, Nambu T, Ogino T: Early detection of osteochondritis dissecans of the capitellum in young baseball players: Report of three cases. *J Bone Joint Surg Am* 1998;80:892-897.
24. Haraldsson S: On osteochondrosis deformans juvenilis capituli humeri including investigation of intra-osseous vasculature in distal humerus. *Acta Orthop Scand* 1959;38(suppl):1-232.
25. Baumgarten TE: Osteochondritis dissecans of the capitellum. *Sports Med Arthrosc Rev* 1995;3:219-223.
26. Woodward AH, Bianco AJ Jr: Osteochondritis dissecans of the elbow. *Clin Orthop* 1975;110:35-41.
27. Baumgarten TE, Andrews JR, Satterwhite YE: The arthroscopic classification and treatment of osteochondritis dissecans of the capitellum. *Am J Sports Med* 1998;26:520-523.
28. Ruch DS, Cory JW, Poehling GG: The arthroscopic management of osteochondritis dissecans of the adolescent elbow. *Arthroscopy* 1998;14:797-803.
29. Holland P, Davies AM, Cassar-Pullicino VN: Computed tomographic arthrography in the assessment of osteochondritis dissecans of the elbow. *Clin Radiol* 1994;49:231-235.
30. Fritz RC, Stoller DW: The elbow, in Stoller DW (ed): *Magnetic Resonance Imaging in Orthopaedics and Sports Medicine*, ed 2. Philadelphia, PA, Lippincott-Raven, 1997, pp 743-849.

31. Peiss J, Adam G, Casser R, Urhahn R, Gunther RW: Gadopentetate-dimeglumine-enhanced MR imaging of osteonecrosis and osteochondritis dissecans of the elbow: Initial experience. *Skeletal Radiol* 1995;24:17-20.

32. Minami M, Nakashita K, Ishii S: Twenty-five cases of osteochondritis dissecans of the elbow. *Rinsho Seikei Geka* 1979;14:805-810.

33. Byrd JW, Jones KS: Arthroscopic surgery for isolated capitellar osteochondritis dissecans in adolescent baseball players: Minimum three-year follow-up. *Am J Sports Med* 2002;30:474-478.

34. Menche DS, Vangsness CT Jr, Pitman M, Gross AE, Peterson L: The treatment of isolated articular cartilage lesions in the young individual. *Instr Course Lect* 1998;47:505-515.

35. Kuwahata Y, Inoue G: Osteochondritis dissecans of the elbow managed by Herbert screw fixation. *Orthopedics* 1998;21:449-451.

36. Harada M, Ogino T, Takahara M, Ishigaki D, Kashiwa H, Kanauchi Y: Fragment fixation with a bone graft and dynamic staples for osteochondritis dissecans of the humeral capitellum. *J Shoulder Elbow Surg* 2002;11:368-372.

37. Kiyoshige Y, Takagi M, Yuasa K; Hamasaki M: Closed-Wedge osteotomy for osteochondritis dissecans of the capitellum: A 7- to 12-year follow-up. *Am J Sports Med* 2000;28:534-537.

38. Takeda H, Watarai K, Matsushita T, Saito T, Terashima Y: A surgical treatment for unstable osteochondritis dissecans lesions of the humeral capitellum in adolescent baseball players. *Am J Sports Med* 2002;30:713-717.

39. Oka Y, Ikeda M: Treatment of severe osteochondritis dissecans of the elbow using osteochondral grafts from a rib. *J Bone Joint Surg Br* 2001;83:738-739..

40. Nakagawa Y, Matsusue Y, Ikeda N, Asada Y, Nakamura T: Osteochondral grafting and arthroplasty for end-stage osteochondritis dissecans of the capitellum: A case report and review of the literature. *Am J Sports Med* 2001;29:650-655.

41. Takahara M, Ogino T, Fukushima S, Tsuchida H, Kaneda K: Nonoperative treatment of osteochondritis dissecans of the humeral capitellum. *Am J Sports Med* 1999;27:728-732.

Epicondylitis in the Athlete

Michael G. Ciccotti, MD

In a simple letter published in *Lancet* in 1882, Henry J. Morris[1] introduced a previously undescribed entity, which he appropriately termed "lawn tennis arm". That brief description has since prompted the mind and pen of numerous orthopaedic researchers, resulting in a vast array of detailed diagnostic and therapeutic reports. However, many questions still remain unanswered with respect to this enigmatic entity called epicondylitis. Most simply defined, it is generally agreed to be an overuse injury of the musculotendinous origins of either the medial or lateral elbow. From that point on, however, debate and speculation continue with respect to many aspects of this disorder.

Etiology

The bulk of the literature on epicondylitis suggests that repetitive stress or overuse is the primary etiology of this disorder.[2–5] However, the occurrence of epicondylitis has also been documented in patients, athletes and nonathletes, after a single traumatic event.[4,5] No definitive etiology has been determined, and it would seem that either mode of injury might lead to this disorder. Epicondylitis has most commonly been associated on the lateral elbow with tennis and on the medial elbow with golf, but a host of sports (baseball, javelin throwing, fencing) and occupational activities (carpentry, plumbing, meat cutting) have also been identified as possible causes.

A variety of risk factors have been proposed for epicondylitis. Because our understanding of these risk factors comes from the study of tennis, they are most often discussed in terms of racquet sports. Improper techniques, such as leading on the groundstroke with a flexed elbow and hitting the ball off center on the racquet, may enhance the occurrence of tennis elbow.[2,6,7] It has been shown that epicondylitis is most common in recreational tennis players, not in elite players, which suggests that technique may very well be a risk factor.[3] The use of poorly sized or inappropriate equipment may also be a key risk factor for epicondylitis.[2,6] Choosing the appropriately sized tennis racquet, golf club, bat, or other equipment has been successful in returning athletes to their sports after being treated for epicondylitis, indicating that inappropriate equipment is also an etiologic risk factor. Certainly, lack of experience has also been identified as a risk factor for this disorder, because a variety of epidemiologic studies of tennis elbow suggest that this entity occurs 7 to 10 times more frequently in less experienced players.[3] This higher rate may be related to improper technique or the choice of poorly fitting equipment. Certainly, there are a variety of risk factors for epicondylitis, all of which lead to repetitive stress or overuse as the most common etiology for this disorder.

Pathophysiology

Since the earliest description of epicondylitis, an abundance of literature has been devoted to its precise pathophysiology, resulting in numerous proposed theories. Early reviews consistently describe this entity as a purely inflammatory process involving such structures as the periosteum, synovium and annular ligament.[8–10] More recently, however, Nirschl and Pettrone[2] and Regan[11] have confirmed histologically that the normal parallel orientation of collagen fibers is disrupted by an invasion of fibroblasts and vascular granulation-like tissue, with a paucity of acute or chronic inflammatory cells. It may very well be that the early stages of epicondylitis have an inflammatory or synovitic component, which in later stages parallels the degenerative changes in the tendon substance. These degenerative changes, which have been identified as possible microtearing, with a subsequent, aborted neurovascular response, have been termed "angiofibroblastic hyperplasia" by Nirschl and Pettrone[2] and occur either medially or laterally. On the lateral side, they have most often been identified within the substance of the extensor carpi radialis brevis. On the medial side, these changes have been noted within the flexor carpi radialis or pronator teres. Thus, although no distinct, universal pathophysiology has been determined for epicondylitis, it is generally agreed that this entity represents a microtearing of either the medial or lateral tendon origin, with a subsequent failed healing response that alters the normal musculotendinous biomechanics.

Diagnosis

Epicondylitis is characterized by pain at either the lateral or medial epicondyle, which often radiates into the forearm. The severity of this pain varies greatly from patient to patient. Range of motion is most often full except in chronic severe cases, in which patients may lack full extension. The neurovascular status of the upper extremity is normal in pure epicondylitis.

Lateral epicondylitis results in tenderness over the conjoined tendon origin, most often localized to the extensor carpi radialis brevis. The area of maximum tenderness lies approximately 5 mm distal and anterior to the midpoint of the lateral epicondyle, and the pain is worsened with resisted wrist extension while the elbow is in full extension. This tenderness is in contradistinction to that seen with posterior intraosseous nerve syndrome (PIN) or intra-articular radiocapitellar disease (arthrosis/osteochondritis dessicans). PIN, an entrapment of the posterior interosseous branch of the radial nerve at the arcade of Frohse, may be confused with epicondylitis. The discomfort noted with PIN is more diffuse, and it usually occurs anterolaterally. It is worsened by resisted forearm supination and is rarely identifiable by electromyography or nerve conduction velocity testing. Intra-articular disease involving the radiocapitellar joint usually results in pain and clicking with elbow motion. Swelling of the joint is often present, and plain radiographs, computed tomography, or magnetic resonance imaging (MRI) will identify the lesion.

Medial epicondylitis results in tenderness most often over the flexor carpi radialis and pronator teres origins. The area of maximal tenderness is approximately 5 mm distal and anterior to the midpoint of the medial epicondyle, and the pain is worsened by resisted wrist flexion and forearm pronation. In cases of suspected medial epicondylitis, it is essential to consider primary ulnar neuropathy or medial collateral ligament instability. Ulnar neuritis can be identified by the elbow flexion test. This test is performed by placing the elbow in maximum flexion and the wrist in extension for approximately 30 to 60 seconds, resulting in medial elbow pain and numbness or tingling in the ring and little fingers. Ulnar collateral ligament instability is best identified with valgus stress testing at 30°, which produces pain along the course of the ligament, or by the milking test, which is performed by pulling on the thumb with the elbow flexed the and forearm supinated and which illicits pain along the medial collateral ligament.

Radiographs of the affected elbow are usually normal, but 20% to 25% of patients may have soft-tissue calcification about the epicondyle.[2] On the lateral side, this calcification appears to have no prognostic implications, but on the medial side this calcification, if present within the ulnar collateral ligament, may suggest concomitant instability. MRI may show increased signal within the musculotendinous structures but rarely adds to the diagnostic or therapeutic decision-making process. An MRI, however, may be of use in diagnosis of the throwing athlete with confounding lateral or medial symptoms, for more precise identification of the source of pathology.

These straightforward principles suggest that epicondylitis should pose no diagnostic dilemma, however, as with any disorder, a multitude of other conditions may mimic epicondylitis. The most common or challenging ones include posterior interosseous nerve syndrome and radiocapitellar articular disease on the lateral elbow and ulnar neuropathy and medial collateral ligament instability on the medial elbow. It is also essential to consider cervical disease with radiculopathy in the differential diagnosis.

Nonsurgical Treatment

Certainly, consensus would suggest that nonsurgical treatment is the cornerstone of care for epicondylitis, because volumes of orthopaedic articles have proposed the success of nonsurgical measures for this disorder. But what exactly constitutes nonsurgical treatment? A closer look at the literature available indicates that this aspect of epicondylitis is also controversial and that there are a wide range of nonspecific measures. The general principles of nonsurgical treatment include initial relief of pain, followed by guided rehabilitation and return to previous activities.

Initial Phase

Relief of pain is the primary goal of the first phase of nonsurgical treatment. If a particular activity can be identified as causing the epicondylitis, this activity should be either modified or avoided. Complete inactivity or immobilization, however, should be discouraged to avoid disuse atrophy, which can compromise later rehabilitation. Ice is recommended for its local vasoconstrictive and anesthetic effects. An oral anti-inflammatory medication is often administered for a 10 to 14 day period, if the patient has no medical contraindication to the use of such drugs. But if one assumes that epicondylitis is a degenerative process and not inflammatory, why is there benefit from use of anti-inflammatory medications? It has been proposed that because this disorder often results in an accompanying synovitis, the anti-inflammatory medication may be effective in relieving the pain associated with the synovitis. If the patient does not respond to these initial therapeutic measures or if night pain is present, use of a corticosteroid injection has traditionally been proposed. As with the oral anti-inflammatory medications, the benefits of corticosteroid are most likely related to the accompanying synovitis that occurs with epicondylitis. The choice of dose and steroid preparation have remained arbitrary, because no carefully controlled prospective comparison of commonly used agents has been carried out.[12] The appropriate technique of injection requires instilling the mixture deep to the extensor carpi brevis on the lateral side and the flexor pronator mass on the medial side. Care should be taken to avoid injection into the superficial tissues, which may result in subcutaneous atrophy, or into the tendon, which may result in irreversible ultrastructural tendon changes. Is there therapeutic benefit from corticosteroid injections? Several short-term studies have indicated that pain relief occurs in 55% to 59% of patients receiving these injections, but recurrence of symptoms has been noted in 18% to 54% of those who initially experienced relief.[12]

In addition to oral and injectable anti-inflammatory medications, a variety of physical therapy modalities, such as ultrasound and high voltage galvanic stimulation, have been used to relieve the pain of epicondylitis. Although reports exist citing the success of each of these modalities, no prospective, randomized, controlled studies exist to demonstrate their efficacy. Therefore, although these modalities are recommended as part of the initial nonsurgical program, they should be discontinued if symptomatic relief is not obtained soon after their initiation.[13]

What treatment for sports-related injury would be complete without some form of bracing? Counterforce bracing was first introduced by Ilfeld in 1965. Theoretically, this type of brace inhibits full muscular expansion and thus decreases the force experienced by sensitive or injured muscular tissue proximal to the brace. Several studies have indicated that there is some benefit to the use of these supportive devices. Groppel and Nirschl[14] demonstrated with 3-dimensional cinematography and surface electromyography that lower extensor muscle activity was produced by the use of counterforce bracing during the tennis serve and one-handed tennis backhand. Snyder-Mackler and Epler,[15] using the more sensitive indwelling electromyographic technique, noted a significant reduction in muscle activity in the extensor carpi radialis brevis and extensor digitorum communis of healthy subjects during maximum voluntary isometric contraction while using an airbladder type of brace. Thus, if the athlete does not find these braces too cumbersome or too restrictive, they seem to have the benefit of decreasing symptoms during the athlete's return to activity.

Second Phase

Once the pain and discomfort of epicondylitis is eased by oral anti-inflammatory medications, injections, modalities, and counterforce bracing, a rehabilitation program is carried out for the involved arm. This begins with wrist extensor or flexor stretching and progressive isometric exercises. Initially these exercises may be done with the elbow flexed to minimize pain, then, as symptoms allow, the exercises are done with the elbow in progressively greater extension. As flexibility and strength improve, concentric and eccentric resistive exercises are performed. When the patient is capable of sprint repetitions to fatigue without significant elbow pain, a sports stimulation is staged. If successfully completed, the patient is reinitiated into his or her sport by gradually increasing the duration and intensity of exposure.

Upon return to sport, it is essential that the athlete and the athlete's coaches or trainers identify any inadequacies in equipment that may have led to the development of epicondylitis. The proper equipment, especially in the racquet sports, is essential to allow athletes to return to their sport and prevent subsequent episodes of epicondylitis.[16] Proper racquet grip size is assessed by measuring from the proximal palm crease to the tip of the ring finger, along its radial border. Lighter racquets, though providing less momentum, allow ease of positioning for impact. Frames of low vibration materials, such as graphite and epoxies, dampen impact forces imparted to the flexor and extensor origins. Using racquets that are less tightly strung or that have a higher string count per unit area and playing on slower surfaces, such as clay courts, will diminish the loads transmitted to the elbow. In golf, selection of clubs with proper weight, length, and grip can also significantly reduce the forces generated in the elbow.

As with equipment, proper technique is essential to allow the athlete to return to his or her sport safely.[16] If the athlete uses aberrant techniques in the sport, these should be identified and corrected through the guidance of coaches and trainers. For example, in tennis, the forehand stroke should allow the player to hit the ball in front of the body with the wrist and elbow extended. This allows the torso and the upper arm, rather than the wrist extensors, to provide most of the stroke power. The two-handed backhand stroke allows a distribution of forces between the upper extremities, and thus greatly diminishes force at the leading lateral epicondyle.[16]

As the athlete returns to sport, the conditioning of the involved elbow as well as the entire body is essential. Conditioning is best carried out with a slow, structured interval program that allows the athlete to return to the sport under the guidance of the coach, trainer, and physician. This conditioning should include flexibility, strength, and endurance training.

Although most authors report that the majority of patients with epicondylitis respond to nonsurgical care, there is a true paucity of clinical data on the long-term outcome of nonsurgical treatment. The available literature suggests that 5% to 15% of patients will suffer a recurrence of symptoms, but the majority of these patients with relapses will not have been fully rehabilitated or will have prematurely discontinued the preventive measures suggested.[16] In one such prospective review of nonsurgical treatment, Binder and Hazleman[13] noted that 26% of patients had a recurrence of symptoms, and over 40% had prolonged minor discomfort. Consequently, the previously documented rates of 85% to 90% for successful nonsurgical treatment may be somewhat optimistic, and persistent or recurrent symptoms may occur more frequently than has been reported in the past. Nonetheless, most clinical reports agree that nonsurgical management remains the mainstay of treatment for epicondylitis.

Surgical Treatment

The main indications for surgical treatment of epicondylitis include: (1) persistent, severe pain at the epicondylar region, (2) no response to a well-coordinated nonsurgical program spanning a minimal of 3 to 6 months, and (3) the exclusion of other diagnoses.

Historical Treatment

Historically, the surgical treatment for epicondylitis spans nearly three quarters of a century. For lateral epicondylitis, a host of techniques varying in popularity have been proposed, ranging from release of the extensor aponeurosis,[10] through transection of the annular ligament,[10,17] to open Z-plasty lengthening of the distal extensor carpi radialis brevis tendon.[18] Historically, very little has been written on the surgical treatment of medial epicondylitis. Various techniques, from percutaneous epicondylar release to epicondylectomy, have been vaguely reported.[16] Currently, the most widely accepted surgical procedure for lateral or medial epicondylitis involves: (1) excision of the pathologic portion of the tendon, (2) repair of the resulting defect, and (3) a firm reattachment of any elevated tendon origin back to the epicondyle.

Technique for Lateral Epicondylitis

With the patient supine and the arm supported on an arm board, a tourniquet is applied to the upper arm. A 5 to 7 cm oblique incision centered just anterior to the lateral epicondyle is created. The interval between the extensor carpi radialis longus and the extensor communis is identified and entered, revealing the underlying extensor carpi radialis brevis origin (Fig. 1, *A*). This origin is split longitudinally, and the area of pathology is carefully identified and then sharply debrided (Fig. 1, *B*). The lateral epicondyle is then rongeured to remove any fibrous tissue and to provide a bleeding surface for extensor reattachment. Although the extensor carpi radialis brevis is intimately attached to the underside of the longus, it is felt that adequate debridement may necessitate elevation of the majority of the brevis attachment from the epicondyle, and that a firm reattachment should be carried out. This is done by using a 5/64-inch drill bit to create a V-shaped tunnel, drilled perpendicular to the long access of the extended arm (Fig. 1, *C*). A heavy suture is then passed through the posterior leaf of elevated extensor tendon, through the bony tunnel from posterior to anterior, and then through the anterior leaf of elevated extensor tendon (Fig. 1, *D*). A side-to-side repair of the remaining extensor tendon is performed (Fig. 1, *E*). Routine subcutaneous and skin closures are carried out.

Technique for Medial Epicondylitis

With patient supine and the arm resting on an arm board, a tourniquet is applied. A 5 to 7 cm oblique incision is made centered just anterior to the medial epicondyle. The common flexor origin is incised at the pronator teres-flexor carpi radialis interval, either longitudinally (if the pathology is well localized) or transversely (if the tendon changes are diffuse or not easily identifiable) (Fig. 2, *A*). The

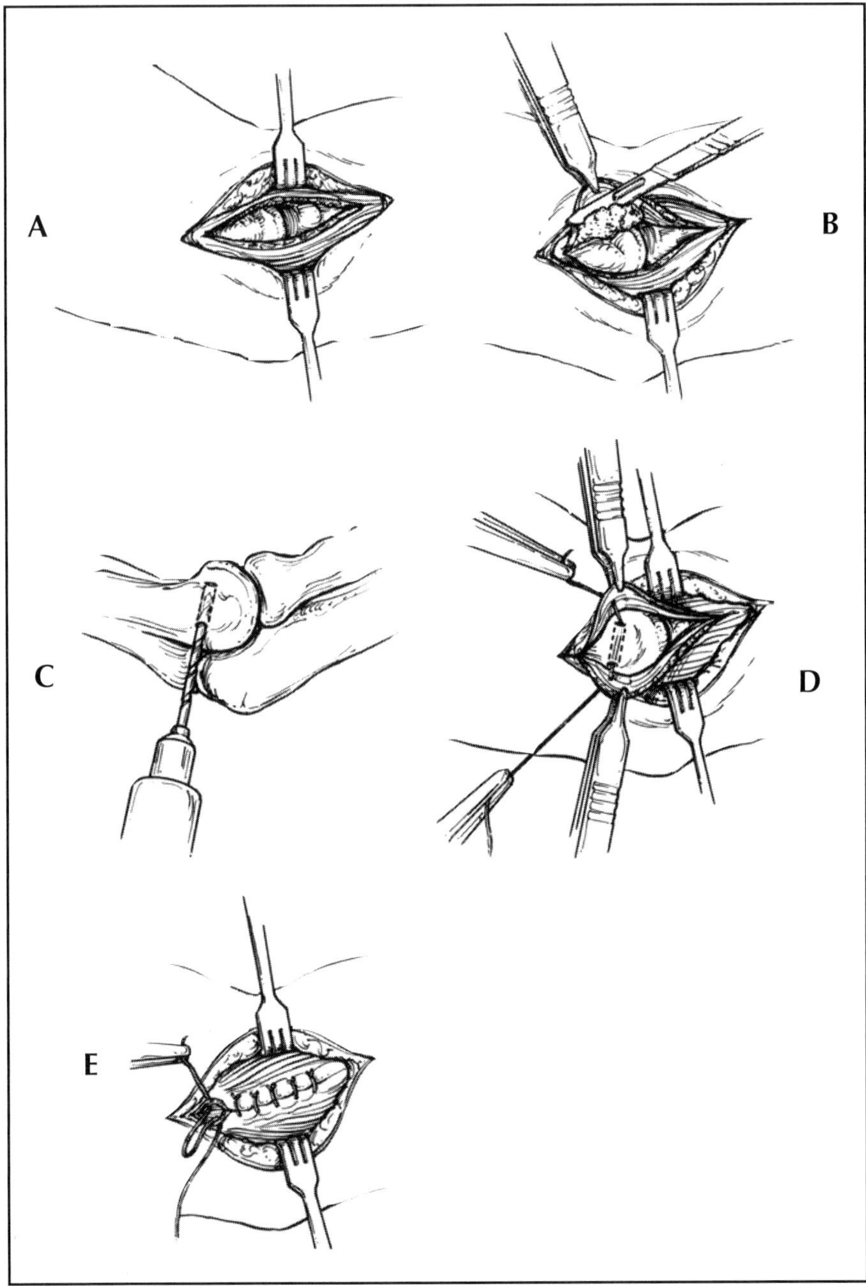

Fig. 1 Technique for surgical treatment of lateral epicondylitis. **A,** Skin incision and development of extensor interval. **B,** Excision of pathologic tissue. **C,** Drilling of lateral epicondylar bone tunnel. **D,** Reattachment of extensor origin to lateral epicondyle. **E,** Side-to-side repair of extensor origin. (Reproduced with permission from Ciccotti MG, Lombardo SJ: Lateral and medial epicondylitis, in Jobe FW (ed): *Operative Techniques in Upper Extremity Injuries in Sports.* St. Louis, MO, CV Mosby, 1996, pp 431–446.)

medial collateral ligament and the ulnar nerve are identified, assessed for pathology, and protected during the procedure. The pathologic tissue is then sharply excised, and the epicondyle is prepared by rongeuring any fibrous tissue (Fig. 2, *B*) and by drilling small multiple holes in the medial epicondyle to create a vascular bed. The common flexor pronator origin is then reattached to the bleeding surface with interrupted sutures (Fig. 2, *C*). Routine subcutaneous and skin closures are carried out.

Postoperative Care

The postoperative care is similar for both lateral and medial epicondylitis. A posterior plaster splint is applied in the operating room. The splint and skin sutures are removed at 7 to 10 days postoperatively. Gentle passive and active elbow, wrist, and hand exercises are begun. Gentle isometrics are initiated at 3 to 4 weeks postoperatively, and more vigorous resistive exercises, including resisted wrist extension for lateral epicondylitis and resisted wrist flexion and forearm pronation for medial epicondylitis, are begun at 6 weeks postoperatively. A progressive strengthening program follows, and return to activity is generally attained by 3 to 4 months postoperatively.

Surgical Results

Of patients who undergo surgical treatment of lateral epicondylitis, 85% to 90% return to full activity without pain.[2,16] Approximately 10% to 12%, however, are noted to have some improvement but still have pain during aggressive activities. In approximately 2% to 3%, no appreciable improvement is obtained. In those patients with persistent symptoms, the other previously mentioned causes of lateral elbow pain should be pursued again. At the Kerlan-Jobe Orthopaedic Clinic,[4,16] 1,140 of 1,200 patients (95%), in whom lateral epicondylitis was diagnosed over a 10-year period, were successfully treated with nonsurgical measures. Sixty patients (5%) were unresponsive to nonsurgical treatment, and subsequently underwent extensor debridement and repair. Thirty-nine of these

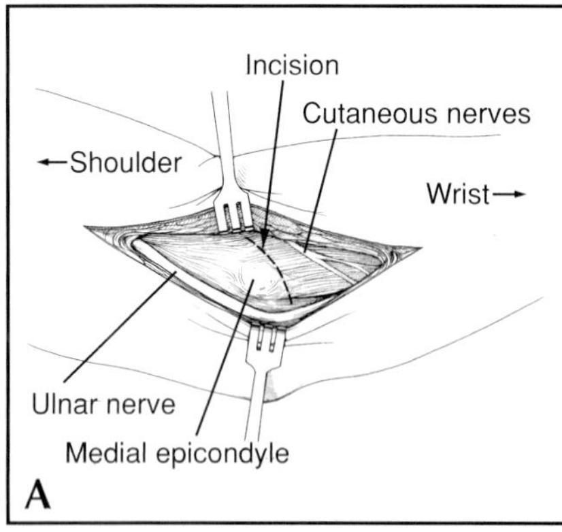

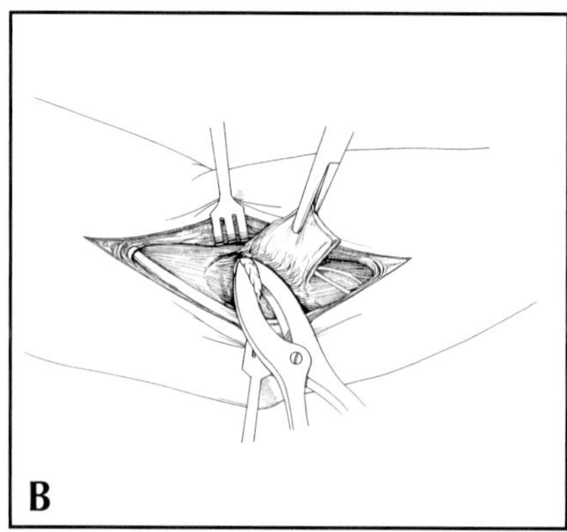

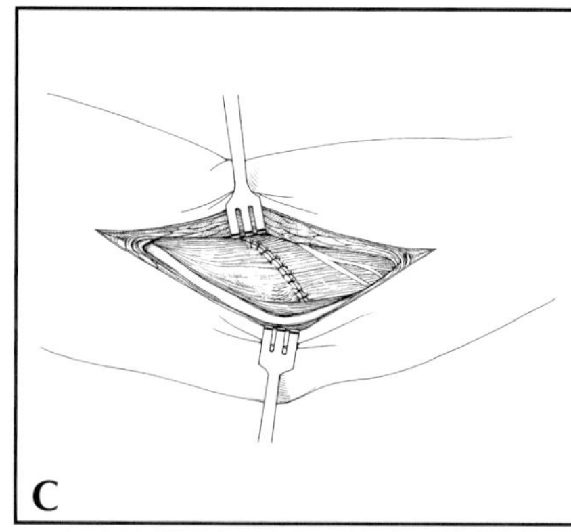

Fig. 2 Technique for surgical treatment of medial epicondylitis. **A,** skin incision and intended incision of common flexor-pronator origin. **B,** Distal reflection of common flexor-pronator origin with debridement of pathologic tissue. **C,** reattachment of common flexor-pronator origin to medial epicondyle. (Reproduced with permission from Jobe FW, Ciccotti MG: Lateral and medial epicondylitis of the elbow. *J Am Acad Orthop Surg* 1994;2:1–8.)

patients (65%) were seen 2.5 to 10 years after the procedure. Ninety-four percent of the patients reported dramatic improvement in symptoms. The objective outcome measures showed that 36% had limitations with heavy lifting, 50% had grip-dynamometer deficits, and 100% had some degree of isokinetic deficit. In our review at the Rothman Institute and Thomas Jefferson University, 24 patients were treated surgically for recalcitrant lateral epicondylitis over a 5-year period. Ninety-six percent showed overall good to excellent results with respect to pain relief and return to functional activity. All patients had significant strength improvement postoperatively as compared to preoperative hand grip-dynamometer measurements, but 12% were noted to have up to a 15% residual strength deficit. All athletes in the study returned to their preinjury level of sports competition within 6 months postoperatively.

With respect to medial epicondylitis, Vangsness and Jobe[19] reviewed 35 patients with recalcitrant medial epicondylitis treated surgically; they noted 97% good or excellent results and 98% subjective pain relief. Eighty-six percent had no limitation in the use of the elbow. Grip-strength testing revealed no significant side-to-side differences postoperatively. All of the 20 athletically active patients returned to their sport. In general, surgical treatment of epicondylitis results in high patient satisfaction with reliable pain relief. Some residual strength deficits may exist, but these do not seem to interfere with functional activities.

Arthroscopy

Does arthroscopy have a place in the surgical treatment of epicondylitis? Several authors have proposed that an adequate arthroscopic debridement of the extensor carpi radialis brevis with subsequent decortication of the lateral epicondyle can be performed.[20] This procedure uses standard elbow arthroscopic techniques and has been previously described. Opponents have suggested that this technique may not allow thorough debridement and decortication of the epicondyle, that the lateral ulnar collateral ligament is at risk for detachment during the procedure, and that the released extensor carpi radialis brevis, which is not reattached by this arthroscopic technique, may produce a functional deficit in the athlete's arm. Baker and Cummings[20] have shown in a cadaveric study that adequate decortication and debridement of the extensor carpi radialis brevis, without violation of the later ulnar collateral ligament, can be carried out arthroscopically. Their clinical results also suggest a high rate of success with this arthroscopic technique.[20] However, because of the paucity of clinical data available on arthroscopic treatment of epicondylitis, this technique remains controversial and has not yet gained wide support.

Summary

Since the first description of epicondylitis of the elbow in 1882, there have been volumes of descriptive, diagnostic, and therapeutic reports detailing every aspect of this entity. It is now known that epicondylitis can be caused both by occupational and sports-related activities, that its diagnosis may be confused with a variety of other pathologic entities affecting the elbow, that the majority of patients will respond favorably to well-guided nonsurgical treatment, and that in those patients whose persistent symptoms make them unable to return to their activities, surgical treatment results in reliable pain relief and return to preinjury level of activity.

References

1. Morris H: The rider's sprain. *Lancet* 1882;2:133–134.
2. Nirschl RP, Pettrone FA: Tennis elbow: The surgical treatment of lateral epicondylitis. *J Bone Joint Surg* 1979;61A:832–839.
3. Gruchow HW, Pelletier D: An epidemiologic study of tennis elbow: Incidence, recurrence, and effectiveness of prevention strategies. *Am J Sports Med* 1979;7:234–238.
4. Ciccotti MG, Lombardo SJ: Lateral and medial epicondylitis of the elbow, in Jobe FW, Pink MM, Glousman RE, Kvitne RS, Zemel NP (eds): *Operative Techniques in Upper Extremity Sports Injuries*. St. Louis, MO, Mosby-Year Book, 1996, pp 431–446.
5. Leach RE, Miller JK: Lateral and medial epicondylitis of the elbow. *Clin Sports Med* 1987;6:259–272.
6. Bernhang AM, Dehner W, Fogarty C: Tennis elbow: A biomechanical approach. *J Sports Med* 1974;2:235–260.
7. Kelley JD, Lombardo SJ, Pink M, Perry J, Giangarra CE: Electromyographic and cinematographic analysis of elbow function in tennis players with lateral epicondylitis. *Am J Sports Med* 1994;22: 359–363.
8. Runge F: Zur genese und behandlung des Schreibekrampfes. *Berliner Klin Wochenschr* 1873;10:245–248.
9. Trethowan WH: Editorial: "Tennis elbow." *Br Med J* 1929;2:1218–1224.
10. Bosworth DM: The role of the orbicular ligament in tennis elbow. *J Bone Joint Surg* 1955;37A:527–533.
11. Regan W, Wold L, Coonrad R, Morrey B: Microscopic histopathology of chronic refractory lateral epicondylitis. *Am J Sports Med* 1992;20:746–749.
12. Price R, Sinclair H, Heinrich I, Gibson T: Local injection treatment of tennis elbow: Hydrocortisone, triamcinolone and lignocaine compared. *Br J Rheumatol* 1991;30: 39–44.
13. Binder AI, Hazleman BL: Lateral humeral epicondylitis: A study of natural history and the effect of conservative therapy. *Br J Rheumatol* 1983;22:73–76.
14. Groppel JL, Nirschl RP: A mechanical and electromyographical analysis of the effects of various joint counterforce braces on the tennis player. *Am J Sports Med* 1986;14:195–200.
15. Snyder-Mackler L, Epler M: Effect of standard and Aircast tennis elbow bands on integrated electromyography of forearm extensor musculature proximal to the bands. *Am J Sports Med* 1989;17:278–281.
16. Jobe FW, Ciccotti MG: Lateral and medial epicondylitis of the elbow. *J Am Acad Orthop Surg* 1994;2:1–8
17. Newman JH, Goodfellow JW: Fibrillation of head of radius as one cause of tennis elbow. *Br Med J* 1975;2:328–330.
18. Garden RS: Tennis elbow. *J Bone Joint Surg* 1961;43B:100–106.
19. Vangsness CT Jr, Jobe FW: Surgical treatment of medial epicondylitis: Results in 35 elbows. *J Bone Joint Surg* 1991;73B:409–411.
20. Baker CL Jr, Cummings PD: Arthroscopic management of miscellaneous elbow disorders. *Op Tech Sports Med* 1998;6:16–21.

Biceps Tendon Injury

Bernard F. Morrey, MD

Other than epicondylitis, isolated injury to the muscles or tendons about the elbow is rather uncommon.[1-5] Distal biceps tendon injury, most commonly avulsion from the radial tuberosity, although rare, is the most common tendinous injury in this region. The biceps muscle-tendon complex may be injured at the musculotendinous junction by an in-continuity tear of the tendon, and by a complete or partial tear or avulsion from the radial tuberosity.

A tear of the musculotendinous junction or an in-continuity tear of the tendon are very rare. These conditions have been seen in weightlifters and in association with anabolic steroid use. Surgical treatment is not predictable, but I have used a ligament augmentation device (LAD)™ to assist in the repair/reconstruction. Recovery is slow and incomplete. Simple plication of the stretched tendon is not reliable.

By far the most common injury is tendon avulsion, and complete avulsion is much more common than partial rupture. Even so, until recently this has been considered a rather uncommon injury.

Incidence

The rarity of the condition is exemplified by the fact that of the 355 surgeons responding to a questionnaire by Dobbie in 1941, only 51 cases were reported.[6] By 1956, there were 152 reported cases in the literature.[7] Currently the injury is well known, and either its incidence is increasing or it is becoming recognized.[8-15]

Over 80% of the reported cases have involved the right dominant upper extremity, usually in a well developed man,[16,17] who has an average age of about 50 years,[6,18,19] ranging between 21 and 70 years.[6,17]

Mechanism of Injury

In virtually every reported case,[6,19] the mechanism of injury is a single traumatic event, often involving 40 kg or more of extension force with the elbow in about 90° of flexion. This mechanism and the tendency for anabolic steroid abuse in well conditioned, healthy, competitive weightlifters accounts for the surprisingly common occurrence of injury in this group. Preexisting degenerative changes in the tendon make rupture more likely.[20]

Etiology

The etiology of the injury has been discussed by several authors.[20,21] During pronation and supination, inflammation and degeneration of the biceps tendon are initiated by irritation from the irregularity of the radial tuberosity. Spurring of the radial tuberosity is common and is consistent with the degenerative nature of this injury. An interesting recent study on the etiology has also implicated a hypovascular zone of tendon near its attachment as a cause or contributing factor to the injury.[21] Acute pain, as in the antecubital fossa, is noted immediately. Rarely, a patient complains of a second episode of acute pain several days later. Such a history suggests the possibility of an initial partial rupture or of secondary failure of the lacertus fibrosus.[10,22] Forearm pain has been reported but is not considered common.

Presentation

Subjective Complaints

The common symptom of distal biceps tendon rupture is a sudden, sharp, tearing pain followed by discomfort in the antecubital fossa or in the lower anterior aspect of the brachium. Activity is possible, but difficult, immediately after the injury. If the injury is not repaired with surgery, however, chronic pain with activity is common in the antecubital fossa and proximal forearm.[23] Flexion weakness of about 15% is inevitable, but it tends to decrease with time.[24] Loss of supination strength (about 40%) has been reported and is the source of considerable dysfunction. Diminution of grip strength also has been reported.[8,19]

Objective Findings

Ecchymosis is present in the antecubital fossa[6] and occasionally over the proximal ulnar aspect of the elbow joint.[25] Extensive bleeding is uncommon. With elbow flexion, the muscle contracts proximally, and a visible, palpable defect of the distal biceps muscle is obvious (Fig. 1). Local tenderness is present in the antecubital

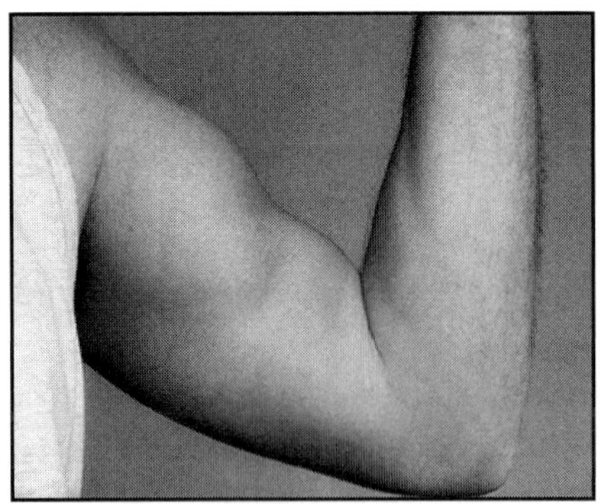

Fig. 1 Proximal migration, when present, allows the diagnosis to be readily made. (Reproduced with permission from the Mayo Foundation, Rochester, MN.)

fossa. The defect may be palpable; if not, and symptoms are otherwise consistent with the diagnosis, a partial rupture may have occurred. With partial rupture, crepitus or grinding is noted with forearm rotation.[10] Motion is not altered except possibly as a result of pain at the extremes of flexion, extension, and supination. Flexion weakness is usually and supination weakness invariably detectable by routine clinical examination.

Radiographic Changes

The routine use of the MRI has been recommended to make or confirm the diagnosis.[13] Although helpful occasionally, routine MRI is not necessary (Fig. 2).

Surgical Findings

The tendon will have recoiled into the muscle or be found to lie loosely curled in the antecubital fossa. Invariably, there is clean separation from the radial tuberosity.[6,16,19,24] The lacertus fibrosus may be attenuated, but is usually not completely torn. After several months, the tendon has retracted into the substance of the biceps muscle, making retrieval and reattachment impossible. In this instance, the lacertus fibrosus is usually torn and retracted.

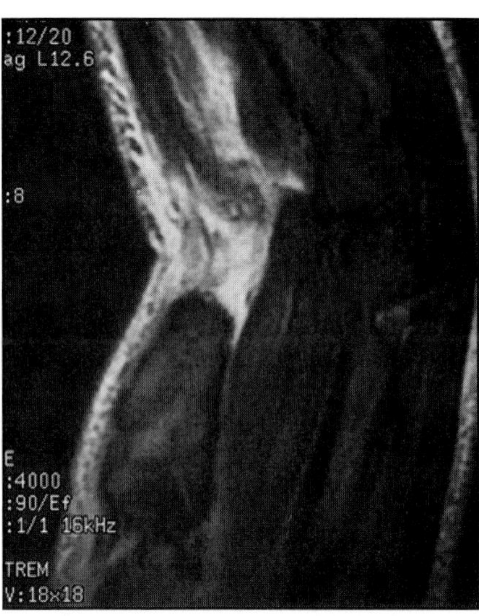

Fig. 2 Magnetic resonance imaging scan of the arm 4 days after injury. This study was of value in demonstrating retraction of the tendon and absence of tendon in the cubital fossa. (Reproduced with permission from the Mayo Foundation, Rochester, MN.)

Treatment

The functional superiority of surgical treatment is obvious when the results of cases treated with and without surgical intervention are reviewed.[19] The recent literature offers overwhelming documentation of the excellent results with early repair.[8,9,14,26] With a partial rupture, there is less functional loss or the tear may heal; hence, surgical management may not always be necessary.

Suture Anchor

Reattachment of the tendon to the radius by any one of several techniques[15,16,18,27] is clearly the treatment of choice. The difficulty of the anterior exposure needed to avoid radial nerve injury has prompted the development of a second incision placed over the dorsal aspect of the forearm.[25] It is of paramount importance to understand that the original 2-incision Boyd/Anderson technique has been modified at the Mayo Clinic to lessen the likelihood of the development of ectopic bone between the radius and ulna.[27]

Because of concern over the development of ectopic bone associated with the 2-incision technique and with the advent of suture anchors, the anterior exposure using these anchors is gaining in popularity. If the procedure is done promptly, the tract of the biceps tendon is still present and is easily identified. If performed late (more than 2 weeks after injury), this tract may be obliterated, making the exposure more difficult.

I have no personal experience with these devices for distal biceps tendon rupture. The specific technique varies according to 3 variables: exposure, type of anchor used, and method of reattachment. The exposure is usually via a limited anterior approach. Two or 3 suture anchors are most often used directly into the unprepared tuberosity. Both the screw and barb designs have been described for use at the medial tuberosity (Fig. 3).

Two-Incision Technique (Mayo Clinic)

With the patient in the supine position, the extremity is prepared and draped in the usual fashion using an elbow table. A tourniquet is applied to the arm. A limited 3-cm transverse incision is performed in the cubital crease (Fig. 4). The arm is grasped and milked distally to deliver the biceps tendon. Most of the time, the tendon is readily retrieved with this maneuver. The tendon is inspected and is invariably found to have avulsed cleanly from the radial tuberosity. The distal 5 to 7 mm of degenerative tendon is resected, and two No. 5 nonabsorbable Bunnell or whip stitch (Krackow) sutures are placed in the torn tendon (Fig. 4).

The tuberosity is palpated with the index finger and a blunt, curved hemostat is carefully inserted into the space previously occupied by the biceps tendon. The instrument slips past the tuberosity and is advanced below the radius and ulna so that the tip of the instrument may be palpated on the dorsal aspect of the proximal forearm. A second incision is made over the instrument. The tuberosity is exposed by a *muscle-splitting* incision with the forearm maximally pronated. The ulna is never exposed.[28] A high-speed burr is used to evacuate a 1.5-cm wide and 1-cm deep defect in the radial tuberosity. The tendon is carefully introduced into the excavation formed in the tuberosity, and with the forearm in the neutral position the sutures are pulled tight and secured. The wounds are closed in layers, with a suction drain inserted both anteriorly and posteriorly in the depths of the wound. The elbow is placed in 90° of flexion with forearm rotation between neutral and supination. A compressive dressing is applied.

Postoperative Care The splint and surgical dressing are removed in 4 or 5 days and passive motion begun. Passive forearm rotation is encouraged as tolerated. Active flexion and extension and forearm rotation are begun at 7 to 10 days. Full active motion is attained by 3 to 4 weeks. Light weights, for example, 0.5 to 1 kg, are allowed at 4 to 6 weeks with progression as tolerated. Dynamic splints or prolonged protection are no longer used. Full activity is allowed after the third month as tolerated.

Results Strength restoration approached normal in flexion and supination. Nontreated distal biceps rupture results in a loss of about 20% flexion and 40% supination strength.[19] On the other hand, restoration of normal strength has been reported,[19] and reaffirmed by Agins and associates[8] using Cybex testing for both strength and endurance. However, these authors and others[12] have observed restoration of normal strength only to the dominant extremity and a residual 20% to 30% weakness if the nondominant side was involved.

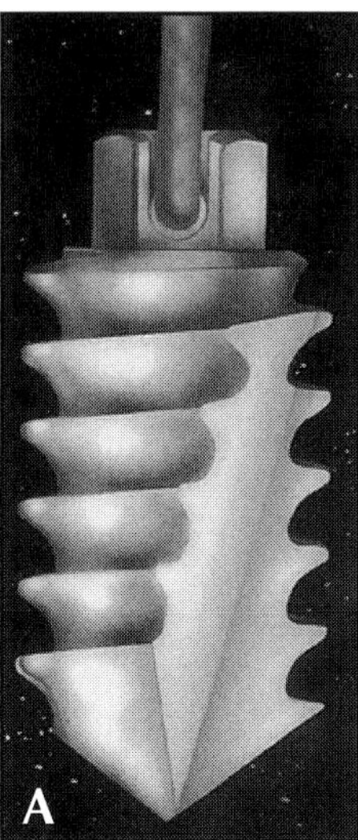

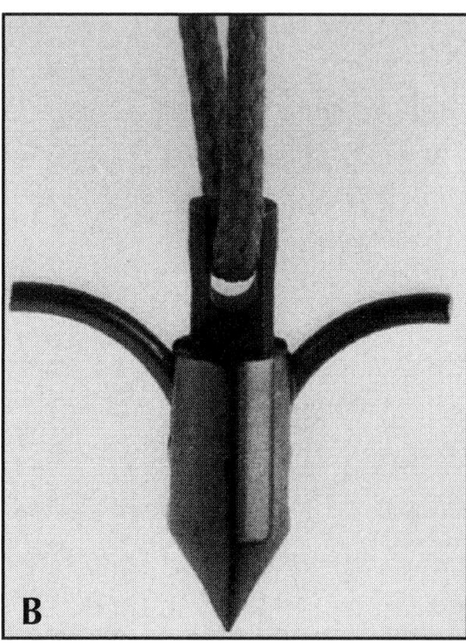

Fig. 3 Both the screw (**A**) and barbed tip (**B**) suture anchor designs had been used for biceps tendon attachment. (Reproduced with permission from the Mayo Foundation, Rochester, MN.)

Complications To my knowledge, there are no individual reports specifically dealing with the complications of surgical treatment for distal biceps tendon rupture in the English literature. Transient radial nerve palsy with reattachment to the tuberosity has been and continues to be occasionally noted.[6,14,26,29] A delayed posterior interosseous palsy has also been reported after repair.[30] As mentioned, the use of suture anchors has become of interest to prevent injury to the nerve. Strauch and associates[15] reports 3 instances of successful treatment using a limited anterior approach and suture anchors.

Reattachment of the tendon through an anterior approach with a pullout suture to avoid ectopic bone also has received recent support.[26] In 2 recent series with 24 combined cases, this approach resulted in excellent restoration of function. There was, however, 1 musculocutaneous nerve injury and 2 temporary radial nerve palsies, which have been well documented to be associated with an anterior surgical approach for this condition.

The possibility of ectopic bone formation after the 2-incision approach is well known. We have not had a complete bridge in our practice. The possibility of this complication is lessened but continues to exist, even with suture anchors (Fig. 5). If the 2-incision technique is used, it must be emphasized that the tuberosity is exposed by a muscle-splitting approach and the ulna is never visualized (Fig. 6).

If an osseous bridge does develop, successful resection can be undertaken about 8 to 9 months after the initial surgery.[31] Some cases of extensive involvement of the interosseous space as well as site of attachment pose rather significant challenges of treatment. In some instances the biceps repair may be intimately associated with the ectopic bone. Removing the osseous bar resulted in detachment of

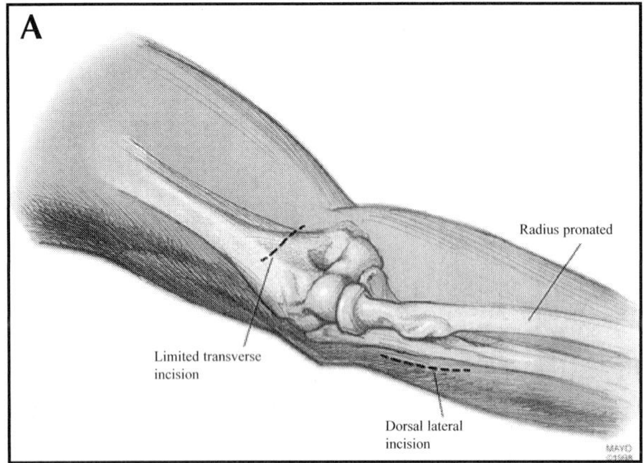

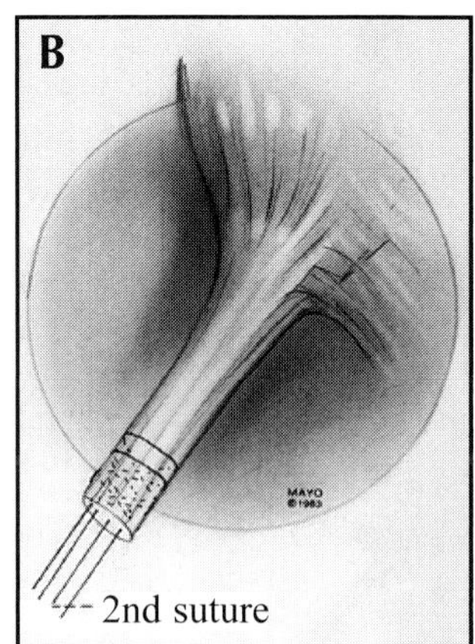

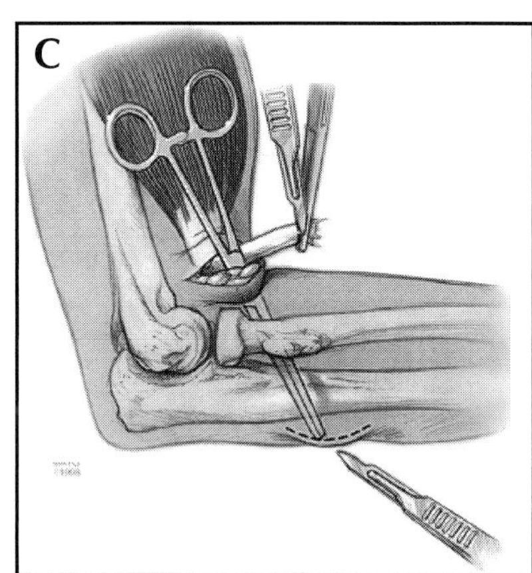

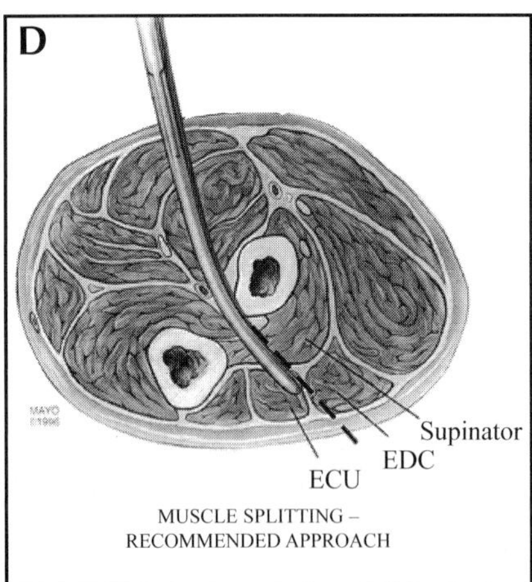

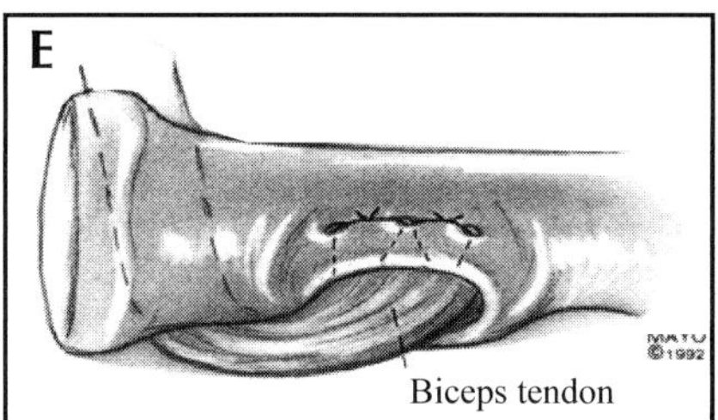

Fig. 4 A, A 3- to 4-cm transverse incision is made in the cubital space. **B,** Two heavy, nonabsorbable Bunnel sutures are placed in the end of the tendon. **C,** A blunt instrument is introduced in the tract of the biceps tendon, and the skin is indented on the volar aspect of the proximal forearm. An incision is made over this instrument. **D,** The common extensor and supinator muscles are then split to expose the radial tuberosity. The ulna is not exposed. Full pronation of the forearm brings the tuberosity into the field. **E,** The radial tuberosity is excavated using a high-speed bur and the biceps tendon is brought through its previous tract and reinserted into the radial tuberosity with the 2 nonasorbable sutures. (Reproduced with permission from the Mayo Foundation, Rochester, MN.)

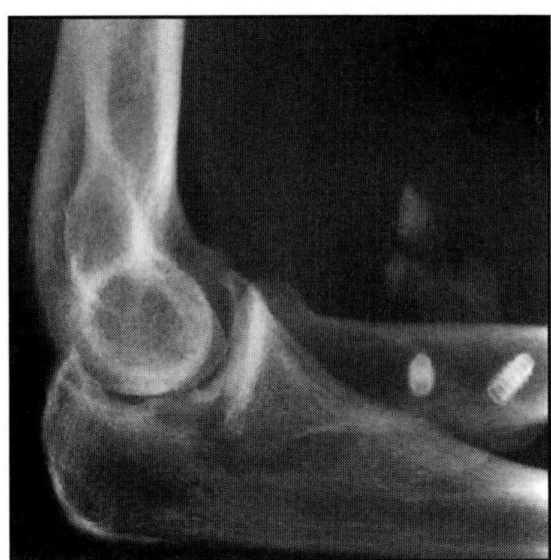

Fig. 5 Ectopic ossification associated with use of suture anchors.(Reproduced with permission from the Mayo Foundation, Rochester, MN.)

the biceps tendon, which then required reattachment into the tuberosity (Fig. 7). A good result may be anticipated but the rehabilitation must begin anew. If a bridge is excised, irradiation with 700 cGy may be administered but my experience shows that there is little tendency for recurrence of the ectopic bone.

Recurrence of the avulsion is rarely reported. There is 1 such case in a paralytic man using his arms for transfer and local motion less than 2 months after repair.

Once again, the development of proximal radioulnar synostosis is thought to be associated with exposing the periosteum of the lateral ulna, and can be avoided or at least minimized with a muscle-splitting incision.[28] There is no attempt to expose the ulna. This approach allows adequate exploration of the tuberosity, reliable reattachment of the tendon, and no significant limitation of motion; it continues to be the treatment of choice.[28]

Because of the emergence of the popular suture anchor technique through an anterior approach, over 70 cases treated at the Mayo Clinic have been reviewed. Of these, 70% were treated as described above, with 2 incisions. Only 4 had a minimal amount of ectopic bone or calcification localized in the tendon and not limiting motion. Of the 9 treated with an anterior exposure and secured to the tuberosity, 2 had transient paresthesias of the radial nerve and 1 developed a small amount of ectopic bone with no consequences on motion.

Author's Preferred Treatment Method

If the diagnosis of disruption of the distal biceps tendon is made within the first 7 to 10 days after injury, reattachment to the radial tuberosity using the 2-incision technique is recommended. I have reservations about the initial strength of the suture anchors that would permit early motion.

Late Reconstruction

The individual needs of the patient and the goals of any late surgical procedure must be carefully balanced. If the patient's occupation and residual strength do not require improvement of supination strength, simple reinsertion into the brachialis muscle is performed. Although rarely indicated, this surgical procedure is easy, improves flexion strength, and is essentially free of complications. Postoperative rehabilitation is similar to that previously described except that no limitation is placed on pronation and supination in the early postoperative course.

If, after careful discussion with the patient, improved supination strength is found to be required, several reconstruction methods have been reported. A fascia lata graft has been described by Hovelius and Josefsson.[32] Others have used a free autogenous semitendinous tendon. If the tendon is retracted and shortened, which is typical, some form of breech augmentation is required. Although results were favorable, the LAD™ has been abandoned in favor of an autologous Achilles tendon graft; this tissue is ideally suited for this reconstruction. The fleck of calcaneus bone is trimmed and embedded into excavated radial tuberosity. Then with the elbow flexed 45° to 60°, the Achilles fascia is draped over the biceps muscle and the bone tendon stump is sewn into the muscle. This method offers a very gratifying reconstruction and allows a more aggressive rehabilitation program.

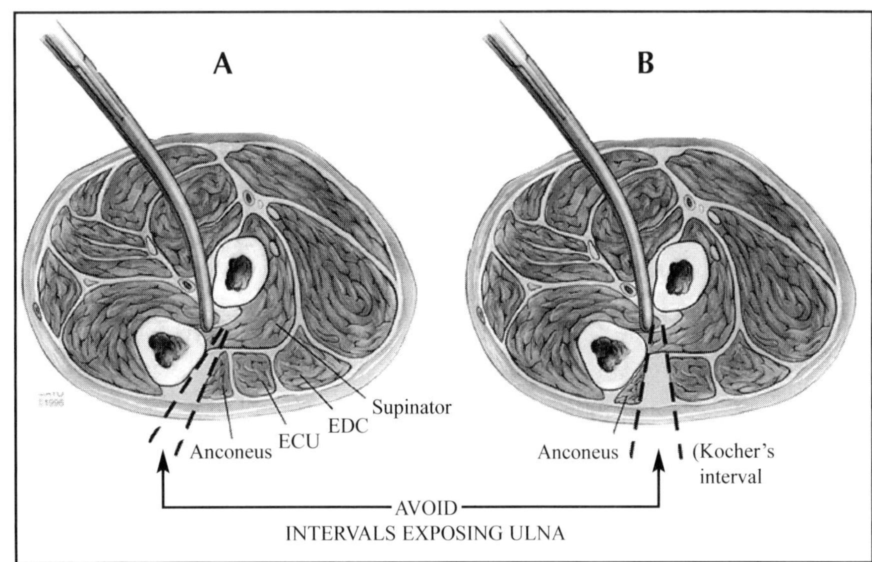

Fig. 6 The curved hemostat passes close to the radius and past the tuberosity, avoiding the ulna (**A**). Curving the instrument toward the ulna is to be avoided (**B**). (Reproduced with permission from the Mayo Foundation, Rochester, MN.)

Partial (Incomplete) Distal Biceps Rupture

Partial rupture of the distal biceps tendon has been reported since the first volume of this book and has been increasingly recognized since then. Nielsen[33] documented a case in which the lacertus fibrosus was thought to have initially ruptured with a secondary elongation of the biceps tendon. Chevallier[22] reported a biceps tendon rupture with secondary stretch of the lacertus fibrosus. My experience suggests that first, a partial rupture of the biceps tendon occurs and the second episode of pain completes the rupture (Fig. 8). A secondary stretch or disruption of the lacertus fibrosis may occur later.

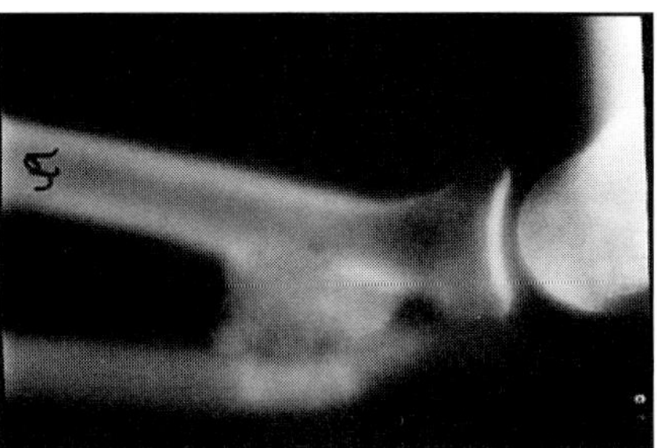

Fig. 7 Ectopic bone resulted from reattachment of an avulsed right biceps tendon to the radial tuberosity using the 2-incision technique of Boyd and Anderson, during which the ulna was exposed. (Reproduced with permission from the Mayo Foundation, Rochester, MN.)

Diagnosis of partial or impending rupture of the biceps tendon is not easy. The history of forced eccentric contracture is typical and overuse may have preceded this event. Pain subsides, but not completely. Weakness and fatigue are prominent and crepitus with forearm rotation is common. Distinction from bicipital tubercle bursitis may be difficult, especially because the 2 conditions

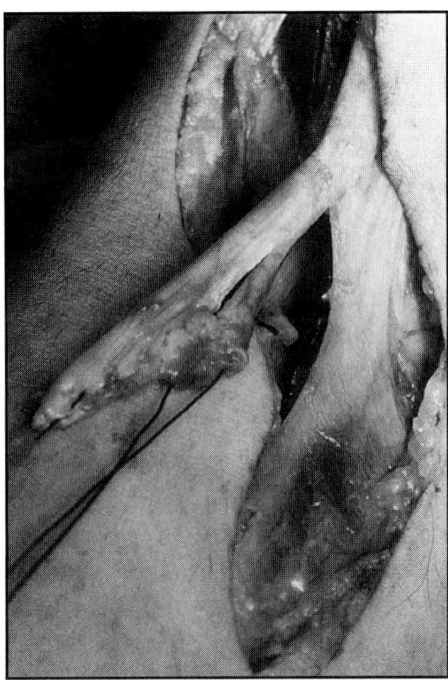

Fig. 8 Surgical photograph showing some fibers of the biceps tendon detached and retracted (lax suture), while others had remained in continuity (taut surface). Note that the lacertus fibrosus is stretched. (Reproduced with permission from the Mayo Foundation, Rochester, MN.)

may coexist. One of the 2 patients with cubital bursitis reported by Karanjia and Stiles[34] was a woman who was noted at surgery to have a distal biceps tendon degeneration in association with the bursitis. It is possible that the cubital bursitis was a reaction to the partial rupture. I have observed this finding in 1 patient in whom the initial exploration through a Henry approach revealed extensive "bursitis;" only after a careful inspection of the biceps tendon was it noted that a 50% disruption had occurred.[10]

The treatment of the partial tendon rupture may best be understood by considering the pathology of a degenerative tendon. Reimplantation of the remaining portion of the tendon to the radial tuberosity does not reliably relieve pain.[3] Complete removal of the remaining fibers, converting the problem to a complete tear, trimming of the distal tendon, and then reattachment as if this were an acute event is the treatment of choice.

References

1. Anzel SH, Covey KW, Weiner AD, Lipscomb PR: Disruption of muscles and tendons: An analysis of 1,014 cases. *Surgery* 1959;45:406–414.
2. Brickner WM, Milch H: Ruptures of muscles and tendons. *Int Clin* 1928;2:94–107.
3. Conwell HE, Alldredge RH: Ruptures and tears of muscles and tendons. *Am J Surg* 1937;35:22–33.
4. Haldeman KO, Soto-Hall R: Injuries to muscles and tendons. *JAMA* 1935;104:2319–2324.
5. Waugh RL, Hathcock TA, Elliott JL: Ruptures of muscles and tendons: With particular reference to rupture (or elongation of long tendon) of biceps brachii with report of fifty cases. *Surgery* 1949;25:370–392.
6. Dobbie RP: Avulsion of the lower biceps brachii tendon: Analysis of fifty-one previously unreported cases. *Am J Surg* 1941;51:662–683.
7. Giugiaro A, Proscia N: Rupture of the distal tendon and of the short head of brachial biceps. *Minerva Orthop* 1957;8:57–65.
8. Agins HJ, Chess JL, Hoekstra DV, Teitge RA: Rupture of the distal insertion of the biceps brachii tendon. *Clin Orthop* 1988;234:34–38.
9. Baker BE, Bierwagen D: Rupture of the distal tendon of the biceps brachii: Operative versus non-operative treatment. *J Bone Joint Surg* 1985;67A:414–417.
10. Bourne MH, Morrey BF: Partial rupture of the distal biceps tendon. *Clin Orthop* 1991;271:143–148.
11. Hang DW, Bach BR Jr, Bojchuk J: Repair of chronic distal biceps brachii tendon rupture using free autogenous semitendinosus tendon. *Clin Orthop* 1996;323:188–191.
12. Leighton MM, Bush-Joseph CA, Bach BR Jr: Distal biceps brachii repair: Results in dominant and nondominant extremities. *Clin Orthop* 1995;317:114–121.
13. Le Huec JC, Moinard M, Liquois F, Zipoli B, Chauveaux D, Le Rebeller A: Distal rupture of the tendon of biceps brachii: Evaluation by MRI and the results of repair. *J Bone Joint Surg* 1996;78B:767–770.
14. Louis DS, Hankin FM, Eckenrode JF, Smith PA, Wojtys EM: Distal biceps brachii tendon avulsion: A simplified method of operative repair. *Am J Sports Med* 1986;14:234–236.
15. Strauch RJ, Michelson H, Rosenwasser MP: Repair of rupture of the distal tendon of the biceps brachii: Review of the literature and report of three cases treated with a single anterior incision and suture anchors. *Am J Orthop* 1997;26:151–156.
16. Bauman GI: Rupture of the biceps tendon. *J Bone Joint Surg* 1934;16:966–967.
17. Postacchini F, Puddu G: Subcutaneous rupture of the distal biceps brachii tendon: A report on seven cases. *J Sports Med Phys Fitness* 1975;15:81–90.
18. Baker BE: Operative vs. non-operative treatment of disruption of the distal tendon of biceps. *Orthop Rev* 1982;11:71.
19. Morrey BF, Askew LJ, An KN, Dobyns JH: Rupture of the distal tendon of the biceps brachii: A biomechanical study. *J Bone Joint Surg* 1985;67A:418–421.
20. Davis WM, Yassine Z: An etiological factor in tear of the distal tendon of the biceps brachii: Report of two cases. *J Bone Joint Surg* 1956;38A:1365–1368.
21. Seiler JG III, Parker LM, Chamberland PD, Sherbourne GM, Carpenter WA: The distal biceps tendon: Two potential mechanisms involved in its rupture. Arterial supply and mechanical impingement. *J Shoulder Elbow Surg* 1995;4:149–156.
22. Chevallier CH: Sur un cas de desinsertion du tendon bicipital inferieur. *Mem Acad Chir* 1953;79:137–139.
23. Jaslow IA, May VR: Avulsion of the distal tendon of the biceps brachii muscle. *Guthrie Clin Bull* 1946;15:124.
24. Lee HG: Traumatic avulsion of tendon of insertion of biceps brachii. *Am J Surg* 1951;82:290–292.
25. Boyd HB, Anderson LD: A method for reinsertion of the distal biceps brachii tendon. *J Bone Joint Surg* 1961;43A:1041–1043.
26. Norman WH: Repair of avulsion of insertion of biceps brachii tendon. *Clin Orthop* 1985;193:189–194.
27. Tendon injuries about the elbow, in Morrey BF (ed): *The Elbow and Its Disorders*, ed 2. Philadelphia, PA, WB Saunders, 1993, pp 492–504.
28. Failla JM, Amadio PC, Morrey BF, Beckenbaugh RD: Proximal radioulnar synostosis after repair of distal biceps brachii rupture by the two-incision technique: Report of four cases. *Clin Orthop* 1990;253:133–136.
29. Meherin JM, Kilgore ES Jr: The treatment of ruptures of the distal biceps brachii tendon. *Am J Surg* 1960;99:636–640.
30. Katzman BM, Caligiuri DA, Klein DM, Gorup JM: Delayed onset of posterior interosseous nerve palsy after distal biceps tendon repair. *J Shoulder Elbow Surg* 1997;6:393–395.
31. Failla JM, Amadio PC, Morrey BF: Post-traumatic proximal radio-ulnar synostosis: Results of surgical treatment. *J Bone Joint Surg* 1989;71A:1208–1213.
32. Hovelius L, Josefsson G: Rupture of the distal biceps tendon. *Acta Orthop Scand* 1997;48:280–285.
33. Nielsen K: Partial rupture of the distal biceps brachii tendon: A case report. *Acta Orthop Scand* 1987;58:287–288.
34. Karanjia ND, Stiles PJ: Cubital bursitis. *J Bone Joint Surg* 1988;70B:832–837.

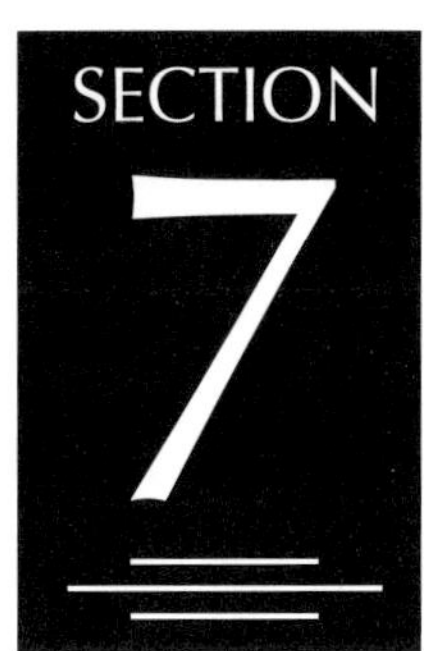

Degenerative Diseases About the Elbow

Degenerative Diseases About the Elbow

Surgical treatment of degenerative diseases about the elbow has been an area of much excitement and recent innovation. Formerly considered a relatively difficult and unforgiving area of the body to treat surgically, the elbow more recently has become an area where degenerative conditions can be successfully and reliably improved through surgical intervention. This section presents five recent articles covering some of the more important advances in surgical treatment of the degenerative elbow.

Jupiter and associates provide a comprehensive review of how to workup, treat, and rehabilitate the stiff elbow. The variety of conditions described ranges from the most simple elbow extrinsic contractures to the most complex, including those with associated heterotopic ossification. Surgical management is detailed as well, specifically open contracture releases from both lateral and medial approaches, as well as more complex arthroscopic techniques.

The authors begin by describing the critical contribution of elbow motion to quality of life. A functional arc of 100° (30°-130° of flexion-extension) is required for common functional tasks involving the hand. Morrey's classification system is highlighted, in which stiffness is divided into two principal groups (extrinsic and intrinsic factors) based on etiology and location. Intrinsic contractures are characterized by intra-articular pathology, and extrinsic factors are extra-articular. Understanding the characteristics of each type facilitates patient assessment. The authors also emphasize that management decisions are appropriately based on the degree of functional impairment and not specifically on any absolute loss of motion or contracture measured by goniometer. Thus, treatment options and surgical indications are highly individualized.

An excellent overview of surgical technique is provided. The authors note that arthroscopic release can be highly difficult in these patients and may require the use of specialized techniques developed for stiff elbows. Specifically, the authors emphasize the importance of using retractors inside the joint through accessory portals to elevate the surrounding soft tissues in an effort to decrease the potential for inadvertent nerve injury. They also note that 50% of lost motion is restored with either arthroscopic or open treatment. At least 90% of patients gain at least 10° of motion arc, and about 80% of patients who undergo either open or arthroscopic release obtain a functional arc of motion.

Heterotopic ossification is addressed in a separate section. The authors state that ossification generally can be removed once subsequent radiographs show maturation of the bone, generally within 3 to 6 months. Once heterotopic bone is removed, low-dose external-beam irradiation given at a single dose of 600-700 cGy can significantly decrease the risk of recurrence. Simple removal of bone is not sufficient; complete capsular release is generally necessary because early, aggressive postoperative rehabilitation to restore motion is important in an effort to reduce the risk of recurrence.

The next article by Morrey addresses nonprosthetic reconstruction of the elbow joint. Two options are described, arthrodesis and interpositional arthroplasty. Arthrodesis generally has very limited indications since elbow motion is so integral to quality of life. He emphasizes that elbow arthrodesis can restrict the most personal of body functions. Thus, interpositional arthroplasty may be a more viable option in patients in the third, fourth, or fifth decades of life who require pain relief, especially the posttraumatic population with ankylosis, and those too young for prosthetic reconstruction. Dr. Morrey, however, emphasizes that use of interpositional arthroplasty requires the presence of the broad contours of the distal humerus. Additional contraindications include active infection and gross instability. Residual instability is a major determinant of outcome; thus, the potential for maintaining stability postoperatively is an important consideration.

A variety of tissue choices is available for interpositional arthroplasty, but Dr. Morrey prefers either cutis or Achilles allograft. Given its low donor morbidity, Achilles allograft is his current tissue of choice. He describes an elegant technique using the allograft in that it not only provides interpositional tissue but also material for collateral ligament reconstruction. The construct is protected by use of a hinged external fixator. Although the literature review of this technique is relatively sparse, several authors have reported reasonably good (70%) results in midterm follow-up.

In the next article, Graham King describes new developments in elbow reconstruction by total elbow arthroplasty (TEA), specifically the important advances made in design and technique that have allowed it to become a very reliable procedure in low-demand individuals such as those with inflammatory arthropathies. He also describes some of the opportunities for design and implant technique refinements to expand the indications for higher demand individuals, such as the younger, more active populations.

The article begins by defining relevant terminology when describing TEA components. Although terms such as constrained, semiconstrained, unconstrained, and resurfacing have been used in the past, Dr. King believes that classifying implants as either linked or unlinked is much simpler and ultimately more helpful. Most modern designs, whether linked or unlinked, are semiconstrained. This design provides for a certain amount of varus and valgus laxity to allow muscle control within the limits of loading of the bones from that interface.

He notes that implant selection depends on the amount of bone destruction, the status of the capsuloligamentous restraints, and surgeon experience with these devices. Unlinked TEA generally is indicated in patients with relatively preserved bony architecture and reasonable soft-tissue stability. Components are implanted with one of the collateral ligaments preserved or with a system that ensures adequate repair of the collateral ligaments. The potential advantage of this design is better long-term wear characteristics. In contrast, Dr. King describes a linked TEA or "loose hinge" design as one in which the indications can be broader, including patients with greater degrees of bone and ligament deficiency. Improvements in TEA design have resulted in survivorship in medium-term follow-up for low-demand individuals to be similar to that for total hip arthroplasty.

A review of the TEA literature generally shows that more than 90% of patients report adequate pain relief and a functional arc of motion. The most troublesome complication of TEA has been infection. Postoperative instability associated with unlinked arthroplasty designs and ulnar nerve neuropathy are also problematic.

The final two articles in this section focus on the increasing use of arthroscopy to treat degenerative conditions about the elbow. As described by Ramsey in the first of these articles, arthroscopy has become an important tool not only for diagnosis but also for treating a variety of elbow disorders. Although technically demanding, elbow arthroscopy has been proved to be safe and effective given adequate experience and familiarity with the setup and technique. He notes that the ideal indication for elbow arthroscopy is a history of pain or mechanical symptoms in the context of radiographic evidence of intra-articular pathology. He also notes that the greater the degree of intra-articular pathology and contracture, the more difficult elbow arthroscopy becomes. These issues must be carefully considered when deciding to pursue arthroscopy. Safe elbow arthroscopy is highly dependent on an understanding of the neurovascular anatomy. Any process that significantly distorts normal elbow anatomy is a relative contraindication to elbow arthroscopy.

Ramsey importantly notes that the key to avoiding complications is to understand the relationship of the neurovascular structures in the elbow to the topographic anatomy. The radial and ulnar nerves, in particular, are in very close proximity to the capsule, and a safe distance can be obtained only with careful portal placement and maximizing the distance between the capsule and bone either by distention or the use of retractors. The multiple portal sites used with the standard elbow arthroscopy are described, followed by an overview of the technique for treating arthritis.

The final article by Norberg and associates discusses arthroscopic treatment of elbow arthritis. Even though the article was written in the relatively early stages of this treatment, the basic principles they describe are still relevant when treating people arthroscopically. Indications for arthroscopic treatment of elbow arthritis include loose bodies, impinging osteophytes off the olecranon and coronoid, and the corresponding "kissing lesions" on the olecronon and coronoid fossa. These problems can be addressed quite well with arthroscopic techniques, given adequate experience. The authors also note that corresponding contracture of the capsule often is present. Thus, a release of these tissues may be necessary.

Complications have been reported in approximately 10% of patients; however, most of these are minor. The authors note that serious nerve injuries, which are the greatest fear associated with advanced arthroscopic techniques, may be underreported. Therefore, they emphasize the importance of ensuring that the distance between the principal nerves and the portals must be maximized. The authors reported that 23 of their 24 patients had satisfactory results with an arthroscopic procedure 2 to 5 years after surgery. Improvements in arc of motion averaged from 50° to 131°. They also reported no neurovascular injuries.

Surgical techniques for degenerative conditions of the elbow have evolved since the publication of the five articles presented in this section. Multiple new designs in prosthetic arthroplasty have been introduced only in the last several years. Many of the areas of opportunity described by Dr. King, including improvements in materials, polyethylene, replication of flexion axis, and more refined surgical instrumentation, have been realized. However, whether these changes will lead to long-term improvements in outcome or expanded indications to younger, more active populations remains to be seen. Initial results appear promising; however, older loose-hinged designs such as the Coonrad-Morrey have an enviable track record and remain the gold standard.

Arthroscopic treatment of degenerative elbow conditions offers promising future opportunities. Several procedures that formerly required extensile, open approaches can now be treated quite successfully by arthroscopic and/or minimally invasive techniques. In particular, the osteocapsular arthroplasty as developed and pioneered by Shawn O'Driscoll appears to be an outstanding procedure for treating early or moderate osteoarthritis of the elbow. The technique offers comprehensive treatment of osteophytes on the coronoid tip, olecranon fascia, radial head fossa, radial head, and olecranon tip; it also addresses any soft-tissue abnormalities, including capsular contractures and the posterior band of the medial collateral ligament. Early results with this procedure appear to compare favorably with open techniques such as the Outerbridge procedure. Arthroscopic release of contractures has become increasingly mainstream as a highly effective and minimally invasive way to treat significant loss of motion. Concurrent treatment of ulnar nerve problems with arthroscopy soon may be possible as well.

Similar to the advancements and rapid innovations made in shoulder treatment over the last 15 years, surgical treatment of degenerative lesions of the elbow will continue to evolve over the next decade. It should prove to be an exciting time for those surgeons treating degenerative lesions of the elbow.

Ken Yamaguchi, MD
Professor of Orthopaedic Surgery
Chief, Shoulder and Elbow Service
Department of Orthopaedic Surgery
Barnes-Jewish Hospital
Washington University School of Medicine

The Assessment and Management of the Stiff Elbow

Jesse B. Jupiter, MD
Shawn W. O'Driscoll, PhD, MD
Mark S. Cohen, MD

Abstract

Posttraumatic loss of elbow motion can cause substantial disability, limiting the ability to put one's hand in the volume of a sphere in space. Although a number of conditions can lead to loss of motion, a greater understanding of the functional anatomy of the elbow has led to advances in surgical management. Elbow stiffness has been classified in a number of ways, but the consistent feature is capsular contracture. Treatment of the stiff elbow begins with clinical evaluation of elbow stiffness and identification of indications for surgical intervention. Techniques of open and arthroscopic elbow contracture release are evolving. Assessment and management of elbow contracture associated with heterotopic ossification, and treatment of distal humerus nonunion should be done early to restore elbow motion.

The function of the elbow is to place the hand within the volume of a sphere in space. This is distinguished from the function of the shoulder, which places the hand on the surface of the same sphere. As the elbow permits the hand to move to and from the center of the sphere, it effectively determines the radius of the sphere of reach of the hand. The volume of the sphere is proportional to the cube of its radius, so that any loss of elbow motion can significantly diminish the volume of reach of the hand.

One or more of the authors or the departments with which they are affiliated have received something of value from a commercial or other party related directly or indirectly to the subject of this chapter.

Posttraumatic conditions that adversely affect the function of the elbow joint represent a wide spectrum of pathologic processes.[1-17] Loss of mobility represents the most common sequelae. A number of factors have been implicated to explain the elbow's propensity to stiffness. These include the intrinsic congruity of the humeroulnar articulation, the presence of three articulations within a synovial-lined cavity, and/or the close interrelationship of the joint capsule to both the intracapsular ligaments and surrounding muscles.[1-3,5,12,13,18-21] Morrey and associates[22] studied 33 normal volunteers using an electrogoniometer designed to measure three-dimensional motion of the elbow in daily activities. Their work demonstrated that most activities could be done within a functional arc of 100° (30° to 130°) of flexion and extension of the elbow and 100° of rotation of the forearm (50° of pronation and supination for each). Yet certain functional tasks may demand greater motion in one direction or another.[22-25] As the upper limb represents an integration of several articulations, the combined loss of elbow extension and supination of the forearm, for example, will have an additive effect on the performance of activities requiring power for total use.[26] Irrespective of the underlying etiologies, elbow stiffness is a threat to the integrated function of the entire upper limb, thus making the restoration of motion a basic goal of most reconstructive efforts following traumatic injury to the elbow.

Classification

Kay[27] established a classification system for the stiff elbow based on the specific components involved: type I is soft-tissue contracture; type II, soft-tissue contracture with ossification; type III, undisplaced articular fracture with soft-tissue contracture; type IV, displaced intra-articular fracture with soft-tissue contracture; and type V, posttraumatic bony bars.

Morrey[12,13] classified elbow stiffness into two major groups on the basis of the etiology and anatomic location of the contracture. Extrinsic factors included contracture of the soft tissues, such as the joint capsule or collateral ligaments, extra-articular malunions, and/or heterotopic ossification. An intrinsic contracture is characterized by intra-articular adhesions, articular malalignment, loss of articular cartilage, or a multifaceted etiology. Contracture resulting from primarily extrinsic causes may be treated with resection of the contracted structures; in contrast, those resulting from intrinsic causes may necessitate alteration of the articular anatomy. As a general rule, intrinsic contractures almost always have an extrinsic component (capsular contracture).

Because more than one anatomic structure is often involved, it is also helpful to classify elbow stiffness on the basis of the structures involved, which can include the overlying skin rendered noncompliant from thermal trauma; muscle contracture resulting from shortening of the muscle-tendon unit or myositis ossificans; capsular contracture; degeneration or loss of the articular cartilage as a result of trauma, incongruity, or nonunion; or heterotopic ossification (R Hotchkiss, MD, personal communication, 1995).

Assessment

To fully assess a patient with a stiff elbow, it is crucial to determine the extent to which the loss of mobility compromises the patient's functional capabilities. Management decisions are more appropriately made on the basis of the degree of functional impairment than on the basis of the absolute loss of motion or joint contracture. The details of the original injury and initial treatment must also be understood. Associated conditions including infection, neurologic dysfunction, or ipsilateral limb injury will also influence management decisions.

Examination of the patient should include assessment of the entire upper limb, in particular the ulnar nerve because of its common involvement in elbow trauma.[28-47] In some instances, a patient may not appreciate subtle changes in ulnar innervated muscle because of a greater focus on the impaired function associated with the elbow. Evaluation of two-point discrimination, pinch strength, intrinsic muscle function, and electrophysiologic parameters is important to document the status of the ulnar nerve before surgery.

Careful radiologic assessment may require CT scanning as well as standard radiographs, especially when there is a question of intra-articular pathology. If there is any actual or potential alteration in the bony or articular anatomy, a lateral tomogram or a CT scan with reconstruction is appropriate. The AP (coronal plane) reconstruction should be performed after scanning the elbow in full extension and supination, while the lateral (sagittal plane) reconstruction should be performed after scanning the elbow in 90° of flexion in neutral forearm rotation (Fig. 1).

In determining when to remove heterotopic ossification, two factors should be considered: maturity of the heterotopic bone (as indicated by a smooth, well-demarcated cortical margin and defined trabecular markings, best appreciated by comparing sequential radiographs) and time since onset of ossification (bone can be removed within 3 to 6 months of its appearance).

Nonsurgical Management

Loss of full mobility often will lead a patient to seek surgical intervention; however, nonsurgical modalities, including splints, serial casting, or physical therapy, may be effective.[5,12,13,48-53] Several authors have noted substantial gains in elbow extension with the use of either turnbuckle splints or serial above-the-elbow casts.[50,53,54] Physical manipulation of the stiff elbow has long been thought to be problematic because of potential adverse sequelae, such as heterotopic ossification.[55] However, Bonutti and associates[48] noted a 30° average increase in elbow motion without adverse effect in 20 patients, and Duke and associates[49] reported favorable results in 6 of 11 patients treated with a single elbow manipulation while under general anesthesia.

Surgical Treatment Options

Surgical treatment for elbow contracture can be performed using open or arthroscopic techniques, or a combination of the two. The indications and methods for arthroscopic release of an elbow contracture are evolving, but arthroscopy has proved to be safe and has good rates of success, especially under less complex conditions.[56]

Indications for Surgical Contracture Release

Indications for surgery include impairment of function and limitation of daily activities. Generally, surgery has been limited to patients with elbow flexion contractures of at least 30° or those who could not flex the elbow beyond 120° or 130°. However, these parameters are of limited value for two reasons. First, some patients require full or nearly full motion for specific lifestyle demands. Second, as techniques of arthroscopic release of elbow contractures evolve, it may be possible to surgically restore even less severe losses of motion with minimal complications.

Definition of "Simple" Stiff Elbow

Before surgical management is begun, it is necessary to distinguish complex cases from simple cases; that is, those that require extensive surgical expertise or have a high likelihood of complications from those that do not. Simple stiff elbow is characterized by contractures that meet all of the following criteria: mild to moderate contracture (range of motion ≤ 80°), no or minimal prior surgery, no prior ulnar nerve transposition, no or minimal internal fixation hardware in place, no or minimal heterotopic ossification, and normal bony anatomy has been preserved. Patients with elbow contractures resulting from primary osteoarthritis or rheumatoid arthritis and adolescents with elbow contractures related to osteochondritis dissecans of the capitellum will usually meet all of these criteria; the majority of patients with posttraumatic stiffness will fail to meet one or more of these criteria.

Open Contracture Release

Surgical Exposure The surgical approach must provide access to the anterior and posterior aspects of the elbow as well as the requirement for anterior and posterior capsulectomies and/or removal of bone. It also includes the possibility of having to identify neurovascular structures in order to protect them or to transpose the ulnar nerve.

As with many surgical approaches, the superficial and deep exposures are considered separately. This is especially true around the elbow. Extensive clinical experience indicates that a posterior midline (just lateral to the tip of the olecranon) skin incision is the most useful approach for the elbow because it permits posteromedial or posterolateral arthrotomies as well as access to the ulnar nerve, the anterior elbow via the deep medial or lateral approaches.[57] The posterior midline skin incision should not cross the tip of the olecranon, especially in patients with olecranon bursitis or rheumatoid arthritis in whom the soft tissues over the olecranon are more susceptible to wound infection or breakdown. Separate medial and/or lateral skin incisions may be more advisable when scars from prior surgeries must be used to avoid skin flap devascularization or when there is a concern about the integrity of the soft tissues over the back of the elbow.

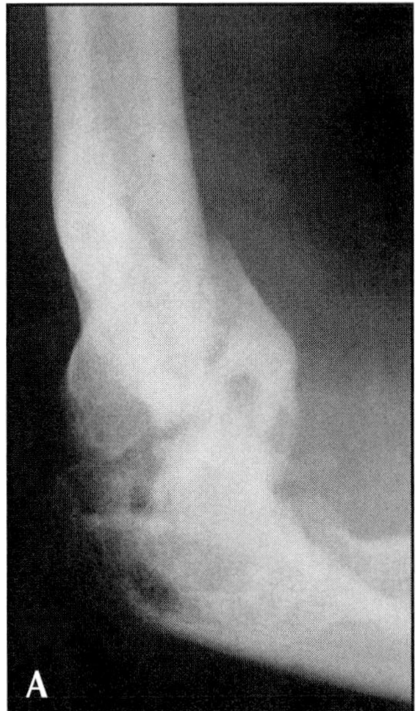

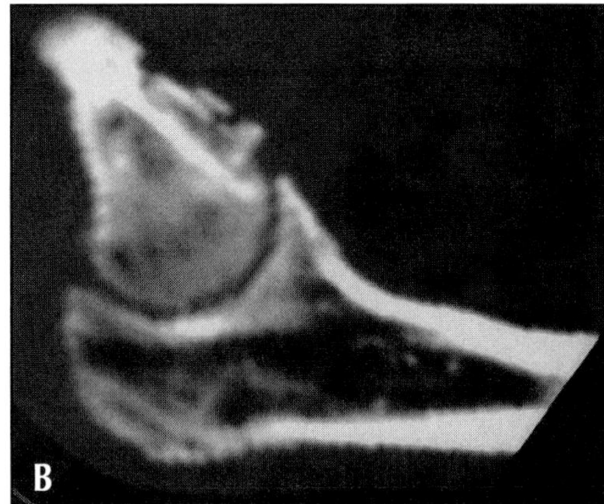

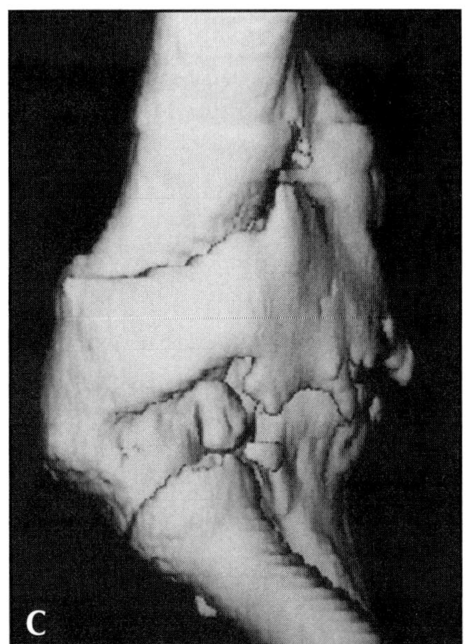

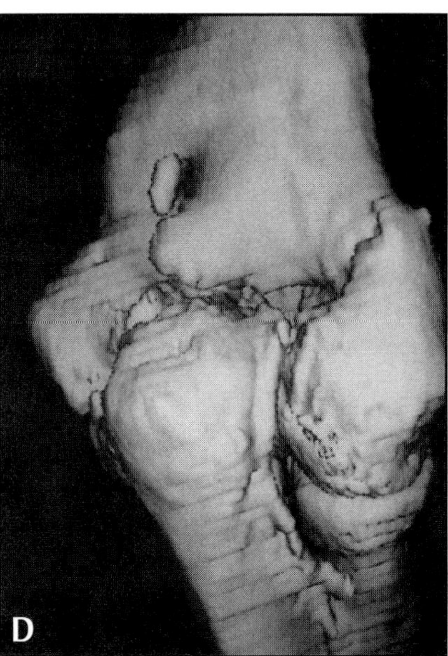

Fig. 1 A, Lateral radiograph of a complex trauma case with a deformity complicated by extensive heterotopic bone. **B,** Sagittal CT section reveals preservation of the ulnohumeral joint. Three-dimensional reconstruction of anterior (**C**) and posterior (**D**) surfaces allows better visualization of the bony detail for planning surgical resection.

Deep exposure to the elbow joint can be accomplished with either a medial or a lateral approach; occasionally, both are required. Although a lateral approach is highly versatile, it is often necessary to expose the ulnar nerve on the medial side to protect it from injury. The medial approach provides direct view of the ulnar nerve but puts the radial nerve at risk at the depth of the exposure on the far side anteriorly. The median nerve is farther from the capsule than the radial nerve; therefore, the likelihood of nerve injury is decreased. No differences in the number of nerve injuries using the medial and lateral approaches have been reported.

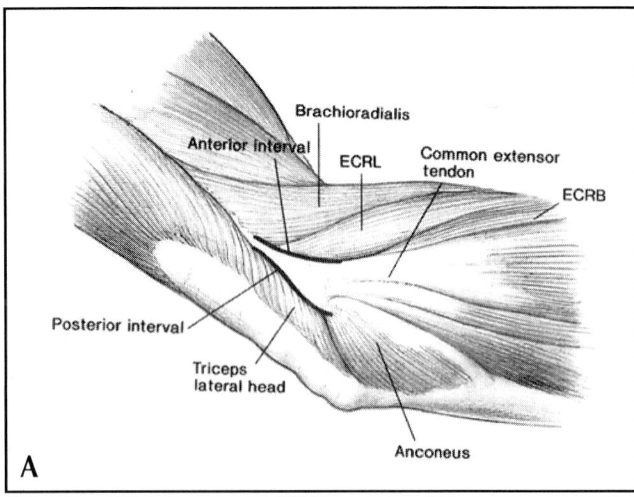

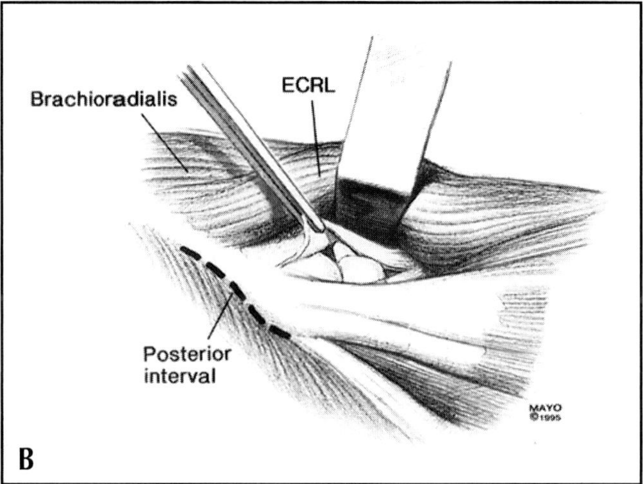

Fig. 2 Lateral column approach. ECRL = extensor carpi radialis longus, ECRB = extensor carpi radialis brevis. (Reproduced with permission from the Mayo Foundation, Rochester, MN.)

The anterior approach, originally described by Urbaniak and associates,[58] is indicated only in the presence of an isolated flexion contracture with normal full flexion of the elbow and when there is no evidence on the preoperative tomograms of bony abnormalities at the olecranon or in the olecranon fossa. This exposure is the most restricted; therefore, its indications are limited. Its use in the presence of a extension contracture (loss of full flexion) is contraindicated because it will not permit improvement in flexion and its use has been associated with a resultant loss of flexion. Therefore, both flexion and extension contractures should be released simultaneously when they are present.

Lateral Column Approach The lateral approach to a stiff elbow can be thought of in an algorithm of steps that have been described by Cohen and Hastings[59] and Mansat and associates,[60,61] who refer to it as a "column" approach. After raising a fasciocutaneous flap, the lateral column of the elbow is exposed as follows and as illustrated in Figure 2. Starting proximally, the lateral supracondylar ridge of the humerus is exposed distally to the epicondyle by subperiosteally reflecting the extensor carpi radialis longus anteriorly off the humerus and the lateral triceps off the humerus posteriorly (Fig. 2, *A*). Next, dissection is continued for 2 to 3 cm distally through the common extensor tendon from the epicondyle in a line toward Lister's tubercle. This generally passes in the interval between extensor carpi radialis longus and extensor carpi radialis brevis, along the anterior edge of the extensor digitorum communis. The entire anterior soft tissues are then reflected anteriorly off the capsule, which can then be excised (Fig. 2, *B*). The release should continue down to the level of the collateral ligaments. When elevating the brachialis off of the scarred anterior capsule, it is safer to dissect from proximal to distal to avoid crossing a nerve that may be embedded in the scar tissue. It is also technically easier to first dissect between the brachialis and the capsule than it is to elevate the capsule off of the humerus and then try to separate the capsule from the brachialis.

Posteriorly, the triceps is raised from the back of the humerus and dissected off of the posterior capsule. The capsule is then elevated from the humerus and the olecranon fossa is cleared of scar tissue and osteophytes. When dissecting medially, the ulnar nerve is at risk. To avoid injury but complete the release, it is often safer to expose the nerve. This can be done through a separate medial exposure (raising a medial skin flap) or underneath the triceps from the lateral side. The nerve runs along the medial border of the triceps adjacent to the intermuscular septum. Following the plane of dissection under the triceps medially to the intermuscular septum, just proximal to the elbow, it is readily exposed between the septum and the triceps. The nerve can then be exposed along its course and retracted while the capsule and scar are excised with the nerve in direct view. Although this approach is quicker and obviates the need for a medial skin flap or separate medial incision, anterior transposition of the nerve may be required to prevent the delayed onset of ulnar neuropathy resulting from stretching and compression of the ulnar nerve in the cubital tunnel with increased flexion postoperatively. This is caused by contraction of the cubital tunnel retinaculum, which lengthens with elbow flexion.[42]

Medial Column Approach If a medial approach is used, the dissection is conceptually similar to that described for the lateral column approach and is illustrated in Figure 3. After transposing the ulnar

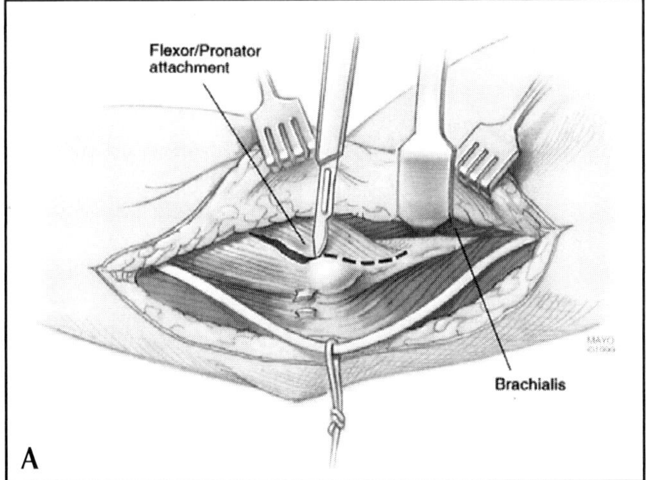

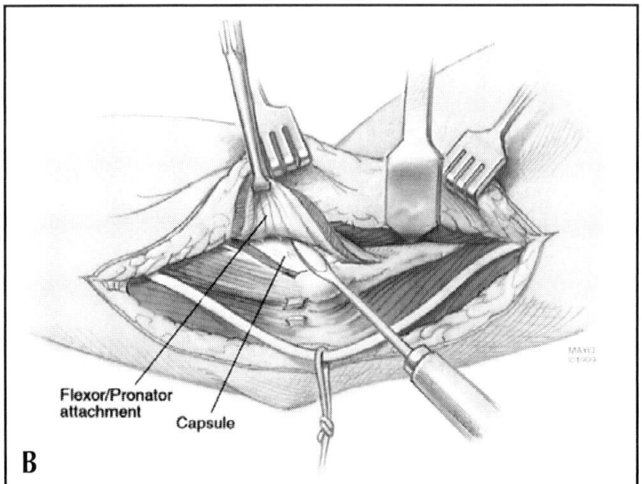

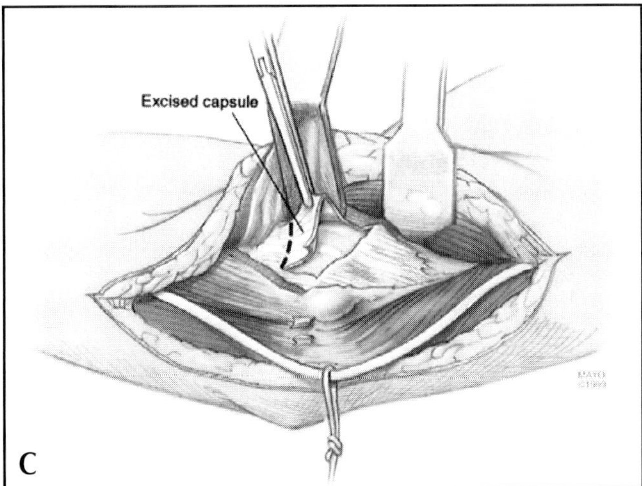

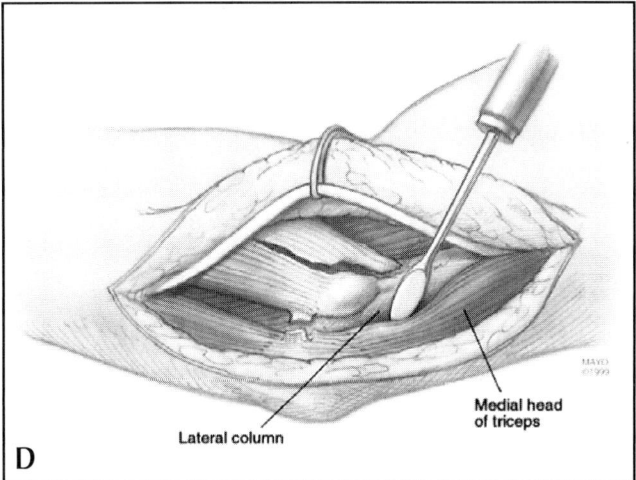

Fig. 3 Medial column approach. (Reproduced with permission from the Mayo Foundation, Rochester, MN.)

nerve, the pronator teres muscle origin is reflected from the medial supracondylar ridge down to the level of the medial epicondyle. From there, the common flexor-pronator tendon is split longitudinally for 2 cm distally. The brachialis and the anterior portion of the flexor-pronator group are dissected subperiosteally off of the anterior humerus and capsule in a proximal to distal direction (Fig. 3, *A* and *B*). The capsule is then excised (Fig. 3, *C*). If there is any question about the safety of the radial nerve, a separate limited exposure can be made on the lateral side as previously described to resect the lateral capsule under direct vision. The posterior release from the medial side is identical to release from the lateral side, except that the ulnar nerve must be first transposed (Fig. 3, *D*). If there is difficulty releasing the posterolateral capsule to restore adequate flexion, a separate lateral exposure may be required.

The collateral ligaments are preserved with both of these approaches, along with the common extensor and flexor-pronator tendons. Doing so greatly facilitates rehabilitation and virtually eliminates the possible complication of instability. Collateral ligament release is required to subluxate the elbow and thereby release intra-articular adhesions or to perform an interposition arthroplasty, which is reserved for those joints with at least 50% of the surface destroyed. In long-standing severe contractures, it may be necessary to partially release portions of the ligaments. Posteriorly, the posterior band of the medial collateral ligament (MCL) and the posterolateral joint capsule need to be released to restore full flexion when it is restricted preoperatively to less than 110° to 120°. The anterior fibers of the MCL and lateral collateral ligament may also need to be released in severe flexion contractures as well.

Upon completion of the release, the common flexor-pronator and/or extensor tendons are reattached to the epicondyle and supracondylar ridge through drill holes. If a sufficient thickness of tissue is

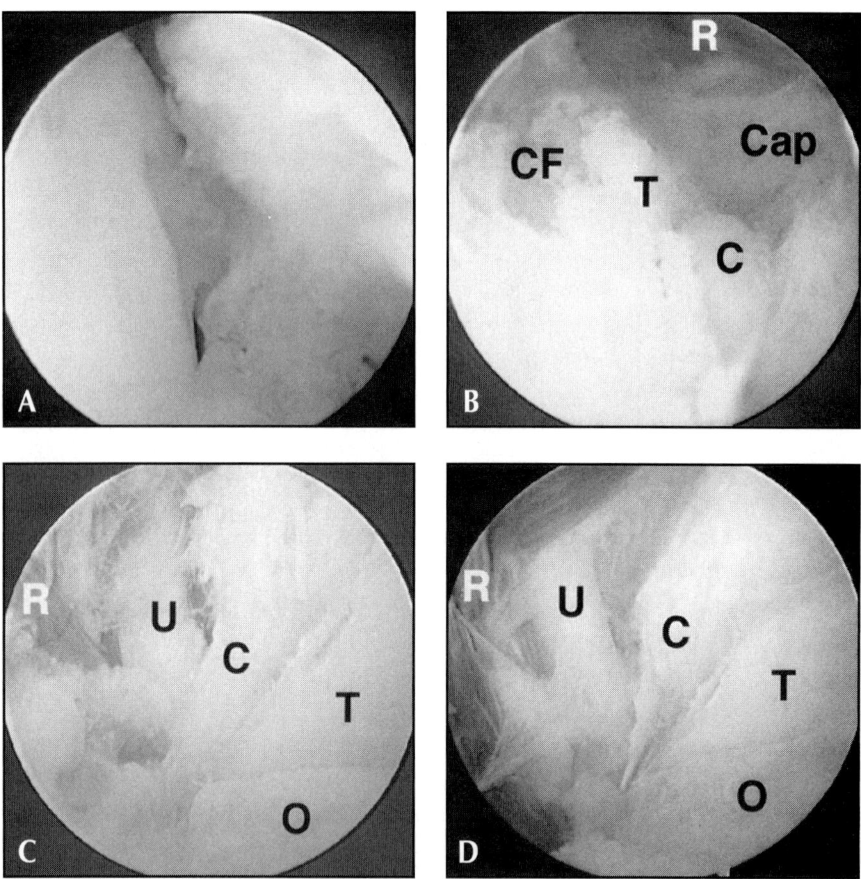

Fig. 4 The use of retractors greatly facilitates arthroscopic work in a stiff elbow and makes it possible to perform procedures safely that otherwise might not be able to be performed. Identical views from the anterolateral portal of a right elbow with posttraumatic contracture before **(A)** and after **(B)** placing a retractor. The space in which to work is dramatically increased. The coronoid (C), trochlea (T), coronoid fossa (CF), capsule (Cap), and retractor (R) are visible. Views of the posteromedial elbow before **(C)** and after **(D)** placing a retractor. The olecranon (O), trochlea (T), and posteromedial capsule (Cap) are seen. The retractor (R) makes it possible to open up the view, retract the triceps muscle, and move the ulnar nerve (U) away from the capsular resection. Two retractors are sometimes necessary to do this effectively.

left on the bone during exposure, drill holes are not necessary. The skin is closed over drains with subcutaneous sutures, then with staples. It is essential that sufficient strength of wound closure be provided to avoid wound breakdown during the aggressive rehabilitation postoperatively.

Arthroscopic Contracture Release

Gallay and associates[62] showed that capsular contracture leads to marked loss of intra-articular volume capacity (a mean of 6 mL in stiff elbows compared with 25 mL in normal elbows).[63] Timmerman and Andrews[64] found that access was so difficult in some cases of arthroscopic release as to prevent visualization altogether; therefore, the surgeon should be aware of special techniques that have been developed for stiff elbows.

The single most important technical factor that facilitates performing a capsular release is the use of retractors inside the joint[65] (Fig. 4). In this regard, the use of retractors permits more complex procedures to be performed without nerve injury. Retractors, which are routinely used in open surgery, are required for adequate visualization and to retract nerves away from motorized and cutting instruments. In addition, by retracting the capsule, pressurized distension is not needed and therefore swelling is less likely to become a serious impediment to progress. Consequently, multiple portals (one for the arthroscope, one for the shaver/cutter, and one to two for retractors) may be required.

Posterior Capsular Release The first objective in arthroscopic posterior capsular release is to establish a view. With the arthroscope in the posterolateral portal and the shaver in the posterior portal (or the arthroscope in the direct midlateral portal and the shaver in the posterolateral portal), a view is established by débriding the olecranon fossa to create a space in which to work. A radiofrequency ablation device can be used to remove dense scar tissue. The capsule can then be elevated from the distal humerus with a shaver or periosteal elevator to further increase working space. A retractor placed in a proximal posterolateral portal is useful to maintain that space. The next step is to perform a synovectomy. The capsule should be preserved until the synovectomy is complete, which makes it easier and safer to perform the capsulectomy. At this stage, the osteophytes are removed, along with loose bodies as they are encountered. Once any abnormal bone or osteophytes have been removed, the posterior capsule is resected. This is most easily performed with a shaver or radiofrequency ablation device through the posterolateral portal. The posterolateral capsule is then resected. Finally, the posteromedial capsule must be released when there is a significant lack of flexion. If the elbow does not flex beyond 90° to 110°, the posterior band of the MCL will likely have to be released to regain that motion. Because this tissue represents the floor of the cubital tunnel, the ulnar nerve is at significant risk of injury (Fig. 5).

The nerve is closer to the epicondyle than the tip of the olecranon, so release of the capsule is safer along the olecranon. A retractor placed in the proximal posterolateral portal, or even in a proximal posterior portal (sometimes using two retractors), is invaluable at this stage. The capsule should be kept on tension as it is divided. As a general rule, posteromedial release should not be performed before the location of the nerve has been identified. One option is to identify the exact location of the nerve, either arthroscopically or using a small, open incision.[65] Arthroscopic nerve exposure is a demanding procedure that should only be performed by experienced surgeons.

Some patients require ulnar nerve transposition along with the capsular release. A subcutaneous ulnar nerve transposition performed before the release permits safer access to the posteromedial capsule and the opportunity for direct visual feedback regarding where the shaver is located in the vicinity of the (transposed) nerve.

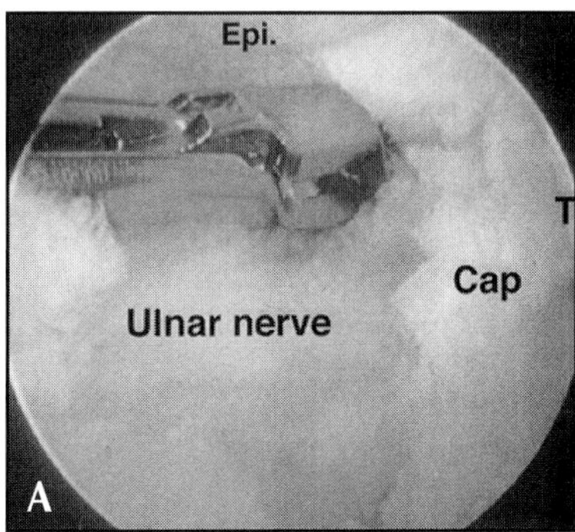

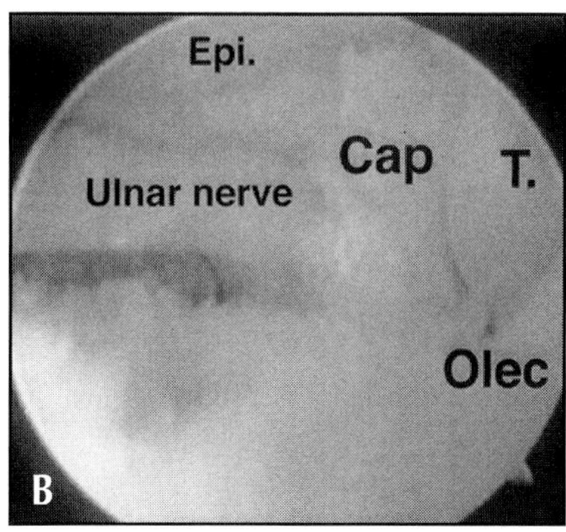

Fig. 5 The ulnar nerve is at significant risk of injury during posteromedial capsular release. **A,** The capsule (Cap) and posterior band of the MCL form the floor of the cubital tunnel, behind which is the ulnar nerve. **B,** The ulnar nerve is closer to the epicondyle (Epi.) than to the tip of the olecranon (Olec) as it passes beside the trochlea (T.); therefore, release of the capsule is safer along the olecranon. During this portion of the release, one or two retractors placed in the proximal posterolateral or proximal posterior portal to keep the capsule under tension and the nerve retracted away from the cutting instrument makes the procedure easier and safer.

Anterior Capsular Release Arthroscopic anterior capsular release can be performed in these steps: capsular stripping from the humerus, capsulotomy, and capsulectomy. Although the risk of nerve injury increases with the extent of capsular excision, it is possible that the efficacy of these three techniques is proportional to the completeness of the capsular excision. This presents a paradox because it appears that the greater the efficacy of the procedure, the greater the risk of nerve injury. As techniques evolve to permit these newer procedures to be performed more safely, capsular release, which began with capsular stripping from the humerus, progressed to capsulotomy and then to capsulectomy.[65,66]

To begin arthroscopic anterior capsular release, the arthroscope should be placed through the anterolateral portal and the shaver through the proximal anteromedial portal.[67-70] Because a retractor will either be necessary or extremely helpful, a retractor should be placed through the proximal anterolateral portal. As with posterior capsular release, a view is established and a space created in which to work. A second retractor can be inserted if necessary (through the anteromedial portal). Once the joint surface is visualized and the landmarks confirmed (coronoid, coronoid fossa), the débridement is initiated, followed by a synovectomy just medial to the midline. The anterior capsule is stripped off of the humerus proximally to permit further anterior retraction of the capsule and enlargement of the working space, and loose bodies are removed as they are encountered; numerous techniques have been described for the removal of large loose bodies.[71-74] A synovectomy and bony recontouring (removal of osteophytes or abnormal bone) are performed prior to removing the capsule. At this point, the capsule is clearly delineated as a structure before it is cut. This facilitates the actual capsulotomy/capsulectomy. The capsular attachments should be resected to the supracondylar ridge. The capsulotomy is best performed with a wide-mouthed duckling punch in a medial to lateral direction because the plane of dissection between the capsule and the brachialis is more distinct on the medial side (Fig. 6). Using a knife to extend the capsulotomy down to the level of the collateral ligaments on each side completes the capsulotomy.

The final step is a capsulectomy during which risk of nerve injury greatly increases. Although outcome efficacy may be better with a complete capsulectomy, this remains to be demonstrated in comparative or randomized studies. The capsulectomy should be performed on the medial side extending from a proximal to distal direction. The lateral capsule should then be excised proximally and distally. This is the most dangerous aspect of the anterior surgery because the radial nerve is not protected behind the capsule but is located just anterior to the radial head, between the brachialis and the extensor carpi radialis brevis.

At the completion of the procedure, two drains are placed—one through the proximal anterolateral portal and one posteriorly, which is brought out through a separate exit wound. Portal wounds are closed with locked horizontal mattress sutures to minimize problems with prolonged drainage. If an incision was used to expose the ulnar nerve, it can be closed with staples.

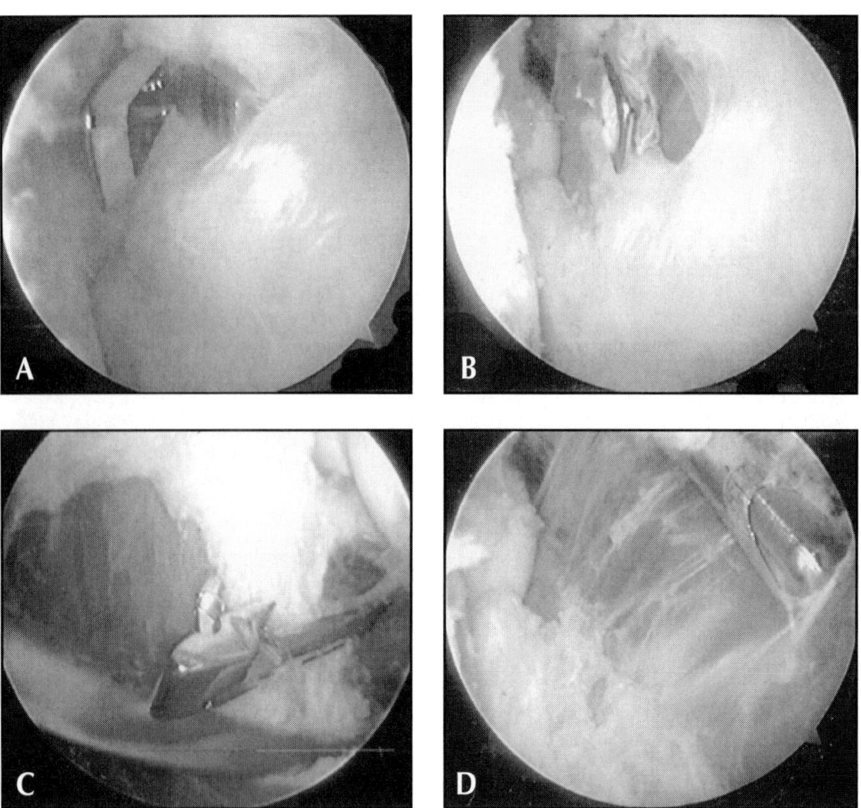

Fig. 6 A and **B,** Anterior capsulotomy. **C,** A reverse-cutting punch can be helpful to complete the release at the lateral side. **D,** Finally, the capsulectomy is performed with a shaver from a medial to lateral direction. Suction is disconnected from the shaver during this step, and the blade is kept facing away from the neurovascular structures.

Postoperative Care

For both open and arthroscopic release, the elbow is lightly wrapped in a bulky bandage with an anterior plaster slab extending from the shoulder to the hand while the elbow is in full extension. This maintains enough tension in the anterior soft tissues and compression against the posterior soft tissues that bleeding and edema of the periarticular soft tissues is minimized in the immediate postoperative period.[75,76] Once a patient's neurologic status is confirmed to be intact, an indwelling axillary catheter is placed for brachial plexus block anesthetic. Continuous passive motion (CPM) is commenced within 1 day after surgery. Because fluid accumulation was responsible for loss of motion before surgery, CPM must be from full flexion to full extension to prevent more fluid accumulation around the elbow. Before CPM is begun, the splint and dressing must be removed and exchanged for a thin, elastic sleeve with absorbent gauze over the wounds. Constrictive or nonelastic dressings are contraindicated with CPM because they cause shearing of the skin during motion. In the first 24 hours, the patient should be allowed out of the CPM device for no longer than 5-minute intervals because bleeding and edema accumulation occur rapidly when the elbow is not in a position of flexion or extension. The duration of these intervals is increased each day, and the patient is usually hospitalized for about 3 days. At the end of the second day, the local anesthetic is changed to a short-acting agent, which is then discontinued early in the morning on the third day. The patient may be discharged from the hospital when an acceptable range of motion can be maintained without severe pain. If not, the brachial plexus block may need to be resumed for another day.

CPM should then be continued at home for 3 to 4 weeks. The total hours that are required each day vary with the pathology, the severity and duration of the contracture before release, and the nature of the surgery. Patient-adjusted static splints are helpful in maintaining the range of motion achieved in surgery and are routinely used by many surgeons.[48,54] The postoperative administration of indomethacin is recommended for those at risk of developing ectopic ossification, although its efficacy in preventing recurrence is unknown. Meticulous surgical technique as well as copious irrigation during surgery may help to decrease the likelihood of heterotopic ossification.

Results

Although to our knowledge there are no published reports in the literature comparing open versus arthroscopic contracture release, several studies have documented the efficacy of each procedure.[8,13,14,56,59-61,64,65,77-84] It is widely reported that after either treatment patients regain about 50% of lost motion. A meta-analysis of the literature suggests that 90% to 95% of patients regain lost motion (defined by at least a 10° increase in the arc of motion) and about 80% obtain a functional arc of motion (defined as ranging from 30° to 130°); another 5% to 10% get to within 5° to 10° at each end of this functional range.[85] Although some believe that the degree of regained motion diminishes immediately after surgery and then gradually increases, this diminution may be prevented by the diligent use of CPM in the immediate postoperative period (Fig. 7).

Complications

The complication rate for open contracture release is reported to be from 10% to

30%, depending on the nature of the underlying pathology and the treatment required, and this rate is lower for "simple" contractures than it is for complex contractures.[13,59-61,77,78,80] The reported complications, in their approximate order of frequency, include wound complications (hematoma, seroma, or ischemia), infection, neuritis or neuropathy, ectopic ossification or excessive scar tissue formation, and pain. In addition, a recently recognized complication, delayed-onset ulnar neuropathy, has caused physicians to rethink the traditional approach to the management of the stiff elbow. A patient whose significant lack of flexion is acutely restored with surgery and maintained postoperatively is at risk of developing irritation or even loss of function of the ulnar nerve, which is caused by compression under the cubital tunnel retinaculum. Normally, this structure is not tight with flexion beyond 120°.[42] However, in patients with loss of flexion, the retinaculum may shorten and become tight in lesser degrees of flexion. Other factors that have been noted anecdotally to be potential contributors to this complication include the presence of an anconeus epitrochlearis muscle, dislocation of the ulnar nerve, and the presence of a medial osteophyte under the nerve. Patients with this complication may lose ulnar nerve function in the first few days postoperatively or pain may simply be too severe to maintain flexion. The pain, localized to the cubital tunnel, may be treated with ulnar nerve transposition. This delayed-onset ulnar neuropathy can be prevented by decompressing or transposing the ulnar nerve prophylactically in patients who present with less than 90° of flexion. Patients with 90° to 100° of flexion should probably have the nerve decompressed or transposed, and those with 100° to 115° of flexion may benefit from the same treatment. Firm recommendations will not be possible until further data have been collected and verified.

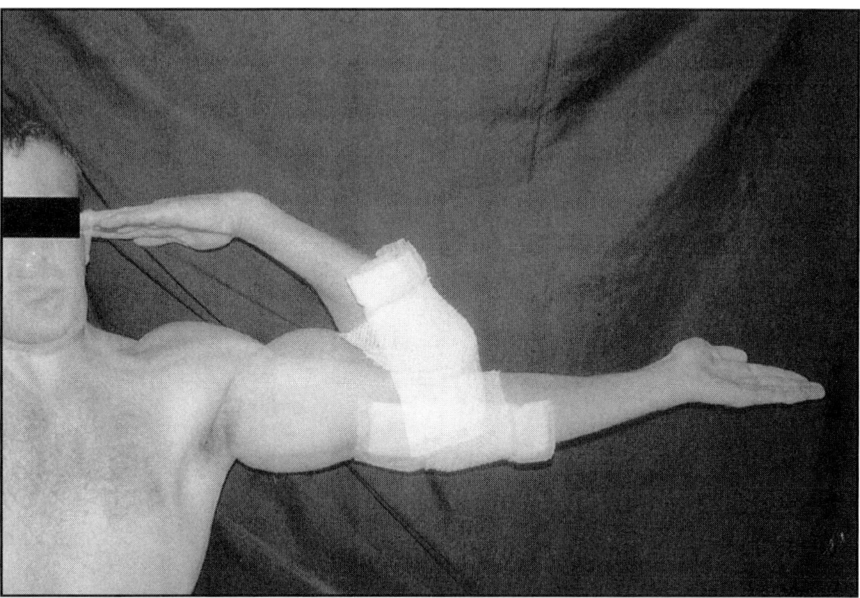

Fig. 7 Three days following capsular release and osteocapsular arthroplasty followed by 3 days of CPM in the hospital, this patient has close to full active motion. His preoperative motion was 30° to 125°. With intensive CPM, patients are able to maintain the ranges of motion obtained immediately after surgery.

Wound problems that occur with CPM should be managed by stopping CPM, elevating and extending the elbow for 1 to 2 days, and then reevaluating the wound. Hematomas and seromas should be washed out surgically because they have a tendency to impede flexion and can become infected.

Nerve injuries have been reported with both open and arthroscopic contracture releases.[57,59,69,83,86,87] The risk of nerve injury with arthroscopic contracture release has anecdotally been considered to be higher than that for open contracture release. Although that may or may not be the case, this belief is probably dependent on a number of factors, including surgeon experience and complexity of the surgery. Most reported nerve injuries occurred early during arthroscopic contracture release. Our experience with over 150 arthroscopic contracture releases suggests that the risk of nerve injuries can be reduced by instituting the following five safety measures: (1) use of retractors; (2) avoiding the use of suction anywhere near a nerve and leaving the shaver outlet open with no tube connected to it; (3) use of a shaver instead of a burr near a nerve to avoid the "power-takeoff" effect in which the burr wraps tissue and pulls the nerve into it; (4) knowledge of where the nerves are and/or actually visualizing and retracting them; and, most importantly, (5) recognizing the limits of surgical expertise and operating within them.

Heterotopic Ossification of the Elbow

The elbow is uniquely predisposed to developing heterotopic ossification, the formation of mature lamellar bone in nonosseous locations. This predisposition appears to be related to the severity of the injury, and heterotopic ossification has been reported in approximately 3% of simple elbow dislocations and in up to 20% of fracture-dislocations.[88,89] It is then most often seen in neural axis trauma, occurring below the level of spinal cord injuries.[90] It also forms in 5% to 10% of patients with isolated closed head trauma, most commonly on the side of involvement in those with hemiplegia.[91,92] The individuals who appear to have the greatest risk for developing heterotopic ossification (76% to 89%) are those with head injury and elbow trauma.[93,94] In addition, heterotopic ossification may occur in the elbow following thermal or electrical burns, and its incidence also appears to be related to the degree and severity of the burn.[95-97] It has also been reported to occur following certain surgical procedures, such as the Boyd approach for distal biceps tendon repair.[98]

Historically, heterotopic ossification was observed following forceful manipulation of the elbow, which led to concern regarding this form of rehabilitation for elbow stiffness. Delaying the treatment of elbow trauma was also once considered a risk factor for heterotopic ossification, but this has not proved to be a valid concern, nor is surgical delay any longer considered to be a significant variable for the development of heterotopic ossification.[99] However, multiple surgical insults within the first 7 to 14 days following trauma appears to be associated with a higher risk for the development of ectopic bone.[100]

The pathophysiology of heterotopic ossification is not completely understood. What is recognized is that the condition is the result of an inappropriate differentiation of pleuripotential mesenchymal stem cells into osteoblastic cell lines. This requires osteogenic precursor cells, an inductive agent (which is thought to most likely be a growth factor), and an environment that is conducive to osteogenesis.[101,102] An increase in circulating osteoblasic growth factors has been identified in patients with closed head injuries.[103] The bone that inappropriately develops is histologically identical to native bone but more metabolically active and without a true periosteal layer. Because heterotopic ossification is seen in association with certain HLA foci, some studies have suggested a genetic predisposition to the condition.[104,105]

Once the process of heterotopic ossification begins, there is, unfortunately, no effective medical management that underscores the importance of prophylaxis in high-risk patients. Although diphosphonates only delay bone mineralization, nonsteroidal anti-inflammatory drugs (NSAIDs) may be effective if administered within approximately 5 days of the inciting event. Indomethacin, ibuprofen, naproxen, and aspirin have all been shown to be beneficial in that they disrupt the prostaglandin pathway and experimentally inhibit the migration and differentiation of stem cells.[101,102] The duration of oral chemotherapy required to prevent heterotopic ossification is not entirely clear, and reports of its effectiveness vary regarding duration of treatment, extending from 5 days to 6 weeks of administration.[82,106]

Low-dose external beam radiation, which is thought to be effective by inhibiting the differentiation of stem cells, is a widely accepted method used to prevent heterotopic ossification. It can be given as a single dose of 600 to 700 cGy, with limited field technique decreasing soft-tissue exposure.[106-108] As with oral medication, it should also be administered within 3 to 4 days of the inciting event to be effective. Radiation-induced sarcoma has not been reported to occur in patients who received doses of external beam radiation less than 3,000 cGy.[109] An additional prophylactic modality is the early active mobilization of the elbow following an inciting event. Although clinical data support this benefit, the mechanism of action for early active mobilization is not entirely clear. [101,110-113] However, instituting active joint therapy early appears to lessen the likelihood of ectopic ossification and allows for a more rapid functional recovery following trauma.

Clinically, heterotopic ossification presents as local soft-tissue swelling, tenderness, warmth, and progressive loss of elbow motion. This inflammation-mediated condition can be mistaken for infection, especially during the perioperative period. Pain is not usually the predominant symptom, but it will be observed at the extremes of motion. Although the actual process begins at the time of the inciting event, it can occur anytime within 2 to 12 weeks thereafter. Laboratory test results reveal a transient fall in serum calcium and an increase in inorganic phosphate levels in patients with heterotopic ossification, and serum alkaline phosphatase levels begin to rise within 2 to 4 weeks and peak at three to four times the normal level at approximately 3 months.[114-116]

When heterotopic ossification develops, technetium bone scans can reveal abnormally increased metabolic activity in the first several weeks, which can remain abnormal for well over 1 year. Serial bone scans have also been used to assess the biologic activity and maturity of the process. Historically, surgical treatment to resect the heterotopic ossification was often delayed until the activity observed on serial bone scans became metabolically quiescent, often at 12 to 18 months; this was done to diminish the potential for recurrence. However, neither laboratory values nor serial bone scan have been shown to provide prognostic information; therefore, these parameters are no longer relied upon for the evaluation and treatment of heterotopic ossification in the elbow.

The most effective way to evaluate heterotopic ossification and follow its progression is to use standard radiography. Within several weeks, a fluffy, ill-defined periarticular density can be identified (Fig. 8). With time, the margins become more distinct with trabeculation. Radiographic maturity, defined as the ability to identify sharp cortical margins, commonly takes 3 to 5 months. It is now recognized that surgical intervention can safely proceed at this time. In children, however, it may be prudent to wait

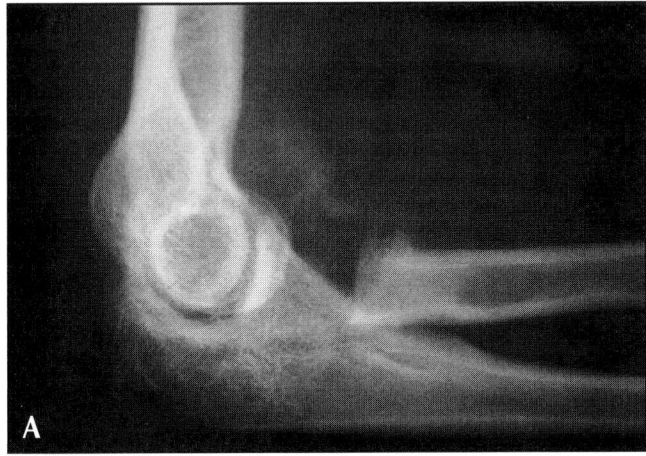

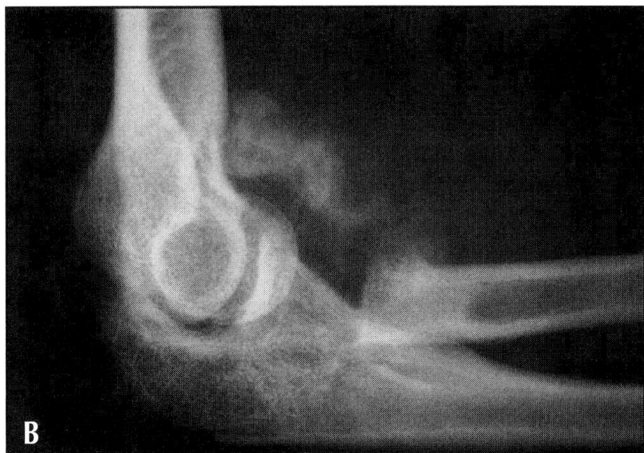

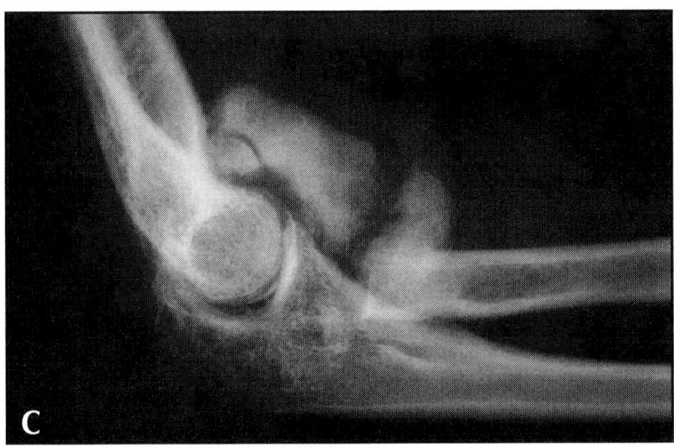

Fig. 8 A, Heterotopic ossification typically begins as a fluffy, ill-defined density as seen in this lateral radiograph 4 weeks after radial head resection. **B,** Lateral radiograph obtained at 8 weeks reveals consolidation of the ectopic bone with poorly defined borders. **C,** At 16 weeks, the process appears mature, with sharp cortical margins.

longer because nonbridging heterotopic bone may resorb over time in skeletally immature individuals.[117]

Heterotopic bone formation can develop in a localized or more diffuse pattern and does not necessarily follow anatomic tissue planes. Furthermore, its development does not necessarily imply a loss of motion or function. Surgical resection is only indicated for functional impairment. When it develops anteriorly, the process most commonly forms beneath the brachialis muscle and is separated from the anterior articular surface by an area of radiolucency. Posterior heterotopic bone often forms in continuity with the joint beneath the triceps. This is the most common pattern leading to complete ankylosis.

In the majority of cases, plain radiographs are adequate to follow heterotopic bone growth and preoperatively plan surgical resection. In complex cases, CT may be helpful to define the status of the ulnohumeral joint and the geometry of the ectopic bone. Three-dimensional reconstructions can be particularly helpful in this regard (Fig. 1). It has been determined that earlier resection of the heterotopic ossification will limit capsular and ligamentous contracture, muscle atrophy, and cartilage degeneration and allow a more rapid functional return. Early surgical intervention may also be technically easier.

The appropriate surgical approach for resection depends, in part, on the location and extent of the ectopic bone. Surgical principles include bony resection with burrs, curettes, osteotomes, and rongeurs, with identification and protection of the radial, median, and ulnar nerves when indicated. Posterior heterotopic ossification requires elevation of the triceps in part or completely from the olecranon. With posteromedial involvement, the ulnar nerve can be totally encased in a shell of bone without preoperative neurologic symptoms (Fig. 9). As there is often no demonstrable difference in the quality and appearance of the heterotopic bone and the host cortex, resection is facilitated with the use of intraoperative fluoroscopy.

In cases of complete posterior ankylosis, the goal is to identify the articular level along the medial or lateral ulnohumeral joint and obtain a jog of motion, which helps identify the appropriate plane for further resection. Care is taken to protect the collateral ligaments, although this is not always possible, especially with extensive posteromedial

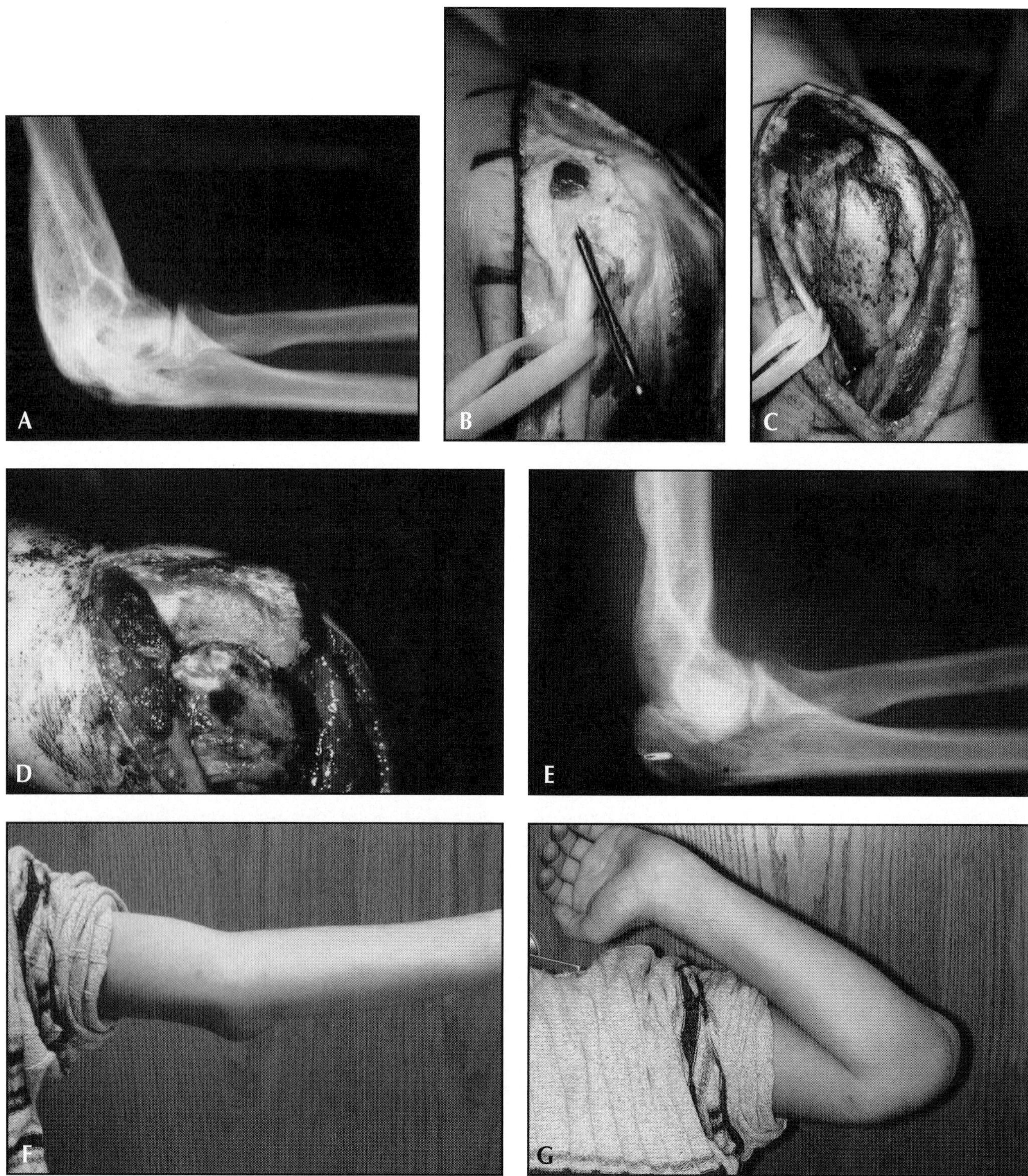

Fig. 9 A, Lateral radiograph of the left elbow of a person following closed head trauma reveals profound posterior heterotopic ossification with complete obliteration of the ulnohumeral joint and ankylosis. **B,** Intraoperative photograph depicts the ulnar nerve encased beneath a shell of bone through a posterior approach. The elevator defines the nerve path. The patient had no preoperative ulnar nerve symptoms. **C,** Medial view following nerve decompression and mobilization. The triceps is reflected laterally revealing the heterotopic bone bridging the olecranon and humerus. **D,** Intraoperative photograph of the ulnohumeral joint following resection of the ectopic bone. The joint cartilage was preserved even several years following injury. **E,** Lateral radiograph following resection. Extension **(F)** and flexion **(G)** of the elbow at follow-up.

involvement. Even in long-standing cases with ulnohumeral joint ankylosis, the articular surfaces are invariably preserved, in which case it may be radiocapitellar joint motion that is responsible for synovial fluid distribution and the maintenance of articular integrity over time.

Anterior heterotopic ossification is most commonly approached from the medial or lateral sides or both in more extensive cases (Fig. 10). Ectopic bone location dictates the approach. The lateral approach allows the radiocapitellar and proximal radioulnar joints to be addressed, and the medial approach allows decompression of the ulnar nerve and ulnohumeral exposure.[59,118,119] The anatomic plane that is chosen will be independent of the skin incision, and both approaches can usually be performed without damaging the collateral ligaments.

Anterior ectopic bone can follow the brachialis, biceps, or capsule or extend proximally off the coronoid. When there is extensive anterolateral ossification, it is often prudent to identify the radial and posterior interosseous nerves. The median nerve is most commonly protected by the brachialis, although care must be taken to keep the plane of dissection beneath this muscle belly. An anatomic plane between the anterior articular surface and the heterotopic bone at the joint level will facilitate the resection. Proximally and distally, the ectopic bone often becomes contiguous with the anterior cortices of the distal humerus and/or bones of the proximal forearm.

After complete heterotopic bone resection, it is often necessary to perform a formal capsular release to obtain full elbow motion. This includes anterior and posterior capsular resection; clearance of any impingement in the coronoid, radial, and olecranion fossae; and tenolysis of the triceps and brachialis in long-standing cases. In patients lacking significant elbow flexion preoperatively or in those with clinical evidence of ulnar nerve irritability

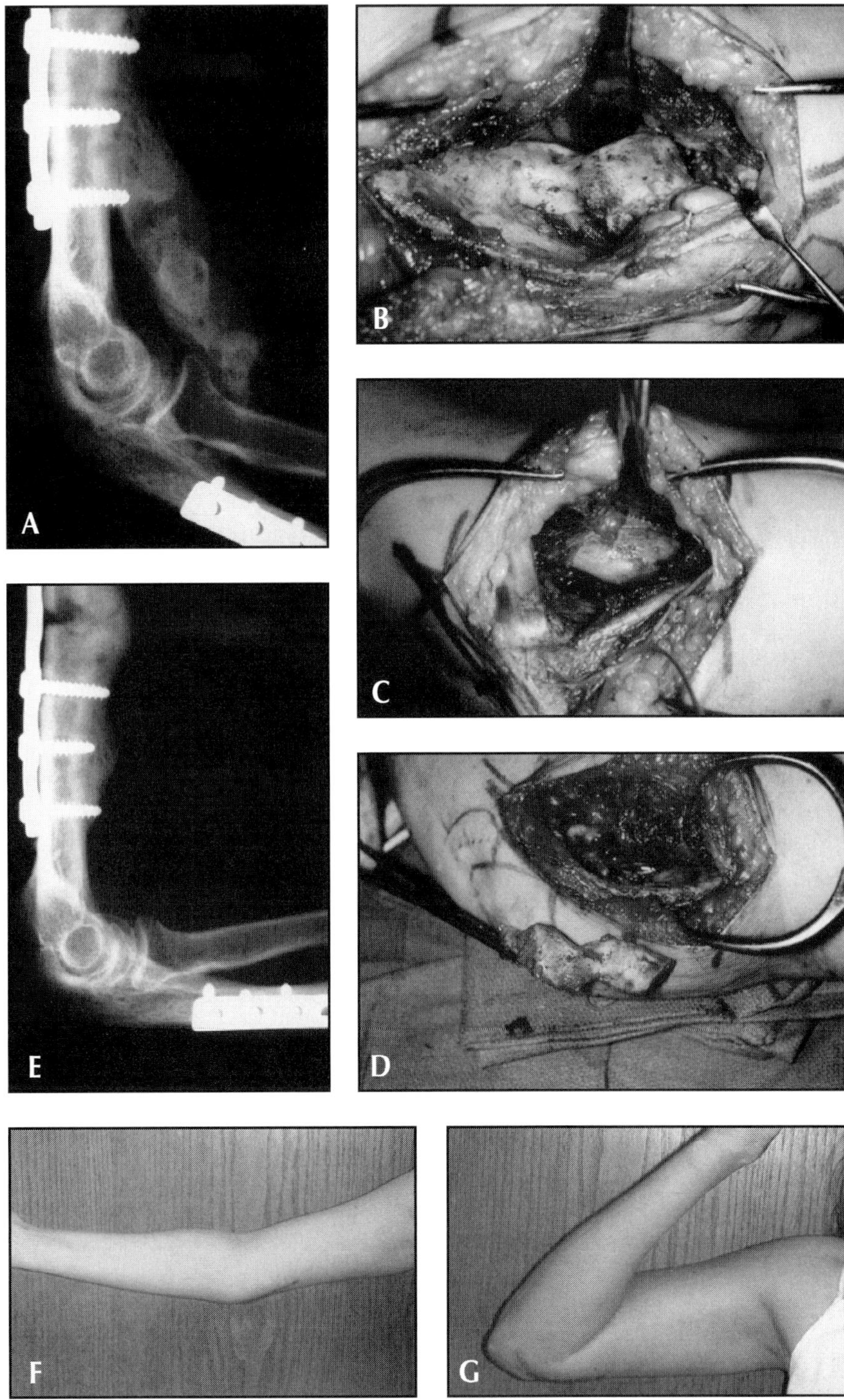

Fig. 10 A, Lateral radiograph of right elbow depicting anterior heterotopic ossification and joint ankylosis in a person with trauma to the humerus and proximal forearm and mild closed head injury. This was resected through both a deep lateral and medial approach to the joint. **B,** Intraoperative photograph revealing deep lateral exposure. Note the anterior aspect of the radiocapitellar joint and the ectopic bone more medially. **C,** Intraoperative photograph of the deep medial approach revealing ectopic bone. **D,** The plane between the bone and the joint is better visualized from the medial side facilitating resection. **E,** Follow-up lateral radiograph. Extension **(F)** and flexion **(G)** of the elbow at follow-up.

preoperatively, transposition of the nerve anterior to the joint axis is indicated to decrease the potential for ulnar nerve tension signs that can occur following rapid recovery of terminal joint flexion.

Postoperatively, as with other elbow-release procedures, long-acting axillary block anesthesia and CPM of the elbow will facilitate rehabilitation. Therapy is begun shortly after surgery and consists of edema control modalities, active and gentle passive motion, low-weighted stretches, and patient-adjusted static elbow splints. Although there is some evidence to suggest that it may not be necessary in all cases, it is common to use some form of prophylaxis (an NSAID or low-dose radiation) in most cases to decrease the potential for recurrence.[113]

Depending on the severity of the initial injury and the resultant heterotopic ossification, resection of heterotopic bone in the elbow can achieve appreciable results. In the majority of patients, functional arc of joint motion can be regained, even in patients with long-standing ulnohumeral joint ankylosis. Negative predictive factors following resection include residual spasticity and incomplete neurologic recovery of the upper extremity, both of which correlate with a higher recurrence rate of heterotopic ossification.[120,121] Although limited partial regrowth of heterotopic bone can occur, regrowth is only clinically significant when it limits elbow motion, and functionally limiting recurrence is rare.

Nonunion of the Distal Humerus

When a fracture of the distal humerus fails to unite, associated synovial pseudarthrosis, loose implants, capular contracture, and an ulnar neuropathy often occur.[122-126] Attempts to gain union are made more complex by sclerotic fracture surfaces, small articular fracture fragments, and poor bone quality, which has led some researchers to suggest that total elbow arthroscopy may be a viable reconstructive option, especially in the older patient.[127] The impact of an associated capsular contracture not only adds to the complexity of surgical treatment of the nonunion, but it will also have a negative impact on the overall functional outcome. Ackerman and Jupiter[122] reported on the internal fixation of 20 distal humeral nonunions, noting a substantially worse functional outcome in those cases in which the fracture, despite successful union, had been interarticular. In that series, no attempt was made to release the contracted elbow capsules.

Nonunion following a distal humeral fracture may vary in the level of the nonunion, the presence of intra-articular deformity, and the degree of underlying osteopenia. Sim and Morrey[128] identified patterns of nonunion seen among patients with distal humeral fractures at the Mayo Clinic. They observed that 50% occurred at the supracondylar level, 30% resulted from a T or Y intracondylar fracture, 10% were lateral condylar nonunions, and 5% were medial condyle nonunions.

The surgical techniques to achieve union are based on an extensile exposure; posterior and anterior capsulectomy; débridement of a synovial pseudarthrosis, if present; removal of any retained hardware; ulnar nerve neurolysis and transposition; realignment and stable internal fixation; and autogenous bone graft, except for those patients in whom total elbow arthroplasty is a possibility. In addition, exposure through an olecranon osteotomy will provide optimal visualization of the joint itself, and elevation of the proximal olecranon will facilitate a complete posterior capsulectomy.

Prior to the osteotomy, it may be preferable to identify the ulnar nerve and mobilize the nerve at least 6 to 8 cm proximal and distal to the cubital tunnel. This places the nerve anterior to the medial aspect of the distal humerus. The results of neurolyses and the subcutaneous transposition of the ulnar nerve in conjunction with reconstructive procedures has been extremely encouraging, with several studies reporting improvement in both sensory and motor function.[34,41,129]

Nonunions associated with instability (flail limb) usually consist of a synovial-lined pseudarthrosis. Thorough débridement of this synovial membrane will be required to obtain realignment of the bone structures and reestablish a vascularized environment. Of particular importance is the fact that what appears on radiographs to be a very small distal fragment may be misleading because the fragment is often flexed in association with a contracted and noncompliant capsule. Excision of both posterior and anterior capsular contracture will facilitate realignment and stable internal fixation (Fig. 11).

Realignment of the bone contours of a synovial pseudarthrosis at the supracondylar level is often complicated by irregularities of the original fracture margins. In some instances, the distal part of the proximal fragment can be contoured into a chevron that is shaped with the apex pointed distally and a corresponding recess created in the distal fragment. This provides a greater surface area of contact of decorticated bone surfaces and enhances the intrinsic stability of the realignment.

When the nonunion also involves articular surfaces, precise realignment may not always be possible. The surgical goal in this instance is the same as that of internal fixation of an articular fracture (for example, to maintain the width of the trochlea). Although uncommon, it may be necessary to place a corticocancellous autogenous bone graft to achieve this.[123] Even in cases in which elbow articulation has been immobile with motion coming more proximally through a synovial pseudarthrosis, once the joint has been released and the nonunion stabilized, excellent mobility can be expected. McKee and associates[129] reported on 13 patients who were treated surgically for a malunited or nonunited intra-articular

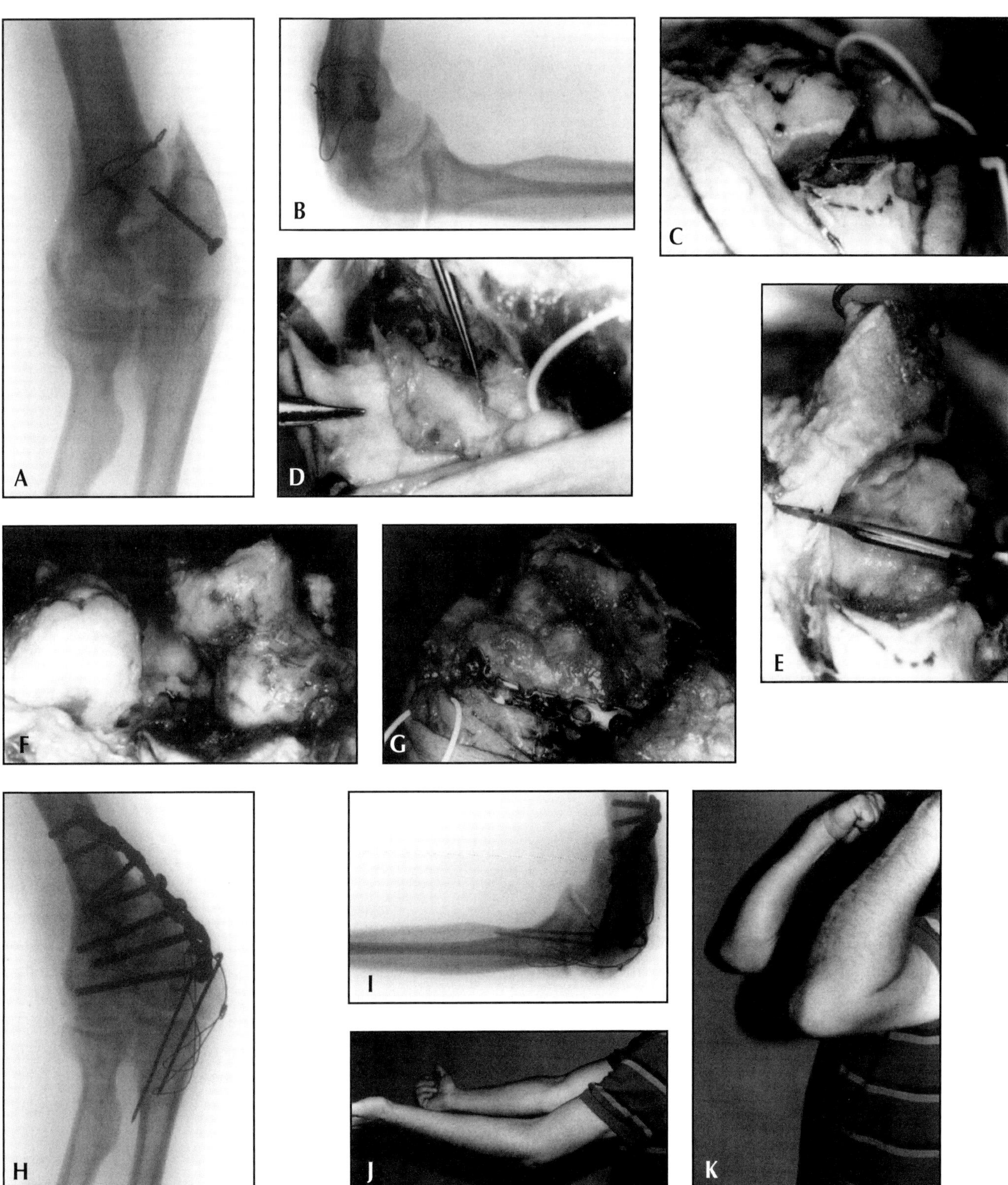

Fig. 11 An intra-articular nonunion of the distal humerus of 7-year duration in a 37-year-old man. AP (**A**) and lateral (**B**) radiographs of the intra-articular nonunion. **C,** The olecranon osteotomy is used to gain exposure of the articular surfaces. **D,** An external neurolysis of the ulnar nerve was performed. **E,** The scarred posterior capsule was sharply excised while the proximal olecranon fragment was elevated. **F,** The anterior capsule could be excised through the articular nonunion. **G,** Stable fixation with a medial band plate. An autogenous iliac crest graft was used to fill the defect. AP (**H**), and lateral (**I**) radiographs of the healed nonunion. Functional elbow flexion (**J**) and extension (**K**) at follow-up.

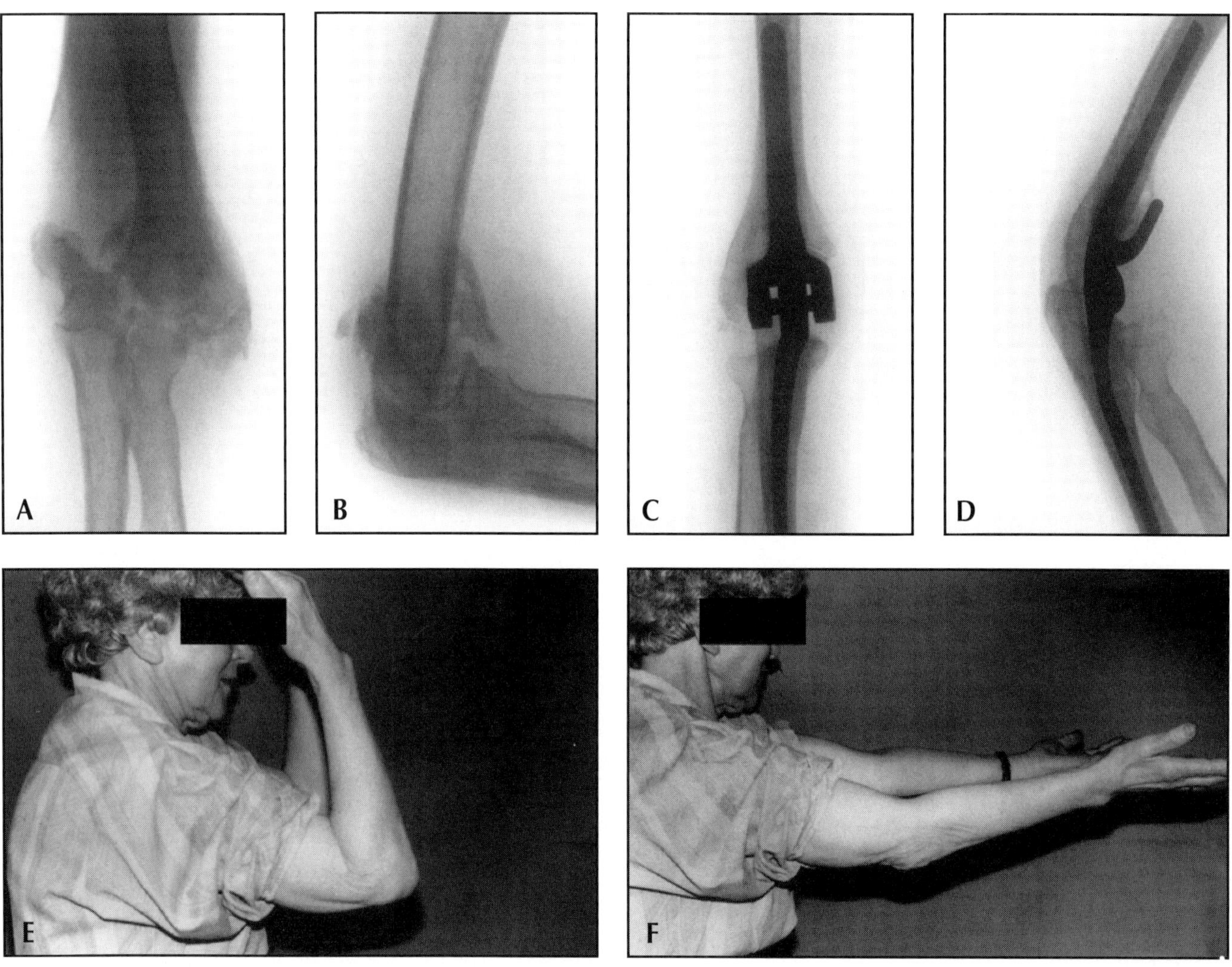

Fig. 12 An intra-articular nonunion in a 64-year-old woman with diabetes and marked collapse of the articular surfaces. AP **(A)** and lateral **(B)** radiographs of the nonunion. Two-year follow-up AP **(C)** and lateral **(D)** radiographs of the total elbow arthroplasty. Functional elbow flexion **(E)** and extension **(F)** at follow-up.

fracture of the distal humerus. An olecranon osteotomy was performed in each case, followed by extensive capsular resection. Autogenous iliac crest bone graft and stable internal fixation achieved successful union in each patient and the mean arc of elbow motion increased from 43° preoperatively to 97° postoperatively.

The techniques for achieving stable internal fixation of both the articular and supracondylar components of a fracture of the distal humerus that has failed to unite mirror those that have proven successful for the treatment of complex intra-articular fractures of the distal humerus.[35,36,130-135] Placing plates and screws at right angles to each other substantially enhances stability. Moreover, Jupiter and Goodman[34] reported the use of a third plate placed along the lateral column (others on the posterior lateral and medial columns) in the management of such nonunions in older patients.

Surgical outcomes of 40 patients with nonuniting fractures of the distal humerus who were treated to gain union were recently reviewed. Thirty-eight of these patients were available for follow-up at a mean of 54 months after surgery. Union after the index procedure was achieved in all but 4 patients. Of the 4 patients whose fractures failed to unite, successful union occurred in one after a second procedure, two underwent total elbow arthroplasty, and one refused further treatment. Additional procedures included a contracture release in one patient, implant removal in eight, and ulnar nerve transposition in two (Fig. 12). The mean arc of motion at final follow-up was 101° (range, 65° to 130°), with a mean flexion of 125° (range, 100° to 140°) and mean flexion contracture of 24° (range, 0° to 45°). Radiographic evaluation revealed no arthrosis in 19 patients, mild arthritis in

16, and moderate arthritis in 2. The Mayo functional score for the 35 patients with healed nonunions was excellent for 7, good for 27, and fair for 1.

Summary

Although the etiologies and associated conditions of stiff elbow vary, the outcomes after surgical contracture release have proved to be rewarding. The use of surgical treatment for elbow contracture offers patients the opportunity to regain a functional limb.

References

1. Akeson WH: An experimental study of joint stiffness. *J Bone Joint Surg Am* 1961;43:1022-1034.
2. Akeson WH, Amiel D, Woo SL: Immobility effects on synovial joints: The pathomechanics of joint contracture. *Biorheology* 1980;17:95-110.
3. Akeson WH, Amiel D, Mechanic GL, Woo SL, Harwood FL, Hamer ML: Collagen cross-linking alterations in joint contractures: Changes in the reducible cross-links in periarticular connective tissue collagen after nine weeks of immobilization. *Connect Tissue Res* 1977;5:15-19.
4. Byrd JW: Elbow arthroscopy for arthrofibrosis after type I radial head fractures. *Arthroscopy* 1994;10:162-165.
5. Cooney WP III: Contractures of the elbow, in Morrey BF (ed): *The Elbow and Its Disorders*, ed 2. Philadelphia, PA, WB Saunders, 1993, pp 464-475.
6. Cooper JE, Shwedy KE, Quanbury AO, Miller J, Hildebrand D: Elbow joint restriction: Effect on functional upper limb motion during performance of three feeding activities. *Arch Phys Med Rehabil* 1993;74:805-809.
7. Figgie MP, Inglis AE, Mow CS, Figgie HE III: Total elbow arthroplasty for complete ankylosis of the elbow. *J Bone Joint Surg Am* 1989;71:513-520.
8. Gates HS III, Sullivan FL, Urbaniak JR: Anterior capsulotomy and continuous passive motion in the treatment of post-traumatic flexion contracture of the elbow: A prospective study. *J Bone Joint Surg Am* 1992;74:1229-1234.
9. Itoh Y, Saegusa K, Ishiguro T, Horiuchi Y, Sasaki T, Uchinishi K: Operation for the stiff elbow. *Int Orthop* 1989;13:263-268.
10. Luppino T, Salsi A, Fiocchi R, Stefanini T, Lagana A: Arthrolysis in the treatment of ankylosis and severe posttraumatic stiffness of the elbow. *Ital J Orthop Traumatol* 1992;18:459-465.
11. Modabber MR, Jupiter JB: Reconstruction for post-traumatic conditions of the elbow joint. *J Bone Joint Surg Am* 1995;77:1431-1446.
12. Morrey BF: Post-traumatic stiffness: Distraction arthroplasty, in Morrey BF (ed): *The Elbow and Its Disorders*, ed 2. Philadelphia, PA, WB Saunders, 1993, pp 476-491.
13. Morrey BF: Post-traumatic contracture of the elbow: Operative treatment, including distraction arthroplasty. *J Bone Joint Surg Am* 1990;72:601-618.
14. Nowicki KD, Shall LM: Arthroscopic release of a posttraumatic flexion contracture in the elbow: A case report and review of the literature. *Arthroscopy* 1992;8:544-547.
15. Oyemade GA: Fascial arthroplasty for elbow ankylosis. *Int Surg* 1983;68:81-84.
16. Seth MK, Khurana JK: Bony ankylosis of the elbow after burns. *J Bone Joint Surg Br* 1985;67:747-749.
17. Wilson PD: Capsulectomy for the relief of flexion contractures of the elbow following fracture. *J Bone Joint Surg* 1944;26:71-86.
18. Motzkin NE, Cahalan TD, Morrey BF, An KN, Chao EY: Isometric and isokinetic endurance testing of the forearm complex. *Am J Sports Med* 1991;19:107-111.
19. Simon WH, Friedenberg S, Richardson S: Joint congruence: A correlation of joint congruence and thickness of articular cartilage in dogs. *J Bone Joint Surg Am* 1973;55:1614-1620.
20. Tucker K: Some aspects of post-traumatic elbow stiffness. *Injury* 1978;9:216-220.
21. Weiss AP, Sachar K: Soft tissue contractures about the elbow. *Hand Clin* 1994;10:439-451.
22. Morrey BF, Askew LJ, An KN, Chao EY: A biomechanical study of normal functional elbow motion. *J Bone Joint Surg Am* 1981;63:872-877.
23. Askew LJ, An KN, Morrey BF, Chao EY: Functional evaluation of the elbow: Normal motion requirements and strength determinations. *Trans Orthop Res Soc* 1981;6:183.
24. Morrey BF: Anatomy and kinematics of the elbow. *Instr Course Lect* 1991;40:11-16.
25. Nicol AC, Berme N, Paul JP: A biomechanical analysis of elbow joint function, in *Joint Replacement in the Upper Limb*. London, England, Institution of Mechanical Engineers, 1977, pp 45-51.
26. Kapandji IA (ed): *The Physiology of the Joints: Annotated Diagrams of the Mechanics of the Human Joints*, ed 5. Edinburgh, Scotland, Churchill Livingstone, 1982, vol 1, pp 72-96.
27. Kay NRM: Arthrolysis of the post-traumatic stiff elbow, in Stanley D, Kay NRM (eds): *Surgery of the Elbow: Practical and Scientific Aspects*. London, England, Edward Arnold, 1998, pp 228-234.
28. Apfelberg DB, Larson SJ: Dynamic anatomy of the ulnar nerve at the elbow. *Plast Reconstr Surg* 1973;51:79-81.
29. Froimson AI, Anouchi YS, Seitz WH Jr, Winsberg DD: Ulnar nerve decompression with medial epicondylectomy for neuropathy at the elbow. *Clin Orthop* 1991;265:200-206.
30. Galbraith KA, McCullough CJ: Acute nerve injury as a complication of closed fractures or dislocations of the elbow. *Injury* 1979;11:159-164.
31. Heithoff SJ, Millender LH, Nalebuff EA, Petruska AJ Jr: Medial epicondylectomy for the treatment of ulnar nerve compression at the elbow. *J Hand Surg Am* 1990;15:22-29.
32. Jobe FW, Fanton GS, Elattrache NS: Ulnar nerve injury, in Morrey BF (ed): *The Elbow and Its Disorders*, ed 2. Philadelphia, PA, WB Saunders, 1993, pp 560-565.
33. Josefsson PO, Johnell O, Gentz CF: Long-term sequelae of simple dislocation of the elbow. *J Bone Joint Surg Am* 1984;66:927-930.
34. Jupiter JB, Goodman LJ: The management of complex distal humerus nonunion in the elderly by elbow capsulectomy, triple plating, and ulnar nerve neurolysis. *J Shoulder Elbow Surg* 1992;1:37-46.
35. Jupiter JB, Mehne DK: Trauma to the adult elbow and fractures of the distal humerus, in Browner BD, Jupiter JB, Levine AM, Trafton PG (eds): *Skeletal Trauma: Fractures, Dislocations, Ligamentous Injuries*. Philadelphia, PA, WB Saunders, 1992, vol 2, pp 1125-1176.
36. Jupiter JB, Morrey BF: Fractures of the distal humerus in the adult, in Morrey BF (ed): *The Elbow and its Disorders*, ed 2. Philadelphia, PA, WB Saunders, 1993, pp 328-366.
37. Laurencin CT, Schwartz JT Jr, Koris MJ: Compression of the ulnar nerve at the elbow in association with synovial cysts. *Orthop Rev* 1994;23:62-65.
38. Manske PR, Johnston R, Pruitt DL, Strecker WB: Ulnar nerve decompression at the cubital tunnel. *Clin Orthop* 1992; 274:231-237.
39. McGowan AJ: The results of transposition of the ulnar nerve for traumatic ulnar neuritis. *J Bone Joint Surg Br* 1950;32:293-301.
40. McKee MD, Jupiter JB: A contemporary approach to the management of complex fractures of the distal humerus and their sequelae. *Hand Clin* 1994;10:479-494.
41. McKee M, Jupiter J, Toh CL, Wilson L, Colton C, Karras KK: Reconstruction after malunion and nonunion of intra-articular fractures of the distal humerus: Methods and results in 13 adults. *J Bone Joint Surg Br* 1994;76:614-621.
42. O'Driscoll SW, Horii E, Carmichael SW, Morrey BF: The cubital tunnel and ulnar neuropathy. *J Bone Joint Surg Br* 1991;73:613-617.
43. Rettig AC, Ebben JR: Anterior subcutaneous transfer of the ulnar nerve in the athlete. *Am J Sports Med* 1993;21:836-840.
44. Sharma RK, Covell NA: An unusual ulnar nerve injury associated with dislocation of the elbow. *Injury* 1976;8:145-147.
45. Uchida Y, Sugioka Y: Ulnar nerve palsy after supracondylar humerus fracture. *Acta Orthop Scand* 1990;61:118-119.
46. Wadsworth TG: The external compression syndrome of the ulnar nerve at the cubital tunnel. *Clin Orthop* 1977;124:189-204.
47. Wang KC, Shih HN, Hsu KY, Shih CH: Intercondylar fractures of the distal humerus: Routine anterior subcutaneous transposition of the ulnar nerve in a posterior operative approach. *J Trauma* 1994;36:770-773.

48. Bonutti PM, Windau JE, Ables BA, Miller BG: Static progressive stretch to reestablish elbow range of motion. *Clin Orthop* 1994;303: 128-134.

49. Duke JB, Tessler RH, Dell PC: Manipulation of the stiff elbow with patient under anesthesia. *J Hand Surg Am* 1991;16:19-24.

50. Green DP, McCoy H: Turnbuckle orthotic correction of elbow-flexion contractures after acute injuries. *J Bone Joint Surg Am* 1979;61:1092-1095.

51. Karachalios T, Maxwell-Armstrong C, Atkins RM: Treatment of post-traumatic fixed flexion deformity of the elbow using an intermittent compression garment. *Injury* 1994;25:313-315.

52. Shewring DJ, Beaudet M, Carvell JE: Reversed dynamic slings: Results of use in the treatment of post-traumatic flexion contractures of the elbow. *Injury* 1991;22:400-402.

53. Zander CL, Healy NL: Elbow flexion contractures treated with serial casts and conservative therapy. *J Hand Surg Am* 1992;17:694-697.

54. Gelinas JJ, Faber KJ, Patterson SD, King GJ: The effectiveness of turnbuckle splinting for elbow contractures. *J Bone Joint Surg Br* 2000;82:74-78.

55. Mohan K: Myositis ossificans traumatica of the elbow. *Int Surg* 1972;57:475-478.

56. Jones GS, Savoie FH III: Arthroscopic capsular release of flexion contractures (arthrofibrosis) of the elbow. *Arthroscopy* 1993;9:277-283.

57. O'Driscoll SW: Elbow reconstruction, in Frymoyer JW (ed): *Orthopaedic Knowledge Update 4: Home Study Syllabus*. Rosemont, IL, American Academy of Orthopaedic Surgeons, 1993, pp 335-352.

58. Urbaniak JR, Hansen PE, Beissinger SF, Aitken MS: Correction of post-traumatic flexion contracture of the elbow by anterior capsulotomy. *J Bone Joint Surg Am* 1985;67:1160-1164.

59. Cohen MS, Hastings H II: Operative capsular release for elbow contracture: The lateral collateral ligament sparing operative technique. *Orthop Clin North Am* 1999;30:133-139.

60. Mansat P, Morrey BF, Hotchkiss RN: Extrinsic contracture: "The column procedure": Lateral and medial capsular releases, in Morrey BF (ed): *The Elbow and Its Disorders*, ed 3. Philadelphia, PA, WB Saunders, 2000, pp 447-456.

61. Mansat P, Morrey BF: The column procedure: A limited lateral approach for extrinsic contracture of the elbow. *J Bone Joint Surg Am* 1998;80:1603-1615.

62. Gallay SH, Richards RR, O'Driscoll SW: Intraarticular capacity and compliance of stiff and normal elbows. *Arthroscopy* 1993;9:9-13.

63. O'Driscoll SW, Morrey BF, An K-N: Intraarticular pressure and capacity of the elbow. *Arthroscopy* 1990;6:100-103.

64. Timmerman LA, Andrews JR: Arthroscopic treatment of posttraumatic elbow pain and stiffness. *Am J Sports Med* 1994;22:230-235.

65. Kelly EW, Morrey BF, O'Driscoll SW: Complications of elbow arthroscopy. *J Bone Joint Surg Am* 2001;83:25-34.

66. O'Driscoll SW: Arthroscopic treatment for osteoarthritis of the elbow. *Orthop Clin North Am* 1995;26:691-706.

67. Lindenfeld TN: Medial approach in elbow arthroscopy. *Am J Sports Med* 1990;18:413-417.

68. Lynch GJ, Meyers JF, Whipple TL, Caspari RB: Neurovascular anatomy and elbow arthroscopy: Inherent risks. *Arthroscopy* 1986;2:190-197.

69. Marshall PD, Fairclough JA, Johnson SR, Evans EJ: Avoiding nerve damage during elbow arthoscopy. *J Bone Joint Surg Br* 1993;75: 129-131.

70. Miller CD, Jobe CM, Wright MH: Neuroanatomy in elbow arthroscopy. *J Shoulder Elbow Surg* 1995;4:168-174.

71. O'Driscoll SW: Elbow arthroscopy: Loose bodies, in Morrey BF (ed): *The Elbow and Its Disorders*, ed 3. Philadelphia, PA, WB Saunders Company, 2000, pp 510-514.

72. O'Driscoll SW: Operative elbow arthroscopy: Part I. Loose bodies and synovial conditions, in Green DP, Hotchkiss RN, Pederson WC (eds): *Green's Operative Hand Surgery*, ed 4. New York, NY, Churchill Livingstone, 1999, pp 235-249.

73. O'Driscoll SW: Loose bodies of the elbow, in Norris TR (ed): *Orthopaedic Knowledge Update: Shoulder and Elbow*. Rosemont, IL, American Academy of Orthopaedic Surgeons, 1997, pp 355-362.

74. O'Driscoll SW: Elbow arthroscopy for loose bodies. *Orthopedics* 1992;15:855-859.

75. Bain GI, Mehta JA, Heptinstall RJ: The dynamic elbow suspension splint. *J Shoulder Elbow Surg* 1998;7:419-421.

76. O'Driscoll SW, Giori NJ: Continuous passive motion (CPM): Theory and principles of clinical application. *J Rehabil Res Dev* 2000;37: 179-188.

77. Husband JB, Hastings H II: The lateral approach for operative release of post-traumatic contracture of the elbow. *J Bone Joint Surg Am* 1990;72:1353-1358.

78. Mih AD, Wolf FG: Surgical release of elbow-capsular contracture in pediatric patients. *J Pediatr Orthop* 1994;14:458-461.

79. Moritomo H, Tada K, Yoshida T: Early, wide excision of heterotopic ossification in the medial elbow. *J Shoulder Elbow Surg* 2001;10: 164-168.

80. Morrey BF: Anterior capsular release for flexion contracture, in Morrey BF (ed): *Master Techniques in Orthopaedic Surgery: The Elbow*. New York, NY, Raven Press, 1994, pp 291-305.

81. Morrey BF: Distraction arthroplasty: Clinical applications. *Clin Orthop* 1993;293:46-54.

82. Viola RW, Hanel DP: Early "simple" release of posttraumatic elbow contracture associated with heterotopic ossification. *J Hand Surg Am* 1999;24:370-380.

83. Cohen AP, Redden JF, Stanley D: Treatment of osteoarthritis of the elbow: A comparison of open and arthroscopic debridement. *Arthroscopy* 2000;16:701-706.

84. Micheli LJ, Luke AC, Mintzer CM, Waters PM: Elbow arthroscopy in the pediatric and adolescent population. *Arthroscopy* 2001;17: 694-699.

85. O'Driscoll SW: Elbow: Reconstruction, in Kasser JR (ed): *Orthopaedic Knowledge Update 5: Home Study Syllabus*. Rosemont, IL, American Academy of Orthopaedic Surgeons, 1996, pp 283-294.

86. Haapaniemi T, Berggren M, Adolfsson L: Complete transection of the median and radial nerves during arthroscopic release of post-traumatic elbow contracture. *Arthroscopy* 1999;15:784-787.

87. Papilion JD, Neff RS, Shall LM: Compression neuropathy of the radial nerve as a complication of elbow arthroscopy: A case report and review of the literature. *Arthroscopy* 1988;4: 284-286.

88. Roberts PH: Dislocation of the elbow. *Br J Surg* 1969;56:806-815.

89. Thompson HC III, Garcia A: Myositis ossificans: Aftermath of elbow injuries. *Clin Orthop* 1967;50:129-134.

90. Stover SL, Hataway CJ, Zeiger HE: Heterotopic ossification in spinal cord-injured patients. *Arch Phys Med Rehabil* 1975;56: 199-204.

91. Garland DE: A clinical perspective on common forms of acquired heterotopic ossification. *Clin Orthop* 1991;263:13-29.

92. Roberts JB, Pankratz DG: The surgical treatment of heterotopic ossification at the elbow following long-term coma. *J Bone Joint Surg Am* 1979;61:760-763.

93. Garland DE, O'Hollaren RM: Fractures and dislocations about the elbow in the head-injured adult. *Clin Orthop* 1982;168:38-41.

94. Sazbon L, Najenson T, Tartakovsky M, Becker E, Grosswasser Z: Widespread periarticular new-bone formation in long-term comatose patients. *J Bone Joint Surg Br* 1981;63:120-125.

95. Hoffer MM, Brody G, Ferlic F: Excision of heterotopic ossification about elbows in patients with thermal injury. *J Trauma* 1978;18:667-670.

96. Holguin PH, Rico AA, Garcia JP, Del Rio JL: Elbow anchylosis due to postburn heterotopic ossification. *J Burn Care Rehabil* 1996;17: 150-154.

97. Peterson SL, Mani MM, Crawford CM, Neff JR, Hiebert JM: Postburn heterotopic ossification: Insights for management decision making. *J Trauma* 1989;29:365-369.

98. Failla JM, Amadio PC, Morrey BF, Beckenbaugh RD: Proximal radioulnar synostosis after repair of distal biceps brachii rupture by the two-incision technique: Report of four cases. *Clin Orthop* 1990;253:133-136.

99. McLaughlin HL: Some fractures with a time limit. *Surg Clin North Am* 1955;35:553-561.

100. Morrey BF: Ectopic ossifcation about the elbow, in Morrey BF (ed): *The Elbow and Its*

Disorders, ed 3. Philadelphia, PA, WB Saunders, 2000, pp 437-446.

101. Ellerin BE, Helfet D, Parikh S, et al: Current therapy in the management of heterotopic ossification of the elbow: A review with case studies. *Am J Phys Med Rehabil* 1999;78:259-271.

102. Summerfield SL, DiGiovanni C, Weiss AP: Heterotopic ossifcation of the elbow. *J Shoulder Elbow Surg* 1997;6:321-332.

103. Bidner SM, Rubins IM, Desjardins JV, Zuckor DJ, Goltzman D: Evidence for a humoral mechanism for enhanced osteogenesis after head injury. *J Bone Joint Surg Am* 1990;72:1144-1149.

104. Garland DE, Alday B, Venos KG: Heterotopic ossification and HLA antigens. *Arch Phys Med Rehabil* 1984;65:531-532.

105. Hunter T, Dubo HI, Hildahl CR, Smith NJ, Schroeder ML: Histocompatibility antigens in patients with spinal cord injury or cerebral damage complicated by heterotopic ossification. *Rheumatol Rehabil* 1980;19:97-99.

106. Hastings H II, Graham TJ: The classification and treatment of heterotopic ossification about the elbow and forearm. *Hand Clin* 1994;10: 417-437.

107. Abrams RA, Simmons BP, Brown RA, Botte MJ: Treatment of posttraumatic radioulnar synostosis with excision and low-dose radiation. *J Hand Surg Am* 1993;18:703-707.

108. McAuliffe JA, Wolfson AH: Early excision of heterotopic ossification about the elbow followed by radiation therapy. *J Bone Joint Surg Am* 1997;79:749-755.

109. Kim JH, Chu FC, Woodard HQ, Melamed MR, Huvos A, Cantin J: Radiation-induced soft-tissue and bone sarcoma. *Radiology* 1978;129:501-508.

110. Crawford CM, Varghese G, Mani MM, Neff JR: Heterotopic ossification: Are range of motion exercises contraindicated? *J Burn Care Rehabil* 1986;7:323-327.

111. Dias DA: Heterotopic para-articular ossification of the elbow with soft tisssue contracture in burns. *Burns Incl Therm Inj* 1982;9:128-134.

112. Jupiter JB: Heterotopic ossification about the elbow. *Instr Course Lect* 1991;40:41-44.

113. Jupiter JB, Ring D: Operative treatment of post-traumatic proximal radioulnar synostosis. *J Bone Joint Surg Am* 1998;80:248-257.

114. Bolger JT: Heterotopic bone formation and alkaline phosphatase. *Arch Phys Med Rehabil* 1975;56:36-39.

115. Furman R, Nicholas JJ, Jivoff L: Elevation of the serum alkaline phosphatase coincident with ectopic-bone formation in paraplegic patients. *J Bone Joint Surg Am* 1970;52:1131-1137.

116. Orzel JA, Rudd TG: Heterotopic bone formation: Clinical, laboratory, and imaging correlation. *J Nucl Med* 1985;26:125-132.

117. Viola RW, Hastings H II: Treatment of ectopic ossification about the elbow. *Clin Orthop* 2000;370:65-86.

118. Cohen MS, Hastings H II: Post-traumatic contracture of the elbow: Operative release using a lateral collateral ligament sparing approach. *J Bone Joint Surg Br* 1998;80:805-812.

119. Kasparyan NG, Hotchkiss RN: Dynamic skeletal fixation in the upper extremity. *Hand Clin* 1997;13:643-663.

120. Garland DE: Surgical approaches for resection of heterotopic ossification in traumatic brain-injured adults. *Clin Orthop* 1991;263:59-70.

121. Garland DE, Hanscom DA, Keenan MA, Smith C, Moore T: Resection of heterotopic ossification in the adult with head trauma. *J Bone Joint Surg Am* 1985;67:1261-1269.

122. Ackerman G, Jupiter JB: Non-union of fractures of the distal end of the humerus. *J Bone Joint Surg Am* 1988;70:75-83.

123. Cobb TK, Linscheid RL: Late correction of malunited intercondylar humeral fractures: Intra-articular osteotomy and tricortical bone grafting. *J Bone Joint Surg Br* 1994;76:622-626.

124. Figgie MP, Inglis AE, Mow CS, Figgie HE III: Salvage of non-union of supracondylar fracture of the humerus by total elbow arthroplasty. *J Bone Joint Surg Am* 1989;71:1058-1065.

125. Helfet DL, Rosen H: The management of non-unions of the lower end of the humerus. *Orthop Trans* 1988;12:679.

126. Helfet DL, Schmeling GJ: Bicondylar intraarticular fractures of the distal humerus in adults. *Clin Orthop* 1993;292:26-36.

127. Morrey BF, Adams RA: Semiconstrained elbow replacement for distal humeral nonunion. *J Bone Joint Surg Br* 1995;77:67-72.

128. Sim FH, Morrey BF: Nonunion and delayed union of distal humeral fractures, in Morrey BF (ed): *The Elbow and its Disorders*, ed 3. Philadelphia, PA, WB Saunders, 2000, pp 331-340.

129. McKee MD, Jupiter JB, Bosse G, Goodman L: Outcome of ulnar neurolysis during post-traumatic reconstruction of the elbow. *J Bone Joint Surg Br* 1988;80:100-105.

130. Holdsworth BJ, Mossad MM: Fractures of the adult distal humerus: Elbow function after internal fixation. *J Bone Joint Surg Br* 1990;72:362-365.

131. Hotchkiss RN, Green DP: Fractures and dislocations of the elbow, in Rockwood CA Jr, Green DP, Bucholz RW (eds): *Fractures in Adults*, ed 3. Philadelphia, PA, JB Lippincott, 1991, pp 739-841.

132. Jupiter JB: The management of multiple fractures in one upper extremity: A case report. *J Hand Surg Am* 1986;11:279-282.

133. Jupiter JB, Neff U, Holzach P, Allgöwer M: Intercondylar fractures of the humerus: An operative approach. *J Bone Joint Surg Am* 1985;67:226-239.

134. Müller ME, Allgöwer M, Schneider R, Willenegger H (eds): *Manual of Internal Fixation: Techniques Recommended by the AO Group*, ed 2. Berlin, Germany, Springer-Verlag, 1979, pp 176-181.

135. Zagorski JB: Complex fractures about the elbow. *Instr Course Lect* 1990;39:265-270.

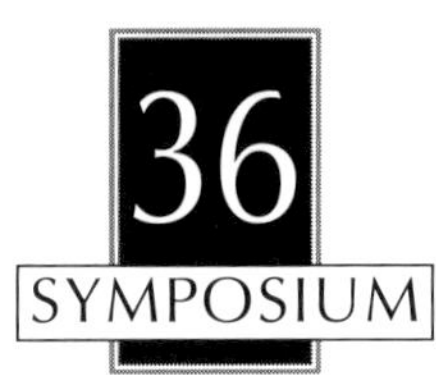

Nonreplacement Reconstruction of the Elbow Joint

Bernard F. Morrey, MD

Arthrodesis

Arthrodesis of the elbow is not commonly indicated. Functionally, a limited range of 100° in midposition is enough for most daily activities, but removing all elbow motion restricts most personal body functions.[1] Most experience with fusion of the elbow has come from spontaneous arthrodesis occurring after infection, trauma, or rheumatic disease of the elbow. In my experience, these patients have great difficulty adjusting to this dysfunction. Hence, in patients older than 45 years with bilateral disease and limited shoulder or wrist motion, interposition arthroplasty is preferred. Arthrodesis may be indicated in younger patients with posttraumatic unilateral arthrosis of an elbow requiring strength and stability.

Complications

Nonunion is the most bothersome problem after arthrodesis but appears to be decreasing in recent years with improved experience.[2] The long lever arm created by elbow fusion causes increased stress along the entire extremity. Fracture through or proximal to the fused or ankylosed joint is not uncommon and occurred in 4 of 17 patients reported by Koch and Lipscomb.[3] In spite of the improved fusion rate with enhanced techniques, the functional limitation is such that I very seldom, if ever, select fusion as a viable alternative to some other form of reconstructive surgical procedure at the elbow.

Interposition Arthroplasty

Interposition arthroplasty, one of the oldest reconstructive procedures, continues to be a viable reconstruction option, especially in young patients and in those unable or unwilling to adjust to the lifting restrictions created by prosthetic replacement.

Indications

The ongoing need to treat severe arthritis in patients in the third, fourth, or fifth decades of life continues to warrant consideration of this alternative procedure to restore motion and relieve discomfort in relatively young adults. Specifically, interposition arthroplasty is especially attractive in the treatment of patients younger than 40 to 50 years of age with posttraumatic ankylosis of the elbow[4] with good motion but severe pain, and in some younger patients with inflammatory arthritis. The anatomic requisite is that the broad contour of the distal humerus must be present. For patients with ankylosis, additional procedures may be necessary, such as extensive soft-tissue release or reconstruction of the distal humerus. Osteosynthesis may be required before or at the time of the interposition procedure. Young adults with stage I or II rheumatoid arthritis with stiff or painful elbows can be successfully treated with this technique.[5]

Contraindications

Arthroplasty procedures are contraindicated in the presence of active infection. Residual instability is a major determinant of outcome, and the grossly unstable rheumatoid or posttraumatic elbow cannot be adequately stabilized by a fascial interposition procedure. Congenital ankylosis of the elbow joint lacks the necessary soft-tissue ligamentous and muscular support to allow soft-tissue interposition. As with other elbow arthroplasty techniques, the patient's need to use the upper extremities in ambulation or transfer from bed to chair is a relative contraindication because excessive loading of the elbow will destabilize the joint. The noncompliant patient should be identified and avoided.

Preferred Tissue

The record of various tissues used as interposition arthroplasty of the elbow is colorful and includes muscle flaps, pig bladder, fat, fascia, chromatized zenografts, and dermis.[6] In general, autogenous skin and fascia and Achilles tendon allografts are currently favored. The cutis is very durable and thick, rapidly adheres to the bone, and has been quite successful in early and more recently reported experiences.[7-9] Cutis harvest techniques are relatively simple and the thin tissue obtained allows easier primary closure than bulkier interposition materials. Harvesting cutis tissue without the epidermis is somewhat more difficult. Fascia also is commonly used;[10,11] it is readily available from the thigh and can be overlapped to ensure adequate bulk. The Achilles tendon allograft is attractive for

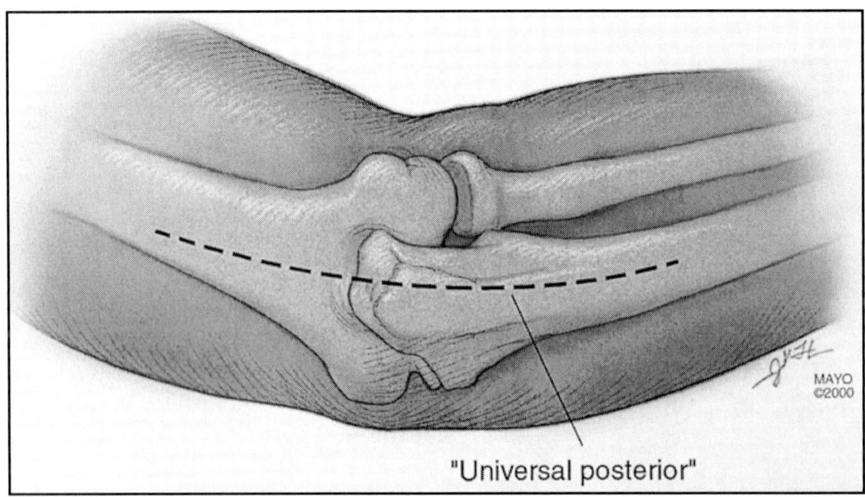

Fig. 1 A universal posterior skin incision is made to allow exposure of both the medial and lateral aspects of the joint. (Reproduced with permission from the Mayo Foundation, Rochester, MN.)

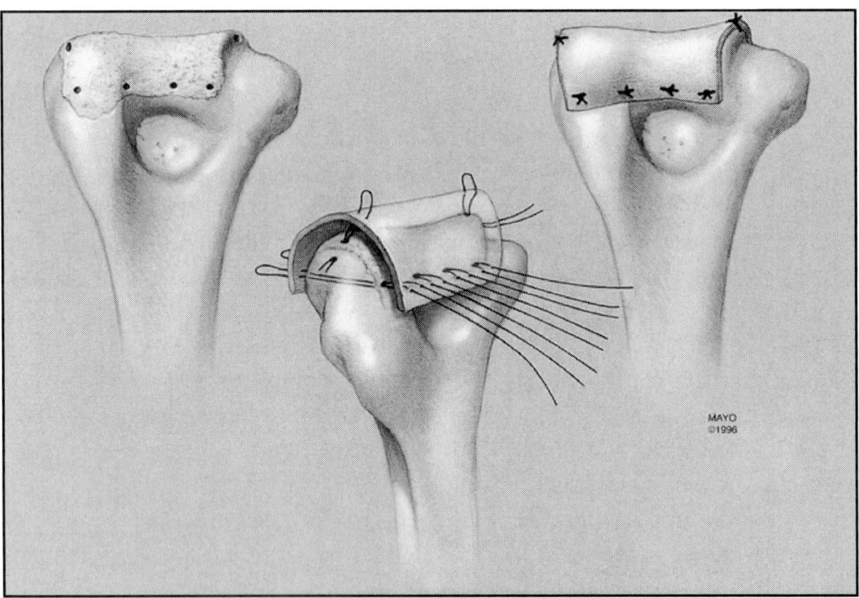

Fig. 2 The distal humerus is exposed and prepared so as to receive the interposed tissue. Sutures from front to back and marginal sutures on the medial and lateral aspects secure the interposed tissue to the distal humerus. (Reproduced with permission from the Mayo Foundation, Rochester, MN.)

its ready availability, absence of donor site morbidity, and large size and thickness; it also provides sufficient material for ligament reconstruction when necessary. The Achilles allograft is my current tissue of choice for interposition arthroplasty.

Assessment

Radiographic determination of adequate bone at both the distal humerus and proximal ulna is essential. Sophisticated MRI or CT is not necessary. Ulnar nerve symptoms should be carefully evaluated before surgery with the intention of addressing the cause of the symptoms at the time of the interposition procedure. Because stability is a major determinant of successful outcomes, the preoperative state of both the medial and lateral collateral ligaments is essential. When there are associated signs or symptoms of compromise of the ipsilateral shoulder and wrist, these regions should also be included in the radiographic studies.

Achilles Tendon Allograft

Technique

Exposure and Preparation The patient is positioned supine and the arm is brought across the chest. A posterior incision is preferable to expose the ulnar nerve (Fig. 1). The elbow is then exposed with an extensile Kocher approach, with possible release of a small portion of the lateral triceps attachment to improve the exposure. The lateral collateral ligament is released and the anterior and posterior capsules excised. The radial head is preserved if at all possible. To allow approximation of the articulating surfaces, it is important to remove bone and deformity to balance the ulnohumeral articulation. Care is taken to remove the ridge (incisura) of the olecranon to allow a flat articulation on the humerus. It is important to remove enough bone for the trochlea and capitellum to accommodate the tendon graft and also to allow a few millimeters of laxity to ensure adequate motion. When possible, a slight ridge of bone left medially and laterally on the humerus helps stabilize the construct.

In the distal humerus three or four holes are drilled from posterior to anterior covering the full width of the humerus (Fig. 2). The Achilles tendon is evaluated to determine the width required to cover the full dimension of the distal humerus. The tendon portion is generally placed anteriorly and the broad fascial portion is

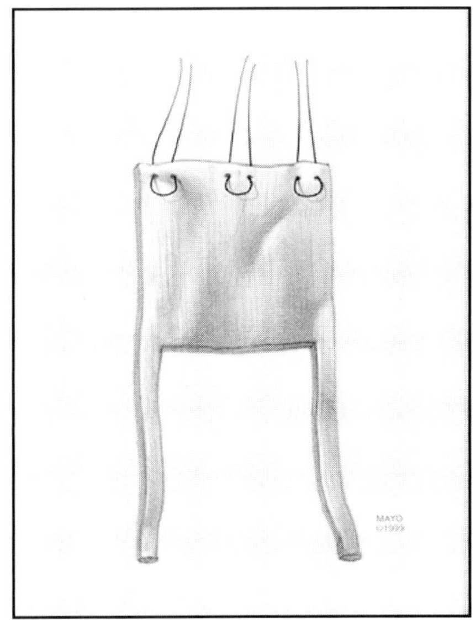

Fig. 3 An Achilles tendon graft provides distal humerus coverage; however, medial and lateral extensions of the graft allow reconstruction of the collateral ligaments. (Reproduced with permission from the Mayo Foundation, Rochester, MN.)

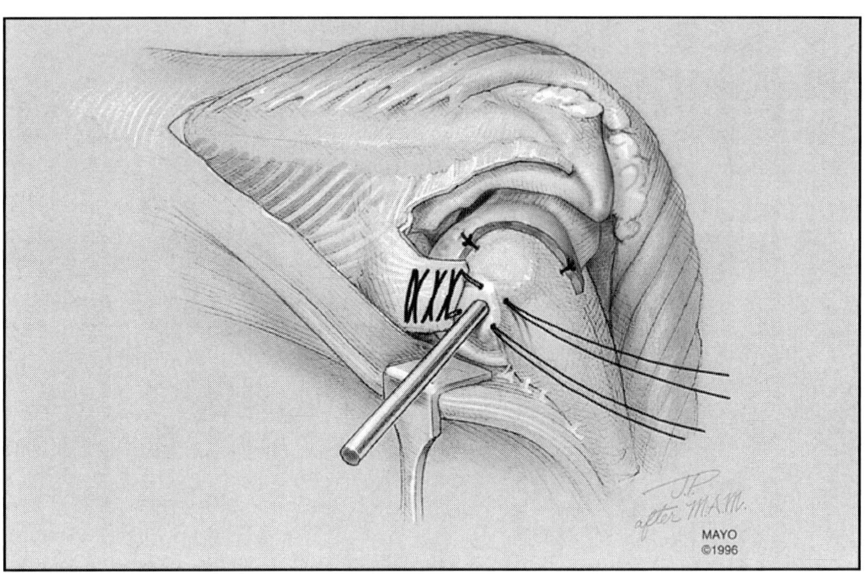

Fig. 4 If the collateral ligaments have been preserved, they are reattached to the anatomic origin around a guide pin to assure that the insertion or removal does not cut or interfere with the ligament attachment. (Reproduced with permission from the Mayo Foundation, Rochester, MN.)

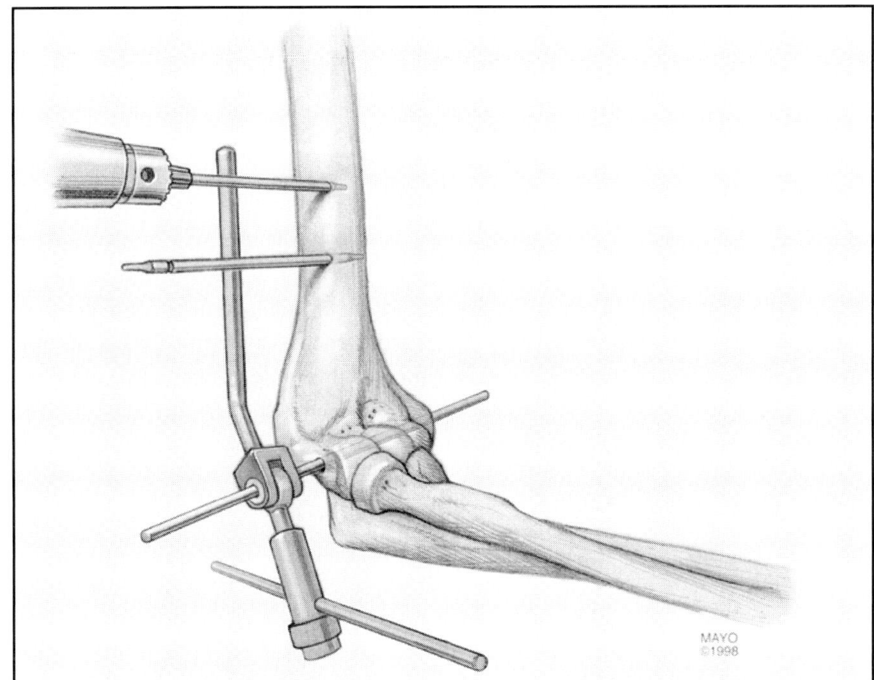

Fig. 5 A half-pin fixator used with the axis pin serves temporarily until the external fixator is secured. The half-pin fixator is then removed. (Reproduced with permission from the Mayo Foundation, Rochester, MN.)

directed posteriorly. This provides the maximum graft thickness anteriorly and makes tissue available for ligament reconstruction posteriorly. The tendon is then situated over the humerus, and the best portion of the graft to cover the humerus is defined. The anterior excess of the graft is transected. The anterior graft is sewn to the anterior humerus with No. 1 nonabsorbable sutures, the graft is pulled taut, and the posterior flap is secured.

If the ligament tissue is not adequate for repair, a strip of Achilles graft is taken medially, laterally, or both, measuring about 0.5 × 6 cm (Fig. 3). For lateral reconstruction, two holes are drilled from anterior to posterior, originating at the axis of rotation. The graft is rotated around the lateral epicondyle and secured with suture. A similar technique can be used medially, with the graft brought under and secured to the medial epicondyle. If both ligaments are to be reconstructed, a tunnel connects the sub-

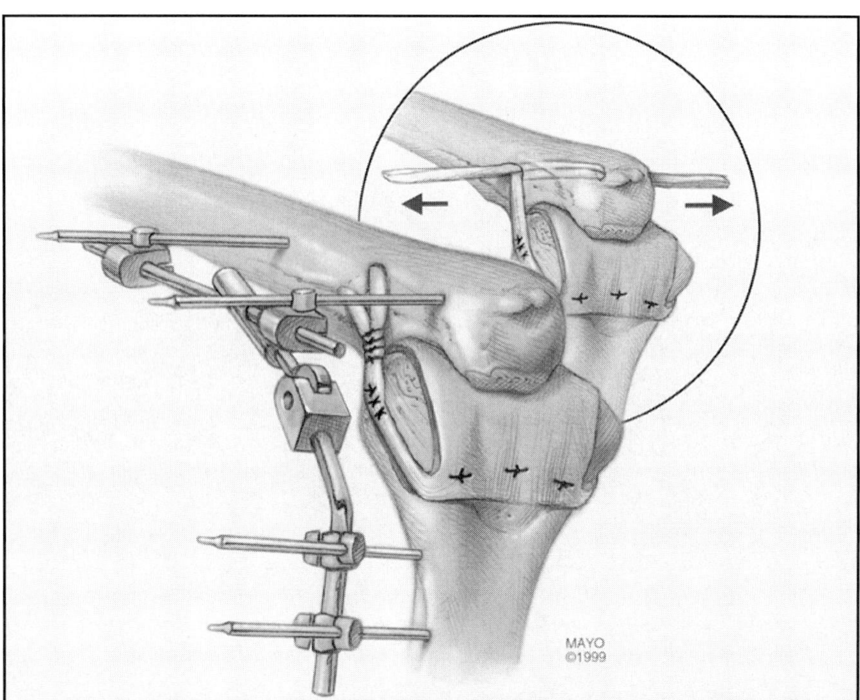

Fig. 6 The Achilles tendon graft in place and the reconstructed lateral collateral ligament with the half-pin external fixator. If both collateral ligaments are deficient (inset) then the ulna insertions are connected with a drill bit, and the medial and lateral arms of the graft are brought across the ulna in a "sling type" of procedure to stabilize the ulna to the humerus. (Reproduced with permission from the Mayo Foundation, Rochester, MN.)

lime tubercle and the crista supernatoris through which each ligament reconstruction is drawn. Once the ligaments have been secured, this construct usually is protected with a half-frame articulated external fixator (Figs. 4 through 6). Before application of the external fixator, the tourniquet is released and hemostasis obtained. The triceps is reattached through dense holes drilled across the proximal ulna, along with the extensor muscle mass to the lateral epicondyle. The extensor muscle mass is reattached, as well. The ulnar nerve is again inspected and if subluxation or constriction occurs with flexion, the nerve is translocated into a subcutaneous pocket. Closure is then routine.

Aftercare Motion is begun on the first postoperative day with a continuous motion machine and maintained for 3 to 4 weeks. The fixator is removed with the patient under anesthesia and elbow motion and stability are examined. Activity is begun and, if the joint is stiff, static splints are prescribed.

Results

Although both rheumatoid and traumatic conditions can be treated with interposition arthroplasty when the proper indications are met,[8,12-16] there are little data regarding outcomes in nonrheumatoid patients.

One review of 37 fascial arthroplasties for rheumatoid arthritis[15] revealed that 26 patients (70%) had excellent or good results. When arthroplasty was used to treat stiff joints with intrinsic pathology (Fig. 7), 80% had satisfactory results. This reflected an improvement of motion arc from 30° to 100°, with minimal pain in 88% of patients.[4] Regarding the outcome for painful, nonankylosing, posttraumatic arthritis, Cheng and Morrey[17] documented 75% satisfactory results in 13 patients with traumatic arthritis a mean of 5 years (range, 2 to 12 years) after fascial arthroplasty using fascia lata. It is notable that 80% of patients without preexisting instability had satisfactory outcomes.

Complications

The complications arising from interposition arthroplasty are considerable and may include bone resorption, heterotopic bone formation, triceps rupture, medial and lateral joint subluxation, infection, and long-term failure.

Bone resorption occasionally occurs at the distal humeral condyles and often causes no difficulty. If significant instability develops as a late sequela, subsequent ligamentous reconstruction may be beneficial if the elbow is painless. I have successfully avoided instability by repairing or reconstructing the collateral ligaments and applying a distraction device, as mentioned earlier.[4] Triceps rupture is an uncommon complication related to the surgical exposure rather than to the procedure itself. Careful attention to the details of repair minimizes this problem.

For superficial infections and cellulitis, the elbow is placed at rest, elevated, and immobilized in a long arm posterior splint while appropriate antibiotics are administered. If the infection involves the deep structures, open drainage and excision of the graft may be required. If bony infection occurs, removal of the implant and osseous débridement are required. The extremity is immobilized and often develops a functional resection arthroplasty. Although this will leave the elbow more unstable, a useful limb often can be salvaged.

Failure of the procedure may occur because of pain, reankylosis, or instability. The result can deteriorate with time,

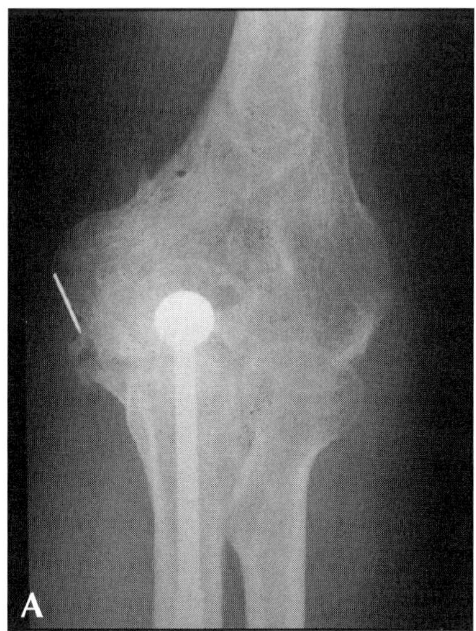

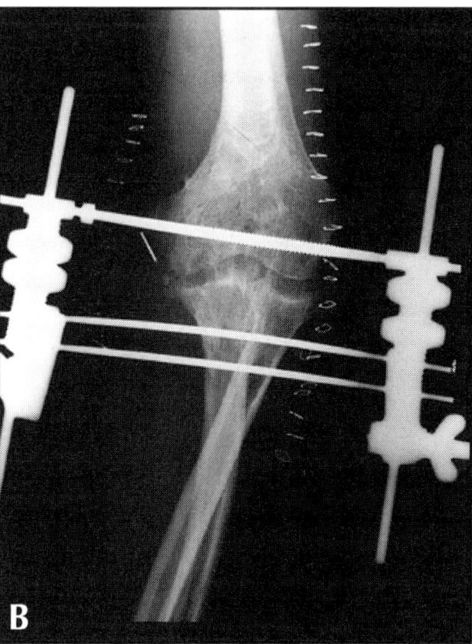

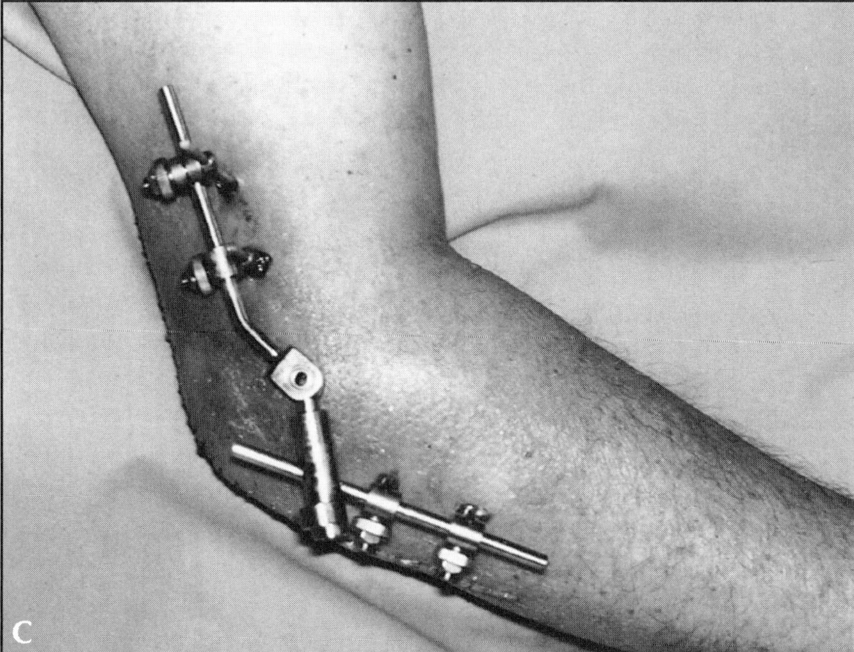

Fig. 7 A, Radiograph of a 50-year-old patient with a failed open reduction and internal fixation with posttraumatic arthritis and stiffness, having an arc of 60° to 90° of motion. **B,** Postoperatively, the joint is protected and distracted with the original external fixator design. **C,** The currently used half-pin fixator. Note that the axis of the rotation pin has been removed.

especially in active individuals. Typically, prosthetic replacement is the salvage procedure of choice. Prosthetic replacement has recently been shown to be successful in 12 of 13 patients with previous interposition arthroplasties.[18]

References

1. Morrey BF, Askew LJ, An KN, Chao EY: A biomechanical study of normal functional elbow motion. *J Bone Joint Surg Am* 1981;63: 872-877.
2. McAuliffe JA, Burkhalter WE, Ouellette EA, Carneiro RS: Compression plate arthrodesis of the elbow. *J Bone Joint Surg Br* 1992;74: 300-304.
3. Koch M, Lipscomb PR: Arthrodesis of the elbow. *Clin Orthop* 1967;50:151-157.
4. Morrey BF: Post-traumatic contracture of the elbow: Operative treatment, including distraction arthroplasty. *J Bone Joint Surg Am* 1990;72: 601-618.
5. Ljung P, Jonsson K, Larsson K, Rydholm U: Interposition arthroplasty of the elbow with rheumatoid arthritis. *J Shoulder Elbow Surg* 1996;5:81-85.
6. Wright PE II, Froimson AI, Morrey BF: Interposition arthroplasty of the elbow, in Morrey BF (ed): *The Elbow and Its Disorders*, ed 3. Philadelphia, PA, WB Saunders, 2000, pp 718-730.
7. Dee R: Elbow arthroplasty. *Proc R Soc Med* 1969;62:1031-1035.
8. Hämäläinen MMJ, Kataoka Y: Late radiographic results after resection skin interposition arthroplasty of the elbow in rheumatoid arthritis. *Rheumatology* 1991;15:42-46.
9. Harris JE: Abstract: Triceps fascial interpositional arthroplasty of the elbow in rheumatoid arthritis. *J Shoulder Elbow Surg* 1997;6: 186-187.
10. Grishin IG, Goncharenko IV, Kozhin NP, Sarkisyan AG, Gobulev AG, Devis AE: Restoration of the function of the cubital joint in extensive defects of bones and soft tissues using endoprosthesis and free skin grafts. *Acta Chir Plast* 1989;31:143-147.
11. Hass J: Functional arthroplasty. *J Bone Joint Surg* 1944;26:297-306.
12. Agrifoglio E, De Benedetti M: Artroplastica con interposizione di lembo cutaneo nelle rigidita e anchilosi del gomito: English version: Arthroplasty with interposition of skin flaps in rigidity and ankylosis of the elbow. *Arch Ortop (Milano)* 1959;72:603-614.
13. Froimson AI, Silva JE, Richey D: Cutis arthroplasty of the elbow joint. *J Bone Joint Surg Am* 1976;58:863-865.
14. Hurri L, Pulkki T, Vainio K: Arthroplasty of the elbow in rheumatoid arthritis. *Acta Chir Scand* 1964;127:459-465.
15. Kimura C, Vainio K: Arthroplasty of the elbow in rheumatoid arthritis. *Arch Orthop Unfallchir* 1976;84:339-348.
16. Uuspaa V: Anatomical interposition arthroplasty with dermal graft: A study of 51 elbow arthroplasties on 48 rheumatoid patients. *Z Rheumatol* 1987;46:132-135.
17. Cheng SL, Morrey BF: Treatment of the mobile, painful arthritic elbow by distraction interposition arthroplasty. *J Bone Joint Surg Br* 2000;82:233-238.
18. Blaine T, Morrey BF: The salvage of failed interposition arthroplasty by total joint replacement. *J Bone Joint Surg Am* (submitted for publication).

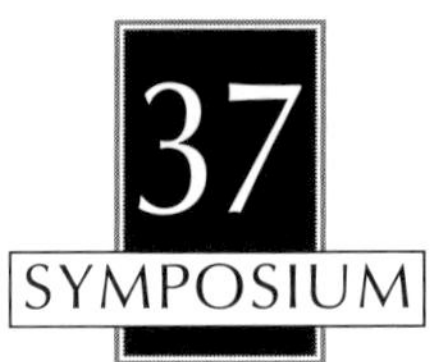

New Frontiers in Elbow Reconstruction: Total Elbow Arthroplasty

Graham J.W. King, MD, FRCSC

Background

Although results with early elbow prostheses were disappointing, improvements in surgical technique and implant design have made total elbow arthroplasty a reliable procedure for many patients. Total elbow arthroplasty relieves pain, provides a functional arc of motion, and improves patients' ability to perform activities of daily living. Further refinements are needed, however, particularly for younger and more active patients in whom mechanical failure and loosening continue to be significant clinical problems.

Indications

The most common indications for total elbow replacement are pain, stiffness, and loss of elbow function due to rheumatoid arthritis. Patients with rheumatoid arthritis who have minimal joint destruction may be candidates for open or arthroscopic synovectomy, with or without radial head excision, as a means to delay arthroplasty. Other forms of inflammatory arthritis, such as hemophilia, are also indications for total elbow arthroplasty. Posttraumatic arthritis and primary osteoarthritis are increasingly common indications for replacement arthroplasty.[1-3] Careful consideration should be given to patient age and functional demands, however, because failure rates have been higher in patients with posttraumatic arthritis and primary osteoarthritis than in patients with inflammatory arthritis.[3] With the advent of newer implant designs, total elbow arthroplasty has been successfully used in the management of selected comminuted distal humeral fractures in elderly patients, distal humeral nonunions, and tumors.[4-11]

Total elbow arthroplasty is contraindicated in patients who are candidates for alternative procedures, such as synovectomy, débridement, and open reduction and internal fixation. Patients with incompetent collateral ligaments should not undergo an unlinked total elbow arthroplasty. Conversion of an elbow arthrodesis to an arthroplasty is challenging and the outcome is unpredictable.[12] Previous infection is a strong relative contraindication; however, recent studies suggest that total elbow arthroplasty can be successfully performed in selected patients using a staged débridement with negative cultures.[13] Patients with inadequate bone stock or soft tissue or muscle function that cannot be reconstructed should not undergo total elbow arthroplasty. Patients with neurologic dysfunction resulting in a Charcot joint and patients who cannot be expected to comply with the postoperative restrictions of a total elbow should not be considered for a joint replacement.

Terminology

Constrained, semiconstrained, unconstrained, and resurfacing are terms that have been used to classify elbow arthroplasty designs. These terms are misleading because even "unconstrained" implants have some intrinsic constraint by virtue of the interlocking shape of their articular surfaces.[14] Most currently used linked implants have some laxity built into the hinge mechanism, so they are not fully constrained. A simplified classification designates implants as either linked or unlinked.

Biomechanics

The function of the elbow is to position and stabilize the hand in space for bimanual activities. The range of elbow motion in the flexion and extension plane varies from approximately 0° to 140°. Of this total arc, only approximately 30° to 130° are necessary to perform most activities of daily living.[15] The motion pathway of elbow flexion-extension has been shown to approximate that of a loose hinge joint. The flexion-extension axis follows a line that can be drawn between the center of the capitellum and the center of curvature of the trochlear groove. External landmarks useful in defining

One or more of the authors or the departments with which they are affiliated have received something of value from a commercial or other party related directly or indirectly to the subject of this chapter.

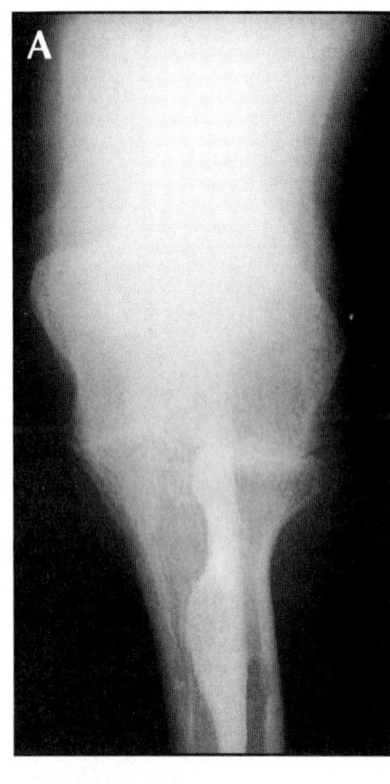

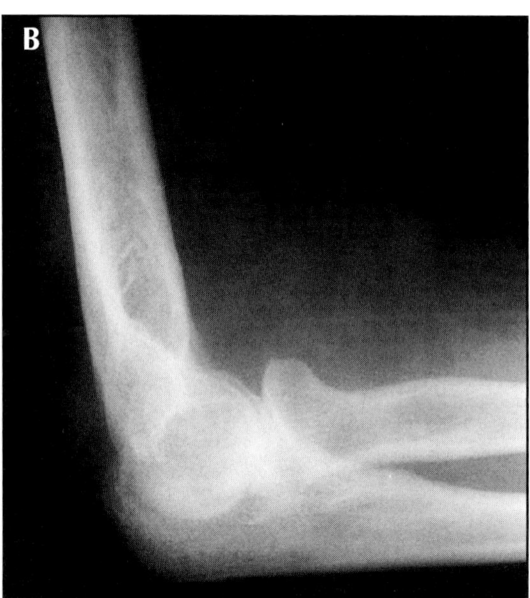

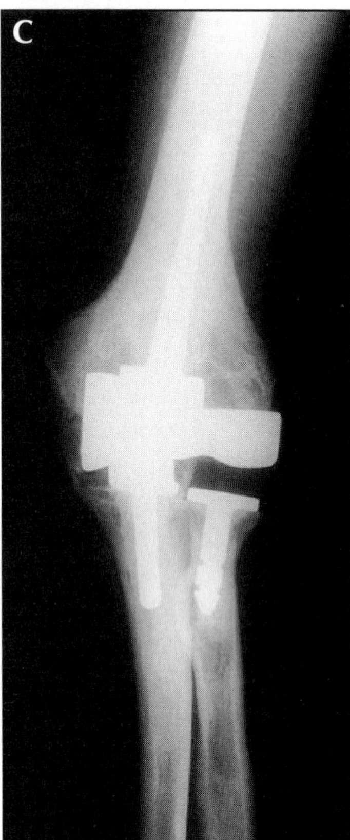

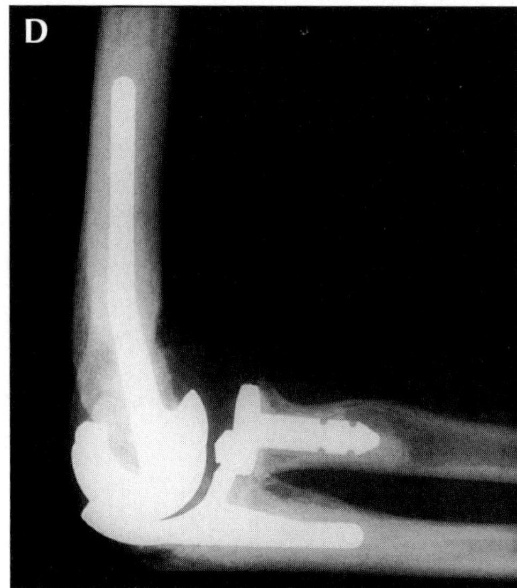

Fig. 1 Sorbie unlinked total elbow arthroplasty for rheumatoid arthritis. **A,** AP radiograph of a 54-year-old woman with polyarticular rheumatoid arthritis of 30 years' duration. Note the complete loss of joint space with relative preservation of bone architecture. **B,** Lateral radiograph. **C,** Three-year postoperative AP radiograph after Sorbie total elbow arthroplasty. The patient had complete relief of pain and restoration of a functional arc of elbow motion. **D,** Lateral postoperative radiograph demonstrates a partial triceps avulsion that was asymptomatic.

this axis are the anteroinferior aspect of the medial epicondyle and the center of the arc of curvature of the capitellum. It has been demonstrated that the locus of instant centers of rotation is small, moving less than 4 mm throughout the arc of elbow flexion-extension.[16] The axis of rotation is approximately 3° to 5° internally rotated relative to the plane of the medial and lateral epicondyles and is in 4° to 8° of valgus with respect to the long axis of the humerus.

Forces across the elbow have been estimated to approach three to four times body weight with certain strenuous activities.[17,18] Halls and Travill,[19] using transducers in the radiocapitellar and ulnotrochlear joints, demonstrated that 57% of the force went through the radiocapitellar joint and 43% through the ulnohumeral joint. Morrey and An[20] demonstrated a similar distribution of forces with the elbow extended.

Laboratory data suggest that muscle activation about the elbow may allow "semiconstrained" linked arthroplasties to function within the laxity of their loose hinge.[21] This limits loading of the bone-cement interface and may explain the lower mechanical loosening rates relative to fixed-hinge devices. Unlinked replacements rely on capsuloligamentous tissues, muscles, and the intrinsic constraint of the implant to maintain joint stability.[14] The intrinsic constraint of an unlinked total elbow arthroplasty depends on the articular shape and congruency of the implant. The greater the intrinsic constraint of the prosthesis, the higher the transfer of loads to the bone-cement interface and hence the greater potential for loosening.[22] Conversely, less constrained devices may have a higher incidence of instability.[14,23] Although many early elbow replacements were designed without stems on either the humeral or ulnar components, a high incidence of mechanical loosening was observed.[24-26] The addition of stems has resulted in improved results of total elbow arthroplasty. An implant that incorporates a radial head replacement should be advantageous with respect to load transfer and, therefore, prosthesis survivorship; however, this has not been confirmed by clinical experience.[27]

Unlinked Total Elbow Arthroplasty

The decision to use an unlinked or a linked arthroplasty depends on the amount of bone destruction, the status of the capsuloligamentous tissues of the elbow joint, and the surgeon's experience with these devices. Numerous unlinked implants have been developed and used.[24-26,28-37] All unlinked designs seek to replicate the axis of motion of the elbow to optimize ligamentous balance and maintain joint stability. Incorrect component placement causes joint maltracking, excessive articular wear, and instability, possibly leading to dislocation.[23,38]

The preferred surgical approach is specific to the implant used. One of the principles of treatment for most unlinked implants is to preserve either the medial or lateral collateral ligament. Currently, most unlinked total elbow arthroplasties are inserted through an extended Kocher approach. The elbow is subluxated on the intact medial collateral ligament to achieve adequate exposure for placement of the components. Management of the ulnar nerve is controversial. Most surgeons recommend identification and protection of the nerve with or without formal transposition. Instrumentation specific to the implant system is used to guide bony resection and ensure optimal implant placement. Before cementing the definitive components, a trial reduction should be performed to ensure congruent tracking of the arthroplasty. The elbow is passively flexed and extended with the forearm maintained in pronation to tension the medial collateral ligament and close the lateral side of the elbow, destabilized by the surgical exposure. If there is maltracking, one or both of the components should be repositioned.[23,39]

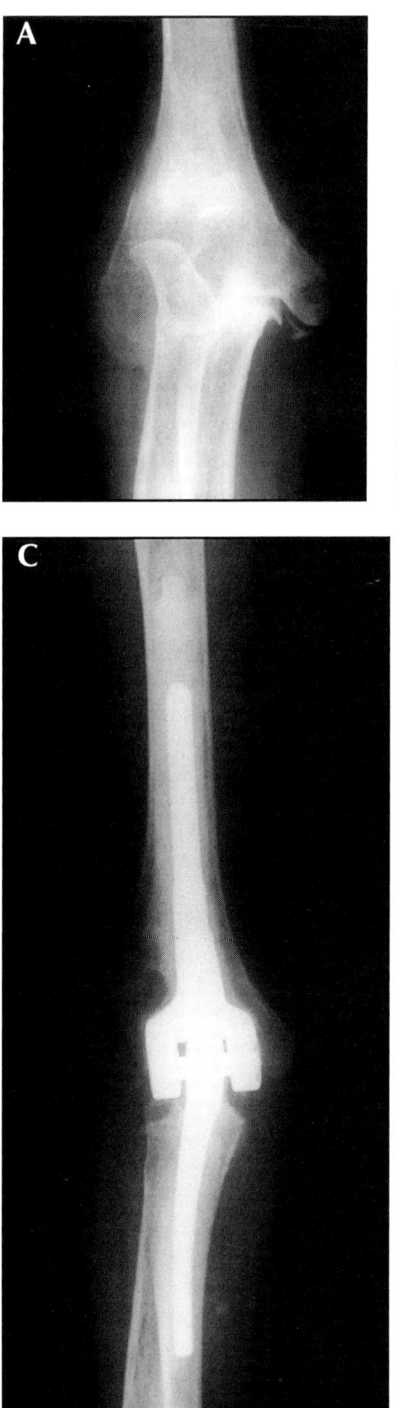

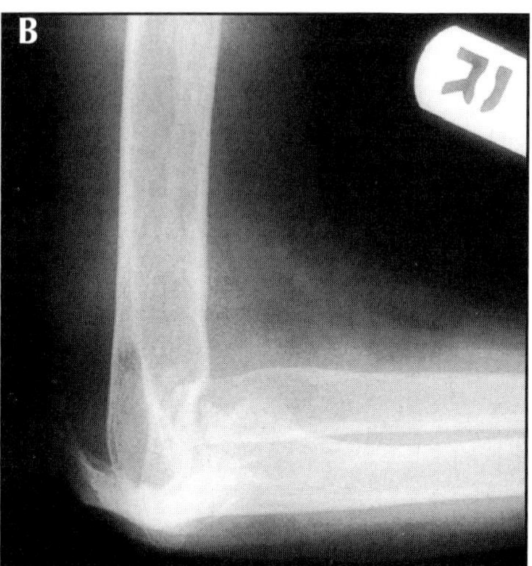

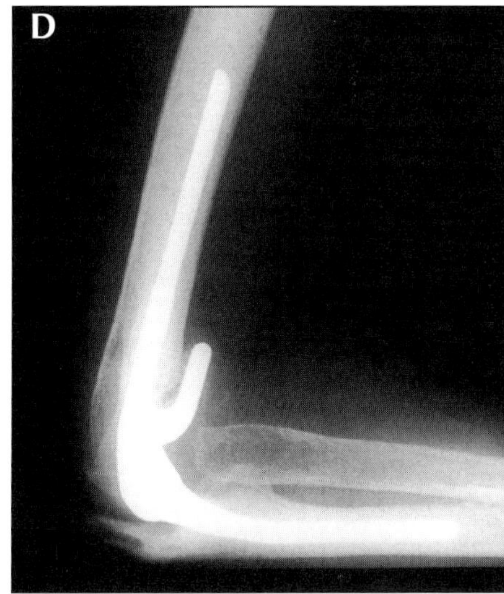

Fig. 2 Coonrad-Morrey linked total elbow arthroplasty for rheumatoid arthritis. **A,** AP radiograph of a 52-year-old woman with polyarticular rheumatoid arthritis of 25 years' duration. The patient had severe pain and moderate instability due to progressive bone resorption. **B,** Lateral radiograph. **C,** Four-year postoperative AP radiograph after a Coonrad-Morrey total elbow arthroplasty. The patient had complete relief of pain and restoration of elbow stability. **D,** Lateral postoperative radiograph demonstrates good cement technique with the use of cement restrictors.

A linked arthroplasty should be done when there is instability due to an incompetent medial collateral ligament or persistent maltracking that cannot be corrected with component repositioning. An unlinked elbow arthroplasty that is unstable or maltracks intraoperatively usually continues to function poorly postoperatively. Careful repair of the lateral collateral ligament complex to the lateral epicondyle is needed to prevent postoperative instability. The fascia of the Kocher interval is closed to augment lateral elbow stabili-

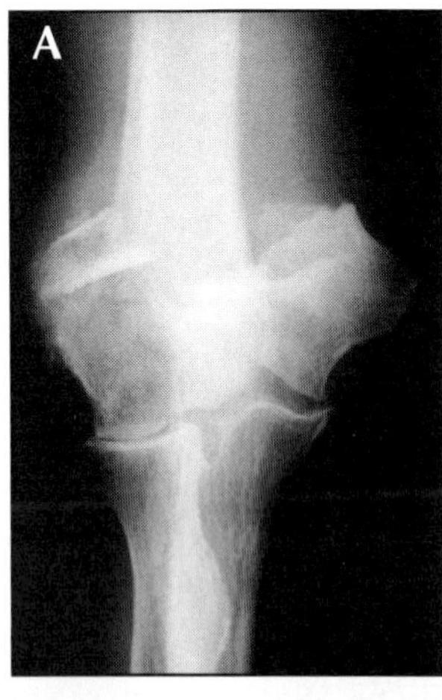

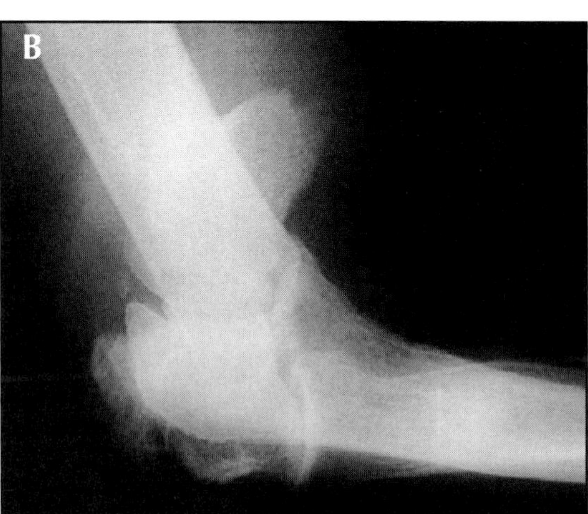

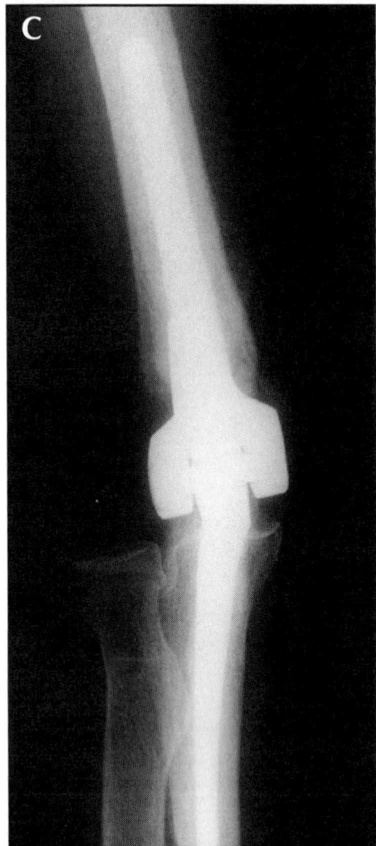

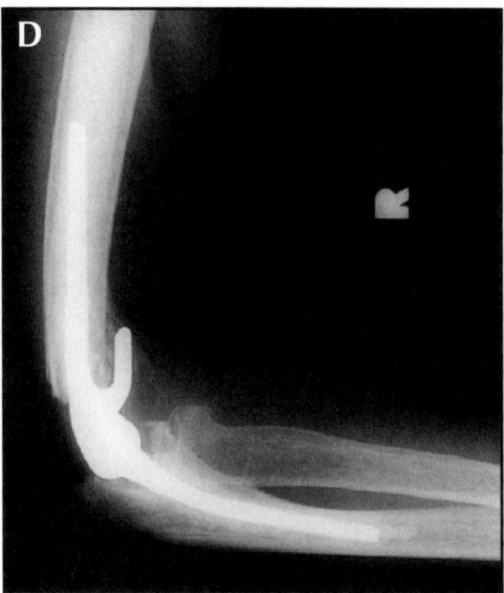

Fig. 3 Coonrad-Morrey linked total elbow arthroplasty for fracture. **A,** AP radiograph of an 81-year-old man with a comminuted intra-articular distal humeral fracture. **B,** Lateral radiograph. **C,** AP radiograph 6 months after a Coonrad-Morrey total elbow arthroplasty placed through a triceps-sparing surgical approach. The patient had complete relief of pain and an arc of motion of from 20° to 140°. **D,** Lateral postoperative radiograph.

ty, as described by Cohen and Hastings[40] (Fig. 1).

Linked Total Elbow Arthroplasty

The initial experience with fully constrained hinged arthroplasty of the elbow had a high mechanical loosening rate.[41-44] The advent of improved loose-hinge linked designs has improved survivorship, equalling that of unlinked elbow arthroplasties at medium-term follow-up[45] (Fig. 2). Linked devices allow the indications for total elbow arthroplasty to be broadened to patients with greater degrees of bone and ligamentous deficiency[1,4,6-10,46] (Fig. 3).

The surgical technique is specific for each implant design. A Bryan-Morrey approach is typically used, elevating the triceps from medial to lateral off the olecranon in continuity with the anconeus muscle to expose the distal humerus.[47] This creates a continuous sling of the extensor mechanism. A triceps-sparing approach has been dev-eloped that has been useful when performing linked total elbow arthro-plasty.[48] Triceps weakness is reduced, and triceps disruption should not occur. Instrumentation is used to facilitate bony resection and implant alignment. After insertion and coupling of the implant, the triceps is reattached to the olecranon with sutures through drill holes.

Rehabilitation

Unlinked elbow arthroplasties are splinted in approximately 60° of flexion, whereas linked arthroplasties are splinted in full extension. The arm is elevated overnight to control edema. Motion begins one day postoperatively, if the soft tissues permit, alternating a sling at 90° with active range of motion. Elbow flexion and extension are performed with the forearm fully pronated for 6 weeks to protect the lateral ligament repair done with unlinked designs.[34,49] Similarly, if the medial collateral ligament has been divided as part of the surgical exposure of an unlinked total elbow arthroplasty, motion should be initiated with the forearm maintained in supination.[36,50] Forearm pronation and supination are permitted only with the elbow at 90° of flexion.

Active assisted flexion and passive gravity-assisted extension protect the triceps tendon repair for a 6-week period. Extension past 30° is avoided in unlinked designs for the first 3 to 4 weeks to avoid posterior subluxation or, worse, dislocation of the elbow. A nighttime resting extension splint is used for 12 weeks after surgery in all linked designs and when sta-

Table 1
Selected Unlinked Total Elbow Arthroplasty Results

Author	Year	Implant	Number of Implants	Diagnosis (%)	Mean Follow-up (yrs)	Infection (%)	Motion (degrees)	Functional Stability (%)	Pain* (%)	Aseptic Loosening (%)	Revision (%)
Kudo et al[24]	1980	Kudo stemless	24	100 RA	3.8	0	42-124	96	96 good	4	8
Lowe et al[25]	1984	Lowe	44	80 RA	3.0	6	37-135	82	84 good	14	36
Souter[28]	1985	Souter-Strathclyde	108	100 RA	3.5	5	143 arc	96	97 good	11	—
Weiland et al[30]	1989	Capitello-condylar	40	45 RA	7.2	5	39-113	71	—	0	0
Poll and Rozing[31]	1991	Souter-Strathclyde	33	100 RA	4.0	3	31-138	81	92 good	15	15
Ewald et al[34]	1993	Capitello-condylar	202	100 RA	5.8	1.5	30-135	98.5	87 good	1.5	3
Kudo et al[36]	1999	Kudo V	43	100 RA	3.8	0	42-133	74 moderate instability	100 good	0	0
Rozing[52]	2000	Souter-Strathclyde	33	95 RA	7.8	4.5	32-132	95.5	—	15	12
Yanni et al[29]	2000	Roper-Tuke	49	100 RA	6.5	6.8	37-130	96.6	84 good	33	8.4

**Multiple methods of grading outcomes were used, which make comparisons impossible between series.*
RA = rheumatoid arthritis
(Adapted with permission from King GJW: Arthroplasty and arthrodesis of the elbow, in Chapman MW (ed): Chapman's Orthopaedic Surgery, *ed 3. Philadelphia, PA, Lippincott Williams & Wilkins, 2001, p 2682.)*

bility is judged to be adequate in unlinked designs. Patients are counseled not to lift more than 5 kg and not to participate in any upper extremity impact sport (eg, golf, tennis) after total elbow arthroplasty.

Results

There are numerous published results of unlinked elbow arthroplasty[29,36] (Table 1). Pain relief and restoration of a functional arc of motion are achieved in more than 90% of patients. The largest reported experience in North America is with the capitellocondylar total elbow prosthesis.[34] The designer of this implant has reported excellent results in patients with rheumatoid arthritis, with only a 1.5% incidence of postoperative dislocation and a low incidence of aseptic loosening.[34] However, other surgeons have noted instability in up to 20% of patients.[30,51] Souter[28] reported good functional results with the Souter-Strathclyde total elbow arthroplasty (Howmedica, Rutherford, NJ) and a low incidence of loosening and instability, although a troubling incidence of humeral loosening with this more constrained, unlinked implant has been reported in recent long-term studies.[35,52]

Pain relief, joint stability, and a functional arc of motion are achieved in more than 90% of patients after linked total elbow arthroplasty[45] (Table 2). The loosening rate of the Coonrad-Morrey device (Zimmer, Warsaw, IN) has been low at medium-term follow-up in patients with rheumatoid arthritis;[45] however, the failure rate has been considerably higher in patients with post-traumatic arthritis.[1] The clinical experience with the Pritchard Mark II hinge device (DePuy, Warsaw, IN) has been less successful.[53] The GSB III (Gschwend-Scheier-Bahler; Sulzer Orthopedics, Austin, TX) implant with a loose-hinge linkage mechanism has been reported to have good clinical and radiologic outcomes.[54-56]

Complications

The most devastating complication of total elbow arthroplasty is infection. Acute infections are managed with urgent surgical débridement if the implant is to be successfully salvaged. Intravenous antibiotics followed by suppressive antibiotics may allow retention of the implant. Late, indolent infections or persistent sepsis in spite of débridement should be managed by removal of the implant and all cement. Reimplantation after an infected elbow arthroplasty remains controversial; however, a staged revision arthroplasty has been reported to be successful in many patients.[13,57]

Postoperative subluxation or dislocation of an unlinked arthroplasty often requires revision to a linked design. The radiographic position of the components is

Table 2
Selected Linked Total Elbow Arthroplasty Results

Author	Year	Implant	Number of Implants	Diagnosis (%)	Mean Follow-up (yrs)	Infection (%)	Motion (degrees)	Functional Stability (%)	Pain* (%)	Aseptic Loosening (%)	Revision (%)
Dee[63]	1973	Dee hinge	30	87 RA	1.5	0	—	100	—	14	7
Garrett et al[43]	1977	GSB hinge	10	100 RA	3	10	25-128	100	70 good	50	20
Johnson et al[44]	1984	Stanmore hinge	44	100 RA	6	5	40-138	100	97 good	7	3
Figgie et al[64]	1987	Triaxial	20	100 OA	4.2	11	30-120	78	89 good	11	11
Kraay et al[65]	1994	Osteonics	113	86 RA	—	6	—	100	—	7	5
Madsen et al[53]	1994	Pritchard II	26	100 RA	6.3	4	27-132	85	94 good	2	27
Cobb and Morrey[4]	1997	Coonrad III	21	Fracture	3.3	0	25-130	100	100 good	0	5
Inglis et al[8]	1997	Triaxial Osteonics custom	21	14 RA, 81 nonunion	5.4	10	105 arc	85	76 good	5	19
Schneeberger et al[1]	1997	Coonrad III	41	100 OA	5.1	5	27-131	100	73 good	0	17
Gill and Morrey[45]	1998	Coonrad III	78	100 RA	8	5	28-131	100	90 good	3	4
Gschwend et al[66]	1999	GSB III	32	88 RA, 12 PTA	13.5	4.6	28-144	86	97 good	4.6	14
Hildebrand et al[3]	2000	Coonrad III	39	50 RA, 50 PTA	4.2	8	31-140	100	90 good	32	3
Schneeberger et al[54]	2000	GSB III	14	64 RA, 36 PTA	6	7	19-140	86	50 good	29	29

**"Good" relief is as described by the authors of each article. Multiple methods of grading outcomes were used, thus making comparisons impossible between series*
GSB = Gschwend-Schneier-Bahler; OA = osteoarthritis; PTA = posttraumatic arthritis; RA = rheumatoid arthritis
(Adapted with permission from King GJW: Arthroplasty and arthrodesis of the elbow, in Chapman MW (ed): Chapman's Orthopaedic Surgery, *ed 3. Philadelphia, PA, Lippincott Williams & Wilkins, 2001, p 2688.)*

evaluated before revision. If one or both components are malpositioned, then repositioning, although difficult, can be considered. If the component position is judged to be adequate, closed reduction and splinting can be used to allow capsule and ligament healing. If the elbow remains unstable after a period of immobilization and the component position is acceptable, repair or reconstruction of one or both of the collateral ligaments may successfully stabilize the arthroplasty. If stability cannot be achieved by component repositioning or ligament reconstruction, revision to a linked arthroplasty should be considered. Revision arthroplasty may be more reliable than soft-tissue procedures for management of an unstable total elbow arthroplasty.

Ulnar neuropathy is common after total elbow arthroplasty.[58] Fortunately, it most often is transient numbness that resolves; however, residual sensory and motor symptoms are frequent. Damage to the ulnar nerve can occur at any time during surgery, particularly if the nerve is not protected and transposed. The nerve may be compressed while the elbow is subluxated to place the components, damaged by power instruments, or sustain thermal injury from extravasated bone cement.

Intraoperative fractures of one or both humeral columns may preclude the successful placement of an unlinked design. Open reduction and internal fixation of the columns can be done in patients with good bone quality and reconstructible fractures; however, conversion to a linked arthroplasty often is advisable. Cortical perforation or fracture can occur due to the small diameter and curving shape of the medullary canals of the humerus and ulna. Careful repair of the triceps tendon to the olecranon is required to prevent triceps disruption and postoperative extension weakness. Triceps insufficiency may require surgical reconstruction because of patient difficulties in performing overhead activities.

Elbow stiffness may occur because of inadequate capsular release during surgery, a delay in postoperative rehabilitation, or heterotopic ossification. Wound-healing problems are uncom-

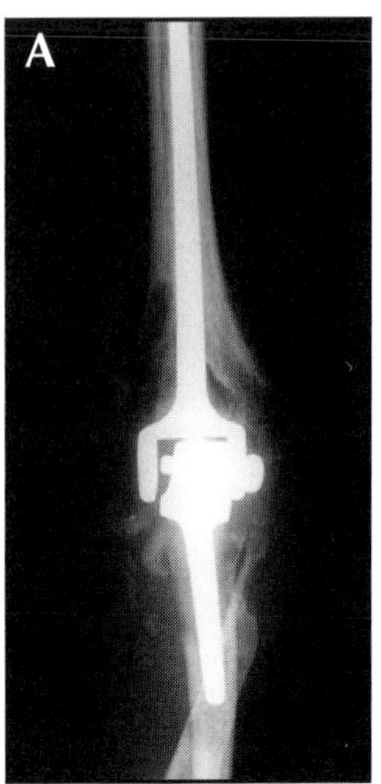

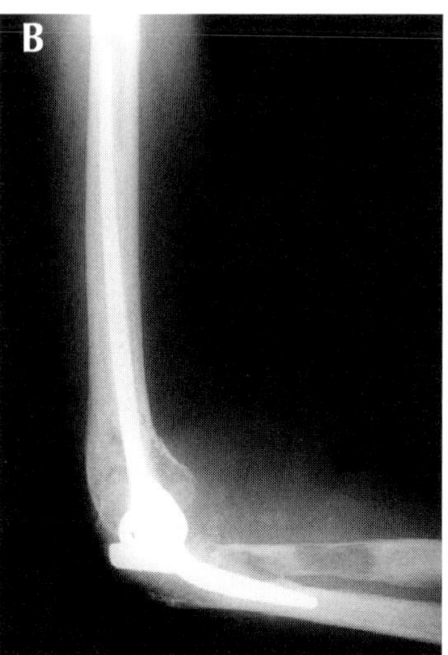

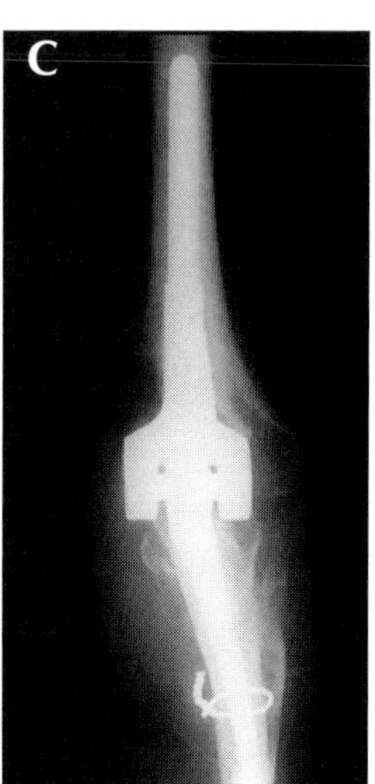

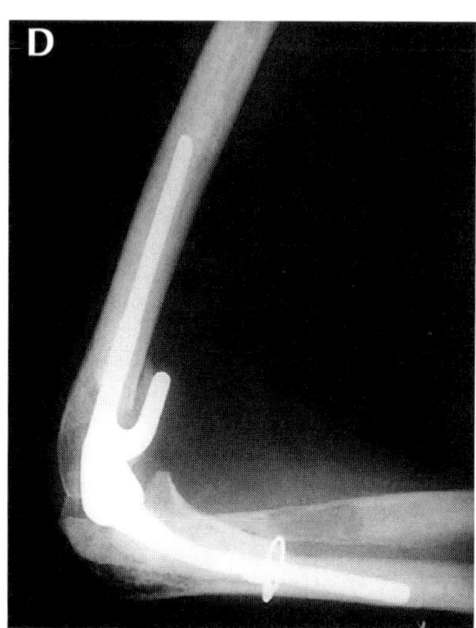

Fig. 4 Osteolysis following Pritchard Mark II total elbow arthroplasty. **A,** AP radiograph of a 49-year-old woman with long-standing rheumatoid arthritis 9 years after Pritchard Mark II total elbow arthroplasty. The patient complained of increasing pain and progressive elbow instability. **B,** Lateral radiograph showing elbow subluxation, disassociation of the linkage mechanism, and osteolysis around the component stems. **C,** Postoperative AP radiograph following an allograft revision to a Coonrad-Morrey total elbow arthroplasty. The patient had minimal pain, a stable elbow, and a functional arc of motion at 6 months' follow-up. The patient sustained a cortical perforation at the tip of the ulnar component. **D,** Lateral radiograph demonstrates the position of the ulnar allograft.

mon with careful tissue handling, postoperative extension splinting, and suction drains. Delayed wound healing occasionally occurs in patients with rheumatoid arthritis, particularly those taking ster- oids. Although delayed mobilization and extension splinting can effectively treat minor areas of superficial dermal necrosis, early surgical débridement, with or without flap coverage, should be considered in patients with full-thickness skin loss.

Aseptic loosening with associated osteolysis is the most common cause of failure of total elbow arthroplasty at longer periods of follow-up, particularly in higher demand patients. Failure of the linkage mechanism due to polyethylene wear has been reported with a number of currently available linked devices (Fig. 4). Although this has been a particular problem for the Triaxial device[59] (Stryker Howmedica Osteonics, Rutherford, NJ), failure of the linkage bearings has also been reported in patients with Coonrad-Morrey, Pritchard-Walker (DePuy), and GSB devices.[1,45,46,53,54] Stem fractures have also been reported, most com-monly occurring after falls or heavy lifting.[45]

Future Advances

The outcome of total elbow arthroplasty has improved markedly over the last 2 decades as a consequence of improved implant design and surgical technique. Recent studies have demonstrated that linked total elbow arthroplasty is now as successful as hip and knee arthroplasty in patients with inflammatory arthritis.[45] Higher demand patients, such as those with osteoarthritis and post-traumatic arthritis, remain problematic because their implant survival rate has been lower.[1,2] Opportunities for improvement include advances in implant design and implantation techniques.

Implant Design

The optimal material for total joint arthroplasty remains unknown. Titanium, cobalt-chrome, and polyethylene are the most common materials currently used for elbow arthroplasty. Whether ceramic or other materials will improve the longevity of total elbow arthroplasty will require extensive investigations, such as are currently underway for total hip arthroplasty. The optimal stem shape and length for total elbow arthroplasty has not been determined. Some implants have smooth stems while others have various surface treatments, which may or may not be beneficial. In one study, a newer surface treatment had a higher incidence of ulnar component loosening than an older design.[3] Prospective outcome studies and joint registries are needed to ensure that advances in implant design or materials result in an improvement in outcome.

Implant alignment is important to the survival of a total elbow arthroplasty.[60,61] Greater attention to restoration of the normal anatomic axis of elbow motion using improved implant designs or instrumentation will more accurately replicate muscle moment arms, improve load distribution and stability, and potentially may increase the longevity of elbow arthroplasty. It is likely that com-

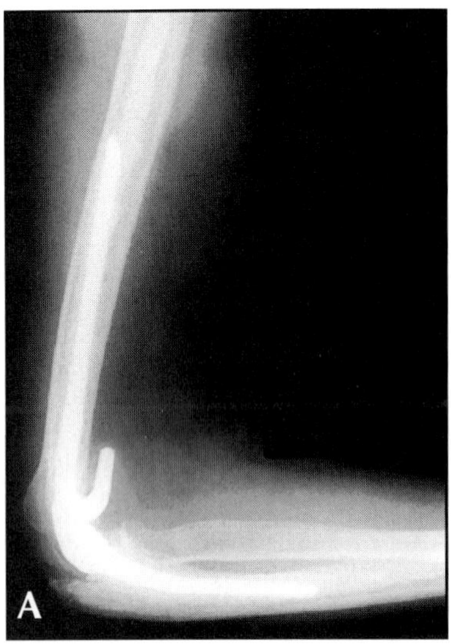

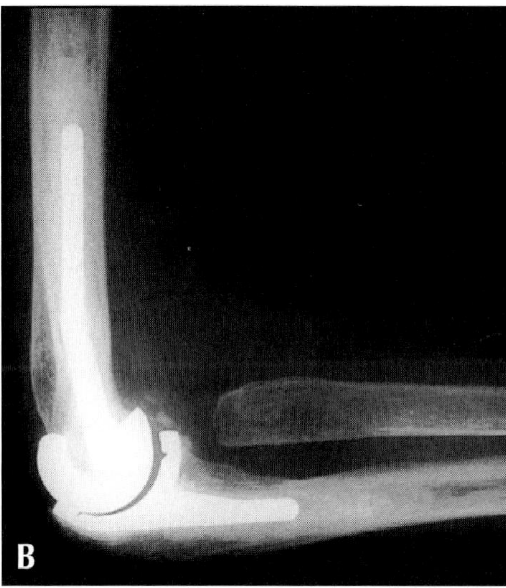

Fig. 5 Cement technique in total elbow arthroplasty. **A,** Lateral radiograph demonstrating poor cement technique following a Coonrad-Morrey total elbow arthroplasty. There is poor containment of cement and an inadequate cement mantle. **B,** Lateral radiograph demonstrating improved cement containment and penetration with the use of cement restrictors and pressurization following a Sorbie total elbow arthroplasty.

puter-assisted surgery will be used in the future to improve the accuracy of implant placement during elbow arthroplasty.

Polyethylene wear is an important clinical problem in the linkage mechanisms of total elbow prostheses, particularly in younger, more active patients.[1,59] Improve-ments in polyethylene durability may be an important contribution to implant survivorship. The development of a reliable radial head replacement should improve load transfer and joint stability and potentially improve the survivorship of elbow arthroplasty that relies exclusively on the ulnar-humeral joint. Given the poor track record of radial head components in total elbow replacements, it remains to be seen whether a radial head component can be developed that will contribute to improved outcome of total elbow arthroplasty.[27] Problems with implant maltracking and soft-tissue tensioning will need to be solved if a radial head component is to be successful.

Surgical Implantation

Advances in instrumentation should improve the accuracy of implant placement and allow better restoration of elbow kinematics and stability. Well-designed instrumentation should reduce surgical times, decrease complications, and improve implant longevity. Advanced cementing techniques using canal restrictors and cement delivery and pressurization systems improve the initial fixation of the implant to bone (Fig. 5). Advanced cementing techniques have been demonstrated to provide a two-fold increase in initial humeral component fixation in the laboratory.[62] This improvement in initial implant fixation has been shown to increase hip arthroplasty longevity; elbow arthroplasty durability also should improve.[54] The development of an expandable cement restrictor to fit within the distal humerus and proximal ulna would also facilitate revision surgery, often made difficult by poorly contained cement that precludes placement of long-stemmed revision components.

References

1. Schneeberger AG, Adams R, Morrey BF: Semiconstrained total elbow replacement for the treatment of post-traumatic osteoarthrosis. *J Bone Joint Surg Am* 1997;79:1211-1222.
2. Kozak TK, Adams RA, Morrey BF: Total elbow arthroplasty in primary osteoarthritis of the elbow. *J Arthroplasty* 1998;13:837-842.
3. Hildebrand KA, Patterson SD, Regan WD, MacDermid JC, King GJ: Functional outcome of semiconstrained total elbow arthroplasty. *J Bone Joint Surg Am* 2000;82:1379-1386.
4. Cobb TK, Morrey BF: Total elbow arthroplasty as primary treatment for distal humeral fractures in elderly patients. *J Bone Joint Surg Am* 1997;79:826-832.
5. Morrey BF: Fractures of the distal humerus: Role of elbow replacement. *Orthop Clin North Am* 2000;31:145-154.
6. Sperling JW, Pritchard DJ, Morrey BF: Total elbow arthroplasty after resection of tumors at the elbow. *Clin Orthop* 1999;367:256-261.
7. Ramsey ML, Adams RA, Morrey BF: Instability of the elbow treated with semiconstrained total elbow arthroplasty. *J Bone Joint Surg Am* 1999;81:38-47.
8. Inglis AE, Inglis AE Jr, Figgie MM, Asnis L: Total elbow arthroplasty for flail and unstable elbows. *J Shoulder Elbow Surg* 1997;6:29-36.
9. Figgie MP, Inglis AE, Mow CS, Figgie HE III: Salvage of non-union of supracondylar fracture of the humerus by total elbow arthroplasty. *J Bone Joint Surg Am* 1989;71:1058-1065.
10. Figgie HE III, Inglis AE, Mow C: Total elbow arthroplasty in the face of significant bone stock or soft tissue losses: Preliminary results of custom-fit arthroplasty. *J Arthroplasty* 1986; 1:71-81.
11. Morrey BF, Adams RA: Semiconstrained elbow replacement for distal humeral nonunion. *J Bone Joint Surg Br* 1995;77:67-72.
12. Mansat P, Morrey BF: Semiconstrained total elbow arthroplasty for ankylosed and stiff elbows. *J Bone Joint Surg Am* 2000;82:1260-1268.
13. Yamaguchi K, Adams RA, Morrey BF: Semiconstrained total elbow arthroplasty in the context of treated previous infection. *J Shoulder Elbow Surg* 1999;8:461-465.
14. King GJ, Glauser SJ, Westreich A, Morrey BF, An KN: In vitro stability of an unconstrained total elbow prosthesis: Influence of axial loading and joint flexion angle. *J Arthroplasty* 1993; 8:291-298.
15. Morrey BF, Askew LJ, Chao EY: A biomechanical study of normal functional elbow motion. *J Bone Joint Surg Am* 1981;63:872-877.
16. An KN, Morrey BF, Chao EY: Carrying angle of the human elbow joint. *J Orthop Res* 1984; 1:369-378.
17. Amis AA, Dowson D, Wright V: Elbow joint force predictions for some strenuous isometric actions. *J Biomech* 1980;13:765-775.
18. Amis AA, Dowson D, Wright V, Miller JH: The derivation of elbow joint forces, and their relation to prosthesis design. *J Med Eng Technol* 1979;3:229-234.
19. Halls AA, Travill A: Transmission of pressures across the elbow joint. *Anat Rec* 1964;150:243-247.
20. Morrey BF, An KN: Articular and ligamentous contributions to the stability of the elbow joint. *Am J Sports Med* 1983;11:315-319.

21. O'Driscoll SW, An KN, Korinek S, Morrey BF: Kinematics of semi-constrained total elbow arthroplasty. *J Bone Joint Surg Br* 1992;74: 297-299.

22. Schneeberger AG, King GJ, Song SW, O'Driscoll SW, Morrey BF, An KN: Kinematics and laxity of the Souter-Strathclyde total elbow prosthesis. *J Shoulder Elbow Surg* 2000;9:127-134.

23. King GJ, Itoi E, Niebur GL, Morrey BF, An KN: Motion and laxity of the capitellocondylar total elbow prosthesis. *J Bone Joint Surg Am* 1994;76:1000-1008.

24. Kudo H, Iwano K, Watanabe S: Total replacement of the rheumatoid elbow with a hingeless prosthesis. *J Bone Joint Surg Am* 1980;62: 277-285.

25. Lowe LW, Miller AJ, Allum RL, Higginson DW: The development of an unconstrained elbow arthroplasty: A clinical review. *J Bone Joint Surg Br* 1984;66:243-247.

26. Ljung P, Jonsson K, Larsson K, Rydholm U: Interposition arthroplasty of the elbow with rheumatoid arthritis. *J Shoulder Elbow Surg* 1996;5:81-85.

27. Trepman E, Vella IM, Ewald FC: Radial head replacement in capitellocondylar total elbow arthroplasty: 2- to 6-year follow-up evaluation in rheumatoid arthritis. *J Arthroplasty* 1991;6:67-77.

28. Souter WA: Anatomical trochlear stirrup arthroplasty of the rheumatoid elbow, in Kashiwagi D (ed): *Elbow Joint*. Amsterdam, Netherlands, Elsevier Science Publishers, 1985, pp 305-311.

29. Yanni ON, Fearn CB, Gallannaugh SC, Joshi R: The Roper-Tuke total elbow arthroplasty: 4- to 10-year results of an unconstrained prosthesis. *J Bone Joint Surg Br* 2000;82:705-710.

30. Weiland AJ, Weiss AP, Wills RP, Moore JR: Capitellocondylar total elbow replacement: A long-term follow-up study. *J Bone Joint Surg Am* 1989;71:217-222.

31. Poll RG, Rozing PM: Use of the Souter-Strathclyde total elbow prosthesis in patients who have rheumatoid arthritis. *J Bone Joint Surg Am* 1991;73:1227-1233.

32. Ruth JT, Wilde AH: Capitellocondylar total elbow replacement: A long-term follow-up study. *J Bone Joint Surg Am* 1992;74:95-100.

33. Sorbie C, Shiba R, Siu D, Saunders G, Wevers H: The development of a surface arthroplasty for the elbow. *Clin Orthop* 1986;208:100-103.

34. Ewald FC, Simmons ED Jr, Sullivan JA, et al: Capitellocondylar total elbow replacement in rheumatoid arthritis: Long-term results. *J Bone Joint Surg Am* 1993;75:498-507.

35. Trail IA, Nuttall D, Stanley JK: Survivorship and radiological analysis of the standard Souter-Strathclyde total elbow arthroplasty. *J Bone Joint Surg Br* 1999;81:80-84.

36. Kudo H, Iwano K, Nishino J: Total elbow arthroplasty with use of a nonconstrained humeral component inserted without cement in patients who have rheumatoid arthritis. *J Bone Joint Surg Am* 1999;81:1268-1280.

37. Davis RF, Weiland AJ, Hungerford DS, Moore JR, Volenec-Dowling S: Nonconstrained total elbow arthroplasty. *Clin Orthop* 1982;171:156-160.

38. King GJ, Itoi E, Risung F, Niebur GL, Morrey BF, An KN: Kinematic and stability of the Norway elbow: A cadaveric study. *Acta Orthop Scand* 1993;64:657-663.

39. Itoi E, King GJ, Niebur GL, Morrey BF, An KN: Malrotation of the humeral component of the capitellocondylar total elbow replacement is not the sole cause of dislocation. *J Orthop Res* 1994;12:665-671.

40. Cohen MS II, Hastings H II: Rotatory instability of the elbow: The anatomy and role of the lateral stabilizers. *J Bone Joint Surg Am* 1997;79: 225-233.

41. Dee R: Reconstructive surgery following total elbow endoprosthesis. *Clin Orthop* 1982;170: 196-203.

42. Morrey BF, Bryan RS, Dobyns JH, Linscheid RL: Total elbow arthroplasty: A five-year experience at the Mayo Clinic. *J Bone Joint Surg Am* 1981;63:1050-1063.

43. Garrett JC, Ewald FC, Thomas WH, Sledge CB: Loosening associated with G.S.B. hinge total elbow replacement in patients with rheumatoid arthritis. *Clin Orthop* 1977;127: 170-174.

44. Johnson JR, Getty CJ, Lettin AW, Glasgow MM: The Stanmore total elbow replacement for rheumatoid arthritis. *J Bone Joint Surg Br* 1984;66:732-736.

45. Gill DR, Morrey BF: The Coonrad-Morrey total elbow arthroplasty in patients who have rheumatoid arthritis: A ten to fifteen-year follow-up study. *J Bone Joint Surg Am* 1998;80: 1327-1335.

46. King GJ, Adams RA, Morrey BF: Total elbow arthroplasty: Revision with use of a non-custom semiconstrained prosthesis. *J Bone Joint Surg Am* 1997;79:394-400.

47. Bryan RS, Morrey BF: Extensive posterior exposure of the elbow: A triceps-sparing approach. *Clin Orthop* 1982;166:188-192.

48. Pierce TD, Herndon JH: The triceps preserving approach to total elbow arthroplasty. *Clin Orthop* 1998;354:144-152.

49. Dunning CE, Zarzour ZD, Patterson SD, Johnson JA, King GJ: Muscle forces and pronation stabilize the lateral ligament deficient elbow. *Clin Orthop* 2001;388:118-124.

50. Armstrong AD, Dunning CE, Faber KJ, Duck TR, Johnson JA, King GJ: Rehabilitation of the medial collateral ligament-deficient elbow: An in vitro biomechanical study. *J Hand Surg Am* 2000;25:1051-1057.

51. Ljung P, Jonsson K, Rydholm U: Short-term complications of the lateral approach for non-constrained elbow replacement: Follow-up of 50 rheumatoid elbows. *J Bone Joint Surg Br* 1995;77:937-942.

52. Rozing P: Souter-Strathclyde total elbow arthroplasty. *J Bone Joint Surg Br* 2000;82: 1129-1134.

53. Madsen F, Sojbjerg JO, Sneppen O: Late complications with the Pritchard Mark II elbow prosthesis. *J Shoulder Elbow Surg* 1994;3:17-23.

54. Schneeberger AG, Hertel R, Gerber C: Total elbow replacement with the GSB III prosthesis. *J Shoulder Elbow Surg* 2000;9:135-139.

55. Bell S, Gschwend N, Steiger U: Arthroplasty of the elbow: Experience with the Mark III GSB prosthesis. *Aust N Z J Surg* 1986;56: 823-827.

56. Gschwend N, Simmen BR, Matejovsky Z: Late complications in elbow arthroplasty. *J Shoulder Elbow Surg* 1996;5:86-96.

57. Yamaguchi K, Adams RA, Morrey BF: Infection after total elbow arthroplasty. *J Bone Joint Surg Am* 1998;80:481-491.

58. Spinner RJ, Morgenlander JC, Nunley JA: Ulnar nerve function following total elbow arthroplasty: A prospective study comparing preoperative and postoperative clinical and electrophysiologic evaluation in patients with rheumatoid arthritis. *J Hand Surg Am* 2000;25:360-364.

59. Matarese W, Stuchin SA, Kummer FJ, Zuckerman JD: Polyethylene bearing component failure and dislocation in the triaxial elbow: A report of two cases. *J Arthroplasty* 1990;5:365-367.

60. Figgie HE III, Inglis AE, Mow C: A critical analysis of alignment factors affecting functional outcome in total elbow arthroplasty. *J Arthroplasty* 1986;1:169-173.

61. Schuind F, O'Driscoll S, Korinek S, An KN, Morrey BF: Loose-hinge total elbow arthroplasty: An experimental study of the effects of implant alignment on three-dimensional elbow kinematics. *J Arthroplasty* 1995;10:670-678.

62. Faber KJ, Cordy ME, Milne AD, Chess DG, King GJ, Johnson JA: Advanced cement technique improves fixation in elbow arthroplasty. *Clin Orthop* 1997;334:150-156.

63. Dee R: Total replacement of the elbow joint. *Orthop Clin North Am* 1973;4:415-433.

64. Figgie HE III, Inglis AE, Ranawat CS, Rosenberg GM: Results of total elbow arthroplasty as a salvage procedure for failed elbow reconstructive operations. *Clin Orthop* 1987; 219:185-193.

65. Kraay MJ, Figgie MP, Inglis AE, Wolfe SW, Ranawat CS: Primary semiconstrained total elbow arthroplasty: Survival analysis of 113 consecutive cases. *J Bone Joint Surg Br* 1994; 76:636-640.

66. Gschwend N, Scheier NH, Baehler AR: Long-term results of the GSB III elbow arthroplasty. *J Bone Joint Surg Br* 1999;81:1005-1012.

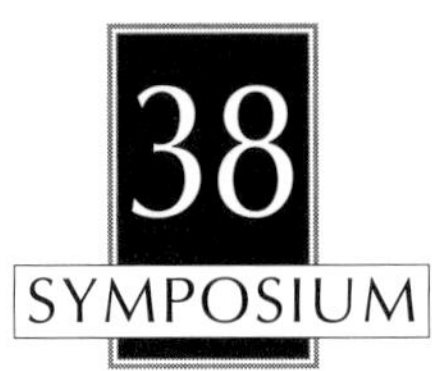

Elbow Arthroscopy: Basic Setup and Treatment of Arthritis

Matthew L. Ramsey, MD

Introduction

Arthroscopic surgery of the elbow has become an important tool in the diagnosis and treatment of a variety of disorders of the elbow. It is safe, effective, and reproducible but also is technically demanding. Elbow arthroscopy is valuable because normal and diseased intra-articular structures can be more easily seen, leading to prompt identification of pathology and treatment options. An understanding of the neurovascular anatomy and attention to detail is critical if complications are to be avoided.

Indications

The ideal indications for arthroscopy of the elbow are a history of pain or mechanical symptoms and a physical examination and radiographic studies that reveal intra-articular pathology. Arthroscopy is rarely used in the diagnosis and treatment of patients who have a history of pain but no physical findings or radiographic studies suggesting intra-articular pathology.[1] In these patients, arthroscopy is sometimes useful to document the absence of intra-articular pathology as the cause of pain.

The established indications for elbow arthroscopy are listed in Table 1. The management of elbow instability (posterolateral rotatory instability) and elbow trauma are yet to be established as indications.

Absolute contraindications to elbow arthroscopy are relatively few. When severe capsular contracture or frank ankylosis prevents the protection of the neurovascular structures through adequate joint distention, arthroscopy is best avoided. Any process that distorts the normal anatomy of the elbow is a relative contraindication to elbow arthroscopy. Congenital anomalies, posttraumatic deformity, or surgical alteration of normal anatomy (for example, ulnar nerve transposition) can affect anatomic relationships to such a degree that the risk of neurovascular injury is unacceptably high.

Surgical Technique

The key to avoiding complications in elbow arthroscopy is understanding the relationship of the neurovascular structures to the topographic anatomy of the elbow. The elbow is a subcutaneous joint with easily palpated bony landmarks, including the medial epicondyle, lateral epicondyle, olecranon process, and radial head. Because these landmarks can be difficult to palpate after joint distention, they should be outlined on the skin before joint distention to assist in portal placement.

Patient Position

Arthroscopy can be done with the patient supine, prone, or in the lateral decubitus position. The supine position described by Andrews and Carson[2] facilitates easy access to the airway for anesthesia and allows excellent access to the anterior aspect of the elbow joint. The joint is anatomically oriented, making arthroscopy less confusing for the novice arthroscopist. Disadvantages include the requirement for an overhead traction device, awkward positioning for access to the posterior aspect of the elbow, and a less stable working base because the arm is suspended in the air.

The prone position, popularized by Poehling and associates,[3] affords easy access to the anterior and posterior compartments of the elbow and allows the surgeon to work from a stable base. Because no accessory traction devices are required, the elbow is easily taken through a full range of motion without restrictions. The disadvantage of this technique is the need to place the patient face down, a position associated with anesthetic difficulties.

The lateral decubitus position alleviates the disadvantages of both the supine and prone positions while maintaining certain advantages.[1] The affected arm is allowed to hang free over a padded support to permit free flexion and extension of the elbow joint (Fig. 1). Conversion to open surgery on the lateral side of the elbow is easily managed. However, open surgery on the medial side of the elbow can be somewhat difficult. Elbow arthroscopy as described herein is done with the patient in the lateral decubitus position, but general principles are applicable to arthroscopy done with the patient prone or supine.

Arthroscopy Setup

A general anesthetic is administered and the patient is placed in the lateral decubitus position with the involved extremity facing upward. The arm is supported and stabilized on a padded bolster, with the

Table 1
Established Indications for Elbow Arthroscopy

Loose body removal
Synovectomy
Degenerative arthritis
Posttraumatic arthritis
Lateral epicondylitis
Osteochondral lesions
Contracture release

shoulder abducted to 90° and the elbow flexed to 90°.

The extremity is prepped and draped free to allow intraoperative manipulation. The forearm is wrapped with an elastic bandage from the fingers to just below the portal sites to minimize fluid extravasation into the forearm. The topographic anatomy of the elbow and the portal sites are marked on the skin before joint distention. Distending the joint before establishing arthroscopic portals increases the distance between the bony landmarks of the elbow and the neurovascular structures about the elbow.

An 18-gauge spinal needle is inserted into the joint through the lateral "soft spot" bounded by the lateral epicondyle, radial head, and olecranon process. The elbow is distended with 15 to 25 mL of sterile saline. Distention of the joint with more than 15 to 25 mL of fluid risks capsular rupture and fluid extravasation during arthroscopy.[4] Free backflow of fluid is confirmed after joint distention.

Portal Placement

The risk of injury to the neurovascular structures exists at all levels of portal placement from the skin incision to joint penetration, regardless of the portal used. Experiences with a variety of anterior and posterior portals have been described[1-3,5-7] as surgeons have sought to decrease the risks of cutaneous and deep neurovascular injury while providing adequate intra-articular visualization of the elbow joint.

Anterolateral Portal Andrews and Carson[2] originally described the anterolateral portal as being located 3 cm distal and 1 cm anterior to the lateral epicondyle. This portal location places the radial nerve at significant risk for injury.[8] Several authors[5,6,9] have stressed the importance of avoiding the distal placement of this portal in favor of a more proximal location. Recent studies indicate that more proximal placement of the anterolateral portals increases the margin of safety with respect to the radial nerve.[6]

Midanterolateral Portal Field and associates[6] described a midanterolateral portal that is analogous to the more proximally placed anterolateral portal advocated by Morrey[9] and Boe.[5] This portal is placed in the sulcus and can be palpated between the radial head and capitellum anterior to the lateral epicondyle.

Proximal Anterolateral Portal Field and associates[6] also described a proximal anterolateral portal 1 to 2 cm proximal to the lateral epicondyle directly on the anterior humerus. Proximal placement of this portal brings the arthroscope into the lateral aspect of the joint at an angle that allows excellent visualization not only of the medial joint but also of the radiocapitellar joint and lateral gutter. In practice, anterior portal placement from the lateral side of the elbow can occur anywhere from the sulcus between the radial head and capitellum to a point 2 cm proximal to the lateral epicondyle along the anterior aspect of the humerus without placing the radial nerve at increased risk. In fact, as the portal moves proximally, the risk of neurovascular injury diminishes.[6]

Anteromedial Portal The anteromedial portal was described by Andrews and Carson[2] and is located 2 cm anterior and 2 cm distal to the medial epicondyle. This portal traverses the flexor-pronator muscle mass and places the medial antebrachial cutaneous nerve at risk, allowing excellent visualization of the lateral elbow joint as well as of the proximal capsular insertion. The anteromedial portal is used primarily to augment the proximal anteromedial portal when instrumentation of the medial gutter is required.

Proximal Anteromedial The proximal anteromedial portal popularized by Poehling and associates[3] is located 2 cm proximal to the medial epicondyle and just anterior to the intramuscular septum. The ulnar nerve is located approximately 3 to 4 mm from this portal posterior to the intramuscular septum. Palpating the septum and making sure that the portal is established anterior to the septum minimizes the risk of injury to the nerve. This portal has an advantage over the anteromedial portal in that it allows excellent visualization of the joint while maintaining the medial neurovascular structures at a safer distance from the arthroscope.[7]

Posterocentral Portal The posterocentral portal is located 3 cm proximal to the tip of the olecranon in the midline. It pierces the triceps muscle just above the musculotendinous junction and provides excellent visualization of the entire posterior compartment of the elbow including the medial and lateral gutters.

Proximal Posterolateral Portal The proximal posterolateral portal is classically located 3 cm proximal to the tip of the olecranon and lateral to the triceps tendon. This serves as an accessory posterior portal that in combination with the posterocentral portal provides complete access to the posterior compartment.

Accessory Posterolateral Portals The posterolateral anatomy of the elbow allows for portal placement anywhere from the proximal posterolateral portal to the lateral soft spot. Altering the portal position along the line between the proximal posterolateral and lateral soft spot portals changes the orientation of the portal relative to the joint. These portals are particularly useful to gain access to the posterolateral gutter.

Soft Spot Portal The lateral soft spot portal is located at the center of the triangle defined by the radial head, lateral epicondyle, and olecranon process. Some authors advocate the use of this portal as the initial visualization portal for diagnostic arthroscopy.[1,10] It allows excellent visualization of the inferior aspect of the capitellum and the inferior portion of the radioulnar articulation and is a necessary component to a complete arthroscopic examination of the elbow.

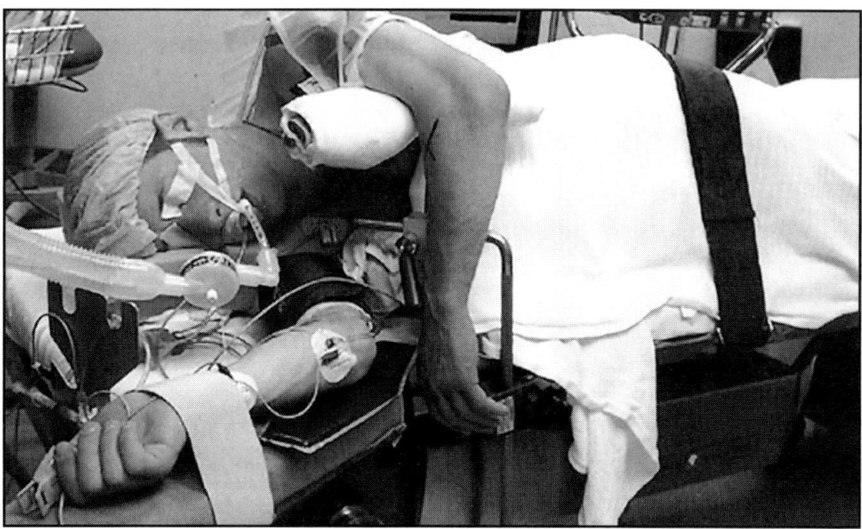

Fig. 1 Lateral decubitus position for elbow arthroscopy. Note that the shoulder is abducted 90° and the elbow is able to freely flex and extend.

Management of Elbow Arthritis

Inflammatory Arthritis

The elbow is commonly involved in inflammatory disorders, including rheumatoid arthritis. Proliferative synovitis results in pain and loss of motion. When synovitis is left unchecked, over time the articular cartilage, periarticular soft-tissue structures, and subchondral bone are progressively affected. When nonsurgical measures fail, synovectomy is a proven treatment for the rheumatoid elbow.

Synovectomy of the elbow is indicated in patients with a symptomatic synovitis with little or no destruction of the joint cartilage that has not responded to nonsurgical management. Radial head resection in association with synovectomy remains controversial. The radial head is critically important in load sharing in the elbow. With a normal-functioning medial collateral ligament, the radial head serves as a secondary stabilizer to applied valgus loads. Attenuation of the medial collateral ligament with disease progression, combined with excision of the radial head, increases stress on the ulnohumeral articulation. This has led some authors[11] to recommend preservation of the radial head to avoid late destruction of the joint.

Arthroscopic synovectomy offers several advantages over open synovectomy, including decreased morbidity, improved visibility of the entire joint, and faster rehabilitation; however, the technical requirements of arthroscopic synovectomy should not be underestimated. Lee and Morrey[12] reported satisfactory results in 93% of 14 patients with rheumatoid arthritis during the early postoperative period after arthroscopic synovectomy, but these results deteriorated substantially by 42 months postoperatively. In a review of 46 patients treated with arthroscopic synovectomy for inflammatory arthritis, all patients had improved motion and decreased pain over a 5-year period.[13] Unfortunately, no long-term results are available for comparison with open synovectomy.

The indication for arthroscopic radial head resection in conjunction with synovectomy is pain determined to originate from the radiocapitellar joint. Patients with instability as a result of destruction of the bony or ligamentous restraints are at risk for increased instability or secondary joint destruction after radial head resection. All options should be considered in these patients before proceeding with radial head resection.

Radial head excision is done with the arthroscope in the proximal anteromedial portal and the shaver initially in the midanterolateral portal. The radial head is resected from lateral to medial by sweeping the burr proximal to distal. Resection should proceed to the level of the annular ligament, and care should be taken not to violate the anterolateral capsule to avoid radial nerve injury.[14] As resection proceeds posteriorly, the burr can be moved to the soft spot portal to complete resection of the radial head. Pronation and supination of the forearm assist in delivering the radial head into the field of vision for resection.

Degenerative Arthritis

Degenerative conditions of the elbow are appropriate for arthroscopic management. Loose bodies can be found in isolation or, more commonly, associated with degenerative changes of the elbow, including osteophyte formation of the coronoid and olecranon processes and in their respective fossae. These periarticular manifestations of degenerative arthritis result in limitation of range of motion, pain at the extremes of motion, and mechanical symptoms of locking, clicking, or catching of the elbow.

The most common indication for elbow arthroscopy is for the removal of loose bodies. Isolated loose bodies can occur in the absence of other manifestations of degenerative arthritis, and patient response to arthroscopic excision is good.[1,5,15,16] When loose bodies are associated with osteophyte formation, simple loose body excision is insufficient to manage all of the patient's symptoms. Osteophyte impingement in flexion and/or extension limits range of motion and causes pain with forced motion at the allowable extremes. In this situation, débridement of the osteophytes from the olecranon and coronoid processes and recreation of the radial, coronoid, and olecranon fossae depth are necessary. These technical requirements for successful surgery require advanced arthroscopic skills and a keen awareness of the potential neurovascular risks to avoid potentially devastating complications.

Removal of anterior compartment osteophytes from the tip of the coronoid process and re-creation of the coronoid and radial fossae require the use of several anterior arthroscopic portals. As mentioned previously, proximal portals on the medial and lateral sides of the joint provide the greatest margin of safety with respect to the surrounding neurovascular structures. The proximal anteromedial and anterolateral portals position the arthroscope ideally for management of osteophytes in the coronoid and radial fossae and facilitate capsular release from the humeral insertion. Excision of osteophytes from the coronoid tip is possible through proximal portals and is assisted by flexing the elbow to deliver the coronoid tip. Occasionally, a midanterolateral portal more appropriately positions the instruments for osteophyte excision from the coronoid fossa.

Several authors have reported successful arthroscopic management of degenerative arthritis of the elbow,[17-19] although range of motion was not improved in some studies, presumably because capsular release was not done in conjunction with débridement of the elbow.[18] The results of the management of degenerative conditions of the elbow must be viewed in the context of the underlying pathology to be corrected at the time of arthroscopy. Arthroscopic loose body excision has proved to be an effective therapeutic tool.[1,5,10,15,16,20] As previously mentioned, however, patients with other features of degenerative arthritis beyond loose bodies do not benefit from loose body excision alone; their surgery must also include osteophyte excision.[1,16,20]

References

1. O'Driscoll SW, Morrey BF: Arthroscopy of the elbow: Diagnostic and therapeutic benefits and hazards. *J Bone Joint Surg Am* 1992;74:84-94.
2. Andrews JR, Carson WG: Arthroscopy of the elbow. *Arthroscopy* 1985;1:97-107.
3. Poehling GG, Whipple TL, Sisco L, Goldman B: Elbow arthroscopy: A new technique. *Arthroscopy* 1989;5:222-224.
4. O'Driscoll SW, Morrey BF, An KN: Intraarticular pressure and capacity of the elbow. *Arthroscopy* 1990;6:100-103.
5. Boe S: Arthroscopy of the elbow: Diagnosis and extraction of loose bodies. *Acta Orthop Scand* 1986;57:52-53.
6. Field LD, Altchek DW, Warren RF, O'Brien SJ, Skyhar MJ, Wickiewicz TL: Arthroscopic anatomy of the lateral elbow: A comparison of three portals. *Arthroscopy* 1994;10:602-607.
7. Lindenfeld TN: Medial approach in elbow arthroscopy. *Am J Sports Med* 1990;18:413-417.
8. Lynch GJ, Meyers JF, Whipple TL, Caspari RB: Neurovascular anatomy and elbow arthroscopy: Inherent risks. *Arthroscopy* 1986; 2:190-197.
9. Morrey BF: Arthroscopy of the elbow. *Instr Course Lect* 1986;35:102-107.
10. O'Driscoll SW, Morrey BF: Arthroscopy of the elbow, in Morrey BF (ed): *The Elbow*. New York, NY, Raven Press, 1994, pp 21-34.
11. Rymaszewski LA, Mackay I, Amis AA, Miller JH: Long-term effects of excision of the radial head in rheumatoid arthritis. *J Bone Joint Surg Br* 1984;66:109-113.
12. Lee BP, Morrey BF: Arthroscopic synovectomy of the elbow for rheumatoid arthritis: A prospective study. *J Bone Joint Surg Br* 1997;79: 770-772.
13. Thal R: Arthritis, in Savoie FH, Field LD (eds): *Arthroscopy of the Elbow*. New York, NY, Churchill Livingstone, 1996, pp 103-116.
14. Jones GS, Savoie FH III: Arthroscopic capsular release of flexion contractures (arthrofibrosis) of the elbow. *Arthroscopy* 1993;9:277-283.
15. McGinty JB: Arthroscopic removal of loose bodies. *Orthop Clin North Am* 1982;13:313-328.
16. O'Driscoll SW: Elbow arthroscopy for loose bodies. *Orthopedics* 1992;15:855-859.
17. Ogilvie-Harris DJ, Gordon R, MacKay M: Arthroscopic treatment for posterior impingement in degenerative arthritis of the elbow. *Arthroscopy* 1995;11:437-443.
18. Redden JF, Stanley D: Arthroscopic fenestration of the olecranon fossa in the treatment of osteoarthritis of the elbow. *Arthroscopy* 1993;9: 14-16.
19. Savoie FH III, Nunley PD, Field LD: Arthroscopic management of the arthritic elbow: Indications, technique, and results. *J Shoulder Elbow Surg* 1999;8:214-219.
20. Ogilvie-Harris DJ, Schemitsch E: Arthroscopy of the elbow for removal of loose bodies. *Arthroscopy* 1993;9:5-8.

Arthroscopic Treatment of Arthritis of the Elbow

Frank B. Norberg, MD
Felix H. Savoie III, MD
Larry D. Field, MD

Introduction

The role of arthroscopy for treatment of elbow disease is a rapidly developing area in orthopaedics. In recent years, the advantage of direct visualization of the entire joint with minimal soft-tissue disruption has been used for a number of elbow conditions. Compared with open procedures, arthroscopy allows more rapid rehabilitation and reduces the amount of scarring and capsular contracture, important factors in treatment of the arthritic elbow.

Treatment of arthritis of the elbow has ranged from conservative modalities in mild cases to fusion and arthroplasty in more severe cases. Synovectomy has also been effective in the treatment of inflammatory disease. Elbow arthroplasty has not been as successful as joint replacement of the knee or hip. Arthroscopy serves as an intermediate step between conservative treatment and joint replacement, allowing the surgeon to perform lavage, debridement, spur excision, loose body removal, and synovectomy.

Inflammatory Arthritis

The elbow is commonly involved in systemic inflammatory disease. Patients with rheumatoid arthritis will have elbow involvement in 20% to 50% of cases.[1,2] Spontaneous improvement may occur, but is unlikely. The synovium is affected, causing patients to maintain the arm in a flexed position, resulting in a flexion contracture.

Conservative treatment of these chronic debilitating disorders is standard. The usual approach consists of medications to control systemic inflammation and symptoms. Flare-ups in individual joints may be treated with splinting, gentle physiotherapy, and occasional steroid injections. Synovectomy may be considered if these measures fail to control symptoms.

Open synovectomy may be performed and is an accepted procedure with good results.[1-4] Debate continues regarding the best approach to the elbow, although the lateral Kocher approach was most commonly used in recent series.[1,5-7] Controversy also exists regarding the excision of the radial head. Rymaszewski and associates[6] cite excision of the radial head as a main cause of failure due to instability and increased lateral ulnohumeral arthritis. Other studies report good results with radial head resection in selected patients and resection is recommended when appropriate.[6,8-10] Range of motion after open synovectomy will improve in approximately 40% of cases and decrease somewhat in 15%; in the remaining 45%, range of motion will be unchanged.[5] Complications include loss of motion, along with transient and permanent neurologic injury. Permanent neurologic injury to both the ulnar and radial nerves has been reported.[1,11]

Degenerative Arthritis

Primary osteoarthritis of the elbow is an uncommon problem, accounting for only 1% to 2% of patients presenting with degenerative arthritis.[12,13] Patients will typically present in their third to eighth decade. Those presenting at younger ages tend to have arthritic changes secondary to athletic injuries or osteochondritis dissecans. The usual presentation is pain at the limits of motion with a mechanical block of both flexion and extension (Fig. 1). Patients will often report pain when carrying any object with the elbow in extension. Radiographs of the elbow commonly show osteophytes of the olecranon and coronoid, as well as osteophytes of the olecranon and coronoid fossae (Fig. 2). Loose bodies are not uncommon.

Conservative management of elbow arthritis is usually successful.[14] For those patients who fail to respond to conservative treatment or whose decreased range of motion interferes with their daily activities, arthroscopy should be considered. Morrey and associates[15] have shown that a 100° arc of motion, from 30° to 130° of flexion, is adequate for performance of 90% of activities of daily living. A greater range of motion may be required by those involved in athletics and for certain occupations. Removal of osteophytes from the olecranon and coronoid as well as from the olecranon

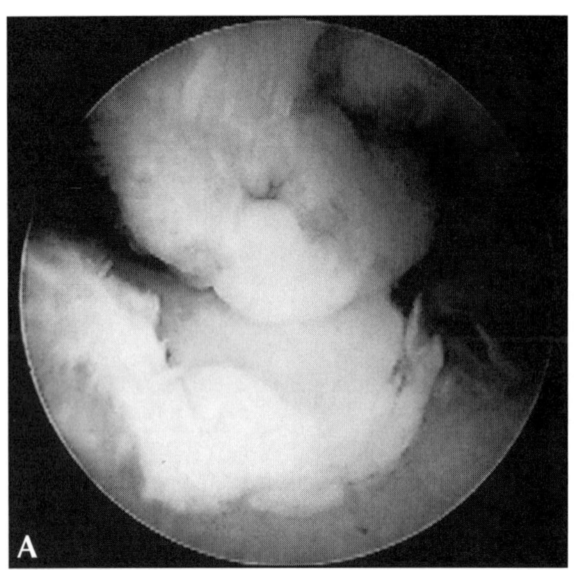

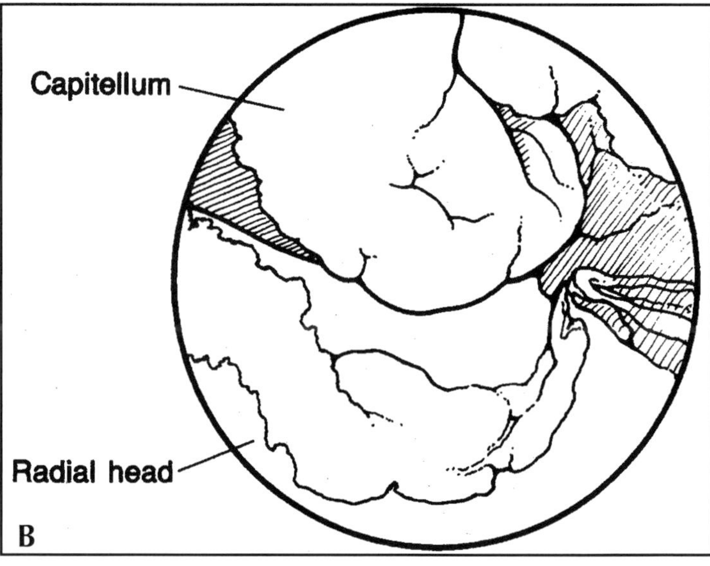

Fig. 1 Capitellar osteophytes, an anatomic feature described in the osteoarthritic elbow. **A,** Arthroscopic view. **B,** Line drawing. (Reproduced with permission from Thal R: Arthritis, in Savoie FH, Field LD (eds): *Arthroscopy of the Elbow.* Philadelphia, PA, Churchill Livingstone, 1996, p 107.)

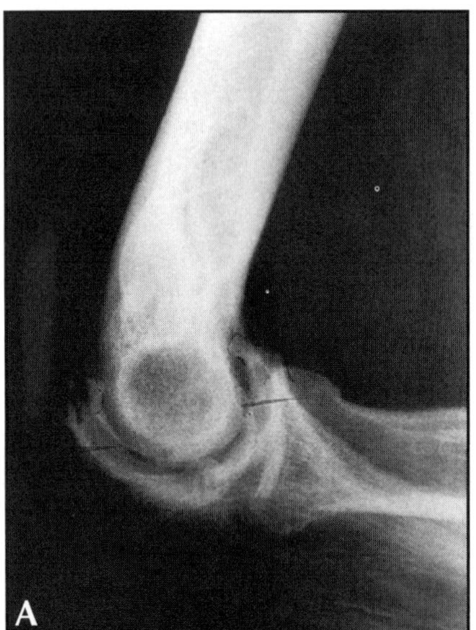

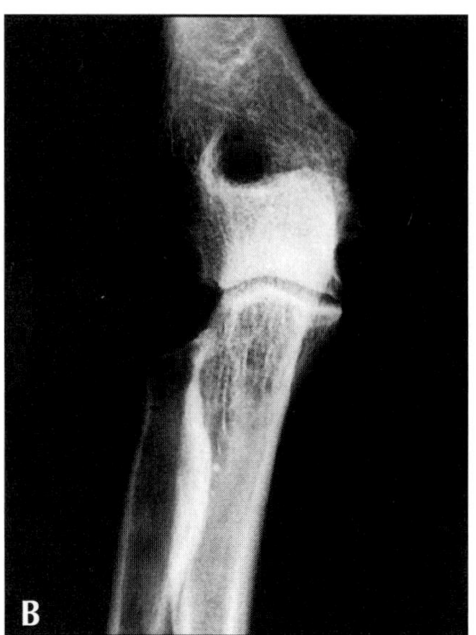

Fig. 2 A, Lateral radiograph of an arthritic elbow with lines indicating planned osteophyte resection. **B,** Anteroposterior radiograph of elbow after radial head resection and olecranon fossa fenestration.

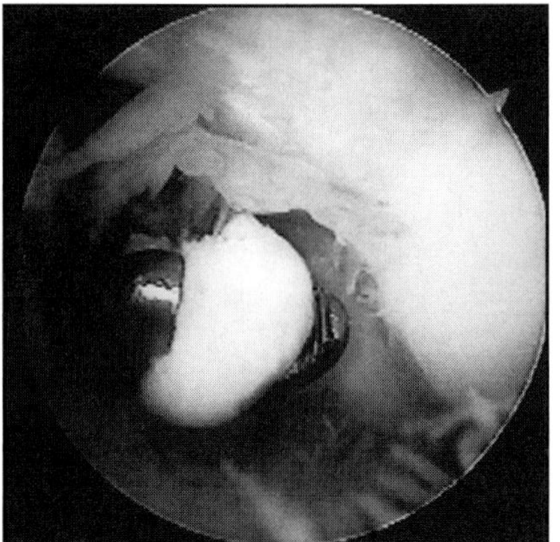

Fig. 3 Loose body in the anterior compartment. (Reproduced with permission from Thal R: Arthritis, in Savoie FH, Field LD (eds): *Arthroscopy of the Elbow.* Philadelphia, PA, Churchill Livingstone, 1996, p 57.)

and coronoid fossae has been shown to be effective in the management of early primary degenerative arthritis.[16-18]

Loose Bodies

Loose bodies are formed as a result of osteoarthritis, osteochondritis dissecans, trauma, and overuse, and occasionally are idiopathic. Arthritic debris and loose bodies are removed using the motorized synovial resector and occasionally arthroscopic graspers (Fig. 3). Standard radiography will typically underestimate the incidence of loose bodies found on arthroscopy.[19-23] Careful inspection of the joint is necessary to locate all fragments, and both the 30° and 70° scopes can be very useful. However, arthritic conditions are seldom improved by simply removing loose bodies.[19-21, 24-26]

Arthrofibrosis

A flexion contracture of the elbow may

be caused by fractures, dislocations, burns, head injury, spasticity, and arthritis. Capsular contracture is not usually a major part of the pathology of the arthritic elbow in our experience. Yet, some patients will continue to have significant flexion contractures after the resection of bony spurs, ulnohumeral arthroplasty, and debridement of loose bodies. These patients may benefit from capsular release. O'Driscoll and Morrey[17] have recommended capsular release of the anterior capsule from the humeral attachment using a blunt periosteal elevator or similar instrument. We prefer to perform an arthroscopic resection of the proximal 1 to 2 cm of the anterior capsule from its origin at the humerus. **(CD-24.1)**

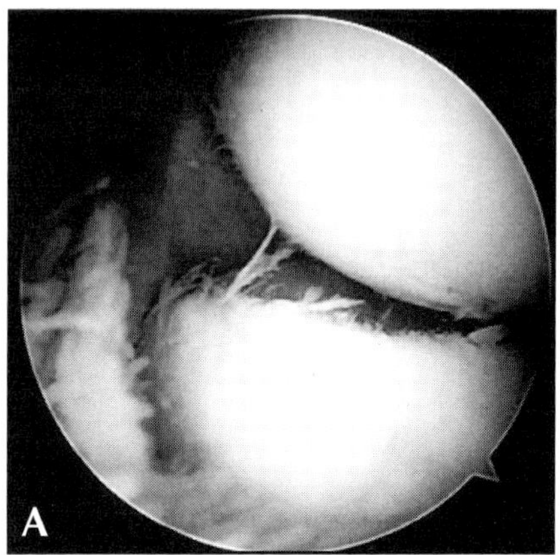

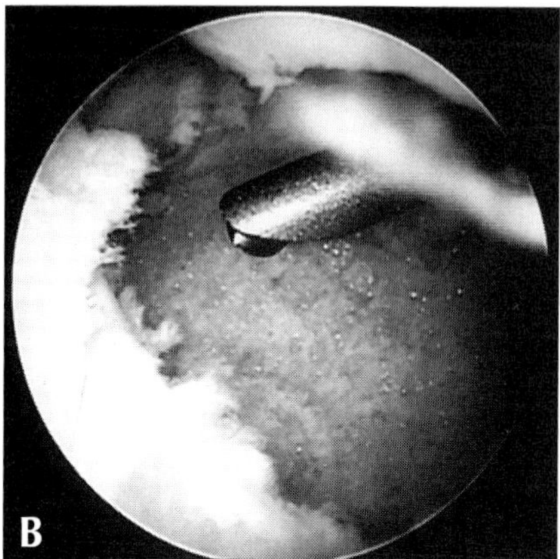

Fig. 4 A, Anterior view of degenerative radial head. **B,** Same view following resection with the shaver in the lateral soft spot portal.

Contraindications

Contraindications to elbow arthroscopy include severe arthrofibrosis or ankylosis, which prevents entry into the joint. Patients who have had previous surgery will also be at higher risk of neurovascular complications and may be better served by open procedures with direct visualization of the neurovascular structures. Capsular contracture decreases the working space and visualization in the joint. More importantly, it decreases joint distention and the distance to the overlying neurovascular structures. Ulnar nerve subluxation has been documented in 16% of the population.[27] Prior ulnar nerve transposition or a subluxated ulnar nerve is a relative contraindication to placement of an anteromedial portal, but not to arthroscopy.

Technique

Initially most arthroscopic procedures were performed with the patient in the supine position. The prone or lateral decubitus positions are now chosen because of the improved access and ease of surgery. The prone position allows better access to the elbow; the lateral decubitus position allows the anesthesiologist better access to the patient. We place the patient in the prone position for elbow arthroscopy. A block is placed under the arm so that it is elevated away from the arm board, and the forearm and hand are allowed to hang free with the elbow flexed at 90° to allow maximum intra-articular volume. The forearm and hand should be wrapped with Coban compressive wrapping to restrict swelling and the space for fluid extravasation during the procedure; afterward, the space available for extravasated fluid will be increased when the wrapping is removed. The elbow capsule is distended by injecting with an 18-gauge spinal needle placed in the area of the posterior portal into the olecranon fossa. The "soft spot" portal is also commonly used for joint distention. Typically, as the capsule of the elbow is distended, the arm will slightly extend and supinate. Blunt trocars are used when establishing portals to decrease the risk of injury to the joint and neurovascular structures.[28,29] All portal positions are checked with an 18-gauge spinal needle prior to placement of the trocar and cannula. When establishing portals, care is taken to only incise the skin with the scalpel. The elbow is initially entered through an anterior proximal medial portal, 2 cm proximal and just anterior to the intermuscular septum, as described by Poehling and associates.[30] Then, an anterior proximal lateral instrument portal is established, after checking the position with the 18-gauge needle, 2 cm proximal and 1 cm anterior to the lateral epicondyle, under direct visualization as described by Field and associates.[31] The lateral portal has various uses (for example, synovectomy, radiocapitellar joint debridement, excision of coronoid osteophytes, and deepening of the coronoid fossa) depending on the pathology observed via the proximal anteromedial portal. Instruments passed through the medial portal are used to excise spurs from the trochlea, complete the debridement, and perform the lateral half of the anterior capsular release when indicated.

Osteoarthritic spurs are debrided from the coronoid process with a shaver in the lateral portal. If radial head excision is necessary because of radiocapitellar degeneration, the anterior aspect of the radial head is then excised (Fig. 4). It is important to keep the cutting surface of the shaver facing posterior because the posterior interosseous nerve lies adjacent to the anterior capsule at this level. Penetration of the capsule in this area will damage the nerve. The arthroscope is left in the proximal medial portal and the posterior soft spot (straight lateral) portal is then used for instrumentation, sweeping the shaver medially, and laterally

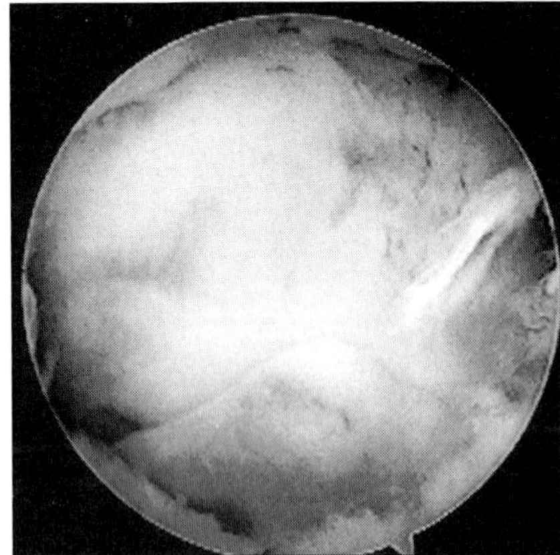

Fig. 5 Posterior view of the elbow showing olecranon spurring and thickening of the olecranon fossa with loss of depth.

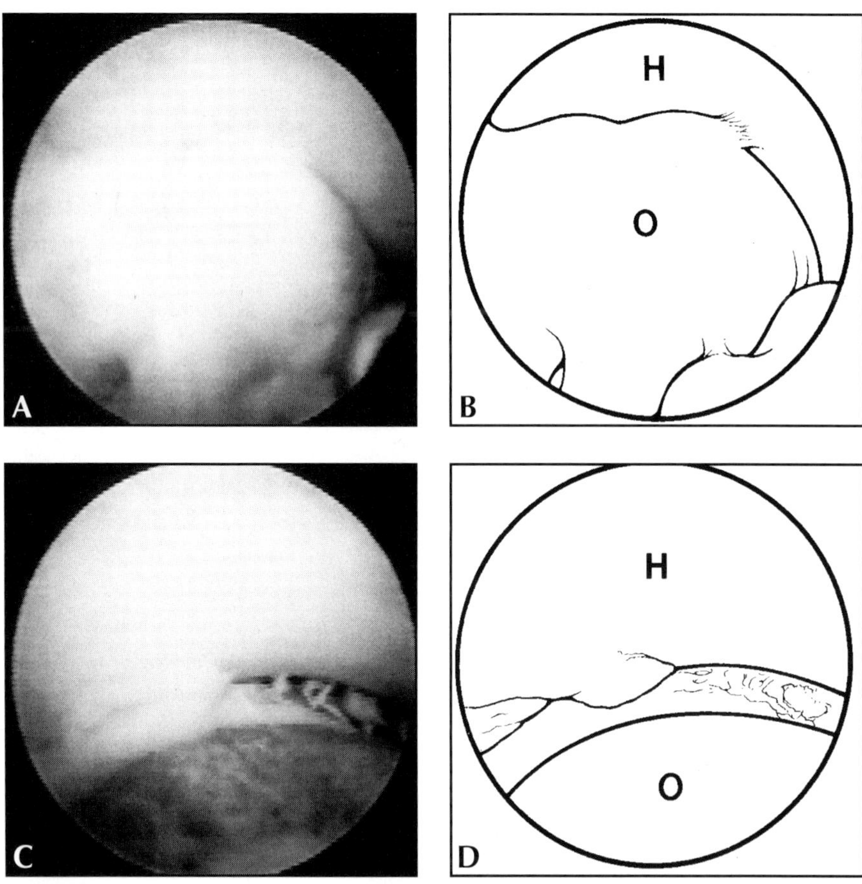

Fig. 6 A, Posterior view of the elbow demonstrating olecranon spurring. **B,** Corresponding line drawing. H = humerus; O = olecranon. **C,** View after resection of olecranon spurring. **D,** Corresponding line drawing.

excising the radial head until adequate clearance is obtained, usually 5 to 8 mm. The proximal radial ulnar joint is assessed; if further debridement is necessary, additional bone is removed. This can be aided by pronating and supinating the forearm while resection is performed. The extent of radial head excision is evaluated by fluoroscopy periodically at this point to avoid an oblique resection of the radial head. Once an adequate debridement of the anterior aspect of the elbow joint, including excision of coronoid process spurs, debridement of the coronoid fossa and excision, if necessary, of the radial head, has been accomplished, the instrumentation is switched to the posterior aspect of the elbow. In a recent review, 13 of 14 patients who had a radial head resection had successful results. The single failure was a debridement with partial radial head resection. Capsular release is usually not necessar, because bony spurs are typically the source of motion loss. When necessary, resection of the proximal 1 to 2 cm of the anterior capsule is performed arthroscopically to prevent immediate scarring of the capsule. This is begun at the coronoid fossa and brought laterally with the shaver in the proximal anteromedial portal. The scope and shaver positions are then reversed and the medial portion of the capsule is resected to the medial border of the humerus. The resection will allow visualization of the brachialis muscle fibers that are protecting the overlying neurovascular structures.[12] Care must be exercised to avoid catastrophic complications. Direct visualization must be maintained while resecting the capsule, and care should be taken to keep the shaver against the anterior humerus. Adhesions around the radial head and coronoid should also be debrided. After anterior release, any posterior adhesions should then be addressed. One posterior interosseous nerve disruption was reported in the initial series and remains the only significant complication encountered with this procedure.[32]

The inflow is left anteriorly in the proximal medial portal and the arthroscope introduced through a standard posterolateral portal. The posterior central portal is then used initially for instrumentation, and the olecranon fossa debrided of arthritic spurs and loose bodies (Fig. 5). Loose bodies will quite commonly have soft-tissue attachments or be imbedded in the synovium. These can be removed with a shaver or burr. The tip of the olecranon and associated spurs are then excised until 0° to -5° of extension can be achieved (Fig. 6). The medial gutter is debrided of synovium with care taken to always keep the blunt aspect of the shaver toward the ulnar nerve and medial capsule. No suction is used in this area. The lateral gutter is then debrided with excision of the posterolateral plica.

A 5-mm drill bit is placed in the center of the olecranon fossa and drilled from posterior to anterior connecting the olecranon and coronoid fossae. The drill is centered in the olecranon fossa and angled toward the center of the coronoid fossa. The intersection of the long axis of the humerus with the inflow cannula in the anterior proximal medial portal provides a guide as to the proper orientation of the drill. After assessing the location and depth of this channel connecting the 2 fossae, a motorized burr is used to enlarge the hole to at least 1 cm in diameter or until full (135° or more) flexion and extension (-5° or less) can be achieved. The goal of the procedure is contact with the medial or lateral columns of the distal humerus (Fig. 7). **(CD-24.2)**

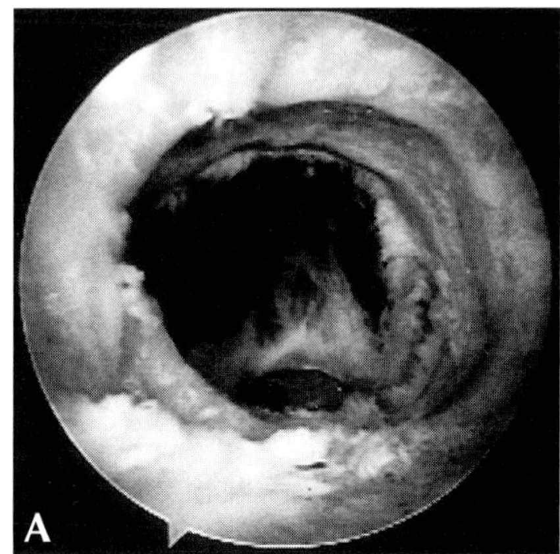

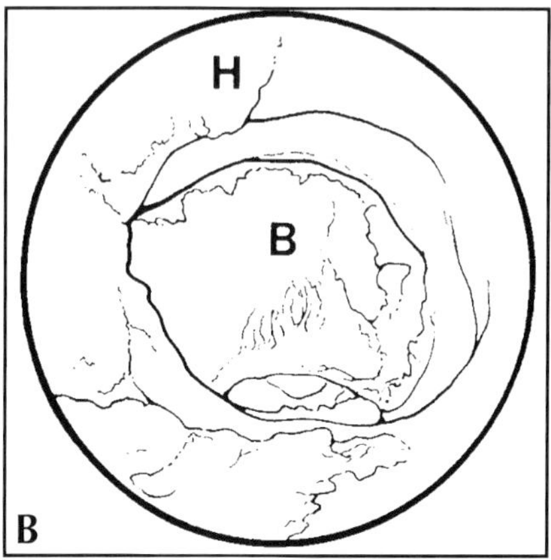

Fig 7 A, Posterior view of the elbow after ulnohumeral arthroplasty. **B,** Line drawing. H = humerus; B = brachialis and anterior capsule.

When performing arthroscopy of the elbow the need to work quickly and efficiently must be stressed. The repeated inadvertent removal and replacement of cannulae through the capsule results in rapid fluid extravasation and results in difficulty manipulating instruments and decreased working space. A concise preoperative plan, adequate familiarity with the procedure, and appropriate equipment will allow a large amount of work to be performed in a short time.

Once the procedure has been completed, suction drains are placed anteriorly and posteriorly as needed. Continuous passive motion (CPM) is initiated in the recovery room and continued during the first 1 to 3 weeks of home care. Patients are usually discharged the day after surgery. All patients receive physical therapy instructions for home exercise while in the hospital.

Discussion

Most patients with mild to moderate arthritis of the elbow do well with conservative treatment.[12,33] However, once the condition becomes disabling there are relatively few procedures to improve function and decrease pain. Smith[34] recommended open debridement of the arthritic elbow after failure of conservative treatment but recognized this as a temporizing measure. Open distraction arthroplasty has been described with encouraging results.[35] This procedure may require significant dissection and is associated with a more complicated postoperative course. Distraction arthroplasty also requires the use of an expensive and bulky external fixator; the patient must be highly motivated so that good results can be achieved.

Kashiwagi[36,37] has described the Outerbridge-Kashiwagi procedure using a Cloward drill to trephinate the olecranon fossa. Morrey[35] has reported on 15 patients with 2-year follow-up using a modification of the Outerbridge-Kashiwagi procedure where the triceps is elevated off the olecranon from the medial side instead of the previously described triceps splitting approach. Fourteen of 15 patients had good relief of pain. Elbow extension improved 11° and flexion improved 10°.

Redden and Stanley[18] recommended a similar procedure for arthroscopic fenestration of the olecranon fossa. They reported good to excellent pain relief but no improvement in range of motion. The lack of increased range of motion may be related to the lack of anterior release. Savoie and associates[38] studied 24 patients who underwent arthroscopic ulnohumeral arthroplasty, with good results. Twenty-three of 24 patients were satisfied with the procedure 2 to 5 years after surgery. The average total arc of elbow motion improved from 50° preoperatively to 131° postoperatively, an improvement of 81°. Radial head resection was performed in 18 of the 24 cases. No neurovascular complications were encountered. Ward and Anderson[22] reported results in 35 athletes who were treated for loose bodies or osteophytes of the elbow with arthroscopic loose body removal and debridement. Improvement in pain and function was seen in approximately 90% of patients, and 34 of 35 believed that the surgery was worthwhile.

Arthroscopy of the arthritic elbow has several advantages. Removal of intra-articular debris, thickened synovial fluid and inflamed synovium may decrease symptoms and temporarily retard the arthritic process. Removal of bone spurs and loose bodies may relieve pain and restore motion and function, allowing more rapid rehabilitation. Arthroscopic treatment of osteoarthritis of the elbow represents a valuable adjunct and with time may become the standard treatment.

Complications

Complications in elbow arthroscopy have been reported in approximately 10% of cases, and the majority of them are minor. Complications reported include persistent drainage, stiffness, iatrogenic cartilage damage, tourniquet complications, hematoma formation, transient nerve palsies, and injuries to the cutaneous or major nerves.[11,12,20,29,32,39,40] Few reports have looked at major neurologic complications.[11,21,24,32,39,40] Reports of major nerve injuries would appear to be underreported based on numerous anecdotal reports from around the country. Ogilvie-Harris and Schemitsch[21] reported in 1986 a single radial nerve injury in 1,569 cases in a retrospective study by the members of the Arthroscopy Association of North America. A more recent review of 465 cases showed a complication rate of 3.6% (16 reported nerve injuries: 7 transient and 9 permanent). A review of 247 patients treated by us from 1990 through 1993 revealed 15 complications for a rate of 6% (2.4% major and 3.6% minor). Major complications were classified as those resulting in decreased function of the elbow or the need for reoperation. Minor complications occurred in 9 patients. Seven had hematoma formation or swelling that resolved without surgery. One synovial fistula (posterolateral soft spot portal) was seen following synovectomy for rheumatoid arthritis; 1 transient neurapraxia resolved spontaneously. Major complications occurred in 6 patients. There were 3 neurologic injuries requiring additional surgical intervention: 2 posterior interosseous nerve injuries and 1 ulnar nerve injury. Two patients developed arthrofibrosis that required repeat arthroscopy, and 1 patient developed significant scar formation requiring reoperation.

The distances between the major nerves and the anterior portals are increased with joint distention with the elbow flexed 90°.[39] The intracapsular volume has been shown to be decreased from the average 25 ml in the normal elbow to 12.5% or less.[41] This may place the arthritic or arthrofibrotic elbow at greater risk of neurovascular injury. These patients require careful screening and a ready conversion to open procedures if difficulties are encountered.

Based on experience, the following recommendations can be made. Significant heterotopic ossification or displaced radial head fractures, where the posterior interosseous nerve may be at risk without exploration and protection, are contraindications to arthroscopy. Arthroscopic debridement of an arthritic elbow should be limited to a single medial portal. Drains should also be used liberally after extensive debridement, and posterolateral portals should always be sutured to decrease the risk of synovial fistulas.

Conclusion

The surgical technique of elbow arthroscopy, although demanding and requiring a skilled technician, results in better pain control and improved range of motion. Arthroscopy represents a valuable adjunct in the treatment of the arthritic elbow. There may be an increased risk of neurovascular injury due to the abnormal anatomy and the limited capsular distention of the arthritic elbow. However, careful attention to the described technique, knowledge of the elbow anatomy, and a ready willingness to convert to open procedures can prevent complications.

References

1. Ferlic DC, Patchett CE, Clayton ML, Freeman AC: Elbow synovectomy in rheumatoid arthritis: Long-term results. *Clin Orthop* 1987;220: 119-125.
2. Inglis AE, Ranawat CS, Straub LR: Synovectomy and debridement of the elbow in rheumatoid arthritis. *J Bone Joint Surg* 1971;53A: 652-662.
3. Brattstrom KH: Synovectomy of the elbow in rheumatoid arthritis. *Acta Orthop Scand* 1975;46: 744-750.
4. . Eichenblat M, Hass A, Kessler I: Synovectomy of the elbow in rheumatoid arthritis. *J Bone Joint Surg* 1982;64A:1074-1078.
5. Laine V, Vainio K: Synovectomy of the elbow, in Hijmans W, Paul WD, Herschel WH (eds): *Early Synovectomy in Rheumatoid Arthritis*. Amsterdam, The Netherlands, Excerpta Medica Foundation, 1969, pp 117-118.
6. Rymaszewski LA, Mackay I, Amis AA, Miller JH: Long-term effects of excision of the radial head in rheumatoid arthritis. *J Bone Joint Surg* 1984;66B:109-113.
7. Tulp NJ, Winia WP: Synovectomy of the elbow in rheumatoid arthritis: Long-term results. *J Bone Joint Surg* 1989;71B:664-666.
8. Copeland SA, Taylor JG: Synovectomy of the elbow in rheumatoid arthritis: The place of excision of the head of the radius. *J Bone Joint Surg* 1979;61B:69-73.
9. Mackay I, FitzGerald B, Miller JH: Silastic radial head prosthesis in rheumatoid arthritis. *Acta Orthop Scand* 1982;53:63-66.
10. Swett P: A review of synovectomy. *J Bone Joint Surg* 1970;51A:371.
11. Thomas MA, Fast A, Shapiro D: Radial nerve damage as a complication of elbow arthroscopy. *Clin Orthop* 1987;215:130-131.
12. Collins DH (ed): *The Pathology of Articular* and *Spinal Diseases*. London, England, E Arnold, 1949.
13. Huskisson EC, Dieppe PA, Tucker AK, Cannell LB: Another look in osteoarthritis. *Ann Rheum Dis* 1979;38:423-428.
14. Doherty M, Preston B: Primary osteoarthritis of the elbow. *Ann Rheum Dis* 1989;48:743-747.
15. Morrey BF, Askew LJ, An KN, Chao EY: A biomechanical study of normal functional elbow motion. *J Bone Joint Surg* 1981;63A: 872-877.
16. O'Driscoll SW, Bell DF, Morrey BF: Posterolateral instability of the elbow. *J Bone Joint Surg* 1991;73A:440-446.
17. O'Driscoll SW, Morrey BF: Master techniques in orthopaedic surgery, in Morrey BF (ed): *The Elbow: Arthroscopy of the Elbow*. New York, NY, Raven Press, 1994, pp 21-34.
18. Redden JF, Stanley D: Arthroscopic fenestration of the olecranon fossa in the treatment of osteoarthritis of the elbow. *Arthroscopy* 1993;9: 14-16.
19. O'Driscoll SW: Elbow arthroscopy for loose bodies. *Orthopedics* 1992;15:855-859.
20. O'Driscoll SW, Morrey BF: Arthroscopy of the elbow: Diagnostic and therapeutic benefits and hazards. *J Bone Joint Surg* 1992;74A:84-94.
21. Ogilvie-Harris DJ, Schemitsch E: Arthroscopy of the elbow for removal of loose bodies. *Arthroscopy* 1993;9:5-8.
22. Ward WG, Anderson TE: Elbow arthroscopy in a mostly athletic population. *J Hand Surg* 1993;18A:220-224.
23. Ward W, Belhobek GH, Anderson TE: Arthroscopic elbow findings: Correlation with preoperative radiographic studies. *Arthroscopy* 1992;8:498-502.
24. Andrews JR, Carson WG: Arthroscopy of the elbow. *Arthroscopy* 1985;1:97-107.

25. Boe S: Arthroscopy of the elbow: Diagnosis and extraction of loose bodies. *Acta Orthop Scand* 1986;57:52-53.

26. Woods GW: Elbow arthroscopy. *Clin Sports Med* 1987;6:557-564.

27. Clarke RP: Symptomatic, lateral synovial fringe (plica) of the elbow joint. *Arthroscopy* 1988;4: 112-116.

28. Burman MS: Arthroscopy of the elbow joint: A cadaver study. *J Bone Joint Surg* 1932;14: 349-350.

29. Carson WG Jr: Arthroscopy of the elbow, in Bassett FH III (ed): *Instructional Course Lectures XXXVII*. Park Ridge, IL, American Academy of Orthopaedic Surgeons, 1988, pp 195-201.

30. Poehling GG, Whipple TL, Sisco L, Goldman B: Elbow arthroscopy: A new technique. *Arthroscopy* 1989;5:222-224.

31. Field LD, Altchek DW, Warren RF, O'Brien SJ, Skyhar MJ, Wickiewicz TL: Arthroscopic anatomy of the lateral elbow: A comparison of three portals. *Arthroscopy* 1994;10:602-607.

32. Jones GS, Savoie FH III: Arthroscopic capsular release of flexion contractures (arthrofibrosis) of the elbow. *Arthroscopy* 1993;9:277-283.

33. Chess D: Osteochondritis, in Savoie FH III, Field LD (eds): *Arthroscopy*. New York, NY, Churchill Livingstone, 1996, pp 77-86.

34. Smith FM (ed): *Surgery of the Elbow*, ed 2. Philadelphia, PA, WB Saunders,. 1972.

35. Morrey BF: Primary degenerative arthritis of the elbow: Treatment by ulnohumeral arthroplasty. *J Bone Joint Surg* 1992;74B:409-413.

36. Kashiwagi D: Intra-articular changes of the osteoarthritic elbow, especially about the fossa olecrani. *J Jpn Orthop Assoc* 1978;52:1367-1382.

37. Kashiwagi D: Osteoarthritis of the elbow joint: Intraarticular changes and the special operative procedure: Outerbridge-Kashiwagi method (O-K method), in Kashiwagi D (ed): *Elbow Joint*. Amsterdam, The Netherlands, Elsevier Science, 1985, pp 177-188.

38. Savoie FH, Nunley PD, Field LD: Arthroscopic management of the arthritic elbow: Indications, technique, and results. *J Shoulder Elbow Surg* 1999;8:214-219.

39. Lynch GJ, Meyers JF, Whipple TL, Caspari RB: Neurovascular anatomy and elbow arthroscopy: Inherent risks. *Arthroscopy* 1986;2: 191-197.

40. Papilion JD, Neff RS, Shall LM: Compression neuropathy of the radial nerve as a complication of elbow arthroscopy: A case report and review of the literature. *Arthroscopy* 1988;4: 284-286.

41. Gallay SH, Richards RR, O'Driscoll SW: Intraarticular capacity and compliance of stiff and normal elbows. *Arthroscopy* 1993;9:9-13.

Reference to Video

Savoie FH III: Advances in Elbow Arthroscopy. Jackson, MS, Mississippi Sports Medicine and Orthopaedic Center, 1998.

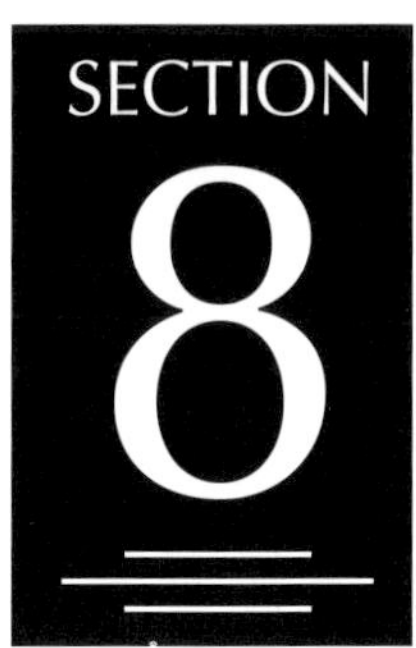

Trauma About the Elbow

Trauma About the Elbow

This section provides an overview of traumatic conditions about the elbow, beginning with a review of soft-tissue conditions resulting in elbow instability, progressing through complex instability, and finishing with difficult fractures of the elbow.

Yadao and associates provide an excellent overview of posterolateral rotatory instability (PLRI). Their review of the history of PLRI highlights the lack of appreciation of the presentation of this condition. Earlier articles described the pathoanatomy, physical examination, and surgical management of this condition. In this article, the bony and soft-tissue anatomy of the elbow is reviewed, but the discussion focuses principally on the lateral ligament complex. The elements of the lateral ligament complex are described, and the importance of the lateral ulnar collateral ligament to PLRI is highlighted. The history, physical examination, and diagnostic evaluation also are detailed. The authors stress the subtlety of the physical findings in these patients. A variety of provocative tests to assist in diagnosing PLRI are described, including the pivot-shift test and the prone and seated push-up tests. The role of radiographic imaging is reviewed, and the arthroscopic features of PLRI are described. The authors conclude with a discussion of surgical technique, rehabilitation, and results. The reader should come away with an appreciation of the importance of the lateral ligament complex to the rotatory stability of the elbow. This article provides a foundation for later sections that focus on bony and soft-tissue injuries.

In the next article, Ball and associates build on the groundwork established by Yadao and associates, beginning with an overview of the anatomic aspects underlying elbow stability. The osteology of the elbow joint and its role in elbow stability are reviewed, as are the capsuloligamentous structures contributing to elbow stability. The role of the medial collateral ligament (MCL), specifically the anterior bundle, is detailed. The anatomy of the lateral collateral ligament (LCL) and treatment of PLRI also are described; this discussion is an extension of the concepts outlined in Yadao and associates.

Treatment of acute MCL injuries is compared with that of partial and complete chronic MCL injuries. Some authors advocate repair of the MCL in acute injuries, but these authors point out that most of these ligament tears heal anatomically, without surgical repair. However, surgical reconstruction is indicated for a complete MCL rupture in a high-performance athlete who wishes to return to competition. Several surgical techniques are described, including the classic Jobe reconstruction, the docking procedure, and other techniques using suture anchors or interference screws. The surgical techniques for LCL reconstruction are reviewed as well.

O'Driscoll and associates review complexities of elbow instability in the next article, beginning with isolated soft-tissue injuries and then progressing to complex and recurrent instability. The stages of soft-tissue disruption, beginning on the lateral side of the elbow, which occurs with simple dislocation, are emphasized. The primary static constraints to instability, as well as the secondary static and dynamic constraints, are reviewed. Fracture patterns encountered in complex instability are described, specifically coronoid and radial head fractures, and the importance of addressing soft-tissue injuries associated with these fractures is emphasized. The indications for hinged external fixation are listed for both acute and chronic injuries.

In the final article in the section, O'Driscoll and colleagues, who represent the thought leaders in this field, present their views of the management of what they term "difficult" elbow fractures. The review begins with a discussion of comminuted distal humerus fractures. The section on surgical technique details the strategy for managing complex elbow fractures, beginning with issues at the articular surface and progressing to how to achieve stable fixation between the articular segment and the distal humeral diaphysis. The authors also highlight the advantages of precontoured anatomic distal humerus plates over straight plates bent at the time of surgery. They prefer medial and lateral plate fixation over the accepted standard of 90-90 plating and explain why they believe 90-90 plating is suboptimal in its current form. Other topics include fractures of the distal articular surface (coronal shear fractures of the capitellum and trochlea) and the importance of recognizing injury patterns combined with the difficulty in managing these injuries. Specifically, they comment on the challenges associated with obtaining stable fixation of fracture fragments, which can consist of small articular pieces with subchondral impaction. The article concludes with a discussion of complex elbow instability.

The final article in this section is the most comprehensive of the group. The authors also discuss many other complex problems, including: (1) olecranon fracture-dislocations, which may result in ulnohumeral instability; (2) the need to carefully evaluate potential involvement of the coronoid process and the need for anatomic reduction of the fragment in the fixation construct; and (3) fracture patterns of the coronoid process. The authors propose a classification system for coronoid fractures that considers fracture patterns outside of the axial plane fractures used in the Regan and Morrey classification.

Bony and soft-tissue injuries associated with coronoid fractures are described in detail, as are anteromedial coronoid fractures and their mechanism of injury (ie, varus posteromedial rotation with axial loading). This injury pattern is associated with tensile disruption of the LCL complex, which can create a subtle instability pattern that is difficult to identify. More recognizable patterns of complex instability also are addressed, including coronoid fractures, radial head fractures, and soft-tissue disruption of the LCL and possibly the MCL resulting from dislocation (known as the terrible triad). Technical strategies for dealing with each of these injury patterns are discussed.

Matthew L. Ramsey, MD
Associate Professor of Orthopaedic Surgery
Chief, Shoulder and Elbow Service
Penn Orthopaedic Institute
University of Pennsylvania School of Medicine
Philadelphia, Pennsylvania

Posterolateral Rotatory Instability of the Elbow

Melissa A. Yadao, MD
Felix H. Savoie III, MD
Larry D. Field, MD

Abstract

Posterolateral rotatory instability (PLRI) of the elbow is recurrent elbow instability caused by injury to the radial ulnohumeral ligament or lateral ulnar collateral ligament. Deficiencies of the radial ulnohumeral ligament and laxity of the lateral capsule allow the proximal radioulnar joint to rotate and the radial head to subluxate posteriorly when stressed. Whether isolated or in conjunction with other injuries, PLRI represents the initial stage in the pathology of the unstable elbow. The diagnosis of PLRI can be difficult because the provocative tests are challenging to perform. Diagnostic arthroscopy is an excellent tool to demonstrate this instability. Treatment options include bracing for acute injuries, and primary repair or reconstruction for chronic injuries. Although arthroscopic plication and repair have been as effective as open techniques, the clinician should be prepared for open reconstruction if needed.

In 1991, O'Driscoll introduced the term posterolateral rotatory instability (PLRI) to describe elbow instability caused by injury to the radial ulnohumeral ligament (RUHL) or lateral ulnar collateral ligament (LUCL).[1] Since then, PLRI and elbow instability in general have gained much attention. The functional anatomy of the lateral collateral ligament complex has been closely examined. The diagnosis and treatment of this condition have evolved with good results. It is now recognized that PLRI plays an important, initial role in the pathology of the unstable elbow, which encompasses a spectrum of injuries ranging from instability to frank dislocation.

O'Driscoll originally reported on a group of patients with symptoms of valgus instability after trauma who did not exhibit typical clinical findings of a deficient medial collateral ligament complex. In these patients, the radial head rotated and subluxated posteriorly when the elbow was forced into valgus from a supinated and extended position. This instability was attributed to the incompetence of posterolateral structures, specifically the RUHL. Although these patients had responded poorly to the standard treatment of valgus instability, they did well after plication or reconstruction of this ligament. O'Driscoll subsequently developed the posterolateral rotatory instability test or pivot-shift test, which is one of the most helpful tools for diagnosis.

Background

PLRI is not a new problem, as a few studies and case reports before O'Driscoll and associates classic article seem to describe this condition under the guise of recurrent dislocations of the elbow and radial head.[1-5] In 1966, Osborne and Cotterill[2] reported on a group of patients with posterior subluxations of the radial head; physical examination was normal in 3 of 30 patients. These authors believed that laxity in the posterolateral capsule caused this problem and successfully treated their patients with plication or repair of the lateral ligament complex.

In 1975, Symeonides and associates[3] and Hassman and associates[4] separately reported cases of recurrent elbow dislocations that were difficult to treat, probably representing examples of what is now recognized as PLRI. One patient studied by Hassman and associates had a clinically stable ulnohumeral joint despite a history of multiple dislocations.[4] Other case reports described posttraumatic subluxations of the elbow that could be reproduced with ma-

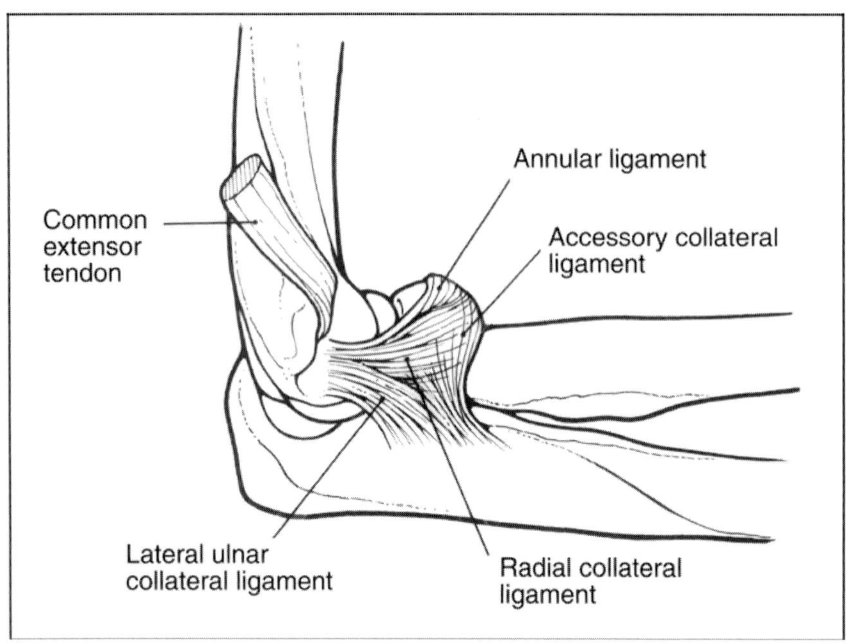

Figure 1 Anatomy of the lateral ligamentous complex of the elbow. Lateral ulnar collateral ligament = radial ulnohumeral ligament.

neuvers similar to the pivot-shift test.[1,5] The patients reported locking and snapping of the elbow. Stress radiographs showed typical findings of PLRI: widening of the ulnohumeral joint space and posterior subluxation of the radial head.[5]

Anatomy

The elbow is one of the most inherently stable joints because of its bony articulations and soft-tissue stabilizers. The three bony articulations include the radiocapitellar joint, the proximal radioulnar joint, and the ulnohumeral joint. With the trochlea cradled by the olecranon posterior and the coronoid anterior, the ulnohumeral joint provides the primary static restraint to varus/valgus, anterior/posterior, as well as rotatory motion at the elbow.[6] The radiocapitellar joint is an important secondary stabilizer, accepting up to 60% axial loads when the elbow is extended.[7]

The medial and lateral ligament complexes are the major static soft-tissue stabilizers of the elbow. Three major components make up the medial or ulnar ligament complex: the anterior medial bundle, the posterior medial bundle, and the transverse oblique bundle. While the proximal fibers have been described as distinct structures, distally they resemble more the ligaments of the shoulder as capsular thickenings.[8,9] The medial ligament complex protects the elbow against valgus stress with the forearm in pronation.[1,9-11] Biomechanical studies have shown that only the anterior and posterior bundles play important roles in elbow stability.[7]

The lateral or radial ligament complex is made up of four components: the RUHL or LUCL, the radial collateral ligament (RCL), the annular ligament, and the accessory lateral collateral ligament[8] (Figure 1). Unlike the medial structures, these individual ligaments are often difficult to differentiate proximally where they originate as a broad band from the lateral epicondyle deep to the extensor wad.[12-14] Distally, the fibers either remain as a single broad band or split into two bands,[10] with the RCL comprising the more anterior band and the RUHL the posterior band.[13] The annular ligament sweeps over the radial head and is thought to be a stabilizer of the proximal radioulnar joint. The RCL primarily restrains varus stress.[1,7]

The RUHL has been shown to play a key role in PLRI. The RUHL originates from the posterior inferior aspect of the lateral epicondyle and inserts on the supinator crest of the ulna.[1] It is often difficult to distinguish proximally and is more easily identified at its distal insertion.[10,14] Positioning the arm in varus and supination may help differentiate the RUHL from the RCL.[12]

Other soft-tissue structures of the elbow such as the capsule and musculature act as important dynamic stabilizers of the elbow. The capsule augments the strength of both the medial and lateral ligaments. With the elbow extended, the anterior capsule acts as a powerful restraint against varus and valgus stresses.[9,10] Surgical techniques to restore stability incorporate the capsule with ligament plication.[1,2,15] The anconeus and extensor wad are important dynamic restraints laterally while the flexor-pronator mass strengthens stability medially.[9]

Pathophysiology

Studies by O'Driscoll and associates[1] have shown that deficiencies of the RUHL and laxity of the lateral capsule allows the proximal radioulnar joint to rotate and the radial head to subluxate posteriorly when stressed, leading to PLRI. Recent investigations have questioned the exact role of the entire lateral collateral ligament complex.

In patients with PLRI, the radial head subluxates, and on rare occasion, can dislocate posteriorly depending on the position of the elbow. With the forearm supinated and slightly flexed, valgus stress applied to the elbow causes rotation of the ulnohumeral joint, compression of the radiocapitellar joint, and posterior subluxation of the radial head.[1,10,15] Extreme supination of the forearm stresses the posterolateral structures while flexion of the elbow releases the olecranon tip from the olecranon fossa, allowing rotation of the ulnohumeral joint.[16]

The proximal radioulnar joint must remain intact for PLRI to occur. During posterolateral rotation, the proximal forearm rotates as a unit so that the coronoid passes under the trochlea as the radial head moves posterior. In O'Driscoll and associates'[1] anatomic studies, the annular ligament was intact in all specimens. The integrity of this joint distinguishes PLRI from other instabilities such as recurrent dislocations of the radial head and elbow where disruption of this joint was thought necessary for dislocation to occur.[1,17]

Recent biomechanical studies have attempted to define the functional anatomy of the entire lateral collateral ligament complex and its relation to PLRI. Cohen and Hastings[10] have shown that injury to the RUHL alone was not sufficient to cause instability. The entire lateral ligament complex as well as the lateral musculature played significant roles.[10] Similarly, Dunning and associates[12] demonstrated that both the RUHL and the RCL needed to be cut before PLRI occurred. On the other hand, Olsen and associates[13] and Seki and associates[14] found that transection of either the RUHL or the RCL created this instability.

Although there is still much disagreement over the exact roles of the lateral ligament complex, PLRI is considered to be the first phase of elbow instability that can develop into frank dislocation. As proposed in several studies,[17-19] the mechanism leading to an unstable elbow is a progressive disruption of the ring of soft-tissue stabilizers beginning laterally and sweeping medially. The first injured structure is the RUHL, resulting in PLRI that can reduce spontaneously. Further injury tears anterior and posterior capsules resulting in ulnohumeral subluxations. Complete dislocation occurs when the medial structures are disrupted, although the anterior band of the medial collateral ligament may be only minimally injured.

Clinical Evaluation

History

Most patients will describe a history of trauma. Although elbow dislocation is the inciting event in 75% of patients younger than 20 years old, varus extension stress without true dislocation is more likely the initiating event in older patients.[15] PLRI can occur secondary to repetitive stresses on the elbow such as cubitus varus and recurrent valgus instability from medial collateral ligament tears.[20,21] Some patients with lateral epicondylitis may also have PLRI. Repetitive motion may produce laxity in the lateral ligamentous complex, leading to secondary lateral epicondylitis. On the other hand, lateral epicondyle release can cause iatrogenic instability, which has been found in 25% of patients in one study (SW O'Driscoll, MD, personal communication, 2003). PLRI has also been reported following radial head excision.[9]

Symptoms vary from obvious instability to subtle reports of pain and discomfort. Occasionally patients will report clicking, popping, snapping, or locking. True dislocations tend to be rare. Rather, patients describe the elbow slipping in and out of the joint, particularly when the arm is supinated and slightly flexed.[1,2,15,19]

Physical Examination

PLRI may be difficult to diagnose on routine examination of the elbow. A thorough upper extremity examination is necessary to rule out other pathology. Differential diagnosis includes lateral epicondylitis, radial tunnel syndrome, valgus instability, and pure proximal radial head dislocation. Standard stability tests are often normal. Valgus instability should be tested with the forearm in supination and pronation. With valgus loads, pronation of the forearm tests the medial collateral ligamentous complex, whereas supination stresses posterolateral structures, in particular the RUHL.[1,10]

Several provocative tests, including the PLRI test or pivot-shift test, can help make the diagnosis. The pivot-shift test for the elbow resembles the pivot-shift test for the anterior cruciate ligament deficient knee (Figure 2). With the patient supine, the arm is raised overhead, stabilizing the humerus to prevent external rotation. With the forearm fully supinated and the elbow extended, a valgus-supination force is applied to the elbow while slowly flexing it from an extended position. As a result, the ulnohumeral joint rotates and the radiohumeral joint subluxates posteriorly, sometimes even dislocating (Figure 2, *A*). Dimpling of the skin may be seen proximal to the subluxating radial head. As the elbow is flexed more than 40°, the clinician may hear or feel the radiohumeral joint suddenly reduce.[1]

This test is not easy to perform on

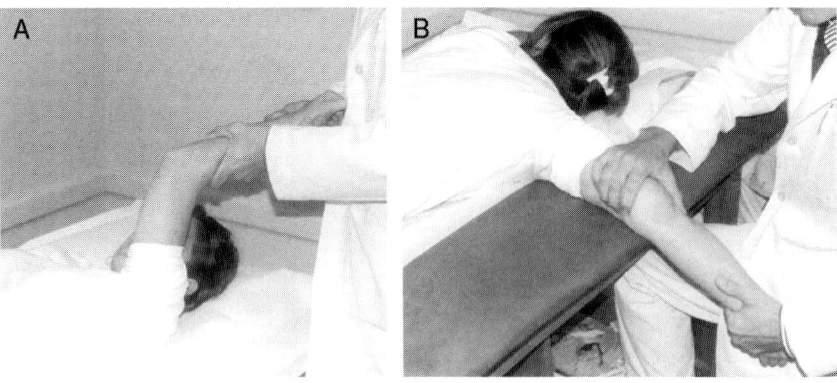

Figure 2 PLRI test or pivot-shift test. **A,** Performing the test in the supine position maximally externally rotates the arm and allows the examiner to use both hands to manipulate the elbow. **B,** Performing the test with the patient prone stabilizes the humerus and frees one hand to more easily palpate the radiohumeral joint.

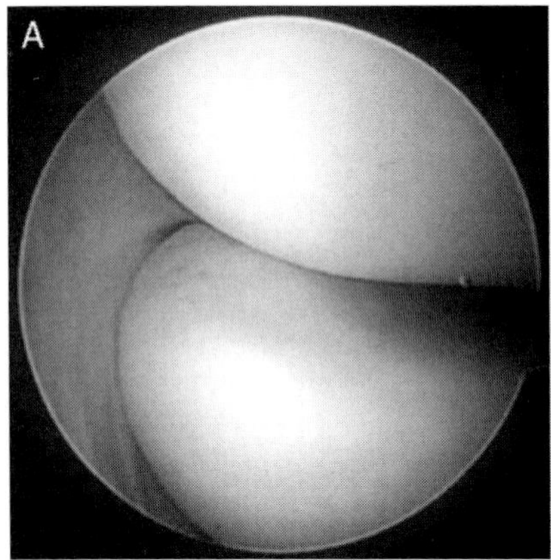

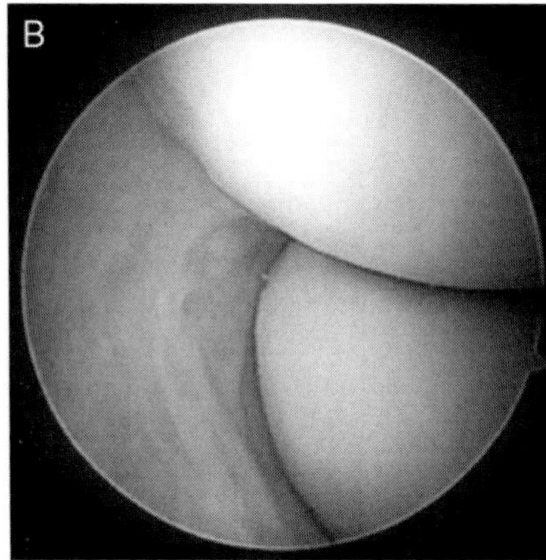

Figure 3 Arthroscopic findings of PLRI. **A,** The view from the anteromedial portal shows the normal position of the radial head with the forearm in pronation. **B,** During the PLRI or pivot-shift test, the radial head can be seen to subluxate posteriorly. In a stable elbow, the radial head would rotate but not translate posteriorly.

the awake patient. Feelings of pain or apprehension are considered a positive result in such patients in the absence of instability.

The pivot-shift test can be performed with the patient prone. Resting the arm over the edge of the table stabilizes the humerus, allowing the examiner to more easily palpate the radiohumeral joint during the examination[16] (Figure 2, *B*).

Two other provocative maneuvers designed by Regan simulate the pivot-shift test. The first requires the patient to push up from a prone or wall position with the forearms maximally pronated with the thumbs turned toward each other. The test is repeated with forearms maximally supinated. PLRI occurs when the arms are supinated, not pronated. Another test requires a patient to push up out of a chair using the armrests. With palms facing inward, essentially placing them in supination, pushing up will produce similar symptoms of pain (J Regan, MD, personal communication, November 1999).

Diagnostic Evaluation

Radiology Standard AP and lateral radiographs of the elbow should be obtained but are often normal. Bony avulsions following ligament injury can be identified. On lateral views, typical PLRI radiographic findings include widening of the ulnohumeral joint space with posterior subluxation of the radial head. These are best illustrated with radiographic or fluoroscopic stress views while performing the pivot-shift test with the patient under anesthesia.[1,15] Late sequalae of degenerative changes can also be seen.

Currently MRI plays a limited role in diagnosis. Injuries to the RUHL and other structures have been identified on MRI using special sequencing that requires operator experience.[22]

Arthroscopy Diagnostic arthroscopy can demonstrate PLRI in a patient in whom instability is suspected. The pivot-shift test should be performed while viewing from the anteromedial portal. The radial head will rotate and translate posterior if PLRI is present; with a competent ligament, the radial head will rotate but not translate[16] (Figure 3). In addition, while viewing from the posterolateral portal, the arthroscope easily can be driven through the lateral gutter and into the lateral aspect of the ulnohumeral joint if instability is present. This situation is described as the elbow drive-through sign, resembling the drive-through sign in shoulder instability.

Treatment

The most efficacious treatment of posterolateral rotatory instability is protection at the time of initial trauma. The clinician should be suspi-

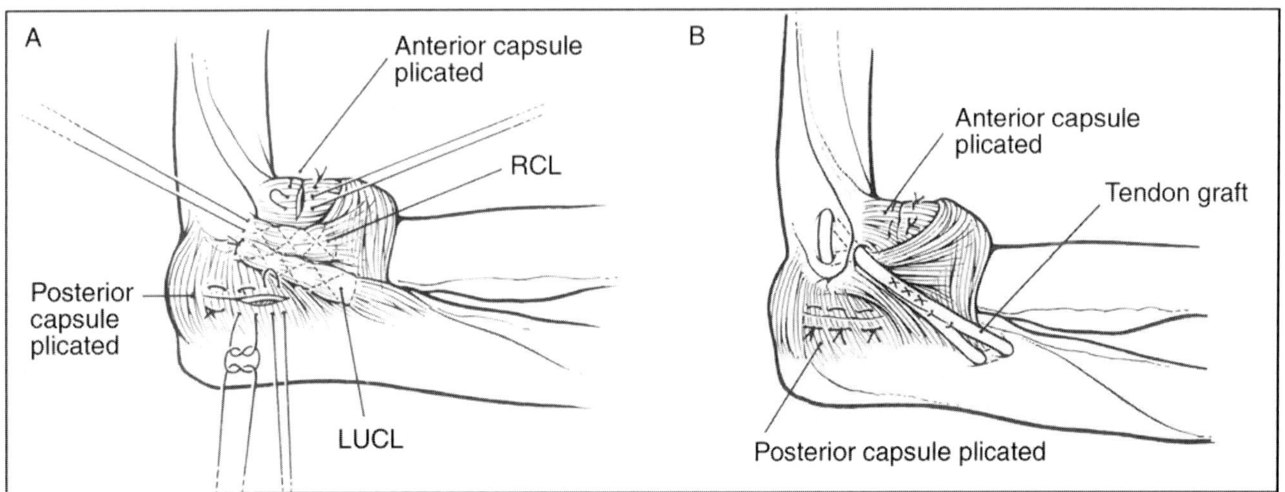

Figure 4 Open lateral reconstruction for PLRI as described by O'Driscoll and associates.[1] **A,** Repair of the RUHL by imbricating the ligament and reattaching it to its insertion point on the lateral epicondyle. The redundant posterolateral capsule is also plicated. **B,** Reconstruction of the ligament with a free tendon graft. It is essential to place the ligament in its correct anatomic position on the humeral epicondyle and supinator crest of the ulna. The posterolateral capsule is also plicated.

cious of injury to the lateral ligament complex following an acute elbow dislocation. If the lateral structures are found to be disrupted upon careful examination, the elbow should be stabilized with the arm in pronation in a hinged brace for 4 to 6 weeks to promote healing and prevent instability.[17,19,23]

Unfortunately, chronic ligament insufficiencies do not appear to stabilize with conservative modalities. Surgery remains the treatment of choice for symptomatic patients. Both open and arthroscopic techniques have been described in detail, with early results showing similar success.

Open Technique

An open technique to plicate, repair, and reconstruct the RUHL has been described in the literature.[1,15,19] With the patient supine, the elbow is entered through a modified Kocher approach, exposing the entire lateral ligament complex from the lateral epicondyle to the supinator crest. The pivot-shift test is performed to identify laxity in the lateral capsule and insufficiencies of the RUHL. An attenuated or detached ligament can be repaired by reattaching the ligament through bone to the posterior inferior lateral epicondyle. The ligament can be advanced or imbricated as needed. The loose capsule is plicated with sutures tied following completion of the repair (Figure 4, *A*).

Reconstruction with tendon autograft may be necessary if the ligament tissue is of poor quality. Drill holes are placed through the anatomic insertion sites of the ligament. Two ulnar holes are first drilled in the proximal and distal portion of the supinator crest and the isometric point of insertion on the lateral epicondyle is determined before establishing the humeral drill holes. The graft is passed through the ulnar tunnels, through the isometric point of the humerus, and then sewn back onto itself with the elbow positioned in 40° flexion and the forearm fully pronated[1,15,19] (Figure 4, *B*).

Palmaris graft is most commonly used. Single or double limbs of the graft can be passed through the isometric origin of the lateral epicondyle.[1,19] However, a recent study by King and associates[24] has shown that no biomechanical differences exist between single or double strand grafts.

A screw technique can be used for reconstruction of the lateral collateral ligamentous complex that tensions the graft through the ulnar tunnel. Palmaris tendon is used as a double- or quadruple-strand graft. A single tunnel is drilled lateral to posteromedial through the ulna at midportion of the supinator crest. Using sutures as a guide, the isometric point on the lateral epicondyle is determined and a single drill hole is placed. The graft is first passed through the humerus and stabilized using the docking technique.[25] The two free ends of the graft are then retrieved through the tunnel in the ulna. The sutures/graft are pulled tightly and stabilized by interference screw placement (Figure 5).

One alternative technique is to drill completely through the lateral epicondyle. The graft is then passed

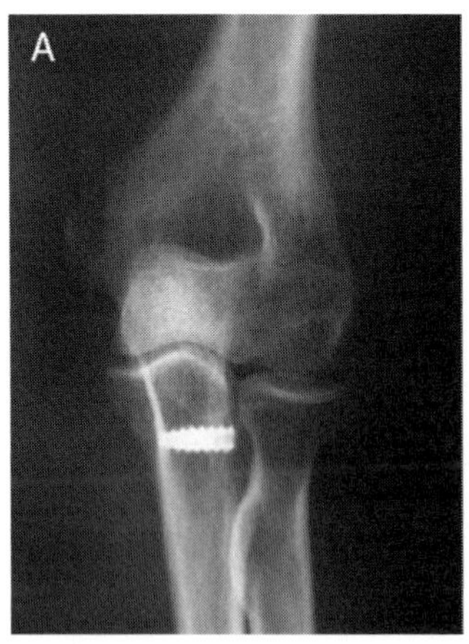

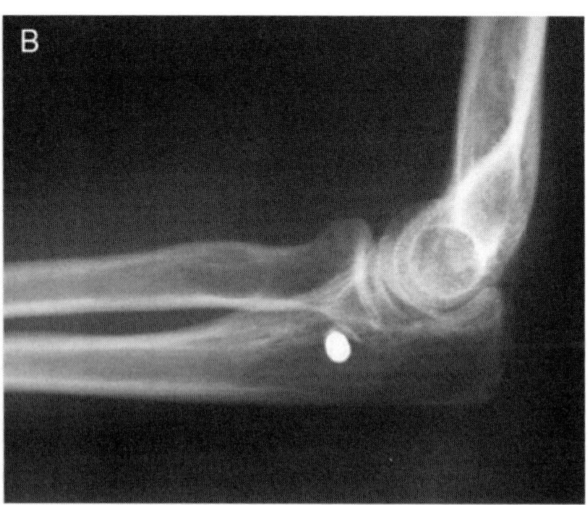

Figure 5 AP (**A**) and lateral (**B**) radiographs demonstrating open screw technique for lateral collateral ligament reconstruction. Although bioabsorbable screws can be used, the metal screw shown here demonstrates the correct anatomic position of the ulnar tunnel at the supinator crest.

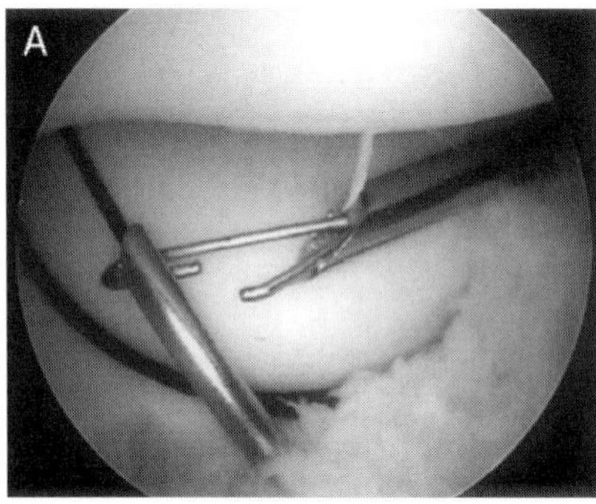

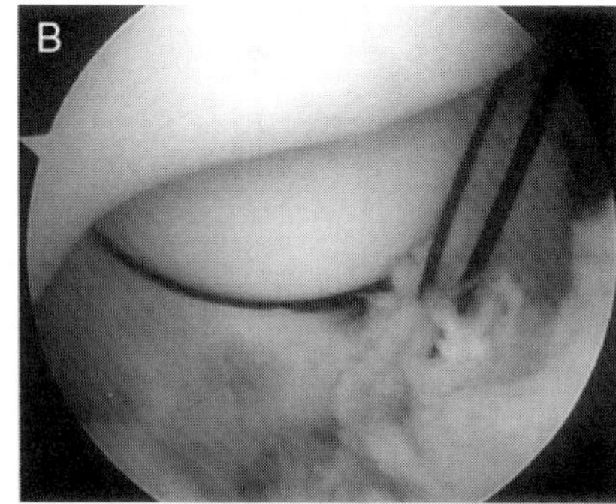

Figure 6 Arthroscopic lateral reconstruction for PLRI. **A,** An absorbable suture is placed into the lateral gutter through a spinal needle and retrieved with a suture retriever. **B,** The needle and retriever are placed specifically to recreate the path of the RUHL. Tensioning the sutures tightens the posterolateral structures and decreases the volume of the lateral gutter.

through this tunnel, leaving four free ends. All four ends are then pulled into the ulnar tunnel and stabilized via screw placement.

Arthroscopy

Arthroscopic techniques have recently been developed to plicate or repair the RUHL. As mentioned earlier, PLRI can be diagnosed by findings of a posterior subluxating radial head during a pivot-shift test or seeing a drive-through sign. While viewing through the posterolateral portal, an absorbable suture is passed into the joint through a spinal needle placed into the joint directly adjacent to the lateral aspect of the proximal ulna at the level of the supinator crest (Figure 6, *A*). This first suture pierces the annular ligament. The suture is retrieved adjacent to the posterior inferior aspect of the lateral epicondyle. Four to seven sutures can be passed, starting distal to proximal (Figure 6, *B*). The two ends of each suture are brought out together through a lateral incision and are tied separately in the same order.[16] By pulling the sutures before tying, the lateral structures will tighten and the lateral gutter space will collapse.

If significant insufficiency is found, the repair can be augmented with a suture anchor. Through a small incision, the anchor is placed at the isometric point onto the posterior aspect of the lateral epicondyle. One limb is passed into the joint, lassoing all the plication sutures before being retrieved near the ulna. Tying this suture subcutaneously further tightens the lateral structures, essentially reattaching the entire ligament complex to the lateral epicondyle.[16]

Rehabilitation

Postoperative rehabilitation is similar following either technique. Patients are immediately immobilized in a splint with the elbow flexed 70° to 90° with the arm in full pronation. After 1 to 2 weeks, limited flexion of 45° to 90° is initiated with the elbow protected in a double-hinged elbow brace. Full range of motion in the brace is allowed at 3 weeks. Full painless range of motion should be achieved by 6 weeks, followed by wrist and elbow strengthening exercises in the brace. At 10 to 12 weeks, the brace can be removed if the patient can perform all strengthening exercises in the brace pain-free.[19,26]

Results

Few results following surgical management of PLRI exist in the literature. In O'Driscoll and associates' first study, four of five patients were assessed for 15 to 30 months. None had recurrence of instability and all achieved full range of motion.[1] In a follow-up study by Nestor and associates,[15] 3 of 11 patients underwent repair and 7 underwent ligament reconstruction with palmaris graft. Stability was achieved in 10 patients, with 7 having an excellent functional result.[15]

Upon reviewing his series of patients, O'Driscoll and associates found 90% satisfaction with no subluxations if the radial head is intact and no degenerative articular changes are present. Patient satisfaction decreases to 67% to 75% in the face of radial head excision or arthritis. Mild flexion contracture (10°) is accepted as it protects against instability. Recurrent laxity or redislocation has been reported, but it usually occurs after reinjury involving significant stress.[19]

In an unpublished study (D Gurley, MD; F Savoie, MD; Jackson, MS, unpublished data, 2002), 54 patients with an average follow-up of 41 months (range, 12 to 103 months) underwent surgical management of PLRI. Diagnostic arthroscopy confirmed PLRI in all patients. Thirty-seven patients were treated with open techniques; 34 had ligament repair, and 3 had reconstruction with tendon graft. Seventeen patients were treated with arthroscopy; 11 had ligament plication alone, while 6 required an anchor to augment the repair.

Twenty-five percent of the 54 patients had a previous history of lateral epicondyle release. Indications for open rather than arthroscopic repair included having concurrent procedures such as lateral epicondyle release, open extensor mass avulsion repairs, and release of the posterior interosseous nerve.

Overall Andrew-Carson scores improved significantly for all repairs, from 145 to 180 ($P < 0.0001$). Subjective scores improved from 57 to 85 ($P < 0.0001$) and objective scores from 88 to 95 ($P = 0.008$). Open repairs improved from 146 to 176 ($P = 0.0001$) and arthroscopic repairs from 144 to 182 ($P < 0.001$). Overall, open and arthroscopic techniques were shown to be equally effective (D Gurley, MD; F Savoie, MD; Jackson, MS, unpublished data, 2002).

Summary

PLRI should be considered in a patient who reports vague elbow pain and giving way, with a history of an elbow dislocation or previous lateral elbow surgery. Although the topic is currently debated, the RUHL does play an important role in this instability. Future investigations will help determine the exact role of the lateral collateral ligament complex in the unstable elbow. Indeed, PLRI is part of a continuum of injury from instability to frank dislocation.

The diagnosis of PLRI can be difficult as the provocative tests are challenging to perform and radiographic studies are not helpful. Early recognition following acute trauma and attention to detail during open elbow procedures provide the best prevention of PLRI. Diagnostic arthroscopy is an excellent tool to demonstrate this instability. Although arthroscopic plication and repair have been as effective as open techniques, the clinician should be prepared for open reconstruction if needed.

References

1. O'Driscoll SW, Bell DF, Morrey BF: Posterolateral rotatory instability of the elbow. *J Bone Joint Surg Am* 1991;73:440-446.
2. Osborne G, Cotterill P: Recurrent dislocation of the elbow. *J Bone Joint Surg Br* 1966;48:340-346.
3. Symeonides PP, Paschaloglou C, Stavrou Z, et al: Recurrent dislocation of the elbow: Report of three cases. *J Bone Joint Surg Am* 1975;57:1084-1086.
4. Hassman GC, Brunn F, Neer CS II: Recurrent dislocation of the elbow. *J Bone Joint Surg Am* 1975;57:1080-1084.
5. Burgess RC, Sprague HH: Post-traumatic posterior radial head subluxation: Two case reports. *Clin Orthop* 1984;186:192-194.
6. Guerra JJ, Timmerman LA: Clinical anatomy, histology, and pathomechanics of the elbow in sports. *Oper Tech Sports Med* 1996;4:69-76.
7. An KN, Morrey BF: Biomechanics of the elbow, in Morrey BF (ed): *The Elbow and Its Disorders*, ed 3. Philadelphia, PA, WB Saunders, 2000, pp 43-60.
8. Morrey BF: Anatomy of the elbow joint, in Morrey BF (ed): *The Elbow and Its Disorders*, ed 3. Philadelphia, PA, WB Saunders, 2000, pp 13-42.
9. Morrey BF, An KN: Articular and ligamentous contributions to the stability of the elbow joint. *Am J Sports Med* 1983;11:315-319.
10. Cohen MS, Hastings H II: Rotatory instability of the elbow: The anatomy and role of the lateral stabilizers. *J Bone Joint Surg Am* 1997;79:225-233.
11. Morrey BF, An KN: Functional anatomy of the ligaments of the elbow. *Clin Orthop* 1985;201:84-90.
12. Dunning CE, Zarzour ZD, Patterson SD, Johnson JA, King GJ: Ligamentous stabilizers against posterolateral rotatory instability of the elbow. *J Bone Joint Surg Am* 2001;83:1823-1828.
13. Olsen BS, Sojbjerg JO, Neilsen KK, Vaesel MT, Dalstra M, Sneppen O: Posterolateral elbow joint instability: The basic kinematics. *J Shoulder Elbow Surg* 1998;7:19-29.
14. Seki A, Olsen BS, Jensen SL, Eygendaal D, Sojbjerg JO: Functional anatomy of the lateral collateral ligament complex of the elbow: Configuration of Y and its role. *J Shoulder Elbow Surg* 2002;11:53-59.
15. Nestor BJ, O'Driscoll SW, Morrey BF: Ligamentous reconstruction for posterolateral rotatory instability of the elbow. *J Bone Joint Surg Am* 1992;74:1235-1241.
16. Smith JP III, Savoie FH III, Field LD: Posterolateral rotatory lateral instability of the elbow. *Clin Orthop* 2001;20:47-58.
17. O'Driscoll SW: Elbow dislocations, in Morrey BF (ed): *The Elbow and Its Disorders*, ed 3. Philadelphia, PA, WB Saunders, 2000, pp 409-420.
18. O'Driscoll SW, Morrey BF, Korinek S, et al: Elbow subluxation and dislocation: A spectrum of instability. *Clin Orthop* 1992;280:186-197.
19. O'Driscoll SW, Jupiter JB, King GJ, Hotchkiss RN, Morrey BF: The unstable elbow. *Instr Course Lect* 2001;50:89-100.

20. Abe M, Ishizu T, Morikawa J: Posterolateral rotatory instability of the elbow after post-traumatic cubitus varus. *J Shoulder Elbow Surg* 1997;6:405-409.

21. Eygendaal D, Verdegaal SHM, Obermann WR, Van Guyt AB, Poll RG, Rozing PM: Posterolateral dislocation of the elbow joint: Relationship to medial instability. *J Bone Joint Surg Am* 2000;82:555-560.

22. Potter HG, Weiland AJ, Schatz JA, Paletta GA, Hotchkiss RN: Posterolateral rotatory instability of the elbow: Usefulness of MR imaging in diagnosis. *Radiology* 1997;204:185-189.

23. Cohen MS, Hastings H II: Acute elbow dislocation: Evaluation and management. *J Am Acad Orthop Surg* 1998;6:15-33.

24. King GJ, Dunning CE, Zarzour DS, Patterson SD, Johnson JA: Single-strand reconstruction of the lateral ulnar collateral ligament restores varus and posterolateral instability of the elbow. *J Shoulder Elbow Surg* 2002;11:60-64.

25. Rohrbough JT, Altchek DW, Hyman J, Williams RJ III, Botts JB: Medial collateral ligament reconstruction of the elbow using the docking technique. *Am J Sports Med* 2002;30:541-548.

26. Morrey BF: Acute and chronic instability of the elbow. *J Am Acad Orthop Surg* 1996;4:117-128.

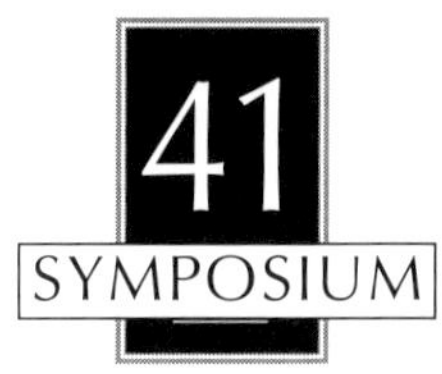

Elbow Instability: Treatment Strategies and Emerging Concepts

Craig M. Ball, MD, FRACS
Leesa M. Galatz, MD
Ken Yamaguchi, MD

Introduction

Significant progress has been made during the past decade in the diagnosis and treatment of elbow instability. Crucial to this progress has been increased understanding of the functional anatomy of the elbow and its relation to stability. In this chapter, the functional anatomy of the elbow will be reviewed and emerging concepts in the evaluation and treatment of the unstable elbow discussed.

Anatomic Considerations

The maintenance of normal elbow stability relies on a complex interaction between the articular surfaces and both static and dynamic soft-tissue constraints.

Bony Articulation

Osteology The elbow is classified as a trochoginglymoid joint and is one of the most congruous joints in the body.[1] The ulnohumeral articulation resembles a hinge that allows flexion and extension. The radiohumeral and proximal radioulnar articulations allow axial rotation or a pivoting type of motion.

The spool-shaped trochlea of the distal humerus forms a highly conforming articulation with the greater sigmoid notch of the ulna. The two surfaces are separated by the trochlear sulcus, which lies slightly medial to the central axis of the humerus and courses in a helical fashion from anterolateral to posteromedial. The greater sigmoid notch of the ulna forms an ellipse with an arc of approximately 190°. Its longitudinal guiding ridge articulates with the apex of the trochlear sulcus in all degrees of elbow flexion, resulting in significant inherent stability.

The capitellum, almost spheroidal in shape, is separated from the trochlea by a groove in which the rim of the radial head articulates. The radial head is a concave disk that is offset from the neck of the radius. The neck in turn is angulated approximately 15° from the radial shaft. The radial head is not usually a circular structure but is more often elliptical in shape. Approximately 240° of the outside circumference of the radial head articulates with the ulna at the lesser sigmoid notch.

Role in Stability The bony contribution to elbow stability has not been fully characterized but is uniformly considered to be important. The congruent nature of the ulnohumeral articulation confers significant inherent stability. Because of this congruity, elbow joint motion has been considered primarily a hinge type. However, the position of the axis of elbow flexion follows an irregular course.[2] From a practical point of view, this deviation in the center of rotation is minimal, and the ulnohumeral joint can be assumed to move as a uniaxial articulation except at the extremes of flexion and extension. The axis of rotation can be defined as passing through the center of the arcs formed by the trochlear sulcus and the capitellum.[3]

The joint articulation provides approximately 55% of the stabilizing contribution to varus stability in extension and up to 75% in 90° of flexion.[4] Valgus stability is equally divided among the medial collateral ligament (MCL), the anterior capsule, and the bony articulation in full extension. At 90° of flexion, the contribution of the articulation to valgus stability does not change.[4] These values represent pure varus and valgus stresses, however, and do not account for the rotational forces that usually are present with instability.

The olecranon process of the ulna contributes a significant amount to varus and valgus stability of the elbow, providing inherent stability after reduction of a simple elbow dislocation. Removal of the olecranon process disrupts the greater sigmoid notch, which is key to this bony stability. Incremental excision of the olecranon process leads to a linear decrease in combined stability, both in extension and at 90° of flexion.[5] Valgus stress is primarily resisted by the proximal half of the greater sigmoid notch, whereas varus stress is resisted primarily by the distal half.

The coronoid process provides an anterior bony buttress to resist the posteriorly directed forces that occur from both the flexor and extensor musculature (Fig. 1). The forward flexion of the distal humeral

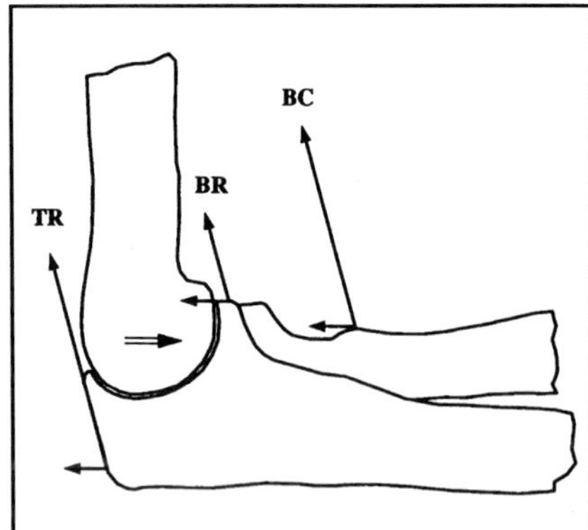

Fig. 1 The coronoid process resists the tendency for posterior ulnar translation with both flexion and extension movements. BC = biceps; BR = brachioradialis; TR = triceps. (Reproduced with permission from Morrey BF, O'Driscoll SW: Complex instability of the elbow, in Morrey BF (ed): *The Elbow and Its Disorders*, ed 3. Philadelphia, PA, WB Saunders, 2000, pp 421-430.)

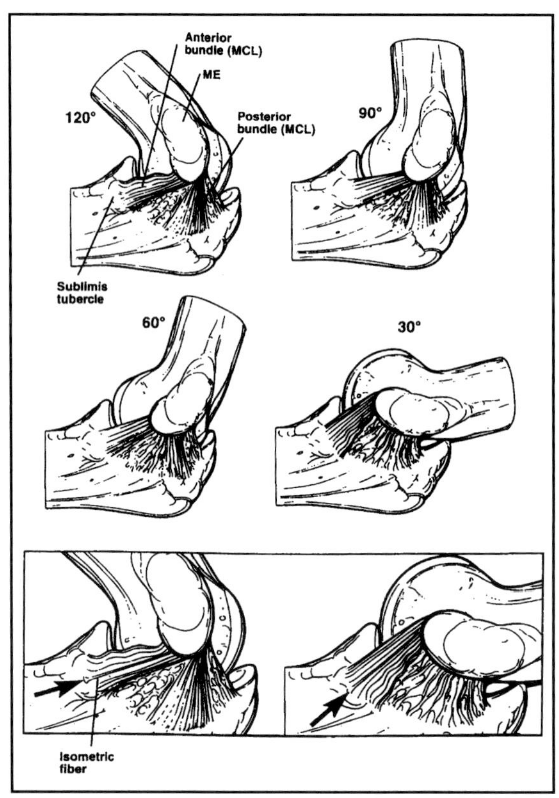

Fig. 2 Sequential tightening of the anterior bundle fibers occurs as the elbow is flexed and extended. At least some of the fibers are isometric. (Reproduced with permission from Callaway GH, Field LD, Deng X-H, Torzilli PA, et al: Biomechanical evaluation of the medial collateral ligament of the elbow. *J Bone Joint Surg Am* 1997;79:1223-1231.)

articulation and the 30° posterior opening of the greater sigmoid notch also may be important in this regard. Regan and Morrey[6] showed a correlation between coronoid fracture fragment size and the tendency for dislocation, which was particularly evident in the absence of a radial head. Cage and associates[7] later described the soft-tissue attachments of the coronoid process and correlated these insertion loci with coronoid fractures. They found that type I fractures were intra-articular, whereas the capsule was attached to type II fracture fragments. Only in type III fractures was the insertion of the anterior bundle of the MCL involved.

The importance of the radial head to elbow stability has become increasingly recognized. Early reports showed that its contribution to valgus stability may be as high as 30%, even with an intact MCL.[8] With disruption of the MCL, the radial head becomes a critical secondary stabilizer of the elbow, with up to 75% of the resistance to a valgus stress seen in the radial head.[9] Additionally, up to 60% of a longitudinally applied force is normally transmitted through the radial head.[10]

Capsuloligamentous Structures

Capsule A thin and almost translucent, regular orientation of fibrous bands within the elbow joint capsule provides significant strength and an important stabilizing effect when taut in extension.[11] Morrey and An[4] showed that the anterior capsule was a significant stabilizing element to pure varus stress (accounting for 32% of stability) and valgus stress (38%) in extension, but not at 90° of flexion (13% varus stress and 10% valgus stress at 90° of flexion). The soft-tissue resistance (85%) to distraction in extension also primarily originates from the anterior capsule, but virtually no resistance (8%) is offered at 90° of flexion.

Medial Collateral Ligament The MCL complex comprises three components: the anterior bundle, the posterior bundle, and the transverse bundle.[9] Biomechanically, the anterior bundle is the most important portion of the MCL, originating in the lateral two thirds of the anteroinferior aspect of the medial epicondyle.[12] It inserts on the medial aspect of the coronoid process at the sublime tubercle,[13] an average of 18 mm distal to the coronoid tip.[7] The anterior bundle is the strongest and stiffest portion of the MCL, with an average load to failure of 260 N.[14] It is taut throughout most of the entire arc of flexion, with sequential tightening of the fibers as the elbow flexes. At least some of the fibers originate from the axis of rotation of the joint and are therefore isometric[15] (Fig. 2).

The anterior bundle of the MCL is the primary restraint to valgus stress, contributing 55% to 70% to valgus stability.[4] Excision results in gross valgus instability at all degrees of flexion short of full extension, at which position the radial head and anterior capsule become important secondary stabilizers.[4,16] The posterior bundle of the MCL is much less differentiated from the capsule and does not contribute significantly to valgus stability except near terminal flexion.[14] The transverse fibers contribute little to elbow stability because they originate from and insert on the ulna.

Lateral Collateral Ligament The lateral collateral ligament (LCL) complex consists of four components: the annular ligament, the radial collateral ligament, the lateral ulna collateral ligament (LUCL), and the accessory LCL.[13] The LCL complex originates from the lateral epicondyle at a point through which the center of rotation passes. This complex therefore is isometric throughout the normal range of flexion and extension. The radial collateral ligament terminates indistinguishably in the annular ligament, which stabilizes the proximal radioulnar joint. The LUCL blends with the fibers of the annular ligament but also arches superficial and distal to it to insert on the tubercle of the supinator crest of the ulna.[17]

In 1991, O'Driscoll and associates[18] first described posterolateral rotatory instability of the elbow. The cause for this condition was thought to be a laxity of the LUCL, which allows a transient rotatory subluxation of the ulnohumeral joint and a secondary dislocation of the radiocapitellar joint. Ordinarily the LCL complex maintains these joints in a reduced position when the elbow is loaded in supination. A mechanism for elbow subluxation and dislocation was then described in which there was increasing ligamentous and capsular damage progressing from lateral to medial across the joint.[19] Dislocation was the final of three sequential stages of elbow instability resulting from posterolateral rotation.

The LCL complex also resists varus forces, an important concept given that these are the predominant forces on the elbow during many activities of daily living. Additionally, the LCL complex is farther away from the varus-valgus axis of the elbow joint than is the MCL, thus allowing greater excursions to occur with dysfunction of the ligament when it is put under stress (Fig. 3). Both factors highlight how critical lateral ligament integrity is to overall elbow stability. Among the primary restraints to elbow stability, portions of the LCL complex may be the most important.

Dynamic Stability Dynamic stability of the elbow joint is in part related to the flexor and extensor muscles providing compression across the joint, increasing the inherent stability provided by the highly congruent articular surfaces. In addition, the extent of instability of the elbow after simple elbow dislocations appears to have a direct association with the amount of muscular damage at the medial and lateral epicondyles.[20] Further stability may be imparted because of a bulk effect: the brachialis and triceps muscles in particular have broad cross-sectional areas, and their insertions are close to the axis of joint rotation. The role of the anconeus muscle remains unclear, but its location suggests that it may be an important dynamic constraint to varus and posterolateral rotatory instability.

The overall effect of muscle contraction on stability is likely to be important, but the magnitude of this effect has yet to be determined. In an early electromyographic study, Funk and associates[21] found that when varus and valgus stresses were applied to the elbow joint, most muscles were relatively quiet. Morrey and associates,[9] in contrast, found that muscle activity did occur and lessened the valgus laxity caused by MCL release.

On the medial side of the elbow, the flexor carpi ulnaris, specifically the humeral head, is the predominant musculotendinous unit overlying the MCL, particularly at higher degrees of elbow flexion.[22] The flexor digitorum superficialis is the only other significant contributor. These muscles, because of their position and bulk, are the best suited to provide medial elbow support and may augment the stability of the MCL. The principal dynamic restraints on the lateral side of the elbow are the extensor muscle origins with their fascial bands and intermuscular septa.[23] In supination, these serve to support the forearm unit and prevent it, by virtue of their course alone, from laterally rotating away from the humerus. The LUCL adheres closely to the supinator, anconeus, and extensor muscles and their intermuscular fascia.[24]

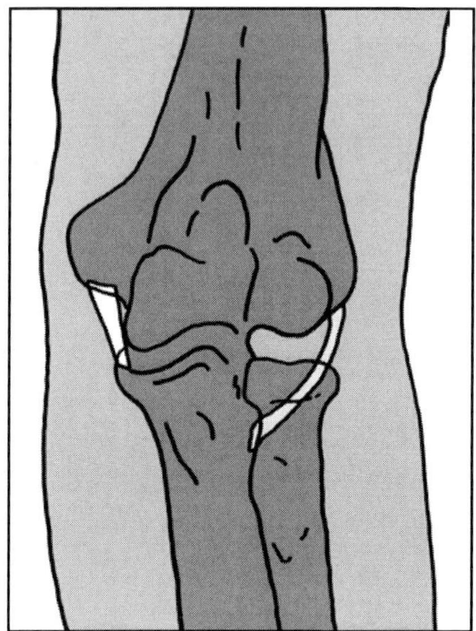

Fig. 3 The lateral collateral ligament must pass around the radial head to reach the ulna. (Reproduced with permission from O'Driscoll SW, Hori E, Morrey BF, Carmichael S: The anatomy of the lateral ulnar collateral ligament. *Clin Anat* 1992;5:296-303.)

Clinical Evaluation

Medial Instability

Symptoms of recurrent medial instability usually are associated with chronic overuse from athletic activities that involve throwing. Throwing applies a significant valgus stress to the elbow, resulting in repetitive microtrauma to the MCL.[25] Attenuation and even rupture of the ligament can result. Acute MCL ruptures that occur with elbow dislocation generally heal well and seldom result in valgus instability, except in athletes.[26] This is probably because of the limited valgus stress imposed on the elbow in daily life. If persistent valgus instability does occur after elbow dislocation, it may be associated with a worse overall clinical and radiographic result.[27]

During the throwing motion, valgus stress occurs primarily during late arm cocking and early acceleration. Tremendous tensile forces can be generated,[28] which are probably dissipated through a combination of the MCL, the flexor-pronator muscles, and the bony articulation. Valgus forces exceeding the tensile strength of the MCL may be produced,[29] highlighting the importance of these bony and dynamic contributions to stability.

Acute ruptures of the ligament usually cause a "pop" and pain and swelling over the medial aspect of the elbow.[30,31] Patients with recurrent medial elbow instability usually have pain and tenderness over the medial aspect of the elbow that is aggravated during and after throwing. With a tear of the ligament, pain may not occur until 70% to 80% of throwing effort is reached. Ulnar nerve symptoms may occur with medial instability because of compression by inflammation of the ligament within the tunnel or traction from repeated valgus loading.[32] These symptoms can be present in up to 40% of patients.[33]

On physical examination, patients may have point tenderness over the insertion of the anterior bundle of the MCL, 2 cm distal to the medial epicondyle. Elbow motion usually is normal, and the instability itself is difficult to demonstrate. In 1981, Norwood and associates[30] described the abduction stress test as a means to evaluate the integrity of the MCL. Performed with the forearm supinated and in 15° to 20° of elbow flexion to unlock the olecranon from its fossa, a positive test reproduces the athlete's symptoms. It is now recognized that this test is better performed with the forearm in full pronation because with the forearm supinated, pseudovalgus instability can occur from unrecognized posterolateral rotatory instability.[18]

The milking maneuver[34] and the moving valgus stress test (SW O'Driscoll, MD, Rochester, MN, personal communication, 2001) also can be used to assess MCL integrity. These tests apply a valgus stress to the elbow during flexion and extension in an attempt to elicit pain or demonstrate joint line opening. The difference in valgus rotation between intact elbows and those in which the anterior bundle of the MCL is deficient has been shown to be significantly greater at 70° to 90° of flexion than at 30°.[35-37] Clinical testing therefore also should be performed at these higher degrees of flexion. Detection of partial ruptures of the anterior bundle based on medial joint opening and increased valgus movement generally is not possible.[37]

Recurrent medial instability is primarily a clinical diagnosis, but a valgus stress radiograph may help to confirm the diagnosis. A normal stress radiograph, however, does not rule out symptomatic ligament attenuation. Valgus stress radiography can be performed manually or with the gravity stress radiograph.[33] Plain radiography also may demonstrate abnormalities that can be associated with recurrent MCL instability, including marginal osteophytes, loose bodies, ligament calcification, or heterotopic bone formation.

Rijke and associates[38] performed a stress radiography study in 42 injured athletes and 4 healthy athletes using a Telos GA-IIE stress device (Telos Medical, Fallston, MD). They reported that all complete and large partial tears were correctly diagnosed when the increase in joint space width was larger than 0.5 mm in the affected elbow compared with the opposite, normal elbow. Significant ulnohumeral gapping can occur in subjects with normal elbows, so comparisons should always be made with the contralateral side.[39] Clinical experience in overhead athletes has shown that a side-to-side difference of more than 2 mm is a better standard for making the diagnosis.

MRI is currently the imaging modality of choice for evaluating the MCL. Published series have described excellent results for the detection of complete ligament tears[40-42] but poorer results for partial tears. Partial tears usually occur on the inner surface of the ulna attachment of the MCL;[43] for these, the use of MRI with intra-articular gadolinium may provide information.[44,45] The role of ultrasound remains to be determined.

Lateral Instability

Most patients with lateral elbow instability present with symptoms after an elbow dislocation. Less commonly, there is a history of surgery to the lateral side of the elbow. Although most studies have indicated that both the MCL and LCL complexes are disrupted after an acute elbow dislocation,[20] residual instability more commonly involves the lateral side.

The clinical presentation is quite variable, although the typical patient presents with a history of recurrent painful clicking, catching, or snapping of the elbow, or a feeling that the elbow is slipping in and out of joint. Sometimes the patient has noticed only pain on the lateral side of the elbow. Symptoms typically occur in the extension portion of the motion arc with the forearm in supination, so that symptoms that occur with flexion and pronation are likely related to reduction of the subluxation. The classic activity that reproduces the patients' symptoms is pushing down on the armrests when rising from a chair.

The physical examination usually is unremarkable. Motion is typically normal, but the patient may be apprehensive with the elbow in full supination and extension. Pseudovalgus instability may be present, with apparent valgus instability in supination but not in pronation. A posterolateral rotatory drawer test has been described,[46] but the most sensitive test reported is the lateral pivot shift apprehension test.[18] However, reproducing the actual subluxation and the "clunk" that occurs with reduction usually is accomplished only with the patient under general anesthesia. Olsen and associates[47] reported that disruption of the entire LCL complex was necessary for elbow joint laxity to occur with the pivot shift test. They also reported that posterolateral instability was best detected at between 70° and 110° of flexion.[48]

Plain radiographs usually are normal, but stress radiographs may be helpful to confirm the diagnosis (Fig. 4). Continuous screening with an image intensifier is preferable, but plain radiographs taken during the application of a varus, valgus, or pivot shift stress also can be used. Malrotation can make these static stress radiographs difficult to interpret, however. It should also be remembered that a varus stress radiograph can be entirely normal even in the presence of clinically significant LCL insufficiency. Side-to-side comparisons should always be performed.

MRI may also be helpful in the diagnosis of posterolateral rotatory instability.[49] With the use of appropriate pulse sequences, identification of abnormalities within the LCL complex is possible. The administration of gadolinium into the elbow joint also may allow a clearer depiction of undersurface tears, which are poorly demonstrated by conventional MRI.[44]

Treatment

Medial Instability

Surgical Indications Surgical repair of the MCL after a simple elbow dislocation has not proved to be better than nonsurgical treatment.[20,50] Although acute repair of the MCL has been recommended,[30] the ligament is known to heal well in most patients. Isolated acute tears of the MCL are uncommon. Originally described in javelin throwers,[51] acute tears are more commonly seen in throwing athletes. Recently, Kenter and associates[52] reported satisfactory return to function at an elite level in National Football League players after nonsurgical treatment of acute MCL injuries. However, in high-demand throwing athletes, immediate repair or reconstruction is required to enable a return to throwing.

Chronic MCL injuries occur almost exclusively in the young athletic population. These patients are reluctant to accept prolonged periods of rest and activity modification, and surgical indications need to be individualized. Recreational, low-demand athletes do not necessarily need reconstruction. For the high-performance overhead athlete who desires to return to competitive sport, a complete tear of the anterior bundle of the MCL is an indication for surgery. Surgical treatment is also considered for symptomatic partial-thickness tears after a minimum of 3 months of supervised nonsurgical treatment. Fluoroscopically-assisted valgus stress testing of the elbow is helpful in this situation, with a side-to-side difference of 2 mm or more considered abnormal.

Finally, some athletes cannot return to successful performance at a high level despite a negative valgus stress test and MRI. These patients present a treatment dilemma, and arthroscopic examination of the elbow has been recommended in such cases.[43] Although some individuals may return to throwing using a modified technique, continued throwing with an unstable elbow can lead in time to posteromedial olecranon impingement and arthritic changes in the joint.[43]

Surgical Technique Primary repair of a torn MCL is generally not recommended, except in an acute tear related to a defined traumatic event. Reconstruction is preferable for ruptures that occur from throwing in association with an attenuated MCL.[33,52] The ligament can still be repaired with suture, but the repair should always be augmented with a graft reconstruction. For partial-thickness tears, the ligament is preserved but augmented with a graft reconstruction.

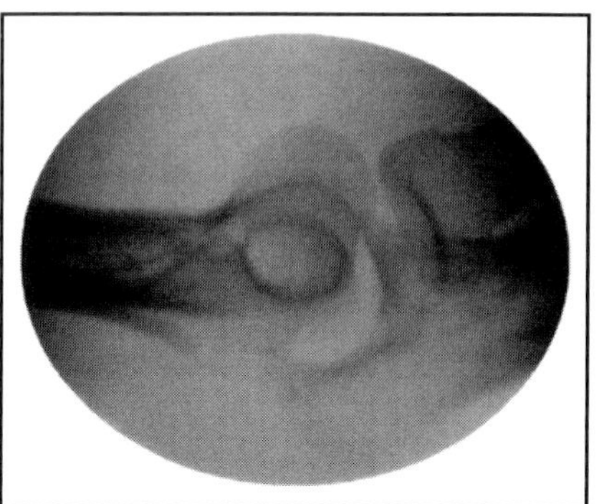

Fig. 4 Lateral stress radiograph showing posterolateral rotatory instability.

The technique of MCL reconstruction has been well described.[52-58] The palmaris longus tendon, with a strength of 357 N,[14] has been the most common graft for reconstruction. Graft site morbidity seems to be minimal.[52] If the palmaris longus is absent, other graft options include the plantaris, the gracilis or semitendinosus, a strip of the flexor carpi radialis, a long toe extensor, or allograft tissue.

Jobe and associates[54] were the first to describe reconstruction of the MCL using a tendon graft, placing this through bone tunnels in the humerus and ulna. Their technique involved dividing the flexor pronator origin and performing a submuscular transposition of the ulnar nerve. Because of a high incidence of complications related to the nerve, their procedure was subsequently modified to use a muscle-splitting approach without transposition of the nerve. In 1996, the "safe zone" for MCL exposure through a muscle-splitting approach was reported.[55] This safe zone extends from the medial epicondyle to approximately 1 cm distal to the insertion of the anterior bundle of the MCL on the sublime tubercle. Enough exposure can be obtained with a muscle split through the posterior third of the common flexor mass that MCL reconstruction can be performed without

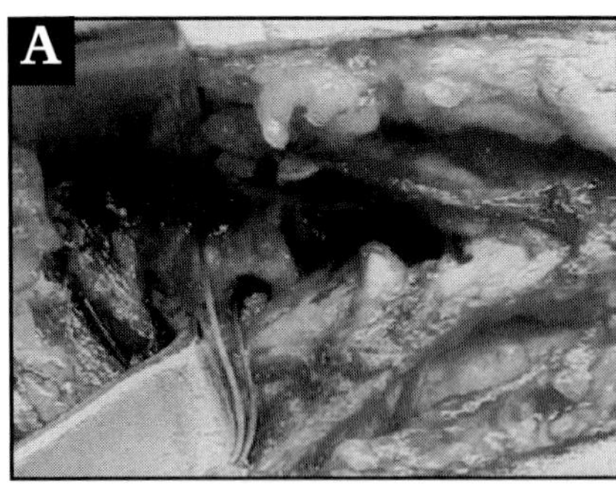

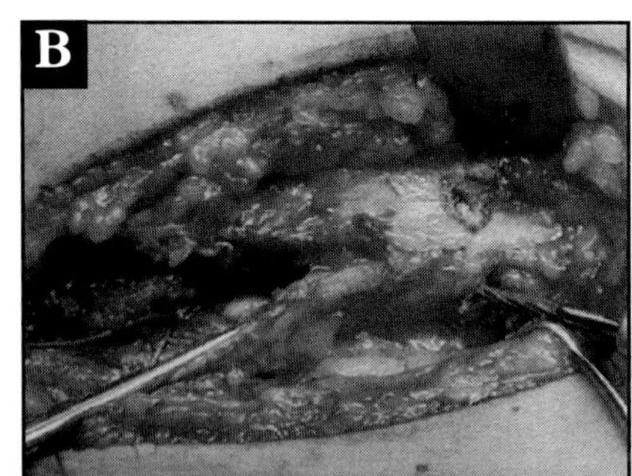

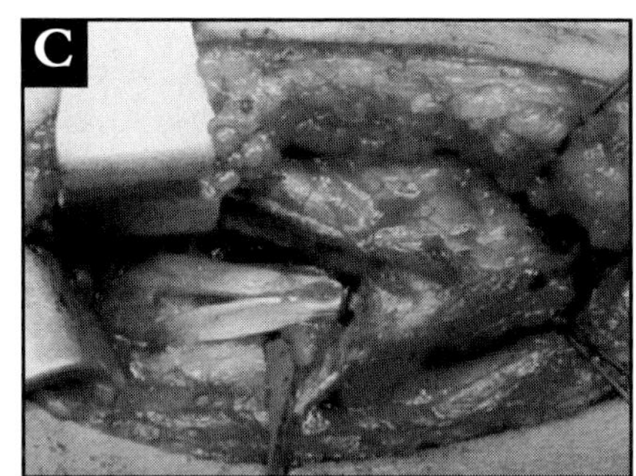

Fig. 5 The docking technique for reconstruction of the anterior bundle of the MCL. **A,** The sublime tubercle is exposed through a muscle-splitting approach and bone tunnels are created. **B,** Drill holes are made to allow passage of the sutures and docking of the graft into the humeral tunnel. **C,** The graft is sequentially seated and tensioned before the sutures are tied.

takedown of the flexor pronator muscles or transposition of the ulnar nerve.

A method of MCL reconstruction using a docking procedure has also been described.[59] In this technique, only one bone tunnel is required on the humeral side of the reconstruction. The two limbs of the graft are sequentially seated into this tunnel, simplifying graft passage and allowing accurate graft tensioning and fixation (Fig. 5). The yoke technique is an alternative method that involves a combination of docking one limb of the graft with a standard figure-of-8 reconstruction of the other.[60]

New methods of ligament reconstruction that eliminate the graft weave are also being investigated. Double docking allows in-line tensioning on both limbs of a two- or three-ply graft through single bone tunnels, with the ulnar end of the graft secured by tying between drill holes on the subcutaneous border. Alternatively, bone anchors can be used for graft fixation.[56] Reconstruction techniques using interference screws for graft fixation also are being explored.

Regardless of the reconstruction method chosen, several key factors should be considered: (1) The flexor pronator origin should be preserved by using a muscle-splitting approach. (2) Associated intra-articular pathology should be treated. (3) Calcification should be removed prior to reconstruction. (4) Bone tunnels should be placed to allow isometric positioning of the graft, with the number of tunnels kept to a minimum. (5) The graft should be securely placed in the bone tunnels and adequately tensioned. (6) The ulnar nerve and medial antebrachial cutaneous nerves should be preserved, with transposition of the ulnar nerve only if required. **(CD- 6.1)**

Results In 1986, Jobe and associates[54] reported that 10 of 16 athletes who had undergone MCL reconstruction returned to their previous levels of competition. In 1992, Conway and associates[33] reported that of 56 overhand athletes who had undergone MCL reconstruction, 80% of the patients had good or excellent results at an average follow-up of 6.3 years, with 68% having returned to their previous levels of sports participation. In 14 additional patients who had undergone a primary repair, 50% returned to their previous levels of competition. Prior elbow surgery was associated with a decreased chance of return to previous sport level.

In 1995, Andrews and Timmerman[61] reported on 11 professional pitchers with MCL injuries. Nine underwent a reconstruction of the ligament and two had a primary repair. Seven athletes, all of whom had had a reconstruction, returned to competition. More recently, Azar and associates[53] reported on 59 MCL reconstructions and 8 repairs at an average follow-up of 35.4 months. Overall, 79% of patients had successful outcomes; 81% of patients with a reconstruction and 63% with repairs returned to their previous levels of competition, with an average time for return to competitive throwing of 9.8 months.

Nonsurgical treatment of MCL insufficiency has only recently been reported.[62] Following a minimum of 3 months' rest with rehabilitation exercises, only 42% of athletes returned to their previous levels of competition.

The duration of recovery is long after MCL reconstruction. High forces occur in the ligament during throwing,[63] so this activity must be delayed until mature biologic healing of the graft into the bone tunnels has occurred. The most important surgical complications associated with MCL reconstruction include medial antebrachial cutaneous nerve injury, ulnar nerve injury, and fracture of the ulnar tunnel, all of which can be avoided with careful surgical technique. Postoperative ulnar neuropathy can occur in up to 21% of patients.[33] Newer techniques that use a muscle-splitting approach and avoidance of routine ulnar nerve transposition have significantly reduced this complication.

Lateral Instability

Surgical Indications Most LCL complex injuries that occur with simple elbow dislocations do not require surgical treatment. With recurrent LCL instability, the need or justification for surgical reconstruction is less well defined. In some patients, recurrent instability associated with LCL insufficiency may significantly interfere with daily function. When incompetent, the ligament does not become stable with time.[64] Patients who present with a history suggestive of LCL instability and who have a positive lateral pivot shift apprehension test may be considered for LUCL reconstruction. Confirmatory imaging studies, although helpful in difficult cases, are not always required. Alternative elbow pathology that could account for the patient's symptoms must be excluded. For the less active patient who is prepared to modify his or her activities and accommodate elbow symptoms, nonsurgical management may be more appropriate.

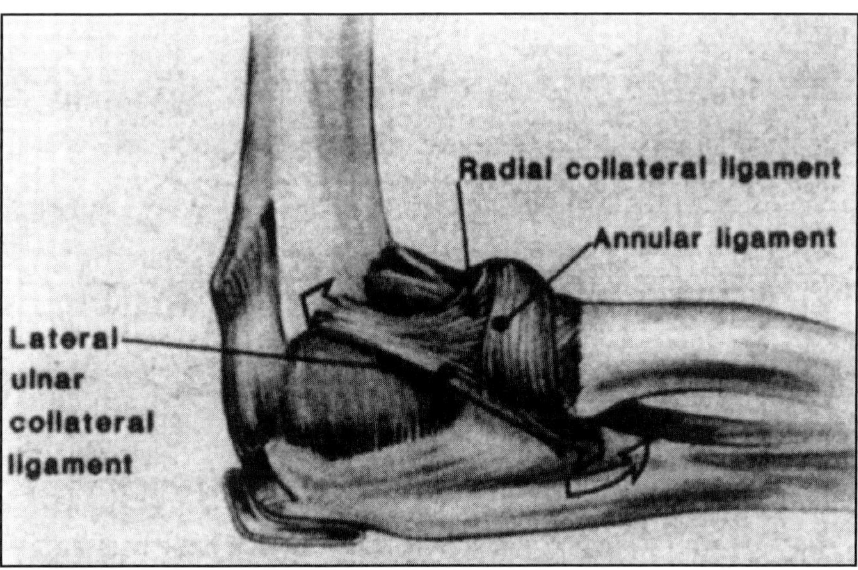

Fig. 6 The orientation and attachment of the lateral ulnar collateral ligament stabilizes the ulna to resist varus and rotatory stresses. (Reproduced with permission from An KN, Morrey BF: Biomechanics of the elbow, in Morrey BF (ed): *The Elbow and Its Disorders*, ed 3. Philadelphia, PA, WB Saunders, 2000, pp 43-60.)

Surgical Treatment Osborne and Cotterill[65] first described repair of the lateral capsuloligamentous structures of the elbow for recurrent dislocation. They postulated that the essential lesion was in the posterolateral ligaments and capsular structures, which were torn or overstretched during the initial dislocation. Durig and associates[66] reported that the surgical findings in acute traumatic dislocations were similar and used the same type of capsuloligamentous repair when there was gross instability. Today, acute ligament repair is recommended only for gross instability after reduction of the elbow or in conjunction with open reduction of fracture dislocations, particularly where internal fixation of the radial head and/or coronoid process has been performed.[64] In such cases, the ligamentous and muscular origins have usually been avulsed from the lateral epicondyle and can be repaired directly back down to bone, thereby reestablishing lateral elbow stability.

Acute repairs usually should be augmented with a heavy suture in the path of the LUCL,[67] which stress-shields the repair during the early postoperative period. The LCL complex also can be augmented using three fan-shaped arcades of suture secured through holes drilled in the lateral epicondyle.[68] The first arcade follows the path of the LUCL, the second follows the path of the LCL and engages the annular ligament, and the third engages the posterior capsule and anconeus muscle. As a result, the normal anatomic restraints to posterolateral rotation of the radioulnar complex are repaired and reinforced.

For patients with recurrent lateral instability, reconstruction of the LUCL using a free tendon graft is recommended.[69] The graft must originate at the isometric origin of the LCL, which lies at the center of rotation of the elbow joint, and attach to the tubercle of the supinator crest of the ulna, several millimeters posterior to the proximal radioulnar joint. In this position, the tendon graft supports the proximal ulna in its relation to the humerus and provides posterolateral restraint to the radial head (Fig. 6). It is critical that the graft be placed at the isometric point of the elbow or the reconstruction will constrain normal motion. Again, the palmaris longus tendon can be harvested for the graft if it is present. Otherwise, the plantaris, the gracilis or semitendinosus, a long toe extensor, or allograft tissue can be used.

The technical aspects of exposure and bone tunnel preparation have been well described.[53,68,69] Most authors favor a three-ply passage of the graft across the joint, as described originally by Nestor and associates,[69] or one of its modifications. Alternatively, docking procedures, as described for MCL reconstruction, can be used.[58] Arthroscopic techniques of reconstruction and the use of interference screws for fixation of the graft also are being investigated. Whatever technique is chosen, the joint should always be inspected for chondral defects and loose bodies, and the arthrotomy should be closed and imbricated underneath the graft.

Results Osborne and Cotterill[65] reported that eight patients treated for recurrent elbow dislocation by imbrication and reattachment of the LCL had no recurrences. Data on the long-term results of treatment for recurrent posterolateral rotatory instability is scant. O'Driscoll and associates[18] briefly mentioned results in five patients in their initial description of the condition. In 1992, Nestor and associates[69] reported on 11 patients at an average follow-up of 42 months. Stability was obtained in 10 patients, with 7 having an excellent functional result. The four patients with less than excellent results had all had previous elbow surgery. If the radial head has been excised or if there is degenerative arthritis of the joint, the satisfactory result decreases, although stability usually can be achieved.[64]

Delayed laxity, redislocation, and reinjury have been observed after LCL reconstruction of the elbow. Complications associated with graft harvesting are also possible. Iatrogenic fracture of the bony tunnels can be avoided with careful surgical technique. A mild flexion contracture can be accepted because the most vulnerable position of instability is full extension. The duration of postoperative splinting depends on a number of variables, including patient compliance, strength of the reconstruction, and response to previous immobilization.[68] Rehabilitation must be progressive, with full activity not allowed for at least 6 months.

Summary

Elbow stability relies on a complex interaction between the bony articulations of the elbow joint, the capsuloligamentous structures, and dynamic muscle restraints. Understanding the functional anatomy of the elbow and the relative contribution of the various elements to elbow stability is important in developing a strategy for diagnosis and management. Elbow instability presents a spectrum from minor subluxation to dislocation. The treatment of an acute dislocation is determined by the stability of the elbow after reduction and the fixation of associated fractures. Isolated acute tears of the LCL are uncommon and are generally treated nonsurgically. On the medial side, augmented repair is required for return to throwing sports. Chronic MCL insufficiency results in valgus instability, which usually is a problem only for the throwing athlete. Chronic LCL insufficiency may lead to symptomatic posterolateral joint subluxation. Free tendon graft reconstruction can be successful on both sides of the joint, with a return of stability and improved elbow function.

References

1. Simon WH, Friedenberg S, Richardson S: Joint congruence: A correlation of joint congruence and thickness of articular cartilage in dogs. *J Bone Joint Surg Am* 1973;55:1614-1620.
2. Morrey BF, Chao EY: Passive motion of the elbow joint. *J Bone Joint Surg Am* 1976;58:501-508.
3. London JT: Kinematics of the elbow. *J Bone Joint Surg Am* 1981;63:529-535.
4. Morrey BF, An KN: Articular and ligamentous contributions to the stability of the elbow joint. *Am J Sports Med* 1983;11:315-319.
5. An KN, Morrey BF, Chao EY: The effect of partial removal of proximal ulna on elbow constraint. *Clin Orthop* 1986;209:270-279.
6. Regan W, Morrey B: Fractures of the coronoid process of the ulna. *J Bone Joint Surg Am* 1989;71:1348-1354.
7. Cage DJ, Abrams RA, Callahan JJ, Botte MJ: Soft tissue attachments of the ulnar coronoid process: An anatomic study with radiographic correlation. *Clin Orthop* 1995;320:154-158.
8. Morrey BF, Askew L, Chao EY: Silastic prosthetic replacement for the radial head. *J Bone Joint Surg Am* 1981;63:454-458.
9. Morrey BF, Tanaka S, An KN: Valgus stability of the elbow: A definition of primary and secondary constraints. *Clin Orthop* 1991;265:187-195.
10. Halls AA, Travill A: Transmission of pressures across the elbow joint. *Anat Rec* 1964;150:243-247.
11. King GJW, Morrey BF, An KN: Stabilizers of the elbow. *J Shoulder Elbow Surg* 1993;2:165-174.
12. O'Driscoll SW, Jaloszynski R, Morrey BF, An KN: Origin of the medial ulnar collateral ligament. *J Hand Surg Am* 1992;17:164-168.
13. Morrey BF, An KN: Functional anatomy of the ligaments of the elbow. *Clin Orthop* 1985;201:84-90.
14. Regan WD, Korinek SL, Morrey BF, An KN: Biomechanical study of ligaments around the elbow joint. *Clin Orthop* 1991;271:170-179.
15. Ochi N, Ogura T, Hashizume H, Shigeyama Y, Senda M, Inoue H: Anatomic relation between the medial collateral ligament of the elbow and the humero-ulnar joint axis. *J Shoulder Elbow Surg* 1999;8:6-10.
16. Hotchkiss RN, Weiland AJ: Valgus stability of the elbow. *J Orthop Res* 1987;5:372-377.
17. O'Driscoll SW, Horii E, Morrey BF, Carmichael SW: Anatomy of the ulnar part of the lateral collateral ligament of the elbow. *Clin Anat* 1992;5:296-303.
18. O'Driscoll SW, Bell DF, Morrey BF: Posterolateral rotatory instability of the elbow. *J Bone Joint Surg Am* 1991;73:440-446.
19. O'Driscoll SW, Morrey BF, Korinek S, An K-N: Elbow subluxation and dislocation: A spectrum of instability. *Clin Orthop* 1992;280:186-197.
20. Josefsson PO, Johnell O, Wendeberg B: Ligamentous injuries in dislocations of the elbow joint. *Clin Orthop* 1987;221:221-225.
21. Funk DA, An K-N, Morrey BF, Daube JR: Electromyographic analysis of muscles across the elbow joint. *J Orthop Res* 1987;5:529-538.
22. Davidson PA, Pink M, Perry J, Jobe FW: Functional anatomy of the flexor pronator muscle group in relation to the medial collateral ligament of the elbow. *Am J Sports Med* 1995;23:245-250.
23. Cohen MS, Hastings H II: Rotatory instability of the elbow: The anatomy and role of the lateral stabilizers. *J Bone Joint Surg Am* 1997;79:225-233.
24. Imatani J, Ogura T, Morito Y, Hashizume H, Inoue H: Anatomic and histologic studies of lateral collateral ligament complex of the elbow joint. *J Shoulder Elbow Surg* 1999;8:625-627.
25. Wilson FD, Andrews JR, Blackburn TA, McCluskey G: Valgus extension overload in the pitching elbow. *Am J Sports Med* 1983;11:83-88.
26. Kuroda S, Sakamaki K: Ulnar collateral ligament tears of the elbow joint. *Clin Orthop* 1986;208:266-271.
27. Eygendaal D, Verdegaal SH, Obermann WR, van Vugt AB, Poll RG, Rozing PM: Posterolateral dislocation of the elbow joint: Relationship to medial instability. *J Bone Joint Surg Am* 2000;82:555-560.
28. Werner SL, Fleisig GS, Dillman CJ, Andrews JR: Biomechanics of the elbow during baseball pitching. *J Orthop Sports Phys Ther* 1993;17:274-278.
29. Pappas AM, Zawacki RM, Sullivan TJ: Biomechanics of baseball pitching: A preliminary report. *Am J Sports Med* 1985;13:216-222.
30. Norwood LA, Shook JA, Andrews JR: Acute medial elbow ruptures. *Am J Sports Med* 1981;9:16-19.
31. Lesin BE, Balfour GW: Acute rupture of the medial collateral ligament of the elbow requiring reconstruction: Case report. *J Bone Joint Surg Am* 1986;68:1278-1280.
32. Ciccotti MG, Jobe FW: Medial collateral ligament instability and ulnar neuritis in the athlete's elbow. *Instr Course Lect* 1999;48:383-391.

33. Conway JE, Jobe FW, Glousman RE, Pink M: Medial instability of the elbow in throwing athletes: Treatment by repair or reconstruction of the ulnar collateral ligament. *J Bone Joint Surg Am* 1992;74:67-83.

34. Veltri DM, O'Brien SJ, Field LD, Deutsch A, Altchek DW, Potter HG: The milking maneuver: A new test to evaluate the MCL of the elbow in the throwing athlete, in *Programs and Abstracts of the 10th Open Meeting of the American Shoulder and Elbow Surgeons*. Rosemont, IL, American Academy of Orthopaedic Surgeons, 1994.

35. Callaway GH, Field LD, Deng X-H, et al: Biomechanical evaluation of the medial collateral ligament of the elbow. *J Bone Joint Surg Am* 1997;79:1223-1231.

36. Floris S, Olsen BS, Dalstra M, Sojbjerg JO, Sneppen O: The medial collateral ligament of the elbow joint: Anatomy and kinematics. *J Shoulder Elbow Surg* 1998;7:345-351.

37. Eygendaal D, Olsen BS, Jensen SL, Seki A, Sojbjerg JO: Kinematics of partial and total ruptures of the medial collateral ligament of the elbow. *J Shoulder Elbow Surg* 1999;8:612-616.

38. Rijke AM, Goitz HT, McCue FC, Andrews JR, Berr SS: Stress radiography of the medial elbow ligaments. *Radiology* 1994;191:213-216.

39. Lee GA, Katz SD, Lazarus MD: Elbow valgus stress radiography in an uninjured population. *Am J Sports Med* 1998;26:425-427.

40. Timmerman LA, Schwartz ML, Andrews JR: Preoperative evaluation of the ulnar collateral ligament by magnetic resonance imaging and computed tomography arthrography: Evaluation in 25 baseball players with surgical confirmation. *Am J Sports Med* 1994;22:26 32.

41. Schwartz ML, Al-Zahrani S, Morwessel RM, Andrews JR: Ulnar collateral ligament injury in the throwing athlete: Evaluation with saline enhanced MR arthrography. *Radiology* 1995;197:297-299.

42. Nakanishi K, Masatomi T, Ochi T, et al: MR arthrography of elbow: Evaluation of the ulnar collateral ligament of elbow. *Skeletal Radiol* 1996;25:629-634.

43. Timmerman LA, Andrews JR: Undersurface tear of the ulnar collateral ligament in baseball players: A newly recognized lesion. *Am J Sports Med* 1994;22:33-36.

44. Cotten A, Jacobson J, Brossmann J, et al: Collateral ligaments of the elbow: Conventional MR imaging and MR arthrography with coronal oblique plane and elbow flexion. *Radiology* 1997;204:806-812.

45. Hill NB Jr, Bucchieri JS, Shon F, Miller TT, Rosenwasser MP: Magnetic resonance imaging of injury to the medial collateral ligament of the elbow: A cadaver model. *J Shoulder Elbow Surg* 2000;9:418-422.

46. Josefsson PO, Gentz C-F, Johnell O, Wendeberg B. Surgical versus non-surgical treatment of ligamentous injuries following dislocation of the elbow joint: A prospective randomized study. *J Bone Joint Surg Am* 1987;69:605-608.

47. Olsen BS, Vaesel MT, Sojbjerg JO, Helmig P, Sneppen O: Lateral collateral ligament of the elbow joint: Anatomy and kinematics. *J Shoulder Elbow Surg* 1996;5:103-112.

48. Olsen BS, Sojbjerg JO, Nielsen KK, Vaesel MT, Dalstra M, Sneppen O: Posterolateral elbow joint instability: The basic kinematics. *J Shoulder Elbow Surg* 1998;7:19-29.

49. Potter HG, Weiland AJ, Schatz JA, Paletta GA, Hotchkiss RN: Posterolateral rotatory instability of the elbow: Usefulness of MR imaging in diagnosis. *Radiology* 1997;204:185-189.

50. Josefsson PO, Gentz C-F, Johnell O, Wendeberg B: Surgical versus nonsurgical treatment of ligamentous injuries following dislocations of the elbow joint. *Clin Orthop* 1987;214:165-169.

51. Waris W: Elbow injuries of javelin-throwers. *Acta Chir Scand* 1946;93:563-575.

52. Kenter K, Behr CT, Warren RF, O'Brien SJ, Barnes R: Acute elbow injuries in the National Football League. *J Shoulder Elbow Surg* 2000;9:1-5.

53. Azar FM, Andrews JR, Wilk KE, Groh D: Operative treatment of ulnar collateral ligament injuries of the elbow in athletes. *Am J Sports Med* 2000;28:16-23.

54. Jobe FW, Stark H, Lombardo SJ: Reconstruction of the ulnar collateral ligament in athletes. *J Bone Joint Surg Am* 1986;68:1158-1163.

55. Smith GR, Altchek DW, Pagnani MJ, Keeley JR: A muscle-splitting approach to the ulnar collateral ligament of the elbow: Neuroanatomy and operative technique. *Am J Sports Med* 1996;24:575-580.

56. Hechtman KS, Tjin-A-Tsoi EW, Zvijac JE, Uribe JW, Latta LL: Biomechanics of a less invasive procedure for reconstruction of the ulnar collateral ligament of the elbow. *Am J Sports Med* 1998;26:620-624.

57. Thompson WH, Jobe FW, Yocum LA: Abstract: Ulnar collateral ligament reconstruction in throwing athletes: Muscle splitting approach without transposition of the ulnar nerve. *J Shoulder Elbow Surg* 1998;7:175.

58. Altchek DW, Hyman J, Williams R, et al: Management of MCL injuries of the elbow in throwers. *Techniques in Shoulder and Elbow Surgery* 2000;1:73-81.

59. Azar FM: Operative treatment of ulnar collateral ligament injuries of the elbow in athletes. *Op Tech Orthop* 2001;11:63-67.

60. Morrey BF, O'Driscoll SW: Lateral collateral ligament injury, in Morrey BF (ed): *The Elbow and Its Disorders*, ed 3. Philadelphia, PA, WB Saunders, 2000, pp 556-562.

61. Andrews JR, Timmerman LA: Outcome of elbow surgery in professional baseball players. *Am J Sports Med* 1995;23:407-413.

62. Rettig AC, Sherrill C, Snead DS, Mendler JC, Mieling P: Nonoperative treatment of ulnar collateral ligament injuries in throwing athletes. *Am J Sports Med* 2001;29:15-17.

63. Dillman CJ, Fleisig GS, Andrews JR: Biomechanics of pitching with emphasis upon shoulder kinematics. *J Orthop Sports Phys Ther* 1993;18:402-408.

64. O'Driscoll SW, Jupiter JB, King GJ, Hotchkiss RN, Morrey BF: The unstable elbow. *J Bone Joint Surg Am* 2000;82:724-738.

65. Osborne G, Cotterill P: Recurrent dislocation of the elbow. *J Bone Joint Surg Br* 1966;48:340-346.

66. Durig M, Muller W, Ruedi TP, Gauer EF: The operative treatment of elbow dislocation in the adult. *J Bone Joint Surg Am* 1979;61:239-244.

67. O'Driscoll SW: Elbow instability. *Hand Clin* 1994;10:405-415.

68. King JC, Spencer EE: Lateral ligamentous instability: Techniques of repair and reconstruction. *Techniques in Orthop* 2000;15:93-104.

69. Nestor BJ, O'Driscoll SW, Morrey BF: Ligamentous reconstruction for posterolateral rotatory instability of the elbow. *J Bone Joint Surg Am* 1992;74:1235-1241.

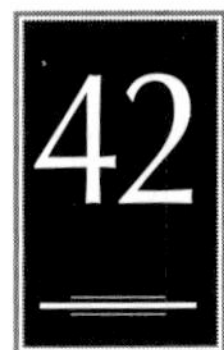

The Unstable Elbow

Shawn W. O'Driscoll, PhD, MD, FRCS
Jesse B. Jupiter, MD
Graham J. W. King, MD, MSc, FRCS
Robert N. Hotchkiss, MD
Bernard F. Morrey, MD

Biomechanics of Elbow Dislocation

Pathoanatomy

The pathoanatomy of an elbow dislocation can be thought of as a disruption of the circle of soft tissue or bone, or both, that begins on the lateral side of the elbow and progresses to the medial side in three stages (Fig. 1, *A*). In stage 1, the lateral collateral ligament is partially or completely disrupted (the ulnar part is disrupted). This disruption results in posterolateral rotatory subluxation of the elbow, which can reduce spontaneously (Fig. 1, *B*). Stage 2 involves additional disruption anteriorly and posteriorly. There is an incomplete posterolateral dislocation of the elbow in which the concave medial edge of the ulna rests on the trochlea. On a lateral radiograph of the elbow, the coronoid process appears to be perched on the trochlea. This dislocation can be reduced with use of minimal force or by the patient manipulating his or her own elbow. Stage 3 is subdivided into three parts. In stage 3A, all of the soft tissues around and including the posterior part of the medial collateral ligament are disrupted, leaving only the important anterior band (the anterior medial collateral ligament) intact. This permits posterior dislocation by a posterolateral rotatory mechanism. The elbow pivots on the intact anterior band of the medial collateral ligament. Reduction is accomplished by gentle manipulation of the elbow beginning with supination and valgus stress, temporarily recreating the deformity, followed by application of traction, varus stress, and pronation simultaneously. The intact anterior medial collateral ligament provides stability if the forearm is kept in pronation to prevent posterolateral rotatory subluxation during valgus stress-testing. Stage 3A instability is most commonly seen in the presence of fractures of the radial head and coronoid process. In stage 3B, the entire medial collateral complex is disrupted. Varus, valgus, and rotatory instability are all present following reduction. In stage 3C, the instability is so severe that the elbow can dislocate even when it is immobilized in a cast in 90° of flexion. This degree of instability occurs because the entire distal aspect of the humerus has been stripped of soft tissues. Usually, reduction can be maintained only by flexing the elbow beyond 90° to 110°. The flexor-pronator and common extensor muscle origins are important secondary stabilizers of the elbow. These pathoanatomic stages all correlate with clinical degrees of elbow instability. Most commonly, elbow dislocations involve disruption of both the medial and the lateral collateral ligament and, therefore, are at least stage 2.[1-3]

Thus, dislocation is the final stage of three sequential stages of elbow instability resulting from posterolateral ulnohumeral rotatory subluxation, with soft-tissue disruption that progresses from the lateral to the medial side. This finding has been confirmed in a study of cadaveric elbows.[4] Twelve of 13 elbows could be dislocated posteriorly with the anterior medial collateral ligament intact. In each stage, the pathoanatomy correlated with the pattern and degree of instability.

This circle of disruption is referred to as the Horii circle and is analogous to the Mayfield spiral of soft tissue or osseous disruption, or both, in carpal instability (Fig. 1, *A*). As disruption progresses from the lateral to the medial side, it may pass through the soft tissues or bone, or both. Therefore, an elbow dislocation is most commonly associated with a torn capsule, but the capsule may be intact if the coronoid process is fractured. Because energy is dissipated with a fracture before the elbow dislocates, the anterior bundle of the medial collateral ligament is often intact when the radial head and coronoid process are both fractured.

This parallel between the pathoanatomy and the degree of displacement explains the spectrum of instability, ranging from posterolateral rotatory

One or more of the authors or the departments with which they are affiliated have received something of value from a commercial or other party related directly or indirectly to the subject of this chapter.

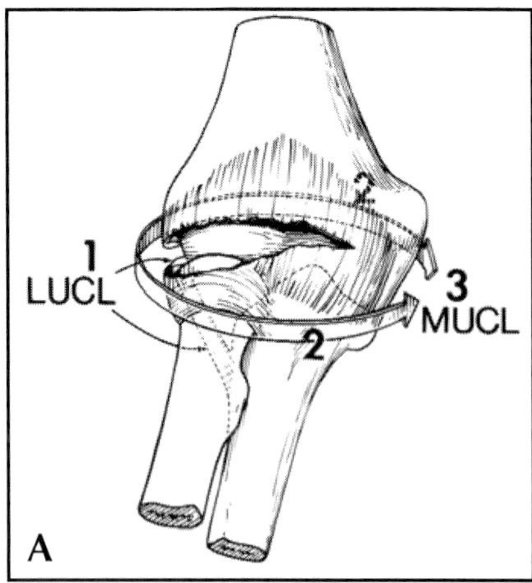

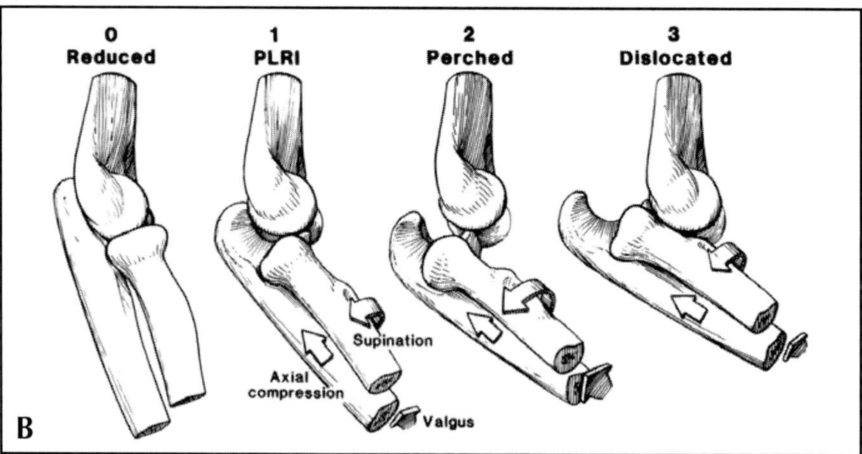

Fig. 1 A, Drawing of the Horii circle of soft-issue injury. The injury progresses from the lateral to the medial side in three stages. In stage 1, the ulnar part of the lateral collateral ligament, the lateral ulnar collateral ligament (LUCL), is disrupted. In stage 2, the other lateral ligamentous structures and the anterior and posterior aspects of the capsule are disrupted. In stage 3, the medial ulnar collateral ligament (MUCL) is either partially disrupted, involving the posterior medial ulnar collateral ligament only (stage 3A), or completely disrupted (stage 3B). The common extensor and flexor origins are often disrupted as well. **B,** Drawings showing the spectrum of elbow instability, from subluxation to dislocation. The three stages correspond with the pathoanatomic stages of capsuloligamentous disruption in **A**. The arrows indicate the forces and moments responsible for displacements. PLRI = posterolateral rotatory instability. (Reproduced with permission from the Mayo Foundation, Rochester, MN.)

instability to posterior dislocation with or without disruption of the anterior medial collateral ligament. Such a posterolateral rotatory mechanism for dislocation would be compatible with those suggested in the 1960s by Osborne and Cotterill[5] and by Roberts.[6]

Constraints to Elbow Instability

The elbow has both static and dynamic constraints, which are analogous to the defenses of a fortress (Fig. 2). The three primary static constraints to elbow instability are the ulnohumeral articulation, the medial collateral ligament, and the lateral collateral ligament, especially the ulnar part of the lateral collateral ligament (also referred to as the lateral ulnar collateral ligament). The secondary constraints include the radial head, the common flexor and extensor origins, and the capsule. The dynamic stabilizers include the muscles that cross the elbow joint and produce compressive forces at the articulation. The anconeus, triceps, and brachialis are the most important muscles in this regard. Originating near the lateral epicondyle and inserting broadly on the ulna in a fan shape, the anconeus seems designed to serve its major function as a dynamic stabilizer, preventing posterolateral rotational displacement of the elbow. A word of caution: the nerve to the anconeus, which enters the muscle proximally, is divided with the traditional olecranon osteotomy for distal humeral fractures.

An elbow with its three primary constraints intact will be stable. If the coronoid process is fractured or lost, the radial head becomes a critical stabilizer. The radial head must not be removed when a dislocated elbow is associated with a fractured coronoid process unless the coronoid process and the ligaments can be securely fixed. The management of injuries to these structures is discussed in the ensuing sections.

Classification of Elbow Instability

Elbow instability can be classified into different types according to five criteria: (1) the articulation or articulations involved (the elbow or the radial head); (2) the direction of displacement (valgus, varus, anterior, or posterolateral rotatory); (3) the degree of displacement (subluxation or dislocation); (4) the timing (acute, chronic, or recurrent); and (5) the presence or absence of associated fractures.[7]

As described in detail in the section on pathoanatomy, elbow instability can be considered a spectrum consisting of three stages (Fig. 1, *B*). In stage 1, the elbow subluxates in a posterolateral direction and the patient has a positive lateral pivot-shift test (Fig. 3). In stage 2, the elbow dislocates incompletely so that the coronoid process is perched on the trochlea. In stage 3, the elbow dislocates fully so that the coronoid process rests behind the humerus. Stage 3 is subclassified into three categories. In stage 3A, the anterior band of the medial collateral ligament is intact and the elbow is stable to valgus stress following reduction. In stage 3B, the elbow dislocates fully and the anterior band of the medial collateral ligament is disrupted so that the elbow is unstable in varus, valgus, and posterolateral rotation. Some flexion (30° to 45°) is usually required to prevent subluxation. In stage 3C, the entire distal aspect of the humerus is stripped of soft tissues, rendering the elbow unstable even in a cast. Reduction can be maintained usually only by flexing the elbow more than 90°. Each stage has specific clinical, radiographic, and pathologic features that are predictable and have implications for treatment. The pathologic characteristics can be predicted from the degree of instability.

Evaluation of Acute Dislocations and Fracture-Dislocations

Acute Elbow Dislocations

Dislocated elbows must be evaluated for functional stability after reduction of the dislocation. Following reduction, instability is assessed by gently moving the elbow through a range of motion. If the elbow appears to subluxate or dislocate, a splint is applied and anteroposterior and lateral radiographs are made. If no subluxation is seen on radiographs, the patient is discharged with the arm in the splint or a sling. The patient should be reevaluated in 5 to 7 days. If the elbow subluxates or dislocates in extension or is noncongruent on the radiographs made at the follow-up visit, the forearm should be pronated and the stability of the elbow should be reassessed. If stability is restored, a hinged brace or cast-brace is applied with the forearm in full pronation. An extension block of 30° is sometimes necessary. If the elbow requires an extension block of more than 30° to 45°, surgical repair should be considered. Extension blocks should be gradually eased so that by 3 weeks the brace allows full motion. At each follow-up examination, the elbow should be reevaluated in exactly the same manner.

Instability may need to be assessed with the patient under general anesthesia, as this is sometimes the only way to adequately examine the joint for stability. This examination is easiest to perform and the findings are easiest to

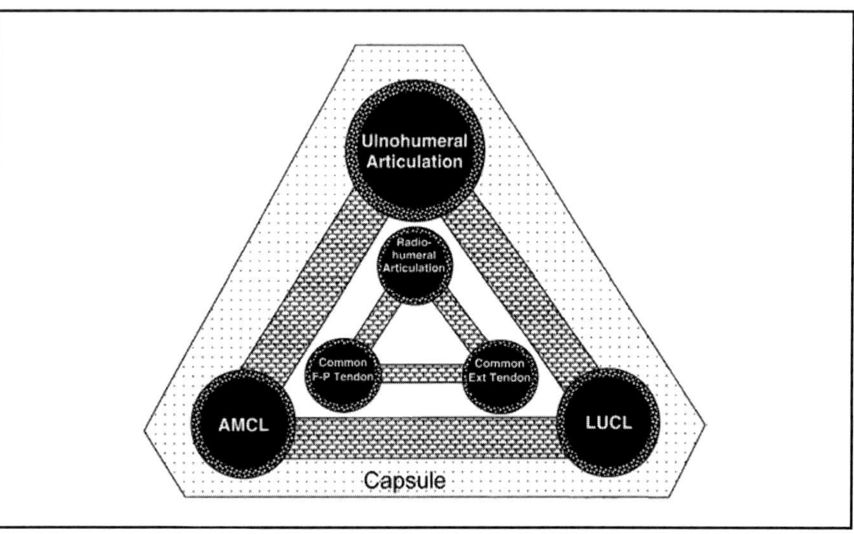

Fig. 2 Drawing showing the static and dynamic constraints to instability, which can be considered analogous to the defenses of a fortress. The three primary static constraints to elbow instability are the ulnohumeral articulation, the anterior medial collateral ligament (AMCL), and the lateral collateral ligament, especially the ulnar part of the lateral collateral ligament, which is also referred to as the lateral ulnar collateral ligament (LUCL). The secondary constraints include the radial head, the common flexor and extensor tendon origins, and the capsule. Dynamic stabilizers include the muscles that cross the elbow joint and produce compressive forces at the articulation. F-P = flexor-pronator. (Reproduced with permission from the Mayo Foundation, Rochester, MN.)

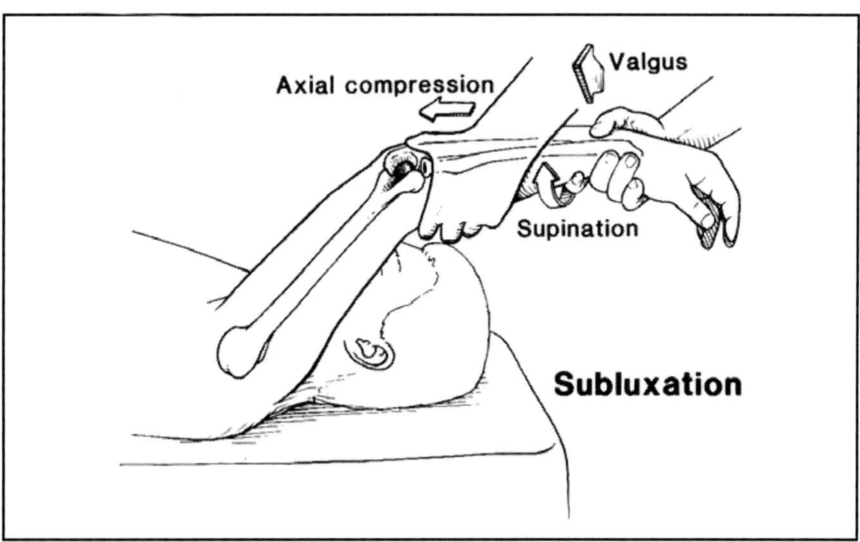

Fig. 3 Drawing showing the lateral pivot-shift test for posterolateral rotatory instability of the elbow, which is performed with the patient's arm overhead. A supination-valgus moment is applied during flexion, causing the elbow to subluxate maximally at about 40° of flexion. Additional flexion causes reduction (with a palpable, visible clunk, if successful). This test creates apprehension in the patient, who notes the sensation that the elbow is about to dislocate. (Reproduced with permission from the Mayo Foundation, Rochester, MN.)

interpret with the arm in the overhead position. The arm then resembles a leg, and the elbow resembles a knee. To most surgeons, this is extremely helpful. The elbow is examined for valgus, varus, and posterolateral rotatory instability. Valgus stress-testing is performed with the forearm fully pronated so that posterolateral rotatory instability is not mistaken for valgus instability.[8] This happens because the ulna and the radius rotate as a unit away from the humerus in response to valgus stress when the lateral collateral ligament is disrupted. Forced pronation prevents posterolateral rotatory instability because the intact medial soft tissues are used as a hinge or fulcrum, just as the periosteum is used for this purpose during the reduction of a supracondylar fracture in a child. Varus stress-testing is easiest to perform with the shoulder fully internally rotated. Both valgus and varus stress-testing are performed with the elbow in full extension and then in about 30° of flexion. Flexion unlocks the olecranon from the olecranon fossa. Posterolateral rotatory instability is diagnosed with use of the lateral pivot-shift maneuver of the elbow. If there is severe soft-tissue disruption, this test can have a false-negative result. With severe soft-tissue disruption, the elbow can sometimes remain dislocated even when it is flexed past 90°. If suspected, this problem can be avoided by the examiner using his or her thumb to prevent the elbow from fully dislocating (or limiting the degree of subluxation during the pivot-shift test).

Lateral Pivot-Shift Maneuver

Currently, the most common method of performing this test is with the patient placed supine on the examining table with the affected extremity overhead[9] (Fig. 3). The elbow is supinated, and a mild to moderate forced valgus stress is applied while the elbow is flexed past approximately 40°. This maneuver results in apprehension or frank subluxation of the radius and the ulna in a rotatory fashion from the humerus. A visible, palpable clunk or an actual pivot shift may be elicited by this maneuver. If instability is not elicited, the test is still positive if there is apprehension, and the diagnosis can be made on this basis. The posterolateral rotatory drawer test involves placing the elbow in approximately 40° of flexion and applying an anterior-posterior force on the ulna and the radius to subluxate the forearm away from the humerus on the lateral side (pivoting on the intact medial ligaments).

Stress radiographs are made in the anteroposterior plane with application of valgus and varus stress and the arm overhead as described above. With the shoulder in 90° of abduction and full external rotation, stress radiographs are also made with the arm in supination and pronation to detect posterolateral rotatory instability and to determine if the medial side opens up with pronation (indicating disruption of the medial soft tissues).

Evaluation and Management of Acute Fracture-Dislocations

The evaluation of a patient who has sustained a fracture-dislocation is very structured, and it is also essential. Stress radiographs should be made, with use of an image intensifier, in the anteroposterior plane with valgus stress and then with varus stress. When valgus stress-testing is performed, the forearm must be held fully pronated with moderated force to prevent posterolateral rotatory subluxation and false-positive valgus instability. With the shoulder in 90° of abduction and full external rotation, lateral stress radiographs are also made with the forearm in supination and pronation to detect posterolateral rotatory instability and to determine if the medial side opens up with pronation (indicating disruption of the medial soft tissues).

The Terrible-Triad Injury

The elbow is one of the most stable articulations in the skeletal system, and when one or more parts of its articular supporting architecture is disrupted in the presence of a dislocation the risk of recurrent instability or arthrosis is substantial.[10-12] The fundamental goal in the management of fracture-dislocation of the elbow (a so-called complex dislocation) is the restoration of the osseous-articular restraints, thereby converting the injury to a so-called simple dislocation, which has been demonstrated in a number of studies to have a generally favorable long-term prognosis.[11,12] Most of the principles of managing complex instability of the elbow can be derived from an understanding of the pathomechanics and treatment of the terrible-triad injury. Hotchkiss[13] used the phrase "terrible triad" for the combination of an elbow dislocation and fractures of the radial head and coronoid process. It received this name because of the major disability that so often results from this injury.[13] The terrible triad often affects young active individuals, and the complications include persistent instability, nonunion, malunion, and osseous proximal radioulnar synostosis. In approaching the management of the terrible-triad injury, the individual injuries to the coronoid process, radial head, and collateral ligaments must be considered.

Fractures of the Coronoid Process

Regan and Morrey[14] classified fractures of the coronoid process into three types. Type I is a small fleck of bone, type II involves 50% of the height of the coronoid process or less, and type III involves more than 50% of the height of the coronoid process. Type I fractures have been incorrectly referred to as avulsion fractures, but Cage and associates[15] showed, in a cadaver study, that they are not, as nothing attaches to the tip of the coronoid process. They represent shear fractures, similar to a Bankart lesion of the shoulder, and they occur during subluxation or dislocation of the elbow.[8] Regan and Morrey[14] found that the prevalence of instability rises, and the prognosis deteriorates, according to the amount of the coronoid process that is fractured.

When the coronoid process is fractured, with or without concomitant fracture of the olecranon, restoration of the intrinsic stability of the elbow depends to a large degree on reestablishment of the anatomic dimensions of the trochlear notch. Fracture of the coronoid process at its base compromises stability in two ways. First, the anterior buttress, which serves to resist the normal posteriorly directed forces occurring with elbow flexion, and second, the anterior band of the medial collateral ligament, the insertion of which is attached to the coronoid fracture fragment, are rendered incompetent.[14-18]

Beredjiklian and associates, in a biomechanical study performed on cadaver, confirmed the role of the coronoid process as a primary stabilizer of the elbow and its critical role in the presence of a radial head fracture and ligament injury (P Beredjiklian, MD, et al, Minneapolis, MN, unpublished data, 1989). O'Driscoll and associates demonstrated, in a cadaveric model simulating the terrible-triad injury, that the coronoid process is a primary stabilizer of the elbow (S O'Driscoll, MD, et al, New Orleans, LA, unpublished data, 1998). Persistent instability was progressively more likely as the amount of coronoid resection increased, even with the radial head present. However, with even a small deficiency in the coronoid process, the radial head became a critically important secondary stabilizer.

The surgical exposures of the coronoid process depend on the associated lesions. A universal posterior skin incision, just lateral to the tip of the olecranon, permits deep access to both the medial and the lateral side of the elbow and provides the versatility needed to treat these injuries. In general, small (type I and many type II) fractures found in association with radial head fractures and dislocated elbows can be approached from the lateral side, as described in the literature.[19] An exception is a medial coronoid fragment (often part of a comminuted type II or type III coronoid fracture), which is more appropriately approached medially. The fractured radial head is retracted gently to permit access to the coronoid process. The medial approach is facilitated when the injury includes avulsion of the origin of the flexor-pronator muscle mass. Elevation of the ulnar origin of the flexor-pronator muscle group allows visualization of the coronoid process. When it is part of a complex proximal ulnar fracture, the coronoid process can occasionally be reduced, and the reduction can be held by exposure through the olecranon fracture itself.[20]

Internal fixation of smaller (type I or type II) fragments may present not only technical problems but also problems that may jeopardize the tenuous blood supply to the coronoid process. We prefer to use the technique in which two braided sutures are passed over the top of the small coronoid fragment, pulled out through drill-holes in the ulna, and tied over the bone[21] (Fig. 4). If the capsule is attached to the fragment, the sutures should be passed through the capsule as well. Reattachment of a fractured coronoid fragment provides important stability through the capsular attachments, just as a volar plate advancement arthroplasty does for an unstable fracture-dislocation of the proximal interphalangeal joint.

Larger (type III and some type II) fractures of the coronoid process require anatomic reduction and stable internal fixation. The best techniques are not yet known, as experience with treating these injuries is limited. However, it is likely that screw fixation and the use of a buttress plate are necessary for most such fractures. This is particularly true for medial coronoid fractures.

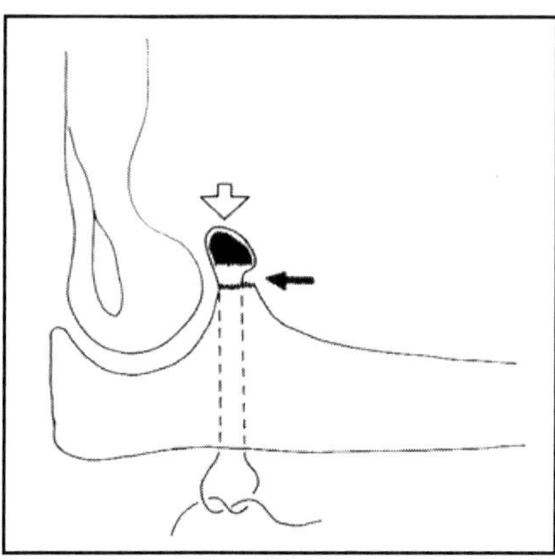

Fig. 4 Drawing showing internal fixation of smaller coronoid fragments (type I or II) with two braided sutures that are passed through the ulna and over the top of the small coronoid fragment and then tied over the bone.[24] If the capsule is attached to the fragment, the sutures should be passed through the capsule as well.

In some instances, the coronoid may not be amenable to fixation because of the size or comminution of the fracture or because of a delay between the injury and the treatment. When the coronoid fracture is associated with a complex fracture of the radial head, a portion of the radial head can be shaped and secured with one or two interfragmentary screws. Alternative sources of osteochondral bone include tricortical iliac crest bone graft, an allograft coronoid, and the proximal tip of the olecranon. If iliac crest bone graft is used, the capsule should be interposed between the graft and the trochlea to prevent direct contact and cartilage erosion.

Results and Complications

To our knowledge, the results of treatment of the terrible-triad injury have not been reported in a single series, but anecdotal experience justifies the name. In a series reviewed by Jupiter (unpublished data) of 56 patients who had a fracture-dislocation that was treated in Boston, 13 patients had a posterior dislocation of the elbow associated with a fracture of the radial head and coronoid process. Ten of the 13 elbows remained unstable following surgical treatment, with early arthrosis seen in all, and only 4 of the 13 patients had a satisfactory outcome. All but one had a type II coronoid fracture, and one had a type III fracture. It is of note that none of the type II lesions had stable internal fixation. It is also noteworthy that 90% of the patients who had removal of the fractured radial head had an unsatisfactory outcome, whereas only one third of the patients in whom the radial head was fixed had an unsatisfactory result.

These data support the concept that the terrible triad is a grave and complex injury and suggest that lesions of both the coronoid process and the radial head need to be stabilized or reconstructed whenever possible.

Fractures of the Radial Head

Fractures of the radial head are commonly associated with dislocation of the elbow and with isolated disruption of the medial collateral ligament, lateral collateral ligament, or interosseous membrane, or all three.[22-24] Fractures of the coronoid process, olecranon, and capitellum are also frequently associated with radial head fractures and may further impair elbow stability.[25,26] The presence of these concomitant injuries has important implications with regard to the management of a radial head fracture.

Anatomy and Biomechanics

The radial head has a concave dish that articulates with the capitellum. The posteromedial two thirds of the radial head articulates with the lesser sigmoid notch of the ulna, whereas the anterolateral one third of the radial head has no articulation. Therefore, internal fixation devices can be placed anterolaterally on the radial head without impingement against the ulna during rotation of the forearm.[27]

The radiocapitellar articulation accounts for as much as 60% of the load transfer across the elbow, and resisted isometric flexion can generate forces up to four times body weight.[28,29] Depressed fractures of the radial head decrease the surface area available for load transfer and decrease elbow stability by virtue of a loss of congruity of the articulating disk of the radial head with the capitellum. The radial head is an important valgus stabilizer of the elbow, particularly in the setting of an incompetent medial collateral ligament, which typically is disrupted in most fracture-dislocations.[2,4,22,24,25,30-36]

Classification

Mason[37] classified radial head fractures into three types. Type I indicates an undisplaced fracture; type II, a fracture with displaced wedge fragments; and type III, a comminuted fracture. Johnson[38] added a fourth type, a radial head fracture associated with an elbow dislocation. More recently, a management-based classification system was developed.[19] Type I indicates a fracture that is undisplaced or minimally displaced (less than 2 mm); type II, a fracture that is displaced but amenable to internal fixation; and type III, a fracture that is not amenable to internal fixation with use of current techniques. The latter classification is preferable because of its implications with regard to treatment.

Imaging

Anteroposterior, lateral, and oblique radiographs of the elbow usually provide sufficient information for the diagnosis and treatment of radial head fractures. Tomography or CT can be useful for evaluating selected fractures that are difficult to classify and can be helpful for preoperative planning. Posteroanterior radiographs of both wrists should be made for patients who have associated wrist pain and for those who have a comminuted fracture of the radial head because such patients have been found to have a higher prevalence of interosseous ligament injury.[22]

Treatment

A concomitant dislocation of the elbow should be reduced, and the radial head fracture should then be managed on its own merits. Decision making is influenced by patient-related factors (age, bone quality, and activity level) and fracture-related factors (fracture size, displacement, and location). For example, an older patient with osteoporosis and a comminuted radial head fracture is a poor candidate for internal fixation, with radial head arthroplasty being the preferred option in the setting of an associated elbow dislocation.

Undisplaced or minimally displaced radial head fractures (Hotchkiss type I) are occasionally seen with elbow dislocations, but displaced radial head fractures are more common when the elbow has been dislocated. As already mentioned, elbow dislocations with a radial head fracture also are typically associated with a coronoid fracture. When the elbow is dislocated and more than one third of the radial head is fractured and displaced greater than 2 mm (Hotchkiss type II), open reduction and internal fixation of the radial head fracture should be attempted when it is technically possible[19,39-41] (Fig. 5).

The management of displaced radial head fractures that are not amenable to internal fixation with use of current techniques (Hotchkiss type III) is controversial. Fragment excision, delayed excision of the radial head, and replacement of the radial head have all been considered. Acute excision of the radial head without replacement is contraindicated when there is concomitant disruption of the medial collateral ligament or the interosseous membrane.[24,31,32] Displaced fractures that block the rotation of the forearm and are too small, comminuted, or osteoporotic for stable internal fixation should be managed with fragment excision. The two prerequisites for fragment excision are evidence that the fragments to be excised do not articulate with the lesser sigmoid notch of the ulna and involvement of less than one third of the radial head. Delayed excision of the radial head can be used for an isolated, comminuted, displaced fracture that involves more than one third of the radial head and does not block forearm rotation, but it is not an option in a patient who has had a fracture-dislocation.[42-44] Arthroplasty of the radial head is indicated for displaced, comminuted radial head fractures when stable internal fixation is not possible and the fracture involves more than one third of the radial head.[45-52]

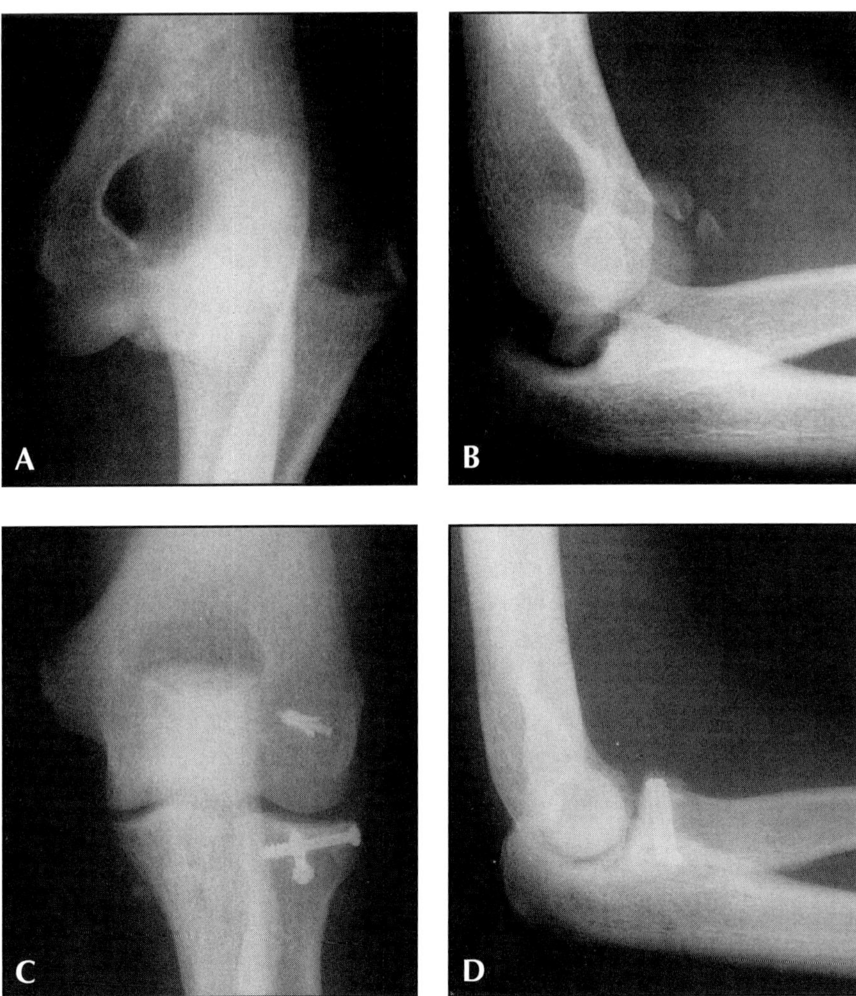

Fig. 5 Radiographs of the elbow of a 24-year-old man who fell off a mountain bike. **A** and **B,** Anteroposterior and lateral radiographs showing dislocation of the elbow with a type II radial head fracture, according to the classification system of Hotchkiss,[13] and a type II coronoid fracture, according to the system of Regan and Morrey.[14] **C** and **D,** Anteroposterior and lateral radiographs demonstrating an anatomic reduction after open reduction and internal fixation of the radial head and repair of the coronoid process with sutures. Early postoperative elbow motion was permitted, and a good result was achieved.

Surgical Techniques

The patient is placed in the supine position on the operating table with a tourniquet in place. Prophylactic antibiotic therapy is administered, and general or regional anesthesia is initiated. As in the case of a coronoid fracture, a posterior elbow incision is used. This approach decreases the risk of a cutaneous nerve injury compared with that associated with a separate medial incision.[53,54] Disruption of the lateral collateral ligament complex and the common extensor muscles from the lateral epicondyle is commonly noted in patients with an elbow dislocation. This approach also simplifies the surgical exposure of the radial head.[2] The interval between the anconeus and the extensor carpi ulnaris (the Kocher interval) is identified and developed. The lateral collateral ligament is incised at the midportion of the radial head, with the surgeon staying anterior to the lateral ulnar collateral ligament.[44,55] The annular ligament often must be divided to improve exposure. **(CD-11.1)**

Internal fixation is performed with use of 1.5-, 2.0-, or 2.7-mm screws and plates or 3.0-mm cannulated screws, depending on the size of the fragment. If plate fixation is used, the plate should be placed on the nonarticular portion of the radial head, which is the lateral part of the radial head when the arm is in neutral rotation.[56] Screws should be countersunk to avoid impingement with the lesser sigmoid notch. Threaded Kirschner wires may be useful for small fragments not amenable to screw fixation. Smooth Kirschner wires should be avoided because of their tendency to migrate during the postoperative period.

A radial head with a fracture that is not amenable to fixation should be replaced with a metallic radial head when there is a medial collateral or interosseous ligament injury.[24,31,32,45] Silicone implants have been used in the past; however, they have a high rate of failure due to fracture and fragmentation.[24,31,32,45,52] The fragmentation of silicone often produces synovitis. Clinical series of patients managed with metallic implants have shown good results.[47,48] Most metallic radial head implants have a monoblock design that makes implantation difficult because a wide surgical exposure is necessary. Recently, modular metallic radial head prostheses have become available. These prostheses have wider sizing options, and they may be easier to implant. A word of caution: the coronoid fragment should not be removed when the radial head is excised.

Following fragment excision, open reduction and internal fixation, or radial head replacement, the lateral collateral ligament complex and the common extensor muscle origins should be carefully repaired back to the lateral epicondyle with use of heavy sutures through drill-holes or suture anchors.[55] The fascial interval between the anconeus and the extensor carpi radialis also should be closed to augment lateral stability of the elbow.[57] The elbow should be carefully evaluated for stability, and concomitant injuries (for example, those involving the medial collateral ligament or the coronoid process) should be repaired when appropriate.

Postoperative Management

Indomethacin (75 mm daily) has been recommended for patients with complex elbow dislocations, to control postoperative pain and to potentially reduce the prevalence of heterotopic ossification.[56,58,59] This medication should be avoided by patients with a history of peptic ulcer disease or a known allergy. An early range of motion within a safe arc should be initiated, depending on associated fractures and ligamentous injuries. An extension-splinting program[60] is initiated as soon as stability improves, and the splint is worn at night for 12 weeks.

Complications

Osteonecrosis might be expected following open reduction and internal fixation of most radial head fractures, as the fragments typically have a precarious blood supply or no blood supply. Fortunately, the fragments usually heal and late collapse is uncommon. Nonunion is usually associated with osteonecrosis and seems to be more common in patients with a fracture involving the radial neck. Malunion is usually a consequence of inadequate fracture fixation or collapse due to osteonecrosis. Osteoarthritis is seen as a consequence of articular cartilage injury from the initial dislocation, late instability, or articular incongruity. Stiffness is a common sequela of a radial head fracture and may be due to capsular contracture or heterotopic ossification. Late axial or valgus instability is uncommon unless the radial head has been excised.

Hinged External Fixation for Unstable Elbows

It is not possible (or wise) to restore stability surgically after all dislocations or fracture-dislocations. In other cases, the constraints may have been repaired, but not securely, and need protection.

Indications

As with most surgical devices and methods, the two most important factors of success are how and when to apply them. This is especially true of hinged fixators about the elbow because of the difficulty and the time that application of the device adds to the procedure and to postoperative care. However, failure to use the device when indicated may result in a stiff and dislocated elbow, the worst of all worlds for a patient with a traumatized elbow.

The three primary indications are: (1) persistent instability in association with an acute fracture-dislocation despite attempted ligament repair and fracture fixation or radial head replacement, or both; (2) gross acute instability in a patient who is not a candidate for surgery; and (3) delayed treatment (approximately 4 weeks or more after the time of injury) of a dislocated and stiff elbow. A relative indication is the need to protect the stability and the fracture reduction during rehabilitation following surgical treatment of an unstable elbow.

The severity of a dislocation is seldom assessed, but it should be evaluated when hinged fixation is considered for the treatment of instability. Gross instability is not a condition that is easily recognized, but there are a few distinguishing features. In most cases, the patient has one or more of the following features: (1) a high-energy injury—that is, an injury sustained in a fall from a considerable height or in a motor-vehicle accident; (2) previous failed attempts at reduction or surgical repair of the dislocation; (3) multidirectional instability on examination after attempted or achieved reduction; and (4) a concomitant fracture of the radial head or the coronoid process, or both (the terrible triad of the elbow). None of these features alone creates a grossly unstable elbow, but if any one is present the others should be looked for.

Hinged fixation is used most commonly as a secondary device to protect surgically repaired or healing structures while permitting and assisting proper kinematic motion. Even if they are not repaired, the medial ligaments usually heal with mechanical integrity if they are protected. Conversely, the lateral ligaments should be repaired or reconstructed, as detailed in other sections.

There are a few situations in which application of the devices alone may be both adequate and optimal. In patients who have polytrauma, time may not permit full anatomic restoration of all structures. In this setting, protecting the elbow in a reduced position before definitive care will assist in the subsequent treatment.

Surgical Technique

At the present time, three very different hinged external fixators for the elbow are commercially available. They each have their own advantages and disadvantages. With two of the devices, the use of a temporary axis pin is crucial to replicate the kinematic axis of the elbow. In earlier reports and designs, the axis pin was left in place in the distal part of the humerus for the duration of use.[59] However, because pin-tract infection at the site of the axis pin led to joint infections, a temporary axis pin is now used with all of the devices. The long-term use of a pin through the axis of rotation at the distal aspect of the humerus is no longer recommended.

In most cases, repair of the fractures and ligaments obviates the need for a fixator. To determine if a fixator is needed, the stability of the joint should be gently tested before application of the fixator, while the ligament sutures are held under tension. If the elbow is stable and the fractures require minimal protection, no fixator is needed.

When the hinged fixator is applied after fixation of the fractures, care must be taken not to disrupt the ligament repair and the delicate fracture fixation. Repair of the coronoid process, so crucial to long-term success yet often quite vulnerable to loading during application of the hinge, must be protected during placement of the device. It is often better to position the sutures for ligament repair without securing them with knots, in anticipation of fixator placement. Because of unfamiliarity with the device or the complexity of fixator application, the repaired ligaments and fractures could be subjected to failure loads, defeating the purpose of the repair efforts. If the sutures for ligament repairs are tied in place after the fixator is applied, tension in the repairs is achieved with confidence that there is no eccentric displacement of the repair.

Technical Tips

The proper technical application of these devices cannot be overemphasized. The most crucial and usually the first step of hinged fixator application is replication of the recognized axis of rotation. If the axis is not replicated or if pin placement in the humerus or ulna impedes motion, the use of the device is entirely compromised and provides little, if any, value. Because the axis of elbow motion is within the distal aspect of the humerus, the frame is attached to the humerus first. A temporary joint-axis pin is placed, and the frame is built from this temporary axis pin. Once the fixator is properly attached to the humerus, the ulna may be reduced and attached to the fixator.

In most cases in which surgery is performed on a grossly unstable elbow, both the medial and the lateral aspect of the distal part of the humerus are exposed and visible. This permits visualization of the instant center of rotation on both sides. The temporary axis pin should penetrate both central points of rotation, ensuring proper function of the hinge. If the distal part of the humerus is not directly visible, the pin and axis must be visualized with fluoroscopic imaging. There are many methods for placement of the axis pin across the distal aspect of the humerus, and these are usually detailed in the instructional materials provided for each particular device. Anterior cruciate ligament drill guides or variations of them may help.

On the medial side, injury to the ulnar nerve is avoided by exposing the nerve anchor or transposing it, or both. The center of rotation from the medial view is slightly distal and anterior to the medial epicondyle. From the lateral view, the center of rotation is in the center of the capitellum. If there is concern about the location on visual inspection, fluoroscopic images should be made. Both the anteroposterior and lateral views are needed to properly ascertain the pin location. As one gains experience, the localization and placement becomes less time-consuming and challenging.

After the axis pin is properly placed in the distal part of the humerus, pin fixation of the frame to the humerus must be done. Adjustment of pin fixation may be necessary if plates on the distal part of the humerus or the proximal part of the ulna interfere with the normal pin position.

Secure fixation of the frame to the distal part of the humerus may require more than just two pins (one medial and one lateral) in the supracondylar region of the humerus. In such cases, an extension can be added onto the frame, with half-pins placed in the humerus more proximally. When pins are placed more proximally in the humerus, the radial nerve should be protected from injury. The half-pins should also be placed to avoid impaling muscle or tendon, because this will impede movement. Placement of pins in the ulna is usually simpler.

Half-pins attached to the fixator should be placed so that there is no skin under tension. The skin tension against the pins should be inspected in all positions of flexion and extension. Skin under tension should be released. Redness, pain, and drainage are avoided by meticulous pin-site care. If skin tension is noted later, it should be released. Antibiotics may be needed if there is erythema and increased pain.

Loss of reduction and mechanical failure can occur. Frequent clinical examination and radiographs to confirm maintenance of the reduction are mandatory. The clamps, nuts, bolts, and frames should be inspected frequently for any loosening during the first few weeks. As rehabilitation activity becomes more vigorous, there is also more stress on the components, which can lead to loosening of the pins in the bone or component failure, or

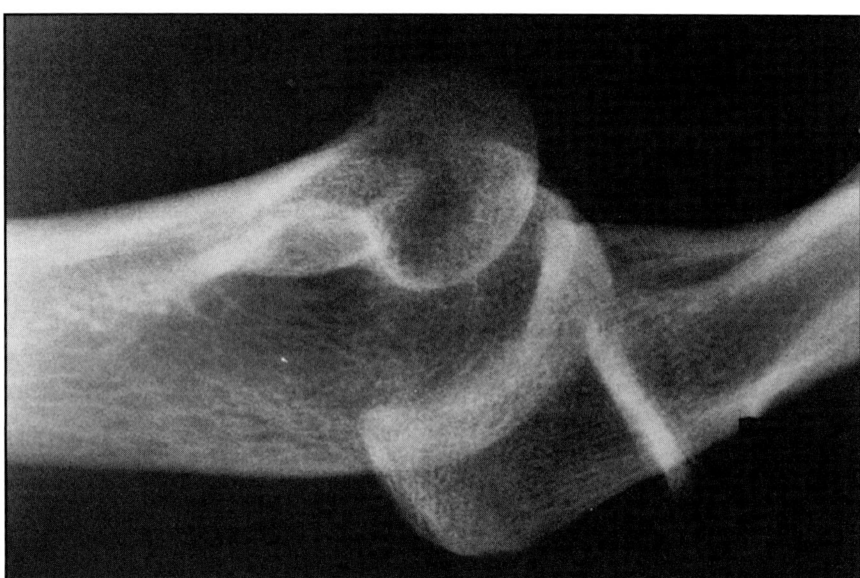

Fig. 6 Lateral radiograph of an elbow with recurrent posterolateral rotatory instability, showing the radial head to be aligned posterior to the capitellum. The ulnohumeral relationship does not appear to be grossly abnormal but, in fact, reveals subtle subluxation.

both. The components should be routinely inspected for signs of fatigue.

Recurrent Elbow Instability

Lateral collateral ligament insufficiency is most commonly seen after elbow dislocation, particularly in young patients. It is the essential lesion leading to elbow instability.[35] While most studies have indicated that both the medial and the lateral collateral ligament complex are acutely disrupted with an elbow dislocation, the residual insufficiency most commonly involves the lateral collateral ligament complex for reasons that have not yet been elucidated. This insufficiency gives rise to recurrent posterolateral rotatory instability.[4]

History

In the vast majority of patients, dislocation with or without fracture accounts for the injury.[61] Sometimes the problem is quite obvious, as the patient is able to demonstrate the instability; however, it may be more subtle. Sometimes the patient has noticed only pain and discomfort and is not aware of instability. Additional symptoms include painful catching, slippage, or clicking with flexion and extension. A feeling of slippage of the joint in and out of place may be reported by the patient. The elbow position most typically associated with symptoms is approximately 40° of flexion with the forearm in supination. The subluxation reduces in pronation. The patient may have noted that specific activity such as pushing on the armrests when rising from a chair reproduces the symptoms of instability.

The physical examination includes the lateral pivot-shift maneuver, the posterolateral rotatory drawer test, and the apprehension test. In some instances, varus stress-testing may suggest a lateral collateral ligament insufficiency. Rising from a chair while pushing on the armrests has been suggested by Morrey and Regan[61] to be particularly helpful, either to demonstrate the instability or as an apprehension-eliciting maneuver.

Radiographs

Classically, the elbow appears normal on anteroposterior radiographs or there is slight widening of the radiohumeral joint. On lateral radiographs, the radial head may appear to be situated post-erior to the capitellum (Fig. 6). Special studies, MRI, and CT have not been necessary or useful in our experience.

Arthroscopy

In some instances, when the presentation does not suggest the injury or the findings on the physical examination are not convincing, or when there is a possiblity of an intra-articular lesion, arthroscopic examination of the elbow may be helpful. Arthroscopy will reveal the laxity of the radiohumeral joint and thus confirm the lesion.

Management

In our experience, the ligament does not become stable over time, except possibly when a patient is seen in the very early stages. By definition, this is a recurrent problem, and it needs a surgical reconstruction or the patient must live with the problem. The latter is rarely acceptable to the patient, as symptoms interfere with daily activity.

Surgical Technique

The patient is placed supine on the operating table, and the arm is brought across the chest. A 10-cm incision is made at the Kocher interval, roughly equidistant proximal and distal to the epicondyle. The dissection proceeds through the Kocher interval, with separation of the anconeus from the extensor carpi ulnaris and identification of the lateral collateral ligament complex, the supracondylar ridge, and the crest of the supinator. The anconeus is further reflected from the margin of the supinator crest and from the lateral face of the proximal part of the ulna. The tubercle of the supinator ridge is palpated. The lateral epicondyle is exposed along with 2 cm of the proximal supracondylar ridge anteriorly and posteriorly. **(CD-11.2)**

The insertion site for the tendon graft is then prepared by creating two

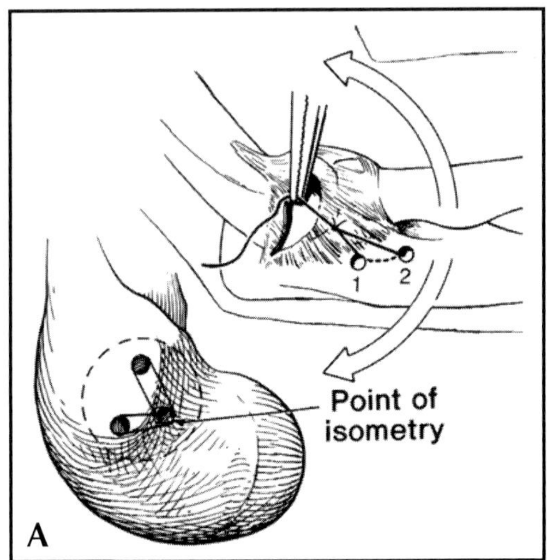

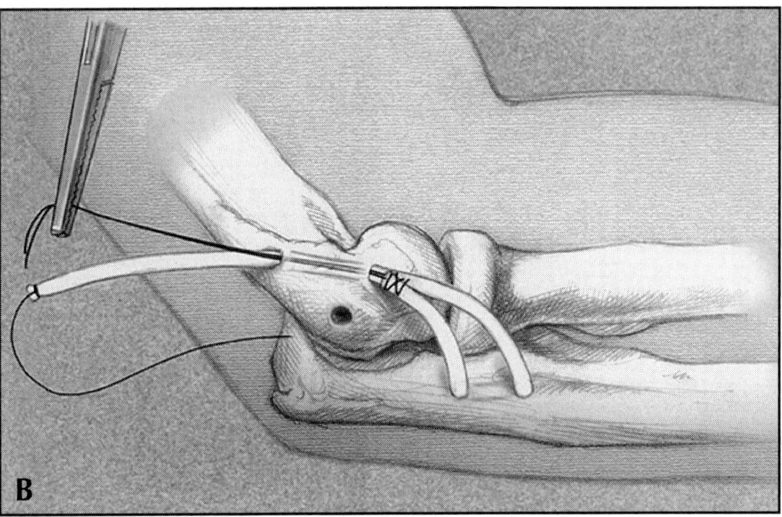

Fig. 7 A, Drawing showing a suture being passed through the osseous tunnels in the ulna distal to the tubercle of the supinator crest. The isometric point is determined by the point at which there is no laxity or increased tension on the suture through the arc of elbow flexion. **B,** Drawing showing a tendon (palmaris longus) graft placed through holes in the ulna and brought into the isometric origin near the lateral epicondyle, out through an exit tunnel proximally, and back into the bone for fixation. (Reproduced with permission from the Mayo Foundation, Rochester, MN.)

drill-holes in the ulna: one near the tubercle on the supinator crest (which is felt by stressing the elbow in varus or supination) and the other, 1.25 cm proximally at the base of the annular ligament (Fig. 7, *A*). A suture is passed through these two holes and tied to itself. It is then pulled toward the lateral epicondyle and grasped with a hemostat at the estimated isometric center of the rotation of the elbow. The isometric ligament origin is then determined by flexion and extension of the elbow to see if the suture moves. No movement occurs when the suture and hemostat are on the isometric point. The isometric point is more anterior than is usually thought to be the case. It is important to remember that instability occurs in extension so the graft must be taut in extension. A Y-shaped tunnel is placed in the lateral epicondyle, with the isometric spot widened in order to accept a three-ply graft. Currently, one of us (BFM) prefers to use the plantaris tendon if a substantial palmaris longus is not present. A 16-cm graft allows a reliable three-ply passage across the joint (Fig. 7, *B*). There are a number of options for fixing the graft into the humerus. One or both limbs of the graft pass into the isometric origin. We prefer to place a stitch in the first two limbs of the graft after the graft is passed through the tunnel in the ulna. Both this stitch (the yoke stitch) and the graft are then passed through one of the tunnels in the humerus. The free end of the graft just reaches the tunnel, ensuring a two-ply passage as the free end of the tendon graft is brought through the holes in the epicondylar region and back down distally across the joint. This end is usually passed back into the ulnar tunnel if sufficient length is present. If not, it is sutured to itself distally near the ulnar tunnel. Once this has been done, the forearm is placed in 40° of flexion and full pronation while axial tension is placed on the yoke stitch, which is then tied. This applies additional tension to the reconstruction.

Rehabilitation

The elbow is placed in 70° to 80° of flexion with the forearm in full pronation. The arm is held in this position for 10 to 14 days, and then the patient is permitted protected motion in a hinged brace for 2 to 6 weeks, with flexion allowed as tolerated. After 6 weeks, the patient may remove the hinged splint for sedentary activities, but otherwise the splint is worn for most activities. At the end of an additional 6 weeks, the use of the splint is discontinued, but conscious protection is recommended for a total of 12 weeks after surgery. Supination is gradually allowed and encouraged, but excessive force is avoided. After 12 weeks, activity is gradually resumed, with 100% activity allowed at 6 months.

Results

Although we are currently reassessing our clinical experience, to date it has been suggested that, if there is no degenerative arthritis and if the radial head is intact, approximately 90% of patients have a satisfactory outcome with no subsequent recurrent subluxation.[62-64] If the radial head is excised or if there is degenerative arthritis of the ulnohumeral joint, the satisfactory result decreases to between 67% and 75%. Delayed laxity, redislocation,

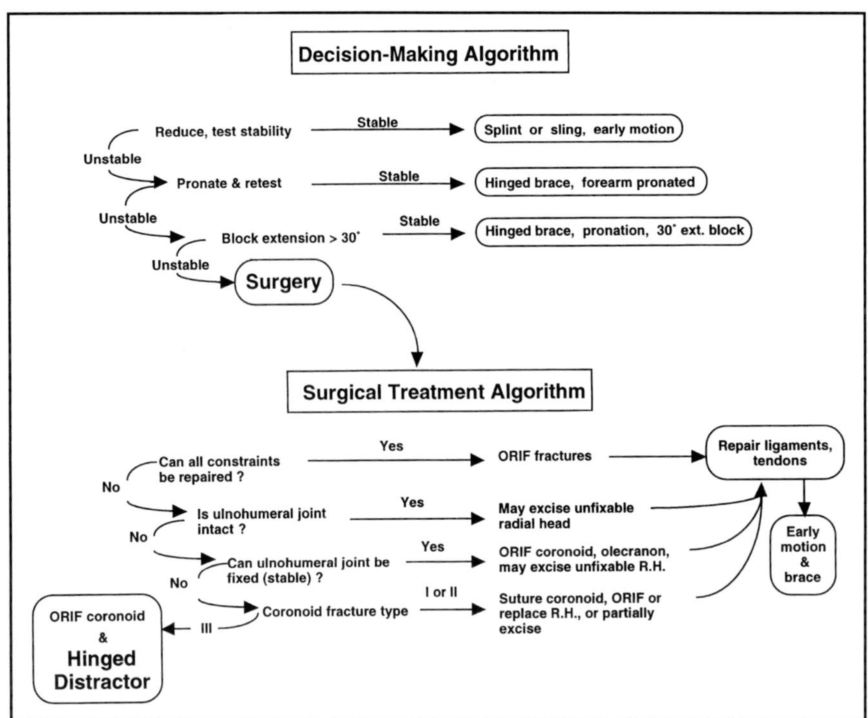

Fig. 8 Chart showing the decision-making algorithm for acute dislocations and fracture-dislocations. The term stable implies functional stability, meaning that the elbow does not apparently subluxate in the functional arc of motion and appears reduced on plain radiographs. ORIF = open reduction and internal fixation; RH = radial head. (Reproduced with permission from the Mayo Foundation, Rochester, MN.)

and reinjury have been observed, usually in association with substantial stress. We accept a mild (10°) flexion contracture, because the most vulnerable position of instability is in full extension.

Summary of Treatment Principles

Reduction of Acute Dislocations and Management After Reduction

The initial treatment of an elbow dislocation without associated fractures is a closed reduction. The reduction should be done with the forearm in supination to clear the coronoid process under the trochlea, thereby minimizing additional trauma to the medial soft tissues that have not yet been disrupted. Essentially, the deformity is recreated in order to make the reduction possible and easy. A simple principle to follow in managing a patient after reduction is to place the elbow in a splint for a brief period (3 to 5 days) and then to start allowing movement unless the elbow tends to subluxate or dislocate. One must be vigilant. Subluxation or dislocation must be detected by careful examination throughout the comfortable range of motion and by radiographic examination, with anteroposterior and lateral radiographs made initially after the reduction and every five to seven days for the first three weeks. If subluxation or dislocation is detected clinically or radiographically at any time, a change of treatment is required.

The so-called stage or degree of instability dictates the treatment. If the elbow feels stable in all positions of forearm rotation, a hinged brace is not necessary. Such stability is usual. When the elbow is stable to valgus stress only with the forearm in pronation (that is, a stage 3A dislocation), the injury is treated immediately in a cast-brace that allows unlimited flexion and extension and holds the forearm in full pronation. A summary of these treatment principles is depicted in Figure 8.

Management of Acute Fracture-Dislocations

The presence of fractures usually changes the management, and almost always these fractures should be treated surgically. In general, the approach to the unstable elbow is to fix the bones internally and then repair the ligaments (particularly on the lateral side) so that early motion can be commenced.

The coronoid process is an important part of the force-bearing surface of the elbow and is important for stability. Type I and type II fractures (those involving 50% of the height of the coronoid process or less) should be fixed if the joint is subluxated or dislocated. Type III fractures (those involving more than 50% of the coronoid process) cause instability and should be fixed. Type III fracture-dislocations have traditionally been associated with a poor prognosis.

Fractures of the radial head associated with an elbow dislocation or subluxation are best managed by internal fixation when technically possible. When the radial head is comminuted and has to be excised, prosthetic replacement is indicated if the elbow is unstable and cannot be rendered stable by ligament reconstruction alone.

Repair of an Acute Ligament Injury

Repair of an acute ligament injury is indicated in all fracture-dislocations requiring internal fixation of the radial head or the coronoid process, or both, and following reduction of a dislocation if gross instability does not allow early protected motion in a cast-brace without subluxation. In such cases, the ligament or ligaments may have been avulsed and can be repaired directly to bone with heavy sutures. In some cases, passing a heavy absorbable suture through the same course as that for a late ligament reconstruction and fixing it to the normal ligament attachments on the epicondyle and the ulna augments the repair.

References

1. Josefsson PO, Gentz CF, Johnell O, Wendeberg B: Surgical versus non-surgical treatment of ligamentous injuries following dislocations of the elbow joint. *Clin Orthop* 1987;214:165-169.
2. Josefsson PO, Gentz CF, Johnell O, Wendeberg B: Surgical versus non-surgical treatment of ligamentous injuries following dislocation of the elbow joint: A prospective randomized study. *J Bone Joint Surg Am* 1987;69:605-608.
3. Josefsson PO, Johnell O, Wendeberg B: Ligamentous injuries in dislocations of the elbow joint. *Clin Orthop* 1987;221:221-225.
4. O'Driscoll SW, Morrey BF, Korinek S, An KN: Elbow subluxation and dislocation: A spectrum of instability. *Clin Orthop* 1992;280:186-197.
5. Osborne G, Cotterill P: Recurrent dislocation of the elbow. *J Bone Joint Surg Br* 1966;48: 340-346.
6. Roberts PH: Dislocation of the elbow. *Br J Surg* 1969;56:806-815.
7. O'Driscoll SW: Classification and spectrum of elbow instability: Recurrent instability, in Morrey BF (ed): *The Elbow and Its Disorders*, ed 2. Philadelphia, PA, WB Saunders, 1993, pp 453-463.
8. O'Driscoll SW: Elbow instability. *Hand Clin* 1994;10;405-415.
9. O'Driscoll SW, Bell DF, Morrey BF: Posterolateral rotatory instability of the elbow. *J Bone Joint Surg Am* 1991;73:440-446.
10. Broberg MA, Morrey BF: Results of treatment of fracture-dislocations of the elbow. *Clin Orthop* 1987;216:109-119.
11. Josefsson PO, Gentz CF, Johnell O, Wendeberg B: Dislocations of the elbow and intraarticular fractures. *Clin Orthop* 1989;246;126-130.
12. Ring D, Jupiter JB: Fracture-dislocation of the elbow. *J Bone Joint Surg Am* 1998;80:566-580.
13. Hotchkiss RN: Fractures and dislocations of the elbow, in Rockwood CA Jr, Green DP, Bucholz RW, Heckman JD (eds): *Fractures in Adults*, ed 4. Philadelphia, PA, Lippincott-Raven, 1996, pp 929-1024.
14. Regan W, Morrey BF: Fractures of the coronoid process of the ulna. *J Bone Joint Surg Am* 1989;71:1348-1354.
15. Cage DJ, Abrams RA, Callahan JJ, Botte MJ: Soft tissue attachments of the ulnar coronoid process: An anatomic study with radiographic correlation. *Clin Orthop* 1995;320:154-158.
16. An KN, Hui FC, Morrey BF, Linscheid RL, Chao EY: Muscles across the elbow joint: A biomechanical analysis. *J Biomech* 1981;14: 659-669.
17. Meeder PJ, Holz U: Replacement-plasty of the coronoid process in unstable elbow joint dislocations with avulsion fracture of the coronoid process and radius head crush fracture. *Aktuelle Traumat* 1985;15:89-90.
18. Stankovi P, Zuhlke V, Persitzky V: Isolated fractures of the coronoid processus of the ulna. *Unfallheilkunde* 1976;79:395-398.
19. Hotchkiss RN: Displaced fractures of the radial head: Internal fixation or excision? *J Am Acad Orthop Surgeons* 1997;5:1-10.
20. McWhorter GL: Fracture of both the coronoid and the olecranon processes of the ulna: Indications for operation and treatment. *J Bone Joint Surg* 1972:767-777.
21. O'Driscoll SW: Olecranon and coronoid fractures, in Norris TR (ed): *Orthopaedic Knowledge Update: Shoulder and Elbow*. Rosemont, IL, American Academy of Orthopaedic Surgeons, 1997, 405-413.
22. Davidson PA, Moseley JB Jr, Tullos HS: Radial head fracture: A potentially complex injury. *Clin Orthop* 1993;297:224-230.
23. Morrey BF (ed): *The Elbow and Its Disorders*, ed 2. Philadelphia, PA, WB Saunders, 1993.
24. Sellman DC, Seitz WH Jr, Postak PD, Greenwald AS: Reconstructive strategies for radioulnar dissociation: A biomechanical study. *J Orthop Trauma* 1995;9:516-522.
25. King GJW, Morrey BF, An KN: Stabilizers of the elbow. *J Shoulder Elbow Surg* 1993;2: 165-174.
26. Regan W, Morrey BF: Classification and treatment of coronoid process fractures. *Orthopedics* 1992;15:845-848.
27. Smith GR, Hotchkiss RN: Radial head and neck fractures: Anatomic guidelines for proper placement of internal fixation. *J Shoulder Elbow Surg* 1996;5:113-117.
28. Amis AA, Dowson D, Wright V: Elbow joint force predictions for some strenuous isometric actions. *J Biomech* 1980;13:765-775.
29. Halls AA, Travill A: Transmission of pressures across the elbow joint. *Anat Rec* 1964;150: 243-247.
30. Frankle MA, Koval KJ, Sanders RW, Zuckerman JD: Radial head fractures associated with elbow dislocations treated by immediate stabilization and early motion. *J Shoulder Elbow Surg* 1999;8:355-360.
31. Hotchkiss RN, Weiland AJ: Valgus stability of the elbow. *J Orthop Res* 1987;5:372-377.

32. King GJ, Zarzour ZD, Rath DA, Dunning CE, Patterson SD, Johnson JA: Metallic radial head arthroplasty improves valgus stability of the elbow. *Clin Orthop* 1999:368;114-125.

33. Mehlhoff TL, Noble PC, Bennett JB, Tullos HS: Simple dislocation of the elbow in the adult: Results after closed treatment. *J Bone Joint Surg Am* 1988;70:244-249.

34. Morrey BF, Chao EY, Hui FC: Biomechanical study of the elbow following excision of the radial head. *J Bone Joint Surg Am* 1979;61:63-68.

35. Morrey BF, Tanaka S, An K-N: Valgus stability of the elbow: A definition of primary and secondary constraints. *Clin Orthop* 1991;265: 187-195.

36. Pribyl CR, Kester MA, Cook SD, Edmunds JO, Brunet ME: The effect of the radial head and prosthetic radial head replacement on resisting valgus stress at the elbow. *Orthopedics* 1986;9:723-726.

37. Mason ML: Some observations on fractures of the head of the radius with a review of one hundred cases. *Br J Surg* 1954;42:123-132.

38. Johnson G: A follow-up of one hundred cases of fracture of the head of the radius with a review of the literature. *Ulster Med J* 1952;31:51-56.

39. Esser RD, Davis S, Taavao T: Fractures of the radial head treated by internal fixation: Late results in 26 cases. *J Orthop Trauma* 1995;9: 318-323.

40. Geel CW, Palmer AK, Ruedi T, Leutenegger AF: Internal fixation of proximal radial head fractures. *J Orthop Trauma* 1990;4:270-274.

41. King GJ, Evans DC, Kellam JF: Open reduction and internal fixation of radial head fractures. *J Orthop Trauma* 1991;5:21-28.

42. Goldberg I, Peylan J, Yosipovitch Z: Late results of excision of the radial head for an isolated closed fracture. *J Bone Joint Surg Am* 1986;68:675-679.

43. Janssen RP, Vegter J: Resection of the radial head after Mason type-III fractures of the elbow: Follow-up at 16 to 30 years. *J Bone Joint Surg Br* 1998;80:231-233.

44. Miki D, Vukadinovi SM: Late results in fractures of the radial head treated by excision. *Clin Orthop* 1983;181:220-228.

45. Carn RM, Medige J, Curtain D, Koenig A: Silicone rubber replacement of the severely fractured radial head. *Clin Orthop* 1986;209:259-269.

46. Gupta GG, Lucas G, Hahn DL: Biomechanical and computer analysis of radial head prostheses. *J Shoulder Elbow Surg* 1997;6:37-48.

47. Harrington IJ, Tountas AA: Replacement of the radial head in the treatment of unstable elbow fractures. *Injury* 1981;12:405-412.

48. Knight DJ, Rymaszewski LA, Amis AA, Miller JH: Primary replacement of the fractured radial head with a metal prosthesis. *J Bone Joint Surg Br* 1993;75:572-576.

49. Morrey BF, Askew L, Chao EY: Silastic prosthetic replacement for the radial head. *J Bone Joint Surg Am* 1981;63:454-458.

50. Stoffelen DV, Holdsworth BJ: Excision or Silastic replacement for comminuted radial head fractures: A long-term follow-up. *Acta Orthop Belg* 1994;60:402-407.

51. Swanson AB, Jaeger SH, La Rochelle D: Comminuted fractures of the radial head: The role of silicone-implant replacement arthroplasty. *J Bone Joint Surg Am* 1981;63:1039-1049.

52. Vanderwilde RS, Morrey BF, Melberg MW, Vinh TN: Inflammatory arthritis after failure of silicone rubber replacement of the radial head. *J Bone Joint Surg Br* 1994;76:78-81.

53. Dowdy PA, Bain GI, King GJW, Patterson SD: The midline posterior elbow incision: An anatomical appraisal. *J Bone Joint Surg Br* 1995;77:696-699.

54. Patterson SD, King GJ, Bain GI: Abstract: A posterior global approach to the elbow. *J Bone Joint Surg Br* 1995;77(suppl 3):316.

55. Morrey BF, An K-N: Articular and ligamentous contributions to the stability of the elbow joint. *Am J Sports Med* 1983;11:315-319.

56. Segstro R, Morley-Forster PK, Lu G: Indomethacin as a postoperative analgesic for total hip arthroplasty. *Can J Anaesth* 1991;38: 578-581.

57. Cohen MS, Hastings H II: Rotatory instability of the elbow: The anatomy and role of the lateral stabilizers. *J Bone Joint Surg Am* 1997;79: 225-233.

58. Kjaersgaard-Andersen P, Ritter MA: Prevention of formation of heterotopic bone after total hip arthroplasty. *J Bone Joint Surg Am* 1991;73:942-947.

59. Knelles D, Barthel T, Karrer A, Kraus U, Eulert J, Kolbl O: Prevention of heterotopic ossification after total hip replacement: A prospective, randomised study using acetylsalicylic acid, indomethacin and fractional or single-dose irradiation. *J Bone Joint Surg Br* 1997;79:596-602.

60. Morrey B, Regan W: Post-traumatic stiffness: Distraction arthroplasty, in Morrey BF (ed): *The Elbow and Its Disorders*, ed 2. Philadelphia, WB Saunders, 1993, pp 472-491.

61. Morrey B, Regan W: Physical examination of the elbow, in Morrey B (ed): *The Elbow and Its Disorders*, ed 3. New York, NY, WB Saunders, 2000.

62. Nestor BJ, O'Driscoll SW, Morrey BF: Ligamentous reconstruction for posterolateral rotatory instability of the elbow. *J Bone Joint Surg Am* 1992;74:1235-1241.

63. Hamilton CD, Glousman RE, Jobe FW, Brault J, Pink M, Perry J: Dynamic stability of the elbow: Electromyographic analysis of the flexor pronator group and the extensor group in pitchers with valgus instability. *J Shoulder Elbow Surg* 1996;5:347-354.

64. Linscheid RL, O'Driscoll SW: Elbow dislocations, in Morrey BF (ed): *The Elbow and Its Disorders*, ed 2. Philadelphia, PA, WB Saunders Company, 1993, pp 441-452.

References to Video

Morrey BF: Distal humerus fractures: Surgical exposure. *Elbow Cadaveric Surgical Demonstration.* Rosemont, IL, American Academy of Orthopaedic Surgeons, Summer Institute, 1999.

Morrey BF: Lateral instability. *Elbow Cadaveric Surgical Demonstration.* Rosemont, IL, American Academy of Orthopaedic Surgeons, Summer Institute, 1999.

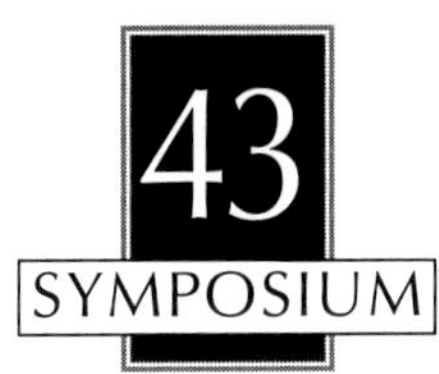

Difficult Elbow Fractures: Pearls and Pitfalls

Shawn W. O'Driscoll, PhD, MD
Jesse B. Jupiter, MD
Mark S. Cohen, MD
David Ring, MD
Michael D. McKee, MD, FRCSC

Abstract

Complex elbow fractures are exceedingly challenging to treat. Treatment of severe distal humeral fractures fails because of either displacement or nonunion at the supracondylar level or stiffness resulting from prolonged immobilization. Coronal shear fractures of the capitellum and trochlea are difficult to repair and may require extensile exposure. Olecranon fracture-dislocations are complex fractures of the olecranon associated with subluxation or dislocation of the radial head and/or the coronoid process. The radioulnar relationship usually is preserved in anterior but disrupted in posterior fracture-dislocations. A skeletal distractor can be useful in facilitating reduction. Coronoid fractures can be classified according to whether the fracture involves the tip, the anteromedial facet, or the base (body) of the coronoid. Anteromedial coronoid fractures are actually varus posteromedial rotatory fracture subluxations and are often serious injuries. These patterns of injury predict associated injuries and instability as well as surgical approach and treatment. The radial head is the bone most commonly fractured in the adult elbow. If the coronoid is fractured, the radial head becomes a critical factor in elbow stability. Its role becomes increasingly important as other soft-tissue and bony constraints are compromised. Articular injury to the radial head is commonly more severe than noted on plain radiographs. Fracture fragments are often anterior. Implants applied to the surface of the radial head must be placed in a safe zone.

Complications such as stiffness, malunion, nonunion, instability, posttraumatic osteoarthritis, and ulnar neuropathy are common following complex elbow fractures. Restoration of stability takes priority over motion because mobility usually can be improved with capsular excision, but instability may damage the articular surface irreversibly.

One or more of the authors or the departments with which they are affiliated have received something of value from a commercial or other party related directly or indirectly to the subject of this chapter.

Comminuted Distal Humeral Fractures

Despite advances in surgical techniques and implants, comminuted fractures of the distal humerus are difficult to treat.[1-4] Because of the complex anatomy of the distal humerus, obtaining and maintaining an anatomic reduction is inherently more challenging than for many other fractures. Factors that increase the complexity of these difficult injuries include open soft-tissue wounds, neurovascular injuries, intra-articular comminution, anterior osteochondral shearing fractures in the coronal plane, metaphyseal comminution, and associated injuries.[5-7] Furthermore, many of these fractures occur in osteoporotic bone, which makes fracture fixation difficult. Although it may not be possible to restore the elbow to normal function, several techniques and methods can be used to optimize outcome. On occasion, especially in severely osteoporotic bone, rigid fixation is not feasible, and elbow arthroplasty may be indicated in the elderly individual.[8] If the fracture involves only the articular bone, a prosthetic hemiarthroplasty can be used to replace the distal humerus only. Otherwise, a linked elbow replacement is required.

Treatment

Surgical Exposure Exposure is critical in the successful treatment of these injuries.[9] It generally is accepted that a posterior surgical approach is optimal for comminuted intra-articular fractures of the distal humerus that require surgical fixation.[1,4,6,10] Typically, exposure is through either an olecranon osteotomy or reflection or splitting of the triceps muscle and tendon. The triceps can be reflected either from side to side[11] or elevated in continuity with the anconeus and reflected proximally as in the triceps-anconeus pedicle (TRAP) approach.[12] Objective muscle strength testing following surgical repair of distal humeral fractures has shown no difference in elbow extension strength after osteotomy or triceps splitting.[10,13] In patients with open intra-articular distal humeral fractures, the shaft of the humerus typically ruptures through the triceps muscle, producing a posterior skin lesion. This defect in the triceps can be easily incorporated into a triceps-splitting approach. These approaches are complementary rather than mutually exclusive; with them the surgeon can be prepared to take advantage of whatever injury is present to facilitate the exposure, be it a large rent in the triceps or an associated olecranon fracture.

An apex-distal chevron-shaped osteotomy is initiated with an oscillating saw and completed by levering it open with a small osteotome. This procedure will create an interdigitating surface to facilitate later repair. The olecranon fragment and triceps are then mobilized proximally. The osteotomy will be repaired with two parallel 0.045-in Kirschner wires (K-wires) drilled obliquely to engage the anterior ulnar cortex distal to the coronoid process and two 22-gauge stainless steel figure-of-8 tension band wires or a precontoured congruent olecranon plate.

Before performing an olecranon osteotomy, it is wise to consider the possibility of having to do a total elbow arthroplasty. In such cases, the olecranon should be preserved. When performing a semiconstrained total elbow arthroplasty for a comminuted distal humeral fracture, it often is possible to preserve the entire extensor mechanism by releasing the triceps muscle from the distal aspect of the humeral shaft and working on either side of it. Excision of the fractured condyles creates a distal working space that facilitates component insertion.[8] This procedure decreases time in surgery and triceps-related complications, and it enhances rapid restoration of elbow strength and motion. However, it may be more difficult to instrument the ulna with the triceps intact.

Surgical Techniques The most technically challenging aspect of the surgical repair of a comminuted distal humeral fracture is severe intra-articular comminution.[1,5,7] **(DVD-10.1)** Although conventional teaching is to reassemble the articular fragments first and then reattach this construct to the metaphysis, alternate methods may be useful in some situations. If one large fragment of the joint surface can be anatomically reduced to either medial or lateral columns, it can be used to the surgeon's advantage in the setting of severe articular comminution. Once this stable construct has been reestablished, the other articular fragments can be assembled to it. This technique requires the surgeon either to use precontoured plates or to contour them. Fortunately, precontoured anatomically congruent plates are available in a range of sizes for the medial, lateral, and posterolateral aspects of the distal humerus. It is important to maintain the dimensions of the trochlea so that the proximal ulna articulates normally. If there is comminution of the trochlea and lag screw compression is applied, the groove may be narrowed, and the ulna will not seat properly. This problem can be avoided by inserting the 3.5-mm screws typically used for this fixation in a nonlag fashion or by adding an intercalary bone graft to the trochlear defect to maintain its width. One advantage of using the triceps-splitting or TRAP approach is that the proximal ulna remains intact and can be used as a bony template against which the trochlear reduction can be judged.[10]

Although small osteochondral fragments may not have nonarticular areas to which conventional plates and screws can be applied, they are important structurally. The use of Herbert screws countersunk through the articular surface perpendicular to the fracture line has been successful in stabilizing these fragments. The head of the screw is inserted flush with the level of the subchondral bone to maximize purchase and avoid prominence in case of cartilage loss. These screws also can be used to repair anterior fragments fractured in the coronal plane. It is important to remember that the screw itself provides relatively little compression; instead it maintains compressive force obtained through use of fracture-reduction forceps.[5] Alternative fixation options include minifragment 2.0- or 2.7-mm screws countersunk through the articular surface or small diameter threaded wires that can be cut off and then burred down flush with the subchondral bone surface. Disadvantages of these options include a greater amount of cartilage surface area lost and the potential for wire prominence if there is loss of cartilage.

Plate fixation of both the medial and lateral columns is necessary to reestablish stability of the distal humerus in bicondylar fractures (Fig. 1). Despite the many biomechanical and clinical studies on the ideal shape and orientation of the plates, some controversy exists.[1,2,9,14,15] What is clear is that two plates placed directly posteriorly on the medial and lateral columns (in the plane of motion of the joint) are biomechanically suboptimal. However, two parallel plates (one on each side) approximately in the sagittal plane are just as strong as two plates perpendicular to each other (ie, one medial and one posterolateral). Stronger 3.5-mm compression plates or plates designed specifically for the distal humerus are preferable. One-third tubular plates are too weak for most distal humerus fractures; they have a higher failure rate, especially when there is metaphyseal comminution in the supracondylar area. Precontoured commercially available plates have proved to be advantageous because they cradle the distal fragments or enable fracture reduction to the plate.[5,9,10] This is useful when severe comminution makes reestablishing the columns difficult. Longer (45 to 70 mm) screws passed through the plates across to the opposite column will also improve fracture construct stability by creating a closed box or triangle effect.

Treatment of severe distal humerus fractures fails either because of nonunion at the supracondylar level (Fig. 2) or stiffness resulting from prolonged immobilization that has been used in an attempt to avoid failure of inadequate fixation. Either way, the limiting factor is fixation of the distal fragments to the shaft. To obtain union and maintain elbow mobility after a severe fracture of the distal humerus, two principles must be satisfied: fixation in the distal fragment must be maximized, and all fixation in the major distal fragments should contribute to stability between the distal fragments and the shaft.[16] There are seven technical objectives by which these principles are met. Every screw in the major distal fragments should: (1) pass through a plate, (2) engage a fragment on the opposite side that also is fixed to a plate, (3) be as long as possible, and (4) engage as many articular fragments as possible. In addition, (5) as many screws as possible should be placed in the distal fragments, and the plates should be applied such that compression (6) is achieved at the supracondylar level for both columns and (7) is strong enough to resist failure before union occurs at the supracondylar level. Severe metaphyseal comminution and/or bone loss can be managed by a supracondylar shortening osteotomy[17] (Fig. 3), which allows restoration of bony contact and functional motion provided the following three guidelines are followed. First, shortening should be limited to 2 cm or less (preferably 1 cm). Second, the distal fragments can be translated laterally or medially with respect to the center of the humeral canal to improve bone contact at the metaphyseal level, but the rotational and varus-valgus alignments of the distal articular surface are carefully restored. Third, the coronoid and olecranon are prevented from impinging on the distal humerus in the functional arc of motion (30° to 130°). A convenient method to provide room for the coronoid and olecranon is to translate the epiphyseal segment anteriorly (to avoid losing flexion) and to sculpt the olecranon fossa with a burr once the fixation is complete (to avoid losing extension). The tip of the olecranon also can be resected to allow extension to at least 20° or 10°. For anatomic repairs, it is important to leave these fossae free of any fixation devices that may impede motion. Intraoperative radiographs will help confirm this is the case.

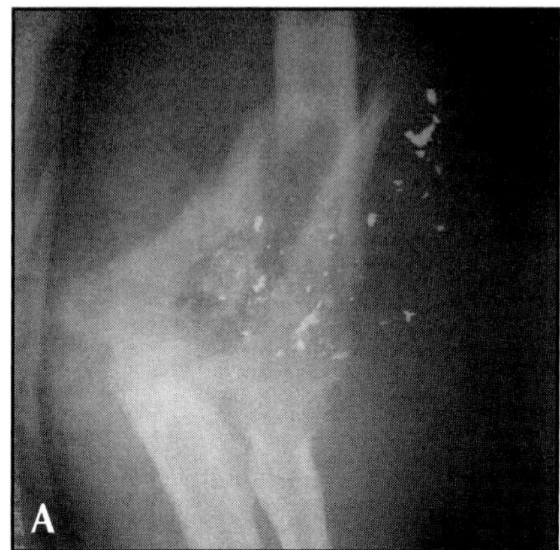

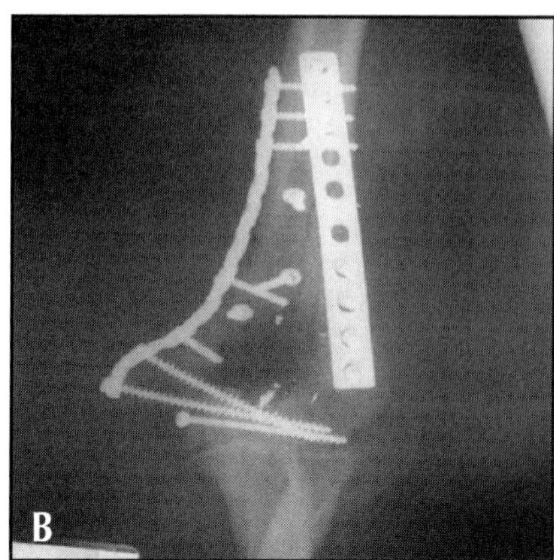

Fig. 1 A, AP radiograph of a comminuted, intra-articular distal humeral fracture caused by a gunshot wound. Fragments of the bullet can be seen in the soft tissues, and by their appearance and the anterior entry and posterior exit wounds a significant defect in the triceps muscle could reasonably be expected. The patient had a complete radial nerve palsy. **B,** This triceps defect was incorporated in the approach, and a triceps split was performed. Rigid fixation with two plates allowed early postoperative motion and enhanced the functional result. The radial nerve was explored and found to be contused but intact. At 1-year follow-up, the fracture had healed, the patient had a 115° arc of flexion-extension, and the radial nerve had recovered fully.

In certain fractures, the combination of articular comminution and osteoporosis may make stable fixation unattainable. In such circumstances, a linked total elbow arthroplasty is indicated if the patient is elderly. This option is reserved for older patients because prosthesis longevity is a concern, and the decision to proceed will depend on the surgeon's experience with both fracture fixation and arthroplasty.[8] If an arthroplasty is contemplated, it is usually necessary to use a linked device, and to preserve the olecranon (important for ulnar component stability) by using a triceps splitting or reflecting approach.

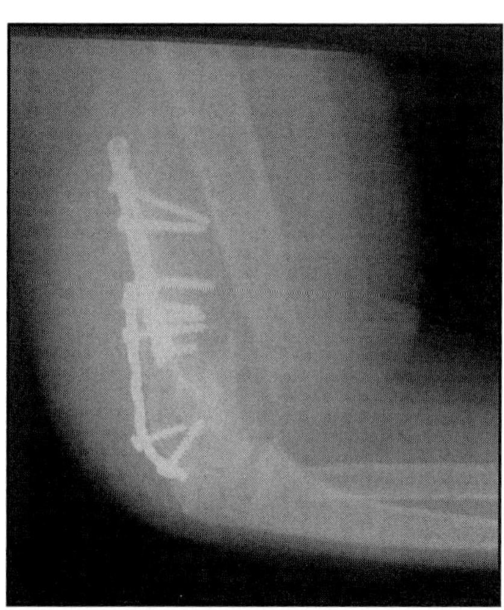

Fig. 2 Fixation failure following surgical repair of a distal humeral fracture. The posterior placement of both plates and lack of screw purchase distal to the fracture contributed to the displacement at the fracture site.

Postoperative Management

Ideally, when repairing comminuted intra-articular distal humeral fractures, sufficient stability is gained surgically to allow early motion of the injured elbow. Prolonged immobilization in an attempt to protect tenuous fixation typically results in stiffness. In a retrospective review, Waddell and associates[9] showed that immobilization for longer than 3

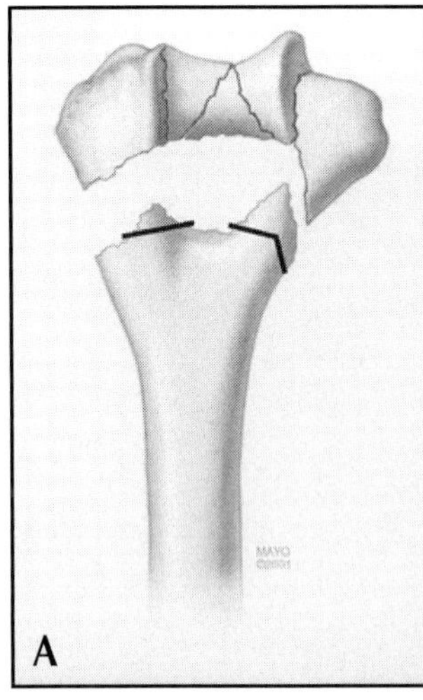

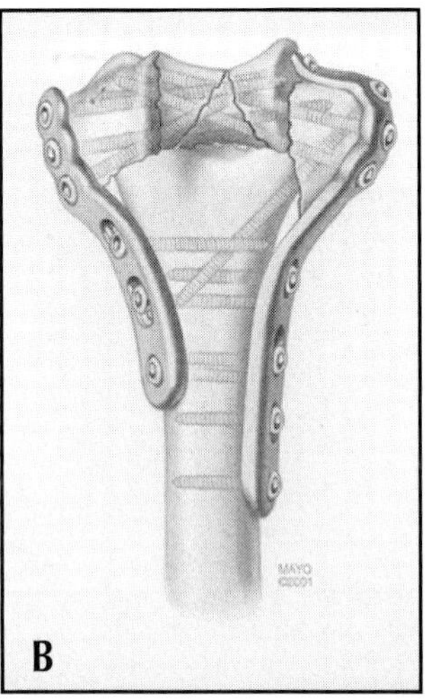

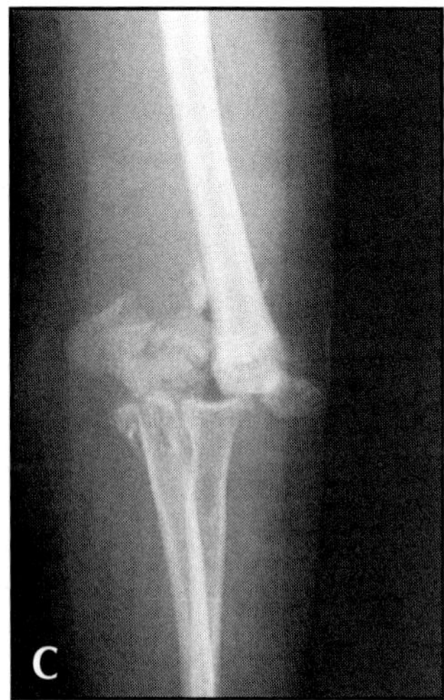

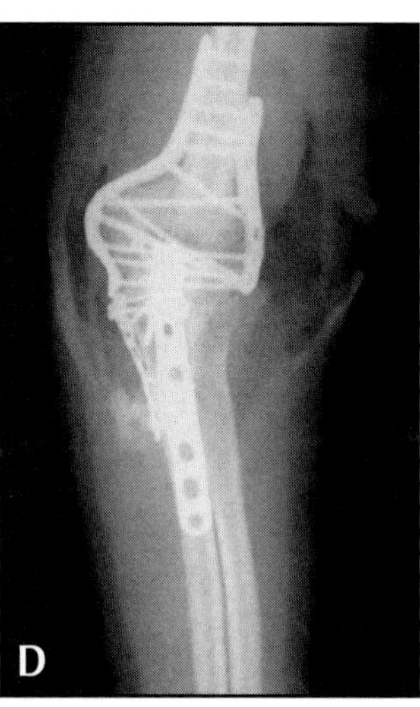

Fig. 3 Supracondylar shortening osteotomy. In cases of supracondylar bone loss and severe comminution, supracondylar shortening osteotomy is a viable option when an anatomic reconstruction is not believed to be possible. **A,** A small amount of bone from the distal end of the shaft is resected (dark lines) (never the articular segments) to enhance and permit compression contact between the distal articular segment and the shaft. **B,** Medial and lateral precontoured plates are placed slightly oblique to the sagittal plane. The distal screws should be as long as possible, passing through as many fragments as possible, and engaging the condyle or epicondyle of the opposite column. The coronoid fossae and radial fossa are best preserved by offsetting the distal segment anteriorly. To preserve terminal extension, the olecranon fossa can be recreated by burring the distal end of the shaft and removing the tip of the olecranon. **C,** Radiographic example of a distal humerus fracture with extensive bone loss and comminution, as well as fractures of the olecranon and coronoid. **D,** A supracondylar shortening osteotomy of 1.5 cm was performed and the fractures rigidly fixed using the Mayo Clinic Congruent Elbow plates (Acumed, Beaverton, OR) that are specially designed for these fractures. All of this patient's fractures healed and final range of motion was 25° to 120°. (Reproduced with permission from the Mayo Foundation, Rochester, MN.)

weeks caused disabling stiffness. Even with optimal surgery and early motion, normal flexion-extension has rarely been reported following this injury. McKee and associates[10] reported a mean flexion-extension arc of 108° (range, 55° to 140°) with a mean flexion contracture of 25° in a recent review of 25 elbows that were splinted for a week after surgical repair of an intra-articular distal humeral fracture and then treated with active range-of-motion (ROM) exercises. To decrease postoperative swelling, the arm should be elevated with the elbow held extended in a well-padded splint. The splint usually is removed 48 hours after surgery in isolated injuries, and active physiotherapy is initiated. The patients are carefully counseled regarding a home exercise program and given an instruction booklet. Some surgeons prefer the patient to use a continuous passive motion device at home for the first 4 weeks. Resisted extension is avoided for the first 6 weeks to protect the extensor mechanism.

The patient is expected to show steady improvement in terms of ROM. Recalcitrant patients are managed with turnbuckle and nighttime extension splinting and flexion strapping. Although prophylactic measures against heterotopic bone may not be used routinely, indomethacin is used in patients with concomitant head injuries (25 mg three times a day orally for 3 weeks).

Although there is a wide range of reported results following this severe injury, the average patient can expect a relatively pain-free, functional,[18] 105° arc of motion, with approximately 75% normal strength if current standards of rigid anatomic fixation and early motion are followed.

Pearls

The surgeon should take advantage of any disruption of the extensor mechanism in the approach (ie, if there is an open fracture and triceps defect, a triceps splitting approach should be considered; if there is an olecranon fracture, it can be used instead of an osteotomy). In addition, the surgeon should make sure that all screws in the major articular fragments also contribute to stability at the supracondylar level. In elderly patients with severe comminution, alternatives to olecranon osteotomy should be considered in case an elbow replacement is required. If a truly unfixable fracture is limited to the articular segment with no supracondylar involvement, replacement can be performed with a distal humeral hemiarthroplasty rather than a total elbow arthroplasty.

Pitfalls

Common complications following surgical intervention for displaced intra-articular fractures of the distal humerus include fixation failure, nonunion, stiffness, elbow weakness, ulnar neuropathy, and infection.[2-4] Fixation failure usually is attributable to inadequate techniques, implants such as thin plates (Fig. 2), or K-wire fixation alone. A common pitfall is prolonged immobilization in an attempt to compensate for such inadequate fixation; severe stiffness is the inevitable result. Another common pitfall is placement of screws in the major articular fragments before plate application, only to find that fixation of those fragments to the shaft is then limited by the number of screws that can be placed into the distal fragments through the plates.

Yet another common pitfall is the placement of hardware adjacent to the ulnar nerve, which then becomes painful and/or impaired as a result of scarring and fibrosis. Ulnar neurolysis and transposition during elbow reconstruction are usually helpful, but nerve recovery may take up to 2 years.[4]

Elbow flexion and extension strength are significantly decreased to about 75% of contralateral strength despite apparently successful fracture treatment.[10,13] This degree of weakness may not be functionally disabling for sedentary individuals, but it may explain the sense of weakness and loss of endurance that more active patients have when they attempt to return to rigorous tasks following this injury.[10]

Table 1
Classification of Articular Shearing Fractures of the Distal Humerus

Type	Description
Type I	A single articular fragment, including the capitellum and a portion of the trochlea; previously described as a coronal shear fracture.
Type II	A shearing fracture of the articular surface, including the lateral epicondyle.
Type III	The shearing articular fragmentation anteriorly, including impaction of the most distal metaphyseal bone of the lateral column.
Type IV	The articular fractures include the anterior and posterior trochlea as separate fragments.
Type V	Involvement of the medial and lateral epicondyles.

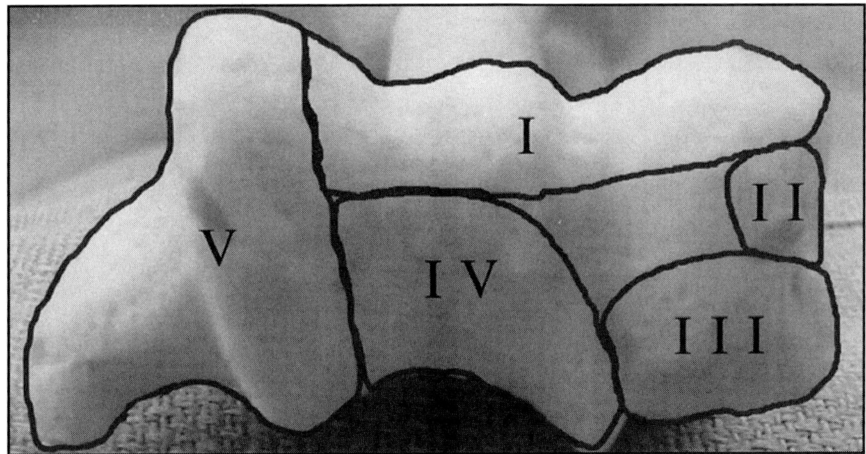

Fig. 4 Patterns of articular shearing fractures of the distal humerus. See Table 1 for descriptions of each pattern.

Coronal Shear Fractures of the Capitellum and Trochlea

A constellation of articular fractures primarily involving the articular surface of the distal humerus has been identified; some of these fractures have little or no supporting metaphyseal subchondral bone.[19] A precise morphologic definition of these different fracture patterns is useful in surgical decision making and choice of surgical techniques and should help in the assessment of outcome in comparisons with alternative techniques such as total elbow arthroplasty.[8]

Patterns of Injury

These fractures have been classified based on involvement of articular surfaces extending from lateral to medial (Fig. 4, Table 1). Although established fracture classifications such as the AO/ASIF include some components of these injuries either in the frontal plane alone or as part of complex multifragmented intercondylar fractures, none depict the variety of patterns that exist with these primarily articular injuries.[20-23] Recognition of the morphology of these complex chondral fractures is critical for preoperative planning and deciding on the most appropriate surgical exposure. Three-dimensional CT has added immeasurably to defining these lesions and, when available, should be considered (Fig. 5).

Chondral articular fractures are difficult to repair because they require extensile surgical exposure, realignment of small and at times impacted articular fragments, and the precise placement of implants that must be countersunk beneath the joint surface. The specific fracture types represent a progression of injury severity extending from an isolated articular component displaced in the frontal plane to combinations of shearing and impaction injury to the capitellum and trochlea with a limited zone of metaphyseal bone support.[1,24-28]

Despite separation from the underlying metaphyseal bone and the complete lack of any soft-tissue attachments, osteonecrosis of these small articular fragments is uncommon, which may be because the stability has been adequate to

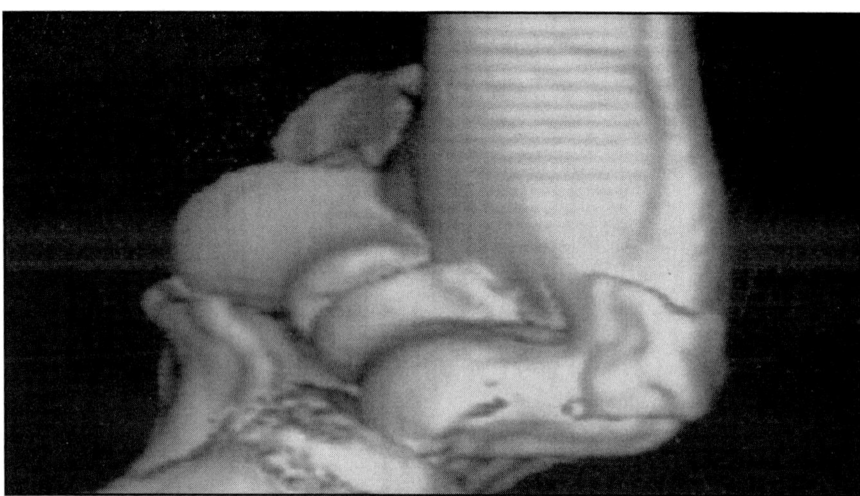

Fig. 5 A three-dimensional CT scan of a chondral shearing fracture.

permit rapid revascularization from the underlying metaphyseal bone support. When osteonecrosis does occur, it can be treated by hemiarthroplasty if the ulna and radial head remain normal.

Treatment

Surgical Exposure Patients whose fractures do not involve the medial epicondyle can be treated using an extensile lateral Kocher exposure. Those fractures extending to involve the medial epicondyle can be treated through an olecranon osteotomy or TRAP approach.[12] For treatment of a fracture of the lateral epicondyle, the lateral exposure is facilitated by elevating and retracting the epicondyle distally along with the attached origins of the wrist and digital extensor muscles and lateral collateral ligament (LCL) complex. The more proximal origins of the radial wrist extensor muscles are elevated from the lateral supracondylar ridge to improve the access to the anterior articular fragments. The exposure is completed by elevating the lateral triceps from the distal humerus and lateral aspect of the proximal olecranon, which permits the elbow joint to be hinged open, providing exposure to the anterior and posterior articular surfaces of the distal humerus.

Surgical Techniques The fracture fragments should be individually identified, repositioned, and provisionally secured with smooth 0.045- or 0.062-in K-wires. Inability to anatomically realign some of the anterior articular fragments may be the result of impaction of the posterior aspect of the lateral bony column or impaction of part or all of the posterior trochlea. Definitive internal fixation of the isolated articular fracture fragments is facilitated using Herbert screws alone or in combination with small threaded K-wires. Alternatively, if an olecranon osteotomy or TRAP approach is used, a lateral precontoured plate in addition to screws from the medial side can be used (Fig. 6).

If it is of sufficient size, the lateral epicondylar fragment is best reattached with a plate and screws. The epicondylar plate and screw fixation can be reinforced with a 22-gauge stainless steel wire placed distally through the soft-tissue insertions and proximally through a drill hole in the distal humerus. A figure-of-8 wire alone will be sufficient when the epicondylar fragment is too small to support screw fixation (Fig. 7).

Patients with a type I single articular fragment require varus distraction but not actual subluxation of the ulnotrochlear articulation for exposure, and the fragment can be reduced and securely stabilized by elevation of the anterior capsule through this lateral approach. If the articular fragment is so comminuted or osteoporotic as to render fixation impossible, prosthetic replacement of the distal humerus is an option.

Postoperative Management

The extremity is splinted in extension overnight, and then active motion is initiated on the first or second postoperative day using gravity to assist flexion.

Pearls

Inability to reduce a coronal shear fracture anatomically usually implies metaphyseal impaction (shortening at the supracondylar level) or impaction of the posterior trochlea. Medial extension to involve the medial epicondyle requires the same exposure as a distal humeral fracture.

Pitfalls

There is a tendency to malreduce the capitellum, leaving it displaced proximally. Ulnohumeral subluxation can impede reduction of a fracture involving the medial trochlea. This subluxation occurs as a result of impingement of the coronoid against the medial trochlear fragment. Such fractures should be reduced through an olecranon osteotomy or a TRAP approach.

Olecranon Fracture-Dislocations

Olecranon fracture-dislocations are complex fractures of the olecranon associated with subluxation or dislocation of the radial head and or the coronoid process (Fig. 8). The fracture of the proximal ulna in an olecranon fracture-dislocation is usually multifragmented.[29,30]

Patterns of Injury

It is useful to distinguish anterior and posterior displacement patterns of olecranon fracture-dislocation. Anterior fracture-dislocations of the olecranon have been described as transolecranon frac-

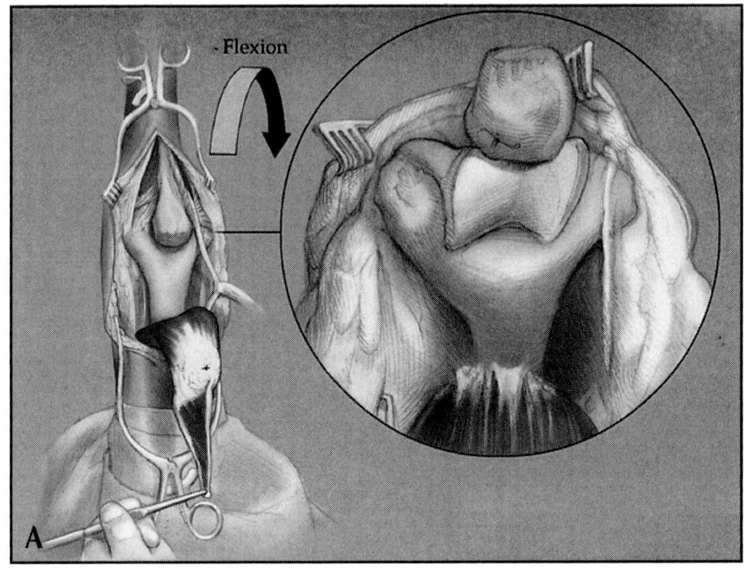

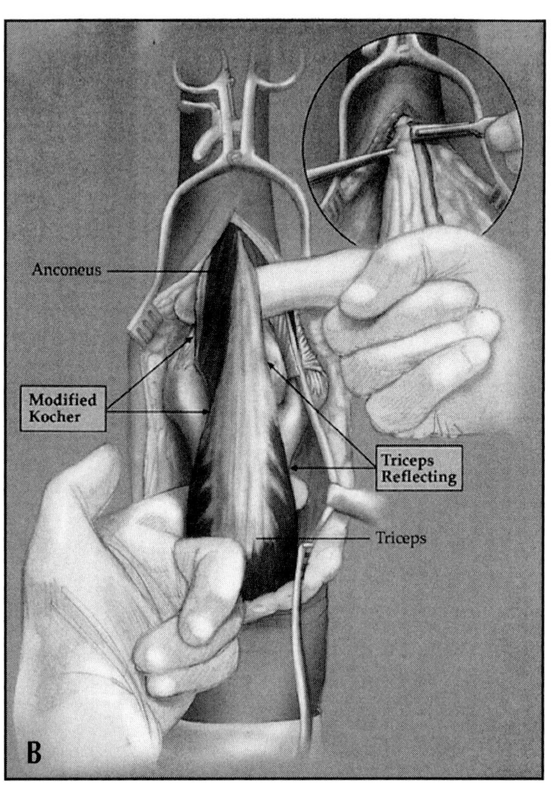

Fig. 6 A and **B**, The TRAP approach involves a combination of a modified Kocher's approach from the lateral side, preserving the LCL complex and posterolateral capsule off of which the anconeus is reflected, and a medial triceps reflecting-approach of Bryan-Morrey. These meet at the distal end of the anconeus. The triceps can then be reflected proximally along with the anconeus pedicle, very much like an olecranon osteotomy reflection. This reflection permits access to the distal humerus similar to that of an olecranon osteotomy except for the midportion of the anterior trochlea, which can be seen by looking in the lateral ulna humeral articulation while retracting the ulna gently. The intact ulna and radial head can be used as a template against which to assemble the articular fragments. (Reproduced with permission from the Mayo Foundation, Rochester, MN.)

ture-dislocations of the elbow[29,31] because the trochlea of the distal humerus appears to have fractured through the olecranon process as the forearm displaced anteriorly (Fig. 8, *A*). Distinction of anterior from posterior fracture-dislocations is straightforward because the radial head is displaced anteriorly rather than posteriorly relative to the capitellum; however, anterior radiocapitellar dislocation often leads to misidentification of this injury as an anterior (Bado type 1[32]) Monteggia fracture-dislocation.[29,30,33] Anterior fracture-dislocations of the olecranon destabilize the ulnohumeral joint, but the radioulnar relationship usually is preserved[29,31,34] (Fig, 8 *B*). In contrast, anterior Monteggia fractures are fracture-dislocations of the forearm in which the ulnohumeral joint is not involved.[33]

Posterior fracture-dislocations of the olecranon can be considered the most proximal injury type among the spectrum of posterior (Bado type 2)[32] Monteggia fractures because the principles and pitfalls of treatment are similar.[30,35] Posterior Monteggia injuries are characterized by an apex posterior fracture of the ulna, posterior dislocation of the radial head with respect to the capitellum, and in about two thirds of injuries, fracture of the radial head[30,32,35-37] (Fig. 8, *B*). These injuries, like more distal posterior Monteggia fractures, threaten both elbow and forearm function.

Fractures of the coronoid process of the ulna are common among both anterior and posterior fracture-dislocations of the olecranon.[29,33] The fracture of the coronoid is usually a basal fracture (see section on coronoid fractures) involving between 50% and 100% of the height of the coronoid process. There can be a single large fragment or comminution (Fig. 9). In some patients, the fracture may be oblique so that it involves the anteromedial facet of the coronoid, particularly in posterior fracture-dislocations of the olecranon.

In some patients with complex fractures of the proximal ulna, the relationship between the radius and ulna and the trochlea may have been restored either spontaneously or by manipulative reduction. The displacement was probably posterior if the radial head is fractured, particularly if some of the fragments remain posterior. The distinction is important because anterior olecranon fracture-dislocations are stable once the alignment of the olecranon and coronoid

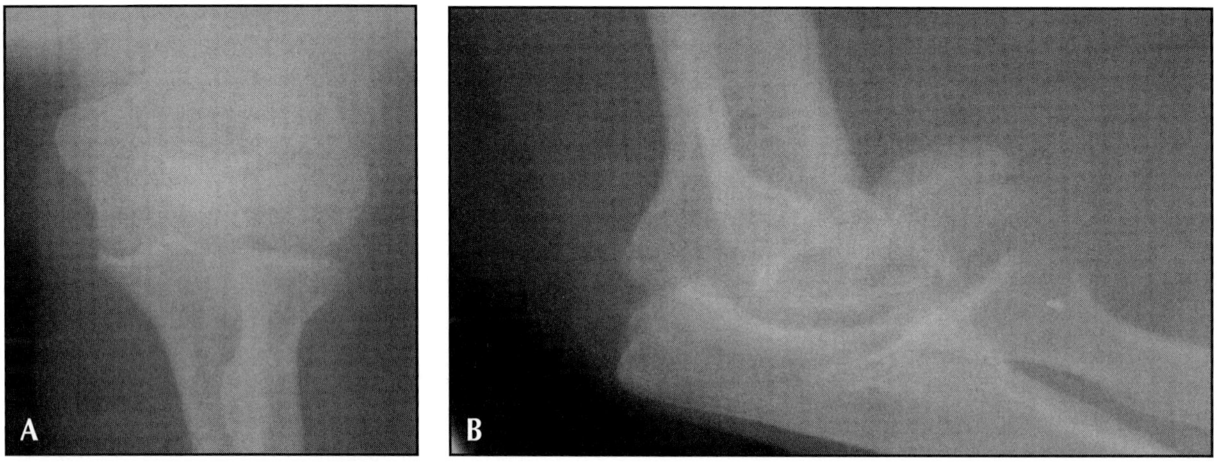

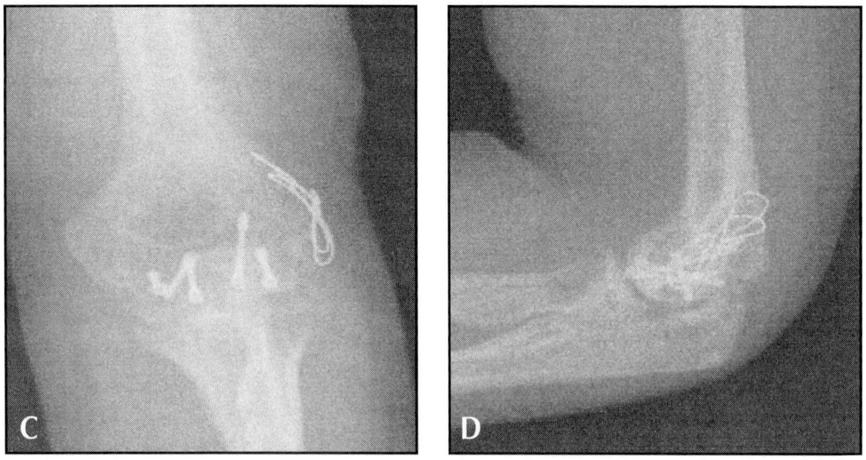

Fig. 7 Type IV chondral shearing fracture in a 46-year-old woman. **A** and **B,** The anterior and lateral radiographs of the fracture. **C** and **D,** AP and lateral radiographs at 6 months. Full elbow and forearm motion was achieved. Note the fixation of the displaced lateral epicondyle with tension wires.

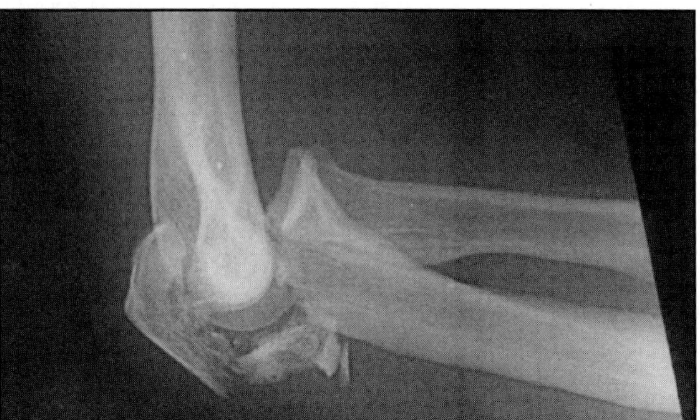

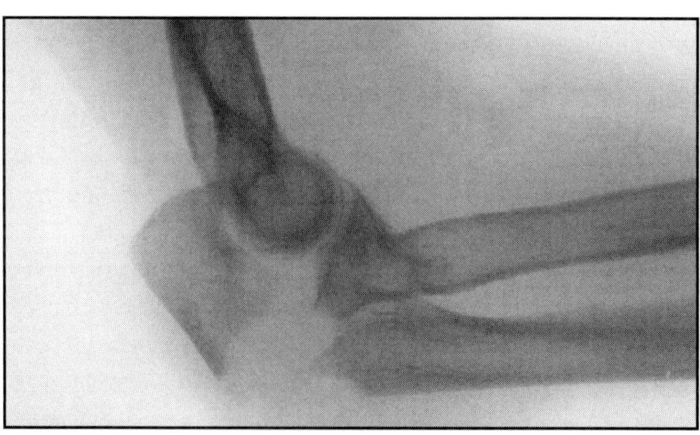

Fig. 8 A, Anterior fracture-dislocations of the olecranon. **B,** Posterior fracture-dislocations of the olecranon.

are restored, and forearm function is rarely in jeopardy.[29] In contrast, ulnohumeral instability is common after posterior olecranon fracture-dislocations, and forearm function often is compromised.[30,33]

Treatment

Surgical Exposure A posterior midline incision is used for exposure.[38,39] The treatment of posterior olecranon fracture-dislocations often requires the creation of a broad lateral skin flap to access the radial head. A medial skin flap can be created if access to the coronoid process from the medial side is required. **(DVD-10.2)**

Exposure of the ulna should preserve periosteal and muscle attachments. A contoured dorsal plate can be applied

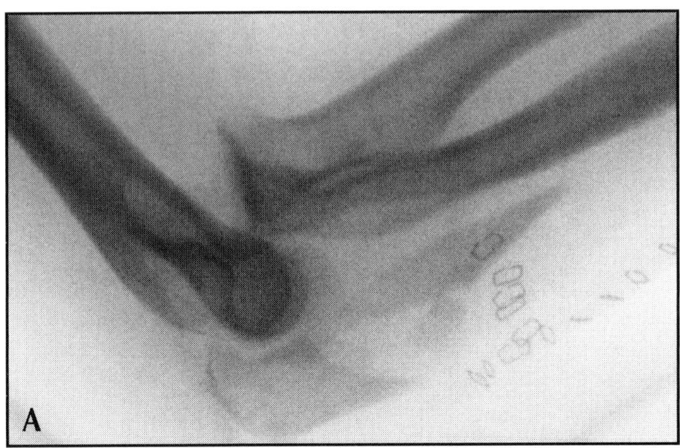

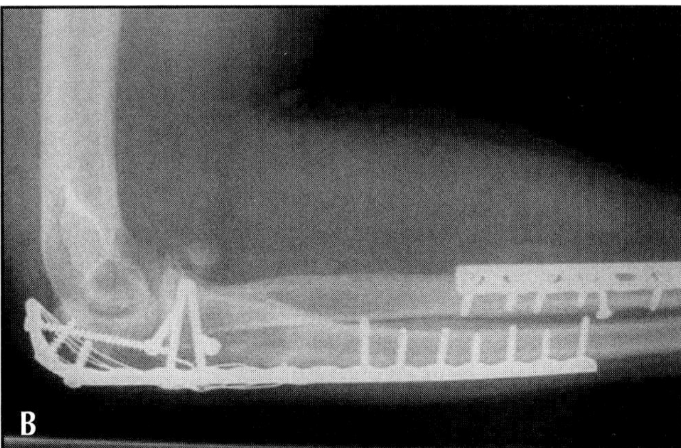

Fig 9 Anterior fracture-dislocations of the olecranon can be so complex that they are not identified as olecranon fracture-dislocations. **A,** Lateral radiograph demonstrates extensive fragmentation extending into the diaphysis. **B,** Six months later the fracture is solidly healed, the elbow is stable, and good elbow function has been restored.

directly over a portion of the triceps insertion at the olecranon and on the apex of the ulnar diaphysis distally without elevating muscle attachments (Fig. 9). This procedure preserves blood supply and optimizes healing. If olecranon comminution is extensive, the plate can be extended proximally through a triceps split to the tip of the olecranon. Despite extensive fragmentation, bone grafts[40] are rarely necessary if the soft-tissue attachments are preserved.

The fractures of the radial head and coronoid process can be evaluated and sometimes definitively treated through the exposure provided by the fracture of the olecranon process.[41-43] With little additional dissection, the olecranon fragment can be mobilized proximally, providing exposure of the coronoid through the ulnohumeral joint (Fig. 9, *B*). If the radial head is fragmented and will be replaced with a prosthesis, replacement can be done through this traumatic exposure in most cases. Doing so, however, makes alignment of the radial head more challenging. If surgical fixation of the radial head with a plate is considered, the use of a separate muscle interval (eg, Kocher's or Kaplan's intervals)[44] rather than further mobilization of the musculature separating the proximal radius and ulna may help limit the potential for synostosis formation.

Posterior olecranon fracture-dislocations often require a lateral exposure to address a fracture of the radial head or coronoid, or to repair the LCL. When the LCL is injured, it may be avulsed at its ulnar insertion or from the lateral epicondyle. This avulsion facilitates both exposure and repair. The LCL origin and common extensor musculature can be mobilized distally. Improved exposure of the coronoid can be obtained by releasing the origins of the radial wrist extensors from the lateral supracondylar ridge and elevating the brachialis from the anterior humerus and by excising the fractured radial head.[43]

A medial exposure (as described in the section on coronoid fractures) may be needed to address a complex fracture of the coronoid, particularly if it involves the anteromedial facet of the coronoid process.

Surgical Techniques The fracture of the coronoid often can be reduced directly through the elbow joint using the limited access provided by the olecranon fracture. However, failure to fix an anteromedial coronoid fragment can seriously jeopardize the result. Provisional fixation can be obtained using K-wires to attach the fragments either to the metaphyseal or diaphyseal fragments of the ulna or to the trochlea of the distal humerus when there is extensive fragmentation of the proximal ulna.[42] An alternative when there is extensive fragmentation of the proximal ulna is the use of a skeletal distractor (a temporary external fixator).[29,45] External fixation applied between a wire driven through the olecranon and up into the trochlea and a second wire in the distal ulnar diaphysis often can obtain reduction indirectly when distraction is applied between the pins. Definitive fixation usually can be obtained with screws applied under image intensifier guidance. The screws are placed through the plate when there is extensive fragmentation of the proximal ulna. The proximal olecranon fragment is grasped with a tenaculum forceps through the triceps insertion and provisionally secured to the trochlea of the distal humerus using a stout, smooth K-wire (usually 5/64 in). **(DVD-10.3)**

A precontoured plate is used, or a long plate is contoured to wrap around the proximal olecranon.[46] The plate can lie directly on a portion of the triceps insertion, or the insertion can be split longitudinally and mobilized slightly so that the plate is in direct contact with the

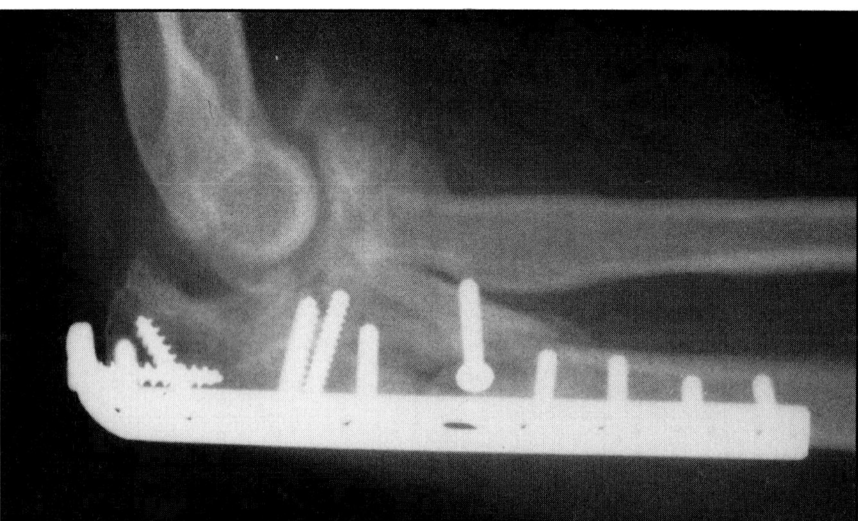

Fig. 10 A radiograph showing a comminuted olecranon coronoid fracture-dislocation in which the anteromedial coronoid fragment remains displaced despite attempts to lag the coronoid fragments in place. This resulted in joint incongruity and early posttraumatic arthritis, requiring a total elbow arthroplasty later.

bone. This proximal contour of the plate makes it possible to insert a greater number of screws in the olecranon fragment and to have those screws interdigitate. In addition, the orthogonal orientation of the most proximal screws to the more distal screws may provide a stronger hold on the fragment. When the olecranon is fragmented, a plate and screws alone may not provide reliable fixation. In this situation, it has proved useful to use ancillary tension-wire fixation through the triceps insertion to control the olecranon fragments.[29]

Direct dorsal placement of the plate is straightforward, requires no soft-tissue stripping, allows more strategic screw placement, and allows the plate to function as a tension band under the influence of the brachialis and triceps muscles. Proximally, a dorsally applied plate rests on the relatively flat surface of the olecranon, but distally it lies directly over the apex of the ulna. In muscular patients, the interval between the flexor carpi ulnaris and the extensor carpi ulnaris must be split to expose the ulna. A very long plate may be needed (between 12 to 16 holes), particularly when there is extensive fragmentation or the bone quality is poor (Fig. 9).

Postoperative Management

In young patients with good bone quality, it is usually possible to obtain fixation secure enough to initiate active gravity-assisted elbow ROM exercises 1 or 2 days after surgery. Patients are also encouraged to use the injured arm for light functional activities.

Posterior olecranon fracture-dislocations are common among older women, and osteoporosis may influence the quality of the fixation. In addition, the coronoid fixation may be somewhat tenuous. In these circumstances, it may prove wise to rest the elbow at 90° of flexion in a removable posterior plastic splint for 4 weeks prior to initiating elbow mobilization. Exercises to prevent digit swelling and stiffness are important during this rest period.

Pearls

Transolecranon fracture-dislocations tend to be intrinsically stable after fracture fixation because the injury is mostly through bone and less through soft tissues. Two key predictors of stability after treatment of a transolecranon fracture-dislocation are the integrity of the LCL complex and that of the anteromedial coronoid. A precontoured plate (commercially available or contoured by the surgeon) that is placed on the posterior surface of the ulna and wraps around the tip of the olecranon should be used. A skeletal distractor can be useful in facilitating reduction.

Pitfalls

Perhaps the most common pitfall is failure to obtain or maintain reduction of the coronoid (Fig. 10). If the coronoid fixation loosens, but the ulnohumeral joint remains stable and concentrically aligned, healing in an adequate position often can be obtained by protecting the elbow in a removable posterior elbow splint for 4 weeks. Stability takes priority over motion because mobility usually can be improved with capsular excision,[29,47,48] but instability may damage the articular surface irreversibly.[49] If the ulnohumeral joint is malaligned, then another attempt to improve coronoid alignment and fixation may be warranted.

Another pitfall to be avoided is placement of the plate on the medial or lateral aspect of the proximal ulna, which provides less fixation than a contoured posterior plate.[30] Failure occurs in these instances by loosening of the screws in the proximal fragment. In contrast, a dorsally applied plate rarely fails by loosening proximally but can loosen from the ulnar diaphysis if the plate is too short or the bone quality is poor. Application of a long plate will ensure correct contouring to prevent malunion. The surgeon should be certain that long plates are available because many commonly used plate and screw sets do not routinely include these longer plates.

Another subtle pitfall is failure to recognize ulnohumeral instability with a posterior olecranon fracture-dislocation.[49] The surgeon should anticipate this problem and ensure that all of the following have been achieved: (1) the radial head has either been repaired or replaced with a prosthesis so that radiocapitellar contact is restored, (2) the ulna has been realigned so that the radial head is aligned with the capitellum, (3) the coronoid has been realigned and secured, and (4) LCL injury has been identified and repaired. If ulnohumeral instability persists even though all of these have been achieved, hinged external fixation of the elbow may be necessary.[49]

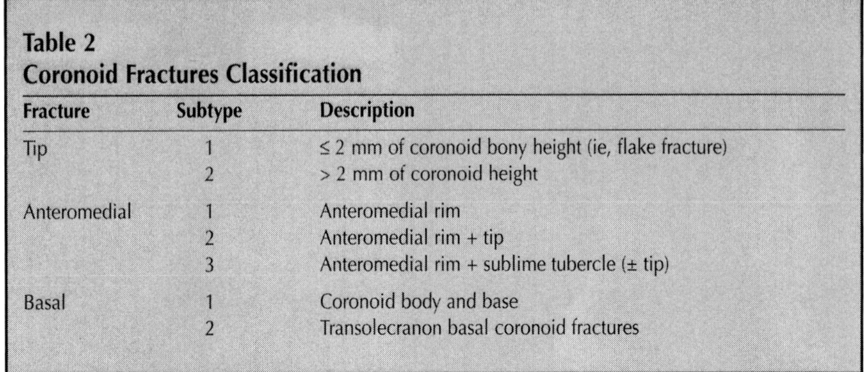

Table 2
Coronoid Fractures Classification

Fracture	Subtype	Description
Tip	1	≤ 2 mm of coronoid bony height (ie, flake fracture)
	2	> 2 mm of coronoid height
Anteromedial	1	Anteromedial rim
	2	Anteromedial rim + tip
	3	Anteromedial rim + sublime tubercle (± tip)
Basal	1	Coronoid body and base
	2	Transolecranon basal coronoid fractures

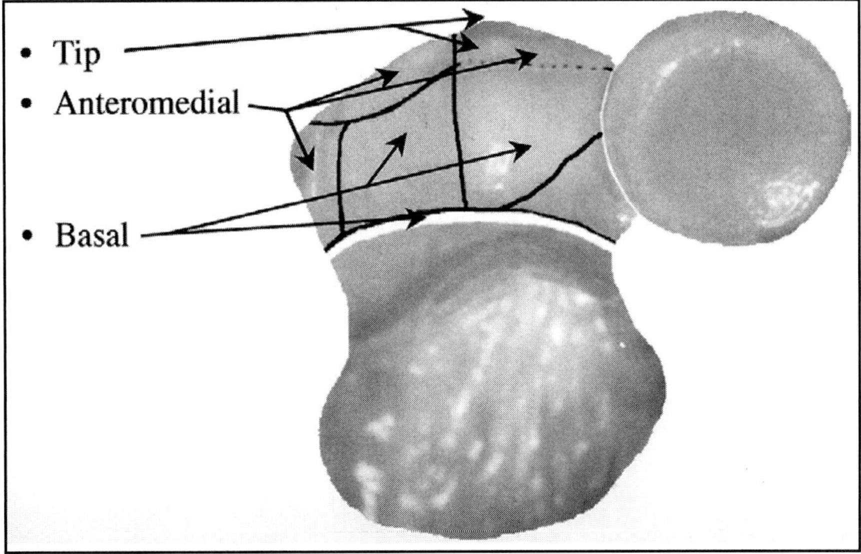

Fig. 11 Schematic showing proposed classification system for coronoid fractures, based on anatomic location with subtypes according to the severity of coronoid involvement, considers the mechanism of injury along with the associated fractures and soft-tissue injuries and dictates surgical approach and treatment (see Table 2 for details).

Coronoid Fractures

Coronoid fractures are most commonly encountered in association with radial head fractures as part of the terrible triad (coronoid fracture, radial head fracture, and elbow dislocation).[50] Less commonly, they are seen either as isolated fractures or as part of complex olecranon fracture-dislocations. Until recently, understanding of these fractures has been lacking; thus, little has been written regarding their management.[51-56]

Patterns of Injury

Regan and Morrey[57] classified these fractures into three types according to the height of the coronoid involved. However, experience has dictated the need for a new classification system. For example, fractures of the anteromedial coronoid may not involve the tip and thus are not classifiable. The patterns of injury that take into account the anatomic location, amount of coronoid fractured, comminution, elbow stability, and associated injuries should be considered (Fig. 11, Table 2). Fortunately, these injury patterns provide a guide to surgical approach and treatment.

Coronoid Tip Fractures The fracture line is in the coronal plane, rarely involves more than about one third of the height of the coronoid, and does not extend medially past the sublime tubercle or into the body of the coronoid. A tip subtype 1 fracture is a small flake off the tip (≤ 2 mm). It may be seen in isolation or as part of a fracture-dislocation. A tip subtype 2 fracture involves a larger segment of the tip (> 2 mm), but does not extend more than about a third of the way into the body of the coronoid or past the sublime tubercle medially. It almost always is seen in association with a radial head fracture in a dislocated elbow, a combination of injuries that has been termed the terrible triad.[50]

Coronoid tip fractures occur as a result of an elbow subluxation or dislocation via a posterolateral rotatory displacement of the ulna under the trochlea.[56,58] The mechanism is a fall onto the outstretched hand, with valgus and supination moments applied to the ulna as it flexes on the humerus during axial loading.[59] The implication of these fractures is that the elbow had subluxated or dislocated, just as a bony Bankart lesion of the glenoid does for anterior shoulder instability.[59,60] Their effect on elbow stability is proportionate to the amount of coronoid lost or fractured. The LCL is disrupted in virtually all instances in which a dislocation has occurred (all of those resulting

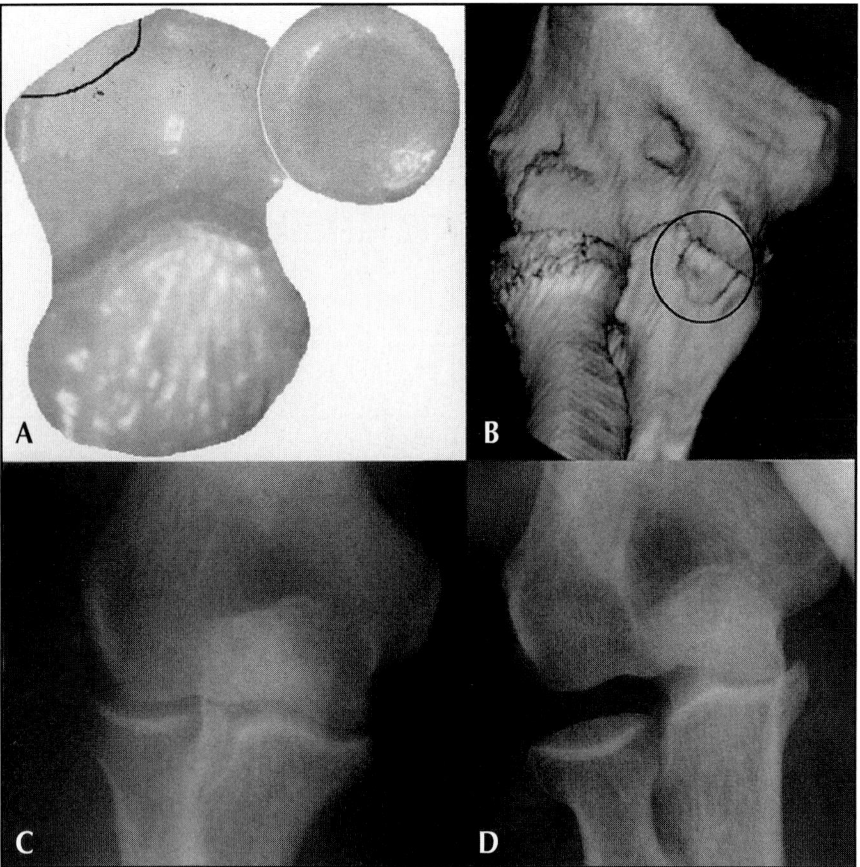

Fig. 12 A and **B,** Location of the anteromedial coronoid fracture fragment shown in a schematic and a three-dimensional CT reconstruction. (Fracture fragment indicated by black outlines.) **C** and **D,** AP radiographs with and without a varus/posteromedial rotatory stress applied contrast show what initially appears to be an almost normal radiograph with one revealing significant varus instability and apparent narrowing of the medial ulnohumeral joint.

from falls), although the medial collateral ligament (MCL) can remain at least partially or functionally intact in these fracture-dislocations.

Anteromedial Coronoid Fractures Anteromedial fractures have not been addressed in the literature. The initial fracture (subtype 1) is located anteromedially, between the tip of the coronoid and the sublime tubercle in an oblique plane between the coronal and sagittal planes (Fig. 12). Medially, the fracture line usually exits the cortex in the anterior half of the sublime tubercle, ie, in the anterior portion of the anterior bundle of the MCL. Laterally, the fracture exits just medial to the tip of the coronoid. Comminution can extend to involve the tip (subtype 2), the sublime tubercle (the attachment site of the anterior bundle of the MCL) (subtype 3), and the body of the coronoid (see section on basal fractures), depending on the energy of the injury.

The mechanism is a varus/posteromedial rotation injury with axial loading. Flexion and abduction torque at the shoulder, while the elbow is flexing under axial load, cause the elbow to go into varus (disrupting the LCL) and the medial trochlea to ride up onto the anteromedial coronoid, which is fractured off by a shearing mechanism (Figs. 12 and 13).

Associated injuries include disruptions of the LCL and posterior band of the MCL. The radial head may be fractured, but usually only in the more severe types (eg, subtype 3). It is safe to assume that in the presence of an anteromedial coronoid fracture the LCL has been disrupted. The LCL usually is avulsed beneath the common extensor tendon origin.

The significance of this injury is that the elbow has a tendency to articulate incongruently under axial load or gravitational varus stress (Fig. 14). On lateral tomograms or sagittal CT reconstructions, the medial trochlea can be seen to articulate with the small coronoid fragment, but not with most of the ulna (Fig. 14, *C*). Instead, there is point loading at the fracture site on the ulna, which causes high stresses on the cartilage of the medial trochlea. This pattern of fracture-subluxation is somewhat analogous to that of a Bennett's fracture-dislocation of the thumb. Joint incongruity such as this naturally can (and does appear to) lead to rapid onset arthritis (Fig. 15). Confirming the incongruity may require lateral tomograms or CT reconstruction. To demonstrate this incongruity, the elbow should be imaged while under normal gravitational force. Patients often present with painful contracture several weeks after a minor coronoid fracture. The ulnar nerve is prone to compressive neuritis because of swelling of the torn posterior band of the MCL.

Closkey and associates[53] may have derived a misleading conclusion concerning the effect of coronoid fractures on elbow stability in a recent biomechanical study. They found that a loss of up to 40% of the coronoid did not change the elbow's resistance to direct posterior subluxation. However, they did not evaluate stability with coupled motions in posterolateral or varus-posteromedial rotation. It has been verified (S O'Driscoll, MD, Rochester, MN, unpublished data, 2002) that simulation of an anteromedial subtype 1 coronoid fracture in a cadaver, in association with LCL detachment, permits varus-posteromedial rotatory instability as seen clinically. The key to considering this diagnosis is to recognize the isolated coronoid fracture, ie, a coronoid fracture without a radial head fracture (especially in the absence of apparent dislocation). This injury may appear benign, but it has a predisposition to rapid posttraumatic arthritis as a result of the persistent slight incongruity of the medial ulnohumeral joint. Thus, these fractures generally should be treated surgically.

Basal Coronoid Fractures Basal fractures involve the body of the coronoid, indicated by at least 50% of the height of the coronoid being fractured. These fractures are usually quite comminuted, but they may result in a single fragment if part of an olecranon fracture-dislocation (see section on olecranon fracture-dislocations). Although elbow congruity and stability may have been severely disrupted, the extent of soft-tissue disruption is often less than that seen with tip fractures; therefore, the prognosis may be good once the fracture has been fixed. The principle distinction between basal subtype 1 and 2 fracture is that the latter involves a fracture of the olecranon.

A basal subtype 1 fracture is comminuted and usually has fragments corresponding to those seen in the anteromedial subtype 3 fractures in addition to a die-punch fragment just dorsal to the anteromedial subtype 1 fracture fragment. Fracture lines extend into the proximal radioulnar articulation as well. The radial head often is fractured with these basal subtype 1 fractures, and the ulnohumeral joint is usually unstable.

A basal subtype 2 fracture through the body or base of the coronoid also involves a fracture of the olecranon. These fractures sometimes have a single large coronoid fragment, and much of the soft tissue still may be preserved, which means that once fracture reduc-

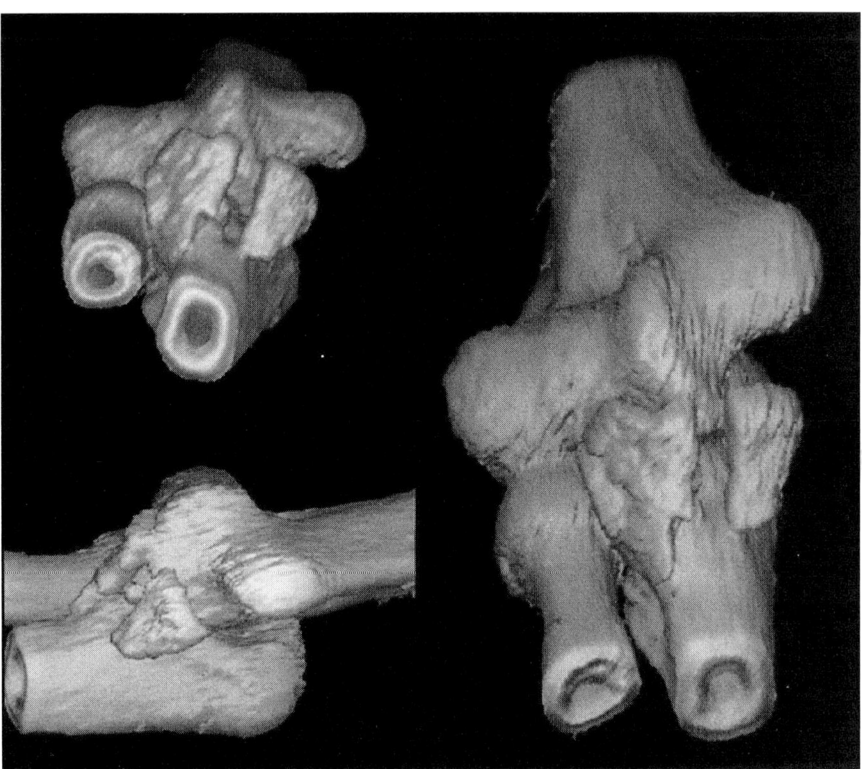

Fig. 13 Mechanism of injury for anteromedial coronoid fractures. Three-dimensional CT reconstruction of an anteromedial subtype 3 coronoid fracture shows involvement of not just the anteromedial fragment but the tip and the sublime tubercle as well. Under varus and axial loads, while the elbow is flexing, flexion and abduction torques at the shoulder cause the medial trochlea to ride up onto the anteromedial coronoid, which is fractured off by a shearing mechanism.

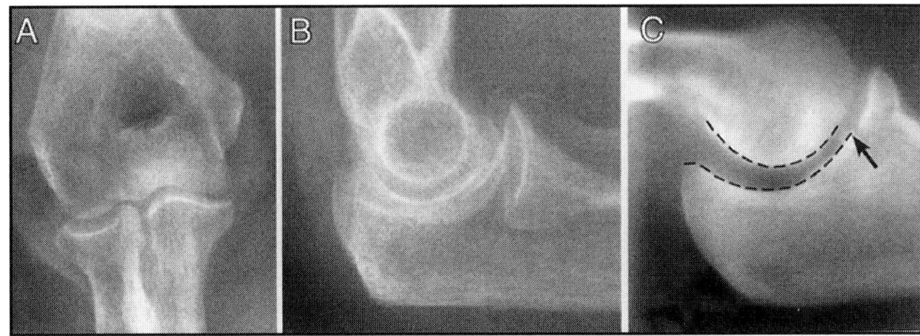

Fig. 14 A and **B,** AP and lateral radiographs of an anteromedial subtype 2 coronoid fracture, showing what appears to be no significant displacement and anatomic joint alignment. **C,** Lateral trispiral tomogram (taken with slight gravitational varus stress on the elbow) through the medial portion of the ulnaohumeral articulation shows an anteromedial subtype 2 fracture (involving the anteromedial coronoid and the tip) with joint incongruity caused by varus posteromedial rotatory subluxation. In this case, the medial trochlea has displaced anteriorly and distally along with the anteromedial coronoid fragment that it displaced and with which it remains congruent. This results in point contact between the medial trochlea and the coronoid at the fracture site (*arrow*), which over the course of a few months leads to medial trochlear erosion. The incongruity is indicated by the ulnohumeral joint being widened posteriorly and converging anteriorly (indicated by converging dotted lines).

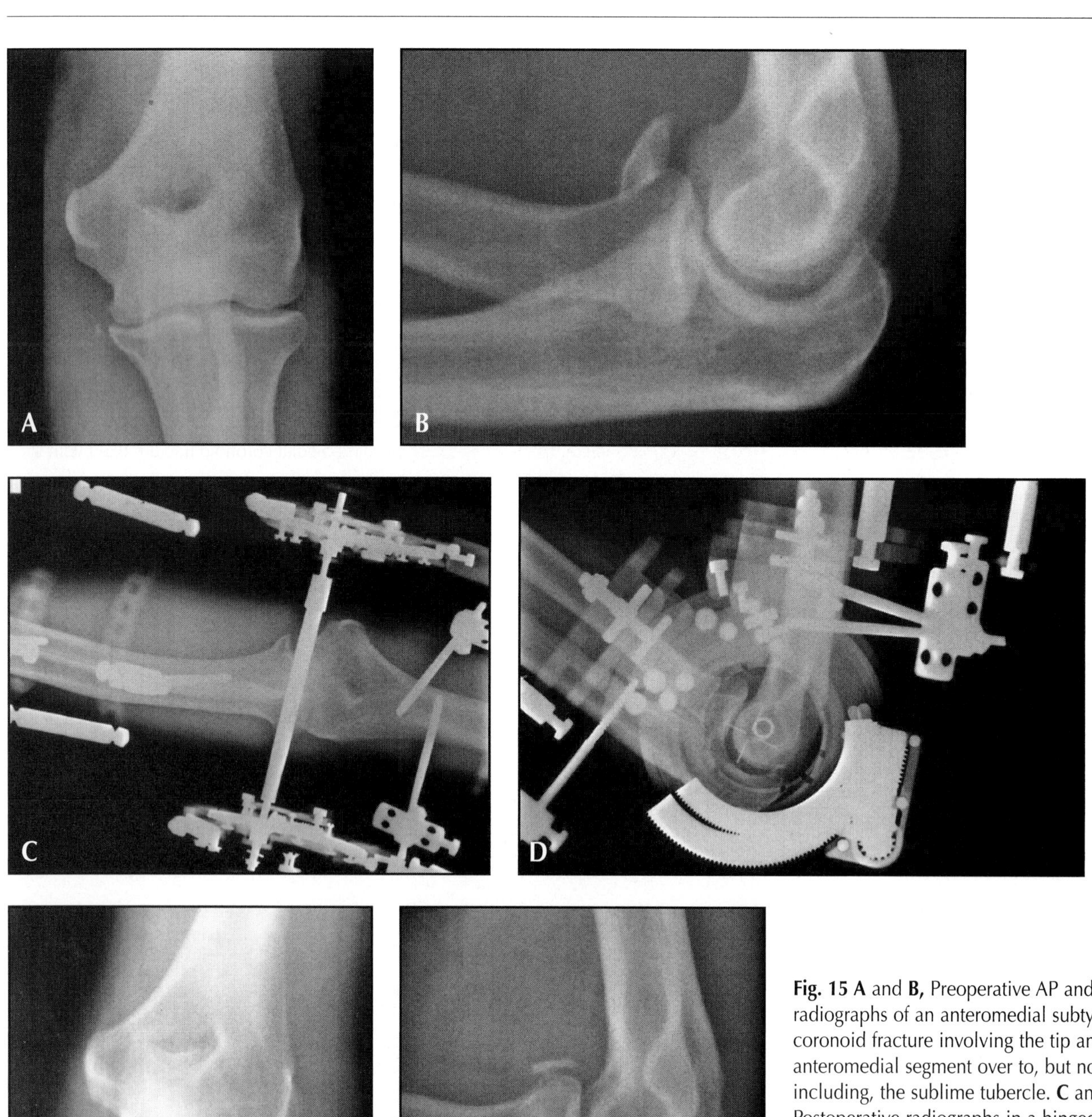

Fig. 15 A and **B,** Preoperative AP and lateral radiographs of an anteromedial subtype 2 coronoid fracture involving the tip and the anteromedial segment over to, but not including, the sublime tubercle. **C** and **D,** Postoperative radiographs in a hinged external fixator after arthroscopic reduction and suture fixation of the fragments, revealing concentric joint alignment and slightly nonanatomic reduction of the fragments. **E** and **F,** AP and lateral radiographs taken 1 year after surgery showing medial ulnohumeral collapse and early arthritis.

tion and stability have been achieved, the prognosis can be quite good.

Treatment

As part of the preoperative evaluation, the presence of a coronoid fracture should be suspected following an elbow dislocation or a fracture of the radial head or olecranon. Clinical examination should include evaluation for tenderness and/or bruising at the origin of the collateral ligament complexes and common flexor and extensor origins, especially on the lateral side where avulsion may not be obvious without an index of suspicion.

Plain AP and lateral radiographs are sometimes adequate, but oblique views can be helpful. CT scans with sagittal and/or three-dimensional reconstruction are also quite helpful in determining the fracture pattern and severity of comminution. Stress radiographs may be necessary to rule out unsuspected instability, especially with anteromedial fractures (Fig. 12).

As is the case for all articular fractures, obtaining and maintaining fracture reduction and joint stability so that early motion can be commenced is the treatment that most predictably assures preservation of function of the joint and limb. Thus, except for stable undisplaced fractures, the treatment of coronoid fractures is usually surgical.

The goal of treatment is to prevent displacement caused by either of the two primary deforming forces: (1) a varus gravitational force with placement of the hand in space and (2) the valgus/posterolateral rotatory stress experienced with axial load across the elbow.

Surgical Exposures The surgical approach depends on the fracture type and the need for other surgery such as ligament repair. A posterior skin incision, just off the midline, permits deep access laterally and medially. Tip fractures can be reduced and fixed through a lateral arthrotomy by retracting the fractured radial head. Anteromedial fractures usually require a medial exposure, which can be obtained either by reflecting a portion of the common flexor-pronator origin or by elevating the flexor carpi ulnaris muscle and tendon origin from the proximal ulna and MCL after transposing the ulnar nerve. If more exposure is required, the entire common flexor-pronator origin can be reflected. The optimum approach remains to be confirmed. An alternative treatment for some of these fractures is to perform an arthroscopic reduction with the fracture under image intensification. Basal subtype 1 coronoid fractures require a medial exposure as just described. However, basal subtype 2 fractures are transolecranon fracture-dislocations; therefore, the coronoid sometimes can be adequately accessed through the olecranon fracture before placing a precontoured posterior plate.

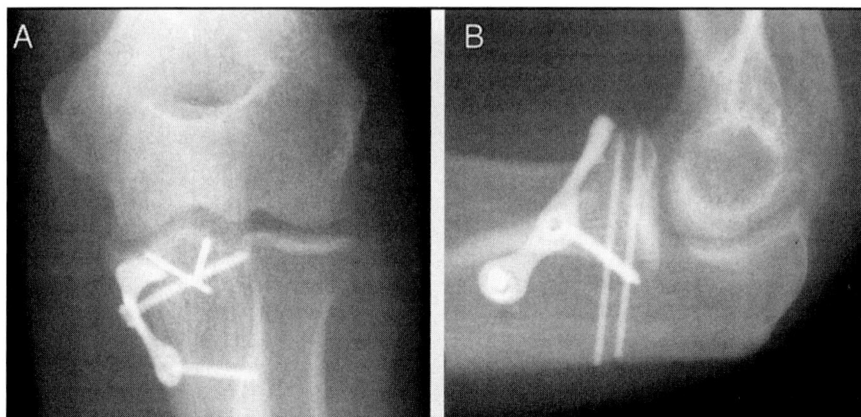

Fig. 16 AP **(A)** and lateral **(B)** radiographs of an anteromedial coronoid fracture fixed with a congruent plate and two fine threaded K-wires.

Surgical Techniques Several options exist for the fixation of coronoid fractures. These include, in various possible combinations, (1) transosseous sutures (or wires) through the ulna, (2) fine threaded K-wires, (3) lag screws, and (4) plate fixation. Neutralization can be achieved either by plate fixation or with a hinged external fixator. The choice of fixation depends on the fracture type, the integrity of the soft tissues, and the presence of associated injuries.

Tip Fractures Tip fractures may not require treatment because they sometimes are very small (≤ 2 mm). Larger tip fractures can be fixed adequately with transosseous sutures and/or fine threaded K-wires. Perfect anatomic reduction of these smaller fragments is not as important as restoration of the anterior buttress, including the capsular insertion of the ulna. Rigid fixation does not seem to be as important with this fracture as it is with an anteromedial or basal coronoid fracture. Two strong sutures or wires are placed through the ulna from the subcutaneous border, emerging at the proximal (articular) edge of the fracture. These are then passed over the coronoid fragment, through the attached capsule, and back down through two separate holes in the ulna just proximal to the distal edge of the fracture and tied tightly. The use of a threaded K-wire pin to position the fracture fragment anatomically, in addition to the two sutures over the top to hold the fragment down, is quite useful. The capsule inserts 4 to 6 mm distal to the tip of the coronoid so it may not be attached to very small fragments.[52] The technique is based on principles similar to those for a volar plate advancement arthroplasty for proximal interphalangeal fracture-dislocations. It is done through the lateral exposure used for treating the radial head fracture. The fractured radial head is simply retracted while working on the coronoid.

Although the optimal treatment of anteromedial coronoid fractures has yet to be determined, these fractures appear to demand surgical treatment, which might include anatomic reduction and either rigid internal fixation or protection with a hinged external fixator. In addition, the LCL must be repaired if a hinged fixator is not being used. One option is anatomic reduction held with threaded 0.062-in K-wires placed through the ulna into the anteromedial fracture fragments and a precontoured buttress plate (Acumed, Beaverton, OR) that has sharp prongs proximally to grasp the fragments (Fig. 16).

Anteromedial Subtype 1 Fractures Anteromedial subtype 1 fractures are deceitfully benign in their presentation, yet appear to have a guarded prognosis. They usually are seen in isolation, without prior dislocation or radial head fracture. Displacement is not great and may be only about 2 mm. Because of their propensity for permitting ulnohumeral incongruity, they may be reduced and fixed and the LCL complex repaired.

Anteromedial Subtype 2 Fractures In anteromedial subtype 2 fractures, the primary fracture is still in an oblique plane from the sublime tubercle but extends laterally in the coronal plane to involve the tip of the coronoid, which also is fractured off (Fig. 11). This fracture must be distinguished from what could mistakenly be thought of as a comminuted fracture of the coronoid tip. These fractures are treated identically to the anteromedial subtype 1 fractures, except that additional threaded 0.062-in Steinmann pins and sometimes sutures are used to hold the tip reduced (Fig. 16). The buttressing of the primary anteromedial fragment or neutralization with a hinged external fixator is still necessary as described above. The LCL is repaired as well.

Anteromedial Subtype 3 Fractures Anteromedial subtype 3 fractures represent a more comminuted version of anteromedial subtypes 1 and 2. In subtype 3 fractures, medial extension occurs in the sagittal plane, fracturing off the sublime tubercle, which represents the insertion of the anterior bundle of the MCL (Fig. 11). These fractures are treated identically to the anteromedial subtype 2 fractures, but they require additional fixation with screws, threaded wires, a second plate, or suture anchors to fix the sublime tubercle. The buttressing of the primary anteromedial fragment is still necessary as described above. The LCL is repaired as well.

Basal Fractures Basal subtype 1 fractures are treated somewhat similarly to anteromedial fractures: the fragments are reduced and held with fine wires or screws and neutralized with a plate placed on the anteromedial surface of the ulna. A key distinction, however, is the need to elevate a depressed medial/central fragment of the coronoid. The elbow also can be neutralized with a hinged external fixator, which is necessary if stable anatomic reduction is not attainable. Any ligamentous disruption (usually the LCL complex or annular ligament) is repaired.

Transolecranon fracture-dislocations (basal subtype 2 fractures) are treated by first attempting a reduction of the coronoid fragment through the olecranon fracture. Special techniques for this reduction are discussed in the section on olecranon fracture-dislocations. A critical factor is to obtain adequate reduction and stability of the anteromedial coronoid fragment. Failure to do so will likely result in joint incongruity and early posttraumatic arthritis (Fig. 10). A posterior contoured plate is used for these fractures.

Postoperative Management

Postoperative management in all cases consists of brief splinting of the elbow in extension for about 36 hours, followed by early motion. A hinged brace offers some protection, but only when the elbow is relatively extended. When the security of fixation is in question, motion is limited to an arc from 30° to 110° for the first 3 to 6 weeks. Stiffness is likely to result if the elbow is immobilized after surgical repair of these fractures, so motion should be started in almost all cases. A hinged external fixator is used to protect the elbow in those cases in which fracture displacement or joint subluxation would be a concern. If for any reason the surgeon is forced to choose between stability and mobility, it is important to realize that a stiff but congruent elbow is less of a problem to correct than an elbow that has been chronically incongruent, as a result of the cartilage erosion that occurs in the latter.

Pearls

An isolated coronoid fracture (ie, no apparent radial head fracture or elbow dislocation) appears benign but is usually a fracture-subluxation with avulsion of the LCL. The LCL injury will be missed unless stress radiographs are taken or the injury explored (including exposing the ligament beneath the common extensor tendon). The anteromedial facet of the coronoid (between the tip and sublime tubercle) is the critical fragment to be buttressed. A dislocated elbow with a radial head fracture usually has an associated coronoid fracture. A coronoid fragment is bigger than it appears on the radiograph because of its cartilage cap.

Pitfalls

Several pitfalls commonly are seen in the treatment of coronoid fractures. Excision of the coronoid fragment, which is mistaken as part of the radial head, can be avoided if the surgeon realizes that any bone fragment sitting in the coronoid fossa on the radiograph is almost always from the coronoid. Another pitfall is the conclusion that small pieces of coronoid are unimportant. However, in patients with terrible triad injury, even small tip fractures are important and should be repaired if the capsule is still attached to them (as it usually is).

A pitfall experienced by most surgeons is misidentification of an anteromedial fracture as a tip fracture. The latter can be treated by near-anatomic reduction and nonrigid fixation if the radial head is replaced or fixed. However, the former must be reduced anatomically and held rigidly (or the elbow neutralized with an external fixator).

The most common complications following coronoid fractures are elbow instability or stiffness. The joint resultant force vector, which is posterior and superior, requires the coronoid to resist posterior displacement of the ulna under the humerus. Thus, the likelihood and severity of such instability is directly related to how much coronoid is lost or displaced. Gravitational varus stress in the postoperative period is probably the major culprit causing displacement of the coronoid. This stress can be avoided by neutralizing the elbow with a hinged external fixator.

Radial Head and Neck Fractures

Fractures of the radial head are the most common skeletal injury in the adult elbow. Most occur in middle-aged individuals between 20 and 60 years of age, with a 2:1 ratio of women to men.[61,62] The most common injury mechanism involves a fall on the outstretched hand with the forearm pronated and the elbow partially extended. Experimentally, axial load applied from 35° to 80° of elbow flexion leads to isolated radial head failure.[51]

The radiocapitellar joint functions in load bearing. The radial head acts as a secondary stabilizer of the MCL to valgus load,[63-65] and together with the coronoid it bears axial load and provides an anterior buttress resisting posterolateral rotatory subluxation of the elbow joint in a secondary capacity.[59,62,66] During strenuous activities, axial force of up to 90% body weight can be transmitted to the radiocapitellar articulation from the hand-forearm unit.[67] Contact forces at this joint are greatest in pronation, which also results in slight anterior translation of the radial head on the capitellum.

The radial head is slightly elliptical in shape with an offset concavity that articulates with the capitellum. The radial head and neck are angulated and offset with respect to the shaft and the neck. The anterolateral third of the head surface lacks thick articular cartilage and strong subchondral support, making this region more susceptible to fracture.

Treatment

Radiographs of the radial head must be centered on and perpendicular to its surface. This is made difficult following fracture because full elbow extension typically cannot be obtained. Studies have shown a high degree of interobserver and intraobserver variability in classifying radial head fractures based on plain radiographs.[68] Oblique views and specialized projections can be helpful.[69] Plain radiographs commonly underestimate the degree of articular involvement and surface depression, and CT scans may be indicated.

Radial head fractures can be complex either as a result of adjacent fractures or of disruption of the ligaments of the elbow and forearm. Joint dislocation is seen in approximately 3% to 10% of radial head fractures.[70] Failure of the interosseous ligament of the forearm with radial head fracture is more rare.[71-74] It is in these settings that all attempts should be made to reconstruct and preserve the radial head or replace it.

Surgical Exposure Internal fixation of comminuted radial head fractures is technically demanding and is predicated on adequate exposure. For most fracture patterns, regardless of the skin incision, deep dissection is centered over the radiocapitellar joint. The white, shiny extensor aponeurosis fascia is split longitudinally in line with its fibers. The midline of the radiocapitellar articulation marks the deep interval between the extensor carpi radialis brevis anteriorly and the extensor digitorum communis posteriorly.[75] Full-thickness flaps are developed in a single plane through the annular ligament and capsule, which are not identifiable as separate structures surgically. Fracture fragments are often anterior; in such cases, it is useful to expose the radial head between the extensor carpi radialis longus and brevis.

For more complex fractures involving the head and neck of the radius, a larger distal exposure is required. One option is simply to split the extensor fascia and tendon origin distally with elevation of the underlying supinator muscle from posterior to anterior exposing the radial neck. The supinator will help protect the posterior interosseous nerve, which is not in direct jeopardy when using a standard 4.0-cm long plate if dissection is not carried distal to the tuberosity.[76,77] However, to avoid a traction neuropathy, care must be taken not to vigorously retract the soft-tissue envelope anteriorly.

If a longer plate is required at and distal to the tuberosity, the posterior interosseous nerve branches must be identified and protected (Fig. 17). Following fracture fixation, a meticulous repair is required, facilitated by large running, locking sutures placed through drill holes in the humerus (or less commonly with suture anchors). These sutures are tied with the forearm in pronation, which reduces the posterolateral joint subluxation.

Surgical Techniques Often the impacted segments of the radial head are covered with an intact periosteal hinge at the radial neck. Central articular depression is not uncommon and can be elevated with fine instruments. The fracture line must be opened gently to remove any interposed osteochondral fragments, which may block reduction. These occasionally include shear fragments off the capitellum[78] (Fig. 18). Once the fracture is reduced, provisional K-wire fixation is helpful.

When the fracture involves only a segment of the radial head, the wires are replaced with small screws for definitive fixation. Two-millimeter and occasionally 1.5-mm implants are used most commonly and are countersunk beneath the articular surface. Alternatively, headless screws can be used. Maximum screw lengths are typically less than 20 to 24 mm in the average adult radial head. Care must be taken to ensure that the screws do not protrude through the opposite cortex. Full rotation of the forearm is documented prior to a careful closure. If the tendon or ligament origins had been torn or avulsed, they must be repaired as well.

It is important to understand that implants applied to the surface of the radi-

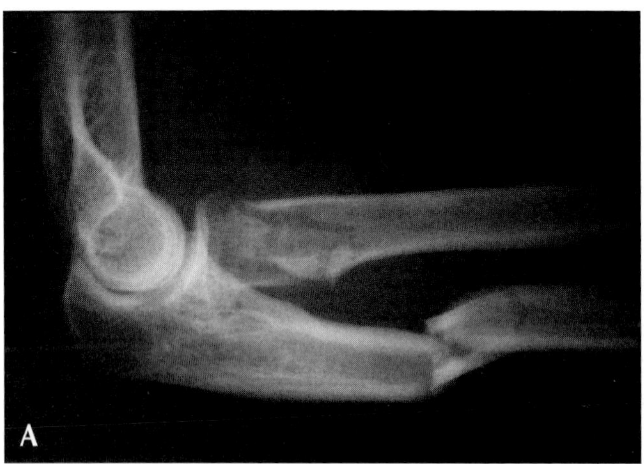

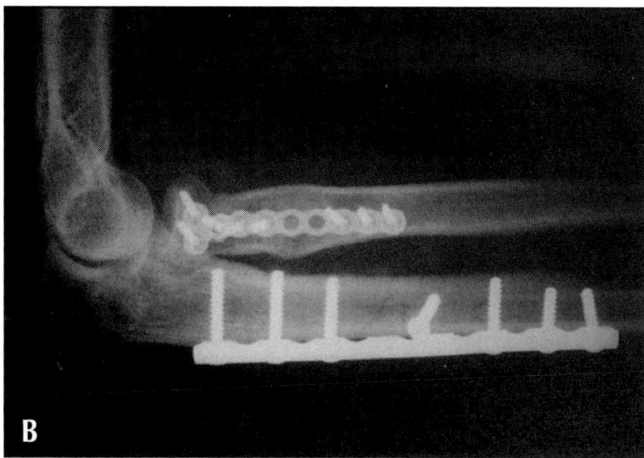

Fig. 17 A, Lateral radiograph depicting comminuted ulnar shaft fracture with associated displaced fracture of the radial neck (Monteggia variant). Note that the radius fracture line extends to nearly the midpoint of the tuberosity. The supinator was retracted anteriorly, protecting the posterior interosseous nerve, and a 2.4-mm plate was applied. Nerve identification is required if dissection is carried out distal to the radial tuberosity. **B,** Final lateral radiograph following internal fixation.

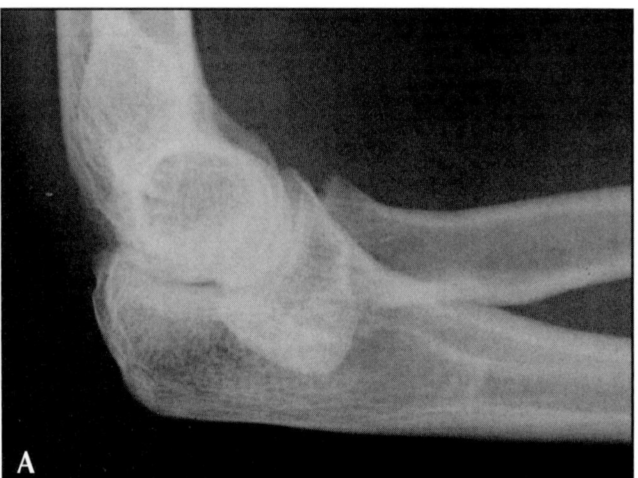

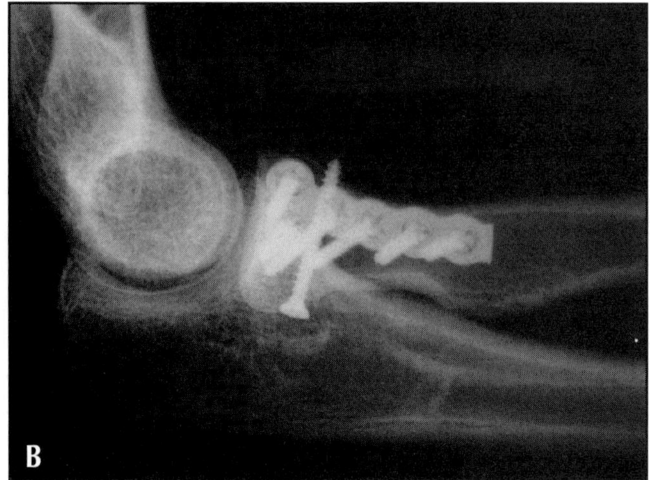

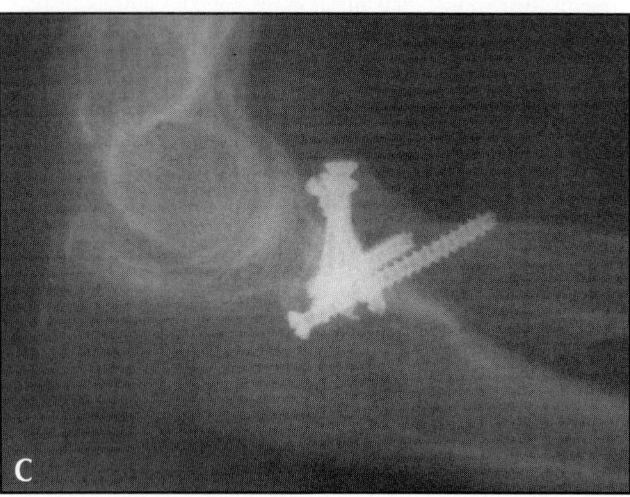

Fig. 18 A, Lateral radiograph of a radial neck fracture with complete displacement. The fracture pattern is oblique in nature, allowing placement of an interfragmentary compression screw. However, it runs from anterior to posterior. (Courtesy of Dr. Graham King, University of Western Ontario, London, Ontario, Canada.) **B,** The plate must still be placed in the safe zone, now functioning in a neutralization mode. A lag screw was applied perpendicular to the main fracture line. **C,** An alternative method of fixing radial head and neck fractures uses crossed cannulated screws.

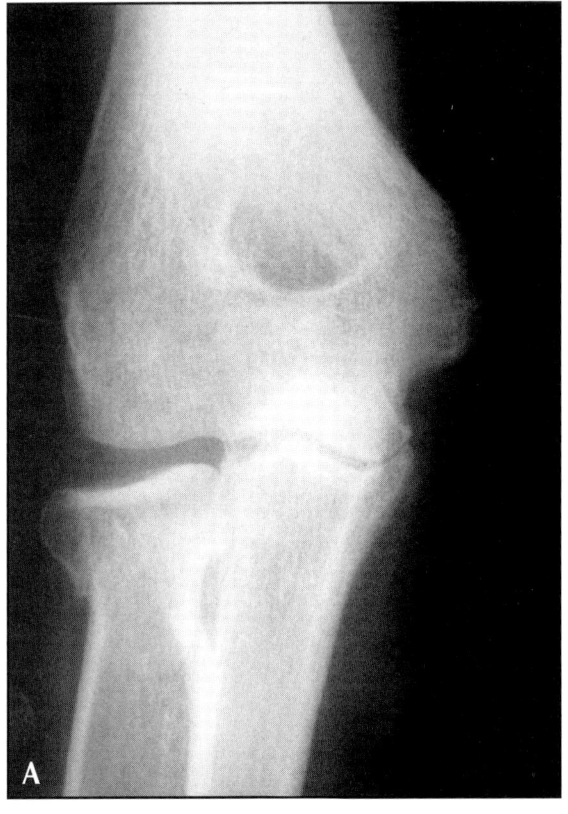

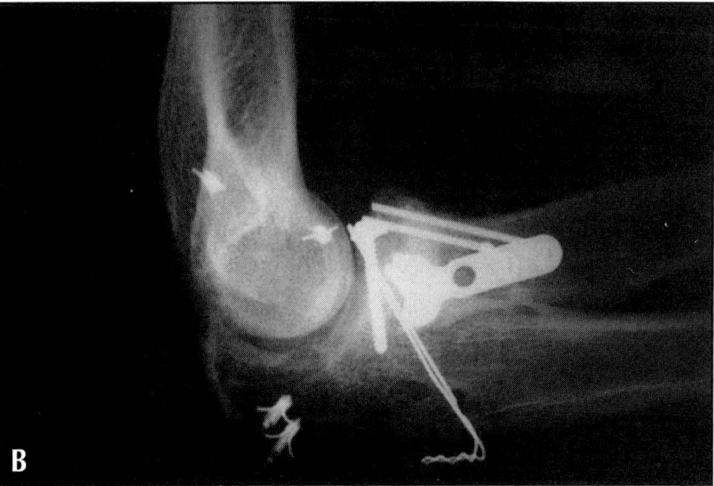

Fig. 19 A, Lateral radiograph depicting malunion of a radial head and neck fracture. In extension, the joint subluxates. **B,** Radial neck and coronoid osteotomies were performed with corticocancellous autograft placed into the radial defect. Note that the plate is not placed in a biomechanically optimal position, sitting approximately 90° to the osteotomy. It must still be applied to the safe zone of the radial head. It was therefore augmented with two threaded K-wires.

al head and neck must be placed in a safe zone so they do not limit forearm rotation. This zone refers to a 110° arc of the head circumference that does not articulate with the radial notch of the ulna.[79,80] The safe zone is perhaps most easily defined as follows: with the forearm in neutral rotation the safe zone is a 90° arc centered on the lateral side of the radial head, with 20° extra added anteriorly (total 110° arc). For fractures involving the radial neck, an interfragmentary compression screw occasionally will be required perpendicular to the fracture line, with a plate then applied as a neutralization device in the safe zone (Fig. 19).

Most commonly, 2.0- and 2.4-mm plates are used to secure and buttress the radial head. Low-profile implants are required because of the close approximation of the annular ligament and overlying soft tissues. These lie in a potential space, and, even if properly placed, implants may impinge on the overlying soft tissues, limiting full forearm rotation. Following fixation, autogenous bone graft often is required to support depressed articular fragments or replace comminuted defects of the radial neck. Graft can be obtained from the distal humerus or the ipsilateral olecranon or distal radial metaphysis.

When radial head fractures are too comminuted to allow for internal fixation with screws, three options are available: (1) fixation with multiple fine threaded K-wires, (2) excision, or (3) replacement. Severely comminuted radial head fractures can sometimes be fixed with good results using five to eight fine threaded K-wires that are cut off and burred down to the cartilage-bone junction. Additional stability can be provided to the radial neck by crisscrossing longitudinal threaded K-wires passed through the rim of the head and down the shaft.

In complex fracture-dislocations, MCL disruption, or forearm interosseous ligament failure, metallic implants are indicated when internal fixation is not possible.[81,82] Silicone arthroplasty is no longer recommended because newer metallic radial head implants are now available.[83-85] The indications and techniques for replacement of the severely fractured head are rapidly evolving. Use of a metal radial head prosthesis restores valgus and axial loading functions of the radius and allows proper healing of the soft tissues. Resection will not result in motion loss but will lead to weakness in grip, rotation, and axial forearm loading.[86-88] If resection is being considered, however, it is important to examine the elbow intraoperatively to rule out occult valgus or axial instability following radial head resection.

Postoperative Management

After surgery, patients are immobilized for 1 or 2 days in a compressive dressing with the elbow extended and elevated.

ROM exercises of the elbow and forearm are then begun with interval protective splinting for comfort and support. Prolonged immobilization is avoided because it is associated with increased stiffness and functional loss.[68,89] A nighttime elbow extension splint may be helpful to decrease the development of a flexion contracture. Terminal elbow extension and full forearm supination are hardest to recover, and therapy should concentrate on these functions. Progressive loading and strengthening are typically not permitted for approximately 6 weeks and often longer depending on the injury and the fixation obtained.

In more severe trauma with extensive soft-tissue injury, some surgeons consider using short-term nonsteroidal anti-inflammatory medication as prophylaxis against heterotopic ossification. This condition is poorly understood but is related, in part, to the severity of the original injury.[90] It also may be associated with a larger surgical dissection, repeated surgical insults to the traumatized elbow, and possibly a delay in surgical intervention.[91]

Pearls

Articular injury to the radial head is commonly more severe than noted on plain radiographs of the elbow. Even simple fractures often involve chondral injury to the capitellum and some degree of collateral ligament trauma. Late symptoms may be attributable to these unrecognized injuries. If the coronoid is fractured, the radial head becomes a critical factor in elbow stability. The role of the radial head becomes increasingly important as other soft-tissue and bony constraints are compromised. Loss of the radial head results in weakness of grip and strength of the forearm both in rotation and axial loading. Implants applied to the surface of the radial head must be placed in a safe zone, which involves a 110° arc of the articular circumference, that is almost directly lateral when the forearm is in neutral rotation. Following radial head injury, loss of terminal elbow extension is more common than loss of forearm rotation. Forearm supination is typically more difficult to recover than pronation. Prolonged immobilization leads to a greater likelihood of joint stiffness.

Pitfalls

Open reduction and internal fixation of radial head fractures is technically difficult and can be fraught with pitfalls and complications. One pitfall is the failure to recognize the need for bone grafting of defects caused by fracture impaction. A low threshold should exist to bone graft areas of comminution, especially in the radial neck, and care must be taken to place internal fixation without excessive stripping of the periosteal sleeve. Another common pitfall is the placement of hardware in positions permitting impingement against the ulna. Provisional fixation of the fracture with K-wires is very helpful to stabilize reduced fragments and allow planning for subsequent definitive fixation in the safe zone.

The complication that occurs most often is loss of motion, especially when plates are used for internal fixation. A common pitfall in attempting to prevent this problem is to provide inadequate protection for patients with nonrigid fixation. The use of a long-arm orthosis between exercises during the early postoperative period may help protect the construct from excessive loads. Occasionally, it is necessary to remove the hardware once union has matured. When problematic, early implant removal is recommended at 4 to 6 months, especially for cancellous injuries. However, this does not always lead to return of full forearm rotation.

Summary

Difficult elbow fractures are defined as those posing challenges in diagnosis, exposure, and treatment or causing serious uncertainty regarding prognosis. These include comminuted fractures of the distal humerus, often with bone loss; complex fracture patterns of the articular surfaces, such as shearing injuries; and certain fractures of the coronoid and the radial head. Improved techniques for achieving adequate stability in complex distal humerus fractures have contributed significantly to advances in treatment. The recent understanding of complex instability patterns, including varus posteromedial rotatory instability, have provided important information on the relevance of the pattern and location of fractures of the coronoid. Anteromedial coronoid fractures can present a benign appearance but pose a serious threat of incongruity and early posttraumatic arthritis. An understanding of the relevant biomechanics (such as the interdependent contributions of the coronoid and radial head) and specific principles of maintaining elbow stability allow the surgeon to treat and appropriately rehabilitate the patient with a difficult elbow fracture while avoiding some of the common pitfalls in the process.

References

1. Jupiter JB, Neff U, Holzach P, Allgower M: Intercondylar fractures of the humerus: An operative approach. *J Bone Joint Surg Am* 1985;67:226-239.
2. Jupiter JB: Complex fractures of the distal part of the humerus and associated complications. *Instr Course Lect* 1995;44:187-198.
3. McKee M, Jupiter J, Toh CL, Wilson L, Colton C, Karras KK: Reconstruction after malunion and nonunion of intra-articular fractures of the distal humerus. *J Bone Joint Surg Br* 1994;76: 614-621.
4. McKee MD, Jupiter JB, Bosse G, Goodman L: Outcome of ulnar neurolysis during post-traumatic reconstruction of the elbow. *J Bone Joint Surg Br* 1998;80:100-105.
5. McKee MD, Jupiter JB: Trauma to the adult elbow and fractures of the distal humerus, in Browner B (ed): *Skeletal Trauma*. Philadelphia, PA, WB Saunders, 1998, vol 2, pp 1455-1522.
6. McKee MD, Kim J, Kebaish K, Stephen DJ, Kreder HJ, Schemitsch EH: Functional outcome after open supracondylar fractures of the humerus. *J Bone Joint Surg Br* 2000;82:646-651.
7. Zagorski JB, Jennings JJ, Burkhalter WE, Uribe JW: Comminuted intraarticular fractures of the distal humeral condyles: Surgical vs nonsurgical treatment. *Clin Orthop* 1986;202:197-204.

8. Cobb TK, Morrey BF: Total elbow arthroplasty as primary treatment for distal humeral fractures in elderly patients. *J Bone Joint Surg Am* 1997;79:826-832.

9. Waddell JP, Hatch J, Richards R: Supracondylar fractures of the humerus: Results of surgical treatment. *J Trauma* 1988;28:1615-1621.

10. McKee MD, Wilson TL, Winston L, Schemitsch EH, Richards RR: Functional outcome following surgical treatment of intra-articular distal humeral fractures through a posterior approach. *J Bone Joint Surg Am* 2000;82:1701-1707.

11. Bryan RS, Morrey BF: Extensive posterior exposure of the elbow: A triceps-sparing approach. *Clin Orthop* 1982;166:188-192.

12. O'Driscoll SW: The triceps-reflecting anconeus pedicle (TRAP) approach for distal humeral fractures and nonunions. *Orthop Clin North Am* 2000;31:91-101.

13. Kasser JR, Richards K, Millis M: The triceps-dividing approach to open reduction of complex distal humeral fractures in adolescents: A Cybex evaluation of triceps function and motion. *J Pediatr Orthop* 1990;10:93-96.

14. Helfet DL, Hotchkiss RN: Internal fixation of the distal humerus: A biomechanical comparison of methods. *J Orthop Trauma* 1990;4: 260-264.

15. Schemitsch EH, Tencer AF, Henley MB: Biomechanical evaluation of methods of internal fixation of the distal humerus. *J Orthop Trauma* 1994;8:468-475.

16. Sanchez-Sotelo J, Torchia ME, O'Driscoll SW: Principle-based internal fixation of distal humerus fractures: *Tech Hand Upper Extrem Surg* 2001;5:179-187.

17. O'Driscoll S, Sanchez-Sotelo J, Torchia ME: Management of the smashed distal humerus. *Orthop Clin North Am* 2002;33:19-33.

18. Morrey BF, Askew LJ, Chao EY: A biomechanical study of normal functional elbow motion. *J Bone Joint Surg Am* 1981;63:872-877.

19. McKee MD, Jupiter JB, Bamberger HB: Coronal shear fractures of the distal end of the humerus. *J Bone Joint Surg Am* 1996;78:49-54.

20. Muller M, Nazarian S, Koch P, Schatzker J (eds): *Comprehensive Classification of Fratures of Long Bones*. New York, NY, Springer, 1990, pp 75-85.

21. Robertson R, Bogart F: Fracture of the capitellum and trochlea combined with fracture of the external humeral condyl. *J Bone Joint Surg Am* 1933;15:206-213.

22. Inoue G, Horii E: Combined shear fractures of the trochlea and capitellum associated with anterior fracture-dislocation of the elbow. *J Orthop Trauma* 1992;6:373-375.

23. Lansinger O, Mare K: Fracture of the capitulum humeri. *Acta Orthop Scand* 1981;52:39-44.

24. Milch L: Fractures and fracture dislocations of the humeral condyles. *J Trauma* 1964;4:592-607.

25. McKee MD, Jupiter JB: A contemporary approach to the management of complex fractures of the distal humerus and their sequelae. *Hand Clin* 1994;10:479-494.

26. Jupiter JB, Neff U, Regazzoni P, Allgower M: Unicondylar fractures of the distal humerus: An operative approach. *J Orthop Trauma* 1988;2: 102-109.

27. Simpson LA, Richards RR: Internal fixation of a capitellar fracture using Herbert screws: A case report. *Clin Orthop* 1986;209:166-168.

28. Grantham SA, Norris TR, Bush DC: Isolated fracture of the humeral capitellum. *Clin Orthop* 1981;161:262-269.

29. Ring D, Jupiter JB, Sanders RW, Mast J, Simpson NS: Transolecranon fracture: Dislocation of the elbow. *J Orthop Trauma* 1997;11:545-550.

30. Ring D, Jupiter JB, Simpson NS: Monteggia fractures in adults. *J Bone Joint Surg Am* 1998;80:1733-1744.

31. Biga N, Thomine JM: Trans-olecranal dislocations of the elbow. *Rev Chir Orthop Reparatrice Appar Mot* 1974;60:557-567.

32. Bado JL: The Monteggia lesion. *Clin Orthop* 1967;50:71-86.

33. Ring D, Jupiter JB, Waters PM: Monteggia fractures in children and adults. *J Am Acad Orthop Surg* 1998;6:215-224.

34. Balakim G, Wippula E: Fractures of the olecranon complicated by forward dislocation of the forearm. *Ann Chir Gyn Fenn* 1971;60:105-108.

35. Jupiter JB, Leibovic SJ, Ribbans W, Wilk RM: The posterior Monteggia lesion. *J Orthop Trauma* 1991;5:395-402.

36. Penrose J: The Monteggia fracture with posterior dislocation of the radial head. *J Bone Joint Surg Br* 1951;33:65-73.

37. Pavel A, Pittman J, Lance E, Wade P: The posterior Monteggia fracture: A clinical study. *J Trauma* 1965;5:185-199.

38. Dowdy PA, Bain GI, King GJ, Patterson SD: The midline posterior elbow incision: An anatomical appraisal. *J Bone Joint Surg Br* 1995;77:696-699.

39. Patterson SD, Bain GI, Mehta JA: Surgical approaches to the elbow. *Clin Orthop* 2000;370:19-33.

40. Ikeda M, Fukushima Y, Kobayashi Y, Oka Y: Comminuted fractures of the olecranon: Management by bone graft from the iliac crest and multiple tension-band wiring. *J Bone Joint Surg Br* 2001;83:805-808.

41. Heim U: Kombinierte verletzungen von radius und ulna im proximalen unterarmsegment. *Hefte Unfallchir* 1994;241:61-79.

42. Hastings H II, Engles DR: Fixation of complex elbow fractures: Part II. Proximal ulna and radius fractures. *Hand Clin* 1997;13:721-735.

43. Ring D, Jupiter JB: Operative fixation and reconstruction of the coronoid. *Tech Orthop* 2000;15.

44. Morrey BF: Surgical exposures of the elbow, in Morrey BF (ed): *The Elbow and Its Disorders*, ed 2. Philadelphia, PA, WB Saunders, 1993, pp 139-166.

45. Mast J, Jokob R, Ganz R: *Planning and Reduction Technique in Fracture Surgery*. New York, NY, Springer-Verlag, 1989, pp 1-254.

46. O'Driscoll SW: Technique for unstable olecranon fracture-subluxations. *Op Tech Orthop* 1994;4:49-53.

47. Mansat P, Morrey BF: The column procedure: A limited lateral approach for extrinsic contracture of the elbow. *J Bone Joint Surg Am* 1998;80:1603-1615.

48. Cohen MS, Hastings H II: Post-traumatic contracture of the elbow: Operative release using a lateral collateral ligament sparing approach. *J Bone Joint Surg Br* 1998;80:805-812.

49. Ring D, Jupiter JB: Reconstruction of posttraumatic elbow instability. *Clin Orthop* 2000;10: 44-56.

50. Hotchkiss RN: Fractures and dislocations of the elbow, in Rockwood CA, Green DP, Bucholz RW, Heckman JD (eds): *Fractures in Adults*, ed 4. Philadelphia, PA, Lippincott Raven, 1996, pp 980-981.

51. Amis AA, Miller JH: The mechanisms of elbow fractures: An investigation using impact tests in vitro. *Injury* 1995;26:163-168.

52. Cage DJ, Abrams RA, Callahan JJ, Botte MJ: Soft tissue attachments of the ulnar coronoid process: An anatomic study with radiographis correlation. *Clin Orthop* 1995;320:154-158.

53. Closkey RF, Goode JR, Kirschenbaum D, Cody RP: The role of the coronoid process in elbow stability: A biomechanical analysis of axial loading. *J Bone Joint Surg Am* 2000;82:1749-1753.

54. Norris TR (ed): *Orthopaedic Knowledge Update: Shoulder and Elbow*. Rosemont, IL, American Academy of Orthopaedic Surgeons, 1997, pp 405-413.

55. Regan W, Morrey B: Fractures of the coronoid process of the ulna. *J Bone Joint Surg Am* 1989;71:1348-1354.

56. O'Driscoll SW: Elbow instability. *Hand Clin* 1994;10:405-415.

57. Regan W, Morrey BF: Classification and treatment of coronoid process fractures. *Orthopaedics* 1992;15:845-848.

58. Frymoyer JW (ed): *Orthopaedic Knowledge Update 4*. Rosemont, IL, American Academy of Orthopaedic Surgeons, 1993, pp 335-352.

59. O'Driscoll SW, Bell DF, Morrey BF: Posterolateral rotatory instability of the elbow. *J Bone Joint Surg Am* 1991;73:440-446.

60. O'Driscoll SW: Classification and spectrum of elbow instability: Recurrent instability, in Morrey BF (ed): *The Elbow and Its Disorders*. Philadelphia, PA, WB Saunders, 1993, pp 453-463.

61. Mason M: Some observations on fractures of the radial head with a review of one hundred cases. *Br J Surg* 1954;42:123-132.

62. Morrey BF: Radial head fracture, in Morrey BF (ed): *The Elbow*, ed 3. Philadelphia, PA, WB Saunders, 2000, pp 341-364.

63. Hotchkiss RN, Weiland AJ: Valgus stability of the elbow. *J Orthop Res* 1987;5:372-377.

64. Morrey BF, An KN: Articular and ligamentous contributions to the stability of the elbow joint. *Am J Sports Med* 1983;11:315-319.

65. Morrey BF, Tanaka S, An KN: Valgus stability of the elbow: A definition of primary and secondary constraints. *Clin Orthop* 1991;265: 187-195.

66. Cohen M, Hastings HS: Rotatory instability of the elbow: The anatomy and role of the lateral stabilizers. *J Bone Joint Surg Am* 1997;79:225-233.

67. Morrey BF, An KN, Stormont TJ: Force transmission through the radial head. *J Bone Joint Surg Am* 1988;70:250-256.

68. Morgan SJ, Groshen SL, Itamura JM, Shankwiler J, Brien WW, Kuschner SH: Reliability evaluation of classifying radial head fractures by the system of Mason. *Bull Hosp Jt Dis* 1997;56:95-98.

69. Greenspan A, Norman A, Rosen H: Radial head: Capitellum view in elbow traima: Clinical application and radiographic anatomic correlation. *AJR Am J Roentgenol* 1984;143:355-359.

70. Bakalim G: Fractures of radial head and their treatment. *Acta Orthop Scand* 1970;41:320-331.

71. Bock GW, Cohen MS, Resnick D: Fracture-dislocation of the elbow with inferior radioulnar dislocation: A variant of the Essex-Lopresti injury. *Skeletal Radiol* 1992;21:315-317.

72. Essex-Lopresti P: Fractures of the radial head with distal radio-ulnar dislocation. *J Bone Joint Surg Br* 1951;33:244-247.

73. Hotchkiss RN, An KN, Sowa DT, Basta S, Weiland AJ: An anatomic and mechanical study of the interosseous membrane of the forearm: Pathomechanics of proximal migration of the radius. *J Hand Surg Am* 1989;14:256-261.

74. Trousdale RT, Amadio PC, Cooney WP, Morrey BF: Radio-ulnar dissociation: A review of twenty cases. *J Bone Joint Surg Am* 1992;74:1486-1497.

75. Cohen M, Romeo A: Lateral epicondylitis: Open and arthroscopic treatment. *J Amer Soc Surg Hand* 2001;3:172-176.

76. Strauch RJ, Rosenwasser MP, Glazer PA: Surgical exposure of the dorsal proximal third of the radius: How vulnerable is the posterior interosseous nerve? *J Shoulder Elbow Surg* 1996;5:342-346.

77. Tornetta P III, Hochwald N, Bono C, Grossman M: Anatomy of the posterior interosseous nerve in relation to fixation of the radial head. *Clin Orthop* 1997;345:215-218.

78. Geel CW, Palmer AK, Ruedi T, Leutenegger AF: Internal fixation of proximal radial head fractures. *J Orthop Trauma* 1990;4:270-274.

79. Hotchkiss RN: Displaced fractures of the radial head: Internal fixation or excision? *J Am Acad Orthop Surg* 1997;5:1-10.

80. Smith GR, Hotchkiss RN: Radial head and neck fractures: Anatomic guidelines for proper placement of internal fixation. *J Shoulder Elbow Surg* 1996;5:113-117.

81. King GJ, Zarzour ZD, Rath DA, Dunning CE, Patterson SD, Johnson JA: Metallic radial head arthroplasty improves valgus stability of the elbow. *Clin Orthop* 1999;368:114-125.

82. Popovic N, Gillet P, Rodriguez A, Lemaire R: Fracture of the radial head with associated elbow dislocation: Results of treatment using a floating radial head prosthesis. *J Orthop Trauma* 2000;14:171-177.

83. Judet T, Garreau de Loubresse C, Piriou P, Charnley G: A floating prosthesis for radial-head fractures. *J Bone Joint Surg Br* 1996;78: 244-249.

84. Knight DJ, Rymaszewski LA, Amis AA, Miller JH: Primary replacement of the fractured radial head with a metal prosthesis. *J Bone Joint Surg Br* 1993;75:572-576.

85. Moro JK, Werier J, MacDermid JC, Patterson SD, King GJ: Arthroplasty with a metal radial head for unreconstructible fractures of the radial head. *J Bone Joint Surg Am* 2001;83:1201-1211.

86. Ikeda M, Oka Y: Function after early radial head resection for fracture: A retrospective evaluation of 15 patients followed for 3-18 years. *Acta Orthop Scand* 2000;71:191-194.

87. Jensen SL, Olsen BS, Sojbjerg JO: Elbow joint kinematics after excision of the radial head. *J Shoulder Elbow Surg* 1999;8:238-241.

88. Morrey BF, Chao EY, Hui FC: Biomechanical study of the elbow following excision of the radial head. *J Bone Joint Surg Am* 1979;61:63-68.

89. Broberg MA, Morrey BF: Results of treatment of fracture-dislocations of the elbow. *Clin Orthop* 1987;216:109-119.

90. Thompson HC III, Garcia A: Myositis ossificans: Aftermath of elbow injuries. *Clin Orthop* 1967;50:129-134.

91. Morrey BF: Ectopic ossification about the elbow, in Morrey BF (ed): *The Elbow,* ed 3. Philadelphia, PA, WB Saunders, 2000, pp 437-446.

Index

F

G

H

I

J

K

L

M

N

O

S

T

U

V

W

Y

Z